Hematopoietic Stem Cell Transplantation
IN CLINICAL PRACTICE

Commissioning Editor: *Timothy Horne*
Development Editor: *Clive Hewat*
Project Manager: *Elouise Ball*
Designer: *Stewart Larking*
Illustrator: *H L Studios*
Illustration Manager: *Merlyn Harvey*

Hematopoietic Stem Cell Transplantation
IN CLINICAL PRACTICE

Edited by

Jennifer Treleaven MD FRCP FRCPath
Consultant Hematologist,
Royal Marsden Hospital, Sutton,
Surrey, UK

A John Barrett MD FRCP FRCPath
Chief, Stem Cell Allotransplantation Section,
National Institutes of Health,
Bethesda, Maryland, USA

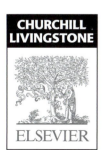

CHURCHILL
LIVINGSTONE

ELSEVIER

Edinburgh London New York Oxford Philadelphia St Louis Sydney Toronto 2009

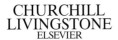

First published 2009

ISBN: 978-0-443-10147-2

British Library Cataloguing in Publication Data
A catalogue record for this book is available from the British Library

Library of Congress Cataloging in Publication Data
A catalog record for this book is available from the Library of Congress

Notice
Knowledge and best practice in this field are constantly changing. As new research and experience broaden our knowledge, changes in practice, treatment and drug therapy may become necessary or appropriate. Readers are advised to check the most current information provided (i) on procedures featured or (ii) by the manufacturer of each product to be administered, to verify the recommended dose or formula, the method and duration of administration, and contraindications. It is the responsibility of the practitioner, relying on their own experience and knowledge of the patient, to make diagnoses, to determine dosages and the best treatment for each individual patient, and to take all appropriate safety precautions. To the fullest extent of the law, neither the Publisher nor the Editors assume any liability for any injury and/or damage to persons or property arising out or related to any use of the material contained in this book.

Neither the Publisher nor the Editors assume any responsibility for any loss or injury and/or damage to persons or property arising out of or related to any use of the material contained in this book. It is the responsibility of the treating practitioner, relying on independent expertise and knowledge of the patient, to determine the best treatment and method of application for the patient.

The Publisher

ELSEVIER your source for books, journals and multimedia in the health sciences

www.elsevierhealth.com

Working together to grow libraries in developing countries

www.elsevier.com | www.bookaid.org | www.sabre.org

ELSEVIER   BOOK AID International   Sabre Foundation

The publisher's policy is to use paper manufactured from sustainable forests

Printed in China

Contents

List of contributors

Douglas R Adkins MD
Associate Professor of Medicine, Division of Oncology, Washington University School of Medicine, St. Louis, Missouri, USA

Jane Apperley FRCP FRCPath
Professor of Hemato-Oncology, Imperial College School of Medicine, Hammersmith Hospital, London, UK

Andrew S Artz MD MS
Assistant Professor of Medicine, Division of Hematology-Oncology, University of Chicago, Chicago, USA

Smita Bahtia MD MPH
Associate Director for Population Research, Division of Population Sciences, City of Hope National Medical Center, Duarte, California, USA

Kristin Baird MD
Assistant Clinical Investigator, Pediatric Oncology Branch, National Cancer Institute, National Institutes of Health, Bethesda, Maryland, USA

A John Barrett MD FRCP FRCPath
Chief, Allogeneic Stem Cell Transplantation Section, Hematology Branch, National Heart, Lung and Blood Institute, Bethesda, Maryland, USA

Michael R Bishop MD
Principal Investigator, Experimental Transplantation and Immunology Branch, Center for Cancer Research, National Cancer Institute, National Institutes of Health, Bethesda, Maryland, USA

Andrew Bodenham FRCA
Consultant in Anesthesia and Intensive Care, Leeds General Infirmary, Leeds, UK

Charles Bolan MD Colonel Retired USA MC
Associate Professor of Medicine, Medical Director, Unrelated Donor Hematopoietic Transplant Program, Hematology Branch, National Heart, Lung and Blood Institute, National Institutes of Health, Bethesda, Maryland, USA

Alan K Burnett MD FRCPath FRCP FMedSci
Professor of Hematology, Cardiff University, Cardiff, UK

Kenneth Carson MD
Fellow, Division of Hematology-Oncology, Feinberg School of Medicine, Northwestern University, Chicago, Illinois, USA

Richard Childs MD CMDR USPHS
Senior Investigator, Hematology Branch, National Heart, Lung and Blood Institute, National Institutes of Health, Bethesda, Maryland, USA

Susan Cleaver BSc(Hons)
Registry Manager, Anthony Nolan Trust, London, UK

Robin P Corbett MRCP FRACP
Clinical Director, South Island Child Cancer Service, Christchurch, New Zealand

Michele Cottler-Fox MD
Director, Cell Therapy and Transfusion Medicine, Department of Pathology, University of Arkansas for Medical Sciences, Little Rock, Arkansas, USA

Charles Craddock FRCP FRCPath
Professor of Hemato-Oncology, Director, Blood and Marrow Transplant Unit, Queen Elizabeth Hospital, Birmingham, UK

H Joachim Deeg MD
Professor of Medical Oncology, Fred Hutchinson Cancer Research Center and the University of Washington, Seattle, USA

Josu de la Fuente MRCPH MRCPath
Consultant Pediatric Hematologist, Department of Hematology, Imperial College Faculty of Medicine, London, UK

William B Ershler MD
Deputy Clinical Director, Clinical Research Branch, National Institute on Aging, National Institutes of Health, Baltimore, Maryland, USA

Stephen O Evans BPharm MRPharmS Dip Clin Pharm
Antimicrobial Pharmacist, Pharmacy Department, Royal Marsden Hospital, Sutton, Surrey, UK

Suzanne Fanning DO
Fellow, Department of Hematology and Medical Oncology, Cleveland Clinic Foundation, Taussig Cancer Center, Cleveland, Ohio, USA

Jürgen Finke MD
Professor, Head Allogeneic Stem Cell Transplantation Section, Division of Hematology and Oncology, Department of Medicine, University Medical Center, Freiburg, Germany

Mary E D Flowers MD
Director, Clinical Long-Term Follow Up, Fred Hutchinson Cancer Research Center, and the University of Washington, Seattle, USA

H Bobby Gaspar BSc MBBS MRCP(UK) PhD MRCPCH
Professor of Pediatrics and Immunology, Molecular Immunology Unit, Institute of Child Health, University College, London, UK

Duncan Gilbert MA MRCP FRCR
Clinical Research Fellow, Institute of Cancer Research, Royal Marsden NHS Foundation Trust, Sutton, Surrey, UK

Eliane Gluckman MD FRCP
Consultant in Hematology, Director of Eurocord, Eurocord-Netcord and European Blood and Marrow Transplant Group, Hôpital Saint Louis, Paris, France

Nicola Gökbuget MD
Head of Study Center, University of Frankfurt, Frankfurt, Germany

John M Goldman DM FRCP FRCPath FMed Sci
Formerly Professor of Hematology, Hammersmith Hospital, London, UK

John G Gribben MD DSc FRCP FRCPath
Director, Stem Cell Transplantation Program, Professor of Experimental Cancer Medicine, Bart's and the London School of Medicine, London, UK

Vikas Gupta MD MRCP MRCPath
Assistant Professor, Department of Medicine, Staff Physician, Leukemia Blood and Marrow Transplant Program, Princess Margaret Hospital, University of Toronto, Toronto, Canada

Rupert Handgretinger MD PhD
Chairman, Department of Hematology/Oncology and General Pediatrics, Children's University Hospital, Tubingen, Germany

Nancy M Hardy MD
Associate Investigator, Experimental Transplantation and Immunology Branch, Center for Cancer Research, National Cancer Institute, Bethesda, Maryland, USA

Carolyn Hemsley MA PhD MRCP FRCPath
Consultant in Microbiology and Infectious Diseases, Guy's and St Thomas's Hospital, London, UK

Louise Henry MSc RD
Senior Dietitian, Royal Marsden Hospital, Sutton, Surrey, UK

Helen E Heslop MD
Professor of Medicine and Pediatrics, Director of the Adult Stem Cell Transplant Program, Center for Cell and Gene Therapy, Baylor College of Medicine, Houston, Texas, USA

Dieter Hoelzer MD
Professor of Internal Medicine, University of Frankfurt, Frankfurt, Germany

Mary Horowitz MD MS
Chief Scientific Director, Center for International Blood and Marrow Transplant Research, Robert A Uihlein Jr. Professor of Hematologic Research, Medical College of Wisconsin, Milwaukee, Wisconsin, USA

Alan Horwich FRCR FRCP PhD FAcadMedSci
Professor of Radiotherapy and Honorary Consultant in Clinical Oncology, Institute of Cancer Research, Royal Marsden Hospital, Sutton, Surrey, UK

Edwin Horwitz MD PhD
Associate Professor and Director of Cell Therapy, Division of Oncology, Philadelphia Children's Hospital, University of Pennsylvania, USA

Gabor Illei MD PhD MHS
Head, Sjögren's Syndrome Clinic, Gene Therapy and Therapeutics Branch, NIDCR, National Institutes of Health, Bethesda, Maryland, USA

Armand Keating MD
Director, Division of Hematology, and Professor of Medicine, Princess Margaret Hospital Ontario Cancer Institute, Toronto, Canada

Hanna Jean Khoury MD FACP
Associate Professor of Hematology/Oncology, Emory University School of Medicine, Atlanta, Georgia, USA

Chris Kibbler MA FRCP FRCPath
Professor of Medical Microbiology, Department of Medical Microbiology, Royal Free Hospital, London, UK

Steven Knapper MA BMBCh DM MRCP FRCPath
Clinical Senior Lecturer in Hematology, Department of Hematology, Cardiff University, Cardiff, UK

Samar Kulkarni MRCP MRCPath
Specialist Registrar in Hematology, Royal Marsden Hospital, Sutton, Surrey, UK

Rifca Le Dieu MRCP MRCPath
Clinical Research Fellow, Bart's and the London School of Medicine, London, UK

Zi Yi Lim MRCP MRCPath
Clinical Lecturer, Department of Hematological Medicine, King's College Hospital, London, UK

Gayle Loader BSc RD
Senior Dietitian, Royal Marsden Hospital, Sutton, Surrey, UK

Chrystal U Louis MD MPH
Instructor, Department of Pediatrics, Section of Hematology-Oncology, Center for Cell and Gene Therapy, Baylor College of Medicine, Houston, Texas, USA

Andreas Lundqvist MD
Hematology Branch, National Institutes of Health, Bethesda, Maryland, USA

Judith Marsh FRCP FRCPath
Professor of Hematology, Division of Cellular and Molecular Medicine, St George's Hospital NHS Trust, London, UK

Jayesh Mehta MD
Professor of Medicine, Director, Hematopoietic Stem Cell Transplant Program, Feinberg School of Medicine, Northwestern University, Chicago, Illinois, USA

Simon Meller MB BS LLB(Hons) FRCP FRCPCh
Center for Medical Law and Ethics, School of Law, King's College, London. Formerly Consultant Pediatric Oncologist, Royal Marsden Hospital, Sutton, Surrey, UK

Stephan Mielke MD
Allogeneic Stem Cell Transplant Center, Division of Hematology and Oncology, Department of Internal Medicine II, Bavarian Julius Maximilian University of Würzburg, Würzburg, Germany

Matthew Montgomery MD
Associate Medical Director, Florida Blood Services, Department of Pathology, University of Arkansas for Medical Sciences, Little Rock, Arkansas, USA

Ghulam J Mufti FRCP FRCPath
Professor of Hematological Medicine, King's College Hospital, London, UK

Tariq I Mughal MD FRCP FACP
Professor of Medicine and Hematology, University of Texas Southwestern School of Medicine, Dallas, Texas, USA

Paolo Muraro MD PhD
Clinical Reader and Honorary Consultant Neurologist, Department of Cellular and Molecular Neuroscience, Imperial College, London, UK

Bijay Nair MD MPH
Fellow in Hematology/Oncology, Myeloma Institute for Research and Therapy, University of Arkansas for Medical Sciences, Little Rock, Arkansas, USA

John Oram MB ChB FRCA
Consultant in Anesthesia and Intensive Care, Leeds General Infirmary, Leeds, UK

Steven Pavletic MD
Head, Graft-versus-Host and Autoimmunity Unit, National Cancer Institute, National Institutes of Health, Bethesda, Maryland, USA

Gavin D Perkins MD MEd MRCP
Associate Clinical Professor in Critical Care and Resuscitation, University of Warwick, UK

Michael Potter FRCP FRCPath
Consultant Hematologist, Royal Marsden Hospital, Sutton, Surrey, UK

Barry Quinn MSc PGCert BD Bacc Phil RN
Senior Nurse Oncology, St George's Hospital, London, UK

Unell Riley MRCPath
Consultant Microbiologist, Royal Marsden Hospital, Sutton, Surrey, UK

Irene A G Roberts MD FRCP FRCPath FRCPCH
Professor of Pediatric Hematology, Department of Hematology, Imperial College Faculty of Medicine, London, UK

Vanderson Rocha MD PhD
Medical Assistant of the HSCT Unit, Eurocord-Netcord and European Blood and Marrow Transplant Group, Hôpital Saint Louis, Paris, France

James A Russell MA MB BChir FRCP(Ed)
Clinical Professor of Medicine and Oncology, University of Calgary, and Director, Alberta Blood and Marrow Transplant Program, Tom Baker Cancer Center, Calgary, Alberta, Canada

Bipin N Savani MD
Assistant Professor of Medicine, Vanderbilt University, and Director of Clinical Research, Veterans Affairs Medical Center Stem Cell Transplant Program, Nashville, Tennessee, USA

Anthony P Schwarer MB BS MD FRACP FRCPA
BMT Physician, Alfred Hospital, Melbourne, Victoria, Australia

Bronwen E Shaw PhD MRCP FRCPath
Consultant in Stem Cell Transplantation, Royal Marsden Hospital and Anthony Nolan Trust, London, UK

Seema Singhal MD
Professor of Medicine, Director, Multiple Myeloma Program, Feinberg School of Medicine, Northwestern University, Chicago, Illinois, USA

Gérard Socié MD PhD
Professor of Hematology and Head, Hematology/Transplantation Center, Hospitalier Universitaire Saint-Louis, Paris, France

Shivani Srivastava MD
Assistant Professor of Medicine, Bone Marrow and Stem Cell Transplantation, Indiana University School of Medicine, Indianapolis, Indiana, USA

John W Sweetenham MD
Professor of Medicine, Cleveland Clinic Taussig Cancer Center, Cleveland, Ohio, USA

Lochie Teague DCH FRACP FRCPA
Clinical Director, Pediatric Hematology/Oncology, Starship Children's Hospital, Auckland, New Zealand

John Theus MD
Assistant Professor, Department of Pathology, University of Arkansas for Medical Sciences, Little Rock, Arkansas, USA

André Tichelli MD
Professor of Hematology, Division of Hematology, University Hospitals, Basel, Switzerland

Jennifer Treleaven MD FRCP FRCPath
Consultant Hematologist, Royal Marsden Hospital, Sutton, Surrey, UK

Jaap van Laar MD PhD
Professor of Clinical Rheumatology, Institute of Cellular Medicine, School of Clinical Medical Sciences, Newcastle University, Newcastle, UK

Frits van Rhee MD PhD MRCP(UK) FRCPath
Professor of Medicine, University of Arkansas for Medical Sciences, Little Rock, Arkansas, USA

Sumithira Vasu MD
Clinical Fellow, Department of Transfusion Medicine, Warren G Magnuson Clinical Center, National Institutes of Health, Bethesda, Maryland, USA

Paul Veys MRCP FRCPath FRCPCH
Reader in Stem Cell Transplantation, Great Ormond Street Hospital for Sick Children, London, UK

Phyllis Warkentin MD
Professor of Pathology and Pediatrics, University of Nebraska Medical Center, Omaha, Nebraska, USA

Alan S Wayne MD
Clinical Director, Pediatric Oncology Branch, National Cancer Institute, National Institutes of Health, Bethesda, Maryland, USA

Daniel Weisdorf MD
Professor of Medicine and Director of the Adult Blood and Marrow Transplant Program, University of Minnesota, Minneapolis, Minnesota, USA

Robert Wynn MD MRCP FRCPath
Consultant Pediatric Hematologist, and Director, Blood and Marrow Transplant Unit, Royal Manchester Children's Hospital, Manchester, UK

FOREWORD

Hematopoietic stem cell transplantation and cellular therapy are rapidly developing, highly effective modalities of treatment for a broad range of hematologic, immunologic, metabolic and malignant diseases. For many disorders, hematopoietic transplantation is potentially curative for what would otherwise be fatal diseases. Hematopoietic transplantation is the most established form of cellular therapy and is a cornerstone of treatment for a broad range of hematologic malignancies.

Hematopoietic transplantation was originally conceived as a means of administering high doses of myelosuppressive chemotherapy and total body radiation, followed by autologous or allogeneic hematopoietic stem cell transplantation to restore hematopoiesis. Much of the benefit, however, is related to an immune graft-versus-malignancy effect mediated by donor immunocompetent cells. Historically, hematopoietic transplantation has been a high-risk form of treatment; life-threatening complications may occur related to drug toxicities, graft rejection, graft-versus-host disease, and infections related to post-transplant immune deficiency.

There has been enormous progress in every aspect of the field. Supportive care has markedly improved and non-myeloablative preparative regimens have been developed which have markedly reduced the toxicity associated with hematopoietic transplantation. The field has been less successful in improving the eradication of malignancy, but there is a plethora of novel strategies currently under investigation.

This book effectively summarizes the progress in ongoing clinical and translational research involving hematopoietic transplantation as well as the clinical issues faced in practice. The history of hematopoietic transplantation and its underlying biology is reviewed. Current considerations for the clinical use of stem cell transplantation are presented and its role versus alternative forms of treatment is discussed. Important practical information is also presented regarding the organization and operation of clinical stem cell units and ethical considerations faced in practice.

Richard Champlin MD 2008

PREFACE

Hematopoietic stem cell transplantation is still a relatively new treatment modality, having been used clinically only since the 1970s. As time has passed, many changes and refinements have been introduced into what was originally an extremely hazardous therapy, and problems have been solved which earlier were not even known to exist. The patient population to which these techniques are applicable has also changed and enlarged as treatment has become safer, with the introduction of improved blood product support, antibiotics and better immunosuppressants, not to mention the expanding role of reduced-intensity conditioned transplantation and an increased repertoire of stem cell sources now that cord blood is available.

Although many of the original difficulties continue to pose problems, advances in the field have occurred so rapidly that it is difficult to keep abreast of all the changes. A regular update is therefore necessary, and it is the aim of this book to provide it. Advances in all fields of transplantation are discussed and an overview of the relevant literature is provided. An attempt has been made to provide a practical approach to problem solving, and where applicable this has been done with tables and lists with the intention of assisting the reader to assess the various options rapidly and effectively.

The book will be of use to healthcare workers in the field of hematopoietic stem cell transplantation, and particularly to those who have day-to-day responsibility for patients, including doctors, nurses, pharmacy staff and many others. It is hoped that students of medicine will also find it readable, and that it will afford them some insight into the options which now face us when dealing with patients undergoing these complicated forms of treatment.

J.T.
J.B.
2008

PART **1**

SETTING THE SCENE

Introduction

Jennifer Treleaven

CHAPTER 1

Stem cell transplantation is now used worldwide in the treatment of many malignant and non-malignant hematologic conditions and in the treatment of various solid tumors. Every year, many hundreds of patients receive an autologous or allogeneic transplant procedure, and the numbers have increased vastly since the pool of allogeneic donors available worldwide widened, enabling a larger number of patients with no sibling donor to undergo an allogeneic transplant prodedure. Figure 1.1 shows the annual number of transplants reported in the International Bone Marrow Transplant Registry and how this increased as stem cell transplantation became a realistic treatment possibility. However, stem cell transplants have only become a therapeutic possibility since the late 1960s. Prior to this, understanding of such topics as human leukocyte antigen matching was rudimentary. The concepts of immunosuppression and graft-versus-host disease were entirely unexplored and little was known about preparative therapies. Early transplants thus invariably met with a woeful lack of success due to problems from regimen-related toxicity, graft-versus-host disease and lack of availability of support measures, including antibiotics and blood products.

As knowledge about these fundamental topics was acquired and methods of identifying a suitable donor improved along with support measures and knowledge about immunosuppression, so did the results of cell transplantation. Since the 1970s, steady progress has been made and stem cell transplantation is now regarded as a routine, rather than an experimental, approach in the treatment of a number of conditions which would have proven fatal earlier on. It is now possible to identify the risk factors which will predict a good or poor outcome in a particular clinical setting, thereby facilitating the decision of whether or not to proceed with the transplant. However, the problems which beset the early transplanters, in particular disease relapse, graft-versus-host disease and overwhelming infection, are still the major causes of treatment failure in spite of the improvements which have been made to support therapies and the immense amount of information now available regarding the cellular and humoral aspects of transplantation and our consequent ability to manipulate and control the microenvironment in the transplant setting. Figure 1.2 depicts some of the milestones in the evolution of stem cell transplantation and therapeutic interventions which have become available in the context of the diseases for which transplantation was attempted early on.

A brief history of bone marrow transplantation

Before the 20th century

One of the earliest references to the therapeutic properties of bone marrow is found in the 8th-century Irish epic tale of the Cattle Raid of Cooley, the *Táin Bó Cúailnge*. The charioteer Cethern, an Ulster warrior, was severely wounded in battle and treated by the healer Fingin. The treatment involved him sleeping in a bath of bone marrow, although its effects were going to be short-lived. Some of his ribs were replaced with chariot parts, and the frame of the chariot was tied to his belly to keep his insides in. According to the legend, this renewed Cethern's strength sufficiently to allow him to resume fighting although he was killed in battle shortly afterwards.[1,2]

In the 19th century it was understood that bone marrow was involved in the formation of blood and the idea arose that bone marrow might have healing properties and could possibly be of use in treating anemia. In 1896, Quine reported that Brown Sequard & D'Arsenoval had administered bone marrow orally in 1891 to treat defective blood formation.[3] Attempts were also made to treat pernicious anemia using a glycerol extract of animal bone marrow administered orally, so there would have been no chance of living cells being transferred and any benefit from the treatment would have derived from the nutritional, rather than cellular, aspect of the mixture.[4,5] Subsequetly, intramedullary injections of marrow were used to treat aplastic anemia, which may have resulted in the transfer of some living cells although they would have remained viable for only a short period of time. Billings in 1894 and Hamilton in 1895 probably correctly attributed any positive effects of treatment to the mineral content of the elixir.[6,7]

Early 20th century: 1920s–1940s

In 1923, Leake & Leake observed some responses in rabbits and dogs with anemia to saline extracts of bone marrow and spleen administered intravenously, particularly when the two were administered as a combination.[8] Daily oral administration of 1% filtered solution of desiccated spleen and powdered red bone marrow in rabbits gave parallel results,[9] depending on whether the extracts were given singly or in combination. Oral administration of a filtered solution of combined powdered red bone marrow and desiccated spleen in dogs caused a marked rise in the number of circulating erythrocytes. The authors concluded that splenic and red bone marrow extracts were more powerful stimulants of erythropoiesis in combination than separately, attributing their action firstly to increasing the rate of production or delivery in existing sites of erythropoiesis, and secondly to causing an increase in the amount of functioning red marrow.

In 1937 Schretzenmayr administered intramuscular injections of freshly aspirated autologous or allogeneic bone marrow to patients suffering from parasitic infections, with limited success. This was the first use of bone marrow administered by a technique likely to result in the transfer of living cells.[10]

A couple of years later, an attempt was made to treat a patient suffering from aplastic anemia. A small quantity of bone marrow from his brother was infused.[11] Prior to this, in 1930, Gloor described the cure of a patient with acute myeloid leukemia by stem cell transplantation.[12] However, stem cell transplantation as an approach for treating leukemia and aplastic anemia was not investigated seriously until the 1960s when it was found that dogs could survive 2–4 times the lethal exposure to irradiation (TBI) if they were given an infusion of bone marrow cells removed and stored prior to the TBI.[13]

In 1948, Jacobson showed that mice could be protected from bone marrow failure by shielding either a portion of marrow in the hindlimb or the spleen,[14] and that provided this were done, a mouse which had received a lethal dose of irradiation would regenerate its blood count. He subsequently showed that bone marrow failure following otherwise lethal doses of irradiation could also be prevented by infusing either spleen cells or bone marrow cells from a litter mate into the animal.[15] At the time, the mechanism involved in this effect was not understood and was thought by some to be due to the transfer of a humoral factor which stimulated or protected the marrow against the effects of irradiation. Others, including Lorenz,[16] believed that transfer of living cells was responsible for the recovery of the marrow.

1950s–1960s

As early as 1956, the idea that allogeneic bone marrow transplants (BMT) might exert a therapeutic immunologic effect against malignancies was proposed by Barnes & Loutit,[17] who observed an antileukemia effect of transplanted spleen cells in experimental murine models.[18] They also observed that animals who had been given allogeneic rather than syngeneic marrow cells died of a 'wasting disease'[19] which would now be recognized as being graft-versus-host disease (GvHD).

In 1954 major advances were made. Ford, using the T6 chromosomal marker which identified the transfused cells, demonstrated that the same marker recurred in all the cells derived from the recovering

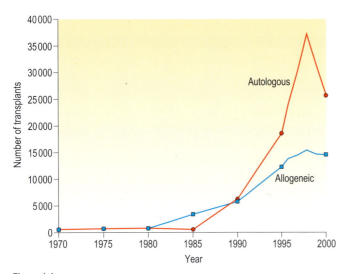

Figure 1.1
Annual numbers of blood and marrow transplants worldwide, 1970–2000, from the CIBMTR.

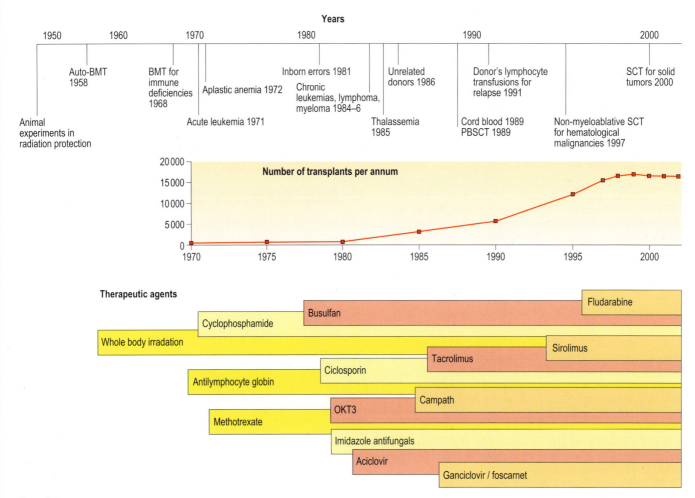

Figure 1.2
Some developmental steps in blood and marrow stem cell transplantation and the introduction of significant therapeutic agents, 1950–2000.

marrow of the lethally irradiated recipient mouse,[20] thereby proving that such cells were donor derived. This proved not only that cellular engraftment had occurred, but also that the transfer of a few cells resulted in complete and stable hematopoietic reconstitution of the recipient. A few years later, in 1961, Till & McCulloch showed that in irradiated mice, marrow repopulation originated from multipotential 'colony-forming units' which could be detected in the spleen.[21] Dosing experiments demonstrated that such colonies must have arisen from the seeding of a single cell – a stem cell. Single colonies isolated from the spleen could reconstitute hematopoiesis in other irradiated recipients, thus demonstating that one stem cell could reconstitute the entire myeloid compartment of a recipient mouse.

However, in spite of various successes with animal models, up to this time almost all attempts to achieve allogeneic grafts in humans had been unsuccessful although it was recognized that marrow transplantation would be of potential use in the treatment of various bone marrow failure syndromes and hematologic disorders. Thomas & Ferrebee had started studies on patients suffering from terminal leukemia, and in 1957 they reported on six such patients who had been treated with irradiation and marrow infusion from a single, normal donor, although only one showed transient marrow engraftment.[22]

Billingham, Brent and Medawar[23] provided much of the early information concerning graft tolerance, using newborn mice which were given allogeneic marrow cells.[24] They went on to make the following observations with regard to allogeneic marrow transfusion.

- Autologous cells did not result in runt disease.
- Allogeneic cells had to persist in the recipient in order for runt disease to develop.
- The severity of runt disease was determined by antigenic differences between the recipient and donor.

In addition to the lack of knowledge at the time concerning tissue typing and HLA compatibility, treatment success was also limited by lack of knowledge of how to administer high-dose therapy and inability to provide adequate supportive care for marrow failure because few antibiotics and antifungal agents were available, and the availability of blood products was very limited.

Georges Mathé was a pioneer in the early development of clinical BMT. In 1958, six physicists were accidentally exposed to large doses of mixed gamma and neutron irradiation at Vinca in Yugoslavia,[25] and were estimated to have received radiation doses of between 600 and 1000 rads. One, who was judged to have received about 700 rads, died. The sixth one survived with no treatment apart from being placed in a 'clean' environment, and he was thought to have received only 400 rads. Mathé gave them multiple allogeneic bone marrow infusions from family members. The men all survived, with eventual autologous marrow recovery, but the allogeneic bone marrow served to protect the patients until this had taken place. Red cell antigen studies of the transfused allogeneic marrow demonstrated that successful but temporary engraftment had taken place, with eventual autologous reconstitution which was evident from the changes seen in the red cell groups in subjects who were not ABO and Rhesus compatible with their donors. Of note was the fact that the red cell output of the donated cells paralleled the amount of marrow initially infused, perhaps indicating that the subjects who received the larger numbers of stem cells experienced enhanced hemopoietic recovery.

In 1963 Mathé published a case report concerning a patient with leukemia who was transfused with a mixture of bone marrow and blood from six family members – mother, father, three brothers and a sister – after preparation with 800 rads of total body irradiation with cobalt-60 preceded by 4 days of mercaptopurine, 300 mg per day. All the donors and the recipient were red cell ABO group O Rh D positive, but because of differences in other red cell antigens between the patient and his donors, it was possible to document engraftment from one of the brothers who had small s and was (Le a+b−), whereas the

patient was big S positive and (Le a−b+). The erythrocyte phenotype remained that of the brother 8 months after transplantation, and the patient was also tolerant of a skin graft from this donor whereas he rejected skin grafts from his other donors at varying lengths of time after transplantation. This paper is probably the first documented case of full donor chimerism to be described after stem cell transfer and it also states that the patient experienced 'secondary disease' with weight loss, digestive disturbances and desquamative erythroderma, now known as graft-versus-host disease.[26]

Mathé continued working on the comparisons in antileukemia effects of allogeneic adult or embryonic hematopoietic grafts conditioned by irradiation and on attempting to control graft-versus-host disease. At this point he was led to observe and describe the graft-versus-leukemia (GvL) effect associated with GvHD and he also observed a specific antileukemia effect of adoptive immunotherapy, resulting in a reduced plasma concentration of the Friend leukemogenic virus.[27] This indicated the possibility that lymphoid elements in the engrafted marrow might react against the malignant cells in the patient to aid in eradicating any remaining malignant cells.[28]

Around the same time, E Donnell Thomas, working on dogs in the USA, defined radiation doses, designed marrow harvesting techniques and ascertained the support required to carry out marrow transplants in man. Dogs can be physically large and have some immunologic similarities to man in terms of the fact that they possess a complex HLA system. The fact that they come in large families enabled experiments to be conducted which relied on the infusion of litter mate marrow to a lethally irradiated recipient, and allowed such issues to be resolved as what constituted a permanently marrow-ablative dose of radiotherapy and the number of cells that it was necessary to infuse to effect marrow reconstitution. The use of autologous marrow as 'rescue' after otherwise lethal irradiation was also documented around this time; marrow from dogs to be irradiated was set aside before the procedure and reinfused after irradiation had taken place. Control dogs which were irradiated and not reinfused with marrow died, whereas those who had received marrow after irradiation experienced autologous reconstitution and lived.[29]

Thomas and colleagues then went on to develop a regimen of posttransplant immunosuppression using methotrexate as GvHD prophylaxis,[30] and they established various facts concerning transplantation which are still valid and which won Thomas the Nobel Prize for Physiology or Medicine in 1990.

Elucidation of the human histocompatibility antigen (HLA) system allowed major steps to be made in the field of transplantation biology, much of the early work having been conducted by Dausset & van Rood who recognized that the HLA system was inherited.[31] They went on to define the nature of various leukoagglutinins found in certain human sera,[32] eventually constructing the major histocompatibility gene map.[33] Again, much of the early work was conducted in dogs. Antisera were subsequently raised in dogs to various HLA antigens so that characterization of the HLA system could be undertaken.[34]

The miniaturization of the matching system by Terasaki and colleagues made HLA typing much more practical,[35] since, with the ability to tissue match donors and recipients, allogeneic transplants could be carried out in humans between HLA identical siblings. One of the first cases to be reported was of an infant with severe combined immune deficiency disease in Leiden, Netherlands.[36] By the end of the 1960s, all the components were in place for developing and expanding a new era of clinical bone marrow transplantation.

1970s–1980s

During the 1970s and 1980s, allogeneic stem cell transfer (SCT) was used to treat many different diseases including congenital immune deficiency syndromes, severe aplastic anemia, and acute and chronic leukemias. Much progress was made in understanding the immunology of transplantation, in controlling the problems associated with transplantation which arose as a consequence of using high-dose chemoradiotherapy, and improved conditioning regimens were worked out. At the same time, progress was made in chemotherapy induction for the acute leukemias, resulting in higher remission rates. Hence, there was renewed interest in autologous BMT for acute leukaemia. By the end of the 1970s, numerous centers worldwide had active BMT programs and two influential multicenter bodies had become established: the International Bone Marrow Transplant Registry and the European Bone Marrow Transplant Group.

The potential of BMT as a means of curing patients with otherwise incurable diseases was clear. However, the shortcomings of the procedure – leukemic relapse, GvHD, graft failure and early toxicity – were still a problem. Improvements were made in conditioning regimes as radiotherapy and various alkylating agents were combined in an attempt to overcome the underlying disease, and dose-limiting toxicities became apparent. Methods of immunosuppressing recipients advanced beyond the use of steroids and methotrexate. Ciclosporin was introduced into the transplant forum in the early 1970s after work had been carried out using dog models. It was initially used in solid organ transplantation,[37,38] where the side-effect of nephrotoxicity was noted, and subsequently in bone marrow transplantation, where it was observed to improve the situation with regard to GvHD, although many side-effects were apparent which resolved when the drug was stopped or the dose reduced.[39,40]

Improvements were also made in infection prophylaxis with the introduction of new antibacterial agents and the antiviral drug aciclovir which had been shown to be active against the herpes virus in animal models.[41] Used on a number of patients who had received treatment for malignant disease or a bone marrow transplant, the drug was noted to arrest the progress of the herpes infections and was found to be most effective when given early. Although some patients showed transient increases in blood urea, possibly the result of aciclovir, the drug was observed to be remarkably non-toxic at the doses used.

The antifungus drug amphotericin was also introduced into the transplant setting around this time,[42] having first been isolated in 1955 from *Streptomyces nodosus*, a filamentous bacterium. Since then, numerous antimicrobials designed to treat a vast array of infecting organisms have become available.

Further strides in stem cell transplantation were possible when understanding of the essentials involved in freezing living cells improved.[43] Obviously, cooling tissue to below 0°C resulted in freezing, which greatly reduced the number of viable cells when these were thawed. As far back as 1949, the discovery had been made that the addition of glycerol to human and bull sperm greatly improved cell viability after freezing to −79° and, using infant mouse spleen cells, Barnes & Loutit later showed that hematopoietic cells would survive low-temperature preservation after slow cooling to −79°C in 15% glycerolized medium.[44] Subsequently, dimethyl sulfoxide was discovered to be a superior cryopreservant to glycerol and it is this agent which is currently used for freezing stem cells[45] in programmed freezers which use liquid nitrogen. Cells could now be stored in liquid nitrogen for an indefinite period, if necessary, prior to reinfusion.

During the 1980s and early 1990s there was rapid expansion of clinical BMT programs worldwide and it became possible to analyze large patient series so as to define specific patient/donor and transplant-related risk factors for various diseases. Antibiotic and antiviral support continued to improve with, for example, the introduction of ganciclovir for the treatment of cytomegalovirus,[46,47] and liposomal amphotericin for the treatment of fungal infections without the nephrotoxicity associated with regular amphotericin.[48,49] There was a consequent reduction in transplant-related morbidity and, as further understanding of the HLA system developed, it was possible to provide

more patients with a suitable matched unrelated donor,[50] particularly in view of the establishment of large, unrelated volunteer donor panels by the Anthony Nolan Research group in London, Europdonor based in Leiden, Holland, and the North American Marrow Donor Pool (NAMDP) in the USA.[51] Blood product support also improved with, for example, the availability of partially HLA-matched platelet transfusions for patients who were failing to increment because of platelet antibodies. The first attempts at transplant engineering were undertaken – the depletion of T-cells from the marrow inoculum to prevent GvHD – although this maneuver, while reducing GvHD, was soon noted to be associated with an increase of both graft rejection and leukemia relapse.[52–54]

The demonstration that patients with chronic myeloid leukemia could be reconstituted with autologous peripheral blood cells[55] heralded the later widespread use of peripheral blood stem cells for transplantation. Autologous transplantation with marrow rescue was used increasingly to treat lymphomas, myeloma and solid tumors[56–58] (see Fig. 1.1), and attempts were made to purge the marrow of malignant cells by various techniques including the use of immunotoxins, complement-conjugated antibodies and magnetic microspheres.[59–61]

The 1990s

The 1990s were a period of rapid development in BMT. Recombinant growth factors had become available, including granulocyte-macrophage colony-stimulating factor (GM-CSF) and granulocyte colony-stimulating factor (G-CSF), which could be used to speed up white cell recovery after chemotherapy or after transplantation, thereby shortening the length of hospital stay.[62–64] The use of peripheral blood stem cells (PBSC) mobilized into the blood by G-CSF virtually replaced the use of bone marrow for transplantation, avoiding the need for a general anesthetic and arguably resulting in more rapid myeloid reconstitution so that it even became feasible to undertake autologous PBSC transplants on an outpatient basis, provided that medical back-up was near at hand.[65]

Cord blood transplantation also started to become popular, following the first successful cord blood stem cell transplant in 1988.[66] Increasing numbers of patients have received cord blood transplants, although their use may have to be restricted to lower body weight recipients because of problems with the cell dose obtainable from a cord in relation to recipient body weight and the possibility of delayed engraftment. However, cord blood stem cell transplants appear to be associated with a relatively low incidence of acute GvHD and their use has greatly expanded the donor pool available worldwide now that both public and private cord blood banks have been established in many countries.[67–69]

New understanding of the pathogenesis of GvHD and of the basic mechanisms involved in alloreactions has dramatically changed the way acute GvHD prevention is being investigated in experimental studies. To prevent GvHD, most therapies rely on the elimination of donor T-cells from the graft or immunosuppression of the host. Unfortunately, these approaches can result in poor engraftment, a loss of GvL activity, and a higher risk of leukemic relapse. Instead of the global immunosuppression conferred by pharmacologic agents and non-selective T-cell depletion methods, new approaches focus on the induction of specific tolerance, which prevents the development of acute GvHD during the establishment of donor immunity. If GvHD does develop, a number of targeted monoclonal antibodies are now available which block the host immune response, such as daclizumab and inolimomab, which are IL-2 receptor blockers,[70–72] and infliximab which is an antitumor necrosis factor antibody (TNF),[73,74] thereby hindering tissue damage.

Another approach is the use of keratinocyte growth factor (KGF), also called fibroblast growth factor 7 (FGF-7).[75] This is important in tissue repair and wound healing and its administration has been shown to be protective against radiation- and bleomycin-induced lung injury in rats,[76] possibly by facilitating repair of DNA damage or increasing time of stem cell survival.

Mesenchymal stem cells have also recently been shown to be of use in treatment therapy-refractory GvHD in humans,[77,78] and probably act by inhibiting proliferation and cytokine secretion of primary T-cells in response to mitogens and allogeneic T-cells.[79,80]

It first became accepted in the 1980s that GvL was a clinical as well as an experimental reality, and since that time, much progress has been made in understanding and characterizing the GvL reaction.[81] While the separation of GvL from GvHD is theoretically possible and has, in limited circumstances, been achieved clinically, lack of ability to identify antigens promoting leukemia-specific alloresponses remains the biggest single obstacle to improving the strength and specificity of GvL in clinical practice. However, reduced-intensity conditioned allogeneic transplants are now in widespread use, relying for efficacy on the graft-versus-tumor effect rather than the conditioning therapy to eliminate disease. An additional advantage of this approach is that, because conditioning is less intensive, older and less fit patients who would not previously have been considered suitable for transplantation have now become eligible.

Advances in the field of molecular biology have made it possible to transfect genes into human cells using an adenovirus vector. With this technique, a new gene is inserted into an adenovirus vector which has been genetically altered to carry normal human DNA, and which is then used to introduce the modified DNA into a human cell. If the treatment is successful, the new gene will make a functional protein. This approach has already been used successfully to treat metastatic melanoma, with killer T-cells genetically retargeted to attack the cancer cells,[82] and it has also been successfully used to treat X-linked granulomatous disease in two adults.[83]

Gene therapy has numerous applications in the field of marrow transplantation: correction of inherited genetic disorders using the patient's own stem cells or lymphocytes as the vehicle to deliver life-long gene replacement, modification of malignant cells to render them more susceptible to immune or chemotherapeutic control, and modification of immune cells to make them more effective. Several gene therapy trials have been initiated in other congenital disorders affecting stem cells. However, the problem of achieving adequate and sustained gene expression has yet to be solved.

The future

It can be anticipated that stem cell transplantation procedures will continue to become safer, thereby allowing us to safely extend curative treatments to elderly patients, patients only partially matched with the donor and conditions that are not immediately life-threatening, such as is already the situation regarding transplantation for certain autoimmune disorders and hemoglobinopathies.

The techniques that can make these developments possible are already under investigation. Current areas of research include the delivery of measured large doses of CD34+ cells to achieve rapid and stable engraftment even in mismatched donor–recipient combinations. It may eventually become possible to expand stem cells in vitro, thus extending the opportunity to increase the size of the transplant. Such an approach may prove of use in the cord blood transplant setting, enabling larger cell doses to be provided in accordance with the recipient's body weight. Using this approach, cord blood banks could be expanded even further to allow a larger number of patients to undergo a stem cell transplant. With the development of all the clinically important growth factors required to stimulate proliferation of stem cells, granulocytes, erythrocytes and megakaryocytes, and their

availability as long-acting preparations, it should be possible not only to significantly reduce the need for transfusion support and eliminate neutropenic episodes, but also to mobilize larger numbers of stem cells for autologous or allogeneic donation.

Progress can be expected in the control of T-cell recovery by depletion, and add-back techniques of T-cells selected to avoid GvHD, the use of vaccines or adoptively transferred T-cells to induce antitumor and antiviral responses in the donor or the autograft recipient, and the use of gene therapy for selection or elimination of designated lymphocyte cell populations. Improvements have already been made in the field of tissue typing, with molecular typing rather than serologic allowing much more precise characterization of the MHC genes in donors and recipients. It has thus become possible to match unrelated donors to a degree not previously achievable, thereby permitting a much wider range of transplants to take place with relative safety.

Continuing improvement in support therapies, including more sophisticated antimicrobial agents and more refined and safer blood product support, will allow transplants to be undertaken more safely, and monoclonal antibodies targeting the biologic mechanisms involved in the graft-versus-host reaction will hopefully also further reduce transplant-related morbidity. Finally, with the development of targeted therapies such as tyrosine kinase, FLT-3 inhibitors and so on, it may be possible that fewer patients with hematologic malignancies will rely upon stem cell transplantation to cure their disease and that this will be achievable with drug therapy.

References

1. O'Rahilly C (ed & trans). Táin Bó Cúailnge, from the Book of Leinster. Dublin Institute for Advanced Studies, 1967, 234–239
2. Kinsella T. The Tain. Oxford University Press, Oxford, 1970, 212
3. Quine WE. The remedial application of bone marrow. JAMA 1896;26:1012–1013
4. Fraser TR. Bone marrow in the treatment of pernicious anaemia. BMJ 1894;i: 1172–1174
5. Danforth IN. Pernicious anaemia: a new method of treatment. Chicago Clin Rev 1894;4:1
6. Billings JS. Theraputic use of extract of bone marrow. Bull Johns Hopkins Hosp 1894;5:115
7. Hamilton AM. The use of medullary glyceride in conditions attended by paucity of red blood corpuscles and haemoglobin. New York Med J 1895;61:44
8. Leake CD, Leake BW. The erythropoietic action of red bone marrow and spleen extracts. J Pharmacol Exper Ther 1923;22:75–88
9. Minot GR, Murphy WP. Treatment of pernicious anaemia by a special diet. JAMA 1926;87:470–476
10. Schretzenmayr A. Treatment of anaemia by bone marrow injection. Klin Wissenschaftschreiben 1937;16:1010–1012
11. Osgood EE, Riddle MC, Matthews TJ. Aplastic anaemia treated with daily transfusions and intravenous marrow: case report. Ann Int Med 1939;13:357–367
12. Gloor W. Ein Fall von geheiltes Myeloblastenleukaemi. Munchen Med Wochenschreibe 1930;77:1096–1098
13. Mannick JA, Lochte HL, Ashley CA et al. Autografts of bone marrow in dogs after lethal body irradiation. Blood 1960;15:255–266
14. Jacobson LO, Simmons EL, Marks EK et al. The role of the spleen in radiation injury and recovery. J Lab Clin Med 1950;35:746–751
15. Jacobson LO, Simmons EL, Bethard WF. Studies on hematopoietic recovery from radiation injury. J Clin Invest 1950;29:825
16. Lorenz E, Congdon CC, Uphoff D. Modification of acute irradiation injury in mice and guinea pigs by bone marrow injections. Radiology 1952;58:863–877
17. Barnes DWH, Loutit JF. Treatment of murine leukaemia with X-rays and homologous bone marrow. BMJ 1956;2:626–627
18. Barnes DWH, Loutit JF. What is the recovery factor in spleen? Nucleonics 1954; 12:68–71
19. Barnes DW, Loutit JF, Micklem HS. 'Secondary disease' of radiation chimeras: a syndrome due to lymphoid aplasia. Ann NY Acad Sci 1962;99:374–385
20. Ford CE, Hamerton JL, Barnes DWH, Loutit JF. Cytological identification of radiation chimeras. Nature 1956;177:452–454
21. Till JE, McCulloch EA. A direct measurement of the radiation sensitivity of normal mouse bone marrow cells. Radiat Res 1961;14:213
22. Thomas ED, Lochte HL, Lu WC, Ferrebee JW. Intravenous infusion of bone marrow in patients receiving radiation and chemotherapy. N Engl J Med 1957;257:491–496
23. Billingham RE, Brent L, Medawar PB. 'Actively acquired tolerance' of foreign cells. Nature 1953;172:606
24. Billingham RE. The biology of graft-versus-host reactions. Harvey Lectures. Academic Press, New York. 1966, 21–78
25. Mathé G, Jammet H, Pendic B et al. Transfusions and grafts of homologous bone marrow in humans accidentally irradiated to high doses. Revue Franc Etudes Clin Biol 1959;4:226–229

26. Mathé G, Amiel JL, Schwarzenberg L et al. Adoptive immunotherapy of acute leukaemia: experimental and clinical results. Cancer Res 1965;25:1525–1531

27. Mathé G, Amiel JL. Reduction of the plasma concentration of the Charlotte Friend leukaemogenic virus by adoptive immunotherapy (graft of allogeneic bone marrow). C R Hebd Seances Acad Sci 1964;259:4408–4410

28. Mathé G, Amiel JL, Schwarzenberg L et al. Haematopoietic chimera in man after allogeneic (homologous) bone marrow transplantation (control of secondary symptom-specific tolerence due to chimerism). BM J 1963;2:1633–1635

29. Alpen EL, Baum SJ. Modification of X-irradiation lethality by autologous marrow infusion in dogs. Blood 1958;13:1168–1175

30. Lochte HL, Levy AS, Guenther DM et al. Prevention of delayed foreign marrow reaction in lethally irradiated mice by early administration of methotrexate. Nature 1962;196:1110–1111

31. Daussett J, Rapaport FT, Ivanyi P, Colombani J. Tissue alloantigens and transplantation. In: Balner H, Cleton FJ, Eernisse JG (eds) Histocompatibility testing. Munksgaard, Copenhagen, 1965, 63–78

32. Dausset J. Iso-leuco-anticorps. Acta Haematol 1958;20:156

33. Dausset J, Rapaport FT, Legrand L et al. Skin allograft survival in 238 human subjects: role of the specific relationship at the 4 gene sites of the first and the second HLA loci. In: Terasaki P (ed) Histocompatibility testing. Munksgaard, Copenhagen, 1970, 381–397

34. Epstein RB, Storb R, Ragde H, Thomas ED. Cytotoxic antisera for marrow grafting in littermate dogs. Transplantation 1968;9:215–229

35. Terasaki PI, McLelland JD. Microdroplet assay of human serum cytotoxins. Nature (London) 1964;204:998–1000

36. de Koning J, van Bekkum DW, Dicke KA et al. Transplantation of bone marrow cells and foetal thymus in an infant with lymphopoenic immunological deficiency. Lancet 1969;1:1223–1227

37. Calne RY, Rolles K, White DJ et al. Cyclosporin A initially as the only immunosuppressant in 34 recipients of cadaveric organs: 32 kidneys, 2 pancreases, and 2 livers. Lancet 1979;2:1033–1036

38. Calne RY, White DJ, Thiru S et al. Cyclosporin A in patients receiving renal allografts from cadaver donors. Transplant Proc 1979;11:860–864

39. Powles RL, Barrett AJ, Clink H et al. Cyclosporin A for the treatment of graft-versus-host disease in man. Lancet 1978;2:1327–1331

40. Powles RL, Clink HM, Spence D et al. Cyclosporin A to prevent graft-versus-host disease in man after allogeneic bone-marrow transplantation. Lancet 1980;1:327–329

41. Selby PJ, Powles RL, Jameson B et al. Parenteral acyclovir therapy for herpesvirus infections in man. Lancet 1979;2:1267–1270

42. Medoff G, Dismukes WG, Meades RHI, Moses JM. A new therapeutic approach to candida infections: a preliminary report. Arch Intern Med 1972;130:241–245

43. Smith AU, Polge C. Survival of spermatozoa at low temperatures. Nature 1950;166:668–669

44. Barnes DW, Loutit JF. The radiation recovery factor: preservation by the Polge-Smith-Parkes technique. J Natl Cancer Inst 1955;15:901–905

45. Ashwood-Smith MJ. Preservation of mouse bone marrow at -79°C with dimethyl sulphoxide Nature 1961;190:1204 -1205

46. Winston DJ, Ho WG, Bartoni K et al. Ganciclovir prophylaxis of cytomegalovirus infection and disease in allogeneic bone marrow transplant recipients: results of a placebo-controlled, double-blind trial. Ann Intern Med 1993;118:179–184

47. Emanuel D, Cunningham I, Jules-Elysee K et al. Cytomegalovirus pneumonia after bone marrow transplantation successfully treated with the combination of ganciclovir and high-dose intravenous immune globulin. Ann Intern Med 1988;109:777–782

48. Lopez-Berestein G, Fainstein V, Hopfer R et al. Liposomal amphotericin B for the treatment of systemic fungal infections in patients with cancer: a preliminary study. J Infect Dis 1985;151:704–710

49. Mehta R, Lopez-Berestein G, Hopfer R et al. Liposomal amphotericin B is toxic to fungal cells but not to mammalian cells. Biochim Biophys Acta 1984;770:230–234

50. Bortin MM, Rimm AA. Increasing utilization of bone marrow transplantation. Transplantation 1986;42:229–234

51. Goldman JM, Cleaver S, Warren P. World Marrow Donor Association: a progress report. Bone Marrow Transplant 1994;13:689–691

52. Weiden PL, Flournoy N, Thomas ED et al. Antileukemic effect of graft-versus-host disease in human recipients of allogeneic marrow grafts. N Engl J Med 1979;300:1068–1073

53. Goldman JM, Gale RP, Horowitz MM et al. Bone marrow transplantation for chronic myelogenous leukaemia in chronic phase: increased risk of relapse associated with T-cell depletion. Ann Intern Med 1988;108:806–814

54. Champlin RE. T-cell depletion for bone marrow transplantation: effects on graft rejection, graft-versus-host disease, graft-versus-leukemia, and survival. Cancer Treat Res 1990;50:99–111

55. Brito-Babapulle F, Bowcock SJ, Marcus RE et al. Autografting for patients with chronic myeloid leukaemia in chronic phase: peripheral blood stem cells may have a finite capacity for maintaining haematopoiesis. Br J Haematol 1989;73:76–81

56. Kingston JE, Malpas JS, Stiller CA et al. Autologous bone marrow transplantation contributes to haemopoietic recovery in children with solid tumors treated with high dose melphalan. Br J Haematol 1984;58:589–595

57. Lazarus HM, Herzig RH, Graham-Pole J et al. Intensive melphalan chemotherapy and cryopreserved autologous bone marrow transplantation for the treatment of refractory cancer. J Clin Oncol 1983;6:359–367

58. Dicke KA, Zander A, Spitzer G et al. Autologous bone-marrow transplantation in relapsed adult acute leukaemia. Lancet 1979;1:514–517

59. Feeney M, Knapp RC, Greenberger JS, Bast RC. Elimination of leukemic cells from rat bone marrow using antibody and complement. Cancer Res 1981;41(9 Pt 1):3331–3335

60. Filipovich AH, Vallera DA, Youle RJ et al. Ex-vivo treatment of donor bone marrow with anti-T-cell immunotoxins for prevention of graft-versus-host disease. Lancet 1984;1:469–472

61. Treleaven JG, Gibson FM, Ugelstad J et al. Removal of neuroblastoma cells from bone marrow with monoclonal antibodies conjugated to magnetic microspheres. Lancet 1984;1:70–73

62. Powles R, Smith C, Milan S et al. Human recombinant GM-CSF in allogeneic bone-marrow transplantation for leukaemia: double-blind, placebo-controlled trial. Lancet 1990;336:1417–1420

63. Morstyn G, Campbell L, Lieschke G et al. Treatment of chemotherapy-induced neutropenia by subcutaneously administered granulocyte colony-stimulating factor with optimization of dose and duration of therapy. J Clin Oncol 1989;7:1554–1562

64. Morstyn G, Campbell L, Souza LM et al. Effect of granulocyte colony stimulating factor on neutropenia induced by cytotoxic chemotherapy. Lancet 1988;1:667–672

65. Glück S, des Rochers C, Cano C et al. High-dose chemotherapy followed by autologous blood cell transplantation: a safe and effective outpatient approach. Bone Marrow Transplant 1997;6:431–434

66. Gluckman E, Broxmeyer H, Auerbach AD et al. Hematopoietic reconstitution in a patient with Fanconi's anemia by means of umbilical cord blood from an HLA-identical sibling. N Engl J Med 1989;321:1174–1178

67. McCullough J, Clay ME, Fautsch S et al. Proposed policies and procedures for the establishment of a cord blood bank. Blood Cells 1994;20:609–626

68. Gluckman E. European organization for cord blood banking. Blood Cells 1994;20:601- 608

69. Fisher CA. Establishment of cord blood banks for use in stem cell transplantation: commentary. Curr Probl Obstet Gynecol Fertil 1996;19:55–58

70. Perales MA, Ishill N, Lomazow WA et al. Long-term follow-up of patients treated with daclizumab for steroid-refractory acute graft-vs-host disease. Bone Marrow Transplant 2007;40(5):481–486

71. Bordigoni P, Dimicoli S, Clement L et al. Daclizumab, an efficient treatment for steroid-refractory acute graft-versus-host disease. Br J Haematol 2006;135:382–385

72. Bay JO, Dhédin N, Goerner M et al. Inolimomab in steroid-refractory acute graft-versus-host disease following allogeneic hematopoietic stem cell transplantation: retrospective analysis and comparison with other interleukin-2 receptor antibodies. Transplantation 2005;80:782–788

73. Patriarca F, Sperotto A, Damiani D et al. Infliximab treatment for steroid-refractory acute graft-versus-host disease. Haematologica 2004;89:1352–1359

74. Jacobsohn DA, Hallick J, Anders V et al. Infliximab for steroid-refractory acute GVHD: a case series. Am J Hematol 2003;74:119–124

75. Panoskaltsis-Mortari A, Lacey D, Vallera D, Blazar B. Keratinocyte growth factor administered before conditioning ameliorates graft-versus-host disease after allogeneic bone marrow transplantation in mice. Blood 1998;92:3960–3967

76. Takeoka M, Ward WF, Pollack H et al. KGF facilitates repair of radiation-induced DNA damage in alveolar epithelial cells. Am J Physiol 1997;272:L1174–1180

77. Ringdén O, Uzunel M, Rasmusson I et al. Mesenchymal stem cells for treatment of therapy-resistant graft-versus-host disease. Transplantation 2006;81:1388–1389

78. Fang B, Song YP, Liao LM et al. Treatment of severe therapy-resistant acute graft-versus-host disease with human adipose tissue-derived mesenchymal stem cells. Bone Marrow Transplant 2006;38:389–390

79. Yañez R, Lamana ML, García-Castro J et al. Adipose tissue-derived mesenchymal stem cells have in vivo immunosuppressive properties applicable for the control of the graft-versus-host disease. Stem Cells 2006;24:2582–2591

80. Min CK, Kim BG, Park G et al. IL-10-transduced bone marrow mesenchymal stem cells can attenuate the severity of acute graft-versus-host disease after experimental allogeneic stem cell transplantation. Bone Marrow Transplant 2007;39:637–645

81. Barrett AJ, Malkovska V. Graft-versus-leukaemia: understanding and using the alloimmune response to treat haematological malignancies. Br J Haematol 1996;93:754–761

82. Morgan RA, Dudley ME, Wunderlich JR et al. Cancer regression in patients after transfer of genetically engineered lymphocytes. Science 2006;314:126–129

83. Ott MG, Schmidt M, Schwarzwaelder K et al. Correction of X-linked chronic granulomatous disease by gene therapy, augmented by insertional activation of MDS1-EVI1, PRDM16 or SETBP1. Nat Med 2006;12:401–409

Essential biology of stem cell transplantation

A John Barrett

Introduction

In addition to an all-round knowledge of internal medicine, the practice of clinical stem cell transplantation (SCT) demands an understanding of the hematologic and immunologic principles that form the basis of transplant patient management. Our current knowledge of SCT biology derives from a vast body of experimental data extending back more than 50 years. Here, we describe only the essentials of transplantation science as it pertains to the daily clinical practice of SCT and outline the biologic basis of factors which determine transplant outcome. The reader is referred to the references at the end of this chapter for the more experimental aspects of SCT hematology and immunology.

Cellular components of the transplant (Fig. 2.1)

Long-lived cell lineages

Transplants contain a variety of cell types but the hematopoietic stem cells (HSC), conveniently identified by the CD34 surface antigen, and CD3+ T-lymphocytes, responsible for immunologic memory, are the most important because they can self-replicate and survive a lifetime in the recipient. Cells within the CD34 compartment establish lifelong hematopoiesis and regenerate an entire immune system comprising dendritic cells (including the specialized Langerhans cells), tissue macrophages, B-cells, T-cells and natural killer (NK) cells. In the first few months after transplant, T-cells are derived from transfused mature (post-thymic) T-cells from the donor. Later, CD34-derived prethymic T-lymphocyte precursors requiring maturation in the host thymus repopulate the peripheral T-cell compartment.[1]

In recent years, there has been much interest in the possibility that SCT contain precursors of cells able to develop into non-hemato-poietic cells such as angiocytes, endothelial cells, fibroblasts, neurone and muscle cells. The surface marker characteristics of the precursors of non-hematopoietic tissues and their relationship to HSC are not fully established. Some data suggest that HSC have plasticity to redifferentiate along alternative developmental pathways; other data suggest that small populations of non-hematopoietic stem cells in the transplant inoculm are responsible for repopulating non-hematopoietic tissues. Whatever mechanism is invoked, it appears that the efficiency with which non-hematopoietic tissues are replaced by donor-derived cells is very low and of little significance in routine SCT.[2,3]

Short-lived cell lineages

Other cells with limited capacity to establish long-term engraftment accompanying the stem cells can have immediate effects after transplant: donor B-cells can reactivate Epstein–Barr virus (EBV) and cause lymphoproliferative syndromes and, if ABO mismatched with the recipient, can generate red cell antibodies against host group A or B red cells, leading to massive intravascular hemolysis of host red cells.[4,5] Transplanted natural killer (NK) cells may promote engraftment, and mesenchymal stromal cells (MSC) in bone marrow transplants have immunomodulatory functions.[6,7]

Hematopoietic stem cell sources

Three transplant stem cell sources are in current use: bone marrow (BM), mobilized peripheral blood stem cells (PBSC) and umbilical cord blood (UCB).[8–10] These sources differ considerably both quantitatively and qualitatively, as shown in Table 2.1.

BM harvesting

In infants and children, red marrow is distributed throughout the skeleton, including the long bones. Later, the red marrow recedes to the axial skeleton. The anterior and posterior spines of the pelvis, the upper sternum in adults, and the head of the tibia in infants are the sites most frequently used for marrow harvesting. The process of multiple aspirations from these sites ruptures marrow sinusoids allowing marrow cells to be aspirated along with some bone spicules. BM collections are a mixture of venous blood enriched with marrow cells. The maximum yield is achieved by limiting the volume of each aspiration and performing multiple punctures, a process that lasts 1–2 hours.[11]

Mobilization of PBSC

Circulating HSC are normally present at frequencies 1/00 to1/1000 times lower than they are in the marrow. HSC are retained adherent to the marrow stroma by the binding of CXCR4 on their surface with VCAM-1 on stromal cells. HSC will pass from the stromal compartment into the sinusoids and thence into the circulation if the VCAM-1/CXCR4 adhesion is interrupted. In PBSC collection the hematopoietic growth factor granulocyte colony-stimulating factor (G-CSF) mobilizes HSC by reducing CXCR4 expression. Large numbers of circulating HSC can be collected by apheresis after six daily injections of G-CSF. PBSC collections are heavily mixed with peripheral blood cells and contain about 10-fold more lymphocytes than do BM collections.[12]

UCB collection

At birth, the umbilical vein is rich in HSC but the total volume available for collection is usually less than 100 ml. This is because most

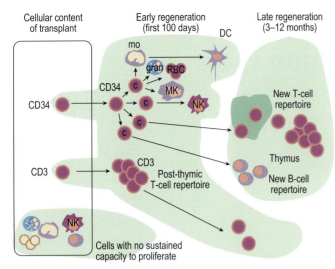

Figure 2.1
Cellular content of the stem cell transplant and fate of long- and short-lived cell lineages in the recipient. CD34, hematopoietic stem cells; CD3, post-thymic T-cells; NK, natural killer cell; B, B-cell; mo, monocyte; gran, granulocytes; MK, megakaryocytes; DC, dendritic cells; c, committed progenitor cells; RBC, red blood cells.

Table 2.1 Bone marrow, peripheral blood and umbilical cord blood stem cell sources compared

Property	BM	PBSCT	UCB
Collection	Multiple aspirates	G-CSF mobilization	Placental blood
HSC minimum for graft ×10⁶/kg recipient wt	1.0	1.0	0.1
Neutrophils > 500/µl Median days post SCT	14	12	21
Platelets > 20,000/µl Median days post SCT	21	18	28
Immunologic characteristics GvHD risk (for equivalent match)	++	+++	+

of the placental blood must be allowed to drain into the newborn infant before cutting the cord, to avoid anemia. Cord blood HSC have strong proliferative potential which partly compensates for the very much lower cell numbers collected. UCB lymphocytes are largely naïve (non-antigen experienced) but have strong proliferative potential. UCB collections also contain endothelial cells.[10]

Cryopreservation

HSC and lymphocytes can be readily stored frozen in liquid nitrogen – for years if necessary – and retain their viability on thawing. Cryopreservation requires slow, controlled-rate freezing and the addition of an agent (usually dimethyl sulfoxide – DMSO) which prevents intracellular ice crystal cell damage. When the cells are required for transplantation they must be rapidly thawed, and rapidly transfused to minimize toxicity from DMSO.[11]

Hematopoietic stem cell homing, engraftment and reconstitution of hematopoiesis[13]

Following intravenous infusion, HSC circulate and accumulate in the lungs before homing within 24 h to hematopoietic sites. Stem cell homing involves endothelial rolling within marrow sinusoids, passage through the endothelium of the sinusoid and lodging in a stem cell niche. Within the niche, the HSC can proliferate and establish foci of hematopoiesis as well as self-replicate (Fig. 2.2).

The localization of HSCT in the marrow is directed by specific adhesion molecule interactions. Endothelial rolling, which is the first step to immobilization of the HSC and its passage through the endothelial wall, is controlled by interaction between selectins such as vascular cell adhesion molecule-1 (VCAM-1) on the endothelial cell, and integrins, sialomucins and CD44 on the HSC. Stromal-derived factor 1 (SDF1) is a chemokine produced by stromal cells which enhances adhesion and transendothelial migration of the HSC through expression of its receptor on HSC CXCR4. Despite the well-established practice of giving the SCT intravenously, animal experiments suggest that the process is relatively inefficient, with only a proportion of transfused HSC reaching their niches.[13] Hematologic recovery (>500 neutrophils/µl) takes about 10 days following SCT from BM and PBSC, while UCB transplants require a median of 21 days.

To engraft in the recipient, HSCT must overcome both immunologic and non-immunologic barriers. The most important factor determining engraftment of *allotransplanted* stem cells is a favorable immune environment: predominance of donor T-cells promotes eventual engraftment of the donor's stem cells. HSC engraftment can be blocked by circulating host antibodies, alloreacting NK cells and donor-specific cytotoxic T-cells. In *autologous* SCT, engraftment depends on the vigor of the autologous stem cells, which may have been compromised by previous chemotherapy and radiotherapy, leading to incomplete hematopoietic reconstitution. HSC may fail to engraft in a marrow full of malignant cells or damaged by fibrosis or chemotherapy. A large spleen can trap circulating HSC, leading to delayed and incomplete engraftment. Once engrafted, human HSC appear to maintain hematopoiesis over many years and with follow-up of some patients transplanted more than 30 years ago, there are no reports of late graft failure from stem cell exhaustion.

Reconstitution of immunity

Recovery of immunity involves the reconstitution of a diverse family of cells and molecules: the innate immune system of the NK cell, the adaptive immunity of the T- and B-cells, the regeneration of antigen-presenting cells and the production of antibodies. We now understand much more about the process of immune reconstruction in both autologous and allogeneic SCT, which show some similarities. However, engraftment of an allogeneic immune system into the recipient introduces further complexities.[14,15]

Recovery of innate immunity

In both autologous and allogeneic SCT, NK cells are the first immune cells to reach normal blood levels, often overshooting in the first month after SCT. Increased production of lymphocyte growth factors, especially IL-12 and IL-15, stimulates rapid neogenesis of NK cells from CD34 cells.[15,16] Antigen-presenting cells (APC) derived from CD34 cells include monocyte-macrophages, dendritic cells (myeloid and plasmacytoid), Langerhans cells and B-cells. Recovery of transplant-origin APC begins within weeks of transplantation and is complete within about 6 months of transplant.[16]

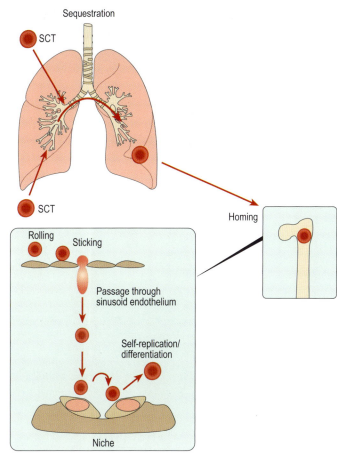

Figure 2.2
Steps in stem cell engraftment.

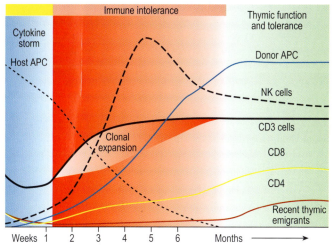

Figure 2.3
Immune recovery after stem cell transplantation. The first few weeks are characterized by a period of lymphopenia followed by rapid recovery of NK cells and a slower recovery of T-cells which are mainly CD8+. In the first few months the T-cell recovery is irregular with numerous clonal expansions as well as defects in the repertoire. A year or more after transplant thymic function restores CD4 leves and broadens the T-cell repertoire with new thymic-derived T-cells. B-cell recovery and restoration of immunoglobulin levels begin in the first year.

Recovery of adaptive immunity

Immediate T-cell immune reconstitution following SCT derives from transfused post-thymic T-cells (largely a memory T-cell compartment) and later from T-cell precursors generated from the CD34 cells in the marrow and processed by the recipient thymus to form a new immune repertoire. The recovery of CD8+ T-cells outpaces the CD4+ T-cells, with an associated deficiency of cell-mediated immunity. After transplant, there is rapid proliferation of grafted lymphocytes, driven by the release of lymphocyte growth factors IL-2, IL-12, IL15, and IL-18 in response to lymphopenia.[15,16] Studies of immune responses to cytomegalovirus after SCT show that in transplants from donors previously exposed to CMV, memory cells expand rapidly and can control reactivating CMV within a few weeks after SCT. Conversely, the acquisition of immunity against reactivating CMV following transplantation from a donor not previously exposed to CMV is much slower, sometimes taking months to generate immune competence.[15] Engrafting T-cells have special functions after allo SCT – they interact with recipient APC and cells of skin, gut and liver as well as residual host T-cells and marrow cells, resulting in GvHD, and the establishment of space for the graft through a graft-versus-marrow effect. Importantly, engrafting T-cells also recognize and kill malignant cells through the so-called graft-versus-leukemia or graft-versus-tumor effect (Fig. 2.3).[13–17]

Humoral immunity

Full reconstitution of antibody production follows the generation of new B-cell precursors from engrafted stem cells. Humoral immunity after transplant is slow to recover, with immunoglobulin levels reaching the normal range at between 6 and 12 months, often longer for IgA and for patients who develop chronic GvHD.[18]

The preparative regimen

The preparative or conditioning regimen has three functions.
  1 It is used to treat the patient's malignant disease intensively and reduce disease burden to minimal levels.
  2 It immunosuppresses the recipient to allow engraftment of the donor hematopoietic and immune system.
  3 It makes space for incoming stem cells in hematopoietic niches in the marrow.

The requirement for one or all of these three functions according to the specific patient–donor situation determines choice of regimen.[19] The intensity of the regimen can also be selected according to the ability of the patient to tolerate the regimen.[20] Thus, older or debilitated patients may be given reduced-intensity regimens to prevent mortality from high-dose treatment but which are nevertheless sufficiently immunosuppressive to ensure engraftment. While the three functions are distinct, the agents used in the regimens (for example, cyclophosphamide) often have overlapping properties of myelosuppression and immunosuppression (see Fig. 2.4).

Treatment to control malignant disease

Some regimens are specific to the particular malignant disease but many regimens use total body irradiation to a dose of 12–15 Gy or busulfan up to 12 mg/kg iv over 2–4 days in association with immunosuppressive agents such as cyclophosphamide, fludarabine or anti-CD52 (Campath) monoclonal antibody, or antilymphocyte globulin (ATG).

Immunosuppression

Immunosuppression is required to achieve engraftment in all allogeneic SCT patients, with the exception of recipients with severe combined immunodeficiency disease who cannot reject an allograft, or recipients of stem cells from an identical twin. Patients who have been sensitized by prior transfusions and children who have greater ability

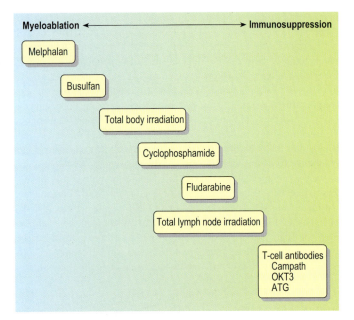

Myeloablation ◄─────────────────────► Immunosuppression

- Melphalan
- Busulfan
- Total body irradiation
- Cyclophosphamide
- Fludarabine
- Total lymph node irradiation
- T-cell antibodies
  Campath
  OKT3
  ATG

Figure 2.4
Agents used in preparative regimens sorted by their relative ability to immunosuppress or myelosuppress.

Table 2.2 Comparison of T-cells and NK cells

	T-cells	NK cells
Origin	CD34 cells – prethymic precursors	CD34 cells
	Mature in thymus	Mature in marrow
Development	Naive ↓ Central memory ↓ Effector memory ↓ End effector	Recognition/activation ↓ Limited expansion ↓ Death
Stimulator cells	APC (DC, B-cells, monocytes)	Hematopoietic cells
Target cells	Any MHC class I/II expressing cell	Hematopoietic cells
Recognition structures	MHC class I and II	MHC class I
	+9–15 mer peptides	Non-classic MHC (MicA/B)
Receptors	T-cell receptor complex	KIR molecules (inhibitory)
	CD4 + CD8+ costimulatory molecules	NKG2D and others (activating)
Receptor diversity	Very high (10^{11-12} TCR sequences)	Low (18 KIR types)
Clinical impact: GvHD GvL Engraftment	+ + +	None + (myeloid leukemias) +

to reject transplants may need more intensive immunosuppression to ensure engraftment.

Myelosuppression

Complete myeloablation is not required to achieve full engraftment but it is usually a consequence of high-dose treatment used to treat malignant disease prior to transplant. Myeloablation is often avoided in patients receiving reduced-intensity transplants. These patients show rapid initial recovery of autologous hematopoiesis, followed several months later by a T-cell mediated elimination of host hematopoiesis and a switch to donor hematopoiesis.[21] Thus, in an allogeneic SCT there is no prerequisite for the conditioning regimen to 'make space' for engrafting donor stem cells as long as cellular immunity has switched to that of the donor.

The basis of alloimmune reactions

Alloimmunity describes the immune interaction between genetically distinct individuals. Because of genetic diversity, all allografts have the potential for donor-versus-host or host-versus-donor immune responses which can cause graft-versus-host disease (GvHD), graft rejection or more favorable graft-versus-leukemia (GvL) responses. Allorecognition involves an adaptive immune response by CD3+ T-cells and an innate immune response mediated by CD16+ CD56+ NK cells. The two immune systems are contrasted in Table 2.2.

The adaptive immune response

The adaptive immune response involves the interaction of T-lymphocytes with antigens from the other individual.[22] Upon antigen recognition, T-cells become activated and proliferate to generate expanded clones of effector and helper cells reacting to the cells bearing the antigen. Once established, these immune responses remain in the T-cell memory, and further contact with the antigen initiates a new wave of effector and helper cell generation. T-cell recognition of alloantigens involves engagement of the T-cell receptor molecule with an HLA-peptide molecular complex on the surface of cells from another individual. All cells express MHC class I HLA molecules (HLA-A, B

and C), but only some cells (including professional antigen-presenting cells) express MHC class II molecules (HLA-DR, DP, DQ). Antigenic peptides presented by class I MHC molecules represent the 'self' of the cell. They are derived from cellular proteins which are degraded into short peptide sequences during the course of protein turnover by the proteasome. Antigens presented by MHC class II molecules are derived from exogenous proteins as well as some self proteins. They are degraded into peptides in lysosomal vacuoles. Endogenous and exogenous peptides complex with MHC class I molecules in the endoplasmic reticulum and with MHC class II molecules in lysosomal vacuoles. The T-cell receptors of CD8+ T-cells engage mainly with MHC class I molecules, while those of CD4+ T-cells interact with MHC class II molecules. The peptide in the MHC molecule is called a minor histocompatibility antigen (mHag) while the MHC is the major antigen. Minor histocompatibility antigens are important because in HLA identical sibling transplants, disparity between host and donor mHag alone can cause lethal GvHD, graft rejection or powerful GvL effects. The molecular basis of antigen presentation is illustrated in Figure 2.5.[23]

The innate immune response

Although the NK repertoire is clonal, its diversity is much less than that of the T-cell. Unlike T-cells, which can only be effective if there is clonal expansion of the relevant antigen-specific T-cell clones, NK immune effects on their target cells occur without prior clonal expansion. NK cells interact with other cells through inhibitory and activation pathways. The activating interactions are mediated through a number of molecules, notably NKG2D encountering the non-classic MHC class I molecules MIC A/B on the target.[24] An activated NK cell kills its target cell by lysis through perforin-granzyme release. To prevent autoimmune attack by self NK cells against self tissues, NK cells also have a predominating inhibitory interaction with other cells.

Inhibition of NK activation occurs when one of a family of killer immunoglobulin-like receptors (KIR) on the NK cell engages with a

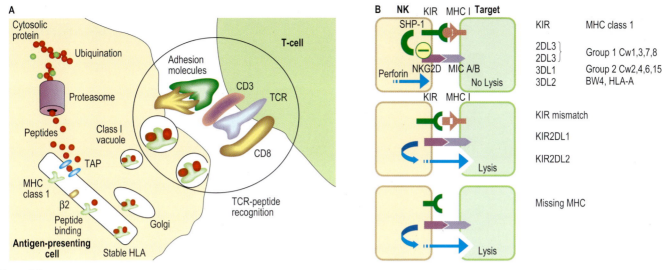

Figure 2.5
Molecular basis of alloreactivity. (a) Adaptive immunity: generation of self peptides from intracytoplasmic degradation of self protein by ubiquination and digestion in the proteasome. Short peptides are actively pumped into the endoplasmic reticulum, where they become incorporated into HLA class I molecules, undergo glycosylation in the golgi and reach the cell surface in a class I vacuole to be scrutinized by passing CD8 T-cells which bind to the MHC molecule through a weak interaction via CD3 and CD8, and a strong interaction between the peptide and T-cell receptor (TCR) hypervariable region. (b) Innate immunity: positive and negative signals control NK reactivity. When KIR groups are matched with an appropriate MHC ligand, SHP-1 is upregulated and blocks the process of perforin-granzyme release, otherwise induced by the NKG2D/MICA/B activating interaction. When there is a KIR mismatch or the target T-cell lacks MHC class I molecules, there is no negative signal to control NK-mediated lysis.

relevant class I MHC molecule on the target, delivering an inhibitory signal to the cell and blocking activation of its lytic machinery. NK-target compatibility involves many KIR types interacting with many HLA class I molecules, but the most important functionally appears to be the inhibitory interaction between KIR group 1 and HLA-C1,-3, -7, -8 and KIR group 2 and HLA-C2,-4,-6,-15. The behavior of an individual NK cell with its target depends on the balance between surface-expressed effector and inhibitory molecules characterizing that particular NK clone. The conditions required for NK alloreactivity are fulfilled when the responder NK cell fails to engage with an inhibitory MHC class I molecule – either because the molecule is not expressed or because it belongs to a non-compatible group. NK allo-reactivity is well characterized for HLA mismatched transplants, but may also occur between HLA identical donor–recipient pairs because KIR groups are inherited differently from the MHC complex. Thus, the donor may lack the KIR group corresponding to that of the recipient, or the recipient may not express MHC molecules compatible with the donor's KIR groups.[25]

NK cells differ from T-cells in their alloimmune responses in important ways. Critically, NK cells predominantly recognize cells of hematopoietic lineage. This explains the importance of NK cells in engraftment: host NK cells can destroy an incoming graft, while donor NK cells facilitate engraftment by eliminating residual host hemato-poietic and lymphoid cells.[26] A second consequence of the hematopoietic specificity of NK cells is that they do not directly cause GvHD. In fact, their ability to deplete host antigen-presenting cells reduces the ability of the host to stimulate alloresponses in donor T-cells.[25]

Tissue typing

The MHC locus is highly polymorphic, representing over 800 alleles described to date, and new molecules continue to be described. The reason for this diversity is believed to be the evolutionary pressure on genetic change required for adapting molecules to emerging variations in micro-organisms encountered during the human diaspora into new environmental niches over the last 100,000 years. HLA typing involves

molecular or serologic typing of blood leukocytes to determine HLA A, B, C (MHC class I) and DR, DP, DQ types (MHC class II). Clinical transplant results clearly show the advantage, in both related and unrelated donor searches, of finding the closest HLA identity possible. In HLA identical siblings, identity at HLA- A, B and DR is sufficient to determine HLA compatibility between donor and recipient, because the MHC complex is inherited from parent to child in a single raft of genes constituting the parental haplotype. So closely are these genes arrayed that only rarely (<2% of cases) do crossovers occur during meiosis, creating mismatches, usually at the A locus. In unrelated donors the situation is different because, while haplotypes tend to be generally conserved, genetic recombination over many generations leads to a legacy of rearrangements through crossovers not shared between patient and donor. To fully define HLA compatibility in unrelated donors, further typing for HLA-C, DQ, and DP is also per-formed (Fig. 2.6).

HLA typing was originally performed on lymphocytes using a panel of antibodies with defined reactivity to certain MHC molecules (serotyping). HLA typing is now increasingly performed by molecular typing, which provides high definition characterization of individual MHC molecules.[27–29]

Functional tests of compatibility

While selecting the best matched (or fully matched) donor is the first step in limiting potential alloreactivity between donor and recipient, it is clear from the preceding description of the alloresponse that HLA typing does not exclude alloreactions occurring from mHag disparities and KIR-MHC incompatibility. Functional compatibility tests can complement HLA typing by identifying alloreactions between donor and recipient without the need to characterize the genetic disparity. The classic test is the mixed lymphocyte reaction (MLR) which mea-sures proliferative response of the donor lymphocytes to the recipient in a 4–6 day assay. It is relatively easy to perform, but suffers from wide variability and requires careful controls. Furthermore, the test

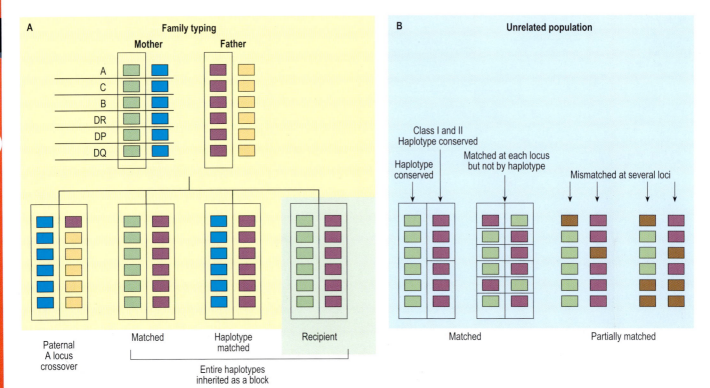

Figure 2.6
Differences in HLA genetics between family typing and unrelated donor search. HLA identity within a family also implies matching of complete MHC region haplotypes whereas this degree of compatibility is not assured in unrelated HLA-matched donors unless there is conservation of ancestral haplotypes between donor and recipient.

has limited applicability – it is not sensitive to incompatibility between HLA-matched individuals, since the MLR is unreactive, although it can be useful to confirm non-reactivity.

More recently, measurement of helper (H) or cytotoxic (C) T-lymphocyte precursor frequencies (TLPf) was introduced. These limiting dilution assays are extremely difficult to establish and operate, and again have limited applicability. In the hands of some investigators, HTLP or CTLP have been found to be predictive for GvHD/rejection in both matched and mismatched settings.[30] A more direct functional assay for GvHD is the skin explant test. A histologically cut skin biopsy from the recipient is cultured with donor lymphocytes. After incubation, the skin biopsy is examined for apoptotic damage, giving a fairly reliable prediction of GvHD in matched and mismatched settings. The technique is difficult to set up and requires a dedicated technician.

In summary, despite much research into functional compatibility testing, none of these tests is in general use.[31]

Cure of disease by stem cell transplantation

Advances in stem cell biology and immunology have greatly broadened the application of both autologous and allogeneic SCT as a curative approach for a wide range of malignant and non-malignant, genetic and acquired disorders. Broadly, SCT has been used as a means of normalizing hematopoietic function, repairing non-hematopoietic states or for its immunologic functions (Table 2.3).

Autologous SCT for malignant disease

The original context of using SCT to permit the use of myeloablative doses of anticancer treatment is still relevant today in the treatment of malignant diseases by autologous SCT. The principle behind the use of myeloablative treatment and stem cell rescue is that some tumors can be eradicated if treated with doses of radiation and chemotherapy that require stem cell rescue. An extension of this strategy, widely used in the treatment of multiple myeloma, is to apply it with two consecutive transplants to further reduce the disease burden. The limitations of autologous SCT are that only some diseases such as lymphomas and some solid tumors can be reduced to a sufficiently low bulk before transplant to make a single or double transplant approach effective at preventing disease recurrence. An early concern with autologous SCT, especially for leukemia and lymphoma, was the risk that malignant cells contaminating the autograft would reseed in the treated recipient. This gave rise to stem cell purging technology to eliminate malignant cells from the transplant. However, in a pioneering gene-marking study in autologous SCT for leukemia, the contribution of transplanted malignant cells to later disease relapse appeared to be minor, and no clearly established advantage for stem cell purging in autologous SCT has been identified.[32]

Gene therapy using autologous SCT

The first successes in gene therapy for severe combined immunodeficiency from adenosine deaminase deficiency were proof of the principle that hematologic and immunologic diseases due to a single known gene mutation could be corrected by gene insertion into autologous hematopoietic stem cells. Unfortunately, the field has been slow to move forward because of difficulties in sustaining large enough populations of gene-modified cells and, more ominously, because of the risk of leukemia from mutagenesis caused by random gene insertion. Nevertheless, it is likely that in the future gene-modified stem cell technology will improve and become safer, opening the way for correction of a wide variety of genetic disorders currently treated by allogeneic SCT.[33]

Table 2.3 Most frequent diseases treated by stem cell transplantation

	Autologous	Allogeneic
Immunodeficiency diseases		
Severe combined immunodeficiency	*	+
Wiskott-Aldrich disease	−	+
Autoimmune diseases		
Immune thrombocytopenic purpura (ITP)	+	−
Lupus and rheumatoid arthritis	+	+
Scleroderma	+	+
Inflammatory bowel disease	+	+
Multiple sclerosis	+	+
Bone marrow failure		
Acquired: aplastic anemia and radiation injury	−	+
Inherited: reticular dysgenesis, Fanconi anemia	*	+
Pure red cell aplasia	−	+
Hemoglobinopathies and other inherited marrow disorders		
Thalassemia syndromes	−	+
Sickle cell anemia	−	+
Chronic granulomatous disease	−	+
Glanzmann's thromboasthenia	−	+
Non-hematologic inherited disorders		
Mucopolysaccharidoses and other liposomal disorders	−	+
Gaucher's disease	−	+
Globosidoses	−	+
Pompé disease	−	+
Hematologic malignancies		
Myeloid : AML, CML, MDS, MPD	+	+
Lymphoid: ALL, CLL, NHL, HD, myeloma	+	+
Non-hematologic malignancies		
Renal cell carcinoma	+	+
Breast cancer	+	+
Neuroblastoma	+	(+)
Germ cell tumors	+	(+)
Sarcomas	+	(+)
Other	+	(+)

Key: +, tried with efficacy; (+), tried with unclear efficacy; −, not attempted; *, gene therapy using autologous stem cells; AML, acute myeloid leukemia; CML, chronic myeloid leukemia; MDS: myelodysplastic syndromes, MPD, myeloproliferative disorders; ALL, acute lymphoblastic leukemia; CLL, chronic lymphocytic leukemia; NHL, non-Hodgkin's lymphoma; HD, Hodgkin's disease.

Autologous or allogeneic SCT for autoimmune diseases

The treatment of autoimmune diseases is the focus of ongoing clinical research. Both autologous and allogeneic SCT can produce spectacular responses, but the underlying mechanisms of cure are still being investigated. The rationale for allogeneic SCT for treating autoimmune disease is relatively straightforward: clinical observation has taught us that autoimmune diseases such as rheumatoid arthritis and psoriasis respond completely to allogeneic SCT given to treat hematologic malignancies. Secondly, severe aplastic anemia (SAA), now recognized as an autoimmune disorder in the majority of patients, is readily correctable by SCT. Thus, autoimmune disorders, whether involving cell-mediated or antibody-driven immune damage, can be corrected by supplanting the immune system of the patient with that of a healthy donor. Autologous SCT has also been effective in some autoimmune disorders, most notably immune thrombocytopenic purpura (ITP) and multiple sclerosis. While it is clear that the preparative regimen can provide powerful immunosuppression to block the autoimmune process, the function of the transplant is less clear. It is possible that the SCT can simply 'reboot' the immune system, with transplanted CD34 cells reshaping the immune system through the generation of new B- and T-cell lineages. For this reason, some autologous SCT are CD34 selected.

Results of treatment vary widely according to type of disease and transplant approach used. Reasons for treatment failure (relapse or failure to respond) are numerous. First, the transplant may not have eradicated the long-lived memory T- and B-cell clones responsible for the autoimmune process. It is well known from conventional allogeneic SCT that recipient memory immune function is most resistant to elimination by the preparative regimen or by incoming donor immune cells. Second, tissue damage caused by the autoimmune process may already be irreparable (consider, for example, type I diabetes mellitus or autoimmune thyroiditis which result in rapid organ failure). Third, the new immune system may re-establish the autoimmune process (especially in an autologous setting). Much still remains to be understood about the mechanism of cure of autoimmune diseases by SCT.[34,35]

Allogeneic SCT for bone marrow failure disorders

SCT is an effective treatment for severe aplastic anemia, whether or not the disease is immune mediated. The curative effect of SCT in SAA relies on the restoration of missing stem cell function, while the preparative regimen making way for the establishment of donor immune function arrests the autoimmune process causing marrow failure.[36]

SCT has also been used to treat victims of non-therapeutic irradiation causing bone marrow failure. In practice, this strategy has limited use because irradiated victims may have received supralethal doses of irradiation to non-hematopoietic tissue, have associated burns or blast injury or they may remain contaminated with radioactive materials that continue to damage the transplanted marrow.[37]

Allogeneic SCT for genetic diseases of HSC

There are numerous genetic bone marrow disorders resulting in failure of production or function of one or all hematopoietic lineages. The list includes the hemoglobinopathies, pure red cell aplasia, agranulocytosis, chronic granulomatous disease, Glanzmann's thrombasthenia, Fanconi aplasia, and reticular dysgenesis. By substitution of a healthy HSC, the transplant corrects the genetic defect.[38]

Allogeneic SCT to correct immune deficiencies

Transplantation of pluripotent lymphohematopoietic progenitors also provides the cells necessary to correct congenital and acquired immune deficiencies. Reconstituted immunity is derived from both post-thymic T-cells given with the transplant, and lymphocytes generated by donor-derived CD34 cells, maturing in the thymus and B-cell developmental areas, to generate a new adaptive immune system. A wide spectrum of T- and B-cell immune deficiencies is correctable by SCT, but notably, SCT has been ineffective in treating immune deficiency from HIV infection because the transplant rapidly acquires the virus.[39]

SCT to repair non-hematopoietic tissues

Replacement of the recipient lymphohematopoietic system with that of a healthy donor also provides a means of correcting genetic errors of metabolism due to defective enzymes (storage diseases, mucopolysaccharidoses, etc.). Correction relies upon the penetration of non-hematopoietic tissue by enzyme-competent donor-derived macrophages, dendritic cells and glial cells, which deliver enzyme to affected cells by diffusion and pinocytosis, or by direct cell–cell exchange.[40]

Allogeneic SCT to treat malignant disease – the graft-versus-malignancy effect

It is now well established that the cure of malignant disease by SCT relies on both the conditioning regimen, which can provide an antitumor effect from myeloablative doses of chemotherapy or radiotherapy, and the graft-versus-malignancy (GvM) (or more specifically in hematologic malignancies, the graft-versus-leukemia (GvL)) effect provided by donor T-cells and NK cells. The effect is sufficiently powerful for a single transfusion of donor lymphocytes to cause disease regression. So powerful is the alloimmune attack on the malignancy that some diseases can be eradicated with transplant conditioning that does no more than immunosuppress the recipient to allow full donor engraftment and the GvM effect.

Malignant diseases have different susceptibilities to eradication by GvM effects. Most sensitive are chronic myelogenous leukemia, chronic lymphocytic leukemia, low-grade B-lymphoproliferative disorders, mantle cell lymphoma and EBV lymphoproliferative disorders. Most other hematologic malignancies have intermediate sensitivity to GvL effects, with decreasing susceptibility in diseases with rapid proliferation rates and advanced or chemorefractory disease.[41] More recently, reduced-intensity conditioned SCT has been used to treat metastatic solid tumors. Responses can occur, notably in renal cell cancer and breast cancer, but complete remissions are uncommon.[42]

Mechanism of the GvL effect

Both T-lymphocytes and NK cells participate in the GvL response. It is believed that cytotoxic T-cells recognize several classes of antigens on leukemia cells: mHag, ubiquitously present throughout the tissues of the recipient leading to GvH and GvL effects, mHag restricted to hematopoietic tissues and leukemia-restricted antigens, normal (non-alleleic) self proteins which are overexpressed by the leukemia such as proteinase-3 and elastase, and tumor-specific antigens such as Wilms' tumor-1 and fusion proteins such as the BCR-ABL fusion specific to chronic myelogenous leukemia and Ph-positive acute lymphoblastic leukemia.[43] NK cells use the perforin-granzyme pathway to kill their targets, but are only activated when inhibitory signals from self-MHC class I molecules on the target are missing or overcome by powerful activating signals through their NKG2D receptor. This can occur when the NK cells are alloreactive, when the malignant cell downregulates MHC class I, or when the malignant cell overproduces MICA/B, leading to NKG2D activation. There is increasing evidence that NK cell-mediated GvL is an important mechanism of GvL against acute and chronic myeloid leukemias, but it is not clear whether NK cells mediate significant GvM effects against other malignancies.[44]

Complications of stem cell transplantation

Graft failure

The graft can fail to generate sustained hematopoiesis either because the stem cells transplanted are defective or because the graft is rejected immunologically. *Non-immunologic graft failure* is more often seen after autologous SCT in patients who have received prior chemotherapy which has damaged the stem cell pool, often in association with deficient stem cell numbers collected prior to transplant. Very rarely, donor stem cells can be defective because the related donor and patient both share a stem cell defect which has led to aplastic anemia in the recipient but has not resulted in a reduction in blood counts in the donor. Other causes of stem cell failure include faulty cryopreservation and damage from the dimethyl sulfoxide cryopreserving agent caused by prolonged intervals between thawing and administration.

Immunologic causes for graft failure occur immediately after transplant causing complete failure of engraftment, or later after the blood counts have fully recovered. Immediate graft rejection can be antibody-, NK cell- or T-cell-mediated. Graft failure can sometimes be detected in the first few days after transplant with a brief rise in circulating atypical lymphocytes. These cells have been shown to be T-cells with donor-specific cytotoxicity. Factors predisposing to early graft rejection are inadequate immunosuppression by the conditioning regimen, younger recipient age, HLA-mismatched transplantation, T-cell depletion, and prior sensitization of recipient to random blood products or from donor transfusions. Engraftment followed by graft rejection implies a change in the balance between donor and host immunity in favor of host immune recovery. After initial engraftment, the blood counts begin to fall and bone marrow shows worsening aplasia. Chimerism analysis will show predominance of recipient T-lymphocytes and falling donor lymphoid chimerism. Withdrawal of immunosuppression tends to favor host immune dominance, while further immunosuppression accompanied by donor lymphocyte infusion can sometimes reverse the process. Patients who reject their transplant may recover autologous hematopoiesis, especially those transplanted for aplastic anemia or those receiving non-myeloablative regimens. Patients rejecting their transplant often successfully engraft after a second transplant from the same donor or a different donor, provided the conditioning regimen is sufficiently immunoablative.

Acute and chronic GvHD

Acute GvHD occurs when recipient antigen-presenting cells present 'non-self' antigens to donor T-cells. The immunologic conditions for acute GvHD require HLA major or mHag mismatching, donor immune dominance and presence of host APC, and are favored by a proinflammatory milieu such as pertains immediately after conditioning (the cytokine storm) or during infections. Since host APC persist only weeks to months after transplant, the risk of acute GvHD from a transfusion of donor lymphocytes falls as time elapses post transplant. Acute GvHD causes systemic illness but the target tissues are very specific, involving the epithelium of the gastrointestinal tract and its continuation into the biliary tree, the skin, conjunctiva, and exocrine glands, leading to the classic triad of gastroenteritis, skin rashes and a mixed obstructive-hepatitic pattern of hepatic involvement. Curiously, the renal tract is spared, as is the vascular endothelium, neural, muscular and bone tissue. The acute GvHD process is characterized by a rather scanty lymphocyte infiltrate and single cell apoptosis of the normally self-renewing cells of the endothelium or epithelium.[45,46]

Chronic GvHD develops around 3 months after transplant. Acute GvHD is the strongest precipitating factor, but chronic GvHD also occurs without prior acute GvHD. The immunology of the condition is not completely understood but involves alloactivated donor CD4 and CD8 T-cells, and autoantibody production leading to tissue damage, fibrosis and immune incompetence. Chronic GvHD has scleroderma-like features: target tissues are the skin and integument, exocrine glands, the lungs, and the musculoskeletal system which is affected by a deep dermal and fascial fibrosis. Hematopoiesis is impaired, and thrombocytopenia is common.[47] A full description of the pathophysiology of GvHD is given in Chapters 38 and 39.

Prevention of GvHD

All allotransplants, except those between identical twins and related donor transplants for infants with severe combined immunodeficiency, require some approach to preventing GvHD. It is known from historical studies that in the absence of immunosuppression even HLA-identical sibling transplants experience an 80% risk of significant GvHD. Acute GvHD can be largely prevented by T-cell depletion of the graft to deliver T-cell doses of less than 10^4 CD3 cells/kg. Interestingly, such recipients can still develop chronic GvHD, but to a lesser extent. Such T-cell depleted transplants suffer from delayed immune reconstitution. This has led to transplant approaches where T-cells are given when host APC have been eliminated and there is no 'cytokine storm'. Delayed lymphocyte transfusions have a low risk of causing severe acute GvHD. The alternative to T-cell depletion is to administer immunosuppression post transplant. The most successful regimens use a calcineurin inhibitor (ciclosporin or tacrolimus) together with either methotrexate, cyclophosphamide or antilymphocyte antibodies in the first week after transplant. The initial intensification may remove newly alloactivated donor T-cells, while the calcineurin inhibitors block cytokine-driven lymphoproliferation of allosensitized lymphocytes. In mismatched transplants, which carry a greater risk of causing GvHD, combinations of T-cell depletion with post-transplant immunosuppression may be required.

DNA viral reactivations

The DNA viruses CMV, BKV, HSV, VZV, EBV, human papillomavirus (HPV), and possibly some adenoviruses, have the ability to persist in the host once established. Normally, the initial immune response to the acute infection establishes a memory pool of competent T-cells which either completely suppress reactivation, as in the case of EBV and CMV, or restrict the site of reactivation, as in VZV or HSV, to the region around nerve endings. After stem cell transplantation, when the T-cell repertoire is defective, these viruses can reactivate and cause life-threatening illness. While antiviral agents such as aciclovir, ganciclovir and cidofovir have done much to limit mortality from viral reactivation, recovery of viral-specific T-cell immunity, typically beyond the third month from transplant, is central to limiting the risk.[48]

Opportunistic infections

Transplanted patients are prey to infection from bacteria, fungi, viruses and protozoa. These are discussed in detail in Chapters 41–44, so here, only the provocative factors for infection will be listed, which include the neutropenic period after transplant, the period of cell-mediated immune incompetence and defective antibody production in the first 6–12 months after transplant, disruption to the integument, permitting bacterial invasion from mucositis in the GI tract, tunneled catheters, and the negative impact of GvHD and immunosuppressive treatment on lymphoid and marrow function.[49]

Relapse of malignant disease

The commonest cause of treatment failure following SCT for malignant disease is disease recurrence. Relapse risk for leukemias and myelodysplasia varies from 10% to 60% depending on whether the disease is transplanted electively (first remission or early-phase disease) or later as a salvage procedure (relapsed or refractory or advanced disease). Disease relapse is thought to occur either because the disease has simply grown back from a low residual after the conditioning regimen, or because a low level of residual disease has broken free from regulation by a GvL effect. Early relapse within the first few months of transplant and relapse after autologous SCT probably represent the unchecked regrowth of disease, while relapse occurring months to years after transplant is more likely to be due to a failure of immune control. Indeed, there are well-documented cases of patients relapsing as immunosuppression is introduced, and of disease recession as immunosuppression is stopped.

Relapse usually arises in the bone marrow, but can also occur in unusual extramedullary sites, possibly due to immune escape from patroling lymphocytes. Studies of relapse after allotransplantation for

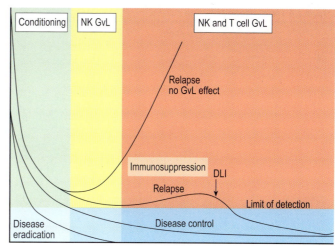

Figure 2.7
Patterns of residual disease and relationship with cure or relapse after transplantation.

myeloma, where the relapsing clone often represents a different idiotype to that of the pretransplant disease, suggest that a more resistant clone is selected from a pool of mutated malignant cells, under the new immunologic conditions of the allograft. Little is known about the ability of the leukemias to escape from immune control by further mutation, but one study suggests that leukemia cells may escape immune regulation by downregulating class I molecules to avoid T-cell recognition, or by developing resistance to NK cells.[50]

The cause of relapse may be different in different malignancies. In CML, unlike AML, relapses have been documented many years after transplant, suggesting that the disease is never fully eradicated but remains mostly contained by the donor immune control, similar to the way in which DNA viruses are prevented from reactivating. Somewhat baffling are the rare occasions when the malignancy recurs in donor cells. This phenomenon may represent an environmental predisposition to leukemic change, perhaps coupled with a genetic predisposition to develop leukemia. Patterns of disease control and relapse after SCT are illustrated in Figure 2.7.

Damage to non-hematopoietic tissues

Preparative regimens using high doses of chemotherapeutic agents or radiotherapy can cause significant toxicity to non-hematopoietic tissues. The effects range from reversible damage such as mucositis to life-threatening permanent damage to major organs such as lungs (interstitial fibrosis), liver (veno-occlusive disease) and heart (myocardial damage). The side-effects of radiation and alkylating agents and other commonly used preparative regimen agents are well described in later chapters and are not detailed here. Patients with pre-existing organ damage are at a higher risk of developing fatal complications from the preparative regimen, but it is possible to avoid major organ toxicity by appropriate choice of conditioning agents and selection of a reduced-intensity regimen.

Factors determining transplant outcome

Clinicians measure transplant outcome by the major endpoints of relapse-related and non-relapse related mortality which together factor into the outcomes, survival and disease-free survival. These endpoints are themselves derived from intermediate 'biologic' endpoints of GvHD, GvL, engraftment, measures of immunologic and hematologic competence, as well as events such as infection or regimen-related organ toxicity. Many factors directly predictive of outcome are now

Table 2.4 Factors affecting transplant outcome

	Favorable	Unfavorable
Patient		
Status of disease prior to transplant	Early Non-malignant In remission/controlled	Advanced Malignant Refractory/progressing
Performance score (Karnofsky)	90–100%	<90% (increased TRM)
Age (years)	Under 20	Over 55 (increased TRM)
Immune recognition of donor	None	Antidonor T-cells/abs (rejection)
Donor		
Immune memory for infectious agents (CMV, etc.) for tumor antigens for recipient antigens (pregnancy, transfusion)	+ + +	– (more risk – from – infection)
Regulatory T-cell frequency	High	Low (more GvHD)
Donor–recipient match		
HLA class I and II match	Less GvHD	Less GvL
mHag match	Less GvHD	Less GvL
KIR match		More relapse/GvHD
KIR mismatch	More GvL, less GvHD	
Transplant characteristics		
CD34 cell dose	High	Low (see Table 2.1)
Standard-intensity preparative regimens	Less relapse	More toxicity
Reduced-intensity preparative regimens	Less toxicity	More relapse
Intensive GvHD prevention (T-cell depletion)	Less GvHD risk	More relapse
Reduced GvHD prophylaxis	Less relapse	More GvHD risk
Post-transplant characteristics		
Day 30 lymphocyte and NK count	High	Low (high TRM + relapse)
Non-MHC genetic factors	See Table 2.5	

Table 2.5 Gene factors affecting transplant outcome

	Donor	Recipient
Cytokine promotor genes TNF-alpha IL-10 IL-6 IL-1 Ra	 +	 + + +
Miscellaneous Vitamin D receptor Estrogen receptor		 + +
Genes associated with infection Mannose binding lectin Myeloperoxidase	 + +	 +

Mismatching at HLA-A, B, C, DR, DP and DQ loci have all been implicated equally in causing alloreactivity and affecting outcome. However, it has recently become appreciated that simply scoring the number of compatible loci between unrelated donor–recipient pairs (e.g. '10/10 match') does not fully describe compatibility, because the individual MHC haplotype must also be considered. Donors who also mirror at least one HLA-A, B, C, DR haplotype of the recipient are better biologic matches than are those where the HLA genes are arranged in the donor differently to the recipient. It should be borne in mind, however, that while mismatching carries risks, it can also protect against disease relapse. Thus, identical twin transplants have significantly higher relapse rates but low TRM, whereas in transplants for advanced disease, the high TRM of a mismatched SCT is offset by a more powerful GvL effect. As a consequence, there is less difference in *overall survival* whether the donor is matched or mismatched.

Prognostic value of individual HLA types

A number of studies have sought to identify whether particular HLA types in HLA-matched transplants confer a better or worse outcome. With the notable exception of HLA-DR15, no correlation has been identified. DR15 is associated with immune reactivity; it is increased in autoimmune disease, predicts for a hematologic response to immunosuppression in aplastic anemia and myelodysplastic syndromes (MDS) and is associated with less acute GvHD but slightly more relapse in HLA-matched sibling transplant.[51]

KIR matching

One of the most important discoveries in recent years has been the impact of NK alloreactivity on transplant outcome. As discussed above, alloreacting NK cells have the useful property of eliminating host APC, reducing GvHD, eliminating residual recipient immune cells, promoting marrow engraftment and exerting cytotoxicity to myeloid leukemias. HLA haploidentically matched transplants and unrelated but T-cell depleted SCT with KIR ligand MHC class I mismatching have better survivals, less GvHD and lower relapse rates for myeloid leukemias. There is also intriguing evidence that NK alloreactivity favorably affects transplant outcome in HLA-identical sibling transplants, similarly to the effect in mismatched SCT.[52,53]

Cytokine gene polymorphisms

Immune reactivity is genetically regulated. Very crudely, the sum of actions of a number of cytokine genes can determine whether the individual's immune system operates more in a proinflammatory or an anti-inflammatory mode. Production of proinflammatory cytokines, such as tumor necrosis factor (TNF), IFN-gamma and IL-1, and anti-inflammatory cytokines, such as IL-10, IL-4, is controlled by promoters which vary in their efficiency according to their precise genetic

known. Some are clearly biologically linked to intermediate events and others may be surrogates for unknown factors. Most useful are predictive factors for outcome that can be discerned from the potential donor, the genetic match between patient and donor, and the characteristics of the patient prior to transplant. Knowledge of these risk factors allows the transplanter to modify the regimen in favor of the particular circumstances. Other factors predicting outcome are only apparent after transplant. Factors predictive of transplant success or failure span genetic, hematologic and immunologic issues, as well as simple but powerful clinical characteristics of patient and donor (Table 2.4).

MHC locus matching

As described above, compatibility at the MHC locus is a major determinant of likely transplant success. There is almost a direct relationship between increase in GvHD and transplant-related mortality (TRM) with the number of mismatched genetic loci, beginning with identical twin transplants which share not only MHC but mHag genes, and progressing through HLA-matched siblings, unrelated but HLA-matched donors to 5/6, 4/6 3/6 and completely mismatched pairs.

sequence. Ongoing studies associating transplant outcome with individual polymorphisms of patient and donor have revealed some powerful genetic polymorphisms which significantly impact on transplant outcome. The effect is enhanced when the gene is homozygous, and most cytokine gene polymorphisms affecting outcome reside in the recipient. An important exception is an IL-1 receptor alpha polymorphism in the donor which impacts upon GvHD, survival and relapse. The study of cytokine gene polymorphism is still in its infancy and much work remains to be done to discover the most important factors (Table 2.5).[54]

Other gene polymorphisms

Distinct from cytokine gene polymorphism (CGP) is an increasing list of genes affecting drug metabolism (thereby affecting immunosuppression), granulocyte function, gastrointestinal function and many other factors that impact upon transplant outcomes by unknown mechanisms (e.g. estrogen receptor, androgen receptor, vitamin D receptor polymorphisms).[54–56]

Racial origin

Several analyses of large transplant databases have sought to identify differences in outcome according to racial mix. These studies inevitably suffer from wrongly attributing differences in outcome to genetic rather than environmental differences. However, there is fairly convincing evidence that Oriental racial groups, especially Japanese, have less GvHD than other racial groups, possibly due to a smaller population gene pool with fewer polymorphisms.[57]

Donor immunologic characteristics

Immunologic characteristics of the donor have a strong influence on the manner in which the new donor immune system develops in the recipient. Donors can influence SCT outcome by the transfer of memory for viral antigens, GvH and GvL targets. Thus, the donor's history of exposure to infectious agents is highly significant for the ability of the recipient to respond to a particular infection. Donor immunity to CMV, VZV, HSV and EBV is a critical factor for the development of early protection against viral reactivation (in recipient tissues) after SCT. For example, patients receiving transplants from donors naïve to CMV are at significantly greater risk from prolonged CMV reactivation and disease than are those who are transplanted from a CMV-immunocompetent donor. Conversely, female donors, especially those who have been sensitized to male (H-Y) antigens during pregnancy, cause a higher incidence of GvHD in male recipients. Multiparous females may become sensitized and develop memory T-cells against a variety of autosomally inherited mHag, leading to a greater incidence of GvHD in recipients of either sex. Donor memory to antigens expressed by leukemia cells such as WT1 and PR1 is also transferred from the donor to the recipient.[54]

Other characteristics of donor immune function also appear to be transferred to the recipient. For example, donors with lower than average circulating regulatory T-cell frequencies give transplants with lower frequencies of Treg in the early post-transplant period and a correspondingly higher potential to develop acute GvHD.[58]

Transplant composition

Stem cell dose

It is now clear that the composition and dose of specific cellular components in the graft strongly modify transplant outcome through engraftment, GvHD and GvL mechanisms. The threshold dose of CD34 cells for engraftment differs according to the stem cell source and the transplant type. Thus, for autologous SCT from PBSCT, a

threshold of 1×10^6 CD34 cells/kg is a safe minimum for engraftment. For PBSCT and BM allotransplants, survival is optimal at CD34 doses above 3×10^6 kg, and higher doses may be necessary for best results in mismatched SCT. CD34 cell doses of 6×10^6/kg or higher also appear to benefit outcome by reducing risk of relapse, possibly through more rapid generation of NK cells.[9] Intriguingly, higher total nucleated cell doses also favor reduced relapse in identical twin SCT for myeloid leukemias.[59] UCB transplants only achieve CD34 doses a log lower. However, stem cells from UCB appear to have a greater potential to engraft, and CD34 doses above 3×10^5 kg appear to be a safe threshold for engraftment.[10]

T-cell dose

While it is clear that T-cell depletion modifies post-transplant immune recovery and thereby affects outcome (less GvHD, more infection and relapse), a clear interaction between T-cell dose and outcome has not been defined. One study found that in T-cell depleted SCT, T-cell doses of less than 1×10^5 kg were associated with a significantly diminished incidence and severity of chronic GvHD, but the threshold for such an effect probably varies according to the method of T-cell depletion and other regimen-specific factors.[54] It is known that CD4+ and CD8+ T-cells contribute differently to GvHD. Transplants that are CD8+ depleted have a small but significantly lower risk of causing GvHD.[60] Also, there are strong data from animal experiments and early human trials that GvHD (but possibly also GvL) is diminished by transplants containing higher frequencies of Treg cells and those containing a preponderance of Th2 Tc2 (anti-inflammatory cytokine-biased T-cells).[61] In mice, GvHD is conferred largely through transfer of naïve post-thymic T-cells. It has yet to be shown whether the transplant of donor T-cells depleted of naïve cells could favorably affect immune reconstitution by transferring only useful donor memory cells.[62]

Patient and donor age

Patient age has a major impact on the transplant outcome for immunologic and non-immunologic reasons. As it ages, the immune system undergoes several significant changes that can affect transplant outcome. Young children and infants have robust but relatively naïve immune systems compared to older individuals. They have intact and functioning thymuses which make it possible after transplant for newly emerging donor-derived prethymic T-cells to passage through the recipient thymus and become fully tolerant to the host. Over the age of about 30 years, the thymus is atrophied and thymic regeneration post transplant is slower and incomplete, leading to a prolonged period post transplant when cellular immunity is provided by transplanted post-thymic T-cells. Older adults appear to function more and more on a limited repertoire of post-thymic T-cells. In addition, they have much lower frequencies of regulatory T-cells.[63,64] This latter feature may predispose recipients of transplants from older donors to develop more GvHD.

Immunologic considerations aside, younger recipient age always favors better transplant outcome; younger individuals and children in particular withstand the effects of conditioning regimens and GvHD better than do older patients. TRM rises progressively by decade but increases substantially between the second and third decade, rising more slowly thereafter to the age of around 60 years. TRM for patients over 60 years is less clearly characterized, because relatively few patients have been treated and the regimens they receive are usually of reduced intensity, which may reduce immediate TRM but leave them more prone to disease relapse. Co-morbidities begin to rise in patients older than 60 years, with cardiovascular disease, renal and pulmonary insufficiency becoming increasingly important co-factors for survival after transplant.[65] There is little evidence that donor age has much impact on patient outcome. However, because donor and recipient age in matched sibling SCT are closely linked, studies evaluating donor age independently of patient age are limited to unrelated donor transplants where some impact has been found.

Nature of the disease at transplantation

SCT is rarely the first treatment for the disease that the patient receives. Patients usually come to transplant with a legacy of effects from prior treatment and the progress of the disease, all of which can reduce the chances of a successful outcome. For example, transplant outcome for patients with thalassemia depends upon the degree of iron overload from multiple transfusions and hepatic damage, although modifications to preparative regimens for such patients have improved survival. Patients with malignant diseases have an increased risk not only of relapse, but also of non-relapse mortality as their disease evolves. Transplants carried out electively, early in the course of disease, consequently have a lower risk of TRM. For malignant and non-malignant diseases alike, the interval between diagnosis and transplant remains an almost universal determinant of survival.

Transplant-related variables

Variation of the transplant regimen to suit the particular circumstances is a critical factor in optimizing transplant outcome. The transplanter can select the dose, cell content and stem cell source for the transplant as well as having a more limited choice in identifying a suitable donor–recipient match. When comparable HLA-matched donors are available, the donor can be chosen for other attributes such as sex, parity, CMV exposure and NK alloreactivity. The choice of conditioning regimens is wide – regimens can be selected for their antileukemia intensity or for their safety, but in transplants for malignant disease a compromise has to be struck between risking higher relapse rates from reduced intensity and higher TRM rates with higher intensity. Ultimately, the final disease-free survival may differ markedly because the different adverse effects of high or low intensity tend to cancel out. The transplanter has a similar set of choices concerning GvHD prevention: low-intensity immunosuppression favors progression-free survival but can risk more GvHD, while intensive T-cell depletion risks leukemic relapse while preventing GvHD. An optimal 'middle way' can, however, be possible – studies have shown that reduced ciclosporin dosing to achieve levels about half the normal therapeutic range results in significantly lower disease relapse but without increased GvHD.[54]

Post-transplant predictive factors

A number of studies of transplant survival have identified the early recovery of the lymphocyte count to be strongly predictive for subsequent survival. It appears that the effect is related to the degree of recovery of NK cells, such that patients achieving NK cell counts over a threshold of 150/μl 1 month after SCT have significantly lower relapse rates, less GvHD and better disease-free survivals.[66,67]

References

1. Shiruzu JA, Negrin RS, Weissman IL. Hematopoietic stem and progenitor cells: clinical and preclinical regeneration of the hematolymphoid system. Ann Rev Med 2005;56: 509–538
2. Orlic D. BM stem cells and cardiac repair: where do we stand in 2004? Cytotherapy 2005; 7:3–15
3. Quesenberry PJ, Colvin GA, Abedi M et al. The stem cell continuum. Ann NY Acad Sci 2005;1044:228–235
4. Gottschalk S, Rooney CM, Heslop HE. Post-transplant lymphoproliferative disorders. Ann Rev Med 2005;56:29–44
5. Lapierre V, Oubouzar N, Auperin A et al. Societe Francaise de Greffe de Moelle. Influence of the hematopoietic stem cell source on early immunohematologic reconstitution after allogeneic transplantation. Blood 2001;97:2580–2586
6. Passweg JR, Stern M, Koehl U et al. Use of natural killer cells in hematopoetic stem cell transplantation. Bone Marrow Transplant 2005;35:637–643
7. Keating A. Mesenchymal stromal cells. Curr Opin Hematol 2006;13:399–406
8. Couban S, Barnett M. The source of cells for allografting. Biol Blood Marrow Transplant 2003;9:669–673
9. Schmitz N, Barrett J. Optimizing engraftment – source and dose of stem cells. Semin Hematol 2002;39:3–14
10. Laughlin MJ. Umbilical cord blood for allogeneic transplantation in children and adults. Bone Marrow Transplant 2001;27:1–6
11. Pamphilon D. Stem-cell harvesting and manipulation. Vox Sang 2004;87(suppl 1): 20–25
12. Lapidot T, Petit I. Current understanding of stem cell mobilization: the roles of chemokines, proteolytic enzymes, adhesion molecules, cytokines, and stromal cells. Exp Hematol 2002;30:973–981
13. Chute JP. Stem cell homing. Curr Opin Hematol 2006;13:399–406
14. Barrett AJ, Rezvani K. Neutrophil granule proteins as targets of leukemia-specific immune responses. Curr Opin Hematol 2006;13:15–20
15. Peggs KS. Reconstitution of adaptive and innate immunity following allogeneic stem cell transplantation in humans. Cytotherapy 2006;8:427–436
16. Guimond M, Fry TJ, Mackall CL.Cytokine signals in T-cell homeostasis. J Immunother 2005;28:289–294
17. Barber LD, Madrigal JA. Exploiting beneficial alloreactive T-cells. Vox Sang 2006;91:20–27
18. Storek J. B-cell immunity after allogeneic hematopoietic cell transplantation. Cytotherapy 2002;4:423–424
19. Barrett AJ, Savani BN. Stem cell transplantation with reduced-intensity conditioning regimens: a review of ten years experience with new transplant concepts and new therapeutic agents. Leukemia 2006;20:1661–1667
20. Barrett AJ. Conditioning regimens for allogeneic stem cell transplants. Curr Opin Hematol 2000;7:339–342
21. Childs R, Clave E, Contentin N et al. Full donor T lymphocyte chimerism predicts for graft-vs-host disease, graft-vs marrow and graft-vs-malignancy effects following a non-myeloablative preparative regimen. Blood 1999;94:3234–3241
22. Rudolph MG, Stanfield RL, Wilson IA. How TCRs bind MHCs, peptides, and coreceptors. Annu Rev Immunol 2006;24:419–466
23. Goulmy E. Minor histocompatibility antigens: from transplantation problems to therapy of cancer. Hum Immunol 2006;67:433–438
24. Murphy WJ, Koh CY, Raziuddin A et al. Immunobiology of natural killer cells and bone marrow transplantation: merging of basic and preclinical studies. Immunol Rev 2001;181:279–289
25. Ruggeri L, Mancusi A, Burchielli E et al. Natural killer cell recognition of missing self and haploidentical hematopoietic transplantation. Semin Cancer Biol 2006;16:404–411
26. Barao I, Murphy WJ. The immunobiology of natural killer cells and bone marrow allograft rejection. Biol Blood Marrow Transplant 2003;9:727–741
27. Hansen JA, Choo SY, Geraghty DE, Mickelson E. The HLA system in clinical marrow transplantation. Hematol Oncol Clin North Am 1990;4:507–515
28. Petersdorf EW, Malkki M. Human leucocyte antigen matching in unrelated donor hematopoietic cell transplantation. Semin Hematol 2005;9:173–180
29. Tiercy JM. Molecular basis of polymorphism: implications in clinical transplantation. Transpl Immunol 2002;10:205–214
30. Jeras M. The role of in vitro T-cell function tests in the selection of HLA matched and mismatched haematopoietic stem cell donors. Transpl Immunol 2002;10:205–214
31. Wang XN, Collin M, Sviland L et al. Skin explant model of human graft-versus-host disease: prediction of clinical outcome and correlation with biological risk factors. Biol Blood Marrow Transplant 2006;12:152–159
32. Brenner MK, Rill DR, Moen RC et al. Gene marking and autologous bone marrow transplantation. Ann NY Acad Sci 1994;716:204–214
33. Puck JM, Malech HL. Gene therapy for immune disorders: good news tempered by bad news. J Allergy Clin Immunol 2006;117:865–869
34. van Laar JM, Tyndall A. Adult stem cells in the treatment of autoimmune diseases. Rheumatology 2006;45:1187–1193
35. Scheinberg P. Stem-cell transplantation for autoimmune diseases. Cytotherapy 2003; 5:243–251
36. Young NS, Calado RT, Scheinberg P. Current concepts in the pathophysiology and treatment of aplastic anemia. Blood 2006;108:2509–2519
37. Weisdorf D, Chao N, Waselenko JK et al. Acute radiation injury: contingency planning for triage, supportive care, and transplantation. Biol Blood Marrow Transplant 2006;12: 672–682
38. Storb RF, Lucarelli G, McSweeney PA, Childs RW. Hematopoietic cell transplantation for benign hematological disorders and solid tumors. Hematol Am Soc Hematol Edu Program 2003;372–397
39. Friedrich W, Muller SM. Allogeneic stem cell transplantation for treatment of immunodeficiency. Springer Semin Immunopathol 2004;26:109–118
40. Hobbs JR. Displacement bone marrow transplantation for some inborn errors. J Inherit Metab Dis 1990;13:572–596
41. Kolb HJ, Schmid C, Barrett AJ, Schendel DJ. Graft-versus-leukemia reactions in allogeneic chimeras. Blood 2004;103:767–776
42. Lundqvist A, Childs R. Allogeneic hematopoietic cell transplantation as immunotherapy for solid tumors: current status and future directions. J Immunother 2005;28:281–288
43. Barrett AJ, Malkovska V. Graft-versus-leukaemia: understanding and using the alloimmune response to treat haematological malignancies. Br J Haematol 1996;93:754–761
44. Farag SS, Fehniger TA, Ruggeri L et al. Natural killer cell receptors: new biology and insights into the graft-versus-leukemia effect. Blood 2002;100:1935–1947
45. Ferrara JL, Reddy P. Pathophysiology of graft-versus-host disease. Semin Hematol 2006;43:3–10
46. Ferrara JL, Yanik G. Acute graft versus host disease: pathophysiology, risk factors, and prevention strategies. Clin Adv Hematol Oncol 2005;3:415–419

47. Cutler C, Antin JH. Chronic graft-versus-host disease. Curr Opin Oncol 2006;18: 126–131

48. Maeda Y, Teshima T, Yamada M, Harada M. Reactivation of human herpesviruses after allogeneic peripheral blood stem cell transplantation and bone marrow transplantation. Leuk Lymphoma 2000;39:229–239

49. Einsele H, Hebart H. Cellular immunity to viral and fungal antigens after stem cell transplantation. Curr Opin Hematol 2002;9:485–489

50. Dermime S, Mavroudis D, Jiang YZ et al. Immune escape from a graft-versus-leukemia effect may play a role in the relapse of myeloid leukemias following allogeneic bone marrow transplantation. Bone Marrow Transplant 1997;19:989–999

51. Battiwalla M, Hahn T, Radovic M et al. Human leukocyte antigen (HLA) DR15 is associated with reduced incidence of acute GVHD in HLA-matched allogeneic transplantation but does not impact chronic GVHD incidence. Blood 2006;107:1970–1973

52. Bignon JD, Gagne K. KIR matching in hematopoietic stem cell transplantation. Curr Opin Immunol 2005;17:553–559

53. Cook MA, Milligan DW, Fegan CD et al. The impact of donor KIR and patient HLA-C genotypes on outcome following HLA-identical sibling hematopoietic stem cell transplantation for myeloid leukemia.Blood 2004;103:1521–1526

54. Barrett AJ, Rezvani K, Solomon S et al. New developments in allotransplant immunology. Hematology Am Soc Hematol Educ Program 2003;372–397

55. Dickinson AM, Charron D. Non-HLA immunogenetics in hematopoietic stem cell transplantation. Curr Opin Immunol 2005;17:517–525

56. Charron D. Immunogenetics today: HLA, MHC and much more. Curr Opin Immunol 2005;17:493–497

57. Oh H, Loberiza FR Jr, Zhang MJ et al. Comparison of graft-versus-host-disease and survival after HLA-identical sibling bone marrow transplantation in ethnic populations. Blood 2005;105:1408–1411

58. Rezvani K, Grube M, Brenchley JM et al. Functional leukemia-associated antigen-specific memory CD8+ T-cells exist in healthy individuals and in patients with chronic myelogenous leukemia before and after stem cell transplantation. Blood 2003;102: 2892–2900

59. Barrett AJ, Ringden O, Zhang MJ et al. Effect of nucleated marrow cell dose on relapse and survival in identical twin bone marrow transplants for leukemia. Blood 2000;95:3323–3327

60. Meyer RG, Britten CM, Wehler D et al. Prophylactic transfer of CD8-depleted donor lymphocytes after T-cell depleted reduced-intensity transplantation. Blood 2007;109:374–382

61. Fowler DH. Shared biology of GVHD and GVT effects: potential methods of separation. Crit Rev Oncol Hematol 2006;57:225–244

62. Chen BJ, Deoliveira D, Cui X et al. Inability of memory T-cells to induce graft-versus-host disease is a result of an abortive alloresponse. Blood 2007;109(7):3115–3123

63. Hakim FT, Gress RE. Reconstitution of thymic function after stem cell transplantation in humans.Curr Opin Hematol 2002;9:490–496

64. Mackall CL, Gress RE. Thymic aging and T-cell regeneration. Immunol Rev 1997; 160:91–102

65. Artz AS, Pollyea DA, Kocherginsky M et al. Performance status and comorbidity predict transplant-related mortality after allogeneic hematopoietic cell transplantation. Biol Blood Marrow Transplant 2006;12:954–964

66. Powles R, Singhal S, Treleaven J et al. Identification of patients who may benefit from prophylactic bone marrow transplantation for acute myeloid leukemia on the basis of lymphocyte recovery early after transplantation. Blood 1998;91:3481–3486

67. Savani BN, Rezvani K, Mielke S et al. Factors associated with early molecular remission after T-cell-depleted allogeneic stem cell transplantation for chronic myelogenous leukemia. Blood 2006;107:1688–1695

PART 2

THE ROLE OF STEM CELL TRANSPLANTATION IN TREATMENT

Acute myeloid leukemia

Alan K Burnett and Steven Knapper

CHAPTER 3

Around 80% of patients with acute myeloid leukemia (AML) who are under 60 years of age will enter complete remission (CR) of their disease with most of the widely used induction chemotherapy combinations.[1,2] The major issue therefore is how to prevent relapse. The median age of presentation is 68 years, however, so there remains a majority of older patients who, if subjected to conventional induction therapy, will only achieve CR in 50–60% of cases, and even if they do, 85% will relapse within 3 years.[2,3] The current role of stem cell transplantation is to prevent relapse. Numerous controlled and uncontrolled studies have led to the conclusion that this approach is the most effective way to prevent disease recurrence, whether it be by permitting myeloablative treatment or exploiting a graft-versus-leukemia effect, or both.[4,5]

The situation is, however, much more complex. In spite of its significant antileukemic effect, transplantation is associated with an apparently unavoidable treatment-related mortality which, when coupled with the prospect that some patients who do relapse can be salvaged, makes its use as a standard approach to consolidation in first remission much less clear. AML is a heterogeneous disease from morphologic, immunophenotypic, cytogenetic and molecular points of view, and this is reflected in a wide variation in the risk of relapse. The consequence is that the evaluation of stem cell transplantation (SCT) as a treatment option requires an estimate of relapse risk to be taken into account. A further complication is that in younger patients the results of chemotherapy are improving such that historical data may no longer be applicable. Similarly, developments in transplantation such as more availability of unrelated donors and reduced-intensity transplantation increase the relevance of this approach.

The possibility of cure without stem cell transplantation

Several prospective multicenter trials indicate that 75–85% of patients under 60 years will achieve complete remission; of these, around 40–50% will survive 5 years.[6–8] Most relapses will have taken place within 3 years, so patients who reach this point have a high chance of cure. For patients who relapse, second remissions are achievable in around 40% of cases but these will be short-lived and, as a general rule, shorter than the first remission, with only 10–15% surviving long term.

Prognostic factors

There has been considerable interest in developing and exploiting prognostic factors to guide postinduction treatment. It is accepted that

the major independent predictors of relapse are cytogenetics, age, morphologic response to induction treatment, de novo or secondary disease and white count at presentation.

Cytogenetics

The relationship between the cytogenetic lesion present in leukemic blasts and response to treatment has been known for many years. However, as treatment results have improved, the ability to delineate relapse risk has become clear from more contemporary collaborative group studies.[9–11] These observations are also prognostic for the risk of relapse after transplant. It is recognized that acute promyelocytic leukemia (APL), which is characterized by the t(15;17) translocation, is a separate entity since the introduction of all trans-retinoic acid and more recently other effective agents such as arsenic trioxide, and the immunoconjugate gemtuzumab ozogamicin.[12,13] Recent results indicate that 85–90% of patients are cured, and of those who are not, at least half perish during induction. There are some higher risk situations in this disease such as presentation with a high white count (>10 $\times$ 10^9/l), persistence or recurrence of molecular evidence of residual disease or frank hematologic relapse. In these situations, arsenic trioxide or gemtuzumab ozogamicin is effective, so patients will only be candidates for SCT in this relatively rare circumstance, although such evidence as exists suggests that autograft may be the preferred option.[14] The other favorable risk group includes patients with t(8;21) or inv(16) who have a 70–75% cure with chemotherapy alone in most series. All three favorable groups may have additional cytogenetic abnormalities but it does not appear that these detract from the favorable outlook.

More recently, mutations of the FLT-3 receptor have been found in AML. FLT-3 mutations are frequent in APL and are closely correlated with a high white cell count but do not independently predict an adverse prognosis in this AML subgroup. Recently, it has been documented that approximately 30% of t(8;21) and inv(16) cases have a mutation of cKit, which significantly increases the risk of relapse.[15] About 15% of younger patients will have abnormalities which, by consensus, have a high risk of relapse and short remissions. Abnormalities of chromosome 5 or 7, 3q-, t(9:22), and complex (>3) abnormalities will have an 80% incidence of relapse with chemotherapy alone. Unlike other cytogenetic risk groups, there is little evidence that there has been any improvement in these patient groups in the last 20 years. All other abnormalities, in addition to those with a normal karyotype, which comprise 60% of younger patients, are regarded as of intermediate risk with a relapse risk of 50–55%.

There is a relationship between age and karyotype, with a tendency for the more favorable groups to be associated with younger age and vice versa for older patients, but age independently predicts outcome. Children now have a 65% rate of cure with chemotherapy. A minority

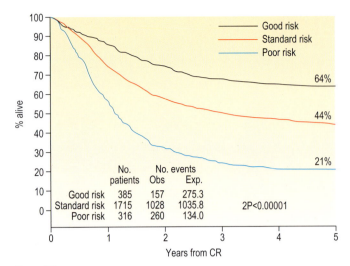

Figure 3.1
MRC AML10 and 12. Survival from CR by risk group.

of patients fail to clear the marrow blasts after the first induction course, but do subsequently enter CR. However, the morphologic response to course 1 is a surrogate marker for resistant disease, and these patients have a higher risk of subsequent relapse and can therefore be categorized as high risk. In the large MRC trials, three risk groups were identified and prospectively validated.[16] Patients in the high-risk category were the unfavorable karyotype and/or patients who had >15% blasts in the bone marrow after course 1 (Fig. 3.1).

Molecular lesions

Risk assessment has become more complex due to the observation that the presence of certain mutations has prognostic impact. Mutations of RAS occur in 12–15% of cases, but do not influence outcome.[17] Mutations of FLT-3 occur in about 30% of patients and occur in two forms.[18–21] The majority (~25–30%) occur as internal tandem duplications (ITD) in the juxtamembrane domain of the receptor, and around 7% occur as point mutations in the activation loop. It is clear from several publications that the presence of an ITD is highly predictive of relapse. There may be a prognostic relationship between the number of duplications and outcome. Paradoxically, TK mutations may confer a favorable prognosis. ITDs are not randomly distributed across the AML subtypes and appear to be more frequent in APL, normal karyotype and trisomy 8 patients.[19] The prognostic impact of cytogenetics can be augmented by FLT-3 mutation information. A large study on behalf of the MRC[19] indicated that the relapse risk for patients with high-risk cytogenetics with or without a mutation was 100% versus 78%; for standard-risk and good-risk groups the respective differences were 74% vs 48% and 39% vs 30%.

More recently, it has been discovered that 50% of patients with a normal karyotype will have a mutation of the nucleophosmin 1 (NPM1) gene.[22] If occurring alone this confers a favorable outcome. It frequently co-exists with a mutation of FLT-3 where it neutralizes the adverse prognosis.[23,24] Mutations of the CEBPα gene occur in around 15% of cases with a normal karyotype and appear to predict a better prognosis.[25] Several other mutations and aberrant expressions are likely to emerge as the number of fully analyzed cases accumulates.

Treatment failures

If a patient relapses, the likelihood of achieving a second remission, and the duration of the second remission, depend more on their age, the duration of first remission and the original cytogenetic risk group

than the reinduction treatment used. A recently reported risk score has confirmed these beliefs.[26]

The contribution of allogeneic transplantation

Registry and other data published over the last 25–30 years clearly demonstrate that patients who undergo allogeneic transplant in CR1 will have a risk of relapse of 20% (±5%), which is apparently better than consolidation using chemotherapy.[4,5] However, this is inevitably associated with a 20–25% rate of non-leukemic death so the expectation of survival is 50–60%. In the MRC database of more than 1000 recipients, the survival at 5 years is 55% several years after the introduction of allograft as the treatment of choice. However, there was a recognition that there was a clear selection bias in favor of patients who actually received the transplant.[27] Patients had to survive in remission and be in acceptable clinical condition to receive the transplant which often did not take place for 2–6 months into remission and would obviously exclude early relapsers. When 'time-censoring' adjustments were made to chemotherapy patient cohorts, there remained evidence for a reduced relapse risk in the transplanted patients, but it was much less clear whether there was a survival advantage. This stimulated the major collaborative group prospective studies aimed at comparing either autologous or allogeneic transplantation with intensive consolidation or in addition to intensive consolidation. Since true randomization was not acceptable, the preferred method of assessment was based on genetic randomization of 'donor versus no donor' where it was assumed that as a surrogate for an intent to treat comparison, the intention was to transplant a patient who had a donor.

Comparative trials

Four major study groups – the EORTC-GIMEMA, GOELAM, the US Intergroup and the UK Medical Research Council – undertook pivotal studies in the late 1980s and during the 1990s.[28–31] In general, the design was similar in that patients who had a donor were expected to undergo a standard allogeneic transplant, while those who did not were randomized between chemotherapy (usually high-dose Ara-C) or autologous transplantation of bone marrow cells which were only subjected to chemical in vitro purging in the US Intergroup Trial (Fig. 3.2). The MRC trials were of a slightly different design in that the transplant was being evaluated in addition to, rather than with, intensive consolidation. In a successor trial (AML12), the MRC conducted the only truly randomized evaluation of allogeneic transplantation, in that patients were randomized to transplant or not, and those allocated to transplant received an allograft if there was a donor available and an autograft if there was not.[32] In all of these studies approximately 1200 patients were randomized in the autograft comparison and the overall observation was that autograft resulted in a reduced risk of relapse, but no consistent overall survival benefit because the reduction in relapse risk was balanced by small treatment-related mortality effects associated with the autograft and the superior ability to salvage in patients who relapsed after chemotherapy. In a landmark analysis of 2-year survivors in the MRC trial, there was a significant survival benefit in the autograft arm. These four published collaborative group trials delivered 924 patients with a donor and 1321 with no donor for comparative study (Table 3.1). The disease-free survival was only significantly superior in the donor group in the EORTC-GIMEMA trial but not in the other three trials. There was no significant survival difference at 4 years in any of the four trials.

These trials are based on clinical experience of 10–15 years ago and may be of less clear relevance in the current generation of patients.

Table 3.1 Results of allogeneic SCT trials in adults

Trial	Study population Donor vs Chemo		Relapse risk (%) Donor vs Chemo	Disease-free survival (%) Donor vs Chemo	Overall survival (%) Donor vs Chemo
EORTC-GIMEMA	295	377	NA	46 vs 33*	48 vs 40
GOELAM	88	157	25 vs 37	44 vs 38	53 vs 53
MRC	428	870	33 vs 51**	47 vs 40	53 vs 46
US Intergroup	113	117	29 vs 62	43 vs 36	46 vs 52****

NA, not available; chemo; chemotherapy
*p = 0.01; **p = 0.02; ***p = 0.04

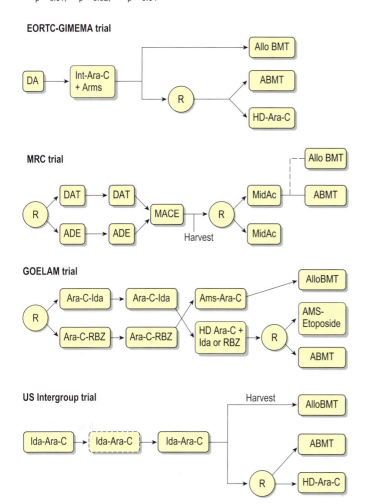

EORTC-GIMEMA trial

MRC trial

GOELAM trial

US Intergroup trial

Figure 3.2
Schema of collaborative group trials.

Table 3.2 Transplant outcomes in good-risk patients

Trial	Relapse risk (%) Donor vs Chemo	Disease-free survival (%) Donor vs Chemo	Overall survival (%) Donor vs Chemo
EORTC-GIMEMA	39 vs 49*	57 vs 45	61 vs 56
GOELAM	NA	61 vs 51	71 vs 67
MRC	26 vs 36	61 vs 60	71 vs 73
US Intergroup	NA	NA	66 vs 35

NA, not available. Risk definitions – EORTC-GIMEMA: CR course 1 with French-American-British (FAB) type M2/M3 and M4 eo; CR course 1 without FAB M1/M4 and WBC < 25 × 10⁹/l. GOELAM: FAB M2 or M3 with WBC < 30 × 10⁹/l, MRC: FAB M3; t(15;17) t(8;21) inv(16). US Intergroup as for MRC but excluding associated del (9q) or complex.
*p = 0.01.

Transplant in relation to relapse risk

A detailed analysis of the MRC AML10 trial[28] indicated that there was no apparent benefit for allografting patients with good-risk cytogenetics even with respect to relapse reduction. Although the numbers were small, the risk of relapse in a donor versus no donor comparison of 49 and 92 patients showed an identical relapse risk of 30% (Table 3.2). In subsequent studies allografting has been omitted in this group without detriment to overall survival. Of interest in this study was the observation that there was an overall reduction in relapse risk in good-risk patients, but this was accounted for only by the APL subset (22% vs 43%). These data were accumulated before all trans-retinoic acid (ATRA) was introduced into APL treatment.

The reduction in relapse risk in AML10 was highly significant in standard-risk patients (36% vs 56%) which translated to a significant survival advantage (54% vs 44%). In patients with an adverse karyotype there was no evidence that the availability of a donor reduced the risk of relapse (80% vs 75%) or improved overall survival (14% vs 27%). The overall conclusion from this trial conducted between 1988 and 1995 was that the addition of transplant to consolidation treatment was of benefit only to patients with standard or intermediate cytogenetic risk disease.

In the successor unpublished AML12 trial, two questions related to transplant were posed. First, should it be given as course 5, that is, in addition to chemotherapy as in the AML10 study, or as course 4? Second, in each case was it superior to chemotherapy? The assessment was a true randomization in that patients were randomized to transplant or not, and if so allocated and a matched (sibling) donor was available, they received an allograft – if not they received an autograft. The results of this trial have not yet been published in full, but there was no overall survival benefit in any risk subgroup.[28] The benefit for standard-risk patients observed in AML10 was not apparent because the outcome with chemotherapy had improved (Fig. 3.3).

It has been possible to reanalyze the other major series based on risk assessment, although there are intertrial differences on definitions, with only the MRC US Intergroup and HOVON studies predominantly based on cytogenetics with similar categorization. In good-risk patients

They are open to some criticism. First, of patients with a donor only 71% actually received the allograft and the rest were denied the antileukemic benefit of the allograft but also avoided the associated mortality and negative impact on quality of life.[33,34] Advocators of transplantation make the justifiable point that it is unfair to judge an intervention where 30% do not receive the allocated treatment.[35]

A more recent report comes from HOVON-SAKK collaborative group[36] where patients were entered in three consecutive trials between 1987 and 2004. The total experience was of 326 patients with a donor and 599 for whom a donor was not found. Of those who had donors, 82% received the transplant. As in previous studies the relapse risk was significantly reduced (32% vs 59%) with an improvement in disease-free survival (48% vs 37%). However, the difference in overall survival (54% vs 46%) failed to reach significance even when limited to standard- and poor-risk patients. They also demonstrated that no benefit was apparent in patients over 40 years of age.

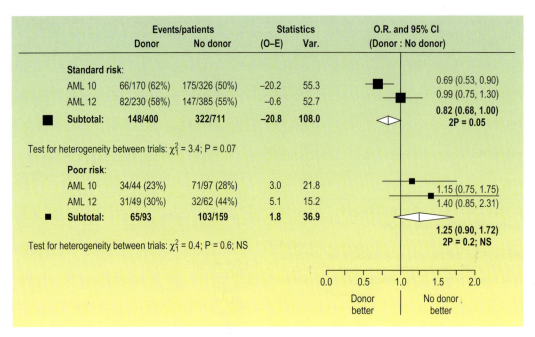

Figure 3.3
AML10 and 12. Donor versus no donor comparisons. Overall survival stratified by risk group.

there was a significant survival advantage in the US Intergroup trial (66% vs 35%) (see Table 3.2). This is inconsistent with the MRC10 trial, in which patients were defined on the same basis, and with the EORTC-GIMEMA and GOELAM trials, which had different good-risk criteria. An explanation may be the unexpectedly poor outcome for the chemotherapy-only arm. Excluding the MRC10 trial, none of the three trials showed a survival benefit for standard-risk (Table 3.3) patients and in poor-risk patients, only the US Intergroup showed a similar advantage (42% vs 15%) (Table 3.4).

These trials have influenced clinical practice in that it is generally accepted that patients with favorable cytogenetics should not receive an allograft as part of first-line treatment. There is less concordance on refraining from transplantation in standard-risk cases, but there is an argument to continue to evaluate its use in the context of a clinical trial where other information will be available. For such patients to be transplanted as standard care, other factors need to be considered. To this end a risk score based on readily available characterization – cytogenetics, age, white count, response to course 1, de novo or secondary disease – has been suggested as a more precise method of identifying patients who will benefit from transplantation in CR1.[37] In a retrospective analysis of the MRC database this scoring system had the effect of identifying as high risk a cohort of patients who, on cytogenetic criteria, were standard risk. This had the effect of increasing the high-risk proportion from 17% to 27%. A small number of patients migrated from high risk to standard risk. When the donor versus no donor criterion was reapplied, there was a significant survival benefit for patients defined by the new criteria as high risk.

Since the toxicity of transplantation using a standard myeloablative approach increases with age, it is important to explore the upper age at which any benefit may disappear. In an analysis of the MRC AML10 and 12 trials using remission duration as the endpoint, the cut-off age is 35 years. The reason for failure above this age is predominantly a result of increased treatment-related mortality. New molecular knowledge is providing new prognostic factors. The most studied is mutation of the FLT-3 receptor. There is a tendency to assume that any poor-risk characteristic means that patients will benefit from allogeneic transplant. Where cytogenetic risk stratification, which has been developed in the context of chemotherapy treatments, has been applied to the

Table 3.3 Transplant outcomes in standard-risk patients

Trial	Relapse risk (%) Donor vs Chemo	Disease-free survival (%) Donor vs Chemo	Overall survival (%) Donor vs Chemo
EORTC-GIMEMA	47 vs 66*	42 vs 29	46 vs 38
GOELAM	NA	34 vs 38	41 vs 57
MRC	34 vs 56**	53 vs 39***	57 vs 45****
US Intergroup	NA	NA	52 vs 55

NA, not available. Risk definitions – EORTC-GIMEMA: CR with course 1 with unfavorable FAB or WBC <25 × 10⁹/l or CR > course 1 with favorable FAB and WBC >25 × 10⁹/l, MRC not good or poor risk. US Intergroup: normal cytogenetics, +8, +9 +6 or del (12p).
* p = 0.00002; ** p = 0.05; *** p = 0.003; **** p = 0.02

Table 3.4 Transplant outcomes in poor-risk patients

Trial	Relapse risk (%) Donor vs Chemo	Disease-free survival (%) Donor vs Chemo	Overall survival (%) Donor vs Chemo
EORTC-GIMEMA	69 vs 87*	22 vs 12	28 vs 22
GOELAM	NA	27 vs 22	41 vs 30
MRC	71 vs 78	22 vs 21	23 vs 25
US Intergroup	NA	NA	42 vs 15†

NA, not available. Risk definitions – EORTC-GIMEMA: CR > course 1; FAB M5,M6, M7; FAB M1, M2, M3 with WBC >25 × 10⁹/l. GOELAM, FAB all except M3 plus WBC >30 × 10⁹/l. MRC -5/del 5q, del 5q, del (7q), 3q-, complex, blasts >15% after course 1. US Intergroup -5/del 5q.
* p = 0.03; † No p-value available.

recipients of allogeneic transplantation, the same impact is observed.[9–11] FLT-3 mutation has also been shown to be a negative risk factor in transplanted patients. In an intent to treat analysis on a large number (>1100) of characterized patients, it was not possible to be sure that the prognosis for patients with a FLT-3 mutation was improved by transplantation.[38] As mentioned previously, not all patients with a FLT-3 mutation have the same relapse risk because of the modulating effect of associated NPM1 mutations. Although the presence of a cKit mutation identifies a subgroup of patients in the favorable cytogenetic risk group with a higher risk of relapse, it is far from clear that such patients will benefit from transplantation – a prospect which will be complicated by the introduction of small molecules with anti-Kit activity.

Assessment of benefit

Since randomized trials have not generally been possible, a donor versus no donor analytical report has been adopted as the next best method of evaluating transplantation. This has the benefit of providing a common time starting point, but it is based on the assumption that if matching is undertaken and a donor found then a transplant is given. In fact, only about 70% of patients with donors receive a transplant. There are a number of reasons for this. First, the physician may just be explaining potential options. For example, in an older patient there may be no real intention to transplant in CR1 but rather, plans in the event of treatment failure are being laid. As indicated earlier, concern has been expressed that it is unfair to assess a treatment which 35% of patients do not receive.[35] On the one hand, the powerful antileukemia effect is only provided by the 50% who receive the transplant, but conversely the same group suffer most of the fatal events. It should also be recognized that prospective evaluations of quality of life do not favor allogeneic transplantation over either autograft or chemotherapy.[33,34]

An alternative statistical approach is the use of the Mantel-Byar technique. Here all patients start on the life table together and when a transplant is delivered the patient joins the transplant survival line. This approach ensures that only patients who receive a transplant are evaluated. However, it tends to favor transplantation because patients who relapse or are considered unfit for transplantation remain on the chemotherapy arm. A retrospective analysis of the MRC database using this test persisted in failing to show a benefit for transplantation in any of the cytogenetic risk groups. The benefit was seen, however, in patients with a high-risk score as referred to above.

Who should be transplanted in CR1?

The major prospective trials have been difficult to undertake and have been useful in providing data to demonstrate that selecting patients for transplantation in CR1 is complicated. There is little doubt that patients with core binding factor leukemia (t(8;21) and inv(16)) do not benefit from a sibling allograft in CR1. If these patients relapse they have a high second remission rate, and thus reserving transplantation for patients who relapse is justified. Whether the subset with cKit mutations should be transplanted in CR1, reinduced with chemotherapy and then transplanted or whether they are capable of being salvaged with molecularly targeted treatment is not known.

The evidence from the collaborative group trials to recommend transplantation in patients with high-risk cytogenetics is mixed. However, by better defining these patients using a score based on several adverse factors, supportive evidence is available. The difficult decision relates to the other 60% of patients in the intermediate- or standard-risk category. None of the trials showed an overall survival benefit for this group. However, newer methods of characterization by molecular markers make this a fluid situation. If patients in this category are to be transplanted this should ideally be done in the context of a clinical trial where some of these difficult issues can be resolved in due course.

Transplantation beyond first remission

When a patient relapses chemotherapy is unlikely to be curative. However, the prognosis depends on age, length of CR1, cytogenetic risk group and FLT-3 mutation status. In a retrospective study of the MRC database[39] there were 3495 patients who avoided transplantation in CR1; 48% relapsed, of whom 44% (n = 751) entered a second remission. Of 293 patients with good-risk cytogenetics who relapsed, 212 (72%) achieved a second remission. On a donor versus no donor analysis there was an advantage for the donor arm (65% vs 36%). Of 931 standard-risk patients who relapsed, 396 (43%) achieved a second remission and the donor arm had a superior survival (40% vs 23%). Poor-risk patients have a limited chance of achieving a second remission, 54 of 213 (25%), and somewhat disappointingly it appears that the prospect of survival is remote (donor 0% vs no donor 19%). Similarly, patients who relapsed after a short first remission (<6 months) had a subsequent survival of 19% whether or not they had a transplant. Transplantation of older patients who are in second remission may have more appeal since they have a poor prospect with chemotherapy. In the retrospective study this appears to be confirmed with a survival of 33% versus 18% in patients over 40 years of age.

These data suggest that there is little doubt that when a patient relapses the aim should be to deliver a transplant. Some patients will fail to reach transplant because they fail to enter CR, become unfit or do not have a donor. Although there is evidence to suggest that transplantation as the treatment of relapse is a viable strategy aimed at getting more people to transplantation, logistic considerations make this an impractical option. The ability to deliver a transplant after relapse is heavily influenced by cytogenetic risk group. For example, in the MRC database 53% of good-risk, 27% of standard-risk, and 16% of poor-risk patients who relapsed got to transplantation. Overall survival from sibling allografts (54%) was superior to unrelated (38%) or autologous (34%) transplants.

The new paradigm

New developments in both chemotherapy and transplantation continue to emerge. Recent preliminary data suggest that the addition of the immunoconjugate Mylotarg to chemotherapy can reduce the risk of subsequent relapse.[40] If confirmed on longer follow-up and accepted as a new standard of care, it means that the comparative studies already described become less relevant. However, this development with Mylotarg does not appear to benefit high-risk patients. Some reservations have been expressed about the use of Mylotarg either before or after allografting where the risk of veno-occlusive disease of the liver may be as much as 15%. This was further suggested to be time related in that the risk is greatest if the Mylotarg is administered within 115 days of the transplant.[41] In the MRC trial experience where a lower Mylotarg dose (3 mg/m^2) was given, no veno-occlusive disease was reported even in patients who received the transplant within 115 days. A US study conducted by the ECOG group is evaluating the role of adding Mylotarg to the preparative protocol for autologous transplantation.

The new molecular knowledge will continue to identify patients at greater or lesser risk than indicated by currently used prognostic factors. Whether these patients should avoid or would benefit from transplantation will take years of careful study to determine.

All five of the major collaborative studies have indicated that although there is a significant reduction in relapse risk in patients over 35 years of age, there is no survival benefit because of increased treatment-related mortality. The development of reduced-intensity allografting clearly offers a potentially important contribution to older patients in whom the disease is more prevalent and the relapse risk greater.

Reduced-intensity conditioning strategies

Over the last decade reduced-intensity conditioning (RIC) approaches have emerged as a strategy to enable HSCT to be offered to AML patients who, due to age or co-morbidity, would not previously have been considered eligible. These approaches aim to exploit donor cell-mediated graft-versus-leukemia (GvL) effects rather than relying on high doses of cytotoxic agents to eradicate residual disease.

RIC regimens include a wide range of protocols of varying intensities, divided broadly into two fundamental strategies. 'Minimally intensive' or 'non-myeloablative' conditioning regimens have evolved from pioneering preclinical canine studies[42] and rely on an almost exclusively immunosuppressive approach to allow engraftment of donor stem cells. These regimens cause little or no cytopenia, and use low-dose total body irradiation (TBI) either alone or in combination with the purine analog fludarabine; this is followed by immunosuppression, usually with ciclosporin and mycophenolate mofetil. The second major strategy involves the addition of varying degrees of myelosuppression, usually using fludarabine in combination with an alkylating agent such as busulfan, melphalan or cyclophosphamide. These more intensive regimens, which meet the more strict recent definition of 'reduced-intensity conditioning', cause variable degrees and durations of cytopenia and form part of a continuum with standard myeloablative conditioning.[43]

The rationale for these 'less than myeloablative' transplant approaches lies in maximizing the GvL effect. GvL may be more easily established in the reduced-intensity setting due to the persistence of host dendritic cells capable of presenting minor host-specific peptides to the incoming donor T-cells.[44] The GvL effect takes time to develop, however, and due to the lower cytotoxicity of these regimens, with the achievement of full donor chimerism frequently being delayed, early relapse is a potential problem, particularly in rapidly progressive conditions such as AML where the rate of onset of GvL may potentially be outpaced by the rapid tempo of the underlying disease.

Clinical experience in AML

The use of RIC regimens has increased rapidly in recent years to the point where this approach now accounts for more than 40% of allogeneic HSCT activity in Europe.[45] This development has occurred largely in the absence of rigorous prospective clinical trials and many of the existing efficacy data are based on retrospective single-institution analyses. Table 3.5 summarizes the results of published trials of RIC-HSCT which included 20 or more AML patients, most of which were conducted between 1998 and 2004. Direct comparison of these studies is limited by the heterogeneity of the patient groups involved in terms of age, risk group, extent of disease and prior therapy, donor factors (stem cell source, proportion of related and unrelated donors, degree of matching in unrelated HSCT), variable durations of patient follow-up and the plethora of different conditioning, T-cell depletion and immunosuppressive protocols employed.

Despite these limitations, some important conclusions may be drawn. In general, reduced-intensity procedures proved feasible in the patient groups studied (median ages 47–60 years), with relatively low procedural mortality and morbidity. Engraftment failure was infrequent with several studies reporting no graft failures at all. One study reported a 19% rate of graft failure with truly non-ablative conditioning in comparison with only 3% failed engraftment with a reduced-intensity regimen.[45] Treatment-related mortality in these studies was generally in the 10–20% range, lower than typically reported in this age range in conventional allogeneic HSCT, although the Co-operative German Transplant Study Group reported 53% 2-year non-relapse mortality, with an even higher rate when analysis was restricted to unrelated donor transplants.[46] A number of the studies provide evidence of relatively low rates of infectious complications, hepatic veno-occlusive disease, mucositis and transfusion requirements in the RIC setting. Overall, GvHD rates were not dissimilar to those seen with traditional myeloablative regimens.

Relapse and GvHD are the major causes of death after RIC-HSCT in AML, with efforts to reduce them usually being offset by increased rates of the other. Comparing a minimal-intensity regimen with a reduced-intensity regimen, de Lima et al reported reduced rates of both grade II–IV acute GvHD (25% vs 39%) and chronic GvHD (27% vs 39%) with minimal-intensity conditioning, but this was achieved at the expense of a much higher rate of relapse (61% vs 30%).[47] Across the trials of RIC in AML, relapse rates were generally high and exceeded 30% in eight of the 14 evaluable studies. Rates of leukemia-free survival and overall survival were, however, generally favorable in the context of the patient groups being studied. More detailed subgroup analysis in several of the larger studies unsurprisingly demonstrated differing outcomes according to patient and disease characteristics: Hamaki et al[48] noted 1-year overall survival rates of 85% in low-risk and 64% in high-risk patients, while patients transplanted in first complete remission showed better rates of overall and leukemia-free survival than did those transplanted in later remissions or with evidence of residual disease.[49,50] It can be postulated that, for patients with more advanced disease, conditioning intensity remains important, with GvL effects alone being insufficient to overcome the inherently high relapse risk.

Comparisons of conventional myeloablative conditioning with RIC

Direct comparison between myeloablative and reduced-intensity conditioning strategies in AML using currently available data is difficult, as RIC has typically been used in patients not eligible for conventional allografting due to advanced age or co-morbidity. The European Blood and Marrow Transplantation (EBMT) group recently attempted a retrospective comparative analysis of 722 AML patients aged over 50.[51] Four hundred and seven had received conventional myeloablative conditioning (defined as 10 Gy or more of TBI or more than 8 mg/kg busulfan), while 315 had received RIC (fludarabine in combination with less than 3 Gy TBI or less than 8 mg/kg busulfan). The two cohorts were not statistically different in terms of karyotype, FAB group, presenting white cell count or disease status at the time of transplant. Rates of both acute and chronic GvHD were significantly higher in the myeloablative-treated patients. Non-relapse mortality was significantly lower in the RIC group (18% vs 32%, $p < 0.001$), but this was offset by a higher relapse rate (41% vs 24%, $p < 0.0001$). As a result, there was no significant difference in 2-year leukemia-free survival or overall survival between the two groups. Other smaller retrospective studies have reported broadly similar findings.[52,53] Improved long-term outcomes with reduced-intensity conditioning were reported, however, in a retrospective Japanese study comparing 70 RIC patients with 137 receiving myeloablative treatment.[54] Here, non-relapse mortality was again significantly lower in the RIC group (15% vs 31%, $p = 0.006$) but there was also superior 2-year leukemia-free and overall survival (56% vs 30% and 69% vs 39%, respectively).

RIC transplants in AML – current status and future directions

Despite a lack of prospective randomized controlled trial evidence, the use of RIC regimens in AML has grown exponentially in recent years. Long-term cure rates in AML patients over the age of 55 are no greater than 15% using chemotherapy alone, and this figure is significantly exceeded in the RIC literature to date, albeit in self-selected patient groups deemed fit for allogeneic procedures. Table 3.6 summarizes the potential benefits and drawbacks of the use of a reduced-intensity strategy in this context. The ad hoc way in which RIC

Table 3.5 Reduced-intensity conditioning hematopoietic stem cell transplantation in AML: summary of trials including at least 20 patients

Reference	No. patients AML/(total)	Median age (range)	Conditioning regimen	Donor type (related/ unrelated)	Graft failure	TRM/NRM	Acute GvHD (II–IV)/ chronic GvHD	Relapse	LFS/PFS	OS
Giralt et al 2001[59]	43 (86)	52 (22–70)	Flu/Mel or 2-CDA/Mel	46 / 40	n/a	37% (100-day)	49% / 68%	27%	23% (2-yr)	28% (2-yr)
Sayer et al 2003[46]	113	51 (16–67)	Flu/Cy/Bu or TBI (4–8 Gy)/Flu	51 / 62	5%	53% (2-yr)	42% / 33%	n/a	29% (2-yr)	32% (2-yr)
Hamaki et al 2004[48]	24 (36)	55 (27–67)	2-CDA or Flu/Bu ± ATG	24 / 0	3%	3% (100-day)	48% / 82%	22%	85% (1-yr) low-risk 64% (1-yr) high-risk	n/a
Ho et al 2004[60]	23 (62)	53 (22–70)	Flu/Bu/Campath	7 / 16	3%	15% (1-yr)	n/a	n/a	62% (1-yr)	74% (1-yr)
Gomez-Nunez et al 2004[61]	20 (145)	54 (19–67)	Flu/Mel or Flu/Bu	20 / 0	n/a	20% (1-yr)	34% / 41% (1-yr)	n/a	52% (1-yr)	60% (1-yr)
de Lima et al 2004[47]	68 (94)	54 (22–75) FM 61 (27–74) FAI	Flu/Mel (FM) or Flu/ AraC/Ida (FAI)	65 / 29	3% FM 19% FAI	26% (100-day) FM 13% (100-day) FAI	39% / 39% FM 25% /27% FAI	30% FM 61% FAI	32% (3-yr) FM 19% (3-yr) FAI	35% (3-yr) FM 30% (3-yr) FAI
Hallemeier et al 2004[49]	32	47 (32–60)	Cy/TBI (5.5 Gy)	29 / 3	0%	28%	3%[a] / 54%	22%	57% (3-yr) CR1 39% (3 yr) CR2+	55% (3-yr) CR1 39% (3 yr) CR2+
Aoudjhane et al 2005[51]	315	57 (50–73)	Flu/Bu or Flu/TBI (<3 Gy)	315 / 0	n/a	18% (1-yr)	22% / 48% (2-yr)	41%	40% (2-yr)	47% (2-yr)
Baron et al 2005[62]	46 (322)	54 (5–72)	TBI (2 Gy) ± Flu	192 / 130	7%	n/a	58% / 56%	34%	39% (3-yr)	50% (3-yr)
van Besien et al 2005[63]	41 (52)	52 (17–71)	Flu/Mel/Campath	27 / 25	4%	33% (2-yr)	33% / 18% (1-yr)	40% (2-yr)	31% (2-yr)	39% (2-yr)
Tauro et al 2005[64]	56 (76)	52 (18–71)	Flu/Mel/Campath	35 / 41	3%	19% (1-yr)	28% / 11%	36%	37% (3-yr)	41% (3-yr)
Schmid et al 2005[65]	75	52 (19–66)	Sequential Flu/AraC/ Amsa then Cy/TBI(4 Gy)/ATG	31 / 44	7%	33% (1-yr)	49% / 35%	17%	40% (2-yr)	42% (2-yr)
Claxton et al 2005[66]	23	59 (28–72)	Flu/Cy/Sirolimus ± ATG	6 / 17	0%	8%	43% / 77%	n/a	n/a	50% (2-yr)
Mohty et al 2005[67]	25 (35)	52 (26–55)	Flu/Bu/ATG	25 / 0	n/a	12%	n/a	12% (4-yr)	62% (4-yr)	n/a
Hegenbart et al 2006[50]	122	57 (17–74)	TBI (2 Gy) ± Flu	58 / 64	5%	16% (2-yr)	40% / 36%	39% (2-yr)	44% (2-yr)	48% (2-yr)
Platzbecker et al 2006[68]	26	49 (17–68)	Flu/Mel or Flu/Bu	11 / 15	n/a	15% (2-yr)	54% / 64%	11%	63% (3-yr)	63% (3-yr)
Scott et al 2006[52]	20 (38)	62 (40–72)	TBI (2 Gy) ± Flu	26 / 12	12%	39% (3-yr)	54% / 55% (2-yr)	31% (3-yr)	27% (3-yr)	28% (3-yr)
Shimoni et al 2006[69]	56 (67)	50 (17–70)	Flu/Bu (either FB2: Bu 6.4 mg/kg or FB4: Bu 12.8 mg/kg)	29 / 38	7% FB2 4% FB4	8% (2-yr) FB2 & FB4	8%[a]/ 31% FB2 8%[a]/ 59% FB4	49% FB2 43% FB4	43% (2-yr) FB2 49% (2-yr) FB4	47% (2-yr) FB2 49% (2-yr) FB4

Abbreviations: 2-CDA, cladribine; Amsa, amsacrine; AraC, cytosine arabinoside; ATG, antithymocyte globulin; Bu, busulfan; CR1, first complete remission; CR2+, second or subsequent complete remission; Cy, cyclophosphamide; Flu, fludarabine; GvHD, graft-versus-host disease; Gy, gray; Ida, idarubicin; LFS, leukemia-free survival; Mel, melphalan; n/a, not available; NRM, non-relapse mortality; OS, overall survival; PFS, progression-free survival; TBI, total body irradiation; TRM, transplant-related mortality; yr, year.
[a] Grade III–IV acute graft-versus-host disease.

approaches have been incorporated into clinical practice has spawned a great diversity of conditioning regimens, with little consensus on which patient subgroups are likely to benefit most from RIC transplantation. No AML-specific prospective trials comparing results of RIC and conventional myeloablative HSCT have yet been published although this situation appears set to be remedied by the major co-operative oncology groups. In order to best identify which transplant approach works best in different patient subpopulations, it is crucial that the design of future prospective trials takes into account a wide range of patient, donor and disease-specific variables.

A great deal of interest has focused on the development of more accurate co-morbidity scoring systems to help the clinician to tailor the choice of conditioning intensity to an individual patient. A Seattle group has recently modified the traditional Charlson Co-morbidity Index (CCI) by using detailed statistical analysis to determine which co-morbidities were most important in predicting non-relapse

Table 3.6 Potential advantages and disadvantages of a reduced-intensity conditioning strategy compared to conventional myeloablative conditioning in AML

Advantages of RIC
• Reduction in treatment-related mortality
• Reduction in peritransplant morbidity including mucositis, hepatic veno-occlusive disease and infection
• Shorter duration of neutropenia
• Reduced transfusion requirements
• Possible lower incidence of both acute and chronic GvHD
• Transplant may be performed wholly or partly in an outpatient setting
• Potential financial savings
• Extension of eligibility for allogeneic transplant to individuals previously excluded on the grounds of age and/or co-morbidity

Disadvantages of RIC
• Potentially increased rate of failed engraftment
• May be inappropriate in individuals with advanced or rapidly proliferating disease due to slower onset of graft-versus-leukemia effect
• Potential requirement of donor lymphocyte infusions for full engraftment
• Increased late relapse rate

mortality in HSCT patients.[55] The resulting 'Hematopoietic cell transplantation co-morbidity index' (HCT-CI) proved more sensitive in predicting survival and non-relapse mortality than the CCI. AML/myelodysplastic syndrome patients, for example, with a HCT-CI score of two or more who received non-myeloablative conditioning had a significantly lower non-relapse mortality (NRM) than similar patients who received conventional myeloablative conditioning.

A number of additional strategies to augment RIC transplant regimens without concomitantly increasing transplant-related mortality remain under investigation. Agents such as [131]I -labelled anti-CD45 monoclonal antibodies or the anti-CD33 monoclonal antibody conjugate Mylotarg have the potential of delivering targeted therapy, while sparing extrahematopoietic organs from toxicity.[56,57] Donor lymphocyte infusions (DLI) used in the context of disease relapse have proved less effective in AML than in chronic myeloid leukemia,[58] but the value and optimum scheduling of prophylactic DLI following RIC-HSCT in AML have not yet been fully established. Other strategies under investigation include antileukemic vaccinations and cytotoxic T-cell infusions.

In summary, RIC regimens provide a feasible, potentially curative option for AML patients who, due to age or co-morbidity, were previously considered ineligible for allogeneic HSCT. Limited studies to date have confirmed relatively low rates of transplant-related mortality with RIC, but at the expense of higher relapse rates. Ultimately, for patients in first complete remission there may be little or no advantage in using conventional myeloablative regimens. In advanced disease, however, conditioning intensity is likely to remain important in preventing relapse. Many questions remain to be answered in future prospective studies.

References

1. Lowenberg B, Downing JR, Burnett A. Acute myeloid leukemia. N Engl J Med 1999; 341:1051–1062
2. Goldstone AH, Burnett AK, Wheatley K et al. Attempts to improve treatment outcomes in acute myeloid leukemia (AML) in older patients: the results of the United Kingdom Medical Research Council AML11 trial. Blood 2001;98:1302–1311
3. Hiddemann W, Kern W, Schoch C et al. Management of acute myeloid leukemia in elderly patients. J Clin Oncol 1999;17:3569–3576
4. Clift RA, Buckner CD, Thomas ED et al. The treatment of acute non-lymphoblastic leukemia by allogeneic marrow transplantation. Bone Marrow Transplant 1987;2:243–258
5. Gale RP, Buchner T, Zhang MJ et al. HLA-identical sibling bone marrow transplants vs chemotherapy for acute myelogenous leukemia in first remission. Leukemia 1996;10:1687–1691
6. Hann IM, Stevens RF, Goldstone AH et al. Randomized comparison of DAT versus ADE as induction chemotherapy in children and younger adults with acute myeloid leukemia. Results of the Medical Research Council's 10th AML Trial (MRC AML 10). Blood 1997;89:2311–2318
7. Bishop JF, Lowenthal PM, Joshua D et al. Etoposide in acute non-lymphoblastic leukemia. Blood 1990;75:27–32
8. Berman E. Chemotherapy in acute myelogenous leukemia: higher dose, higher expectations? J Clin Oncol 1995;13:1–4
9. Grimwade D, Walker H, Oliver F et al. The importance of diagnostic cytogenetics on outcome in AML: analysis of 1,612 patients entered into the MRC AML: 10 Trial. Blood 1998;92:2322–2333
10. Slovak M, Kopecky K, Cassileth PA et al. Karyotypic analysis predicts outcome of prerR-emission and postremission therapy in adult acute myeloid leukemia: a Southwest Oncology Group/Eastern Cooperative Oncology Group Study. Blood 2000;96:4075–4083
11. Ferrant A, Doyen C, Delannoy A et al. Karyotype in acute myeloblastic leukemia: prognostic significance in a prospective study assessing bone marrow transplantation in first remission. Bone Marrow Transplant 1995;15:685–690
12. Soignet SL, Maslak P, Wang Z-G et al. Complete remission after treatment of acute promyelocytic leukemia with arsenic trioxide. N Engl J Med 1998;339:1341–1348
13. Petti MC, Pinazzi MB, Diverio D et al. Prolonged molecular remission in advanced acute promyelocytic leukemia after treatment with gemtuzumab ozogamicin (Mylotarg CMA-676). Br J Haematol 2001;115:63–65
14. Meloni G, Diverio D, Vignetti M et al. Autologous bone marrow transplantation for acute promyelocytic leukemia in second remission: prognostic relevance of pretransplant minimal residual disease assessment by reverse-transcription polymerase chain reaction of the PML/RARa fusion gene. Blood 1997;90:1321–1325
15. Paschka P, Marcucci G, Ruppert AS et al. Adverse prognostic significance of KIT mutations in adult acute myeloid leukemia with inv(16) and t(8;21): a Cancer and Leukemia Group B Study. J Clin Oncol 2006;24:3904–3911
16. Wheatley K, Burnett AK, Goldstone AH et al. A simple, robust, validated and highly predictive index for the determination of risk-directed therapy in acute myeloid leukemia derived from the MRC AML 10 trial. United Kingdom Medical Research Council's Adult and Childhood Leukemia Working Parties. Br J Haematol 1999;107:69–79
17. Bowen DT, Frew ME, Hills R et al. RAS mutation in acute myeloid leukemia is associated with distinct cytogenetic subgroups but does not influence outcome in patients younger than 60 years. Blood 2005;106:2113–2119
18. Nakao M, Yokota S, Iwai T et al. Internal tandem duplication of the flt3 gene found in acute myeloid leukemia. Leukemia 1996;10:1911–1918
19. Kottaridis PD, Gale RE, Frew ME et al. The presence of a Flt3 mutation in AML adds important prognostic information to cytogenetic risk group and response to the first cycle of chemotherapy: analysis of 854 patients from the MRC AML10 and 12 Trials. Blood 2000;96:825a
20. Meshinchi S, Woods WG, Stirewalt DL et al. Prevalence and prognostic significance of Flt3 internal tandem duplication in pediatric acute myeloid leukemia. Blood 2001; 97:89–94
21. Levis M, Small D. FLT3. ITD does matter in leukemia. Leukemia 2003;17:1738–1752
22. Dohner K, Schlenk RF, Habdank M et al. Mutant nucleophosmin (NPM1) predicts favorable prognosis in younger adults with acute myeloid leukemia and normal cytogenetics: interaction with other gene mutations. Blood 2005;106:3740–3746
23. Verhaak RGW, Goudswaard CS, van Putten W. Mutations in nucleophosmin NPM1 in acute myeloid leukemia (AML): association with other genetic abnormalities and previously established gene expression signatures and their favorable prognostic significance. Blood 2005;106:3747–3754
24. Thiede C, Koch S, Creutzig E et al. Prevalence and prognostic impact of NPM1 mutations in 1485 adult patients with acute myeloid leukemia (AML). Blood 2006;107:4011–4020
25. Liang DC, Shih LY, Huang CF et al. CEBPalpha mutations in childhood acute myeloid leukemia. Leukemia 2005;19:410–414
26. Breems DA, van Putten WL, Huijgens PC et al. Prognostic index for adult patients with acute myeloid leukemia in first relapse. J Clin Oncol 2005;23:1969–1978
27. Gray R, Wheatley K. How to avoid bias when comparing bone marrow transplantation with chemotherapy. Bone Marrow Transplant 1991;7(suppl 3):9–12
28. Burnett AK, Wheatley K, Goldstone AH et al. The value of allogeneic bone marrow transplant in patients with acute myeloid leukemia at differing risk of relapse: results of the UK MRC AML 10 trial. Br J Haematol 2002;118:385–400
29. Zittoun RA, Mandelli F, Willemze R et al. Autologous or allogeneic bone marrow transplantation compared with intensive chemotherapy in acute myelogenous leukemia. European Organization for Research and Treatment of Cancer (EORTC) and the Gruppo Italiano Malattie Ematologiche Maligne dell'Adulto (GIMEMA) Leukemia Cooperative Groups. N Engl J Med 1995;332:217–223
30. Harousseau JL, Cahn JY, Pignon B et al. Comparison of autologous bone marrow transplantation and intensive chemotherapy as postremission therapy in adult acute myeloid leukemia. Blood 1997;90:2978–2986
31. Cassileth PA, Harrington DP, Appelbaum F et al. Chemotherapy compared with autologous or allogeneic bone marrow transplantation in the management of acute myeloid leukemia in first remission. N Engl J Med 1998;339:1649–1656
32. Burnett AK, Wheatley K, Goldstone AH et al. MRC AML12: a comparison of ADE vs MAE and S-DAT vs H-DAT + retinoic acid for induction and four vs five total courses using chemotherapy or stem cell transplant in consolidation in 3459 patients under 60 years with AML. Blood 2002;100:155a
33. Watson M, Buck G, Wheatley K et al. Adverse impact of bone marrow transplantation on quality of life in acute myeloid leukemia patients: analysis of the UK Medical Research Council AML10 Trial. Eur J Cancer 2004;40:971–978
34. Zittoun R, Suciu, S, Watson M et al. Quality of life in patients with acute myelogenous leukemia in prolonged first complete remission after bone marrow transplantation

(allogeneic or autologous) or chemotherapy: a cross-sectional study of the EORTC-GIEMEMA AML 8A trial. Bone Marrow Transplant 1997;20:307–315

35. Frassoni F. Commentary and randomised studies in acute myeloid leukemia: the double truth. Bone Marrow Transplant 2000;25:471–473

36. Cornelissen JJ, van Putten WL, Verdonck LF et al. Myeloablative HLA-identical sibling stem cell transplantation in first remission acute myeloid leukemia in young and middle aged adults: benefits for whom? Results of a HOVON/SAKK donor versus no donor analysis. Blood 2007;109(9):3658–3666

37. Hills RK, Kell WJ, Burnett AK. Treatment of AML in the elderly: who is 'fit' for intensive chemotherapy? Blood 2006;108:559a

38. Gale RP, Hills R, Kottaridis PD et al. No evidence that FLT3 status should be considered as an indicator for transplantation in acute myeloid leukemia (AML): an analysis of 1135 patients, excluding acute promyelocytic leukemia, from the UK MRC AML10 and 12 trials. Blood 2005;106:3658–3665

39. Burnett AK, Hills R, Goldstone AH et al. The impact of transplant in AML in 2nd CR: a prospective study of 741 in the MRC AML10 and 12 trials. Blood 2004;104:179a

40. Burnett AK, Kell WJ, Goldstone AH et al. The addition of gemtuzumab ozogamicin to induction chemotherapy for AML improves disease free survival without extra toxicity: preliminary analysis of 1115 patients in the MRC AML15 trial. Blood 2006;108:8a

41. Wadleigh M, Richardson PG, Zahrieh D et al. Prior gemtuzamab ozogamicin exposure significantly increases the risk of veno-occlusive disease in patients who undergo myeloablative allogeneic stem cell transplantation. Blood 2003;102:1578–1582

42. Storb R, Yu C, Wagner JL et al. Stable mixed hematopoietic chimerism in DLA-identical littermate dogs given sublethal total body irradiation before and pharmacological immunosuppression after marrow transplantation. Blood 1997;89:3048–3054

43. Bacigalupo A. Second EBMT workshop on reduced intensity allogeneic hemopoietic stem cell transplants (RI-HSCT). Bone Marrow Transplant 2002;29:191–195

44. Storb R. Nonmyeloablative preparative regimens: how relevant for acute myelogenous leukemia? Leukemia 2001;15:662–663

45. Gratwohl A, Baldomero H, Passweg J, Urbano-Ispizua A. Increasing use of reduced intensity conditioning transplants: report of the 2001 EBMT activity survey. Bone Marrow Transplant 2002;30:813–831

46. Sayer HG, Kroger M, Beyer J et al. Reduced intensity conditioning for allogeneic hematopoietic stem cell transplantation in patients with acute myeloid leukemia: disease status by marrow blasts is the strongest prognostic factor. Bone Marrow Transplant 2003;31:1089–1095

47. de Lima M, Anagnostopoulos A, Munsell M et al. Nonablative versus reduced-intensity conditioning regimens in the treatment of acute myeloid leukemia and high-risk myelodysplastic syndrome: dose is relevant for long-term disease control after allogeneic hematopoietic stem cell transplantation. Blood 2004;104:865–872

48. Hamaki T, Kami M, Kim SW et al. Reduced-intensity stem cell transplantation from an HLA-identical sibling donor in patients with myeloid malignancies. Bone Marrow Transplant 2004;33:891–900

49. Hallemeier C, Girgis M, Blum W et al. Outcomes of adults with acute myelogenous leukemia in remission given 550 cGy of single-exposure total body irradiation, cyclophosphamide, and unrelated donor bone marrow transplants. Biol Blood Marrow Transplant 2004;10:310–319

50. Hegenbart U, Niederwieser D, Sandmaier BM et al. Treatment for acute myelogenous leukemia by low-dose, total-body, irradiation-based conditioning and hematopoietic cell transplantation from related and unrelated donors. J Clin Oncol 2006;24:444–453

51. Aoudjhane M, Labopin M, Gorin NC et al. Comparative outcome of reduced intensity and myeloablative conditioning regimen in HLA identical sibling allogeneic haematopoietic stem cell transplantation for patients older than 50 years of age with acute myeloblastic leukemia: a retrospective survey from the Acute Leukemia Working Party (ALWP) of the European Group for Blood and Marrow Transplantation (EBMT). Leukemia 2005;19:2304–2312

52. Scott BL, Sandmaier BM, Storer B et al. Myeloablative vs nonmyeloablative allogeneic transplantation for patients with myelodysplastic syndrome or acute myelogenous leukemia with multilineage dysplasia: a retrospective analysis. Leukemia 2006;20:128–135

53. Alyea EP, Kim HT, Ho V et al. Comparative outcome of nonmyeloablative and myeloablative allogeneic hematopoietic cell transplantation for patients older than 50 years of age. Blood 2005;105:1810–1814

54. Kojima R, Kami M, Kanda Y et al. Comparison between reduced intensity and conventional myeloablative allogeneic stem-cell transplantation in patients aged between 50 and 59 years. Bone Marrow Transplant 2005;36:667–674

55. Sorror ML, Maris MB, Storb R et al. Hematopoietic cell transplantation (HCT)-specific comorbidity index: a new tool for risk assessment before allogeneic HCT. Blood 2005;106:2912–2919

56. Pagel JM, Appelbaum FR, Sandmaier BM. 131I-anti-CD45 antibody plus fludarabine, low-dose total body irradiation and peripheral blood stem cell infusion for elderly patients with advanced acute myeloid leukemia (AML) or high-risk myelodysplastic syndrome (MDS). Blood 2005;106:119

57. Roman E, Cooney E, Harrison L et al. Preliminary results of the safety of immunotherapy with gemtuzumab ozogamicin following reduced intensity allogeneic stem cell transplant in children with CD33+ acute myeloid leukemia. Clin Cancer Res 2005;11:7164s–7170s

58. Collins RH Jr, Shpilberg O, Drobyski WR et al. Donor leukocyte infusions in 140 patients with relapsed malignancy after allogeneic bone marrow transplantation. J Clin Oncol 1997;15:433–444

59. Giralt S, Thall PF, Khouri I et al. Melphalan and purine analog-containing preparative regimens: reduced-intensity conditioning for patients with hematologic malignancies undergoing allogeneic progenitor cell transplantation. Blood 2001;97:631–637

60. Ho AY, Pagliuca A, Kenyon M et al. Reduced-intensity allogeneic hematopoietic stem cell transplantation for myelodysplastic syndrome and acute myeloid leukemia with multilineage dysplasia using fludarabine, busulphan, and alemtuzumab (FBC) conditioning. Blood 2004;104:1616–1623

61. Gomez-Nunez M, Martino R, Caballero MD et al. Elderly age and prior autologous transplantation have a deleterious effect on survival following allogeneic peripheral blood stem cell transplantation with reduced-intensity conditioning: results from the Spanish multicenter prospective trial. Bone Marrow Transplant 2004;33:477–482

62. Baron F, Maris, MB, Sandmaier BM et al. Graft-versus-tumor effects after allogeneic hematopoietic cell transplantation with nonmyeloablative conditioning. J Clin Oncol 2005;23:1993–2003

63. van Besien K, Artz A, Smith S et al. Fludarabine, melphalan, and alemtuzumab conditioning in adults with standard-risk advanced acute myeloid leukemia and myelodysplastic syndrome. J Clin Oncol 2005;23:5728–5738

64. Tauro S, Craddock C, Peggs K et al. Allogeneic stem-cell transplantation using a reduced-intensity conditioning regimen has the capacity to produce durable remissions and long-term disease-free survival in patients with high-risk acute myeloid leukemia and myelodysplasia. J Clin Oncol 2005;23:9387–9393

65. Schmid C, Schleuning M, Ledderose G et al. Sequential regimen of chemotherapy, reduced-intensity conditioning for allogeneic stem-cell transplantation, and prophylactic donor lymphocyte transfusion in high-risk acute myeloid leukemia and myelodysplastic syndrome. J Clin Oncol 2005;23:5675–5687

66. Claxton DF, Ehmann C, Rybka W. Control of advanced and refractory acute myelogenous leukemia with sirolimus-based non-myeloablative allogeneic stem cell transplantation. Br J Haematol 2005;130:256–264

67. Mohty M, de Lavallade H, Ladaique P et al. The role of reduced intensity conditioning allogeneic stem cell transplantation in patients with acute myeloid leukemia: a donor vs no donor comparison. Leukemia 2005;19:916–920

68. Platzbecker U, Thiede C, Fussel M et al. Reduced intensity conditioning allows for up-front allogeneic hematopoietic stem cell transplantation after cytoreductive induction therapy in newly-diagnosed high-risk acute myeloid leukemia. Leukemia 2006;20:707–714

69. Shimoni A, Hardan I, Shem-Tov N et al. Allogeneic hematopoietic stem-cell transplantation in AML and MDS using myeloablative versus reduced-intensity conditioning: the role of dose intensity. Leukemia 2006;20:322–328

Chronic myeloid leukemia

John M Goldman and Tariq I Mughal

Introduction

Chronic myeloid leukemia (CML) is a rare leukemia in which the initiating event appears to be the acquisition at the level of a hematopoietic stem cell of a *BCR-ABL* fusion gene usually associated with a Ph chromosome (designated 22q-). This leads to gradual expansion of the Ph-positive clone at the expense of Ph-negative (presumably normal) hematopoiesis. Multiple lines of evidence suggest that at the time of diagnosis residual Ph-negative stem cells survive, probably in normal number, in a 'quiescent' or 'deep G_0 state', but they can be resuscitated if the Ph-positive population can be selectively inhibited.[1]

Principal landmarks in our understanding of the biology of CML were the discovery of the Ph chromosome in 1960, the demonstration in 1973 that it was associated with a reciprocal translocation involving chromosomes 9 and 22, the discovery in 1984 of the breakpoint cluster region (BCR) on chromosome 22q, the characterization in 1986 of the *BCR-ABL* fusion mRNA and the demonstration in 1990 that the human disease could be simulated in a murine model system by retroviral-mediated transfer of the *BCR-ABL* gene into murine hematopoietic stem cells.[2]

Although the treatment algorithm for newly diagnosed patients with CML in chronic phase (CP) has changed substantially over the past decade, at present allogeneic stem cell transplantation (SCT) remains the only proven therapy which offers the possibility of long-term remission and probably of cure in most long-term survivors. Table 4.1 summarizes the history of CML treatment. This was revolutionized in 1998 by the introduction of imatinib mesylate (IM), the original tyrosine kinase inhibitor (TKI), and a variety of other TKIs have entered clinical practice since that time. IM substantially reduces the number of CML cells and probably confers a survival benefit in most, if not all subjects. The incidence of complete molecular response is initially low, but increases with time in patients who respond well[3] (see Fig. 4.2). However, most patients do relapse sooner or later if the drug is discontinued, which makes it probable that leukemia stem cells persist in the body in most, if not all patients. Despite this conclusion, IM has displaced allo-SCT as a first-line treatment for the newly diagnosed patient. However, allogeneic SCT retains an important role for patients who fail IM, or who fail IM and also a second-generation TKI.[4] In this chapter we discuss some aspects of the changing treatment paradigm and assess the current and future role of allo-SCT in the 'era of tyrosine kinase inhibitors'.

Cytogenetics and molecular biology

The defining feature for CML is today the identification of a *BCR-ABL* fusion gene which is usually, but not always, located on the Ph chromosome. A small percentage of patients have a *BCR-ABL* fusion gene on an apparently normal chromosome 22, and are designated Ph-negative, *BCR-ABL*-positive CML. Their clinical course and response to IM seem to be indistinguishable from those of patients with Ph-positive disease. The *BCR-ABL* gene expresses a *BCR-ABL* transcript which can be readily detected in the blood and marrow of untreated patients with a reverse transcriptase PCR, and an oncoprotein of MW 210 kD, usually designated p210(Bcr-Abl). The acquisition of a *BCR-ABL* fusion gene is thought to be the first step in the pathogenesis of CML, but how exactly the oncoprotein, which is restricted to the leukemia cell cytoplasm, transmits a leukemogenic signal to the nucleus remains an enigma. The presence of the *BCR-ABL* fusion gene and its product seems to increase the susceptibility of the leukemia clone to acquisition of further genetic change, a status known as genomic instability.[5,6]

Natural history and prognosis

It is generally believed that the initial lesion in CML occurs some years before the disease is diagnosed. In the past, patients frequently presented with various symptoms attributable to a greatly expanded myeloid mass, namely enlarged spleens, high leukocyte counts and anemia, and this constellation of features is still often seen in developing countries. In more developed countries, however, the diagnosis is made with increasing frequency, perhaps greater than 60%, in patients who are entirely asymptomatic. Before the introduction of IM, the disease characteristically presented in chronic phase and then proceeded inexorably to an advanced phase. Progression to advanced phase involved either progression first to an accelerated phase followed by blastic transformation, or direct progression from chronic phase to blastic transformation. Median survival from diagnosis was 5–6 years but with a wide range. The median survival for patients treated with IM, and perhaps other TKIs, is likely to be very much longer than that achievable with older non-transplant treatments. Indeed, comparison of survival of IM-treated patients with survival of patients treated in an earlier period with interferon-alfa or interferon-containing regimens supports the conclusion that IM prolongs overall survival substantially.[7,8]

Many attempts have been made to predict duration of survival based on factors ascertainable at the time of diagnosis. Sokal and colleagues performed multivariate statistical studies on 813 patients treated predominantly with busulfan or hydroxycarbamide (hydroxyurea) and derived four factors, namely age, spleen size, percentage of circulating blasts and platelet count, from which a hazard ratio could be derived that predicted survival with reasonable precision.[9] Subsequently, Hasford and colleagues studied patients treated predominantly with

Table 4.1 Time of introduction of new therapeutic strategies for CML

19th century	Arsenic
Early 20th century	Radiation therapy
1960s	Busulfan
1970s	Hydroxycarbamide (hydroxyurea)
1980s	Interferon-alfa Allogeneic stem cell transplantation
1990s	Reduced-intensity conditioning transplants
1998	Imatinib mesylate

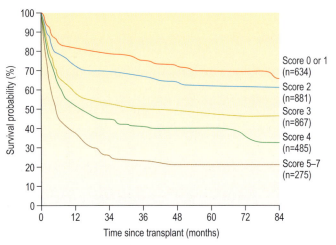

Figure 4.1
Probability of survival according to the prognostic score developed by Gratwohl et al[12] for the European Group for Blood and Marrow Transplantation (EBMT).

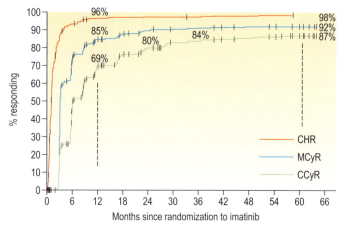

Figure 4.2
Cumulative best responses for patients with CML in CP randomized to receive imatinib as primary therapy for newly diagnosed chronic phase CML in the IRIS study.[3] CHR, complete hematologic response; MCyR, major cytogenetic response; CCyR, complete cytogenetic response.

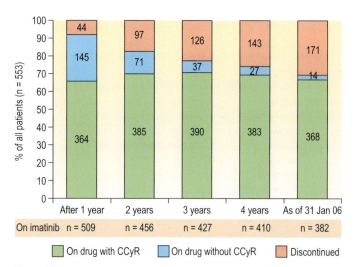

Figure 4.3
Rates of complete cytogenetic response at different time-points in patients who received imatinib mesylate as primary treatment for CML in chronic phase. (Data from Novartis Pharmaceuticals, unpublished data reproduced with permission.)

interferon-alfa and derived a similar prognostic score based on the same features as identified by Sokal et al but with the addition of basophil and eosinophil counts.[10] Interestingly, the Sokal score is valid in predicting response to IM, which suggests that it is an indirect measure of the 'aggressiveness' of the disease, independent of the point at which the disease is diagnosed.[11]

Gratwohl and colleagues made a very important contribution to our understanding of the factors that predict for outcome after allogeneic SCT, based on outcome for 3142 patients with CML transplanted between 1984 and 1994 whose clinical data were entered into the European Group for Blood and Marrow Transplantation (EBMT) database[12] (Fig. 4.1). They developed a scoring system that takes account of (a) patient age, (b) donor type, (c) disease phase, (d) duration of disease from diagnosis, and (e) gender of donor for male recipients. On this basis, patients with low scores, i.e. 0 or 1, had a much better 5-year survival than did those with high scores (6 or 7). The validity of this scoring system has been confirmed in another allo-SCT data set.[13]

Non-transplant options

In the 1990s, the standard treatment for patients with CML presenting in CP who were not eligible for allogeneic SCT was interferon-alfa or the combination of interferon plus cytarabine.[14,15] Survival was prolonged modestly in comparison with earlier therapies, usually busulfan or hydroxycarbamide.[16] Soon after IM became available, a prospective study was begun that compared IM with the combination of interferon and cytarabine for newly diagnosed patients with CP disease. The 5-year update for the patients treated with IM as primary

therapy has been published recently.[3] The cumulative best hematologic response was 98%, and the cumulative best cytogenetic response was 87% (Fig. 4.2). These values do not take into account patients who achieved but subsequently lost their response. It appears, however, that about 67% of newly diagnosed patients were still taking IM and in complete cytogenetic response at 5 years, with evidence that for responders the annual risk of progression was declining with each year on IM (Fig. 4.3). For patients who become resistant to IM, the newer TKIs, dasatinib and nilotinib, clearly have some value and indeed, one of them could replace IM as first-line therapy in the future.[17,18] Based on these data, most adults who present with CML in CP are now offered IM rather than allo-SCT as primary therapy (see below).

Transplant methodology

A number of variables that operate at the time of transplant may influence the chance of success. These include, among others, choice of donor, source of the cells used for transplantation, details of the conditioning employed, and the methods employed to minimize graft-versus-host disease (GvHD).

In the 1980s, transplants for CML were carried out predominantly with bone marrow-derived stem cells collected from HLA-identical siblings. More recently, considerable experience has been gained with transplants using stem cells obtained from unrelated donors, but the degree to which the patients and donors were HLA matched has varied quite considerably.

Type of donor

The original success of transplantation for patients with CML in chronic phase involved the use of stem cells harvested from the patient's identical twin. In 1979, the Seattle transplant group was able to report results of four patients with CML (three in CP and one in advanced phase) who were treated with SCT from a genotypically identical twin donor. All four patients received a conditioning regimen consisting of cyclophosphamide and total-body irradiation (TBI). Following the transplant, the patients had continuing Ph-negative hematopoiesis for 22, 23, 26 and 31 months, respectively.[19] Other transplant teams then performed transplants for patients with genetically HLA-identical siblings,[20,21] and thereafter transplants were performed with marrow collected from volunteer donors whose HLA type matched that of the recipient as well as could be established with contemporary tissue typing techniques.[22,23] A small number of transplants have also been performed with cord blood stem cells.

Stem cell sources

Throughout the 1980s, the only source of stem cells for allogeneic transplants was bone marrow. In the early 1990s it became clear that donors pretreated with hematopoietic growth factors, notably granulocyte colony-stimulating factor (G-CSF), could mobilize large numbers of CD34+ cells and simultaneously large numbers of T-lymphocytes into the peripheral blood. For a time peripheral blood was the preferred source of stem cells in many transplant centers, despite an increased risk in grade 3–4 acute and chronic GvHD. This was based on the notion of peripheral blood stem cells being associated with faster engraftment and improved progression-free survival and a reduction in the relapse risk of patients with advanced disease.[24,25] However, long-term follow-up suggests that results for patients with CML in first CP are significantly better with marrow-derived stem cells; in contrast, the results obtained for patients in the more advanced phases of CML continue to be better with peripheral blood-derived stem cells[26] (Fig. 4.4).

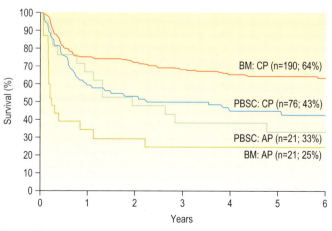

Figure 4.4
Survival after allogeneic SCT performed with peripheral blood or bone marrow stem cells for patients with CML in chronic phase or accelerated phase. BM, bone marrow; PBSC, peripheral blood stem cells; CP, chronic phase; AP, accelerated phase. (Data from the Center for International Blood and Marrow Transplant Research, reproduced with permission.)

Conditioning regimens

Early experience with allo-SCT for CML was based largely on the use of high-dose cyclophosphamide followed by 'supralethal' doses of TBI which was designed to eradicate all leukemia cells. The cyclophosphamide was usually administered at a dose of 60 mg/kg on two consecutive days and the TBI was given as a single dose, often 1000 cGy, or in 200 cGy fractions.[20,21,27,28] The combination of cyclophosphamide and busulfan without TBI was used in some centers and gave broadly comparable results.[29] The introduction of dose-adjusted busulfan appeared to reduce the toxicity of the two-drug combination.[30]

Reduced-intensity conditioning (RIC) regimens

The gradual recognition that disease eradication depended as much, or even more, on the graft-versus-leukemia (GvL) effect mediated by the T-lymphocytes in the donor inoculum as on the chemoradiotherapy preceding the transplant led to the concept of a reduced-intensity conditioning (RIC) allogeneic SCT, also referred to as reduced-intensity transplants, non-myeloablative transplants or mini-transplants.[31,32] In general, it was proposed that the conditioning protocol should emphasize immunosuppression and reduce the intensity of myelosuppression, with the objective of maximizing the GvL effect. For this purpose, most regimens incorporated fludarabine, but in other respects there has been great heterogeneity. One multicenter study has used fludarabine in conjunction with low-dose TBI (i.e. 200 cGy × 1). Table 4.2 lists some of the agents used in reduced-intensity conditioning regimens for transplantation in CML.

T-cell depletion

In the 1980s, studies with experimental animals provided preclinical support for the notion that removal of T-cells from the harvested marrow might abrogate GvHD, and clinical studies showed that this was indeed the case. Thus, treating donor marrow ex vivo with monoclonal antibodies such as OKT3 (anti T-cell) or Campath (CD52, antilymphoid, now termed alemtuzumab)[27] or mechanical removal of T-cell by elutriation was highly effective at minimizing or totally abrogating acute and chronic GvHD but was associated with delayed immune reconstitution, increased risk of infection and also a substantially increased risk of relapse.

Graft-versus-leukemia and principles of donor lymphocyte infusions (DLI)

Although it was widely accepted in the 1980s that patients who developed GvHD had a lower risk of leukemia relapse than those without GvHD, the concept that a GvL effect played a major role in the eradication of CML was most strongly supported by the observation that T-cell depletion greatly increased the risk of relapse[27] and that

Table 4.2 Some chemotherapy and chemoradiotherapy regimens used in reduced-intensity conditioning transplantation for CML

Fludarabine and low-dose total-body irradiation
Fludarabine and busulfan
Fludarabine and melphalan
Fludarabine, melphalan and cyclophosphamide
Fludarabine, cyclophosphamide and other
Cyclophosphamide and thiotepa

From Crawley et al.[46]

recipients of syngeneic marrow had a higher risk of relapse than did recipients of allogeneic cells.[33] The importance of a GvL effect was even more convincingly demonstrated in 1989 by the report from Munich that three patients who relapsed after allografting for CML in chronic phase were restored to complete remission by infusion of leukocytes collected from their respective transplant donors.[34] In fact, these patients also received interferon-alfa but subsequent studies showed that the interferon played no role in induction of the remissions.[35] In 1995, the transplant group at the Sloan Kettering Cancer Center in New York showed that the side-effects engendered by these donor lymphocyte infusions, mainly GvHD and the induction of marrow hypoplasia, could largely be prevented by giving donor lymphocytes on an escalating dosage schedule starting with relatively low cell numbers and increasing subsequent doses in the absence of a discernible response.[36]

Autografting

The notion that stem cells could be collected from a patient's bone marrow at diagnosis, cryopreserved and stored in liquid nitrogen for some years and then used as part of a regimen for treating CML in blastic transformation was developed in the 1970s. In the late 1970s it was shown that marrow-regenerating stem cells were also present in large numbers in the peripheral blood of new CML patients before treatment.[37] Marrow function could indeed be restored with cells from either source in patients who received high doses of chemotherapy for blastic transformation, but the ensuing 'second' chronic phases were usually short, and survival was not greatly prolonged. Subsequent studies suggested that some patients treated with chemotherapy and autografting in chronic phase could achieve durable Ph-negative hematopoiesis.[38] However, autografting has largely fallen from favor since the introduction of tyrosine kinase inhibitors,[16] although it could theoretically prove useful in the management of patients resistant to TKIs.

Outcome after allogeneic stem cell transplantation

Outcome after conventionally conditioned transplantation according to disease phase

The most important determinants of success or failure of allogeneic SCT for CML are patient age and disease phase when the transplant is carried out. Thus, in general most transplant units operate with an upper age limit of 50 years, or thereabouts, for patients who are otherwise eligible for conventionally conditioned transplantation. For the younger patient who undergoes an allogeneic SCT in chronic phase, the probability of survival at 5 years is around 80%, although if one groups together patients of all ages, usually with the upper age limit as mentioned above, the figure is nearer 70%. Single centers have reported better results[39] (Fig. 4.5). If GvHD prophylaxis comprises methotrexate and ciclosporin, the relapse incidence within 3 years is of the order of 20%. GvHD prophylaxis based on T-cell depletion is associated with a higher incidence of relapse.

Patients in chronic phase who receive a transplant from a 'matched' unrelated donor have a 5-year survival of around 60%. These patient groups may not be strictly comparable with patients who receive a sibling donor transplant because some units operate with a lower age limit for patients receiving unrelated donor transplants. Moreover, the degree of HLA matching is undoubtedly different in different series.

Patients transplanted in advanced-phase disease with a sibling or matched unrelated donor have much lower survivals than do those transplanted in chronic phase. The 5-year survival for patients trans-

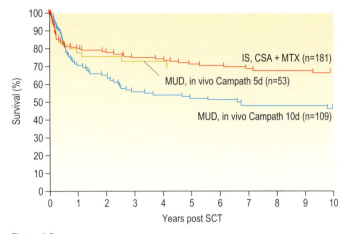

Figure 4.5
Survival after conventional allogeneic SCT for CML in chronic phase at a single center (Hammersmith Hospital, London, UK). IS, HLA-identical sibling donor; MUD, matched unrelated donor; CSA, ciclosporin; MTX, methotrexate.

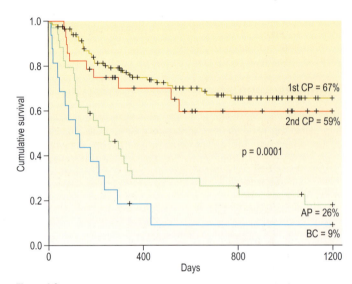

Figure 4.6
Survival after reduced-intensity conditioning transplants for CML in first chronic phase (1st CP), second chronic phase after treatment for advanced phase (2nd CP), accelerated phase (AP) or blastic crisis (BC). (Data reproduced from Crawley et al.[46])

planted in accelerated phase is of the order of 35%, and survival for patients transplanted in blastic transformation is in the range of 5–10%.

In general, patients who survive 5 years without evidence of relapse have an extremely low risk of relapse at a later date. Occasional patients do relapse even after allogeneic SCT in chronic phase, and the latest reported relapse has occurred at 18 years after transplantation for CML in chronic phase.[40,41]

Reduced-intensity conditioned transplants

The results of transplants using reduced-intensity conditioning are difficult to interpret, partly because no controlled clinical studies comparing conventional and RIC transplant have been undertaken.[42–45] Indeed, to date in most reported series, patients undergoing RIC transplantation have often been older than those receiving conventional transplants, and some have had concomitant diseases that would have rendered them ineligible for conventional transplantation. As with full-intensity conditioned transplants, survival again appears to relate to disease phase at the time of transplantation (Fig. 4.6) It does, however, seem that the 100-day mortality attributable to a RIC transplant is substantially lower, and in some series zero, compared to a conventional transplant.

Moreover, the variation in conditioning regimens has been very extensive, in terms of the intensity of both myelosuppression and immunosuppression, and currently there is no consensus as to what constitutes a RIC transplant.[46] This makes a comparative analysis difficult. With this caveat, early comparison of the various studies in patients with CML suggested that the disease-free and overall survivals obtained following RIC SCT were similar compared to conventional SCT.[12] GvHD is, however, no less severe than after a conventional transplant, and this has led some groups to undertake RIC transplants preceded by treatment with intravenous antibodies (for example, alemtuzumab or antithymocyte globulin) designed to achieve some level of donor T-cell depletion. This, is turn, is associated with a high level of persisting or relapsing leukemia that has necessitated the use of DLI.

Monitoring and relapse

The majority of patients who receive conventionally conditioned allogeneic SCT for CML have Ph-positive metaphases demonstrable in their bone marrow for some months after the procedure, and it has become conventional, therefore, to delay monitoring until 6 months after the procedure. In the 1980s, patients were monitored primarily with bone marrow cytogenetics but the introduction of techniques for identifying BCR-ABL transcripts in the peripheral blood[47] and subsequently the capacity to quantitate such transcripts have largely replaced the use of bone marrow cytogenetics. In most patients *BCR-ABL* transcripts have become undetectable by 1 year post transplant,[48] and in many cases they are never again detected during the duration of follow-up. In other cases, BCR-ABL transcripts may be detected intermittently at a low level. The Hammersmith transplant group has proposed criteria for defining molecular relapse, namely the finding of transcripts in excess of 0.02% on three consecutive studies, or transcripts in excess of 0.05% on two consecutive studies.[41] The clinical value of this proposal has not yet been confirmed by others. Above these relatively low levels, a rising number of *BCR-ABL* transcripts is usually an indication that without therapeutic intervention the patient will sooner or later proceed to cytogenetic, and eventually to hematologic, relapse.

Management of relapse

Because of variation in methodology for monitoring patients in different centers, relapse has, in practice, been diagnosed at different levels. It was conventional in the 1980s to offer patients in relapse a second allogeneic SCT, usually from the same donor as was used originally, but the results of second transplants were generally poor. After the 1990s, most patients in relapse were treated with donor lymphocyte infusions (DLI). Patients who received DLI for treatment of molecular relapse had an 80–90% response rate, whereas patients treated in hematologic relapse had a lower response rate.[49] The principal complications associated with single dose or 'bulk dose' DLI were the occurrence of GvHD or the occasional induction of bone marrow hypoplasia.[50] With the introduction of escalating dose DLI, GvHD may still occur but its incidence is very greatly reduced.[36] Once a patient who received DLI has achieved molecular remission, such second remissions may be very durable and may exceed the duration of the first remission in length. This suggests that DLI may, on occasion, effect the cure that did not occur after the original transplant. Patients who relapse after allogeneic SCT for CML in advanced phase respond less well to DLI than do those whose disease relapses as CP. Nonetheless, some patients transplanted in accelerated phase have derived benefit from DLI.

In the last 8 years, a number of patients who relapse have been treated with IM.[51] This agent is highly effective at restoring molecular negativity, but discontinuation of IM has frequently been associated with recurrent disease at the molecular or cytogenetic levels. Others have used interferon-alfa to treat relapse after allogeneic SCT in chronic phase. It is likely that combining a tyrosine kinase inhibitor with DLI could be the most effective therapy.

Decisions and algorithms for 2008

Until the year 1999 it was standard practice to recommend allo-SCT to all patients with newly diagnosed CML in CP provided they had a suitable HLA-identical sibling or 'matched' unrelated donor and provided they were relatively young (less than 50 years of age). Patients presenting with advanced-phase disease usually received some form of combination chemotherapy and allo-SCT if a 'second' CP could be achieved. When it became apparent that IM could induce complete cytogenetic remission in a high proportion of patients presenting in chronic phase, the recommended practice changed.[52]

Many investigators proposed that the majority of new patients should be treated initially with IM at 400 mg/daily, with the possible exception of the few patients who may be eligible to receive an allo-SCT. With 5 years of follow-up for patients who received IM as primary therapy for newly diagnosed CP disease, it has now become standard practice to initiate therapy with IM for all adults with newly diagnosed CML in CP.

Clearly, the notion of considering an allo-SCT for patients irrespective of response to IM would require a randomized study which would not be practical. Efforts have therefore focused on the identification of individual patients for whom the anticipated results of SCT are such that it might be best to offer them an allo-SCT. A retrospective analysis from the International Bone Marrow Transplant Registry (IBMTR) and the EBMT suggests that for adult patients, including those at low risk for transplant-related mortality by EBMT criteria, it is not possible to identify a cohort who would clearly benefit from an immediate SCT versus continuing IM, irrespective of the outcome from IM. The outcome for children, those with a potential syngeneic donor and possibly those with high-risk disease by Sokal or Hasford criteria is uncertain.[13] The current EBMT experience, however, suggests that patients with high-risk disease and a low transplant risk should probably still be considered for an early allo-SCT.[53] Such a cohort, if treated with IM in the first instance, should probably not receive a second TKI on relapse but rather proceed to SCT. With regard to children, many pediatric hematologists still recommend initial treatment by allo-SCT for patients under the age of 16 who have an HLA-identical sibling, largely because of a lack of adequate data pertaining to the use of IM as first-line therapy in children.

About 25% of patients either demonstrate primary resistance to imatinib or respond initially but subsequently lose their reponse and so satisfy criteria for failure.[54] It would be logical to offer such patients treatment by allo-SCT if they are relatively young and have a suitable sibling or matched unrelated donor. In practice, many such patients opt for treatment with one or other of the available new TKIs, namely dasatinib or nilotinib. If such alternative drugs are offered, it is probably reasonable to aim for a complete cytogenetic response or major molecular response by predetermined time points and to offer an allo-SCT graft to patients who do not achieve the landmarks.

Patients who proceed to transplantation after prior treatment with imatinib appear to have a higher relapse incidence than do those who have not previously received IM;[55] this is not surprising since they have presumably been selected for their relatively resistant disease. Preliminary data based on relatively small numbers of patients do not, however, suggest that prior treatment with imatinib increases the probability of transplant-related mortality.[55,56] Moreover, in a small series, patients with kinase domain mutations appeared to fare as well post transplant as those lacking such mutations.[57]

The experience with allo-SCT after initial treatment of advanced-phase disease with IM is still limited. It does, however, appear logical that patients who present with accelerated-phase disease or blastic transformation should be treated initially with IM and then proceed to allo-SCT if possible. In a study of 229 patients with myeloid blast crisis, IM at 400–600 mg daily doses induced complete hematologic responses in 31%, and major cytogenetic responses in 16%, with a median survival of only 6.9 months.[58] Because the response to tyrosine kinase inhibitors is short-lived, an allo-SCT should if possible be performed as soon as the patient is restored to chronic phase, because this will otherwise not be maintained. Post-SCT maintenance with a tyrosine kinase inhibitor may be useful.

Future developments

The precise role of allo-SCT in the management of CML during the next 5 or 10 years is difficult to predict. Although in most cases patients who respond to IM appear to show reducing numbers of BCR-ABL transcripts in their peripheral blood over subsequent years and many eventually achieve a BCR-ABL transcript undetectable status, there is considerable uncertainty as to whether leukemia stem cells are actually eliminated in any patient. This raises the possibility that even good responders might eventually relapse, a situation that might be prevented by allo-SCT with its associated potent GvL effect. Alternatively, the capacity of IM to reduce the number of residual leukemia stem cells to a low level or, rather, the number of leukemia cells susceptible to acquisition of new genetic change might be compatible with long-term freedom from relapse or disease progression. Conversely, any significant advance in the technology of allogeneic SCT, such as the ability to prevent GvHD without abrogation of GvL, would restore allogeneic SCT as an attractive option for the newly diagnosed patient who might otherwise have to continue to take a tyrosine kinase inhibitor for life.

References

1. Goldman JM, Gordon M. Why do CML stem cells survive allogeneic stem cell transplantation or imatinib? Does it really matter? Leuk Lymphoma 2006;47:1–8
2. Goldman JM, Daley GQ. Chronic myeloid leukemia – a brief history. In: Melo JV, Goldman JM (eds) Myeloproliferative disorders. Springer, New York, 2007, 1–13
3. Druker BJ, Guilhot F, O'Brien SG et al. Five-year follow up of patients receiving imatinib for chronic myeloid leukemia. N Engl J Med 2006;355:2408–2417
4. Mughal TI, Goldman JM. Optimal management of patients with newly diagnosed chronic phase chronic myeloid leukemia in 2007. Clin Lymphoma Myeloma 2007;7:S95–S101
5. Mughal TI, Goldman JM. Why does CML evolve from a chronic phase to blast phase? Front Biosci 2006;1:198–208
6. Melo JV, Barnes D. Chronic myeloid leukemia – biology of advanced phase. In: Melo JV, Goldman JM (eds) Myeloproliferative disorders. Springer, New York, 2007, 37–58
7. Roy L, Guilhot J, Krahnke T et al. Survival advantage from imatinib compared with the combination of interferon-alpha plus cytarabine in chronic-phase chronic myelogenous leukemia: historical comparison between two phase 3 trials. Blood 2006;108:1478–1484
8. Kantarjian HM, Talpaz M, O'Brien S et al. Survival benefit with imatinib mesylate versus interferon alfa-based regimens in newly diagnosed chronic-phase chronic myeloid leukemia. Blood 2006;108:1835–1840
9. Sokal JE, Cox EB, Baccarani M et al. Prognostic discrimination in good-risk chronic granulocytic leukemia. Blood 1984;63:789–799
10. Hasford J, Pfirrmann M, Hehlmann R et al. A new prognostic score for survival of patients with chronic myeloid leukemia treated with interferon-alpha. J Natl Cancer Inst 1998;90:850–858
11. Goldman JM, Lu D-P. Chronic granulocytic leukemia – origin, prognosis and treatment. Semin Hematol 1982;19:241–256
12. Gratwohl A, Hermans J, Goldman JM et al. Risk assessment for patients with chronic myeloid leukemia before allogeneic blood or marrow transplantation. Chronic Leukemia Working Party of the European Group for Blood and Marrow Transplantation. Lancet 1998;352:1087–1092
13. Passweg JR, Walker I, Sobocinski KA et al. Validation and extension of the EBMT Risk Score for patients with chronic myeloid leukemia (CML) receiving allogeneic hematopoietic stem cell transplants. The Chronic Leukemia Study Writing Committee of the International Bone Marrow Transplant Registry. Br J Hematol 2004;125:613–620
14. Tura S, Baccarani M, Zuffa E et al. Interferon alfa-2a as compared with conventional chemotherapy for the treatment of chronic myeloid leukemia. N Engl J Med 1994;330:820–828
15. Guilhot F, Chastang C, Michallet M et al. Interferon alfa-2b combined with cytarabine versus interferon alone in chronic myelogenous leukemia. N Engl J Med 1997;337:223–229
16. Chronic Myeloid Leukemia Trialists' Collaborative Group. Interferon alpha versus chemotherapy for chronic myeloid leukemia: a meta-analysis of seven randomized trials. J Natl Cancer Inst 1997;89:1616–1620
17. Talpaz M, Shah NP, Kantarjian H et al. Dasatinib in imatinib-resistant Philadelphia chromosome positive leukemias. N Engl J Med 2006;354:2531–2541
18. Kantarjian H, Giles F, Wunderle L et al. Nilotinib in imatinib-resistant Philadelphia chromosome-positive leukemias. N Engl J Med 2006;354:2542–2551
19. Fefer A, Cheever MA, Thomas ED et al. Disappearance of Ph1-positive cells in four patients with chronic granulocytic leukemia after chemotherapy, irradiation and marrow transplantation from an identical twin. N Engl J Med 1979;300:333–337
20. Clift RA, Buckner CD, Thomas ED et al. Treatment of chronic granulocytic leukemia in chronic phase by allogeneic marrow transplantation. Lancet 1982;2:621–623
21. Goldman JM, Baughan ASJ, McCarthy DM et al. Marrow transplantation for patients in the chronic phase of chronic granulocytic leukemia. Lancet 1982;2:623–625
22. Hansen JA, Gooley TA, Martin PJ et al. Bone marrow transplants from unrelated donors for patients with chronic myeloid leukemia. N Engl J Med 1998;338:962–968
23. Mackinnon S, Hows JM, Goldman JM et al. Bone marrow transplantation for chronic myeloid leukemia: the use of histocompatible unrelated volunteer donors. Exper Hematol 1990;18:421–425
24. Elmaagacli AH, Beelen DW, Opalka B et al. The risk of residual molecular and cytogenetic disease in patients with Philadelphia-chromosome positive first chronic phase chronic myelogenous leukemia is reduced after transplantation of allogeneic peripheral blood stem cells compared with bone marrow. Blood 1999;94:384–389
25. Stem Cell Trialists' Collaborative Group. Allogeneic peripheral blood stem-cell compared with bone marrow transplantation in the management of hematologic malignancies, an individual patient data meta-analysis of nine randomized trials. J Clin Oncol 2005;23:5074–5087
26. Giralt S. Allogeneic hematopoietic progenitor cell transplantation for the treatment of chronic myelogenous leukemia in the era of tyrosine kinase inhibitors: lessons learned to date. Clin Lymphoma Myeloma 2007;7:S102–S104
27. Goldman JM, Apperley JF, Jones L et al. Bone marrow transplantation for patients with chronic myeloid leukemia. N Engl J Med 1986;314:202–207
28. Thomas ED, Clift RA, Fefer A et al. Marrow transplantation for the treatment of chronic myelogenous leukemia. Ann Intern Med 1986;104:155–163
29. Slattery JT, Clift RA, Buckner CD et al. Marrow transplantation for chronic myeloid leukemia: the influence of plasma busulfan levels on the outcome of transplantation. Blood 1997;89:3055–3060
30. Radich JP, Gooley T, Bensinger WC et al. HLA-matched related hematopoietic cell transplantation for chronic phase CML using a targeted busulfan and cyclophosphamide preparative regimen. Blood 2003;102:31–35
31. Giralt S, Estey E, Albtar M et al. Engraftment of allogeneic hematopoietic progenitor cells with purine analog-containing chemotherapy: harnessing graft-versus-leukemia without myeloablative therapy. Blood 1997;89:4531–4537
32. Slavin S, Nagler A, Naparstek E et al. Nonmyeloablative stem cell transplantation and cell therapy as an alternative to conventional bone marrow transplantation with lethal cytoreduction for the treatment of malignant and nonmalignant hematologic disease. Blood 1998;91:756–763
33. Gale RP, Horowitz MM, Ash RC et al. Identical-twin bone marrow transplants for leukemia. Ann Intern Med 1994;120:646–652
34. Kolb H, Mittermuller J, Clemm C et al. Donor leukocyte transfusions for treatment of recurrent chronic myelogenous leukemia in marrow transplant patients. Blood 1990;76:462–465
35. Cullis JO, Jiang YZ, Schwarer AP et al. Donor leukocyte infusions in the treatment of chronic myeloid leukemia in relapse following allogeneic bone marrow transplantation (letter). Blood 1992;79:1379–1381
36. Mackinnon S, Papadopoulos EP, Carabasi MH et al. Adoptive immunotherapy evaluating escalating doses of donor leukocytes for relapse of chronic myeloid leukemia following bone marrow transplantation: separation of graft-versus-leukemia responses from graft-versus-host disease. Blood 1995;86:1261–1267
37. Goldman JM, Catovsky D, Hows J et al. Cryopreserved peripheral blood cells functioning as autografts in patients with chronic granulocytic leukemia in transformation. BMJ 1979;i:1310–1313
38. Mughal T, Hoyle C, Goldman JM. Autografting for patients with chronic myeloid leukemia. Stem Cell 1994;11:20–22
39. Radich JP, Gooley T, Bensinger W et al. HLA-matched related hematopoietic stem cell transplantation for chronic-phase CML using a targeted busulfan and cyclophosphamide preparative regimen. Blood 2003;102:31–35
40. Mughal TI, Yong A, Szydlo R et al. Molecular studies in patients with chronic myeloid leukemia in remission 5 years after allogeneic stem cell transplant define the risk of subsequent relapse. Br J Hematol 2001;115:569–574
41. Kaeda J, Syzdlo RM, O'Shea D et al. Serial measurements of BCR-ABL transcripts in the peripheral blood after allogeneic stem cell transplantation for chronic myeloid leukemia: an attempt to define patients who may not require therapy. Blood 2006;107:4171–4176
42. Uzunel M, Mattsson J, Bruce M et al. Kinetics of minimal residual disease and chimerism in patients with chronic myeloid leukemia after nonmyeloablative conditioning and stem cell transplantation. Blood 2003;101:469–472
43. Sloand E, Childs RW, Solomon S et al. The graft versus leukemia effect of nonmyeloablative stem cell allografts may not be sufficient to cure chronic myelogenous leukemia. Bone Marrow Transplant 2003;32:897–901

44. Or R, Shapira MY, Resnick I et al. Nonmyeloablative allogeneic stem cell transplantation for the treatment of chronic myeloid leukemia in first chronic phase. Blood 2003;101:441–445

45. Weisser M, Schleuning M, Ledderose G et al. Reduced-intensity conditioning using TBI (8 Gy), fludarabine, cyclophosphamide and ATG in elderly CML patients provides excellent results especially when performed in the early course of the disease. Bone Marrow Transplant 2004;34:1083–1088

46. Crawley C, Szydlo R, Lalancette M et al. Chronic Leukemia Working Party of the EBMT. Outcomes of reduced-intensity transplantation for chronic myeloid leukemia: an analysis of prognostic factors from the Chronic Leukemia Working Party of the EBMT. Blood 2005;106:2969–2976

47. Cross NP, Hughes TP, Feng L et al. Minimal residual disease after allogeneic bone marrow transplantation for chronic myeloid leukemia in first chronic phase: correlation with acute graft-versus-host disease and relapse. Br J Haematol 1993;84:67–74

48. Radich JP, Gooley T, Bryant E et al. The significance of bcr-abl molecular detection in chronic myeloid leukemia patients 'late', 18 months or more after transplantation. Blood 2001;98:1701–1707

49. Dazzi F, Szydlo R, Cross N et al. Durability of responses following donor lymphocyte infusions for patients who relapse after allogeneic stem cell transplantation for chronic myeloid leukemia. Blood 2000;96:2712–2716

50. Kolb H, Schattenberg A, Goldman JM et al. Graft-versus-leukemia effect of donor lymphocyte transfusion in marrow grafted patients. Blood 1995;86:2041–2050

51. Olavarria E, Siddique S, Griffiths MJ et al. Posttransplantation imatinib as a strategy to postpone the requirement for immunotherapy in patients undergoing reduced-intensity allografts for chronic myeloid leukemia. Blood 2007;110:4614–4617

52. Goldman JM, Druker BJ. Chronic myeloid leukemia: current treatment options. Blood 2001;98:2039–2042

53. Gratwohl A, Brand R, Apperley J et al. Allogeneic hematopoietic stem cell transplantation for chronic myeloid leukemia in Europe 2006: transplant activity, long-term data and current results. An analysis by the Chronic Leukemia Working Party of the European Group for Blood and Marrow Transplantation (EBMT). Hematologica 2006;91:513–521

54. Baccarani M, Saglio G, Goldman JM et al. Evolving concepts in the management of chronic myeloid leukemia: recommendations from an expert panel on behalf of the European LeukemiaNet. Blood 2006;108:1809–1820

55. Deininger M, Schleuning M, Greinix H et al. The effect of prior exposure to imatinib on transplant-related mortality. Hematologica 2006;91:452–459

56. Oehler VG, Gooley T, Synder DS et al. The effects of imatinib mesylate treatment before allogeneic transplantation for chronic myeloid leukemia. Blood 2007;109:1782–1789

57. Jabbour E, Cortes J, Kantarjian H et al. Allogeneic stem cell transplantation for patients with chronic myeloid leukemia and acute lymphoblastic leukemia after Bcr-Abl kinase mutation-related imatinib failure. Blood 2006;108:1421–1423

58. Sawyers C, Hochhaus A, Feldman E et al. Imatinib induces hematologic and cytogenetic responses in patients with chronic myelogenous leukemia in myeloid blast crisis: results of a phase II study. Blood 2002;99:3530–3539

Acute lymphoblastic leukemia in adults

CHAPTER 5

Nicola Gökbuget and Dieter Hoelzer

Introduction

Until the 1980s, adult acute lymphoblastic leukemia (ALL) was rarely curable, with an overall survival (OS) of less than 10%. After adaptation of pediatric protocols, the outcome improved to 30–40%. A period of stagnation then followed, with improvement only in selected subgroups. Over the last 5 years, however, striking new developments have been noticeable. Progress has been made in the techniques available for diagnosing ALL, standard therapy including stem cell transplantation (SCT) has progressively improved, and a variety of new drugs for ALL is now under evaluation. The prerequisites for comprehensive therapy of ALL are, however, standardized diagnostic techniques with good quality control which will permit rapid diagnosis and classification, and allow identification of prognostic factors. Targets for evaluation of minimal residual disease (MRD) require definition so that therapeutic interventions can be adapted accordingly.

Epidemiology

ALL is the most common neoplastic disease in children, with an early peak at the age of 3–4 years (see also Chapter 6). The incidence in adults ranges between 0.7 and 1.8/100,000 per year, with a second peak in the age group above 75 years.

Natural course of the disease

The uncontrolled proliferation of immature lymphoid blast cells in the bone marrow leads to suppression of normal hematopoiesis with subsequent anemia, thrombocytopenia and granulocytopenia. The white blood cell count (WBC) is usually elevated but a normal or decreased WBC does not exclude ALL. More than 90% of ALL patients exhibit lymphatic blast cells in the peripheral blood. The final diagnosis is made by bone marrow aspiration or biopsy. Other parts of the lymphatic system such as lymph nodes, thymus and spleen are frequently involved and lymphoid blast cells may infiltrate other organs, including the central nervous system (CNS). ALL generally progresses rapidly and survival without treatment is less than 2 months.

Diagnosis

ALL is not a uniform disease but consists of distinct subtypes which display characteristic clinical, biologic and prognostic features. Accurate diagnosis is thus essential, to allow disease classification and an appropriate treatment decision. Techniques for disease assessment should include morphology, immunophenotyping, molecular/cytogenetics, evaluation of minimal residual disease and, to an increasing extent, gene expression analysis and pharmacogenetics.

Morphology

The primary diagnosis is generally made on bone marrow morphology, including cytochemistry. According to the World Health Organization (WHO) classification, ALL is grouped together with lymphoblastic lymphoma as either a precursor B-cell or T-cell neoplasm. B-cell ALL is referred to as precursor B-lymphoblastic leukemia/lymphoma. L3-ALL is classified as Burkitt cell leukemia together with Burkitt lymphoma. T-ALL is grouped together with T-cell lymphoblastic lymphoma as precursor T-lymphoblastic lymphoma/leukemia.[1]

Immunophenotyping

The most important method available for the identification of the biologic subgroups of ALL is immunophenotyping. The blast cells are thereby grouped according to lineage (B- or T-lineage) and stage of maturation from early undifferentiated to mature subtypes. There is unfortunately no uniform classification of the immunophenotypes in ALL. The European Group for the Immunological Characterization of Leukemias (EGIL)[2] made an attempt to define a common immunologic classification. Immunophenotypes in ALL are often associated with certain clinical characteristics such as initial manifestation, course of disease and biologic markers, including cytogenetic and molecular abnormalities. The immunologic subgroups of ALL and the corresponding molecular markers are listed in Table 5.1.

Cytogenetics

The major potential of cytogenetics in ALL is the identification of independent risk factors. Aberrations can be structural or numeric. A hyperdiploid karyotype without additional aberrations identifies a favorable subgroup in childhood ALL, whereas complex aberrations are associated with an unfavorable outcome in adults. The most frequent structural aberration is the t(9;22) translocation which has an incidence of 20–30%, increasing to 50% in older patients. Translocation t(4;11) has an incidence of 6% and is correlated with pro-B-ALL. Both are associated with a particularly unfavorable prognosis.

Molecular genetics

Molecular methods are used for targeted detection of fusion transcripts resulting from translocations, and they have a higher sensitivity. The most important translocations are BCR-ABL, which correlates with

Table 5.1 Immunologic subtypes of ALL and corresponding cytogenetic/molecular markers

Subgroups	Most important markers	Incidence	Cytogenetic/molecular marker**
B-Lineage	HLA-DR+, TdT+, CD19+ a./o. CD79a+ a./o. CD22+	**74%**	
Pro B (B-I)	CD10⁻, no other differentiation markers	11%	6% t(4;11)/ALL1-AF4 (70% in pro B) (20% Flt3 in MLL+)
Common ALL (B-II)	CD10⁺	50%	33% t(9;22)/BCR-ABL (30–50% in c/preB)
Pre B (B-III)	cy IgM⁺	9%	4% t(1;19)/PBX-E2A
Mature B	cy or s kappa or lambda	4%	5% t(8;14) / c-myc-IgH
T-Lineage	cy or s CD3⁺, CD7⁺	**26%**	
Early T	cy CD3⁺, CD7⁺, CD5±, CD2⁻, sCD3⁻, CD1a⁻	6%	5% t(10;14)/HOX11-TCR <5% t(11;14)/LMO-TCR
Cortical (thymic) T	CD2+, CD5+, CD1a⁺, sCD3±	13%	2% SIL-TAL1
Mature T (T-IV)	CD2+, CD5+, sCD3⁺, CD1a⁻	7%	4% NUP213-ABL1 (in T-ALL) 33% HOX11** 5% HOX11L2** 50% Notch1**

Abbreviations: a, and; o, or; cy, intracytoplasmic; s, surface; ** according to GMALL data and ref 3.

the t(9;22) translocation, and ALL1-AF4, which correlates with t(4;11). Microarray analysis is increasingly used to detect gene expression signatures, which are associated with specific subtypes or outcomes. Overexpressed genes or those which have low expression also correlate with prognosis and allow new definitions of prognostic factors.[3]

Minimal residual disease

Polymerase chain reaction (PCR) and multiparameter flow cytometry are used to quantitatively detect residual leukemic blasts after morphologic complete remission (CR) has been obtained. PCR is directed to fusion genes associated with ALL-type translocations or to individual clonal rearrangements of the immunoglobulin (IgH) and T-cell receptor genes (TCR). With multiparameter flow cytometry, individual leukemia-specific phenotypes, i.e. characteristic constellations of surface antigens, can be detected with high specificity and sensitivity.

Standard therapy of acute lymphoblastic leukemia

Standard therapy of ALL consists of intensive chemotherapy starting with induction, followed by consolidation cycles and prolonged maintenance therapy of up to a total duration of 2.5 years. SCT is part of consolidation therapy in most trials. In addition, CNS prophylaxis with intrathecal therapy, systemic high-dose therapy and CNS irradiation are the backbone of treatment in ALL (reviewed in ref 4).

Induction therapy

Standard drugs for induction of adult ALL are, at a minimum, a steroid, vincristine and an anthracycline. In many recent trials, prednisone was replaced by dexamethasone (DEXA), based on results in pediatric trials, which showed a decreased CNS relapse rate and improved survival.[5] The DEXA schedule has to be considered carefully, since continuous use of higher doses may lead to long-term complications[5] and to increased morbidity and mortality due to infections.[6]

The most frequently used anthracycline is daunorubicine (DNR). Many groups have replaced weekly use by higher doses of DNR (45–80 mg/m²) given on a number of consecutive days. However, the promising results of smaller trials have not always been reproducible. One reason for this is the increased hematologic toxicity of such regimens. Thus, it remains to be seen whether intensified anthracycline usage is beneficial in any ALL subgroup, particularly in terms of attaining molecular remission.

The use of cyclophosphamide 'upfront' may also confer benefit,[7] although this has not been confirmed in a randomized trial.[8] The majority of studies now include asparaginase (ASP) in induction therapy. Most use native E. coli asparaginase which is replaced in some trials by prolonged-action pegylated asparaginase. ASP is often given in parallel to steroids during induction in patients with cytopenias and may induce additional toxicities such as coagulation disorders and abnormalities of hepatic function. Supportive care is of increasing importance during induction, and includes the use of G-CSF.[9]

With current regimens, the remission rate in ALL is 85–90% (Table 5.2), with early mortalities of up to 11%, increasing with age. However, morbidities due to prolonged cytopenias may compromise further treatment and dose intensification. Increasing molecular CR rates is the most important goal in adult ALL. This can be defined as a level of minimal residual disease (MRD) below the detection limit of 10^{-4} (0.01%); the frequency of molecular CR in adult ALL ranges from 50% for Ph+ ALL treated with imatinib[10] to 60% for standard risk ALL.[11]

Consolidation therapy

Intensive consolidation therapy is standard in the treatment of ALL, although consolidation cycles in large studies vary and it is impossible to evaluate their individual efficacy. In general, it seems that the use of high-dose methotrexate (HDMTX) is beneficial. However, in adults, doses are probably limited at 1.5–2 g/m² if given as a 24-hour infusion. Otherwise, toxicities, particularly mucositis, may lead to subsequent treatment delays and decreased compliance. There is increasing evidence from pediatric ALL trials that intensified use of ASP leads to improved overall results.[12,13] In adult ALL, this approach appears to be useful, particularly in consolidation, where less toxicity can be expected compared to that seen during induction. The role of HD anthracylines, podophyllotoxins and HD cytarabine in consolidation remains undefined. Overall, in adult ALL, stricter adherence to protocols with fewer delays, dose reductions and omission of drugs due toxicities constitute an important contribution to therapeutic progress.

Table 5.2 Results of large trials in adult ALL*

Study	Year	n	SCT Strategy	CR Rate	Early death	Survival
CALGB 9111, USA[8]	1998	198	Ph+	85%	8%	40% (3 y)
LALA 87, France[25]	2000	572	PO	76%	9%	27% (10 y)
NILG 08/96, Italy[29]	2001	121	PR	84%	8%	48% (5 y)
GMALL 05/93, Germany[30]	2001	1163	PR	83%	n.r.	35% (5 y)
JALSG-ALL93, Japan[26]	2002	263	PO	78%	6%	30% (6 y)
UCLA, USA[31]	2002	84	PR	93%	1%	47% (5 y)
Sweden[32]	2002	153	PR	75%	n.r.	28% (5 y)
GIMEMA 0288, Italy[9]	2002	767	–	82%	11%	27% (9 y)
MD Anderson, USA[14]	2004	288	Ph+	92%	5%	38% (5 y)
EORTC ALL-3, Europe[27]	2004	340	PO	74%	n.r.	36%*(6 y)
LALA 94, France[33]	2004	922	PR	84%	5%	36% (5 y)
GOELAL02, France[34]	2004	198	HR	86%	2%	41% (6 y)
MRC XII/ ECOG E 2993, UK-USA[28]	2005	1521	PO	91%	n.r.	38% (5 y)
GIMEMA 0496, Italy[35]	2005	450	n.r.	80%	n.r.	33% (5 y)
Pethema ALL-93, Spain[36]	2005	222	HR	82%	6%	34% (5 y)
Weighted mean		7262		84%	7%	35%

Abbreviations: Ph+, SCT in Ph+ ALL; PO, prospective SCT in all patients with donor; PR, SCT according to prospective risk model; HR, prospective SCT in a study for HR patients only; n.r. not reported. * Survival of CR patients.

Maintenance therapy

Maintenance even after intensive induction and consolidation is still standard for ALL patients since all attempts to omit it have led to inferior long-term outcome. Therefore, some groups even prolong maintenance therapy beyond 2 years of total treatment duration. MTX, preferably given intravenously (iv), and mercaptopurine (MP) given orally are the mainstays of maintenance. The role of intensification cycles during maintenance remains to be determined.

CNS prophylaxis

In protocols with intensive intrathecal (it) therapy and systemic HD therapy, the rate of CNS relapse in adult ALL is below 5%. Few trials still rely on CNS irradiation. Risk factors for CNS disease such as an elevated WBC or LDH, traumatic lumbar punctures and phenotypes such as mature B-ALL and T-ALL are well known. Therefore, risk-adapted approaches to prophylaxis seem reasonable.[14]

Targeted therapies

Molecular therapy of Ph/BCR-ABL positive (Ph+) ALL

As in chronic myeloid leukemia (CML), the *BCR-ABL* fusion gene is the major pathogenetic factor in Ph+ ALL, based on increased tyrosine kinase (TK) activity. Imatinib is the first specific inhibitor of this mechanism, and its clinical efficacy was first demonstrated in CML. Phase II trials have demonstrated a CR rate of 29% in relapsed/refractory Ph+ ALL with imatinib used as a single agent.[15] Despite the rapid development of relapse which occurs within weeks in many patients, some were able to proceed to SCT.[16] Response to imatinib therapy can be closely controlled by quantitative PCR. Treatment can generally be given on an outpatient basis and is associated with few side-effects. Clinical trials in de novo ALL differ for younger and older patients.

- In *younger patients*, imatinib was first administered between chemotherapy cycles. However, with this approach no molecular remissions were obtained. Studies with parallel use of chemotherapy and imatinib were therefore started, which led to CR rates of 91–96% with molecular CR rates of 38–50%.[10,17–19] All studies reported an improved OS of 55–65%, compared to 15% in studies before the imatinib era. No trial described increased toxicity compared to chemotherapy alone, or a negative effect on subsequent SCT.

- In *older patients* with de novo Ph+ ALL, treatment results were extremely poor, with particularly high induction mortalities. Induction chemotherapy was therefore replaced by single-drug therapy with imatinib. The remission rate was 92% in an Italian trial.[20] The German study group (GMALL) conducted a randomized trial comparing dose-reduced chemotherapy and imatinib monotherapy. After induction, all patients received chemotherapy combined with imatinib. The remission rate for imatinib was 93%, compared to 54% with chemotherapy.[21] Survival was superior to that seen in previous trials without imatinib but in both arms the relapse rate was high and there was no difference in outcome.

Frequent monitoring of MRD often leads to early detection of molecular resistance or molecular relapse. Additional treatment can then be initiated before overt relapse. Nowadays, a search for mutations of the TK domain is also required since these mutations can confer resistance to imatinib and sometimes to the second-generation TK inhibitors dasatinib and nilotinib.[22,23] Both of these drugs have increased efficacy compared to imatinib and are active against the majority of mutations, although not the T315I mutation. Remission rates achieved with these drugs in patients who have failed imatinib are approximately 30%. They are currently being evaluated in the relapse setting, but trials in de novo Ph+ ALL are beginning.

Antibody therapy

ALL blast cells express a variety of specific antigens including CD20, CD19, CD22, CD33 and CD52 which may serve as targets for treatment with monoclonal antibodies (MoAb). MoAb therapy is an attractive approach since it is targeted, subtype specific and, compared to chemotherapy, has different mechanisms of action and side-effects. Its use may be most promising in the situation of MRD positivity. The anti-CD20 antibody rituximab has been successfully integrated into the therapy of mature B-ALL. It is now also being evaluated in several pilot studies for CD20+ B-precursor ALL. In a GMALL protocol for elderly patients, rituximab is added before chemotherapy cycles begin, starting from induction, for a total of eight doses. The combination of the Hyper-CVAD regimen with rituximab in B-precursor ALL also proved feasible and a favorable outcome in CD20+ ALL has been reported (reviewed in ref 24). Several studies using anti-CD52 are also under way, either in relapse or in the situation of MRD positivity.

Results from large acute lymphoblastic leukemia trials

One major question in the treatment of adult ALL is the role of SCT as postremission therapy. Over the past decade, therefore, two groups of prospective trials have mainly been reported for adult ALL (see Table 5.2).

- One group was dedicated to the comparative analysis of the role of allogeneic SCT in patients with a sibling donor.[25–28]
- The other group involved studies focusing on optimizing chemotherapy, using SCT only for subgroups such as Ph+ ALL[8,14] with a particularly poor prognosis, or based on prognostic models.[29–33]

CR rates ranged between 74% and 93% and OS between 27% and 48%. Notably, no difference has been evident for OS in studies focusing on SCT (n = 2696), with a weighted mean of 84% for CR and 35% for OS[25–28] or in studies using risk-adapted approaches (n = 2443), with mean CR rates of 83% and OS of 36%.[8,29–33]

Prognostic factors in acute lymphoblastic leukemia

Age

Age is probably the most important prognostic factor.[37] OS progressively decreases with increasing age, from 34–57% below 30 years to 15–17% above 50 years.[8,9,14,26,28] Some groups have used age above 30–35 years as an indication for SCT in CR1.[34,36] This is probably counterproductive since the outcome of SCT also worsens with age.[38]

White blood cell count (WBC)

An elevated WBC at diagnosis (<30–50,000/μl) is associated with a higher relapse risk.[8,9,14,25,26] It is also considered to be the most adverse prognostic factor in B-precursor ALL, where OS of 19–29% have been found.[28,30] However, in T-ALL WBC was not a significant factor in a GMALL multivariate analysis.[30] In the GMALL studies, patients with B-lineage ALL and high WBC experienced a high relapse rate but also seemed to have a higher mortality with chemotherapy and SCT.[39]

Immunophenotype

Pro-B-ALL and/or t(4;11) positive ALL are considered as poor prognostic subgroups in many trials. They appear to be particularly amenable to SCT, as reported from the GMALL studies.[40] Common(c)/pre-B-ALL is associated with Ph/BCR-ABL positivity, which will be discussed separately. Some groups consider the translocation t(1;19) as an unfavorable feature.[33,34] C/pre-B-ALL can be subdivided into

standard and high-risk groups, with significantly different outcomes. However, even with standard risk B-lineage ALL outcome is poor, and this is the major reason for the slow improvement in overall results in adult ALL. Mature B-ALL is usually treated with short, intensive chemotherapy courses based on HDMTX and fractionated cyclophosphamide.

Many groups have confirmed the superior outcome of T-lineage ALL compared to B-lineage.[28,30] T-ALL comprises the subtypes early T-ALL, thymic (cortical T-ALL) and mature T-ALL. Subtype was the most significant prognostic factor in the GMALL studies, with leukemia-free survival (LFS) of 25%, 63% and 28%, respectively.[30] The biologic importance of immunophenotype was emphasized by the fact that elevated expression of HOX11, HOX11L2, SIL-TAL1 and CALM-AF10 is associated with various subtypes, i.e. maturation states of thymocytes (reviewed in ref 41). Other groups have observed inferior outcomes for early T-ALL,[42,43] co-expression of CD13, CD33 and/or CD34,[42] HOX11L2 and SIL-TAL positive T-ALL.[43] Over-expression of HOX11, which is associated with thymic T-ALL, may confer a favorable prognosis. With current treatment regimens, CR rates of more than 80% and a LFS above 50% can be achieved in T-ALL.

Treatment response and MRD

Beside age, the most significant prognostic factor in ALL is still the achievement of CR. Further prognostic factors related to treatment response are delayed time to CR or response to prednisone therapy. A more accurate approach for assessing individual response is MRD evaluation,[37,40] since this is an independent prognostic factor which reflects primary drug resistance as well as the individual reaction therapy and other, unknown, host factors. Two major aims have been foremost with longitudinal MRD evaluation in adult ALL.

- *Identification of high-risk patients* as candidates for SCT or experimental therapy. After start of consolidation, high MRD ($<10^{-4}$) at any time-point is associated with a high relapse risk of 66–88%[11] and the predictive value increases at later time-points (months 6–9).[44] In the GMALL studies, patients with high MRD ($<10^{-4}$) after induction and first consolidation are identified as high risk and are candidates for SCT in CR1.[45]
- *Identification of low-risk patients* in whom less treatment may be justified. An early and rapid decrease in MRD during induction is associated with a relapse risk of only 8%.[11] However, this is observed in only 10% of patients. In the GMALL studies, patients with a negative MRD status after induction, this being repeatedly confirmed during first year and measured with two sensitive markers, are considered as MRD low risk; 30% of the patients fulfill these criteria.

MRD evaluation also offers the option of assessing *molecular CR*, and thereby evaluating different induction therapies, and of detecting *molecular relapse*. These are two important new aspects for follow-up analysis in adult ALL. 'Molecular relapse' is already an inclusion criterion even in Phase II studies. This is logical, since patients with an increase of MRD of above 10^{-4} after achievement of molecular CR are at high risk of relapse (>80%) and therapeutic action should be taken.[46]

New integrated risk classification

All risk factors are, to a certain extent, specific for a defined treatment protocol and used with variations by different study groups. In addition to established factors (Table 5.3), a variety of molecular markers newly detected by microarray analysis have been proposed as prognostic factors.[3] All these factors cannot possibly be integrated into a

Table 5.3 Adverse prognostic factors in adult ALL

Factor	All subtypes	B-precursor	T-ALL
At diagnosis			
High WBC		>30,000 (20–50)	(>100,000)
Subtype		Pro B-ALL or CD10 negative pre B-ALL	Early T Mature T
Cytogenetics/molecular genetics	Complex karyotype (HOX11)	**t(9;22) / BCR-ABL** **t(4;11) / ALL1-AF4** t(1;19) / PBX1-E2A	(HOX11L2) (BAALC)
Age	**>35, >55, >60**		
During treatment			
Individual response	Steroid response **Late CR (>3–4 wks)** **MRD persistance >10^{-4} for 3–4 months**		

Abbreviations: bold, established; not bold, used by several groups; in brackets, rarely used.

conventional risk model which mainly aims to identify patients for SCT in CR1, but rather, they may prompt analysis of underlying mechanisms, drug targets or design of alternative treatment strategies.

Stem cell transplantation

Stem cell transplantation (SCT) has gained an increasingly important role in the treatment of adult ALL. Although the majority of large prospective studies in adult ALL have addressed the issue of indications for SCT in first CR, scheduling and procedures are still not defined in a satisfactory manner. To circumvent the problem with comparability of SCT and chemotherapy, several groups have designed prospective trials with a 'genetic' randomization, offering allogeneic (allo) SCT in CR1 to all patients with a sibling donor. Study results depend upon comparison with the 'conventional' treatment approach. Some groups scheduled autologous (auto) SCT only, and others a randomized comparison of auto SCT and chemotherapy. This trial design uses an 'intention-to-treat' analysis which compares patients with a donor to those without. This type of analysis is, however, only meaningful if transplantation is realized in a significant proportion of patients.

In the following sections, the impact of SCT on overall outcome and the results of comparative studies will be discussed.

Impact of SCT on overall outcome in adult ALL trials

The hardest outcome parameter is OS of the total patient cohort, which answers the question of whether a SCT-based treatment approach is able to improve overall outcome. Overall survivals in studies using 'genetic randomization' are not superior to those using chemotherapy alone (see Table 5.2), which may partly be due to the fact that allo-SCT could be undertaken in only 11–38% of patients.[25–27,33,34,36,47] Even if allo-SCT had yielded superior results, the impact on OS would not be discernible because of the small number of patients undergoing the procedure,

Outcome of different types of SCT

Results of allo-SCT: sibling donor

First remission

According to the IBMTR registry (1996–2001), survival after allo-SCT from a sibling donor is about 48% in patients above 20 years of

Table 5.4 Results of SCT in adult ALL (pooled from published studies)

Type of SCT	Stage	n	TRM	Relapse rate	LFS
Allogeneic					
– Family donor	CR1	1100	27%	24%	50%
	≥CR2	1019	29%	48%	34%
	Rel/Refr	216	47%	75%	18%
– Unrelated donor	CR1	318	47%	10%	39%
	≥CR2	231	8%	75%	27%
	Rel/Refr*	47	64%	31%	5%
Autologous	CR1	1369	5%	51%	42%
	≥CR2	258	18%	70%	24%
Non-myeloablative	All stages	132	42%	47%	23%

Abbreviations: TRM, transplant-associated mortality; LFS, leukemia-free survival.
*one trial.[53]

age.[48] A literature analysis including 1100 patients reveals a LFS of 50%. Relapse rates (RR) (24%) and transplant-related mortality (TRM) (27%) are similar (Table 5.4). Improved supportive care has reduced the TRM in the more recently reported EBMT registry data from 39% before 1985 to 26% currently.[49] Graft-versus-host disease (GvHD) has an important impact on mortality and morbidity after sibling SCT. On the other hand, RR is lower in patients with limited GvHD.

Age is another important prognostic factor influencing outcome after SCT. LFS is 62% for patients less than 20 years of age, and 48% for those more than 20 years old.[48] Nevertheless, the age limit for undertaking SCT has increased continuously up to 50–55 years. Experience of transplant centers may also have a role, with specialized centers in the US reporting LFS of 61–64% for sibling SCT in ALL in first remission.[50–52]

Later remission or relapse

LFS for SCT after relapse is poorer, with 34% for second remission and 18% for SCT in relapse. This is mainly due to an increased RR (see Table 5.4).

Results of allo-SCT: unrelated donor

First remission

Unrelated donor SCT (matched unrelated donor – MUD) plays an increasingly important role in the treatment of adult ALL. The LFS of published studies is 39%, with a lower RR (10%) compared to allo-SCT, whereas TRM (47%) is higher. Both facts are probably due to the more pronounced GvHD effects. It has to be considered, however, that MUD series generally comprise selected, high-risk patients such as those with Ph/BCR-ABL-positive ALL. According to the IBMRT, survival in patients above 20 years is 42%.[48] Another series showed a LFS of 42% in adults with high-risk ALL transplanted in CR1.[54]

Later remission or relapse

MUD SCT may lead to long-term survivals of 27% in later remissions, whereas outcome after transplantation in relapse is only 5% (see Table 5.4).

Comparison of allogeneic sibling and MUD SCT

Due to improved supportive care, better donor selection and extension of indications beyond very high-risk patients, the results of MUD SCT are nowadays similar to those seen after sibling allo-SCT in large study groups. A large study involving prospective SCT showed survivals of 55% (standard and high-risk ALL) in 321 patients after sibling SCT, and of 46% with MUD SCT in 67 patients with very high-risk (Ph/BCR-ABL positive) ALL.[47] A study from nine German centers had more MUD SCTs (60% versus 27%) in first CR, and there was no difference in LFS (45% versus 42%).[55] An analysis of the prospective GMALL trial 05/93 showed a survival of 34% for sibling SCT compared to 51% for MUD SCT; TRM was similar, whereas the RR was lower after MUD SCT.[56] In prospective trials, the TRM for allo-SCT ranged between 15% and 26%[25–27,33,34,36,47] and reached 35% after MUD-SCT.[47] Several factors may have played a role, including intensity of therapy before SCT, preparative regimens, immunosuppressive therapy after SCT and also the experience and conditions at the transplant centers.

Results of autologous SCT

First remission

According to published studies, the survival rate after auto-SCT is 42%. The major problem is a high RR (51%) (see Table 5.4). Published studies show a broad range of results. In unselected, high-risk patients, survival probably does not exceed 30%. The intensity of previous treatment may have an important impact on outcome of auto-SCT since it leads to a reduction in tumor load. Also, maintenance therapy after SCT, particularly in MRD-positive patients, may be an important issue. The use of mercaptopurine and methotrexate is the standard approach.[57]

Later remission or relapse

Few patients experience long-term survivals after auto-SCT when they are in second or subsequent remission or when they are in relapse. This approach may be considered as interim therapy before an allo-SCT if autologous stem cells have been collected during first CR.

Results of non-myeloablative SCT (NMSCT)

NMSCT is increasingly considered as a treatment option for elderly patients in whom conventional SCT is contraindicated. Early results indicate that stable remissions can be achieved in some patients in first CR.[58] Published results show an LFS of 23% for patients in all disease stages, with 42% TRM and 47% RR (see Table 5.4). According to an EBMT analysis, the LFS in 91 adult ALL patients with a median age of 40 years was 18%, with 24% TRM and 58% relapse.[59] The LFS was considerably higher in both studies if NMSCT was conducted during first remission.[58,59]

Results of umbilical cord blood (UCB) and haploidentical SCT

Experience with UCB transplantation in ALL mainly comes from pediatric patients[60] where a recent retrospective analysis indicated that results were at least as good as those seen after bone marrow stem cell transplantation.[61] In adults, the limited cell dose may prove to be one of the major obstacles. However, the first registry results for younger adults with acute leukemia indicate that single or double UCB can be considered as an alternative source of stem cells if available.[62]

Experience with haploidentical SCT is also mainly restricted to pediatric patients, where it may be considered in patients without a donor and in urgent need of SCT.[63] In adult patients with acute leukemia, a retrospective analysis indicated that, if feasible, auto-SCT is preferable to haploidentical SCT; despite a higher RR, overall outcome was slightly superior.[64] Based on the available experience, UCB and haplo-SCT should be undertaken in specialized centers, be performed within clinical trials and be restricted to advanced disease.

Stem cell transplantation in Ph+ ALL

Due to the poor outcomes seen with intensive chemotherapy, SCT has always been the first choice of treatment for Ph-positive ALL. OS after allo-SCT in first CR has ranged from 27% to 65%.[65] The RR is higher compared to Ph-negative ALL, and the outcome is compromised by TRM due to the higher median age of Ph+ ALL patients. Long-term results with auto-SCT are scarce and indicate that survival rates are below 20% depending on tumor load prior to SCT in the patient and in the graft.

Nowadays, the majority of patients with Ph+ ALL receive imatinib with front-line therapy. There is apparently no increase of TRM if SCT is performed thereafter. In one trial, the RR before SCT was considerably reduced in patients who received imatinib before SCT. Thus, the proportion of patients transplanted in CR1 increased and the LFS after SCT was superior for patients pretreated with imatinib (76% versus 38%).[66]

Outcome after SCT may be influenced by MRD status before and after SCT and by the use of imatinib as part of the post-transplant therapy. In patients who were MRD positive after SCT and who rapidly responded to imatinib, it was demonstrated that survival was significantly superior compared to that seen in those who did not respond.[67] The outcome for patients with high MRD before SCT is poor. MRD status and TK domain mutational status must therefore be known before and after SCT, either to instigate additional treatment to reduce tumor load before SCT or to prevent relapse after SCT.

Trials comparing SCT and other approaches

Table 5.5 summarizes prospective trials including SCT as a predefined part of the study design. Interestingly, in most trials the outcome after allo-SCT was superior to registry results. The reason for this remains unclear. On the other hand, the results of treatments compared, such as auto-SCT or chemotherapy, vary considerably and certainly depend on different factors including pretreatment and timing of auto-SCT as well as upon efficacy and duration of chemotherapy.

Donor versus no donor comparisons

Several trials showed no differences in outcome for patients with (allo-sibling SCT) or without a donor (randomization of auto-SCT and chemotherapy).[26,27,68–70] Only the French BGMT study showed an advantage for allo-SCT (donor) compared to auto-SCT (no donor), with a LFS of 71% versus 30%.[71] The extraordinarily good outcomes of patients with donors in this trial remain unexplained.

Table 5.5 Prospective trials of stem cell transplantation in adult ALL

Author, year	Study	Subgroup	Comparison	n	Age	TRM	LFS	OS
Fiere et al, 1993[68]	LALA-87	All	**Donor (allogeneic)**	116	15–40	16%	45%	48%
Sebban et al, 1994[69]			**No donor (R)**	141	15–40	3%	31%	35%
			– Autologous	95	15–50	4%	39%	49%
			– Chemo	96	15–48	4%	32%	42%
Thomas et al, 2004[33]	LALA-94	HR	**Donor (allogeneic)**	100	15–55	18%	47%	51%
			No donor (R)	159	15–55	7%	34%	n.r.
			– Autologous + Maintenance	70	15–55	0%	39%	44%
			– Chemo	59	15–55	7%	24%	35%
Takeuchi et al, 2002[26]	JALSG-93	All	**Donor (allogeneic)**	34	15–40			46%
			No donor (auto or chemo)	108	15–40			40%
Gupta et al, 2004[70]	Monocenter	All	**Donor (allogeneic)**	34	16–54	19%	40%	46%
			No donor (Chemo)	25	16–52	5%	39%	58%
Ueda et al, 1998[73]	JALSG-90	All	Allogeneic, if donor	17	15–45			41%
			No donor (chemo)	40	14–45			30%
Hunault et al, 2004[34]	GOELAL02	HR	**Donor (allogeneic)**	41	15–50	15%	72%	75%
			No donor (autologous)	115	15–59	3%	33%	39%
Attal et al, 1995[71]	BGMT		**Donor (allogeneic)**	43	15–55	12%	71%	
			No donor (autologous)	77	15–55	2%	30%	
Ribera et al, 2005[36]	PETHEMA93	HR	**Donor (allogeneic)**	84	15–50		33%	35%
			No donor (R)	98	15–50		39%	44%
			– **Autologous**	50	15–50		35%	37%
			– **Chemo**	48	15–50		44%	50%
Labar et al, 2004[27]	EORTC ALL-3	All	**Donor (allogeneic)**	68	15–50	24%	38%	41%
			No donor (R)	116		7%	37%	39%
			– Autologous	24			~35%	
			– Chemo	21			~35%	
Rowe et al, 2006[38]	ECOG-MRC	All	**Donor (allogeneic)**	388	15–50 (55)	39%HR 20%SR	50%	53%
			No donor (R)	527		n.r.	41%	45%
			Autologous	220	15–65	12% HR 7% SR	33%	37%
			Chemo	215	15–65	n.r.	42%	46%
Goldstone et al, 2004[47]			Allogeneic, unrelated (Ph+ ALL)	67	15–50 (55)	35%		46%

Abbreviations: R, randomized – patients without sibling donor were randomized between autologous SCT and chemotherapy; HR, high risk; bold, intent-to-treat analysis donor versus no donor; ~ estimated from curves.

The PETHEMA study for high-risk patients showed a trend towards an advantage for patients without donor.[36] In contrast, several other studies have demonstrated an advantage of SCT in high-risk patients.[33,34,69]

The large ECOG/MRC group recently reported their results comparing patients with a donor (allo sibling-SCT) to those without a donor (randomized comparison of chemotherapy and auto-SCT). The special feature of this trial was the use of age (greater than or less than 35 years) as a prognostic factor. Standard-risk patients were defined as younger than 35 years with a WBC <30,000/μl for B-precursor, and <100,000/μl for T-ALL and CR within 4 weeks. Patients with a donor had a superior OS (53%) compared to those without a donor (45%), mainly due to a lower RR (29% versus 54%). The difference was particularly evident in standard-risk (63% versus 51% OS) but not in high-risk (39% versus 36%) patients.[38] Since younger age was the

major factor for definition of standard risk, this result can be interpreted in two ways.[1] Outcome of SCT is better in younger patients, which is a well-known fact,[2] and outcome for young, standard-risk patients is similarly good with chemotherapy, as shown in other trials.

A third issue is the fact that the number of cases undergoing SCT was limited (321 allo-sibling SCTs out of 1508 evaluable patients) in this trial according to an earlier report.[47] The non-relapse mortality reached 20% even in standard-risk patients, and one should not therefore always undertake SCT in younger, standard-risk patients. This would also be in contrast to all other trials and to the successful pediatric approaches for adolescents and younger adults which mainly rely on intensive chemotherapy and not SCT, due to the acute mortality and long-term effects of the latter approach.[72] For older, high-risk patients, the results of the ECOG/MRC trial are somewhat disappointing, particularly the high mortality in CR of 39% which emphasizes the need to improve conditioning regimens and reduce pretransplant morbidity. The OS of 38% in this trial was similar to that of other studies.[28]

Chemotherapy or allo-SCT versus autologous SCT

No significant difference was detected in the comparison of chemotherapy and autologous SCT in several randomized studies.[25,27,33,36] In the large randomized ECOG/MRC trial, the outcome of auto-SCT was inferior (33%) compared to chemotherapy (42%) in terms of LFS, mainly due to a higher RR.[38] The major advantage of auto-SCT compared to chemotherapy is probably the shorter total therapy duration. Auto-SCT may be appropriate in patients with low MRD after induction or a MRD-negative stem cell graft and it provides the option of giving MRD-based maintenance therapy after auto-SCT.

All comparisons of allo- and auto-SCT show inferior outcomes for auto-SCT. In two trials with an intention-to-treat comparison, the results of auto-SCT were poor (30% and 33%).[34,71]

Indications for SCT in adult ALL

Evidence-based recommendations

A recently published evidence-based review emphasized the finding that SCT offers an advantage compared to chemotherapy in high-risk patients and in those in second remission. Other aspects of the review are summarized in Table 5.6. The analyses also revealed the lack of prospective, controlled trials for SCT in ALL.[74] This is probably due to the fact that every study design which includes SCT has, by definition, too many uncontrollable factors including donor availability, individual patient status and patient wishes. Not surprisingly, a meta-analysis of seven studies[26,27,33,34,36,69,75] showed a broad variation in terms of accomplishing the transplant; for allo-SCT 68–96% and auto-SCT 9–81%. The meta-analysis showed a correlation of outcome with compliance to allo-SCT. Again, OS with SCT was superior to that seen with chemotherapy, with a particular advantage in high-risk patients.[76] Thus, the role of allo-SCT in standard-risk ALL remains undefined.

Indications in clinical trials

Indications for SCT in first remission are not uniformly defined. The advantages of SCT (short treatment duration, favorable outcome in some trials) must be compared with the disadvantages (TRM, late complications, poorer quality of life). The major question is whether all patients with a sibling donor should undergo SCT, or only those with specific risk factors.

- *Risk-adapted* approach. In the majority of trials in Europe at present, SCT indications are based on the presence of adverse prognostic factors including MRD. Allo-sibling SCT and MUD SCT are considered in a similar way.
- *Fewer SCTs in young* adults. Although outcome after SCT is better in younger patients, there is a trend towards treating adolescents with pediatric-type intensive chemotherapy protocols and less transplantation.
- *MRD-based* indications. MRD status is of increasing importance when deciding whether SCT is indicated. Further studies will decide whether SCT is really a favorable option for patients with a high MRD load and whether patients with high-risk features but negative MRD status should still be candidates for SCT.
- *SCT after* relapse. There is general agreement that all patients in second or subsequent remission are candidates for SCT. Depending on donor availability and general condition of the patient, experimental procedures such as NMSCT, cord blood SCT and haploidentical SCT may be considered.

Table 5.7 outlines the indications for SCT in the German multicenter study group for adult ALL (GMALL) as an example of a risk-adapted approach.

Factors influencing outcome of SCT in ALL

Procedure-related factors

- The role of *stem cell source* remains open to question. For practical reasons, at present nearly all transplants rely on peripheral blood stem cells (PBSCT) and not bone marrow (BMT). Some data indicate, however, that the incidence of chronic GvHD is higher after PBSCT.[77] Another trial demonstrated better survivals with BMT compared to PBSCT (34% vs 24%).[78]
- There is no standard *preparative regimen* before SCT in ALL. Most regimens are based on total body irradiation (TBI). The usual dose is 12 Gy. TBI is most frequently combined with cyclophosphamide or VP16. A recent analysis of register patients showed no difference for sibling SCT with TBI/VP16 or TBI/cyclophosphamide in CR1. The VP16 combination was associated with a lower RR in second remission,[79] which may be due to superior antileukemia activity. Inferior results have been reported for busulfan-based preparative regimens compared to TBI-based regimens.[55,80] The advantage of TBI has also been reported for Ph+ ALL.[81]
- The *degree of acute and/or chronic GvHD* has an impact on outcome since it increases morbidity and mortality on the one hand and is associated with graft-versus-leukemia (GvL) effects on the other.[82,83] Patients without GvHD have a higher relapse risk, whereas patients with extensive GvHD have a higher TRM. Best results are obtained with limited GvHD.
- The use of female *donors* with male recipients is associated with inferior outcome and this probably also applies to older donors.

Table 5.6 Evidence-based recommendations for SCT in adult ALL[74]

Question	Recommendation
CR1: Allogeneic SCT versus chemotherapy	Comparable results SCT probably superior in high risk No SCT in standard risk
CR2: Allogeneic SCT versus chemotherapy	SCT superior
Autologous SCT versus chemotherapy	Comparable results
Sibling donor versus matched unrelated donor	Comparable results
Conditioning regimen	Data insufficient Advantage for TBI-based regimens
Allogeneic versus autologous SCT	Advantage for allogeneic SCT

Table 5.7 Indications for SCT in the GMALL trials

	Indication	Priorities*
First remission		
High risk	All patients within 3–4 months from diagnosis	1. Allogeneic sibling ** 2. Allogeneic unrelated ** 3. Autologous 4. NMSCT
Standard risk	Molecular non-responders	See above
Relapse, including molecular relapse	All patients in 2nd CR (or good PR or beginning to relapse)	See above (consider cord blood or haploidentical SCT if no donor available)

*Decision depends on age, patient's general condition and donor availability. **Matched or one mismatch.

Table 5.8 Prognostic factors for outcome after SCT

Prognostic factor	Favorable	Unfavorable
Risk group	Pro B-ALL* T-ALL*	B-Lineage-ALL with WBC >30,000* Ph/BCR-ABL+ ALL
Age	<35 years	>35 years
Stage of disease	First remission	Primary refractory ALL Relapsed ALL >= CR2
Minimal residual disease	MRD-negative	MRD-positive before SCT MRD-positive after SCT
GvHD post transplantation	Moderate	No GvHD Severe GvHD

* GMALL experience.

Table 5.9 Options for improvement of all SCT results in ALL

Allogeneic	
Reducing relapse rate	Optimized preparative regimen Use of GvL effects, e.g. by donor lymphocytes Therapy post transplantation based on MRD, e.g. monoclonal antibodies, chemotherapy, imatinib
Reduction of TRM	Improved prophylaxis of infections and GvHD Donor selection
Alternative approaches	Cord blood or hapoloidentical SCT in younger patients without a donor NMSCT in patients with contraindications

Autologous	
Reducing relapse rate	Optimized preparative regimen Intensified prior chemotherapy to reduce tumor load Maintenance therapy after transplantation

- The degree of *HLA compatibility* is associated with outcome with regard to TRM and RR. The lowest TRM is observed in syngeneic SCT from identical twins, although the relapse rate is higher in this situation.[84] Although no difference in outcome is expected for patients with fully matched donor compared to those with a one-antigen mismatch, TRM increases with the number of further mismatches.

Disease course after SCT

After transplantation, regular evaluation of *chimerism* and *MRD* is recommended in order to monitor the disease course. The degree of chimerism correlates with long-term outcome since an increasing amount is associated with the start of relapse.[85] The same is true for MRD analysis, where increasing MRD positivity is associated with impending overt relapse. At the start of relapse, immunologic treatments such as reduction in GvHD prophylaxis and/or administration of donor lymphocytes are promising approaches in the prevention of overt relapse.[86]

Host factors

Additional, transplant-specific factors may be defined which are associated with increased RR or TRM, aside from the factors which originally indicated SCT.

- *Higher age* is an unfavorable factor in all SCT studies. Nevertheless, there are no clear age cut-off points for sibling or unrelated SCT, which may be performed up to the age of 55 years, or even more with dose-reduced conditioning.
- *Advanced disease stage* (refractory/relapsed) is an unfavorable factor. For SCT in second or later remission outcome is inferior, as is the case for patients with early compared to late relapse.
- *Subgroups of ALL* result in differences in outcome. Whereas no overall difference in outcome can be observed for SCT in T-cell as compared to B-cell lineage ALL, the GMALL trials revealed significant survival differences for subgroups of high-risk ALL. The survival rates ranged between 18% for high-risk B-precursor ALL and 74% for pro-B-ALL,[39] and several trials have shown inferior results for Ph/BCR-ABL positive ALL.[65]

The most important prognostic factors for outcome of ALL after SCT are summarized in Table 5.8.

Future requirements for SCT

Large national and even international study groups are committed to the development of chemotherapy schedules and general treatment strategies for adult ALL. Similar multicenter trials are urgently required to prospectively evaluate the optimum integration of SCT into front-line therapy. One important point is the balance between efficacy and toxicity of treatment and the preparative regimen before SCT, in order to reduce TRM. The optimum timing of SCT must also be defined.

For an improvement of outcome after allogeneic SCT, reductions in RR as well as TRM are required. For patients without donor or with contraindications to conventional SCT, alternative approaches need to be explored.

MRD evaluation before and after SCT is essential, particularly in order to decide whether to give maintenance therapy, or immunotherapy such as donor lymphocyte infusions. The prophylactic use of donor lymphocytes may be considered in patients with no or low-level GvHD. They have also been successfully used in pediatric patients with increased MRD and/or a decrease in chimerism.[87] In adults who would be expected to have a poor outcome, long-term remissions have been obtained.[88] These and other options are summarized in Table 5.9.

References

1. Harris NL, Jaffe ES, Diebold J et al. The World Health Organization classification of neoplastic diseases of the haematopoietic and lymphoid tissues: Report of the Clinical Advisory Committee Meeting, Airlie House, Virginia, November 1997. Histopathology 2000;36:69–86
2. European Group for the Immunological Characterization of Leukemia (EGIL), Bene MC, Castoldi G et al. Proposals for the immunological classification of acute leukemias. Leukemia 1995;9:1783–1786
3. Armstrong SA, Look AT. Molecular genetics of acute lymphoblastic leukemia. J Clin Oncol 2005;23:6306–6315
4. Gökbuget N, Hoelzer D. Treatment of adult acute lymphoblastic leukemia. Hematol Am Soc Hematol Educ Program 2006;133–141
5. Mitchell CD, Richards SM, Kinsey SE et al. Benefit of dexamethasone compared with prednisolone for childhood acute lymphoblastic leukemia: results of the UK Medical Research Council ALL97 randomized trial. Br J Haematol 2005;129:734–745
6. Gökbuget N, Baur K-H, Beck J et al. Dexamethasone dose and schedule significantly influences remission rate and toxicity of induction therapy in adult acute lymphoblastic leukemia (ALL): results of the GMALL pilot trial 06/99. Blood 2005;106:1832
7. Kantarjian HM, O'Brien S, Smith TL et al. Results of treatment with hyper-CVAD, a dose-intensive regimen, in adult acute lymphocytic leukemia. J Clin Oncol 2000;18:547–561
8. Larson RA, Dodge RK, Linker CA et al. A randomized controlled trial of filgrastim during remission induction and consolidation chemotherapy for adults with acute lymphoblastic leukemia: CALGB study 9111. Blood 1998;92:1556–1564
9. Annino L, Vegna ML, Camera A et al. Treatment of adult acute lymphoblastic leukemia (ALL): long-term follow-up of the GIMEMA ALL 0288 randomized study. Blood 2002;99:863–871
10. Wassmann B, Pfeifer H, Gökbuget N et al. Alternating versus concurrent schedules of Imatinib and chemotherapy as front-line therapy for Philadelphia-positive acute lymphoblastic leukemia (Ph+ALL). Blood 2006;108:1469–1477
11. Bruggemann M, Raff T, Flohr T et al. Clinical significance of minimal residual disease quantification in adult patients with standard-risk acute lymphoblastic leukemia. Blood 2006;107:1116–1123
12. Pession A, Valsecchi MG, Masera G et al. Long-term results of a randomized trial on extended use of high dose L-asparaginase for standard risk childhood acute lymphoblastic leukemia. J Clin Oncol 2005;23:7161–7167
13. Moghrabi A, Levy DE, Asselin B et al. Results of the Dana-Farber Cancer Institute ALL Consortium Protocol 95–01 for children with acute lymphoblastic leukemia. Blood 2007;109:896–904

14. Kantarjian H, Thomas D, O'Brien S et al. Long-term follow-up results of hyperfractionated cyclophosphamide, vincristine, doxorubicin, and dexamethasone (Hyper-CVAD), a dose-intensive regimen, in adult acute lymphocytic leukemia. Cancer 2004;101:2788–2801

15. Ottmann OG, Druker BJ, Sawyers CL et al. A phase II study of imatinib mesylate (Glivec) in patients with relapsed or refractory Philadelphia chromosome-positive acute lymphoid leukemias. Blood 2002;100:1965–1971

16. Wassmann B, Pfeifer H, Scheuring U et al. Therapy with imatinib mesylate (Glivec) preceding allogeneic stem cell transplantation (SCT) in relapsed or refractory Philadelphia-positive acute lymphoblastic leukemia (Ph+ALL). Leukemia 2002;16:2358–2365

17. Thomas DA, Kantarjian H, Cortes J et al. Outcome with the Hyper-CVAD and imatinib mesylate regimen as frontline therapy for adult Philadelphia (Ph) positive acute lymphocytic leukemia (ALL). Blood 2006;108:284

18. Yanada M, Takeuchi J, Sugiura I et al. High complete remission rate and promising outcome by combination of imatinib and chemotherapy for newly diagnosed BCR-ABL-positive acute lymphoblastic leukemia: a phase II study by the Japan Adult Leukemia Study Group. J Clin Oncol 2006;24:460–466

19. de Labarthe A, Rousselot P, Huguet-Rigal F et al. Imatinib combined with induction or consolidation chemotherapy in patients with de novo Philadelphia chromosome-positive acute lymphoblastic leukemia: results of the GRAAPH-2003 study. Blood 2007;109:1408–1413

20. Vignetti M, Fazi P, Cimino G et al. Imatinib plus steroids induces complete remissions and prolonged survival in elderly Philadelphia chromosome-positive acute lymphoblastic leukemia patients without additional chemotherapy: results of the GIMEMA LAL0201-B protocol. Blood 2007;109(9):3676–3678

21. Ottmann OG, Wassmann B, Pfeifer H et al. Imatinib compared with chemotherapy as front-line treatment of elderly patients with Philadelphia chromosome-positive acute lymphoblastic leukemia (Ph+ALL). Cancer 2007;109:2068–2076

22. Kantarjian H, Giles F, Wunderle L et al. Nilotinib in imatinib-resistant CML and Philadelphia chromosome-positive ALL. N Engl J Med 2006;354:2542–2551

23. Talpaz M, Shah NP, Kantarjian H et al. Dasatinib in imatinib-resistant Philadelphia chromosome-positive leukemias. N Engl J Med 2006;354:2531–2541

24. Gökbuget N, Hoelzer D. Rituximab in the treatment of adult ALL. Ann Hematol 2006;85:117–119

25. Thiebaut A, Vernant JP, Degos L et al. Adult acute lymphocytic leukemia study testing chemotherapy and autologous and allogeneic transplantation. A follow-up report of the French protocol LALA 87. Hematol Oncol Clin North Am 2000;14:1353–1366

26. Takeuchi J, Kyo T, Naito K et al. Induction therapy by frequent administration of doxorubicin with four other drugs, followed by intensive consolidation and maintenance therapy for adult acute lymphoblastic leukemia: the JALSG-ALL93 study. Leukemia 2002;16:1259–1266

27. Labar B, Suciu S, Zittoun R et al. Allogeneic stem cell transplantation in acute lymphoblastic leukemia and non-Hodgkin's lymphoma for patients > or =50 years old in first complete remission: results of the EORTC ALL-3 trial. Haematologica 2004;89:809–817

28. Rowe JM, Buck G, Burnett AK et al. Induction therapy for adults with acute lymphoblastic leukemia: results of more than 1500 patients from the international ALL trial: MRC UKALL XII/ECOG E2993. Blood 2005;106:3760–3767

29. Bassan R, Pogliani E, Casula P et al. Risk-oriented postremission strategies in adult acute lymphoblastic leukemia: prospective confirmation of anthracycline activity in standard-risk class and role of hematopoietic stem cell transplants in high-risk groups. Hematol J 2001;2:117–126

30. Gökbuget N, Arnold R, Buechner Th et al. Intensification of induction and consolidation improves only subgroups of adult ALL: analysis of 1200 patients in GMALL study 05/93. Blood 2001;98:802a

31. Linker C, Damon L, Ries C, Navarro W. Intensified and shortened cyclical chemotherapy for adult acute lymphoblastic leukemia. J Clin Oncol 2002;20:2464–2471

32. Hallbook H, Simonsson B, Ahlgren T et al. High-dose cytarabine in upfront therapy for adult patients with acute lymphoblastic leukemia. Br J Haematol 2002;118:748–754

33. Thomas X, Boiron JM, Huguet F et al. Outcome of treatment in adults with acute lymphoblastic leukemia: analysis of the LALA-94 trial. J Clin Oncol 2004;22:4075–4086

34. Hunault M, Harousseau JL, Delain M et al. Better outcome of adult acute lymphoblastic leukemia after early genoidentical allogeneic bone marrow transplantation (BMT) than after late high-dose therapy and autologous BMT: a GOELAMS trial. Blood 2004;104:3028–3037

35. Mancini M. An integrated molecular-cytogenetic classification is highly predictive of outcome in adult acute lymphoblastic leukemia (ALL): analysis of 395 cases enrolled in the GIMEMA 0496 Trial. Blood 2001;98:3492a

36. Ribera JM, Oriol A, Bethencourt C et al. Comparison of intensive chemotherapy, allogeneic or autologous stem cell transplantation as post-remission treatment for adult patients with high-risk acute lymphoblastic leukemia. Results of the PETHEMA ALL-93 trial. Haematologica 2005;90:1346–1356

37. Pui CH, Evans WE. Treatment of acute lymphoblastic leukemia. N Engl J Med 2006;354:166–178

38. Goldstone AH, Richards SM, Lazarus HM et al. In adults with standard-risk acute lymphoblastic leukemia, the greatest benefit is achieved from a matched sibling allogeneic transplantation in first complete remission, and an autologous transplantation is less effective than conventional consolidation/maintenance chemotherapy in all patients: final results of the International ALL Trial (MRC UKALL XII/ECOG E2993). Blood 2008;111(4):1827–1833

39. Arnold R, Beelen D, Bunjes D et al. Phenotype predicts outcome after allogeneic stem cell transplantation in adult high risk ALL patients. Blood 2003;102:1719

40. Hoelzer D, Gökbuget N. New approaches in acute lymphoblastic leukemia in adults: where do we go? Semin Oncol 2000;27:540–559

41. Grabher C, von BH, Look AT. Notch 1 activation in the molecular pathogenesis of T-cell acute lymphoblastic leukemia. Nat Rev Cancer 2006;6:347–359

42. Vitale A, Guarini A, Ariola C et al. Adult T-cell acute lymphoblastic leukemia: biologic profile at presentation and correlation with response to induction treatment in patients enrolled in the GIMEMA LAL 0496 protocol. Blood 2006;107:473–479

43. Asnafi V, Buzyn A, Thomas X et al. Impact of TCR status and genotype on outcome in adult T-cell acute lymphoblastic leukemia: a LALA-94 study. Blood 2005;105:3072–3078

44. Mortuza FY, Moreira I, Papaioannou M et al. Immunoglobulin heavy chain gene rearrangement in adult acute lymphoblastic leukemia reveals preference of JH-proximal variable gene segments. Blood 2002;97:2716–2726

45. Gökbuget N, Raff R, Brugge-Mann M et al. Risk/MRD adapted GMALL trials in adult ALL. Ann Hematol 2004;83(suppl 1):S129-S131

46. Raff T, Gökbuget N, Luschen S et al. Molecular relapse in adult standard risk ALL patients detected by prospective MRD-monitoring during and after maintenance treatment data from the GMALL 06/99 and 07/03 trials. Blood 2007;109(3):910–915

47. Goldstone AH, Lazarus HJ, Richards SM et al. The outcome of 551 1st CR transplants in adult ALL from the UKALL XII/ECOG 2993 Study. Blood 2004;104:615

48. Loberiza F. Summary slides 2003 – part III. IMBTR/ABMTR Newsletter 2006;10:6–9

49. Frassoni F, Labopin M, Gluckman E et al. Results of allogeneic bone marrow transplantation for acute leukemia have improved in Europe with time – a report of the Acute Leukemia Working Party of the European Group for Blood and Marrow Transplantation (EBMT). Bone Marrow Transplant 1996;17:13–18

50. Chao MJ, Forman SJ, Schmidt GM et al. Allogeneic bone marrow transplantation for high-risk acute lymphoblastic leukemia during first complete remission. Blood 1991;78:1923–1927

51. Snyder DSN. Fractionated total body irradiation and high-dose etoposide as a preparatory regimen for bone marrow transplantation for 99 patients with acute leukemia in first complete remission. Blood 1993;82:2920–2928

52. Jamieson CH, Amylon MD, Wong RM, Blume KG. Allogeneic hematopoietic cell transplantation for patients with high-risk acute lymphoblastic leukemia in first or second complete remission using fractionated total-body irradiation and high-dose etoposide: a 15-year experience. Exp Hematol 2003;31:981–986

53. Cornelissen JJ, Carston M, Kollman C et al. Unrelated marrow transplantation for adult patients with poor-risk acute lymphoblastic leukemia: strong graft-versus-leukemia effect and risk factors determining outcome. Blood 2001;97:1572–1577

54. Cornelissen JJ, Carston M, Kollman C et al. Unrelated marrow transplantation for adult patients with poor-risk acute lymphoblastic leukemia: strong graft-versus-leukemia effect and risk factors determining outcome. Blood 2001;97:1572–1577

55. Kiehl MG, Kraut L, Schwerdtfeger R et al. Outcome of allogeneic hematopoietic stem-cell transplantation in adult patients with acute lymphoblastic leukemia: no difference in related compared with unrelated transplant in first complete remission. J Clin Oncol 2004;22:2816–2825

56. Arnold R, Bunjes D, Ehninger G et al. Allogeneic stem cell transplantation from HLA-identical sibling donor in high risk ALL patients is less effective than transplantation from unrelated donors. Blood 2002;100:77a

57. Powles R, Sirohi B, Treleaven J et al. The role of posttransplantation maintenance chemotherapy in improving the outcome of autotransplantation in adult acute lymphoblastic leukemia. Blood 2002;100:1641–1647

58. Arnold R, Massenkeil G, Bornhauser M et al. Nonmyeloablative stem cell transplantation in adults with high-risk ALL may be effective in early but not in advanced disease. Leukemia 2002;16:2423–2428

59. Mohty M, Labopin M, Boiron J-M et al. Reduced intensity conditioning (RIC) allogeneic stem cell transplantation (allo-SCT) for patients with acute lymphoblastic leukemia (ALL): a survey from the European Group for Blood and Marrow Transplantation (EBMT). Blood 2005;106:659

60. Tse W, Laughlin MJ. Umbilical cord blood transplantation: a new alternative option. Hematol Am Soc Hematol Educ Program 2005;377–383

61. Eapen M, Rubinstein P, Zhang MJ et al. Outcomes of transplantation of unrelated donor umbilical cord blood and bone marrow in children with acute leukemia: a comparison study. Lancet 2007;369:1947–1954

62. Rocha V, Labopin M, Sanz G et al. Transplants of umbilical-cord blood or bone marrow from unrelated donors in adults with acute leukemia. N Engl J Med 2004;351:2276–2285

63. Klingebiel T, Handgretinger R, Lang P et al. Haploidentical transplantation for acute lymphoblastic leukemia in childhood. Blood Rev 2004;18:181–192

64. Singhal S, Henslee-Downey PJ, Powles R et al. Haploidentical vs autologous hematopoietic stem cell transplantation in patients with acute leukemia beyond first remission. Bone Marrow Transplant 2003;31:889–895

65. Avivi I, Goldstone AH. Bone marrow transplant in Ph+ ALL patients. Bone Marrow Transplant 2003;31:623–632

66. Lee S, Kim YJ, Min CK et al. The effect of first-line imatinib interim therapy on the outcome of allogeneic stem cell transplantation in adults with newly diagnosed Philadelphia chromosome-positive acute lymphoblastic leukemia. Blood 2005;105:3449–3457

67. Wassmann B, Pfeifer H, Stadler M et al. Early molecular response to posttransplantation imatinib determines outcome in MRD+ Philadelphia-positive acute lymphoblastic leukemia (Ph+ ALL). Blood 2005;106:458–463

68. Fiere D, Lepage E, Sebban C et al. Adult acute lymphoblastic leukemia: a multicentric randomized trial testing bone marrow transplantation as postremission therapy. J Clin Oncol 1993;11:1990–2001

69. Sebban C, Lepage E, Vernant J-P et al. Allogeneic bone marrow transplantation in adult acute lymphoblastic leukemia in first complete remission: a comparative study. J Clin Oncol 1994;12:2580–2587

70. Gupta V, Yi QL, Brandwein J et al. The role of allogeneic bone marrow transplantation in adult patients below the age of 55 years with acute lymphoblastic leukemia in first complete remission: a donor vs no donor comparison. Bone Marrow Transplant 2004;33:397–404

71. Attal M, Blaise D, Marit G et al. Consolidation treatment of adult acute lymphoblastic leukemia: a prospective, randomized trial comparing allogeneic versus autologous bone marrow transplantation and testing the impact of recombinant interleukin-2 after autologous bone marrow transplantation. Blood 1995;86:1619–1628

72. Sallan SE. Myths and lessons from the adult/pediatric interface in acute lymphoblastic leukemia. Hematol Am Soc Hematol Educ Program 2006;128–132

73. Ueda T, Miyawaki S, Asou N et al. Response-oriented individualized induction therapy with six drugs followed by four courses of intensive consolidation, 1 year maintenance and intensification therapy: the ALL90 study of the Japan Adult Leukemia Study Group. Int J Hematol 1998;68:279–289

74. Hahn T, Wall D, Camitta B et al. The role of cytotoxic therapy with hematopoietic stem cell transplantation in the therapy of acute lymphoblastic leukemia in adults: an evidence-based review. Biol Blood Marrow Transplant 2006;12:1–30

75. Dombret H, Gabert J, Boiron JM et al. Outcome of treatment in adults with Philadelphia chromosome-positive acute lymphoblastic leukemia – results of the prospective multicenter LALA-94 trial. Blood 2002;100:2357–2366

76. Yanada M, Matsuo K, Suzuki T, Naoe T. Allogeneic hematopoietic stem cell transplantation as part of postremission therapy improves survival for adult patients with high-risk acute lymphoblastic leukemia: a metaanalysis. Cancer 2006;106:1657–1663

77. Ringden O, Labopin M, Bacigalupo A et al. Transplantation of peripheral blood stem cells as compared with bone marrow from HLA-identical siblings in adult patients with acute myeloid leukemia and acute lymphoblastic leukemia. J Clin Oncol 2002;20:4655–4664

78. Garderet L, Labopin M, Gorin NC et al. Patients with acute lymphoblastic leukemia allografted with a matched unrelated donor may have a lower survival with a peripheral blood stem cell graft compared to bone marrow. Bone Marrow Transplant 2003;31:23–29

79. Marks DI, Forman SJ, Blume KG et al. A comparison of cyclophosphamide and total body irradiation with etoposide and total body irradiation as conditioning regimens for patients undergoing sibling allografting for acute lymphoblastic leukemia in first or second complete remission. Biol Blood Marrow Transplant 2006;12:438–453

80. Davies SM, Ramsay NK, Klein JP et al. Comparison of preparative regimens in transplants for children with acute lymphoblastic leukemia. J Clin Oncol 2000;18:340–347

81. Yanada M, Naoe T, Iida H et al. Myeloablative allogeneic hematopoietic stem cell transplantation for Philadelphia chromosome-positive acute lymphoblastic leukemia in adults: significant roles of total body irradiation and chronic graft-versus-host disease. Bone Marrow Transplant 2005;36:867–872

82. Nordlander A, Mattsson J, Ringden O et al. Graft-versus-host disease is associated with a lower relapse incidence after hematopoietic stem cell transplantation in patients with acute lymphoblastic leukemia. Biol Blood Marrow Transplant 2004;10:195–203

83. Yanada M, Naoe T, Iida H et al. Myeloablative allogeneic hematopoietic stem cell transplantation for Philadelphia chromosome-positive acute lymphoblastic leukemia in adults: significant roles of total body irradiation and chronic graft-versus-host disease. Bone Marrow Transplant 2005;36:867–872

84. Gale RP, Horowitz MM, Ash RC et al. Identical-twin bone marrow transplants for leukemia. Ann Intern Med 1994;120:646–652

85. Bader P, Niethammer D, Willasch A et al. How and when should we monitor chimerism after allogeneic stem cell transplantation? Bone Marrow Transplant 2005;35:107–119

86. Schilham MW, Balduzzi A, Bader P. Is there a role for minimal residual disease levels in the treatment of ALL patients who receive allogeneic stem cells? Bone Marrow Transplant 2005;35(suppl 1):S49-S52

87. Bader P, Kreyenberg H, Hoelle W et al. Increasing mixed chimerism is an important prognostic factor for unfavorable outcome in children with acute lymphoblastic leukemia after allogeneic stem-cell transplantation: possible role for pre-emptive immunotherapy? J Clin Oncol 2004;22:1696–1705

88. Massenkeil G, Nagy M, Lawang M et al. Reduced intensity conditioning and prophylactic DLI can cure patients with high-risk acute leukemias if complete donor chimerism can be achieved. Bone Marrow Transplant 2003;31:339–345

Childhood leukemias

Kristin Baird and Alan S Wayne

CHAPTER

6

Introduction

As a group, childhood leukemias represent the most common pediatric malignancy, accounting for approximately 32% of cancer in children younger than 15 years and 25% under 20 years of age (Fig. 6.1). Acute lymphocytic leukemia (ALL) is by far the most common, comprising approximately 23% of childhood cancer with an annual rate of 30–40 new cases per million US children. Acute myeloid leukemia (AML) accounts for approximately 4% of pediatric cancer diagnoses and 20% of childhood leukemia, with an annual rate in the US of 8 per million. Philadelphia chromosome positive (Ph+) chronic myelogenous leukemia (CML) is rare, and accounts for approximately 1% of all pediatric cancer, although it comprises 10% of leukemia in older adolescents. Juvenile myelomonocytic leukemia (JMML) is infrequent, making up about 2% of leukemia and 25% of myelodysplastic syndrome in childhood, three-quarters of which is in children under 3 years of age (Fig. 6.2).[1] Epidemiologic features of leukemia in childhood are summarized in Table 6.1.

Although the majority of pediatric patients with hematologic malignancies are cured, leukemia remains the most frequent cause of death from cancer in children (Fig. 6.3).[1] Allogeneic stem cell transplantation (SCT) plays an important role in the curative management of children with hematologic malignancies. This chapter reviews the approach to transplantation in the treatment of leukemia and myelodysplastic syndrome (MDS) in pediatrics.

Acute lymphocytic leukemia

There are approximately 2400 children and adolescents younger than 20 years diagnosed with ALL each year in the US. The peak incidence of ALL occurs among children aged 2–7 years. An increased risk is associated with several genetic and non-genetic risk factors and conditions (see Table 6.1).[1–5]

Classification

Classification of pediatric ALL was formerly based on morphology according to the French-American-British (FAB) system, which defined three categories (L1, L2, L3).[6] Only the latter is of clinical and prognostic significance, as L3 morphology is indicative of mature B-cell or Burkitt-type ALL. Currently, phenotypic classification is determined by flow cytometry based on lineage and stage of differentiation, as reflected by cell surface markers. The majority of ALL is of precursor B-cell (pre-B) phenotype (CD10, CD19, HLA-DR, TDT +), 10–20% is T-cell (CD2, CD3, CD5 and/or CD7+), and <5% is mature B-cell or Burkitt-type (CD20, surface-IgM+) (Table 6.2).

Prognostic variables and risk stratification

Clinical and biologic features are used to stratify risk and direct treatment (Table 6.3). Initial risk group assignment is based on age, peripheral white blood cell count (WBC), central nervous system (CNS) status, and phenotype determined at diagnosis.[7] CNS status is divided into three categories: CNS-1 (<5 WBC/μl, no blasts), CNS-2 (<5 WBC/μl, with blasts) and CNS-3 ($\geq$5 WBC/μl with blasts). Those patients with a CNS category of 2 or 3 are at increased risk of relapse, including those with a traumatic diagnostic lumbar puncture at diagnosis.[8–12]

Cytogenetic studies are subsequently utilized to further assign risk group. Leukemic blasts usually contain genetic alterations, including recurring chromosomal translocations, gene rearrangements, activating mutations, hyperdiploidy and hypodiploidy. The most common of these is the t(12;21) TEL-AML1 gene fusion, which is found in approximately 25% of cases and is associated with a favorable prognosis.[13–16] 11q23 *MLL* gene rearrangements and the t(9;22) confer extremely poor prognosis.[17–22] The t(1;19) E2A-PBX1 translocation is also associated with an increased risk of relapse, but this can be offset by therapy intensification.[23,24] Hyperdiploidy carries a favorable prognosis,[25,26] as does triple trisomy of chromosomes 4, 10 and 7.[25,27–29] Leukemias that are hypodiploid are at higher risk of treatment failure.[30–33]

The final prognostic indicator used in risk stratification and determination of therapy is that of early response to therapy. Patients with a rapid early response (RER) to therapy, defined as a marrow blast count below 5% within 7–14 days, or clearance of peripheral blasts within 7–10 days, have a better outcome than do those whose response is slower (SER).[34–40]

Recently, cDNA microarray gene expression analysis has been shown to allow further discrimination in regard to risk classification and treatment response prediction.[41]

Treatment

Approximately 80% of children with ALL are cured with chemotherapy.[42] The intensity of treatment is determined by risk assessment of prognostic variables. Treatment for B-precursor and T-cell ALL is stratified based on phenotype and prognostic factors (see Table 6.3) and consists of induction, consolidation/intensification/reinduction, CNS sterilization, and maintenance for a total of 2–3 years.[43–50] This stratified approach has lessened toxicity for patients at lower risk of relapse and improved disease-free survival (DFS) for those in higher risk groups. The majority of patients fall into the standard risk

Table 6.1 Epidemiologic features of childhood leukemia in the US

	ALL	AML	JMML
Male:female	1.3:1 4:1 T-ALL	1:1	2:1
Race	White:black 2:1 Hispanic increased risk	Hispanic increased risk	
Predisposing conditions	Trisomy 21 (15-fold risk); neurofibromatosis-1; chromosomal breakage and immunodeficiency disorders (e.g. ataxia-telangiectasia, Bloom's syndrome, Shwachman–Diamond's syndrome); Langerhans cell histiocytosis; Li-Fraumeni syndrome; Klinefelter's syndrome	Trisomy 21 (50-fold risk AML, 500-fold risk megakaryoblastic), chromosomal breakage and immunodeficiency disorders (e.g. Fanconi anemia 15,000-fold risk, Bloom's syndrome, ataxia-telangiectasia; Shwachman–Diamond's syndrome, Kostmann's syndrome); Klinefelter's syndrome; neurofibromatosis-1; aplastic anemia treated with immunosuppression; paroxysmal nocturnal hemoglobinuria; myelodysplastic syndrome; familial monosomy 7	Neurofibromatosis-1 (500-fold risk); Noonan's syndrome; monosomy-7
Environmental factors	Radiation Higher socio-economic status	Epipodophyllotoxins, alkylating agents, radiation	

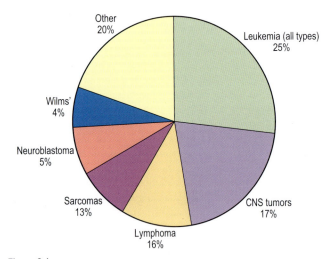

Figure 6.1
Distribution of cancer types in children. Data from NCI SEER Program 1975–1995 for children <20 years of age.[1]

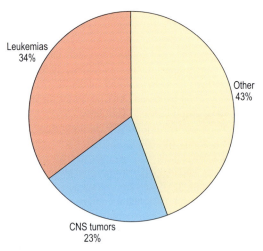

Figure 6.3
Distribution of cancer-associated mortality in children. Data from NCI SEER Program 1975–1995 for children <20 years of age.[1]

Table 6.2 Classification of ALL by cell surface markers by flow cytometry

	CD19	CD10	cIg	sIg	%
Pre pre-B cell	+	–	–	–	5
Early pre-B cell	+	+	–	–	63
Pre-B cell	+	+	+	–	16
Mature B cell	+	+/–	+	+	4
T-cell	–	–	–	–	12

Abbreviations: cIg, cytoplasmic immunoglobulin; sIg, surface immunoglobulin.

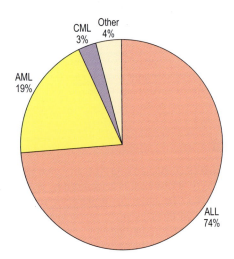

Figure 6.2
Distribution of leukemia subtypes in children. Data from NCI SEER Program 1975–1995 for children <20 years of age.[1]

Table 6.3 Prognostic factors in childhood B-precursor ALL

	Standard risk	High risk	Very high risk
Age (years)	1–9	≥10	<1
WBC	<50,000/µl	≥50,000/µl	
CNS	Negative	Positive	
Chromosomes	t(12;21), Double or triple trisomy 4/10/17	11q23, t(1;19)	t(9;22)
DNA Index	≥1.16 ≤1.60		<1
Initial treatment response	Rapid	Slow	Induction failure

category: age 1–9 years, WBC <50,000 and absence of high-risk chromosomal abnormalities.[7] Therapy for these patients typically consists of a 1-month induction phase with prednisone or dexamethasone, vincristine and L-asparaginase in combination with intrathecal chemotherapy. High-risk patients have an anthracycline and/or cyclophosphamide added to this regimen. The majority of patients, >95%, will go into remission with induction. This is then followed by an approximately 3-month intensification or consolidation phase. There is more variability in treatment regimen at this phase, but typically therapy includes methotrexate (MTX) (high- or intermediate- dose), L-asparaginase, dexamethasone, vincristine, 6-mercaptopurine (6-MP), and intrathecal chemotherapy. This is then followed by a maintenance or continuation phase. Maintenance therapy typically consists of daily oral 6-MP and weekly oral MTX. Patients also receive vincristine and steroid pulses on a monthly basis, as well as continued intermittent intrathecal therapy. Cranial irradiation is reserved for those patients with CNS disease at diagnosis and is usually administered during the consolidation phase of therapy. Males with overt testes involvement require bilateral testicular irradiation.

Finally, individuals with mature B-cell phenotype are treated according to Burkitt lymphoma regimens, which most commonly employ dose- and sequence-intensive, short-course combination chemotherapy.[51–53]

Outcome after relapse

The prognosis for a child with relapsed ALL depends on the timing and site of relapse.[54] Those with a short first remission (CR1) duration (<12–18 months) and those who relapse within the first year of completion of front-line chemotherapy have lower DFS in comparison to those with later relapse. A study from the Children's Oncology Group (COG) evaluated 214 patients with ALL and early marrow relapse within 12 months of completion of primary therapy. More than 50% of patients died, failed reinduction or relapsed within 3 months. Those with B-precursor phenotype and longer CR1 duration had the best DFS. Patients with T-cell ALL and those unable to achieve a second remission had the poorest outcome.[55] The efficacy of chemotherapy in the management of relapse also varies based on the intensity of the initial treatment. Thus, children who receive low-intensity primary therapy and have late relapses are more likely to achieve long-term DFS with chemotherapy.[56,57] Those with isolated extramedullary relapse also fare better than those with marrow relapse.[58,59]

The role of transplantation in ALL

There have been no large, prospective, randomized, controlled clinical trials to definitively evaluate the role of SCT versus chemotherapy in the management of childhood ALL. This is due in part to the success of standard front-line chemotherapy and the inherent variability in stem cell donor availability. Nonetheless, multiple comparative studies indicate that relapse rates are lower after allogeneic SCT in comparison to chemotherapy.[60] Some of this advantage, however, is offset by transplant-associated morbidity and mortality.[61] Consequently, SCT is usually reserved for the management of relapsed ALL and it is rarely employed for children in CR1 except for those with very high risk features, most notably the t(9;22) translocation (see Table 6.3). A suggested approach to the use of SCT in childhood ALL is presented in Figures 6.4 and 6.5, although it is acknowledged that practice will differ in individual cases based on risk/benefit analysis and donor options, as well as financial and technology access considerations. The American Society for Blood and Marrow Transplantation (ASBMT) recently performed an exhaustive review of the published literature and established consensus guidelines for the use of SCT in pediatric ALL (Table 6.4).[18,60–67]

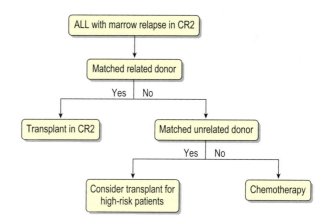

Figure 6.4
ALL: schema for transplantation in second remission. *See text for those patients considered high risk.

Figure 6.5
ALL: schema for transplantation in first remission. *See text and Table 6.3 for those patients considered very high risk.

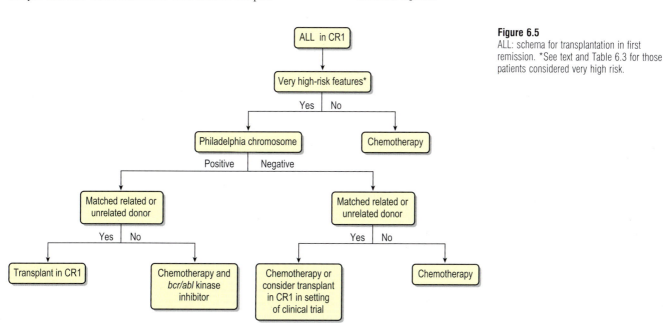

Table 6.4 Treatment recommendations for pediatric ALL[60]

Recommendation	Indication	References
SCT in CR1	Benefit demonstrated for matched related donor SCT for Philadelphia chromosome + only. Not recommended for other high-risk patients, except in the setting of a clinical trial.	Wheeler 2000[62] Chessells 1992[63] Arico 2000[18] Uderzo 1997[64]
SCT in CR2 with prior bone marrow relapse	Recommended for those with matched related donors. Evidence insufficient to recommend unrelated donor SCT.	Barrett 1994[61] Wheeler 1998[65] Uderzo 1995[66] Harrison 2000[67]

Table 6.5 Results of SCT trials for pediatric patients with ALL in second remission

Study group	Dates of study	Patients (n)	Outcome (years)	Reference
BFM	1985–91	51 MRD	52% EFS (5)	Dopfer 1991[68]
IBMTR/POG	1983–91	255 MRD 255 chemo	40% DFS (5) 17% DFS (5)	Barrett 1994[61]
Leiden	1982–91	25 MRD 97 chemo	44% DFS (4) 24% DFS (4)	Hoogerbrugge 1995[69]
AIEOP/GITMO	1980–90	57 MRD 230 chemo	41% DFS (5) 21% DFS (5)	Uderzo 1995[66]
Paris	1983–93	42 MRD	53% (4)	Moussalem 1995[70]
UKALL-X	1985–90	83 MRD, 27 MUD 61 ABMT 261 chemo	40% EFS (5) 34% EFS (5) 26% EFS (5)	Wheeler 1998[65]
UKALL-R1	1991–95	63 MRD 41 MUD 15 ABMT, 89 chemo	46% EFS (5) 54% EFS (5) 43% EFS (5)	Harrison 2000[67]
IBMTR/COG	1991–97	CR1 <36 months 92 MRD + TBI 19 MRD no TBI 110 chemo CR1 ≥36 months 61 MRD + TBI 14 MRD no TBI 78 Chemo	32% OS (8) 44% OS (8) 18% OS (8) 66% OS (8) 63% OS (8) 32% OS (8)	Eapen 2006[71]
COG	1995–98	32 MRD 19 MUD 23 chemo	42% DFS (3) 29% DFS (3) 30% DFS (3)	Gaynon 2006[55]

Abbreviations: chemo, chemotherapy; MUD, matched unrelated donor; MRD, matched related donor; EFS, event-free survival; DFS, disease-free survival; OS, overall survival; ABMT, autologous bone marrow transplant; TBI, total body irradiation.

SCT in CR2

Results of recent studies of SCT for pediatric patients with ALL in second remission are presented in Table 6.5.[55,61,65–71] For children who have an HLA-matched sibling donor, allogeneic SCT in second marrow remission is considered standard. Unrelated donor SCT is usually reserved for those at high risk of relapse with second-line chemotherapy regimens, see below (see Fig. 6.4).

A retrospective matched cohort analysis performed by the COG and International Bone Marrow Transplant Registry (IBMTR) compared matched related marrow transplantation versus chemotherapy for children with ALL in second remission. SCT was superior (leukemia-free survival and relapse rates) to chemotherapy in all patient groups irrespective of the CR1 duration.[61] In a more recent study from the COG and IBMTR, overall survival, leukemia-free survival and treatment-related mortality were superior for transplantation utilizing total body

irradiation (TBI) over both chemotherapy and non-TBI transplant regimens for patients who had experienced an early relapse (<36 months CR1 duration). For those with a late (≥36 months CR1 duration) relapse, survival rates were equivalent in both the chemotherapy and TBI transplant groups. The non-TBI transplant group had inferior outcomes for both early and late relapse.[71]

Despite the apparent reduction in relapse associated with SCT, the overall advantage of this approach must take into account transplant-associated risks of morbidity (e.g. graft-versus-host disease (GvHD)) and mortality, as well as the expected outcome after chemotherapy alone. When relapse occurs late (i.e. >36 months CR1 duration) approximately one-third of patients may achieve long-term DFS using aggressive chemotherapy alone.[55,61,72,73] This, of course, also incurs risks of toxicity.[74] In addition, salvage rates are expected to decline as more effective front-line regimens are employed.

Thus, decisions about the use and timing of SCT for children with relapsed ALL are commonly individualized based on specific biologic, clinical, treatment and donor factors (see Fig. 6.4). Transplant is commonly recommended for children with relapse who have available HLA-matched related donors, irrespective of underlying prognostic factors. However, an alternative approach for those with a long CR1 duration is to reserve SCT for subsequent relapse. The risks of transplant-related morbidity and mortality are increased with alternative donors (unrelated and HLA-mismatched related). Consequently, such transplants are often reserved for those who have other adverse prognostic risk factors. For patients with recurrence in the bone marrow either during front-line therapy or within 6 months of completion of initial therapy, the prognosis for long-term survival is poor using chemotherapy alone and SCT with an alternative donor should be strongly considered. SCT should also be considered for patients with T-cell ALL and marrow relapse at any time. Additional factors that place an individual patient at high risk of subsequent relapse (e.g. Ph+) or that limit the ability to administer chemotherapy (e.g. allergy, organ toxicity) also warrant consideration of SCT.

SCT in CR1

SCT in first remission has not been proven to benefit patients defined as high risk by WBC count and age. However, for those with a low probability of long-term remission (i.e. very high risk) with existing therapy, such as those with t(9;22), hypodiploidy and those with failure to achieve remission with induction therapy, SCT from an HLA-matched sibling is commonly considered (see Fig. 6.5, Table 6.3). In patients with Ph+ ALL, SCT from a matched sibling donor improves outcome in comparison to standard chemotherapy (Table 6.6).[18,62,64,75–79] The role of SCT for the other very high-risk groups is still under debate and should be considered in the setting of a clinical trial.[60] Transplant from an unrelated donor in the very high-risk setting is less certain. However, recent improvements in HLA matching and GvHD prophylaxis have resulted in better outcomes, which might be expected to change risk analysis in the future.[80]

The role of SCT for infants with ALL, and in particular those with MLL-rearrangements, remains somewhat controversial, in part because of the adverse effects of transplant conditioning on these very young patients. Some case series have suggested that outcomes following SCT in first remission may be superior to chemotherapy.[48,81–83] However, others show no definitive benefit when compared to intensive chemotherapy without transplant.[17] Recent studies suggest that distinct risk stratification can be achieved within this group, optimizing treatment choice and outcome.[84] A recent study from Japan found infants with a germline MLL gene to have a 95% event-free survival (EFS) with intensive chemotherapy alone,[85] which is in stark contrast to published experience with unselected infants with MLL-associated ALL.[86,87] In 2006, the IBMTR published results of a study evaluating

Table 6.6 Results of SCT trials for pediatric patients with ALL in first remission

Study group	Dates of study	High risk indicator	Patients (n)	Outcome (years)	Reference
Toronto	1985–2001	t(9;22)	11 MRD, MUD 10 chemo	53% EFS (4)	Sharathkumar 2004[75]
UKALL -X UKALL -XI	1985–90 1990–97	WBC >100,000/μl +/– t(9;22), Near-haploid, Induction failure	76 MRD, 25 MUD 351 chemo	45% EFS (10) 39% EFS (10)	Wheeler 2000[62]
AIEOP/GITMO	1986–94	WBC >100,000/μl BFM risk index >1.7 t(9;22), t(8;11) Steroid resistance T-cell disease, Induction failure	30 MRD 130 chemo	58% DFS (4) 48% DFS (4)	Uderzo 1997[64]
NOPHO	1981–91	WBC >100,000/μl	22 MRD 44 chemo* 405 chemo†	73% DFS (10) 50% DFS (10) 59% DFS (10)	Saarinen 1996[76]
IBMTR	1978–90	t(9;22)	33 MRD	38% DFS (2)	Barrett 1992[77]
Groupe d'Etude de la Greffe de Moelle Osseuse	1980–87	t(9;22) WBC >100,000/μl Induction failure	32 MRD	84% DFS (2.5)	Bordigoni 1989[78]

Abbreviations: chemo, chemotherapy; EFS, event-free survival; DFS, disease-free survival.
* Matched control patients; † unmatched patients.

outcomes of unrelated bone marrow and cord blood in comparison to HLA-matched sibling donor SCT in infants <18 months old. High transplant mortality rates were seen with the unrelated stem cell sources. In particular, cord blood recipients had a TRM rate of 31%. Relapse rates were lower for unrelated donor transplants; however, this advantage was lost for patients with a higher disease burden at the time of transplant. The only factor to correlate with overall survival was disease status at the time of transplant, and 3-year probabilities of leukemia-free survival were 49% and 54% after HLA-matched sibling and unrelated donor transplantation in CR1, respectively.[88]

Conditioning regimens

Several studies indicate that transplant conditioning regimens which include TBI produce higher cure rates for pediatric ALL than chemotherapy-only preparative regimens and this is the recommended approach.[60,71,89,90] However, irradiation has a variety of long-term effects on growth, endocrine function, neurocognitive function and cataract development. Nonetheless, chemotherapy-only regimens (e.g. busulfan/cyclophosphamide) are also associated with a variety of toxicities.[91] Treatment-related mortality from busulfan appears to be less in pediatrics than in adult patients, and monitoring of serum busulfan levels may lead to better outcomes.[92,93] Notably, second SCT using TBI has been successfully employed for patients with relapse following a busulfan-based preparative regimen.[94]

Disease status at the time of transplant

Better results are reported for patients transplanted in remission in comparison to those in relapse or partial remission. In addition, many series report that patients transplanted in earlier remissions fare better than those transplanted after multiple relapses. However, such data are subject to obvious selection bias. Nonetheless, as opposed to other diseases, there would seem to be no role for performing SCT for ALL in the absence of complete remission.[95]

Donor selection

Although there is still some debate, a number of groups have reported equivalent outcomes to HLA-identical sibling donors using alternative donor options including matched unrelated (MUDs), partially matched related, partially mismatched unrelated cord blood, and haploidentical

donors.[96–101] Techniques such as depletion of donor T-cells along with improvements in supportive care, most notably prophylaxis and treatment of infection and GvHD, have improved the outcomes of these transplants. However, T-cell depletion increases the risk of graft rejection, mixed chimerism, and relapse, the latter probably due to a diminished graft-versus-leukemia (GvL) effect.[99] Treatment-associated mortality remains high (>20%) with alternative donor transplants for ALL, due in part to the high-risk nature of patients who have historically been treated with that approach. Reported rates of clinically extensive chronic GvHD (c-GvHD) also remain high after MUD transplants.[97–101]

Second transplants

For patients relapsing after an allogeneic SCT for ALL, a second transplant may be feasible. However, many patients will be unable to undergo a second SCT procedure because of death caused by progressive disease or toxicity related to salvage therapy. Among the selective group of patients able to undergo a second SCT, the outlook is very poor.[102] Although remission can be obtained in as many as 50–70% of patients, the duration is typically short-lived and only 10–30% achieve long-term event-free survival. The prognosis is more favorable for patients with longer duration of remission after the first SCT and for patients who achieve a CR prior to the second transplant.[98,103,104] Donor leukocyte infusion (DLI) has shown limited benefit for patients with ALL who relapse after allogeneic SCT, although successful remission induction with withdrawal of immunosuppression and/or DLI can be achieved in approximately 10% of cases.[105–109]

Acute myelogenous leukemia

AML represents 16% of cases of childhood leukemia under 15 years of age, and 36% of cases in those between 15 and 19 years of age. As with ALL, certain environmental exposures, genetic risk factors, and acquired disorders are associated with an increased risk of developing AML (see Table 6.1).[2,110–114]

Classification

The FAB classification system categorizes AML into subtypes based on morphology and detection of lineage markers, while the newer

World Health Organization (WHO) classification[115] differs slightly (Table 6.7).

Prognostic variables and risk stratification

A variety of clinical and biologic features are known to influence outcome. However, to date most have not been used to modify treatment (see below). A number of recurrent cytogenetic abnormalities are found in AML, and these serve as the main determinants of prognosis (Table 6.8).[116,117] The most significant adverse prognostic factors include internal tandem duplications of Flt3,[118] treatment-associated 11q23 abnormalities,[119] monosomy 7,[120] and secondary AML.[121]

Table 6.7 AML classification

French-American-British system (FAB)
M0: acute myeloblastic leukemia without differentiation
M1: acute myeloblastic leukemia with minimal differentiation but with the expression of myeloperoxidase
M2: acute myeloblastic leukemia with differentiation
M3: acute promyelocytic leukemia (APL)
M4: acute myelomonocytic leukemia (AMML)
M5: acute monocytic leukemia (AMoL)
M6: acute erythroid leukemia (AEL)
M7: acute megakaryocytic leukemia (AMKL)
World Health Organization system
Acute myeloid leukemia with recurrent genetic abnormalities Acute myeloid leukemia with t(8;21)(q22;q22), (AML1/ETO) Acute myeloid leukemia with abnormal bone marrow eosinophils and inv(16)(p13; q22) or t(16;16)(p13;q22), (CBFα/MYH11) Acute promyelocytic leukemia with t(15;17)(q22;q12), (PML/RARα) and variants Acute myeloid leukemia with 11q23 (MLL) abnormalities
Acute myeloid leukemia with multilineage dysplasia
Acute myeloid leukemia and MDS, therapy related
Acute myeloid leukemia, not otherwise categorized Acute myeloid leukemia, minimally differentiated Acute myeloid leukemia without maturation Acute myeloid leukemia with maturation Acute myelomonocytic leukemia Acute monoblastic/acute monocytic leukemia Acute erythroid leukemia (erythroid/myeloid and pure erythroleukemia) Acute megakaryoblastic leukemia Acute basophilic leukemia Acute panmyelosis with myelofibrosis Myeloid sarcoma

Table 6.8 Prognostic factors in childhood AML

	'Lower' risk factors	'Higher' risk factors
Age (years)	≥1	<1
WBC (/μl)	<100,000/μl	≥100,000/μl
CNS	Negative	Positive
Cytogenetics	Trisomy 21, t(15;17), t(8;21), inv(16), t(16;16)	Flt3 internal tandem duplications 11q23 (epipodophyllotoxin related) −7, −5
Subtype	FAB M1, M2, M3, M4 with eosinophilia	FAB M4/5 infant, M6, M7 Secondary AML
Initial treatment response	Rapid	Slow Induction failure

Treatment

The standard approach to AML treatment includes induction, consolidation, and CNS sterilization. The use of all-*trans*-retinoic acid during induction and maintenance for acute promyelocytic leukemia (FAB M3) leads to improved results for this subtype (approximately 80% DFS).[122–125] Young children with AML and Down's syndrome also have excellent outcomes despite the use of less intensive regimens.[126,127] In addition, 10% of infants with trisomy 21 develop a self-limited myeloproliferative disorder, sometimes referred to as 'transient leukemia'. Although chemotherapy may be needed to manage acute life-threatening consequences of blast infiltration and approximately one-third will eventually develop AML, most do not require therapy.[128] The outcome for other subgroups of childhood AML is poor, and only about 50–75% are cured.[129]

The primary objective of most current pediatric AML trials remains to attempt to improve DFS rates through increased treatment intensity. Approximately 75–90% of patients will achieve a CR after initial induction with regimens that commonly consist of cytarabine (Ara-C) and anthracyclines with or without additional agents.[130–135] Increasing the intensity of induction via dose escalation or treatment interval compression improves DFS rates even in the absence of increases in CR rates.[130,136,137] Postremission consolidation is essential, and high-dose Ara-C is commonly used in combination with other agents for 2–3 cycles.[138,139] Randomized trials of standard consolidation regimens versus high-dose chemotherapy with autologous stem cell rescue suggest equivalent results. Autologous rescue lowers relapse rates, but at the expense of treatment-associated mortality, which offsets any survival advantage (Table 6.9).[130–133,140–149]

The role of transplantation in AML

Allogeneic SCT is commonly employed in CR1 for pediatric patients with HLA-matched sibling donors. There have been multiple 'genetic randomization' studies of matched related allogeneic SCT (i.e. individuals with donors assigned to transplant) for consolidation of AML in pediatrics. Allogeneic SCT is clearly associated with lower relapse rates and improved DFS in comparison to chemotherapy with or without autologous rescue (see Table 6.9).[130–133,140–143,145–148] Clinical benefits may be offset in part by transplant-related morbidity and mortality, and such risks may nullify overall survival advantage in low-risk groups.[131,150–153] Consequently, there is some debate as to whether transplantation should be employed in CR1 or CR2 for children with matched sibling donors.[153–155] The ASBMT has recently published consensus guidelines for the use of SCT in pediatric AML (Table 6.10)[141–143,145–147,156,157] and a suggested approach to the use of SCT in childhood AML is presented in Figure 6.6.

SCT in CR1

Allogeneic SCT in CR1 after intensive consolidation is the most common treatment approach in the US for patients who have matched related sibling donors, excluding low-risk groups.[143] These treatment recommendations are largely based on published pediatric series from the Pediatric Oncology Group (POG) and the Children's Cancer Group (CCG). Treatment outcomes were recently published in two reports summarizing the POG experience from 1979 to 1995[117] and the CCG experience from 1981 to 2000.[116] Both groups established the importance of dose-intensified Ara-C and also found superior outcomes for those high- and intermediate-risk patients receiving SCT in CR1. The 5-year overall survival for patients transplanted with a matched sibling donor in CR1 ranges from 52% to 72% (see Table 6.9).[116,117,130–133,143,147] Matched unrelated donor SCT should be considered in CR1 for those patients with higher risk factors (see Table 6.8).

Table 6.9 Postremission therapy for childhood AML in first remission

Study group	Disease free survival			Median follow-up	Reference
	Matched related donor SCT	**Chemotherapy**	**Autologous SCT**		
AML-80	43%	31%	–	6 years	Dahl 1990[140]
AIEOP LAM-87	51%*	27%	21%	5 years	Amadori 1993[146]
CCG-213	54%*	37%	–	5 years	Wells 1994[141]
CCG-251	45%*	32%	–	8 years	Nesbit 1994[142]
POG-8821	52%*	36%	38%	3 years	Ravindranath 1996[145]
MRC AML-10	61%*	46%	68% ^	7 years	Stevens 1998[131]
AML BFM-93	64%	61%	–	5 years	Creutzig 2001[130]
CCG-2891	55%*	47%	42%	8 years	Woods 2001[147]
LAME-89/91	72%*	48%	–	6 years	Perel 2002[132] Aladjidi 2003[133]

Key: * p ≤ 0.05 allogeneic vs others; ^ p ≤ 0.05 autologous vs chemotherapy.

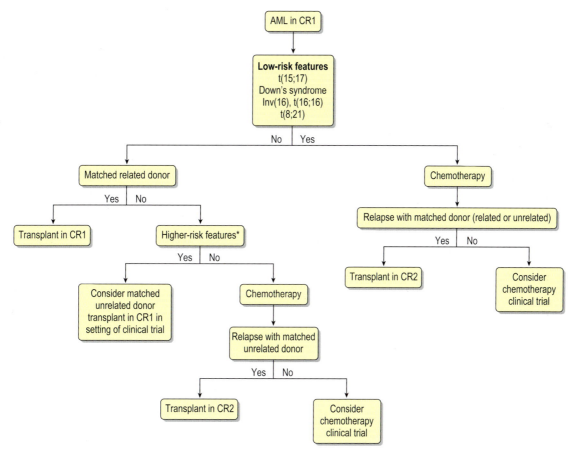

Figure 6.6
AML: schema for transplantation. *See text and Table 6.8 for those patients considered higher risk.

SCT in CR2

As stated above, some recommend reserving SCT for the management of patients who relapse after chemotherapy, especially for low-risk groups.[155] This avoids transplantation for the approximately 30–50% of individuals who might be cured by chemotherapy alone. Long-term survival can be achieved in approximately 30% of patients who are transplanted in CR2 with either matched unrelated or mismatched related donors.[133] The ASBMT consensus guidelines recommend SCT in CR2 for patients with matched related donors only, as evidence supporting an advantage in the unrelated donor setting is lacking.[143]

Conditioning regimens

In studies conducted in adults with AML, preparative regimens containing busulfan and cyclophosphamide compared to TBI and cyclophosphamide were associated with similar DFS, but higher treatment-related mortality rates.[158] Studies comparing these regimens in pediatrics are limited, although no obvious differences are apparent.[159] In general, children tolerate conditioning with busulfan and cyclophosphamide well, and this is the most commonly employed regimen in pediatric AML.

Table 6.10 Treatment recommendations for pediatric AML[143]

Recommendation	Indication	References
SCT in CR1	Benefit demonstrated for matched related donor SCT	Alonzo 2005[156] Woods 2001[147] Ravindranath 1996[145] Wells 1994[141] Nesbit 1994[142] Amadori 1993[146]
SCT in CR2	Recommended for those with matched related donors Evidence insufficient to recommend unrelated donor SCT, except in the setting of a clinical trial	Aladjidi 2003[133] Pession 2000[231] Gorin 1996[232]

Table 6.11 WHO diagnostic criteria for CML

Chronic phase
t(9;22) [p210]
Blasts < 10%
Accelerated phase
One or more of the following additional findings (unrelated or unresponsive to therapy): Blasts 10–19% Basophils ≥20% (peripheral blood) Platelet count <100,000/μl or >1,000,000/μl Progressive splenomegaly and leukocytosis Clonal evolution Megakaryocytic proliferation with fibrosis and/or myeloid dysplasia (suggestive)
Blastic phase
Blasts ≥20% (peripheral blood or bone marrow)
Extramedullary blast proliferation
Blast clusters (bone marrow)

Disease status at the time of transplant

Although some patients with AML in relapse can be salvaged by SCT,[95] patients with a higher marrow blast percentage at the time of transplant have an increased risk of relapse.[121] As in adults, pediatric patients with therapy-related AML or MDS have very poor outcomes after SCT. A study from St Jude reported survival rates of 15% and treatment related mortality rate of 60%.[48]

Donor selection

Selection of donors mismatched for natural killer cell killer immunoglobulin-like receptor (NK KIR) has the potential to improve post-transplant outcome in AML.[160]

Second transplants

As in the setting of ALL, the outcome of second transplants for individuals with AML depends on the interval from prior transplantation.[161]

Chronic myelogenous leukemia

CML represents the most common chronic myeloproliferative disorder in childhood, but it occurs much less frequently than in adults and comprises only approximately 5% of childhood leukemia. Most patients are over 5 years of age and the peak incidence occurs among children older than 16. There are no known inherited, familial or geographic predispositions, although an increased frequency has been seen in individuals exposed to radiation.[162]

Classification

As in adults, CML is a myeloproliferative disorder that involves all hematopoietic cell lineages and is nearly always characterized by the presence of the Philadelphia chromosome, a translocation between chromosomes 9 and 22, t(9;22). In CML the classic fusion product encodes an oncoprotein of 210 kD, whereas in pediatric Ph+ ALL, the fusion results in a protein product of 190 kD. CML has three defined clinical phases: chronic, accelerated, and blast crisis, with most patients presenting with chronic phase disease (Table 6.11). Chronic phase usually presents with signs and symptoms secondary to hyper-leukocytosis such as weakness, fever, night sweats, bone pain, respiratory distress, and splenomegaly. The accelerated phase is characterized by progressive splenomegaly, thrombocytopenia, and an increased percentage of peripheral and bone marrow blast cells, along with an accumulation of karyotypic abnormalities in addition to the Philadelphia chromosome. The risk of transformation to blast crisis is approximately 3–4% per year, which is characterized by bone marrow or peripheral blood with greater than 20% blasts and a clinical picture that is indistinguishable from acute leukemia. Approximately two-thirds of blast crises are myeloid and the remainder lymphoid, usually of B-lineage. Although not completely exclusive, the p210 protein can be useful in distinguishing CML in blast crisis from Ph+ ALL.[163]

Prognostic variables and risk stratification

Response to treatment and survival correlate with phase of disease. Patients with chronic phase CML have the longest survival and best responses to therapy. Treatment responses are short-lived in blast phase. Results and outlook are intermediate for those with accelerated-phase CML.[164] Within chronic phase, the Sokal score has been shown to predict response to therapy and survival. Although this has not been studied specifically in pediatric populations, age represents one of the four prognostic criteria, along with spleen size, platelet count, and blast percentage, in this system.[165]

Treatment

The *bcr/abl* fusion kinase inhibitor imatinib mesylate (Gleevec) has transformed the approach to treatment of patients with CML.[166] This agent induces hematologic and cytogenetic complete remissions in most patients with chronic-phase CML.[167] However, continuous therapy appears to be required and resistance to imatinib may develop.[167,168] Currently, several newer more potent *bcr/abl* kinase inhibitors are undergoing clinical trials,[169] although only one is currently open in the pediatric setting in the US. Thus, although the *bcr/abl* kinase inhibitors are highly effective against CML, there is currently no evidence that they will be curative, and they cannot be recommended as a replacement for allogeneic SCT in children who have an HLA-matched donor.[170] For patients started on imatinib, a number of criteria have been proposed for deciding when to proceed to transplantation, including loss of therapeutic response or failure to achieve a complete hematologic response by 3 months or a substantial cytogenetic response by 3–6 months of treatment.[171]

Role of transplant in CML

As noted above, allogeneic SCT is the only proven cure for CML. Thus, donor availability and transplant options should be considered soon after diagnosis for all children with CML. Post-transplant DFS rates are inversely related to age and exceed 80% for young children with matched sibling donors in first chronic phase.

Conditioning regimens

As with adults, busulfan/cyclophosphamide represents the most common SCT preparative regimen used for pediatric patients with CML. The use of T-lymphocyte depletion to prevent GvHD results in a higher relapse rate and decreased survival. Additionally, regimens that include intensive GvHD prophylaxis and patients who do not develop GvHD are associated with an increased risk of relapse.[172]

Disease status at the time of transplant

Results are best when SCT is performed in first chronic phase and with a shorter diagnosis–transplant interval. Transplantation during accelerated phase or in blast crisis reduces survival substantially, and efforts should be made to induce a second chronic phase.[173,174]

Donor selection

Transplant-related mortality is low in pediatric patients and results with matched unrelated donors are similar to those with matched related donors. This approach is therefore usually recommended for those who lack sibling donors.[166,170,174–177]

Second transplants

Donor lymphocyte infusions have been clearly demonstrated to be effective in the management of post-transplant relapse of chronic phase CML in adult studies and in a small pediatric series.[107] When that approach is unsuccessful, a second transplant might be considered, especially for those who received a T-cell depleted or reduced-intensity regimen.[109]

Myelodysplastic syndromes in children

The myelodysplastic syndromes account for approximately 5% of all malignant hematologic disorders in children and represent a heterogeneous group of disorders characterized by ineffective hematopoiesis, impaired maturation of myeloid progenitors, cytopenias, dysplastic changes, and a propensity for the development of AML.[178,179] Although the majority of patients have normocellular or hypercellular bone marrows, some patients may present with a very hypocellular bone marrow, making the distinction with severe aplastic anemia difficult. Risk factors associated with developing MDS include environmental factors such as exposure to irradiation and alkylating agents, as well as inherited conditions such as Fanconi anemia, Bloom's, Schwachman's and Down's syndrome. As noted below, rare myeloproliferative syndromes that commonly include features of dysplasia are frequently considered within the context of pediatric MDS.

Classification

The FAB and WHO classification systems used for adults with MDS are not completely applicable to children. Thus, modified classification schemes have been employed in pediatrics.[180–182] A restructuring of the WHO classification of myelodysplastic and myeloproliferative diseases for pediatrics was published in 2003. This system recognizes three major diagnostic groups: JMML, myeloid leukemia of Down's syndrome (including MDS, transient myeloproliferative disease, and AML), and MDS occurring de novo and secondary to previous therapy or pre-existing disorders. The main subtypes of MDS encountered in pediatric patients included within this system are: refractory cytopenias (RC) (bone marrow blasts <5%); refractory anemia with excess of blasts (RAEB) (bone marrow blasts 5–20%); and RAEB in transformation (RAEB-T) (bone marrow blasts 20–30%).[180] An alternative

'category, cytology, cytogenetics' (CCC) system that excludes myeloproliferative entities has also been proposed to classify MDS in pediatrics.[181]

Features and diagnostic criteria of juvenile myelomonocytic leukemia (JMML), formerly known as juvenile chronic myeloid leukemia (JCML), are noted in Tables 6.1, 6.12 and 6.13.[115,183,184]

Prognostic variables and risk stratification

In general, pediatric MDS carries a poor prognosis, and clinical variables have little practical utility in guiding therapy. Low blast count and higher platelet count have been associated with longer survival in MDS and JMML, and level of fetal hemoglobin <15% at the time of diagnosis has been reported to be prognostic for longer survival in individuals with JMML who did not undergo SCT.[185,186] Notably, unlike AML, monosomy 7 does not appear to confer adverse risk in children with MDS or JMML.[120,186,187]

Treatment

Few approaches other than SCT have resulted in long-term survival and transplant is considered the only curative treatment for childhood MDS and JMML. Some patients can have an indolent course without therapy for several years, in particular those with RC and RAEB associated with monosomy 7.[120] Cytotoxic therapy has been studied primarily in adults, but small series in children using AML-based

Table 6.12 Common presenting features of JMML

Clinical
Boys (60%)
Age <5 years (95%)
Hepatosplenomegaly (100%)
Upper respiratory infections, pulmonary infiltrates (50%)
Hemorrhage (50%)
Skin rash (60%): xanthogranulomas, café-au-lait spots
Features of NF-1 (15%)
Peripheral blood
Leukocytosis
Anemia
Thrombocytopenia
Immature granulocytes and monocytes
Blasts <5%
Bone marrow
Hypercellular
Myeloid and monocytic precursor expansion
Blasts <20%

Table 6.13 WHO diagnostic criteria for JMML

Peripheral blood monocyte count >1000/μl
Blasts + promonocytes <20% of peripheral WBC and bone marrow nucleated cells
Philadelphia chromosome negative

At least two of the following: WBC >10,000/μl
  Immature granulocytes in peripheral blood
  Clonal cytogenetic abnormality (e.g. monosomy 7)
  In vitro hypersensitivity of myeloid progenitors to GM-CSF
  Hemoglobin-F increased for age

regimens reveal similar outcomes, with low response and high relapse rates.[179] The largest such published trial included 60 patients with MDS (two refractory anemia, 33 RAEB, 26 RAEB-T, 16 patients AML preceded by MDS) treated with AML-type therapy (CCG-2891).[187] Those with RC/RAEB had a poor remission induction rate (48%), while those with RAEB-T (69%) and MDS/AML (81%) had similar remission rates to de novo AML (77%). Six-year survival was poor for those with RC/RAEB (28%) and RAEB-T (30%), while those with MDS/AML had a similar outcome to those with de novo AML (50% vs 45% respectively). Multiple new agents are undergoing study, predominantly in adults with MDS, including antiangiogenic agents and inhibitors of receptor tyrosine kinases, farnesyltransferases, DNA methylation, and histone deacetylases.[179] One recent study evaluated the use of antithymocyte globulin (ATG) and ciclosporin-A in 29 children with hypoplastic refractory cytopenias. The authors report promising results, with overall and DFS rates of 88% and 57% at 3 years.[188]

JMML is resistant to therapy. Chemotherapy may transiently reduce disease burden, but responses are usually short-lived and the disease rapidly progressive, with a median survival of approximately 1 year.[189] The European Working Group of MDS (EWOG-MDS) in Childhood reported a retrospective analysis of 110 cases of JMML. The probability of survival at 10 years was 39% for those who were treated with SCT, and 6% for the non-transplant group.[186] A small pilot study of 13-cis-retinoic acid for 12 patients with JMML revealed that approximately 50% had partial or complete responses with minimal toxicity.[190]

Role of transplant

SCT is considered the only curative treatment for childhood MDS and JMML. Given the low response rates to non-transplant therapies, and because failure rates after SCT appear lower when transplant is performed soon after diagnosis, strong consideration should be given to early transplantation, especially when a matched sibling donor is available. DFS is significantly increased from less than 10% with immunosuppressive or cytoreductive therapy up to 50–64% with transplant. Results of the largest published SCT series for children with MDS and JMML are summarized in Table 6.14.[191–197] Disease subtype, age greater than 4 years, and female gender are recognized poor prognostic indicators. For patients with JMML, those who develop GvHD have a lower incidence of relapse.[178,198]

Conditioning regimens

Busulfan- and TBI- based regimens have both been utilized for pediatric patients with MDS and JMML, and neither has been shown definitively to be superior, although results with second transplants suggest that radiation may be advantageous (see below). Given the risks of radiation in young children, however, busulfan-based regimens are most commonly employed for patients with JMML.

Disease status at the time of transplant

Although definitive recommendations cannot be made given the relative rarity of diagnoses, it would appear that outcome is better when transplant is performed with a lower blast percentage. Thus, pretransplant induction chemotherapy is commonly employed for patients with an elevated blast count.[187,199] Similarly, the role for splenectomy prior to SCT is unclear, although this is sometimes performed for patients with massive splenomegaly due to concerns for the risk of non-engraftment.

Donor selection

Given the poor prognosis without transplant and the favorable results of matched unrelated donor SCT in pediatric patients, this approach is commonly recommended for children who lack an HLA-matched related donor (see Table 6.14).[192,193,196,197]

Second transplants

Management of post-transplant relapse commonly includes withdrawal of immunosuppression and/or DLI, although this is seldom effective. In contrast to other types of leukemia, outcome after second SCT appears to be equivalent to results after first transplant for children with JMML (see Table 6.14).[194] In a recent EWOG-MDS report, most patients received transplants from the same donor, but with reduced intensity of the GvHD prophylaxis in comparison to the first transplant and using a TBI-based regimen with the second versus busulfan-based conditioning with the first transplant. Chronic GvHD was significantly associated with improved DFS after second SCT. Notably, there was no apparent impact of the interval between transplants.[192]

Table 6.14 Results of SCT trials for pediatric patients with MDS and JMML

Patients (n)	Survival (years)					Reference
	RA/RARS	RAEB	RAEB/T	MDS/AML	JMML	
48 MRD 52 MUD					55% EFS (5) 49% EFS (5)	Locatelli 2005[192]
30 MRD, 27 MMRD, 30 MUD, 7 MMUD	59% EFS (3) 74% OS (3)	58%EFS (3) 68% OS (3)	18% EFS (3) 18% OS (3)		27% EFS (3) 33% OS (3)	Yusuf 2004[191]
46 MUD					24% DFS (2)	Smith 2002[197]
9 MUD 3 MMRD					64% EFS (3)	Bunin 1999[196]
131 MRD	52% DFS (5) 57% OS (5)	34% DFS (5) 42% OS (5)	19% DFS (5) 24% OS (5)	26% DFS (5) 28% OS (5)		Runde 1998[195]
60 MRD 19 MUD					36% OS (4) 31% OS (4)	Arico* 1997[193]
14 MRD, 1 MMRD, 7 MUD, 2 MMUD (2nd SCT)					32% DFS (5)	Yoshimi 2007[194]

Abbreviations: MRD, matched related donor; MMRD, mismatched related donor; MUD, matched unrelated donor; MMUD, mismatched unrelated donor.
*Review article.

Special considerations for pediatric patients and stem cell transplantation

General recommendations

Pediatric cancers are uncommon in comparison to adult malignancies. Age-appropriate supportive care is important in the management of complications associated with SCT in children. Consideration must be given to the potential adverse effects of pretransplant conditioning and therapy in general on developing organs. For all these reasons, it is strongly recommended that children and adolescents be treated at centers where there is multidisciplinary pediatric expertise in the transplant setting.

Dosing

Chemotherapy for pediatric patients is usually dosed according to body surface area. However, to decrease the risk of severe toxicity in infants under 1 year of age, certain agents should be dosed on a weight (i.e. per kg) basis.

Reduced-intensity conditioning regimens in pediatrics

The goal of reduced-intensity transplant conditioning (RIT) is to decrease the toxicity associated with fully myeloablative regimens. The experience with RIT in adults with hematologic malignancies has been promising and pilot studies in pediatric cancer patients establishing the feasibility of this approach have recently been initiated.[200] Additional studies have been performed in children with non-malignant diseases. Although acute transplant-related toxicity has been low and early engraftment rates high, several studies have shown a high incidence of subsequent graft failure, particularly in patients with non-malignant disease.[201–204] A recently published study that utilized a preparative regimen consisting of busulfan/fludarabine/ATG was closed secondary to a high rate of graft failure (21%) in patients with non-malignant disorders. Despite these findings, the authors found the regimen to be well tolerated, with an overall survival rate of 89% and EFS of 74% at 2 years.[204]

Stem cell source

Bone marrow remains the predominant stem cell source employed in pediatric transplantation. However, alternative sources have been utilized with increasing frequency.

Peripheral blood stem cells

As in the adult setting, the use of granulocyte colony-stimulating factor (G-CSF) mobilized peripheral blood stem cells (PBSC) has increased in pediatrics.[205,206] In adults, this approach has been associated with decreased treatment-related mortality and improved survival despite an increased incidence of c-GvHD. In children, however, data are less clear. A retrospective IBMTR study reported poorer survival for pediatric patients who received PBSC transplants in comparison to bone marrow, despite similar rates of relapse.[205]

Umbilical cord blood transplant

Because of the relatively limited stem cell doses in umbilical cord blood units, this stem cell source has been most frequently utilized in pediatric patients. Results with this alternative stem cell source are promising, with high engraftment rates (>80%) and a low incidence of acute and chronic GvHD, which allows a greater degree of HLA mismatch.[207–211]

Haploidentical donors

Haploidentical stem cell transplantation is another promising option for children who lack an HLA-matched donor. High engraftment rates have been reported in pediatric patients with hematologic malignancies who received high-dose G-CSF mobilized PBSC transplants (CD34 or CD133 selected). Minimal acute and chronic GvHD have been encountered, and overall survival has varied with the underlying disease status, suggesting that the HLA barrier can be overcome by transplantation of megadoses of highly purified CD34+ PBSC.[212,213]

Chronic graft-versus-host disease

c-GvHD is second only to disease recurrence as the most significant cause of morbidity and mortality following SCT for malignancies.[214] There are limited data and research focused on this condition in pediatrics. The incidence of c-GvHD has increased due to the use of peripheral blood and/or unrelated donors.[215,216] Although the rates of c-GvHD are lower in children than adults, this has also increased in pediatrics.[205,214,217,218] Treatment of c-GvHD in children is challenging. The most commonly used therapies, e.g. corticosteroids, can adversely affect organ development, bone growth and integrity, and hormone balance in the developing child. In addition, chronic immunosuppression can profoundly impair normal immune responses to childhood infections and immunizations.

Late effects

Cancer remains the leading indication for SCT in pediatrics and SCT contributes to 5-year cancer survival rates that exceed 80%. Recent studies estimate approximately 270,000 childhood cancer survivors between the ages of 20 and 39 years[219,220] and clearly demonstrate the major impact of late effects on the lives of these survivors. With improvements in post-transplant DFS rates, acute and long-term toxicities have assumed an ever-increasing impact on organ function, quality of life, and overall survival. As these children reach adulthood with chronic, life-altering post-transplant complications, the implications for both the individual survivors and society are substantial. While progress towards developing less toxic therapies continues, such as non-myeloablative SCT,[218] treating and preventing secondary effects remains a critical adjunct to the care of children requiring transplantation. Special consideration should be given to the potential impact of conditioning regimens on the developing child, including linear growth, fertility, endocrine function, and neurocognitive function.[221–223]

Donor considerations

For many pediatric transplants, the matched sibling donor is also a minor, which raises several unique ethical and medical considerations. Bone marrow continues to be the primary stem cell source from minor donors and complications from marrow harvest are rare.[224] Donations can safely be obtained from children younger than 2 years of age.[225] Many children, especially those <20 kg, donate proportionally large volumes and are more likely than adult donors to require red blood cell transfusion.[226] Transfusion-associated risks must be considered and attempts made to minimize them. For PBSC donation, children mobilize well in response to stimulation with G-CSF, although pain secondary to injections and limitations of venous access need to be considered. When multiple sibling donors are available, it is recommended that the oldest optimum donor be selected. Further, stem cell collection, assessment, and post-harvest care of a minor-aged donor should be performed by healthcare providers with pediatric expertise. Evaluation should also include psychologic assessment. Donor verbal assent, as age appropriate, should be obtained.

To avoid medical conflict of interest, it is recommended that the donor be assigned an independent care provider, separate from that of the transplant recipient. As these young donors are often unable to consent for themselves and are shown to have higher rates of psychologic distress responses than do non-donor siblings,[227] special attention needs to be given to the ethical considerations and the process should be subject to full regulatory review of the relative risks and benefits.[206,224,226]

The future of stem cell transplantation for pediatric leukemias

The future of SCT in the setting of pediatric leukemias will include efforts to deliver less toxic pretransplant conditioning without sacrificing relapse-free survival rates. Advances in clinical and translational research are helping to improve class discovery and[228] risk stratification,[41,229] and to identify novel targeted therapies.[230] Disease-specific targeted therapies will probably be incorporated into SCT regimens with increasing frequency in the future. New HLA-genotyping techniques should lead to improved selection of donor–recipient pairs.[160] Although the pathophysiology of GvHD remains incompletely elucidated, significant advances have been made, which are expected to lead to novel methods of GvHD prevention and treatment. Similarly, novel graft manipulation, immunomodulation, and post-transplant tumor-directed immunotherapy strategies are being developed and evaluated in the pediatric setting. Such advances are likely to lead to continued decreases in transplant-related mortality and long-term toxicities, as well as improvements in relapse-free and overall survival rates after SCT.

References

1. Reis LAG, Smith MA, Gurney JG et al (eds). Cancer incidence and survival among children and adolescents: United States SEER Program 1975–1995. NIH Pub no 99-4649. National Cancer Institute, Bethesda, Maryland, 1999
2. Hasle H, Clemmensen IH, Mikkelsen M. Risks of leukaemia and solid tumours in individuals with Down's syndrome. Lancet 2000;355:165–169
3. Bassal M, La MK, Whitlock JA et al. Lymphoblast biology and outcome among children with Down syndrome and ALL treated on CCG-1952. Pediatr Blood Cancer 2005;44:21–28
4. Zeller B, Gustafsson G, Forestier E et al. Acute leukaemia in children with Down syndrome: a population-based Nordic study. Br J Haematol 2005;128:797–804
5. Whitlock JA, Sather HN, Gaynon P et al. Clinical characteristics and outcome of children with Down syndrome and acute lymphoblastic leukemia: a Children's Cancer Group study. Blood 2005;106:4043–4049
6. Bennett JM, Catovsky D, Daniel MT et al. The morphological classification of acute lymphoblastic leukaemia: concordance among observers and clinical correlations. Br J Haematol 1981;47:553–561
7. Smith M, Arthur D, Camitta B et al. Uniform approach to risk classification and treatment assignment for children with acute lymphoblastic leukemia. J Clin Oncol 1996;14:18–24
8. Mahmoud HH, Rivera GK, Hancock ML et al. Low leukocyte counts with blast cells in cerebrospinal fluid of children with newly diagnosed acute lymphoblastic leukemia. N Engl J Med 1993;329:314–319
9. Gilchrist GS, Tubergen DG, Sather HN et al. Low numbers of CSF blasts at diagnosis do not predict for the development of CNS leukemia in children with intermediate-risk acute lymphoblastic leukemia: a Children's Cancer Group report. J Clin Oncol 1994;12:2594–2600
10. Pui CH, Mahmoud HH, Rivera GK et al. Early intensification of intrathecal chemotherapy virtually eliminates central nervous system relapse in children with acute lymphoblastic leukemia. Blood 1998;92:411–415
11. Burger B, Zimmermann M, Mann G et al. Diagnostic cerebrospinal fluid examination in children with acute lymphoblastic leukemia: significance of low leukocyte counts with blasts or traumatic lumbar puncture. J Clin Oncol 2003;21:184–188
12. Gajjar A, Harrison PL, Sandlund JT et al. Traumatic lumbar puncture at diagnosis adversely affects outcome in childhood acute lymphoblastic leukemia. Blood 2000;96:3381–3384
13. McLean TW, Ringold S, Neuberg D et al. TEL/AML-1 dimerizes and is associated with a favorable outcome in childhood acute lymphoblastic leukemia. Blood 1996;88:4252–4258
14. Borkhardt A, Cazzaniga G, Viehmann S et al. Incidence and clinical relevance of TEL/AML1 fusion genes in children with acute lymphoblastic leukemia enrolled in the German and Italian multicenter therapy trials. Associazione Italiana Ematologia Oncologia Pediatrica and the Berlin-Frankfurt-Munster Study Group. Blood 1997;90:571–577
15. Uckun FM, Pallisgaard N, Hokland P et al. Expression of TEL-AML1 fusion transcripts and response to induction therapy in standard risk acute lymphoblastic leukemia. Leuk Lymphoma 2001;42:41–56
16. Kanerva J, Saarinen-Pihkala UM, Niini T et al. Favorable outcome in 20-year follow-up of children with very-low-risk ALL and minimal standard therapy, with special reference to TEL-AML1 fusion. Pediatr Blood Cancer 2004;42:30–35
17. Pui CH, Chessells JM, Camitta B et al. Clinical heterogeneity in childhood acute lymphoblastic leukemia with 11q23 rearrangements. Leukemia 2003;17:700–706
18. Arico M, Valsecchi MG, Camitta B et al. Outcome of treatment in children with Philadelphia chromosome-positive acute lymphoblastic leukemia. N Engl J Med 2000;342:998–1006
19. Johansson B, Moorman AV, Haas OA et al. Hematologic malignancies with t(4;11)(q21;q23) – a cytogenetic, morphologic, immunophenotypic and clinical study of 183 cases. European 11q23 Workshop participants. Leukemia 1998;12:779–787
20. Pui CH, Frankel LS, Carroll AJ et al. Clinical characteristics and treatment outcome of childhood acute lymphoblastic leukemia with the t(4;11)(q21;q23): a collaborative study of 40 cases. Blood 1991;77:440–447
21. Crist W, Boyett J, Pullen J et al. Clinical and biologic features predict poor prognosis in acute lymphoid leukemias in children and adolescents: a Pediatric Oncology Group review. Med Pediatr Oncol 1986;14:135–139
22. Reaman G, Zeltzer P, Bleyer WA et al. Acute lymphoblastic leukemia in infants less than one year of age: a cumulative experience of the Children's Cancer Study Group. J Clin Oncol 1985;3:1513–1521
23. Crist WM, Carroll AJ, Shuster JJ et al. Poor prognosis of children with pre-B acute lymphoblastic leukemia is associated with the t(1;19)(q23;p13): a Pediatric Oncology Group study. Blood 1990;76:117–122
24. Uckun FM, Sensel MG, Sather HN et al. Clinical significance of translocation t(1;19) in childhood acute lymphoblastic leukemia in the context of contemporary therapies: a report from the Children's Cancer Group. J Clin Oncol 1998;16:527–535
25. Harris MB, Shuster JJ, Carroll A et al. Trisomy of leukemic cell chromosomes 4 and 10 identifies children with B-progenitor cell acute lymphoblastic leukemia with a very low risk of treatment failure: a Pediatric Oncology Group study. Blood 1992;79:3316–3324
26. Moorman AV, Richards SM, Martineau M et al. Outcome heterogeneity in childhood high-hyperdiploid acute lymphoblastic leukemia. Blood 2003;102:2756–2762
27. Charrin C, Thomas X, Ffrench M et al. A report from the LALA-94 and LALA-SA groups on hypodiploidy with 30 to 39 chromosomes and near-triploidy: 2 possible expressions of a sole entity conferring poor prognosis in adult acute lymphoblastic leukemia (ALL). Blood 2004;104:2444–2451
28. Heerema NA, Sather HN, Sensel MG et al. Prognostic impact of trisomies of chromosomes 10, 17, and 5 among children with acute lymphoblastic leukemia and high hyperdiploidy (<50 chromosomes). J Clin Oncol 2000;18:1876–1887
29. Sutcliffe MJ, Shuster JJ, Sather HN et al. High concordance from independent studies by the Children's Cancer Group (CCG) and Pediatric Oncology Group (POG) associating favorable prognosis with combined trisomies 4, 10, and 17 in children with NCI standard-risk B-precursor acute lymphoblastic leukemia: a Children's Oncology Group (COG) initiative. Leukemia 2005;19:734–740
30. Harrison CJ, Moorman AV, Broadfield ZJ et al. Three distinct subgroups of hypodiploidy in acute lymphoblastic leukaemia. Br J Haematol 2004;125:552–559
31. Heerema NA, Nachman JB, Sather HN et al. Hypodiploidy with less than 45 chromosomes confers adverse risk in childhood acute lymphoblastic leukemia: a report from the children's cancer group. Blood 1999;94:4036–4045
32. Raimondi SC, Zhou Y, Mathew S et al. Reassessment of the prognostic significance of hypodiploidy in pediatric patients with acute lymphoblastic leukemia. Cancer 2003;98:2715–2722
33. Pui CH, Carroll AJ, Raimondi SC et al. Clinical presentation, karyotypic characterization, and treatment outcome of childhood acute lymphoblastic leukemia with a near-haploid or hypodiploid less than 45 line. Blood 1990;75:1170–1177
34. Gaynon PS, Desai AA, Bostrom BC et al. Early response to therapy and outcome in childhood acute lymphoblastic leukemia: a review. Cancer 1997;80:1717–1726
35. Steinherz PG, Gaynon PS, Breneman JC et al. Cytoreduction and prognosis in acute lymphoblastic leukemia–the importance of early marrow response: report from the Children's Cancer Group. J Clin Oncol 1996;14:389–398
36. Arico M, Basso G, Mandelli F et al. Good steroid response in vivo predicts a favorable outcome in children with T-cell acute lymphoblastic leukemia. The Associazione Italiana Ematologia Oncologia Pediatrica (AIEOP). Cancer 1995;75:1684–1693
37. Gajjar A, Ribeiro R, Hancock ML et al. Persistence of circulating blasts after 1 week of multiagent chemotherapy confers a poor prognosis in childhood acute lymphoblastic leukemia. Blood 1995;86:1292–1295
38. Rautonen J, Hovi L, Siimes MA. Slow disappearance of peripheral blast cells: an independent risk factor indicating poor prognosis in children with acute lymphoblastic leukemia. Blood 1988;71:989–991
39. Griffin TC, Shuster JJ, Buchanan GR et al. Slow disappearance of peripheral blood blasts is an adverse prognostic factor in childhood T cell acute lymphoblastic leukemia: a Pediatric Oncology Group study. Leukemia 2000;14:792–795
40. Panzer-Grumayer ER, Schneider M, Panzer S et al. Rapid molecular response during early induction chemotherapy predicts a good outcome in childhood acute lymphoblastic leukemia. Blood 2000;95:790–794
41. Holleman A, Cheok MH, den Boer ML et al. Gene-expression patterns in drug-resistant acute lymphoblastic leukemia cells and response to treatment. N Engl J Med 2004;351:533–542
42. Unal S, Yetgin S, Cetin M et al. The prognosis and survival of childhood acute lymphoblastic leukemia with central nervous system relapse. Pediatr Hematol Oncol 2004;21:279–289
43. Nachman JB, Sather HN, Sensel MG et al. Augmented post-induction therapy for children with high-risk acute lymphoblastic leukemia and a slow response to initial therapy. N Engl J Med 1998;338:1663–1671

44. Schrappe M, Reiter A, Ludwig WD et al. Improved outcome in childhood acute lympho-blastic leukemia despite reduced use of anthracyclines and cranial radiotherapy: results of trial ALL-BFM 90. German-Austrian-Swiss ALL-BFM Study Group. Blood 2000;95: 3310–3322

45. Richards S, Burrett J, Hann I et al. Improved survival with early intensification: combined results from the Medical Research Council childhood ALL randomised trials, UKALL X and UKALL XI. Medical Research Council Working Party on Childhood Leukaemia. Leukemia 1998;12:1031–1036

46. Silverman LB, Gelber RD, Dalton VK et al. Improved outcome for children with acute lymphoblastic leukemia: results of Dana-Farber Consortium Protocol 91–01. Blood 2001;97:1211–1218

47. Amylon MD, Shuster J, Pullen J et al. Intensive high-dose asparaginase consolidation improves survival for pediatric patients with T cell acute lymphoblastic leukemia and advanced stage lymphoblastic lymphoma: a Pediatric Oncology Group study. Leukemia 1999;13:335–342

48. Pui CH, Sandlund JT, Pei D et al. Improved outcome for children with acute lymphoblastic leukemia: results of Total Therapy Study XIIIB at St Jude Children's Research Hospital. Blood 2004;104:2690–2696

49. Goldberg JM, Silverman LB, Levy DE et al. Childhood T-cell acute lymphoblastic leuke-mia: the Dana-Farber Cancer Institute acute lymphoblastic leukemia consortium experi-ence. J Clin Oncol 2003;21:3616–3622

50. Reiter A, Schrappe M, Ludwig WD et al. Intensive ALL-type therapy without local radiotherapy provides a 90% event-free survival for children with T-cell lymphoblastic lymphoma: a BFM group report. Blood 2000;95:416–421

51. Magrath I, Adde M, Shad A et al. Adults and children with small non-cleaved-cell lym-phoma have a similar excellent outcome when treated with the same chemotherapy regimen. J Clin Oncol 1996;14:925–934

52. Atra A, Imeson JD, Hobson R et al. Improved outcome in children with advanced stage B-cell non-Hodgkin's lymphoma (B-NHL): results of the United Kingdom Children Cancer Study Group (UKCCSG) 9002 protocol. Br J Cancer 2000;82:1396–1402

53. Bowman WP, Shuster JJ, Cook B et al. Improved survival for children with B-cell acute lymphoblastic leukemia and stage IV small noncleaved-cell lymphoma: a pediatric oncol-ogy group study. J Clin Oncol 1996;14:1252–1261

54. Chessells JM. Relapsed lymphoblastic leukaemia in children: a continuing challenge. Br J Haematol 1998;102:423–438

55. Gaynon PS, Harris RE, Altman AJ et al. Bone marrow transplantation versus prolonged intensive chemotherapy for children with acute lymphoblastic leukemia and an initial bone marrow relapse within 12 months of the completion of primary therapy: Children's Oncol-ogy Group study CCG-1941. J Clin Oncol 2006;24:3150–3156

56. Rivera GK, Buchanan G, Boyett JM et al. Intensive retreatment of childhood acute lym-phoblastic leukemia in first bone marrow relapse. A Pediatric Oncology Group Study. N Engl J Med 1986;315:273–278

57. Rivera GK, Hudson MM, Liu Q et al. Effectiveness of intensified rotational combination chemotherapy for late hematologic relapse of childhood acute lymphoblastic leukemia. Blood 1996;88:831–837

58. Ritchey AK, Pollock BH, Lauer SJ et al. Improved survival of children with isolated CNS relapse of acute lymphoblastic leukemia: a pediatric oncology group study. J Clin Oncol 1999;17:3745–3752

59. Buchanan GR, Boyett JM, Pollock BH et al. Improved treatment results in boys with overt testicular relapse during or shortly after initial therapy for acute lymphoblastic leukemia. A Pediatric Oncology group study. Cancer 1991;68:48–55

60. Hahn T, Wall D, Camitta B et al. The role of cytotoxic therapy with hematopoietic stem cell transplantation in the therapy of acute lymphoblastic leukemia in children: an evidence-based review. Biol Blood Marrow Transplant 2005;11:823–861

61. Barrett AJ, Horowitz MM, Pollock BH et al. Bone marrow transplants from HLA-identical siblings as compared with chemotherapy for children with acute lymphoblastic leukemia in a second remission. N Engl J Med 1994;331:1253–1258

62. Wheeler KA, Richards SM, Bailey CC et al. Bone marrow transplantation versus chemo-therapy in the treatment of very high-risk childhood acute lymphoblastic leukemia in first remission: results from Medical Research Council UKALL X and XI. Blood 2000; 96:2412–2418

63. Chessells JM, Bailey C, Wheeler K et al. Bone marrow transplantation for high-risk child-hood lymphoblastic leukaemia in first remission: experience in MRC UKALL X. Lancet 1992;340:565–568

64. Uderzo C, Valsecchi MG, Balduzzi A et al. Allogeneic bone marrow transplantation versus chemotherapy in high-risk childhood acute lymphoblastic leukaemia in first remission. Associazione Italiana di Ematologia ed Oncologia Pediatrica (AIEOP) and the Gruppo Italiano Trapianto di Midollo Osseo (GITMO). Br J Haematol 1997;96:387–394

65. Wheeler K, Richards S, Bailey C et al. Comparison of bone marrow transplant and che-motherapy for relapsed childhood acute lymphoblastic leukaemia: the MRC UKALL X experience. Medical Research Council Working Party on Childhood Leukaemia. Br J Haematol 1998;101:94–103

66. Uderzo C, Valsecchi MG, Bacigalupo A et al. Treatment of childhood acute lymphoblastic leukemia in second remission with allogeneic bone marrow transplantation and chemotherapy: ten-year experience of the Italian Bone Marrow Transplantation Group and the Italian Pediatric Hematology Oncology Association. J Clin Oncol 1995;13: 352–358

67. Harrison G, Richards S, Lawson S et al. Comparison of allogeneic transplant versus che-motherapy for relapsed childhood acute lymphoblastic leukaemia in the MRC UKALL R1 trial. MRC Childhood Leukaemia Working Party. Ann Oncol 2000;11:999–1006

68. Dopfer R, Henze G, Bender-Gotze C et al. Allogeneic bone marrow transplantation for childhood acute lymphoblastic leukemia in second remission after intensive primary and relapse therapy according to the BFM- and CoALL-protocols: results of the German Cooperative Study. Blood 1991;78:2780–2784

69. Hoogerbrugge PM, Gerritsen EJ, vd Does-van den Berg A et al. Case-control analysis of allogeneic bone marrow transplantation versus maintenance chemotherapy for relapsed ALL in children. Bone Marrow Transplant 1995;15:255–259

70. Moussalem M, Esperou Bourdeau H, Devergie A et al. Allogeneic bone marrow transplan-tation for childhood acute lymphoblastic leukemia in second remission: factors predictive of survival, relapse and graft-versus-host disease. Bone Marrow Transplant 1995;15: 943–947

71. Eapen M, Raetz E, Zhang MJ et al. Outcomes after HLA-matched sibling transplantation or chemotherapy in children with B-precursor acute lymphoblastic leukemia in a second remission: a collaborative study of the Children's Oncology Group and the Center for International Blood and Marrow Transplant Research. Blood 2006;107:4961–4967

72. Buchanan GR, Rivera GK, Pollock BH et al. Alternating drug pairs with or without periodic reinduction in children with acute lymphoblastic leukemia in second bone marrow remis-sion: a Pediatric Oncology Group Study. Cancer 2000;88:1166–1174

73. Sadowitz PD, Smith SD, Shuster J et al. Treatment of late bone marrow relapse in children with acute lymphoblastic leukemia: a Pediatric Oncology Group study. Blood 1993;81: 602–609

74. Pui CH, Cheng C, Leung W et al. Extended follow-up of long-term survivors of childhood acute lymphoblastic leukemia. N Engl J Med 2003;349:640–649

75. Sharathkumar A, Saunders EF, Dror Y et al. Allogeneic bone marrow transplantation vs chemotherapy for children with Philadelphia chromosome-positive acute lymphoblastic leukemia. Bone Marrow Transplant 2004;33:39–45

76. Saarinen UM, Mellander L, Nysom K et al. Allogeneic bone marrow transplantation in first remission for children with very high-risk acute lymphoblastic leukemia: a retrospective case-control study in the Nordic countries. Nordic Society for Pediatric Hematology and Oncology (NOPHO). Bone Marrow Transplant 1996;17:357–363

77. Barrett AJ, Horowitz MM, Ash RC et al. Bone marrow transplantation for Philadelphia chromosome-positive acute lymphoblastic leukemia. Blood 1992;79:3067–3070

78. Bordigoni P, Vernant JP, Souillet G et al. Allogeneic bone marrow transplantation for chil-dren with acute lymphoblastic leukemia in first remission: a cooperative study of the Groupe d'Etude de la Greffe de Moelle Osseuse. J Clin Oncol 1989;7:747–753

79. Balduzzi A, Valsecchi MG, Uderzo C et al. Chemotherapy versus allogeneic transplantation for very-high-risk childhood acute lymphoblastic leukaemia in first complete remission: comparison by genetic randomisation in an international prospective study. Lancet 2005;366:635–642

80. Talano JM, Casper JT, Camitta BM et al. Alternative donor bone marrow transplant for children with Philadelphia chromosome ALL. Bone Marrow Transplant 2006;37:135–141

81. Jacobsohn DA, Hewlett B, Morgan E et al. Favorable outcome for infant acute lympho-blastic leukemia after hematopoietic stem cell transplantation. Biol Blood Marrow Trans-plant 2005;11:999–1005

82. Kosaka Y, Koh K, Kinukawa N et al. Infant acute lymphoblastic leukemia with MLL gene rearrangements: outcome following intensive chemotherapy and hematopoietic stem cell transplantation. Blood 2004;104:3527–3534

83. Silverman LB, Weinstein HJ. Treatment of childhood leukemia. Curr Opin Oncol 1997;9:26–33

84. Luciani M, Rana I, Pansini V et al. Infant leukaemia: clinical, biological and therapeutic advances. Acta Paediatr Suppl 2006;95:47–51

85. Nagayama J, Tomizawa D, Koh K et al. Infants with acute lymphoblastic leukemia and a germline MLL gene are highly curable with use of chemotherapy alone: results from the Japan Infant Leukemia Study Group. Blood 2006;107:4663–4665

86. Pui CH, Behm FG, Downing JR et al. 11q23/MLL rearrangement confers a poor prognosis in infants with acute lymphoblastic leukemia. J Clin Oncol 1994;12:909–915

87. Hilden JM, Dinndorf PA, Meerbaum SO et al. Analysis of prognostic factors of acute lymphoblastic leukemia in infants: report on CCG 1953 from the Children's Oncology Group. Blood 2006;108:441–451

88. Eapen M, Rubinstein P, Zhang MJ et al. Comparable long-term survival after unrelated and HLA-matched sibling donor hematopoietic stem cell transplantations for acute leukemia in children younger than 18 months. J Clin Oncol 2006;24:145–151

89. Davies SM, Ramsay NK, Klein JP et al. Comparison of preparative regimens in transplants for children with acute lymphoblastic leukemia. J Clin Oncol 2000;18:340–347

90. Bunin N, Aplenc R, Kamani N et al. Randomized trial of busulfan vs total body irradiation containing conditioning regimens for children with acute lymphoblastic leukemia: a Pediatric Blood and Marrow Transplant Consortium study. Bone Marrow Transplant 2003; 32:543–548

91. Wingard JR, Plotnick LP, Freemer CS et al. Growth in children after bone marrow trans-plantation: busulfan plus cyclophosphamide versus cyclophosphamide plus total body irradiation. Blood 1992;79:1068–1073

92. Kletzel M, Jacobsohn D, Duerst R. Pharmacokinetics of a test dose of intravenous busulfan guide dose modifications to achieve an optimal area under the curve of a single daily dose of intravenous busulfan in children undergoing a reduced-intensity conditioning regimen with hematopoietic stem cell transplantation. Biol Blood Marrow Transplant 2006;12: 472–479

93. Tran HT, Madden T, Petropoulos D et al. Individualizing high-dose oral busulfan: prospec-tive dose adjustment in a pediatric population undergoing allogeneic stem cell transplanta-tion for advanced hematologic malignancies. Bone Marrow Transplant 2000;26:463–470

94. Shah AJ, Lenarsky C, Kapoor N et al. Busulfan and cyclophosphamide as a conditioning regimen for pediatric acute lymphoblastic leukemia patients undergoing bone marrow transplantation. J Pediatr Hematol Oncol 2004;26:91–97

95. Sullivan KM, Weiden PL, Storb R et al. Influence of acute and chronic graft-versus-host disease on relapse and survival after bone marrow transplantation from HLA-identical siblings as treatment of acute and chronic leukemia. Blood 1989;73:1720–1728

96. Dini G, Valsecchi MG, Micalizzi C et al. Impact of marrow unrelated donor search duration on outcome of children with acute lymphoblastic leukemia in second remission. Bone Marrow Transplant 2003;32:325–331

97. Bunin N, Carston M, Wall D et al. Unrelated marrow transplantation for children with acute lymphoblastic leukemia in second remission. Blood 2002;99:3151–3157

98. Saarinen-Pihkala UM, Gustafsson G, Ringden O et al. No disadvantage in outcome of using matched unrelated donors as compared with matched sibling donors for bone marrow

transplantation in children with acute lymphoblastic leukemia in second remission. J Clin Oncol 2001;19:3406–3414

99. Green A, Clarke E, Hunt L et al. Children with acute lymphoblastic leukemia who receive T-cell-depleted HLA mismatched marrow allografts from unrelated donors have an increased incidence of primary graft failure but a similar overall transplant outcome. Blood 1999;94:2236–2246
100. Oakhill A, Pamphilon DH, Potter MN et al. Unrelated donor bone marrow transplantation for children with relapsed acute lymphoblastic leukaemia in second complete remission. Br J Haematol 1996;94:574–578
101. Fleming DR, Henslee-Downey PJ, Romond EH et al. Allogeneic bone marrow transplantation with T cell-depleted partially matched related donors for advanced acute lymphoblastic leukemia in children and adults: a comparative matched cohort study. Bone Marrow Transplant 1996;17:917–922
102. Bosi A, Laszlo D, Labopin M et al. Second allogeneic bone marrow transplantation in acute leukemia: results of a survey by the European Cooperative Group for Blood and Marrow Transplantation. J Clin Oncol 2001;19:3675–3684
103. Schroeder H, Gustafsson G, Saarinen-Pihkala UM et al. Allogeneic bone marrow transplantation in second remission of childhood acute lymphoblastic leukemia: a population-based case control study from the Nordic countries. Bone Marrow Transplant 1999;23:555–560
104. Sanders JE, Thomas ED, Buckner CD et al. Marrow transplantation for children with acute lymphoblastic leukemia in second remission. Blood 1987;70:324–326
105. Lawson SE, Darbyshire PJ. Use of donor lymphocytes in extramedullary relapse of childhood acute lymphoblastic leukaemia following bone marrow transplantation. Bone Marrow Transplant 1998;22:829–830
106. Atra A, Millar B, Shepherd V et al. Donor lymphocyte infusion for childhood acute lymphoblastic leukaemia relapsing after bone marrow transplantation. Br J Haematol 1997;97:165–168
107. Collins RH Jr, Shpilberg O, Drobyski WR et al. Donor leukocyte infusions in 140 patients with relapsed malignancy after allogeneic bone marrow transplantation. J Clin Oncol 1997;15:433–444
108. Helg C, Starobinski M, Jeannet M et al. Donor lymphocyte infusion for the treatment of relapse after allogeneic hematopoietic stem cell transplantation. Leuk Lymphoma 1998;29:301–313
109. Porter DL, Collins RH Jr, Hardy C et al. Treatment of relapsed leukemia after unrelated donor marrow transplantation with unrelated donor leukocyte infusions. Blood 2000;95:1214–1221
110. Hitzler JK, Cheung J, Li Y et al. GATA1 mutations in transient leukemia and acute megakaryoblastic leukemia of Down syndrome. Blood 2003;101:4301–4304
111. Massey GV, Zipursky A, Chang MN et al. A prospective study of the natural history of transient leukemia (TL) in neonates with Down syndrome (DS): Children's Oncology Group (COG) study POG-9481. Blood 2006;107:4606–4613
112. Deschler B, Lubbert M. Acute myeloid leukemia: epidemiology and etiology. Cancer 2006;107:2099–2107
113. Ohara A, Kojima S, Hamajima N et al. Myelodysplastic syndrome and acute myelogenous leukemia as a late clonal complication in children with acquired aplastic anemia. Blood 1997;90:1009–1013
114. Devine DV, Gluck WL, Rosse WF et al. Acute myeloblastic leukemia in paroxysmal nocturnal hemoglobinuria. Evidence of evolution from the abnormal paroxysmal nocturnal hemoglobinuria clone. J Clin Invest 1987;79:314–317
115. Jaffe E, Harris N, Stein N et al. World Health Organization classification of tumours. Pathology and genetics of tumours of haematopoietic and lymphoid tissues. IARC Press, Lyon, 2001
116. Smith FO, Alonzo TA, Gerbing RB et al. Long-term results of children with acute myeloid leukemia: a report of three consecutive Phase III trials by the Children's Cancer Group: CCG 251, CCG 213 and CCG 2891. Leukemia 2005;19:2054–2062
117. Ravindranath Y, Chang M, Steuber CP et al. Pediatric Oncology Group (POG) studies of acute myeloid leukemia (AML): a review of four consecutive childhood AML trials conducted between 1981 and 2000. Leukemia 2005;19:2101–2116
118. Meshinchi S, Woods WG, Stirewalt DL et al. Prevalence and prognostic significance of Flt3 internal tandem duplication in pediatric acute myeloid leukemia. Blood 2001;97:89–94
119. Hale GA, Heslop HE, Bowman LC et al. Bone marrow transplantation for therapy-induced acute myeloid leukemia in children with previous lymphoid malignancies. Bone Marrow Transplant 1999;24:735–739
120. Hasle H, Arico M, Basso G et al. Myelodysplastic syndrome, juvenile myelomonocytic leukemia, and acute myeloid leukemia associated with complete or partial monosomy 7. European Working Group on MDS in Childhood (EWOG-MDS). Leukemia 1999;13:376–385
121. Woodard P, Barfield R, Hale G et al. Outcome of hematopoietic stem cell transplantation for pediatric patients with therapy-related acute myeloid leukemia or myelodysplastic syndrome. Pediatr Blood Cancer 2006;47:931–935
122. Ortega JJ, Madero L, Martin G et al. Treatment with all-trans retinoic acid and anthracycline monochemotherapy for children with acute promyelocytic leukemia: a multicenter study by the PETHEMA Group. J Clin Oncol 2005;23:7632–7640
123. Testi AM, Biondi A, Lo Coco F et al. GIMEMA-AIEOPAIDA protocol for the treatment of newly diagnosed acute promyelocytic leukemia (APL) in children. Blood 2005;106:447–453
124. De Botton S, Chevret S, Sanz M et al. Additional chromosomal abnormalities in patients with acute promyelocytic leukaemia (APL) do not confer poor prognosis: results of APL 93 trial. Br J Haematol 2000;111:801–806
125. Fenaux P, Chevret S, Guerci A et al. Long-term follow-up confirms the benefit of all-trans retinoic acid in acute promyelocytic leukemia. European APL group. Leukemia 2000;14:1371–1377
126. Ravindranath Y, Abella E, Krischer JP et al. Acute myeloid leukemia (AML) in Down's syndrome is highly responsive to chemotherapy: experience on Pediatric Oncology Group AML Study 8498. Blood 1992;80:2210–2214
127. Gamis AS, Woods WG, Alonzo TA et al. Increased age at diagnosis has a significantly negative effect on outcome in children with Down syndrome and acute myeloid leukemia: a report from the Children's Cancer Group Study 2891. J Clin Oncol 2003;21:3415–3422
128. Massey GV. Transient leukemia in newborns with Down syndrome. Pediatr Blood Cancer 2005;44:29–32
129. Razzouk BI, Estey E, Pounds S et al. Impact of age on outcome of pediatric acute myeloid leukemia: a report from 2 institutions. Cancer 2006;106:2495–2502
130. Creutzig U, Ritter J, Zimmermann M et al. Improved treatment results in high-risk pediatric acute myeloid leukemia patients after intensification with high-dose cytarabine and mitoxantrone: results of Study Acute Myeloid Leukemia-Berlin-Frankfurt-Munster 93. J Clin Oncol 2001;19:2705–2713
131. Stevens RF, Hann IM, Wheatley K et al. Marked improvements in outcome with chemotherapy alone in paediatric acute myeloid leukemia: results of the United Kingdom Medical Research Council's 10th AML trial. MRC Childhood Leukaemia Working Party. Br J Haematol 1998;101:130–140
132. Perel Y, Auvrignon A, Leblanc T et al. Impact of addition of maintenance therapy to intensive induction and consolidation chemotherapy for childhood acute myeloblastic leukemia: results of a prospective randomized trial, LAME 89/91. Leucamie Aique Myeloide Enfant. J Clin Oncol 2002;20:2774–2782
133. Aladjidi N, Auvrignon A, Leblanc T et al. Outcome in children with relapsed acute myeloid leukemia after initial treatment with the French Leucemie Aique Myeloide Enfant (LAME) 89/91 protocol of the French Society of Pediatric Hematology and Immunology. J Clin Oncol 2003;21:4377–4385
134. Buckley JD, Lampkin BC, Nesbit ME et al. Remission induction in children with acute non-lymphocytic leukemia using cytosine arabinoside and doxorubicin or daunorubicin: a report from the Children's Cancer Study Group. Med Pediatr Oncol 1989;17:382–390
135. Wells RJ, Adams MT, Alonzo TA et al. Mitoxantrone and cytarabine induction, high-dose cytarabine, and etoposide intensification for pediatric patients with relapsed or refractory acute myeloid leukemia: Children's Cancer Group Study 2951. J Clin Oncol 2003;21:2940–2947
136. Woods WG, Kobrinsky N, Buckley JD et al. Timed-sequential induction therapy improves postremission outcome in acute myeloid leukemia: a report from the Children's Cancer Group. Blood 1996;87:4979–4989
137. Woods WG, Kobrinsky N, Buckley J et al. Intensively timed induction therapy followed by autologous or allogeneic bone marrow transplantation for children with acute myeloid leukemia or myelodysplastic syndrome: a Childrens Cancer Group pilot study. J Clin Oncol 1993;11:1448–1457
138. Capizzi RL, Poole M, Cooper MR et al. Treatment of poor risk acute leukemia with sequential high-dose ARA-C and asparaginase. Blood 1984;63:694–700
139. Woods WG, Ruymann FB, Lampkin BC et al. The role of timing of high-dose cytosine arabinoside intensification and of maintenance therapy in the treatment of children with acute nonlymphocytic leukemia. Cancer 1990;66:1106–1113
140. Dahl GV, Kalwinsky DK, Mirro J Jr et al. Allogeneic bone marrow transplantation in a program of intensive sequential chemotherapy for children and young adults with acute nonlymphocytic leukemia in first remission. J Clin Oncol 1990;8:295–303
141. Wells RJ, Woods WG, Buckley JD et al. Treatment of newly diagnosed children and adolescents with acute myeloid leukemia: a Children's Cancer Group study. J Clin Oncol 1994;12:2367–2377
142. Nesbit ME Jr, Buckley JD, Feig SA et al. Chemotherapy for induction of remission of childhood acute myeloid leukemia followed by marrow transplantation or multiagent chemotherapy: a report from the Children's Cancer Group. J Clin Oncol 1994;12:127–135
143. Oliansky DM, Rizzo JD, Aplan PD et al. The role of cytotoxic therapy with hematopoietic stem cell transplantation in the therapy of acute myeloid leukemia in children: an evidence-based review. Biol Blood Marrow Transplant 2007;13:1–25
144. Bleakley M, Lau L, Shaw PJ et al. Bone marrow transplantation for paediatric AML in first remission: a systematic review and meta-analysis. Bone Marrow Transplant 2002;29:843–852
145. Ravindranath Y, Yeager AM, Chang MN et al. Autologous bone marrow transplantation versus intensive consolidation chemotherapy for acute myeloid leukemia in childhood. Pediatric Oncology Group. N Engl J Med 1996;334:1428–1434
146. Amadori S, Testi AM, Arico M et al. Prospective comparative study of bone marrow transplantation and postremission chemotherapy for childhood acute myelogenous leukemia. The Associazione Italiana Ematologia ed Oncologia Pediatrica Cooperative Group. J Clin Oncol 1993;11:1046–1054
147. Woods WG, Neudorf S, Gold S et al. A comparison of allogeneic bone marrow transplantation, autologous bone marrow transplantation, and aggressive chemotherapy in children with acute myeloid leukemia in remission. Blood 2001;97:56–62
148. Feig SA, Lampkin B, Nesbit ME et al. Outcome of BMT during first complete remission of AML: a comparison of two sequential studies by the Children's Cancer Group. Bone Marrow Transplant 1993;12:65–71
149. Burnett AK, Goldstone AH, Stevens RM et al. Randomised comparison of addition of autologous bone-marrow transplantation to intensive chemotherapy for acute myeloid leukaemia in first remission: results of MRC AML 10 trial. UK Medical Research Council Adult and Children's Leukaemia Working Parties. Lancet 1998;351:700–708
150. Watson M, Buck G, Wheatley K et al. Adverse impact of bone marrow transplantation on quality of life in acute myeloid leukaemia patients; analysis of the UK Medical Research Council AML 10 Trial. Eur J Cancer 2004;40:971–978
151. Cassileth PA, Harrington DP, Appelbaum FR et al. Chemotherapy compared with autologous or allogeneic bone marrow transplantation in the management of acute myeloid leukemia in first remission. N Engl J Med 1998;339:1649–1656
152. Zittoun RA, Mandelli F, Willemze R et al. Autologous or allogeneic bone marrow transplantation compared with intensive chemotherapy in acute myelogenous leukemia. European Organization for Research and Treatment of Cancer (EORTC) and the Gruppo Italiano Malattie Ematologiche Maligne dell'Adulto (GIMEMA) Leukemia Cooperative Groups. N Engl J Med 1995;332:217–223

153. Burnett AK, Wheatley K, Goldstone AH et al. The value of allogeneic bone marrow transplant in patients with acute myeloid leukaemia at differing risk of relapse: results of the UK MRC AML 10 trial. Br J Haematol 2002;118:385–400
154. Chen AR, Alonzo TA, Woods WG et al. Current controversies: which patients with acute myeloid leukaemia should receive a bone marrow transplantation? An American view. Br J Haematol 2002;118:378–384
155. Creutzig U, Reinhardt D. Current controversies: which patients with acute myeloid leukaemia should receive a bone marrow transplantation? A European view. Br J Haematol 2002;118:365–377
156. Alonzo TA, Wells RJ, Woods WG et al. Postremission therapy for children with acute myeloid leukemia: the children's cancer group experience in the transplant era. Leukemia 2005;19:965–970
157. Egeler RM, Neglia JP, Arico M et al. Acute leukemia in association with Langerhans cell histiocytosis. Med Pediatr Oncol 1994;23:81–85
158. Ferry C, Socie G. Busulfan-cyclophosphamide versus total body irradiation-cyclophosphamide as preparative regimen before allogeneic hematopoietic stem cell transplantation for acute myeloid leukemia: what have we learned? Exp Hematol 2003;31:1182–1186
159. Michel G, Gluckman E, Esperou-Bourdeau H et al. Allogeneic bone marrow transplantation for children with acute myeloblastic leukemia in first complete remission: impact of conditioning regimen without total-body irradiation–a report from the Societe Francaise de Greffe de Moelle. J Clin Oncol 1994;12:1217–1222
160. Hsu KC, Keever-Taylor CA, Wilton A et al. Improved outcome in HLA-identical sibling hematopoietic stem-cell transplantation for acute myelogenous leukemia predicted by KIR and HLA genotypes. Blood 2005;105:4878–4884
161. Meshinchi S, Leisenring WM, Carpenter PA et al. Survival after second hematopoietic stem cell transplantation for recurrent pediatric acute myeloid leukemia. Biol Blood Marrow Transplant 2003;9:706–713
162. Quintas-Cardama A, Cortes JE. Chronic myeloid leukemia: diagnosis and treatment. Mayo Clin Proc 2006;81:973–988
163. Melo JV. The diversity of BCR-ABL fusion proteins and their relationship to leukemia phenotype. Blood 1996;88:2375–2384
164. Quintas-Cardama A, Cortes J. Kinase inhibitors in chronic myelogenous leukemia. Clin Adv Hematol Oncol 2006;4:365–374
165. Sokal JE, Cox EB, Baccarani M et al. Prognostic discrimination in 'good-risk' chronic granulocytic leukemia. Blood 1984;63:789–799
166. Pulsipher MA. Treatment of CML in pediatric patients: should imatinib mesylate (STI-571, Gleevec) or allogeneic hematopoietic cell transplant be front-line therapy? Pediatr Blood Cancer 2004;43:523–533
167. Druker BJ, Guilhot F, O'Brien SG et al. Five-year follow-up of patients receiving imatinib for chronic myeloid leukemia. N Engl J Med 2006;355:2408–2417
168. Shah NP. Loss of response to imatinib: mechanisms and management. Hematol Am Soc Hematol Educ Program 2005:183–187
169. Walz C, Sattler M. Novel targeted therapies to overcome imatinib mesylate resistance in chronic myeloid leukemia (CML). Crit Rev Oncol Hematol 2006;57:145–164
170. Kolb EA, Pan Q, Ladanyi M et al. Imatinib mesylate in Philadelphia chromosome-positive leukemia of childhood. Cancer 2003;98:2643–2650
171. Goldman JM, Marin D. Management decisions in chronic myeloid leukemia. Semin Hematol 2003;40:97–103
172. Goldman J, Gordon M. Why do chronic myelogenous leukemia stem cells survive allogeneic stem cell transplantation or imatinib: does it really matter? Leuk Lymphoma 2006;47:1–7
173. Wassmann B, Pfeifer H, Scheuring U et al. Therapy with imatinib mesylate (Glivec) preceding allogeneic stem cell transplantation (SCT) in relapsed or refractory Philadelphia-positive acute lymphoblastic leukemia (Ph+ALL). Leukemia 2002;16:2358–2365
174. Weisdorf DJ, Anasetti C, Antin JH et al. Allogeneic bone marrow transplantation for chronic myelogenous leukemia: comparative analysis of unrelated versus matched sibling donor transplantation. Blood 2002;99:1971–1977
175. Goldman JM, Druker BJ. Chronic myeloid leukemia: current treatment options. Blood 2001;98:2039–2042
176. Gratwohl A, Hermans J, Goldman JM et al. Risk assessment for patients with chronic myeloid leukaemia before allogeneic blood or marrow transplantation. Chronic Leukemia Working Party of the European Group for Blood and Marrow Transplantation. Lancet 1998;352:1087–1092
177. Silver RT, Woolf SH, Hehlmann R et al. An evidence-based analysis of the effect of busulfan, hydroxyurea, interferon, and allogeneic bone marrow transplantation in treating the chronic phase of chronic myeloid leukemia: developed for the American Society of Hematology. Blood 1999;94:1517–1536
178. Stary J, Locatelli F, Niemeyer CM. Stem cell transplantation for aplastic anemia and myelodysplastic syndrome. Bone Marrow Transplant 2005;35(suppl 1):S13–16
179. Niemeyer CM, Kratz CP, Hasle H. Pediatric myelodysplastic syndromes. Curr Treat Options Oncol 2005;6:209–214
180. Hasle H, Niemeyer CM, Chessells JM et al. A pediatric approach to the WHO classification of myelodysplastic and myeloproliferative diseases. Leukemia 2003;17:277–282
181. Mandel K, Dror Y, Poon A et al. A practical, comprehensive classification for pediatric myelodysplastic syndromes: the CCC system. J Pediatr Hematol Oncol 2002;24:596–605
182. Occhipinti E, Correa H, Yu L et al. Comparison of two new classifications for pediatric myelodysplastic and myeloproliferative disorders. Pediatr Blood Cancer 2005;44:240–244
183. Choong K, Freedman MH, Chitayat D et al. Juvenile myelomonocytic leukemia and Noonan syndrome. J Pediatr Hematol Oncol 1999;21:523–527
184. Stiller CA, Chessells JM, Fitchett M. Neurofibromatosis and childhood leukaemia/lymphoma: a population-based UKCCSG study. Br J Cancer 1994;70:969–972
185. Hasle H, Baumann I, Bergstrasser E et al. The International Prognostic Scoring System (IPSS) for childhood myelodysplastic syndrome (MDS) and juvenile myelomonocytic leukemia (JMML). Leukemia 2004;18:2008–2014
186. Niemeyer CM, Arico M, Basso G et al. Chronic myelomonocytic leukemia in childhood: a retrospective analysis of 110 cases. European Working Group on Myelodysplastic Syndromes in Childhood (EWOG-MDS). Blood 1997;89:3534–3543
187. Woods WG, Barnard DR, Alonzo TA et al. Prospective study of 90 children requiring treatment for juvenile myelomonocytic leukemia or myelodysplastic syndrome: a report from the Children's Cancer Group. J Clin Oncol 2002;20:434–440
188. Yoshimi A, Baumann I, Fuhrer M et al. Immunosuppressive therapy with anti-thymocyte globulin and cyclosporine A in selected children with hypoplastic refractory cytopenia. Haematologica 2007;92:397–400
189. Freedman MH, Estrov Z, Chan HS. Juvenile chronic myelogenous leukemia. Am J Pediatr Hematol Oncol 1988;10:261–267
190. Castleberry RP, Emanuel PD, Zuckerman KS et al. A pilot study of isotretinoin in the treatment of juvenile chronic myelogenous leukemia. N Engl J Med 1994;331:1680–1684
191. Yusuf U, Frangoul HA, Gooley TA et al. Allogeneic bone marrow transplantation in children with myelodysplastic syndrome or juvenile myelomonocytic leukemia: the Seattle experience. Bone Marrow Transplant 2004;33:805–814
192. Locatelli F, Nollke P, Zecca M et al. Hematopoietic stem cell transplantation (HSCT) in children with juvenile myelomonocytic leukemia (JMML): results of the EWOG-MDS/EBMT trial. Blood 2005;105:410–419
193. Arico M, Biondi A, Pui CH. Juvenile myelomonocytic leukemia. Blood 1997;90:479–488
194. Yoshimi A, Mohamed M, Bierings M et al. Second allogeneic hematopoietic stem cell transplantation (HSCT) results in outcome similar to that of first HSCT for patients with juvenile myelomonocytic leukemia. Leukemia 2007;21:556–560
195. Runde V, de Witte T, Arnold R et al. Bone marrow transplantation from HLA-identical siblings as first-line treatment in patients with myelodysplastic syndromes: early transplantation is associated with improved outcome. Chronic Leukemia Working Party of the European Group for Blood and Marrow Transplantation. Bone Marrow Transplant 1998;21:255–261
196. Bunin N, Saunders F, Leahey A et al. Alternative donor bone marrow transplantation for children with juvenile myelomonocytic leukemia. J Pediatr Hematol Oncol 1999;21:479–485
197. Smith FO, King R, Nelson G et al. Unrelated donor bone marrow transplantation for children with juvenile myelomonocytic leukaemia. Br J Haematol 2002;116:716–724
198. Yoshimi A, Bader P, Matthes-Martin S et al. Donor leukocyte infusion after hematopoietic stem cell transplantation in patients with juvenile myelomonocytic leukemia. Leukemia 2005;19:971–977
199. Creutzig U, Bender-Gotze C, Ritter J et al. The role of intensive AML-specific therapy in treatment of children with RAEB and RAEB-t. Leukemia 1998;12:652–659
200. Kletzel M, Jacobsohn D, Tse W et al. Reduced intensity transplants (RIT) in pediatrics: a review. Pediatr Transplant 2005;9(suppl 7):63–70
201. Iannone R, Casella JF, Fuchs EJ et al. Results of minimally toxic nonmyeloablative transplantation in patients with sickle cell anemia and beta-thalassemia. Biol Blood Marrow Transplant 2003;9:519–528
202. Del Toro G, Satwani P, Harrison L et al. A pilot study of reduced intensity conditioning and allogeneic stem cell transplantation from unrelated cord blood and matched family donors in children and adolescent recipients. Bone Marrow Transplant 2004;33:613–622
203. Jacobsohn DA, Duerst R, Tse W et al. Reduced intensity haemopoietic stem-cell transplantation for treatment of non-malignant diseases in children. Lancet 2004;364:156–162
204. Horn B, Baxter-Lowe LA, Englert L et al. Reduced intensity conditioning using intravenous busulfan, fludarabine and rabbit ATG for children with nonmalignant disorders and CML. Bone Marrow Transplant 2006;37:263–269
205. Eapen M, Horowitz MM, Klein JP et al. Higher mortality after allogeneic peripheral-blood transplantation compared with bone marrow in children and adolescents: the Histocompatibility and Alternate Stem Cell Source Working Committee of the International Bone Marrow Transplant Registry. J Clin Oncol 2004;22:4872–4880
206. Grupp SA, Frangoul H, Wall D et al. Use of G-CSF in matched sibling donor pediatric allogeneic transplantation: a consensus statement from the Children's Oncology Group (COG) Transplant Discipline Committee and Pediatric Blood and Marrow Transplant Consortium (PBMTC) Executive Committee. Pediatr Blood Cancer 2006;46:414–421
207. Wagner JE, Kernan NA, Steinbuch M et al. Allogeneic sibling umbilical-cord-blood transplantation in children with malignant and non-malignant disease. Lancet 1995;346:214–219
208. Rocha V, Wagner JE Jr, Sobocinski KA et al. Graft-versus-host disease in children who have received a cord-blood or bone marrow transplant from an HLA-identical sibling. Eurocord and International Bone Marrow Transplant Registry Working Committee on Alternative Donor and Stem Cell Sources. N Engl J Med 2000;342:1846–1854
209. Yu LC, Wall DA, Sandler E et al. Unrelated cord blood transplant experience by the pediatric blood and marrow transplant consortium. Pediatr Hematol Oncol 2001;18:235–245
210. Barker JN. Who should get cord blood transplants? Biol Blood Marrow Transplant 2007;13(suppl 1):78–82
211. Gluckman E, Rocha V, Chevret S. Results of unrelated umbilical cord blood hematopoietic stem cell transplantation. Rev Clin Exp Hematol 2001;5:87–99
212. Lang P, Greil J, Bader P et al. Long-term outcome after haploidentical stem cell transplantation in children. Blood Cells Mol Dis 2004;33:281–287
213. Klingebiel T, Handgretinger R, Lang P et al. Haploidentical transplantation for acute lymphoblastic leukemia in childhood. Blood Rev 2004;18:181–192
214. Higman MA, Vogelsang GB. Chronic graft versus host disease. Br J Haematol 2004;125:435–454
215. Lee SJ, Vogelsang G, Flowers ME. Chronic graft-versus-host disease. Biol Blood Marrow Transplant 2003;9:215–233
216. Akpek G, Lee SJ, Flowers ME et al. Performance of a new clinical grading system for chronic graft-versus-host disease: a multicenter study. Blood 2003;102:802–809

217. Zecca M, Prete A, Rondelli R et al. Chronic graft-versus-host disease in children: incidence, risk factors, and impact on outcome. Blood 2002;100:1192–1200

218. Busca A, Rendine S, Locatelli F et al. Chronic graft-versus-host disease after reduced-intensity stem cell transplantation versus conventional hematopoietic stem cell transplantation. Hematology 2005;10:1–10

219. Oeffinger KC, Mertens AC, Sklar CA et al. Chronic health conditions in adult survivors of childhood cancer. N Engl J Med 2006;355:1572–1582

220. Hewitt M, Rowland JH, Yancik R. Cancer survivors in the United States: age, health, and disability. J Gerontol A Biol Sci Med Sci 2003;58:82–91

221. Brougham MF, Wallace WH. Subfertility in children and young people treated for solid and haematological malignancies. Br J Haematol 2005;131:143–155

222. Phipps S, Dunavant M, Srivastava DK et al. Cognitive and academic functioning in survivors of pediatric bone marrow transplantation. J Clin Oncol 2000;18:1004–1011

223. Woolfrey AE, Gooley TA, Sievers EL et al. Bone marrow transplantation for children less than 2 years of age with acute myelogenous leukemia or myelodysplastic syndrome. Blood 1998;92:3546–3556

224. Horowitz MM, Confer DL. Evaluation of hematopoietic stem cell donors. Hematol Am Soc Hematol Educ Program 2005;469–475

225. Sanders J, Buckner CD, Bensinger WI et al. Experience with marrow harvesting from donors less than two years of age. Bone Marrow Transplant 1987;2:45–50

226. Pulsipher MA, Nagler A, Iannone R et al. Weighing the risks of G-CSF administration, leukopheresis, and standard marrow harvest: ethical and safety considerations for normal pediatric hematopoietic cell donors. Pediatr Blood Cancer 2006;46:422–433

227. Wiener LS, Steffen-Smith E, Fry T et al. Hematopoietic stem cell donation in children: a review of the sibling donor experience. J Psychosoc Oncol 2007;25:45–66

228. Golub TR, Slonim DK, Tamayo P et al. Molecular classification of cancer: class discovery and class prediction by gene expression monitoring. Science 1999;286:531–537

229. Yeoh EJ, Ross ME, Shurtleff SA et al. Classification, subtype discovery, and prediction of outcome in pediatric acute lymphoblastic leukemia by gene expression profiling. Cancer Cell 2002;1:133–143

230. Pastan I, Hassan R, Fitzgerald DJ et al. Immunotoxin therapy of cancer. Nat Rev Cancer 2006;6:559–565

231. Pession ARR, Paolucci P, Pastore G et al. Hematopoietic stem cell transplantation in childhood: report from the bone marrow transplantation group of the Associazione Italiana Ematologia Oncologia Pediatrica (AIEOP). Haematologia 2000;85:638–646

232. Gorin NC, Labopin M, Fouillard L et al. Retrospective evaluation of autologous bone marrow transplantation vs allogeneic bone marrow transplantation from an HLA identical related donor in acute myelocytic leukemia. A study of the European Cooperative Group for Blood and Marrow Transplantation (EBMT). Bone Marrow Transplant 1996;18:111–117

The myelodysplastic syndromes

Zi Yi Lim and Ghulam J Mufti

Introduction

The myelodysplastic syndromes (MDS) are a heterogeneous group of clonal hematologic disorders characterized by bone marrow hyperplasia, together with peripheral blood cytopenias. The clinical course is variable and while a subgroup of patients has an extended period of cytopenia without progression, up to 25% of patients will eventually progress to develop acute myeloid leukemia.[1,2]

MDS is predominantly a disease of the elderly with a median age of onset of 70 years. The incidence of MDS has been estimated to be 2–13 cases per 100,000 of the population, with the incidence approaching 50 cases per 100,000 in patients aged 70 years and older.[3–5] The majority of cases of MDS are idiopathic, although various environmental agents such as age, alcohol, smoking, ionizing radiation, benzene and infections have been implicated as causative factors.[6] A significant proportion of secondary MDS cases is related to prior therapy (therapy-related MDS, t-MDS), be it chemotherapy or radiotherapy. In particular, the risk of t-MDS appears to be significantly increased following previous therapy with alkylating agents, and more recently following exposure to quinolone analogs such as fludarabine. T-MDS is associated with complex chromosomal abnormalities and a poorer prognosis.[7,8]

Classification

In 1982, the French-American-British classification (FAB) was proposed. This classification system was based solely on morphologic features of blood and bone marrow, with five subgroups defined: refractory anemia (RA), refractory anemia with ring sideroblasts (RARS), refractory anemia with excess blasts (RAEB), refractory anemia with excess of blasts in transformation (RAEBt), and chronic myelomonocytic anemia (CMML).[9] While subsequent clinical studies verified the utility of the FAB system, one of the limitations of this classification was that it failed to take into account biologic variables, such as the presence of cytogenetic abnormalities.

As a result, the international prognostic scoring system (IPSS) was introduced in 1997.[10] The IPSS incorporated features from seven previous studies and scoring systems on more than 700 untreated patients with MDS. Four stages were established, based on three critical factors: number of lineages of cytopenias, percentage blasts in the bone marrow, as well as specific cytogenetic abnormalities: low, intermediate-1 (Int-1), intermediate-2 (Int-2) and high. Patients with low-risk MDS had a median survival of 5.7 years, while high-risk MDS had a median survival of 0.4 years with a median time to acute myeloid leukemia (AML) transformation of 0.2 years. Both the FAB and IPSS have been extremely useful in the retrospective and prospec-

tive evaluation of MDS studies, and as clinical tools for assessing prognosis.

Recently, the World Health Organization (WHO) classification has been introduced. Important changes include the substratifying of patients with RA/RARS dependent upon whether there was unilineage dysplasia of the erythroid lineage or multilineage dysplasia. The threshold for defining AML was also lowered to 20%. In addition, patients with isolated 5q minus were recategorized as a distinct category, and patients with CMML were considered in a separate category of myelodysplastic syndromes/myeloproliferative diseases. Several studies have since validated that the WHO classification does have improved prognostic value for the low-grade MDS categories.[11–14] Howe et al demonstrated in a series of 64 patients with low-risk MDS that there was a significant difference in median survival between patients with unilineage dysplasia compared to those with multilineage dysplasia.[13] In addition, the study by Malcovati and colleagues examining 467 patients with de novo MDS identified that patients with only isolated erythroid lineage dysplasia had an extremely low risk of transformation to AML, and that survival in this subgroup was affected more by demographic variables than by disease features.[14] Table 7.1 provides a summary of the FAB and WHO classifications as well as the IPSS.

Non-transplantation treatments

Improvements in understanding of the disease

The last decade has seen tremendous advances in our understanding of the pathogenesis and molecular basis of myelodysplastic syndromes and myeloproliferative disorders. In response, a variety of therapeutic agents has been introduced as potential treatments for MDS. The number of therapies available is vast, and it is beyond the scope of this chapter to individually discuss all of them. Instead, this section will briefly introduce several treatment modalities, some more established and several novel agents, which we believe play a significant part in the treatment of the disease. Table 7.2 gives a more extensive list of current therapeutic agents either in use or undergoing clinical studies.

Supportive care

The main purpose of supportive care is to alleviate peripheral cytopenias and maintain a reasonable quality of life for MDS patients. The majority of patients requires some degree of supportive care, and there is evidence that an improved hemoglobin level provides better independence and quality of life.[15,16] Repeated blood transfusions may,

Table 7.1 Classification of the myelodysplastic syndromes

FAB classification					
Refractory anemia					
RARS					
RAEB					
RAEB-t					
CMML					
WHO classification					
Refractory anemia					
RARS					
RCMD					
RCMD-RS					
RAEB-I					
RAEB-II					
5q minus syndrome					

International Prognostic Scoring System (IPSS)					
Score	0	0.5	1.0	1.5	2.0
Karyotype#	Good	Int	Poor		
Bone marrow blasts	<5%	5–10%		11–20%	21–30%
Number of cytopenias	0/1	2/3			

Composite score	**IPSS risk group**
0	Low
0.5–1.0	Intermediate-1
1.5–2.0	Intermediate-2
≥2.5	High

Good – normal, del 5q, del 20q, -Y.
Poor – chromosome 7 abnormalities, complex cytogenetics (≥3 abnormalities).
Intermediate – other abnormalities.

Table 7.2 List of therapeutic agents for treatment of MDS

Growth factors	Erythropoietin
	G-CSF
Immunosuppressive agents	Antithymocyte globulin
	Etanercept
	Ciclosporin A
Immunomodulatory agents/ antiangiogenesis agents	Lenalidomide
	Thalidomide
	Bevacizumab
	Arsenic trioxide
DNMT	5-Azacitidine
	Decitabine
Histone deacetylase inhibitors	Sodium phenylbutyrate
	Valproic acid
	Suberoylanilide hydroxamic acid
Small-molecule inhibitors Farnesyl-transferase inhibitors	Tipifarnib
	Lonafarnib
FLT-3 inhibitors	PKC412
	MLN518 (tandutinib)
VEGFR tyrosine kinase inhibitors	PTK787/ZK 222584

however, result in iron overload, and despite improvements in blood transfusion safety, there still remains a small but acknowledgeable risk of transfusion-acquired infections.

Malcovati et al have shown that transfusion-dependent MDS patients have a significantly shorter survival than patients who do not require transfusions.[14] In addition, developing secondary iron overload significantly affects survival of transfusion-dependent patients. Armand and colleagues have also published data suggesting that, in a myeloablative setting, a pretransplant serum ferritin raised above 1000 ug/ml is an independent prognostic factor for non-relapse mortality and survival amongst patients with AML or MDS.[17] The current use of iron chelators and introduction of new oral agents such as ICL 670 have helped to reduce the effects of transfusion siderosis,[16,18] although the utility of these agents in the pretransplantation setting remains undefined.

There is currently no evidence that routine prophylaxis with antibiotics or the use of growth factors in MDS patients with either neutropenia or thrombocytopenia improves outcomes, although selected 'low-risk' patients may respond favorably to growth factor therapy.[15,19]

Immunosuppressive therapy

Various authors have identified an association between autoimmune phenomena, such as connective tissue and systemic vasculitic disorders, and the presence of MDS, and clinical and laboratory findings have suggested a T-cell immune-mediated component to the pancyto-

penia and bone marrow failure seen in MDS. Immunosuppressive therapy has been shown to induce sustained hematologic responses in a subset of patients.[20]

Antithymocyte globulin (ATG) is a polyclonal immunoglobulin which has been shown to induce hematologic responses in up to 60% of MDS patients.[20–22] While its precise mechanism of action remains unclear, it is believed to involve the amelioration of lymphocyte-mediated suppression of the bone marrow environment. Molldrem et al demonstrated initially that responsiveness to ATG is associated with a loss of lymphocyte-mediated inhibition of colony forming units-granulocyte/macrophage,[23] and more recently that there is a loss of T-lymphocyte clonal dominance in these patients.[24] The extent of responsiveness of MDS patients to immunosuppression remains unclear. Saunthararajah et al[22] have identified factors such as HLA-DR15, younger age and short duration of red cell transfusion dependence as factors linked with treatment responsiveness.

Targeted therapies

Developments in the understanding of the role of DNA methylation and histone acetylation have led to the successful treatment with demethylating agents, such as azacitidine (Vidaza®, Pharmion Corporation, Boulder, CO), which has been associated with hematologic responses in up to 60% of patients.[25] Similarly, treatment with lenalidomide, a thalidomide analog, has been shown to induce cytogenetic and hematologic remissions in 5q minus syndrome.[26–28] Despite such advances, there is little evidence to date showing that these agents lead to eradication of the underlying dysplastic clone.

Epigenetic targeting

Over the past decade, various groups have identified that promoter methylation of a number of genes, such as CDKN2B, is associated with poor-risk MDS and predicts transformation to AML.[29–31] As a consequence, there has been considerable interest in the potential role of DNA methyltransferase (DNMT) inhibitors in the treatment of MDS.[32] Azacitidine (5-azacitidine; Vidaza®) and decitabine (Dacogen®, SuperGen Inc., Dublin, CA, USA, and MGI Pharma Inc., Bloomington, MN, USA) are approved by the FDA for the treatment of all FAB MDS subtypes, including low- and high-risk diseases.[33]

Results from recent Phase III clinical trials[25,34] have shown that azacitidine can induce significant clinical benefits in high-risk MDS patients. Silverman and colleagues reported on the results of three sequential Cancer and Leukemia Group B (CALGB) trials, which showed that azacitidine significantly prevents or delays transformation to AML overall, and significantly prolongs AML-free survival. Decitabine has also been demonstrated to be efficacious in the treatment of MDS when compared to supportive care, with durable hematologic responses and transfusion independence. In addition, decitabine has been shown to significantly prolong AML-free survival in patients with IPSS Int-2/high groups.[35] Further clinical studies are currently under way to assess the role of these DNMT inhibitors in pretransplant induction and post-transplantation consolidation.

Role of stem cell transplantation

At present, despite the numerous advances in our understanding and approaches to treatment, stem cell transplantation remains the only definitive curative option for patients with MDS. This section will discuss the patient and donor factors that need to be considered prior to transplantation (Fig. 7.1).

Age and co-morbidity

The median age of patients with MDS is between 60 and 70 years, and many have pre-existing co-morbidities. The incidence of poor-risk MDS is proportionally greater in elderly patients, with increased frequency of t-AML, as well as adverse cytogenetic abnormalities.[36,37] Early registry studies have demonstrated that there is a significant co-relationship between advanced age and increased transplant-related mortality (TRM).[36,38–43] A report by the European Group of Blood and Marrow Transplantation (EBMT) compared three groups aged <20 years, 20–40 years and >40 years, illustrating the higher TRM of 30%, 43%, 50% and poorer disease-free survival (DFS) of 45%, 37%, 31% respectively with increasing age.[41]

Recent improvements in conditioning regimens and supportive care have bettered transplantation outcomes and permitted extension of the upper age limit for transplantation. A study by Hsu et al of 59 selected patients aged >50 years compared to patients aged <50 years reported no significant difference in outcomes between groups, suggesting that myeloablative allografts can be offered to selected older patients with good performance status.[44] The more recent introduction of reduced-intensity conditioning regimens has also permitted the allografting of older patients with low toxicity (TRM < 10%) despite the presence of co-morbid factors.[45,46]

In view of the advances in transplantation regimens and patient care, there is an increasing awareness that transplant physicians need to consider both age and the co-existence of other co-morbidities in the evaluation of patient suitability for transplantation. Assessment scores such as the Charlson co-morbidity score or, more recently, the specifically developed hematopoietic cell transplantation-comorbidity index (HCT-CI) may help to improve patient selection. The prognostic utility of these scores has been validated in several studies for AML and MDS patients undergoing myeloablative and non-myeloablative conditioned hematopoietic stem cell transplantation (HSCT).[47–49]

Disease stage and disease status at transplantation

In addition to age and co-morbidity, the other single most important variable that has a prognostic impact on transplantation outcomes in most MDS studies is the disease stage at diagnosis, as well as at time of transplantation. Disease stage has been classified in various ways in different studies: by the FAB classification (with RA and RARS

being low risk, and all other types being high risk), the percentage of BM blasts at transplantation, or the IPSS.

The International Bone Marrow Transplant Registry conducted a retrospective analysis of 452 recipients of HLA-identical sibling transplants for MDS reported from 1989 to 1997. Sixty percent had refractory anemia with excess blasts (n = 136) or excess blasts in transformation (n = 136). The 3-year TRM, relapse and DFS rates were 37%, 23% and 40%, respectively. Multivariate analyses identified young age and platelet counts ($>100 \times 10^9$/l) at transplantation as being associated with lower TRM and higher DFS. Conversely, the relapse incidence was higher in patients with high percentages of BM blasts at transplantation or presentation, with a high IPSS at diagnosis, and with T-cell depleted transplants, suggesting that the best candidates for HLA-matched sibling allografts for MDS are younger patients with a low percentage of blasts and preserved platelet counts.[50]

The Seattle group reported on a total of 251 MDS patients with a median age of 38 years who were transplanted at the Fred Hutchinson Cancer Research Center (FHCRC) from 1981 to 1996. The overall DFS was 40%, with a relapse incidence of 18%. Increasing disease duration, morphology and cytogenetics were significant in predicting relapses. In addition, increasing age, disease morphology and cytogenetics were significant in determining DFS. IPSS score was found to correlate significantly with DFS, with a 5-year DFS of 60%, 36%, and 28% for low and Int-1 risk, Int-2 risk, and high-risk patients, respectively.[51]

Role of induction therapy

Intensive chemotherapy is effective in inducing complete remissions in 15–65% of patients.[52–54] However, these remissions are often short-lived due to subsequent disease relapse. Various studies have identified low disease burden at time of transplantation as an important prognostic factor for transplant relapse. While it may appear logical to pretreat patients with intensive chemotherapy to reduce the disease burden, controversy remains about the effectiveness of this approach, as it is unclear whether intensive chemotherapy merely identifies a subgroup of patients with more chemoresponsive treatment.

A long-term French study showed that patients with secondary MDS who achieved remissions with pretransplant chemotherapy had substantially better relapse-free survivals post transplantation when compared to patients who did not achieve a remission. However, patients who failed to respond to induction chemotherapy had a lower probability of a successful post-transplant course than would be expected in patients not treated pretransplant.[43] In addition, the Fred Hutchinson Cancer Research Center reported on a retrospective analysis of 125 patients with advanced MDS and t-AML with HLA-matched siblings or voluntary unrelated donor (VUD) undergoing myeloablative conditioning, and indicated that while patients receiving induction chemotherapy had a lower incidence of relapse post transplantation, this did not actually equate to an improved disease-free or overall survival.[55]

The EBMT is currently conducting a prospective randomized multicenter Phase III study to evaluate the role of remission-induction and consolidation chemotherapy prior to allogeneic transplantation using HLA-identical siblings in patients less than 50 years of age with MDS.

Cytogenetic status

Cytogenetics studies are an important initial test in any newly diagnosed patient with MDS, and play a major role in confirmation of diagnosis and prediction of clinical outcome in MDS.[10,56–59] This is reflected in the IPSS, as well as to a certain extent in the new WHO classification.

Clonal chromosomal abnormalities are a common occurrence in MDS, being detected in 40–70% of cases of de novo MDS, and in up to 95% of cases of t-MDS.[60] The presence of poor-risk cytogenetic abnormalities has been associated with a significantly poorer outcome post transplantation. Using cytogenetic risk categories defined by the IPSS, Nevill and colleagues retrospectively evaluated the outcomes of 60 patients undergoing BMT in Vancouver, Canada. The 7-year event-free survivals for the poor-risk, intermediate-risk and good-risk groups were 6%, 40% and 51%, respectively, with an actuarial risk of relapse of 82%, 12% and 19%, respectively.[61] Similarly, a French study of 71 MDS patients undergoing HSCT reported a 7-year relapse rate of 83% in patients with complex cytogenetic anomalies.[37] In addition, a Dutch consortium has recently shown that deletion of part or all of chromosomes 5 and/or 7, and complex chromosomal abnormalities are predominant features of t-MDS and are associated with a poor prognosis despite intensive therapy and consolidation with allogeneic stem cell transplantation.[62]

Timing of transplantation

Given the relatively indolent time course of some patients with intermediate- and low-risk MDS, there remains considerable debate as to the optimal time to transplant these patients. In response to these questions, Cutler and colleagues constructed a Markov model to examine three transplantation strategies for patients with newly diagnosed MDS who received an HLA-matched sibling allograft:[63] patients transplanted at diagnosis, patients transplanted at time of leukemic progression, and patients transplanted at an interval from diagnosis but prior to leukemia progression.

For low and Int-1 IPSS groups, delayed transplantation maximized overall survival. Patients transplanted prior to leukemic transformation also had a greater number of life-years when compared to those transplanted at the time of leukemia progression. For intermediate-2 and high IPSS groups, transplantation at diagnosis maximized overall survival. The authors concluded that for low- and intermediate-1-risk MDS, delayed allogeneic transplantation was associated with maximal life expectancy, whereas for intermediate-2-risk and high-risk disease immediate transplantation was associated with maximal life expectancy.

Stem cell source

An EBMT multicenter retrospective study described the outcomes of 234 patients with MDS who underwent transplantation from HLA-identical siblings between 1995 and 1999,[64] comparing the outcomes based on the hematopoietic stem cell source used (bone marrow, BM versus granulocyte colony-stimulating factor-mobilized peripheral blood stem cells – PBSC). While the use of PBSC reduced the median duration of neutropenia and thrombocytopenia, the incidence of acute graft-versus-host disease (GvHD) was similar. However, chronic GvHD was more likely to have occurred with PBSC.

The estimated 2-year DFS was 50% with PBSC, versus 39% with BM, and on multivariate analysis, the outcome was significantly improved with PBSC for all subgroups of MDS except for those with either RA or high-risk cytogenetics. On this basis, the authors suggested that PBSC might be the preferred choice of stem cell source for allogeneic transplantation in MDS patients at high risk for relapse because use of this hematopoietic stem cell source may be associated with a lower treatment failure incidence and improved survival. Further prospective data are required, however, to validate these observations.

Types of stem cell transplantation

Autologous transplantation

There are limited data available on the use of autologous transplantation in MDS. The use of autologous cells has been limited by the inability to obtain adequate numbers of hematopoietic stem cells in a large proportion of patients. There is a high degree of disease relapse, in part due to the absence of the allogeneic graft-versus-leukemia effect. There are also concerns about the possible contamination of cell harvests by malignant cells.

The EBMT reported on the outcomes of 114 patients with MDS and secondary AML who underwent autologous BMT, of which 79 patients were in CR1. The 2-year DFS and relapse rates were 34% and 64%, respectively.[65] This experience has been updated recently.[66] In a cohort of 336 patients transplanted since 1992, the 3-year DFS, relapse and TRM rates were 24%, 61% and 13%, respectively. In addition, the cohort was analyzed according to stem cell source. While there was no difference in outcome between the use of bone marrow or peripheral blood harvested stem cells, earlier studies had suggested that disease relapse was associated with use of PBSC. The authors concluded that, as peripheral blood cells often provide a high cell yield and thus more rapid engraftment post transplantation, peripheral blood stem cell harvests should be the preferred cell source.

Standard conditioning transplantation

The majority of transplant centers have adopted a standard myeloablative conditioning regimen using a combination of cyclophosphamide with either total body irradiation (TBI) or busulfan. Myeloablative HSCT in MDS is associated with an overall DFS of 29–56%, and TRM of 34–54%.[36,37,41,51] Transplant-related complications due to drug resistance,[67] toxicity of conditioning regimens[37] and GvHD are directly proportional to the age of the recipient.[68,69] As up to 75% of patients with MDS are >60 years of age, many with significant medical co-morbidities, the use of myeloablative allografting has been restricted to a select group of patients with MDS.

Conventional myeloablative allografting in MDS has been historically restricted to the younger population due to the high TRM. Registry data from the International Bone Marrow Transplant Registry (IBMTR) on 452 HLA-identical siblings undergoing myeloablative HSCT, with a median age 38 years, cite 3-year TRM and DFS rates of 37% and 40%, respectively.[50] This is consistent with EBMT data on 1378 patients allografted from 1983 to 1998. The 3-year DFS for HLA-matched sibling donor recipients was 36% and for VUD recipients 25%, with a significant TRM of 58% for VUDs.[70]

However, transplant outcomes with myeloablative conditioning have steadily improved over the last decade, attributed to a decrease in TRM, which reflects improvements in conditioning regimens and supportive care.[70] In an attempt to reduce TRM, Deeg and colleagues from Seattle have reported on the use of a myeloablative regimen with targeted-dose oral busulfan and cyclophosphamide, for the treatment of MDS patients with related and unrelated donors. They reported on 109 MDS patients with a median age of 46 years (range 6–66 years), achieving impressive 3-year TRM and DFS of 30% and 59%, respectively. However, grade II–IV acute GvHD occurred in 68% of HLA-matched unrelated donors and 100% of HLA non-identical transplants, and chronic GvHD occurred in 47% of transplants.[71]

More recently, the same group from Seattle added ATG to their dose-adjusted oral busulfan plus cyclophosphamide regimen to reduce the incidence of GvHD. Fifty-six patients with MDS and other myeloid disorders underwent transplantation with PBSC from related (n = 30) or unrelated (n = 26) donors. All but two patients achieved engraftment, and 56% survived in remission beyond 1 year. The incidence of a-GvHD was 50%, and c-GvHD 34%. Among 27 MDS patients who underwent transplantation concurrently with targeted busulfan without thymoglobulin, the incidence of acute and chronic GvHD was 82%.[72]

Reduced-intensity conditioning (RIC) regimens

Within the last decade, it has been demonstrated that reduced-intensity or non-myeloablative conditioning can result in stable donor hemopoietic engraftment, without the toxicity associated with conventional HSCT.[73,74] Disease eradication and control are afforded by the graft-versus-malignancy (GvM) effect and to a lesser extent by transplant conditioning. These protocols involve intensive immunosuppression with combinations of low-dose TBI, fludarabine, ATG and/or alemtuzumab (Campath-1H), followed by infusion of unmanipulated peripheral blood stem cells or bone marrow. Donor–recipient chimera are created, which eventually shift toward full donor hematopoiesis spontaneously, or with escalating doses of donor T-cells.[74]

In some protocols, the initial incidence of severe (grade III–IV) acute (a)-GvHD remains significant at up to 38–60%.[74–76] This led some groups to incorporate T-cell depletion into the conditioning regimen. Alemtuzumab (Campath-1H) is a monoclonal anti-CD52 antibody, and its use as an in vivo T-cell depletion agent has dramati-

cally reduced the incidence of severe a-GvHD in reduced-intensity protocols.[77,78] The long half-life of alemtuzumab results in the depletion of donor CD52+ cells including circulating antigen-presenting dendritic cells following infusion into the recipient.[79,80] While the incidence and morbidity associated with GvHD are significantly reduced, the disadvantage of in vivo purging with alemtuzumab may be a clinically significant reduction in the GvL effect, as well as an increase in post-transplant viral infections due to prolonged immunosuppression also associated with an increased risk of disease relapse.[81–83]

The earlier data on reduced-intensity allografting for MDS are mixed, with a multitude of differing conditioning regimens used by different investigators. Although RIC HSCT has been demonstrated to be safe and feasible as an alternative to standard conditioning, earlier publications have included heterogeneity of disease states that often included lymphoid and other non-myeloid conditions. Table 7.3 lists the results of the larger recent MDS-based RIC studies

Which regimen to use?

Several groups have recently performed retrospective analyses in an attempt to address this question. Alyea and colleagues from the Dana-Faber Institute analyzed the results of 152 patients who were older

Table 7.3 Summary of recent studies including data on RIC in MDS

Study	Patients	Median age (years)	Conditioning	GvHD	Outcome calculated at	NRM (%)	DFS (%)	OS (%)
Martino 2002[42]	AML (17) MDS (20)	57	Fludarabine Busulfan	a-GvHD II-IV 19%; c-GvHD 43%	1 year	5	66	
Taussig 2003[99]	AML (4) MDS (12)	54	Fludarabine Cyclophosphamide	c-GvHD 66%	2 years	6	56	69
de Lima 2004[68]	AML (26) MDS (6)	32	Fludarabine Cytarabine Idarubicin	a-GvHD II-IV 25%; c-GvHD 27%	3 years	15	32	30
de Lima 2004[68]	AML (42) MDS (20)	62	Fludarabine Melphalan	a-GvHD II-IV 39%; cGvHD 39%	3 years	39	19	35
Ho 2004[78]	MDS (62)	53	Fludarabine Busulfan CAMPATH	a-GvHD II-IV 17%; c-GvHD 15%	1 year	15	62	74

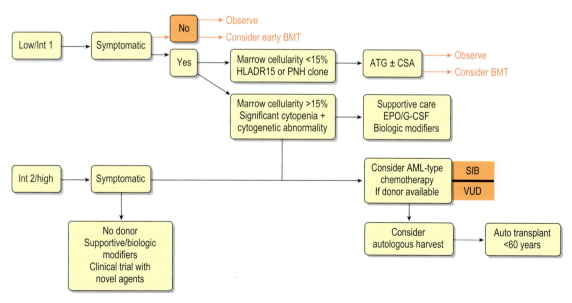

Figure 7.1
Suggested algorithm for the treatment of MDS.

than 50 years undergoing allogeneic HSCT.[84] Seventy-one patients received a non-myeloablative conditioning regimen and 81 patients received a myeloablative regimen. While the non-myeloablative patients were more likely to have unrelated donors, as well as active disease at time of transplantation, the overall survival was improved in this cohort at 1 (51% vs 39%) and 2 years (39% vs 29%). The TRM was lower for the non-myeloablative cohort (32% vs 50%, p = 0.01), with a higher relapse rate (46% vs 30%, p = 0.052).

Investigators from the FHCRC, Seattle, reported on the results of 150 patients receiving allogeneic transplantation for MDS or t-AML.[85] One hundred and twelve patients received a myeloablative regimen and 38 patients received a non-myeloablative regimen. Non-myeloablative patients were older (median age 62 vs 52 years, p < 0.001), more frequently had progressed to t-AML (53% vs 31%, p = 0.06), had higher risk disease by the IPSS (53% vs 30%, p = 0.004), had higher transplant-specific co-morbidity indices (68% vs 42%, p = 0.01) and more frequently had durable complete responses to induction chemotherapy (58% vs 14%). Three-year overall survival (27%/48%, p = 0.56), progression-free survival (28%/44%, p = 0.60), and non-relapse mortality (41%/34%, p = 0.94) did not differ significantly between non-myeloblative/myeloablative conditioning. Overall and progression-free survivals were similar for patients with chemotherapy-induced remissions, irrespective of conditioning intensity.

The EBMT recently reported on a multicenter study of 836 patients with MDS undergoing allogeneic HSCT with HLA-matched siblings, and compared 215 patients receiving RIC with 621 patients receiving myeloablative conditioning. While the 3-year relapse rate was significantly increased in the RIC cohort (HR 1.64; 95% confidence interval (CI) 1.2–2.2, p = 0.001), the 3-year non-relapse mortality was decreased in the RIC group (HR 0.61; 95% CI 0.41–0.91, p = 0.015) with similar overall survival (45% vs 41%, p = 0.8).[86]

Transplantation with unrelated donors

One of the other major limiting factors in allogeneic HSCT is the availability of an HLA-matched donor.[36,69] Less than one-third of patients in Europe or the USA have a suitable HLA-matched sibling.[36] The expansion of donor registries worldwide, as well as the increasing use of umbilical cord stem cells, has increased the probability of finding an HLA-matched VUD.[87,88] However, VUD allografts, particularly in older patients, are associated with an increased risk of graft rejection, GvHD, and TRM.[36,77]

TRM is significantly increased for conventional unrelated allografts; the National Marrow Donor Program (NMDP) reported results of 510 patients with a median age of 38 years (range <1–62 years) and 2-year TRM and DFS of 54% and 29%, respectively.[36] This is consistent with the EBMT experience of 118 unrelated allografts. With a median age of 24 years, the TRM was 57%. In recipients less than 18 years of age, the TRM was 40%, but TRM rose to 81% if the recipient was older than 35 years.[39]

Recent advances in supportive care and conditioning regimens have improved outcomes. As mentioned earlier, the use of targeted-dose busulfan has resulted in a successful reduction in the NRM associated with myeloablative conditioning regimens. In addition, reduced-intensity regimens have now been used with comparable outcomes using both sibling and unrelated donors.[78,85] Most recently, the group from King's College Hospital, London, reported on a prospective study evaluating the outcomes of 75 successive patients receiving a FBC (fludarabine, busulfan, alemtuzumab) RIC protocol for treating MDS patients using VUDs.[89] The median age of the cohort was 52.0 years with a median follow-up of 1038.5 days. Forty-nine patients (65%) had an IPSS stage of ≥Int-2, 35 (46%) had intermediate- or poor-risk cytogenetics, and 23 patients (31%) were HLA mismatched. The actuarial 3-year overall survival, DFS and relapse incidence rates

were 43% (95% CI 37–49), 41% (95% CI 35–47) and 43% (95% CI 36–50), respectively. The incidence of grade III–IV a-GvHD was 26% and the cumulative probability of extensive c-GvHD was 22%.

Use of donor lymphocyte infusions

Donor lymphocyte infusions (DLI) have been used for both mixed donor chimerism and relapsed disease (molecular and clinical relapse) to induce remission in patients with relapsed hematologic malignancies.[38,90] While the allogeneic (GvL) effect of DLI appears most pronounced in patients with chronic myeloid leukemia or multiple myeloma, durable remissions have also been achieved in relapsed MDS/AML patients post transplant.[90–92]

Ho et al have observed that following T-cell depleted RIC, MDS patients who receive DLI for decreasing donor chimerism or cytogenetic relapse have very good responses, with 14/16 reverting to full donor chimerism and 4/4 cytogenetic remission. However, the results following morphologic relapse are poor.[78] At present, uncertainty still remains about the optimum timing and dose of DLI for MDS patients, and given the significant risk of GvHD post DLI, prospective studies evaluating the use of DLI for treating relapse post transplantation are warranted.

On the other hand, Schmid and colleagues have described an approach using sequential intensive chemotherapy, RIC, followed by prophylactic donor lymphocyte transfusions post transplantation in high-risk AML/MDS. RIC consisted of 4 Gy TBI, ATG, and 80–120 mg/kg cyclophosphamide, and prophylactic DLI were given from day +120 in patients who were not receiving immunosuppression and who were free of GvHD.[93] In a prospective study of 75 consecutive patients with a median age of 52 years and a median follow-up of 35 months, the 2-year overall survival and DFS survival were 42% and 40%, respectively. Interestingly, the outcome of patients with refractory disease or with complex cytogenetic aberrations was identical to that of subgroups with a better prognosis.

Umbilical cord blood transplantation

With an increasing number of patients referred for allogeneic HSCT and the difficulty in finding a suitable HLA-matched donor in a significant number of cases, interest in umbilical cord blood (UCB) transplantation has increased. The logistics surrounding the administration of UCB are far fewer than the recruitment of VUDs. However, despite the reduction in the incidence of GvHD and the ability to utilize UCB with increasing HLA disparity, the lower hematopoietic stem cell dose retrieved has led to concern over engraftment in adults and hence limited its use.

The most recent report by the Eurocord and Netcord registries analyzed 682 adults with AML or ALL, 98 of whom received UCB and 584 received bone marrow. A lower incidence of acute grade II–IV GvHD is reported following UCB (26% vs 39%), with 94% receiving UCB from an HLA-mismatched donor, whereas bone marrow recipients were fully HLA matched. No significant difference in TRM, DFS or overall survival was noted between the groups.[88] A multicenter study reported by Laughlin et al compared outcome following UCB from both one (34 patients) and two (116 patients) HLA-antigen mismatched unrelated donors, to recipients of BM from HLA-matched (367 patients) and one antigen-mismatched (83 patients) donors in patients with hematologic malignancies including MDS. Improved outcome was only demonstrated following transplantation using fully compatible BM recipients, with no significant differences between those receiving mismatched UCB or mismatched bone marrow. A higher rate of acute GvHD was identified following HLA-mismatched BM and a higher incidence of chronic GvHD following UCB transplantation.[87]

Ooi et al have recently updated the Japanese experience on UCB transplantation for adults with MDS.[94] Twenty-two patients were treated with a myeloablative regimen consisting of TBI (12 Gy) cytosine arabinoside and cyclophosphamide. The median patient age was 40 years, and the median follow-up 1505 days. The median number of UCB nucleated cells infused was 2.43×10^7 kg, and 21 patients achieved myeloid reconstitution (neutrophil count $>0.5 \times 10^9/l$) at a median time of 22.5 days. The estimated DFS at 4 years was 76%.

Further published reports of adult recipients of UCB consist only of small series of patients with heterogeneous diseases including AML, ALL, CML and few cases of MDS.[94–98] The incidence of grade III–IV acute GvHD is low, reported at 7–27% despite the majority receiving HLA-mismatched units. However, a significant day 100 TRM of 43–56% is documented. Reports to date confirm UCB transplantation as a feasible alternative to BM or PBSC transplantation in patients where a suitable HLA-matched donor is unavailable. Despite low stem cell doses and slow engraftment, similar outcome is observed to that with BM or PBSC allografts using HLA-mismatched donors.

Summary

Allogeneic hematopoietic stem cell transplantation remains a potentially curative therapeutic option for many patients with MDS. Survival outcomes have improved progressively, primarily as a result of the development of more tolerable transplant conditioning regimens such as reduced-intensity regimens. However, the role of the dose intensity of the conditioning regimen remains important, particularly in patients with more advanced disease, as indicated by the higher relapse rates in patients in this subgroup.

The discovery of novel immunomodulatory and disease-modifying agents such as lenalidomide, decitabine and 5-azacytidine has expanded the treatment options for a subset of patients with MDS. The use of these agents, however, does not result in a long-term cure, and future studies are awaited to establish how they may be incorporated into either the pretransplant induction regimen or post-transplantation maintenance protocol, or both.

It is clear that other disease- and patient-specific considerations, such as availability of donor source, patient age, patient co-morbidity status and disease status, need to be considered when assessing patient suitability for transplantation. However, given the increasing choice of options within the field of MDS transplantation, an individualized approach should be adopted in determining specific treatment strategies for a patient with MDS.

References

1. Mufti GJ, Stevens JR, Oscier DG et al. Myelodysplastic syndromes: a scoring system with prognostic significance. Br J Haematol 1985;59:425–433
2. Mufti GJ. Pathobiology, classification, and diagnosis of myelodysplastic syndromes. Best Pract Res Clin Haematol 2004;17:543–557
3. Aul C, Gattermann N, Schneider W. Age-related incidence and other epidemiological aspects of myelodysplastic syndromes. Br J Haematol 1992;82:358–367
4. Aul C, Gattermann N, Schneider W. Epidemiological and etiological aspects of myelodysplastic syndromes. Leuk Lymphoma 1995;16:247–262
5. Aul C, Germing U, Gattermann N, Minning H. Increasing incidence of myelodysplastic syndromes: real or fictitious? Leuk Res 1998;22:93–100
6. Nisse C, Haguenoer JM, Grandbastien B et al. Occupational and environmental risk factors of the myelodysplastic syndromes in the North of France. Br J Haematol 2001;112:927–935
7. Milligan DW, Ruiz De Elvira MC, Kolb HC et al. Secondary leukemia and myelodysplasia after autografting for lymphoma: results from the EBMT. EBMT Lymphoma and Late Effects Working Parties. European Group for Blood and Marrow Transplantation. Br J Haematol 1999;106:1020–1026
8. Rund D, Krichevsky S, Bar-Cohen S et al. Therapy-related leukemia: clinical characteristics and analysis of new molecular risk factors in 96 adult patients. Leukemia 2005;19:1919–1928
9. Bennett JM, Catovsky D, Daniel MT et al. Proposals for the classification of the myelodysplastic syndromes. Br J Haematol 1982;51:189–199
10. Greenberg P, Cox C, LeBeau MM et al. International scoring system for evaluating prognosis in myelodysplastic syndromes. Blood 1997;89:2079–2088
11. Germing U, Gattermann N, Strupp C et al. Validation of the WHO proposals for a new classification of primary myelodysplastic syndromes: a retrospective analysis of 1600 patients. Leuk Res 2000;24:983–992
12. Germing U, Strupp C, Kuendgen A et al. Prospective validation of the WHO proposals for the classification of myelodysplastic syndromes. Haematologica 2006;91:1596–1604
13. Howe RB, Porwit-MacDonald A, Wanat R et al. The WHO classification of MDS does make a difference. Blood 2004;103:3265–3270
14. Malcovati L, Porta MG, Pascutto C et al. Prognostic factors and life expectancy in myelodysplastic syndromes classified according to WHO criteria: a basis for clinical decision making. J Clin Oncol 2005;23:7594–7603
15. Bowen D, Culligan D, Jowitt S et al. Guidelines for the diagnosis and therapy of adult myelodysplastic syndromes. Br J Haematol 2003;120:187–200
16. Greenberg PL. Myelodysplastic syndromes: iron overload consequences and current chelating therapies. J Natl Compr Cancer Netw 2006;4:91–96
17. Armand P, Kim HT, Cutler CS et al. Prognostic impact of elevated pre transplant serum ferritin in patients undergoing myeloablative stem cell transplantation. Blood 2007;109(10):4586–4588
18. Gonzalez FA, Arrizabalaga B, Villegas A et al. [Study of deferoxamine in subcutaneous profusion treatment of iron overload in myelodysplastic syndromes]. Med Clin (Barc) 2005;124:645–657
19. Hellstrom-Lindberg E, Gulbrandsen N, Lindberg G et al. A validated decision model for treating the anemia of myelodysplastic syndromes with erythropoietin + granulocyte colony-stimulating factor: significant effects on quality of life. Br J Haematol 2003;120:1037–1046
20. Molldrem JJ, Leifer E, Bahceci E et al. Antithymocyte globulin for treatment of the bone marrow failure associated with myelodysplastic syndromes. Ann Intern Med 2002;137:156–163
21. Killick SB, Mufti G, Cavenagh JD et al. A pilot study of anti-thymocyte globulin (ATG) in the treatment of patients with 'low-risk' myelodysplasia. Br J Haematol 2003;120:679–684
22. Saunthararajah Y, Nakamura R, Nam JM et al. HLA-DR15 (DR2) is overrepresented in myelodysplastic syndrome and aplastic anemia and predicts a response to immunosuppression in myelodysplastic syndrome. Blood 2002;100:1570–1574
23. Molldrem JJ, Jiang Y, Stetler-Stevenson M et al. Haematological response of patients with myelodysplastic syndrome to antithymocyte globulin is associated with a loss of lymphocyte-mediated inhibition of CFU-GM and alterations in T-cell receptor Vbeta profiles. Br J Haematol 1998;102:1314–1322
24. Kochenderfer JN, Kobayashi S, Wieder ED et al. Loss of T-lymphocyte clonal dominance in patients with myelodysplastic syndrome responsive to immuno-suppression. Blood 2002;100:3639–3645
25. Silverman LR, Mufti GJ. Methylation inhibitor therapy in the treatment of myelodysplastic syndrome. Nat Clin Pract Oncol 2005;2(suppl 1):S12–23
26. List A, Dewald G, Bennett J et al. Lenalidomide in the myelodysplastic syndrome with chromosome 5q deletion. N Engl J Med 2006;355:1456–1465
27. List A, Kurtin S, Roe DJ et al. Efficacy of lenalidomide in myelodysplastic syndromes. N Engl J Med 2005;352:549–557
28. Steensma DP, List AF. Genetic testing in the myelodysplastic syndromes: molecular insights into hematologic diversity. Mayo Clin Proc 2005;80:681–698
29. Au WY, Fung A, Man C et al. Aberrant p15 gene promoter methylation in therapy-related myelodysplastic syndrome and acute myeloid leukemia: clinicopathological and karyotypic associations. Br J Haematol 2003;120:1062–1065
30. Daskalakis M, Nguyen TT, Nguyen C et al. Demethylation of a hypermethylated P15/INK4B gene in patients with myelodysplastic syndrome by 5-Aza-2'-deoxycytidine (decitabine) treatment. Blood 2002;100:2957–2964
31. Uchida T, Kinoshita T, Nagai H et al. Hypermethylation of the p15INK4B gene in myelodysplastic syndromes. Blood 1997;90:1403–1409
32. Fenaux, P. Inhibitors of DNA methylation: beyond myelodysplastic syndromes. Nat Clin Pract Oncol 2005;2(suppl 1):S36–44
33. Kaminskas E, Farrell AT, Wang YC et al. FDA drug approval summary: azacitidine (5-azacytidine, Vidaza) for injectable suspension. Oncologist 2005;10:176–182
34. Silverman LR, McKenzie DR, Peterson B et al. Further analysis of trials with azacitidine in patients with myelodysplastic syndrome: studies 8421, 8921, and 9221 by the Cancer and Leukemia Group B. J Clin Oncol 2006;24:3895–3903
35. Kantarjian H, Issa JP, Rosenfeld CS et al. Decitabine improves patient outcomes in myelodysplastic syndromes: results of a phase III randomized study. Cancer 2006;106:1794–1803
36. Castro-Malaspina H, Harris RE, Gajewski J et al. Unrelated donor marrow transplantation for myelodysplastic syndromes: outcome analysis in 510 transplants facilitated by the National Marrow Donor Program. Blood 2002;99:1943–1951
37. Sutton L, Chastang C, Ribaud P et al. Factors influencing outcome in de novo myelodysplastic syndromes treated by allogeneic bone marrow transplantation: a long-term study of 71 patients Societe Francaise de Greffe de Moelle. Blood 1996;88:358–365
38. Anderson JE, Anasetti C, Appelbaum FR et al. Unrelated donor marrow transplantation for myelodysplasia (MDS) and MDS-related acute myeloid leukemia. Br J Haematol 1996;93:59–67
39. Arnold R, de Witte T, van Biezen A et al. Unrelated bone marrow transplantation in patients with myelodysplastic syndromes and secondary acute myeloid leukemia: an EBMT survey. European Blood and Marrow Transplantation Group. Bone Marrow Transplant 1998;21:1213–1216
40. Copelan EA, Penza SL, Elder PJ et al. Analysis of prognostic factors for allogeneic marrow transplantation following busulfan and cyclophosphamide in myelodysplastic syndrome and after leukemic transformation. Bone Marrow Transplant 2000;25:1219–1222

41. Greenberg P, Anderson J, de Witte T et al. Problematic WHO reclassification of myelodys-plastic syndromes. Members of the International MDS Study Group. J Clin Oncol 2000;18:3447–3452

42. Martino R, Caballero M., Simon JA et al. Evidence for a graft-versus-leukemia effect after allogeneic peripheral blood stem cell transplantation with reduced-intensity conditioning in acute myelogenous leukemia and myelodysplastic syndromes. Blood 2002;100:2243–2245

43. Yakoub-Agha I, de la Salmoniere P, Ribaud P et al. Allogeneic bone marrow transplantation for therapy-related myelodysplastic syndrome and acute myeloid leukemia: a long-term study of 70 patients-report of the French society of bone marrow transplantation. J Clin Oncol 2000;18:963–971

44. Hsu KC, Keever-Taylor CA, Wilton A et al. Improved outcome in HLA-identical sibling hematopoietic stem-cell transplantation for acute myelogenous leukemia predicted by KIR and HLA genotypes. Blood 2005;105:4878–4884

45. Parker JE, Shafi T, Pagliuca A et al. Allogeneic stem cell transplantation in the myelodys-plastic syndromes: interim results of outcome following reduced-intensity conditioning compared with standard preparative regimens. Br J Haematol 2002;119:144–154

46. Shimoni A, Kroger N, Zabelina T et al. Hematopoietic stem-cell transplantation from unrelated donors in elderly patients (age >55 years) with hematologic malignancies: older age is no longer a contraindication when using reduced intensity conditioning. Leukemia 2005;19:7–12

47. Alamo J, Shahjahan M, Lazarus HM et al. Comorbidity indices in hematopoietic stem cell transplantation: a new report card. Bone Marrow Transplant 2005;36:475–479

48. Artz AS, Pollyea DA, Kocherginsky M et al. Performance status and comorbidity predict transplant-related mortality after allogeneic hematopoietic cell transplantation. Biol Blood Marrow Transplant 2006;12:954–964

49. Sorror ML, Maris MB, Storb R et al. Hematopoietic cell transplantation (HCT)-specific comorbidity index: a new tool for risk assessment before allogeneic HCT. Blood 2005;106:2912–2919

50. Sierra J, Perez WS, Rozman C et al. Bone marrow transplantation from HLA-identical siblings as treatment for myelodysplasia. Blood 2002;100:1997–2004

51. Appelbaum FR, Anderson J. Allogeneic bone marrow transplantation for myelodysplastic syndrome: outcomes analysis according to IPSS score. Leukemia 1998;12(suppl 1): S25–29

52. de Witte T, Muus P, de Pauw B, Haanen C. Intensive antileukemic treatment of patients younger than 65 years with myelodysplastic syndromes and secondary acute myelogenous leukemia. Cancer 1990;66:831–837

53. de Witte T, Suciu S, Peetermans M et al. Intensive chemotherapy for poor prognosis myelodysplasia (MDS) and secondary acute myeloid leukemia (sAML) following MDS of more than 6 months duration. A pilot study by the Leukemia Cooperative Group of the European Organisation for Research and Treatment in Cancer (EORTC-LCG). Leukemia 1995;9:1805–1811

54. Parker JE, Pagliuca A, Mijovic A et al. Fludarabine, cytarabine, G-CSF and idarubicin (FLAG-IDA) for the treatment of poor-risk myelodysplastic syndromes and acute myeloid leukemia. Br J Haematol 1997;99:939–944

55. Scott BL, Storer B, Loken MR et al. Pretransplantation induction chemotherapy and post-transplantation relapse in patients with advanced myelodysplastic syndrome. Biol Blood Marrow Transplant 2005;11:65–73

56. Morel P, Hebbar M, Lai JL et al. Cytogenetic analysis has strong independent prognostic value in de novo myelodysplastic syndromes and can be incorporated in a new scoring system: a report on 408 cases. Leukemia 1993;7:1315–1323

57. Toyama K, Ohyashiki K, Yoshida Y et al. Clinical and cytogenetic findings of myelodys-plastic syndromes showing hypocellular bone marrow or minimal dysplasia, in comparison with typical myelodysplastic syndromes. Int J Hematol 1993;58:53–61

58. Toyama K, Ohyashiki K, Yoshida Y et al. Clinical implications of chromosomal abnormalities in 401 patients with myelodysplastic syndromes: a multicentric study in Japan. Leukemia 1993;7:499–508

59. Trost D, Hildebrandt B, Beier M et al. Molecular cytogenetic profiling of complex karyo-types in primary myelodysplastic syndromes and acute myeloid leukemia. Cancer Genet Cytogenet 2006;165:51–63

60. Olney HJ, Le Beau MM. The cytogenetics of myelodysplastic syndromes. Best Pract Res Clin Haematol 2001;14:479–495

61. Nevill TJ, Fung HC, Shepherd JD et al. Cytogenetic abnormalities in primary myelodys-plastic syndrome are highly predictive of outcome after allogeneic bone marrow transplan-tation. Blood 1998;92:1910–1917

62. van der Straaten HM, van Biezen A, Brand R et al. Allogeneic stem cell transplantation for patients with acute myeloid leukemia or myelodysplastic syndrome who have chromo-some 5 and/or 7 abnormalities. Haematologica 2005;90:1339–1345

63. Cutler CS, Lee SJ, Greenberg P et al. A decision analysis of allogeneic bone marrow transplantation for the myelodysplastic syndromes: delayed transplantation for low-risk myelodysplasia is associated with improved outcome. Blood 2004;104:579–585

64. Guardiola P, Runde V, Bacigalupo A et al. Retrospective comparison of bone marrow and granulocyte colony-stimulating factor-mobilized peripheral blood progenitor cells for allo-geneic stem cell transplantation using HLA identical sibling donors in myelodysplastic syndromes. Blood 2002;99:4370–4378

65. de Witte T, van Biezen A, Hermans J et al. Autologous bone marrow transplantation for patients with myelodysplastic syndrome (MDS) or acute myeloid leukemia following MDS. Chronic and Acute Leukemia Working Parties of the European Group for Blood and Marrow Transplantation. Blood 1997;90:3853–3857

66. de Witte T, Brand R, van Biezen A et al. The role of stem cell source in autologous hema-topoietic stem cell transplantation for patients with myelodysplastic syndromes. Haemato-logica 2006;91:750–756

67. Leith CP, Kopecky KJ, Chen IM et al. Frequency and clinical significance of the expression of the multidrug resistance proteins MDR1/P-glycoprotein, MRP1, and LRP in acute myeloid leukemia: a Southwest Oncology Group Study. Blood 1999;94:1086–1099

68. de Lima M, Anagnostopoulos A, Munsell M et al. Nonablative versus reduced-intensity conditioning regimens in the treatment of acute myeloid leukemia and high-risk myelodys-plastic syndrome: dose is relevant for long-term disease control after allogeneic hemato-poietic stem cell transplantation. Blood 2004;104:865–872

69. Demuynck H, Verhoef G, Zachee P et al. Treatment of patients with myelodysplastic syndromes with allogeneic bone marrow transplantation from genotypically HLA-identical sibling and alternative donors. Bone Marrow Transplant 1996;17:745–751

70. de Witte T, Hermans J, Vossen J et al. Haematopoietic stem cell transplantation for patients with myelo-dysplastic syndromes and secondary acute myeloid leukemias: a report on behalf of the Chronic Leukemia Working Party of the European Group for Blood and Marrow Transplantation (EBMT). Br J Haematol 2000;110:620–630

71. Deeg HJ, Storer B, Slattery JT et al. Conditioning with targeted busulfan and cyclophos-phamide for hemopoietic stem cell transplantation from related and unrelated donors in patients with myelodysplastic syndrome. Blood 2002;100:1201–1207

72. Deeg HJ, Storer BE, Boeckh M et al. Reduced incidence of acute and chronic graft-versus-host disease with the addition of thymoglobulin to a targeted busulfan/cyclophosphamide regimen. Biol Blood Marrow Transplant 2006;12:573–584

73. Khouri IF, Keating M, Korbling M et al. Transplant-lite: induction of graft-versus-malignancy using fludarabine-based nonablative chemotherapy and allogeneic blood progenitor-cell transplantation as treatment for lymphoid malignancies. J Clin Oncol 1998;16:2817–2824

74. Slavin S, Nagler A, Naparstek E et al. Nonmyeloablative stem cell transplantation and cell therapy as an alternative to conventional bone marrow transplantation with lethal cytore-duction for the treatment of malignant and nonmalignant hematologic diseases. Blood 1998;91:756–763

75. Giralt S, Thall PF, Khouri I et al. Melphalan and purine analog-containing preparative regimens: reduced-intensity conditioning for patients with hematologic malig-nancies undergoing allogeneic progenitor cell transplantation. Blood 2001;97:631–637

76. Martino R, Caballero MD, Canals C et al. Allogeneic peripheral blood stem cell transplan-tation with reduced-intensity conditioning: results of a prospective multicentre study. Br J Haematol 2001;115:653–659

77. Chakraverty R, Peggs K, Chopra R et al. Limiting transplantation-related mortality follow-ing unrelated donor stem cell transplantation by using a nonmyeloablative conditioning regimen. Blood 2002;99:1071–1078

78. Ho AY, Pagliuca A, Kenyon M et al. Reduced-intensity allogeneic haematopoietic stem cell transplantation for myelodysplastic syndrome and acute myeloid leukemia with mul-tilineage dysplasia using Fludarabine, Busulphan and Alemtuzumab (CAMPATH-1H)(FBC) conditioning. Blood 2004;104:1616–1623

79. Buggins AG, Mufti GJ, Salisbury J et al. Peripheral blood but not tissue dendritic cells express CD52 and are depleted by treatment with alemtuzumab. Blood 2002;100:1715–1720

80. Klangsinsirikul P, Carter GI, Byrne JL et al. Campath-1G causes rapid depletion of circulat-ing host dendritic cells (DCs) before allogeneic transplantation but does not delay donor DC reconstitution. Blood 2002;99:2586–2591

81. Lee SJ, Klein JP, Barrett AJ et al. Severity of chronic graft-versus-host disease: association with treatment-related mortality and relapse. Blood 2002;100:406–414

82. Perez-Simon JA, Caballero D, Diez-Campelo M et al. Chimerism and minimal residual disease monitoring after reduced intensity conditioning (RIC) allogeneic transplantation. Leukemia 2002;16:1423–1431

83. Perez-Simon JA., Diez-Campelo M, Martino R et al. Influence of the intensity of the con-ditioning regimen on the characteristics of acute and chronic graft-versus-host disease after allogeneic transplantation. Br J Haematol 2005;130:394–403

84. Alyea EP, Kim HT, Ho V et al. Comparative outcome of nonmyeloablative and myeloabla-tive allogeneic hematopoietic cell transplantation for patients older than 50 years of age. Blood 2005;105:1810–1814

85. Scott BL, Sandmaier B, Storer B et al. Myeloablative vs nonmyeloablative allogeneic transplantation for patients with myelodysplastic syndrome or acute myelogenous leukemia with multilineage dysplasia: a retrospective analysis. Leukemia 2006;20:128–135

86. Martino R, Iacobelli S, Brand R et al. Retrospective comparison of reduced-intensity con-ditioning and conventional high-dose conditioning for allogeneic hematopoietic stem cell transplantation using HLA-identical sibling donors in myelodysplastic syndromes. Blood 2006;108:836–846

87. Laughlin MJ, Eapen M, Rubinstein P et al. Outcomes after transplantation of cord blood or bone marrow from unrelated donors in adults with leukemia. N Engl J Med 2004;351:2265–2275

88. Rocha V, Labopin M, Sanz G et al. Transplants of umbilical-cord blood or bone marrow from unrelated donors in adults with acute leukemia. N Engl J Med 2004;351: 2276–2285

89. Lim ZY, Ho AY, Ingram W et al. Outcomes of alemtuzumab-based reduced intensity con-ditioning stem cell transplantation using unrelated donors for myelodysplastic syndromes. Br J Haematol 2006;135:201–209

90. Kolb HJ, Schattenberg A, Goldman JM et al. Graft-versus-leukemia effect of donor lymphocyte transfusions in marrow grafted patients. European Group for Blood and Marrow Transplantation Working Party Chronic Leukemia. Blood 1995;86:2041–2050

91. Depil S, Deconinck E, Milpied N et al. Donor lymphocyte infusion to treat relapse after allogeneic bone marrow transplantation for myelodysplastic syndrome. Bone Marrow Transplant 2004;33:531–534

92. Shiobara S, Nakao S, Ueda M et al. Donor leukocyte infusion for Japanese patients with relapsed leukemia after allogeneic bone marrow transplantation: lower incidence of acute graft-versus-host disease and improved outcome. Bone Marrow Transplant 2000;26: 769–774

93. Schmid C, Schleuning M, Ledderose G et al. Sequential regimen of chemotherapy, reduced-intensity conditioning for allogeneic stem-cell transplantation, and prophylactic donor

lymphocyte transfusion in high-risk acute myeloid leukemia and myelodysplastic syndrome. J Clin Oncol 2005;23:5675–5687

94. Ooi J. The efficacy of unrelated cord blood transplantation for adult myelodysplastic syndrome. Leuk Lymphoma 2006;47:599–602

95. Davies SM, Ruggieri L, DeFor T et al. Evaluation of KIR ligand incompatibility in mismatched unrelated donor hematopoietic transplants. Killer immunoglobulin-like receptor. Blood 2002;100:3825–3827

96. Long GD, Laughlin M, Madan B et al. Unrelated umbilical cord blood transplantation in adult patients. Biol Blood Marrow Transplant 2003;9:772–780

97. Rubinstein P, Stevens CE. Placental blood for bone marrow replacement: the New York Blood Center's program and clinical results. Baillière's Best Pract Res Clin Haematol 2000;13:565–584

98. Sanz GF, Saavedra S, Planelles D et al. Standardized, unrelated donor cord blood transplantation in adults with hematologic malignancies. Blood 2001;98:2332–2338

99. Taussig DC, Davies AJ, Cavenagh JD et al. Durable remissions of myelodysplastic syndrome and acute myeloid leukemia after reduced-intensity allografting. J Clin Oncol 2003;21(16):3060–3065

Multiple myeloma

Frits van Rhee and Bijay Nair

CHAPTER 8

Introduction

Surveillance Epidemiology and End Results (SEER) data indicate that there are approximately 54,000 myeloma patients in the USA. It is estimated that approximately 20,000 new patients will be diagnosed with myeloma in 2007. The 5-year survival rate is 34%, and nearly 11,000 patients succumb annually from their disease.[1] Multiple myeloma is the most common indication for autologous stem cell transplantation (AT), and well over 4000 patients are transplanted in the US each year. Myeloma is unique in that AT is performed in most patients before a complete remission (CR) is obtained. In fact, most patients will attain a CR as a direct result of receiving high-dose therapy (HDT) supported by AT. Phase II and randomized Phase III studies, clinical trials, non-randomized comparisons and large reviews all suggest that AT achieves superior survival compared to standard chemotherapy. High-dose therapy with melphalan (MEL) has become the standard of care for younger patients.

In the past decade there have been many new developments in the rapidly changing field of myeloma therapeutics. Several new drugs have been introduced which target the malignant clone not only directly but also indirectly, by suppressing stimulatory signals provided by the bone marrow microenvironment (ME).

However, although approximately 20–30% of patients are alive 10 years after HDT and AT, with a subset remaining in uninterrupted remission, most will eventually relapse. Novel drugs, either alone or in combination, have the potential to overcome alkylator resistance. Important questions are whether novel drugs can replace MEL-based AT or be incorporated into currently used transplant regimens and improve outcome or even achieve cure.

Substantial progress has been made in our understanding of the cytogenetics, genomics and proteomics of myeloma, which has allowed molecular subclassification of myeloma.[2–5] Importantly, these techniques have allowed the identification of patients destined to fare poorly with HDT. Genetics are the principal determinant of heterogeneity in patient outcome, and molecular characterization of myeloma will result in risk-adapted or even individualized therapy for patients.[6,7]

This chapter will discuss single-center and randomized studies of different transplant strategies, the impact of attaining complete remission after AT on long-term outcome, the effect of biologic risk factors on risk stratification for AT and the role of novel agents.

Single autologous transplantation

MEL was first introduced in 1962 for the therapy of myeloma.[8,9] Therapy with MEL and prednisone has been the standard of care for myeloma for several decades, producing median survival rates of less than 3 years.[9–12] Multiagent combination chemotherapy has been extensively explored, but did not yield any significant improvement in survival when compared to MEL and prednisone. This is exemplified by three observations. First, the South Western Oncology Group (SWOG) conducted seven consecutive large Phase III studies and was unable to report improved survival.[13] Second, a meta-analysis of 6633 patients in 27 trials demonstrated no benefit in survival conferred by combination chemotherapy.[12] Lastly, the Nordic Myeloma Group reported no improvement in survival in younger patients with myeloma during the past two decades.[14] Taken together, these data suggested that other therapeutic options deserved exploration.

McElwain and Powles first reported that high-dose MEL had induced complete biochemical and bone marrow responses in three of nine patients.[15,16] It was subsequently reported by Barlogie et al that the prolonged myelosuppression incurred by high-dose MEL therapy could be considerably shortened by infusing autologous bone marrow cells.[17,18] Peripheral blood stem cells have now replaced autologous bone marrow as the source of stem cells, resulting in faster hematologic recovery, with a transplant-related mortality (TRM) of 2–3%, which is similar to the mortality observed during 6 months of standard-dose therapy.[19–21] This prompted numerous Phase I and II studies which reported improved survivals with high-dose MEL therapy in myeloma.[23–42] These studies suggested that high-dose therapy achieves a greater tumor reduction, resulting in longer event-free (EFS) and overall survival (OS). However, selection bias in the aforementioned studies with regard to age, performance status and renal function did not permit valid comparisons with standard-dose therapy (STD).

Two population-based studies and one case–control study reported superior outcome in terms of achieving CR and OS with HDT compared to SDT.[43–45] Several prospective, randomized studies in newly diagnosed patients have now been published addressing the question of whether HDT is indeed superior to STD (Table 8.1). These include studies conducted by the Intergroupe Français du Myélome (IFM), the Medical Research Council of the United Kingdom (MRCVII), the Group Myelome-Autogreffe (MAG), the Programa para el Estudio de la Terapéutica en Hematopatía Maligna (PETHEMA) and the US Intergroup Trial S9321.[46–50] Collectively, the evidence of both retrospective and prospective studies indicates that HDT confers a survival benefit in younger patients (<60 years of age). However, it is difficult to compare these studies directly due to variability in eligibility and conditioning regimens in the HDT arm. Further, the STD therapy arms differed considerably in intensity and duration, and in some studies patients were randomized at diagnosis, whereas in others randomization occurred late. There are also different cross-over rates from STD to HDT arms. Since these studies commenced enrollment in the 1990s, information regarding karyotypic abnormalities and gene expression

Table 8.1 Randomized trials of STD compared to single AT

Author	Group	n	Age (yrs)	Median follow-up (mo)	Regimen	Source of stem cells	CR% (STD vs HDT)	Criteria for defining CR	Median EFS (mo)	Median OS (mo)	Conclusion (based on statistical significance)
Attal[44]	IFM 90	200	=<65	37 STD, 41 AT	VMCP/BVAP vs VMCP/BVAP → MEL (140/TBI)	BM	5 vs 22	Electrophoresis	18 vs 28	44 vs 57	Benefit in EFS & OS
Fermand[46]	MAG	190	55–65	120	VMCP vs VAMP → Bu/ MEL 140 or MEL 200	PBSC	No data	EMBT-IBMTR (IF)	19 vs 25	48 vs 48	Benefit in EFS, but not OS
Child[45]	MRC7	401	<65	32 STD, 40 AT	ABCM vs VAMPC → MEL 200 or MEL 140/ TBI	PBSC	8 vs 44	EMBT-IBMTR (IF)	20 vs 32	42 vs 54	Benefit in EFS & OS
Bladé[47]	PETHEMA	164	=<65	56	VBMCP/VBAD vs VBMCP/ VBAD → MEL 200 or MEL 140/TBI	PBSC	11 vs 30	EMBT-IBMTR (IF)	33 vs 42	66 vs 61	No benefit in OS or EFS
Palumbo[72]	M97G	194	50–70	39 STD, 41AT	MP vs VAD → MEL 100 × 2	PBSC	6 vs 25	Electrophoresis	16 vs 28	43 vs NR	Benefit in OS & EFS
Barlogie[48]	USIG	516	<70	76	HDCTx → VBMCP vs HDCTx → MEL 140 mg/ m² + TBI	PBSC	15 vs 17	EMBT-IBMTR (IF)	22 vs 25	54 vs 62	No benefit in EFS or OS
Segeren[105]	HOVON	261	≤65	33	VAD → MEL 70 × 2 vs VAD → MEL 70 × 2 → Cy60 × 4/TBI	PBSC	13 vs 29	Immunofixation	21 vs 22	50 vs 47	No benefit in EFS or OS

CR, complete remission; EFS, event free survival; OS, overall survival; BM, bone marrow; PBSC, peripheral blood stem cells; IFM, Intergroupe Français du Myelome; MAG, Myelome-Autogreffe; MRC, Medical Research Council; PETHEMA, Programa para el Tratamiento de Hemopatias Malignas; M97G, Italian Multiple Myeloma Study Group trial; USIG, US Intergroup study; HOVON, Hemato-Oncologie voor Volwassenen Nederland. VMCP; vincristine, melphalan, cyclophosphamide, prednisone; BVAP, BCNU [carmustine], vincristine, doxorubicin [adriamycin], and prednisone; Mel 140, Melphalan 140 mg/m²; Mel 200, melphalan 200 mg/m²; Mel 70, melphalan 70 mg/m²; TBI, total body irradiation; VAMP, vincristine, doxorubicin, methylprednisolone; Bu, busulfan; ABCM, doxorubicin; BCNU, cyclophosphamide, melphalan; VAMPC, vincristine, doxorubicin, methylprednisolone, cyclophosphamide; VBMCP, vincristine; BCNU, melphalan, cyclophosphamide, prednisone; VBAD, vincristine; BCNU, doxorubicin, and high-dose dexamethasone; MP, melphalan, prednisone; VAD, vincristine, doxorubicin, dexamethasone; HDCTx, high-dose cyclophosphamide; EMBT-IBMTR, European Bone Marrow Transplant-International Bone Marrow Transplant Registry; IF, immunofixation.

profiles, both powerful predictors of outcome, is largely lacking. Finally, the criteria for defining response were not uniform amongst these studies.

In the IFM90 study,[44] which included patients up to the age of 65 years, the HDT arm induced a higher CR or VGPR rate (38% vs 14%). The 5-year OS and EFS rates in the HDT were also superior (52 vs 12%; p = 0.03 and 28% vs 10%; p = 0.01). The best results were seen in patients <60 years who had a probability of 5-year OS of 70%. One criticism of the IFM study has been that the outcome in the STD arm was particularly poor for patients <65 years, who had, as stipulated by eligibility criteria, good cardiac and renal function. The MRCVII enrolled 407 patients <65 years and also reported higher CR rates (44% vs 8%, p < 0.001). HDT with MEL 200 increased median survival by almost 1 year (54.1 vs 42.3 mths) and significantly improved time to progression.

The MAG, PETHEMA and US Intergroup studies did not show a definite benefit in terms of OS for MEL-based HDT, which can be explained by several factors. The CR rates in the STD and HDT arms in the US Intergroup Trial S9321 were similar (17% vs 15%), but were substantially lower when compared to the IFM and MRCVII studies. It is generally assumed that achievement of CR after HDT correlates with improved survival.[51,52] The lower CR rate in the HDT arm in the Intergroup Trial can be explained by the conditioning used: MEL dose 140 mg/m² and 8 Gy total-body irradiation (TBI), which is inferior to MEL 200 in both historical and randomized comparisons.[53–55] In addition, a large percentage of patients in the STD arm crossed over to receive HDT, which makes interpretation of OS results difficult. Since OS was not different in the two arms, it could be argued that the trial merely showed that upfront HDT and HDT at the time of relapse are equally efficacious. The MAG study compared STD (VMCP) and HDT, comprising MEL 200 or MEL140 mg/m² with busulfan 16 mg/kg in patients between 55 and 65 years old. With a median follow-up of 10 years, there was a trend to better EFS and statistically superior time without treatment or symptoms (TwiSTT) in the HDT arm. However, the OS of 48 months was virtually identical in both arms. It is important to note that 22% of patients in the STD arm received

salvage HDT, which may have contributed to equalizing OS. In the PETHEMA study, randomization was not performed at diagnosis and only patients with chemosensitive disease were randomized to HDT or SDT. Patients refractory to induction chemotherapy are probably most in need of HDT.[56] In addition, the therapy delivered in the STD arm, comprising 12 cycles of VBMP/VBAD, was more intensive than that in the other randomized trials, with the exception of the US Intergroup study. Both factors may have contributed to mitigating any survival benefit conferred by HDT.

In general, most investigators would concur that single HDT is superior to STD chemotherapy in patients less than 65 years. The patients who benefit most from HDT have less aggressive disease and favorable prognostic features, including low beta-2M and no cytogenetic abnormalities (CA) (see below).[54]

Refractory disease

Patients who are resistant to standard regimens derive little benefit from further low-dose therapy and have a dismal median survival of 3–12 months.[57–59] Patients with primary refractory disease do somewhat better than patients with resistant relapse and have a median survival ranging from 15 to 26 months.[60–62] Several investigators have reported that HDT can overcome drug resistance in patients who fail standard remission induction therapies. Vesole et al reported on 135 patients with refractory/relapsed myeloma treated, non-randomized, with three regimens (MEL 90 or 100 mg/m² without AT; TBI/MEL 140 mg/m² or thiotepa 750 mg/m;² MEL 200 mg/m² tandem AT).[61] Dose intensification with tandem MEL 200 mg/m² supported by AT was superior in overcoming drug resistance, thus significantly extending OS and EFS independently of other prognostic variables.

A more recent analysis of 496 patients treated with tandem AT at Arkansas found that 109 patients with primary refractory disease enjoyed better OS and EFS compared to 69 patients who were in resistant relapse (OS 39 vs 25 months, p = 0.008; EFS 23 vs 14 months).[62] The MD Anderson group found that MEL 140 mg/m² TBI followed by single AT prolonged the median survival of 35 patients with primary refractory myeloma from 37 to 83 months compared to historical matched control patients receiving standard care for socioeconomic reasons or who had refused HDT.[58] A recently updated and extended analysis revealed that HDT for primary resistant disease administered later in the disease course resulted in lower response rates and shorter progression-free survival.[63] The principal advantage of HDT in this study appeared to be improving the quality of the response by effecting a combined partial response (PR) and CR rate of 69%. The median survival exceeded 7 years in patients achieving a CR, 4.5 years for patients reaching a PR and 2.2 years for those who had no response.

Investigators from the Mayo Clinic reported a CR rate of 20% and a 1-year progression-free survival rate of 70% in 50 patients receiving HDT for refractory disease. In this study the percentage of patients with abnormal CA was only 34%, which is unusually low for primary refractory disease.[64] The Phase II SWOG S8993 study found that MEL 200 mg/m^2 supported by AT in 66 patients resistant to VAD (vincristine, doxorubicin, dexamethasone) and/or alkylating agents effected a response rate of 65%, with 30% achieving a CR, which is higher than expected in pretreated patients with refractory myeloma.[65] Singhal et al reported the Royal Marsden experience in 222 patients who received remission induction with C-VAMP (cyclophosphamide, vincristine, doxorubicin, methyprednisolone) followed by MEL 200 mg/m^2 AT.[66] Overall, 159 patients (59%) achieved a CR, and importantly, the 5-year OS in these patients was independent of response to C-VAMP induction chemotherapy.

One caveat in interpreting these studies is that it is not always evident if all patients have truly aggressive drug-refractory disease or whether patients with very indolent, slow-cycling myeloma, who are likely to respond only to high-dose MEL, are also included in analyses.[54] However, taken together, these studies support the concept that high-dose therapy can overcome both primary refractory disease and drug-resistant relapse developed during or after cytotoxic therapy, although EFS and OS still remain to be improved. It is also evident that myeloma patients should not be denied access to AT based on inadequate response. Unfortunately, at the time of this writing, Medicare patients in the US still do not have access to AT unless at least a PR is obtained after STD. The introduction of novel agents such as thalidomide, lenalidomide and bortezomib, when applied together with existing agents, may perhaps overcome drug resistance in refractory patients. Other approaches include the use of bone-seeking agents such as [166]holmium DOTMP, and clinical studies of allogeneic transplantation that aim to enhance the graft-versus-myeloma effect without increasing graft-versus-host disease (GvHD). Finally, it is important to realize that there have been no studies comparing AT immediately post diagnosis with AT after remission induction, although it seems reasonable to assume that more efficacious cytoreduction before single or tandem AT will translate into survival benefit.

Older patients

Most of the randomized studies showing the benefit of AT have been performed in younger patients (usually <65 years of age). However, more than 50% of the newly diagnosed cases of myeloma are over 65 years old. Advanced age is considered to be a poor prognostic factor for AT in unselected populations. There have been concerns that chemotherapy and/or AT in the elderly can cause excessive toxicity secondary to impaired drug metabolism and co-existent co-morbidities. The poorer outcomes in older conventional chemotherapy studies have been attributed to decreased dose intensity of therapy rather than intrinsically different myeloma, which has different biologic behavior.[67,68]

Concern about toxicity has thus led to limiting most randomized AT studies to patients younger than 65 or 60 years of age. Nevertheless, in the Total Therapy (TT) trials and other AT studies, age has never been a factor predictive for major endpoints in multivariate analyses.[62] A pairmate analysis of 49 patients with 501 younger patients prepared with MEL 200 mg/m^2 or MEL 140 mg/m^2 with TBI showed that EFS and OS were similar in both groups.[69] The TRM was higher in older patients during the first cycle of HDT (8% vs 2%), but similar with the second AT (Table 8.2). A further study reported that reducing the dose of MEL in the conditioning regimen from 200 mg/m^2 to 140 mg/m^2 reduced TRM from 16% to 2%.[70] In this study, tandem AT effected superior 3-year OS and EFS in older patients (4 vs 1.4 years, and 4 vs 1 year, respectively). Most investigators now use MEL 140 mg/m^2 as the conditioning regimen in patients over the age of 65 years. A study of the Autologous Blood and Marrow Transplant Registry showed no difference in OS, EFS and CR rate between 110 patients ≥65years and 382 patients <60 years.[71] Palumbo et al compared in 80 patients between the age of 65 and 70 years in a multicenter randomized trial six cycles of MEL/prednisone with two cycles of MEL/prednisone followed by two tandem AT with an intermediate dose of MEL 100 mg/m^2 as conditioning. Tandem MEL 100 mg/g^2 improved the OS and EFS from 18% to 31% and 58% to 73% respectively. The median OS was also significantly improved (58 vs 37.2 months).[72] Despite these positive studies, older patients need to be carefully assessed before AT. In this context, co-morbidities and adequate physiologic reserve are more important than chronological age.

The introduction of new drugs such as bortezomib, thalidomide and lenalidomide offers new therapeutic options for elderly patients. A large randomized trial compared MEL, prednisone and thalidomide

Table 8.2 Non-randomized studies comparing AT outcomes across different age groups

Author	Age groups	n	Conditioning regimen	TRM (%)	CR (%)	EFS (mo)	OS (mo)	Conclusion (based on statistical significance)
Siegel[69]	<65	49	MEL 200 × 2	2	43	34	58	No difference in OS/ EFS, TRM higher in elderly
	>=65	49		8%	20%	18	40	
Dumontet[249]	<60	35	MEL +/−TBI	N/A	N/A	24	N/A	EFS is smaller in elderly, OS/TRM not available
	>=60	20				12		
Sirohi[250]	<65	55	MEL 200	11.7	47	23	36	EFS/OS/TRM are similar
	>=65	67		17.6	35.3	24	43	
Reece[71]	<60	52	Various regimens	6	34	27	39	EFS/OS/TRM are similar
	>=60	63		5	33	24	39	
Januten[251]	<65	57	MEL 200	1.4	36	21	66	EFS/OS/TRM are similar, Grade 3–4 oral/GI toxicity is more in the elderly
	>=65	68		0	44	23	57	
Lenhoff[252]	<60	52	MEL 200	0.4	N/A	36	66	EFS/OS are smaller in elderly, TRM are similar
	>60–64	62		1		24	50	

Adapted from Keplin and Hurd, BMT 2006;38:585–592

(MPT) with standard MP in 255 newly diagnosed myeloma patients aged 60–85 years.[73] MPT therapy resulted in significantly higher (n)CR rates (27.9% vs 7.2%) and 2-year EFS (54% vs 27%), although 3-year OS rates were similar in both arms (80% vs 64%). In the MPT arm, there was a higher incidence of early death due to adverse events including infection and thromboembolism, thereby negating any survival benefit. A second study by the IFM reported similar superiority of MPT over MP.[74] The efficacy of the combination of bortezomib, MEL and prednisone was examined in a Phase I/II study in 60 untreated myeloma patients >60 years. Although the follow-up was short, 32% of patients achieved an immunofixation-negative CR and the OS at 16 months was 90%.[75] Interestingly, good responses were also observed in patients with del 17p, t(4;14) and t(14;16) who usually do not do well with AT. The combination of thalidomide, dexamethasone and pegylated doxorubicin has been tested in 50 untreated patients >65 years.[76] At 3 years, EFS and OS were respectively 57% and 75%, which is superior to standard MEL/prednisone.

HDT and AT are certainly feasible and well tolerated with a low TRM in selected elderly patients, especially when MEL is used at doses of 100–140 mg/m². Novel agents will improve the outcome of patients unsuitable for AT, but longer follow-up is necessary to assess durability of responses and to fully appreciate toxicity. Carefully designed studies are required to address the question of whether novel agents are superior to HDT in elderly patients who are transplant candidates.

Renal failure

Renal failure is present in 25–50% of patients with myeloma at the time of diagnosis and 2–3% of myeloma patients require dialysis.[77] Renal failure in myeloma occurs secondary to cast nephropathy, amyloidosis, light chain deposition disease, plasma cell infiltration, hypercalcemia and dehydration, and the side-effects of nephrotoxic medications such as NSAIDs. In our experience complete renal failure is irreversible if present for longer than 6 months.[78] The renal prognosis is best in patients who do not have light chain deposition or amyloidosis. Renal failure is classically considered to be a poor prognostic factor.[79] However, this view has been recently challenged and it is thought that renal failure is caused by a higher tumor burden rather than biologically aggressive disease. The poor outcome seen in renal failure patients may also be secondary to the application of lower doses of chemotherapy and/or higher TRM.[80]

Several studies have shown that renal failure does not hamper the ability to harvest stem cells or time to engraftment.[81–83] HDT with MEL followed by AT can result in improvement of renal function. In one series of 59 dialysis-dependent renal failure patients, nearly one-quarter recovered from dialysis dependency at a median of 4 months post AT.[79] The quality of response of AT (>PR) was a significant determinant of renal recovery. However, the TRM reported in several series varied from 17% to 29%, indicating that myeloma patients with renal failure should only be transplanted in tertiary care centers conversant with managing this complicated patient population.[81,82,84,85] Recovery of renal function is most often accomplished when AT is carried out within 6 months from onset of dialysis.[79] Recovery of renal function is extremely important for quality of life, and patients with renal failure should be promptly referred for possible combination chemotherapy and stem cell collection immediately followed by HDT and AT. In view of the increased TRM with HDT in patients with renal failure, it is important to point out that survival of patients with dialysis-dependent renal failure is extremely poor when managed with STD only.[78,86]

The pharmacokinetics of MEL including $t_{1/2}$, area under the curve and clearance is not adversely affected by renal impairment. However, it has been reported that reducing the dose from MEL 200 mg/m² to

MEL 140 mg/m² or 100 mg/m² in patients with renal failure significantly reduces TRM and mucosal toxicity without compromising outcome.[81,83,87] The reason for the discrepancy between MEL pharmacokinetics being independent of renal function and a MEL dose-dependent toxicity effect in vivo is not clear. One can speculate that renal-dependent clearance of MEL metabolites could be of importance. It has also recently been reported that dosing per mg/m² results in administration of higher doses of MEL calculated in mg/kg in less obese patients, with significantly more mucosal toxicity.[88]

Formal comparisons of appropriately matched patients with and without renal failure have not been conducted. A survey of the literature suggests that renal failure patients do benefit from HDT, but do not enjoy the same survival benefit as patients with normal renal function.[81–83,85]

Tandem autologous transplantation

Total therapies

Total Therapy I, designed for newly diagnosed myeloma, comprised the sequential application of (a) non-cross resistant induction chemotherapy, (b) tandem autologous transplantation and (c) maintenance with interferon-alpha. This trial intended to increase the frequency and duration of complete response, thus extending OS.[89] The concept was inspired by the St Jude's Children's Hospital Total Therapy (TT) programs for acute leukemia which have made unprecedented progress in curing children with both acute lymphoblastic and myeloid leukemias.[90] The 'tandem' transplant idea arose from the observation that (elderly) patients with multiple myeloma (MM) could not tolerate MEL dosing exceeding 200 mg/m² (MEL 200) due to mucositis, which was the dose-limiting toxicity. In addition, a single MEL 200 AT resulted in a CR rate of usually no more than 20%.[18,26,91,92] It was recognized in adult acute leukemia that cures were only obtained when a CR rate of ≥40% was accomplished with single-agent arabinosyl-cytosine.[93] Thus, using CR as a substitute for survival, the underlying hypothesis was that a more marked increase in CR rate from less than 5% with standard MEL-prednisone (MP) to 40% would produce significant prolongation of EFS and OS, and perhaps attain cure.[9]

A pairmate comparison of patients treated with TT and patients treated with standard chemotherapy in SWOG trials showed that TT effected superior EFS and OS.[41] The long-term results of TT1, which enrolled 231 patients, were recently published and the median follow-up was an unprecedented 12 years.[94] At 10 and 15 years respectively, 33% and 17% of patients are alive; 15% and 7% are event free; and 18% and 12% of those achieving CR remain in uninterrupted remission. It is important to realize that it is feasible in myeloma to achieve a long-term survival of >30% at 10 years with high-dose MEL. This also sets a new yardstick against which recently developed newer drugs should be tested. Metaphase cytogenetics comprising hypodiploidy and/or del13, CRP ≥4 mg/dl conferred poorer OS and EFS in multivariate analysis. ISS stage 3 and beta-2M ≥4 mg/dl were associated with decreased OS, whilst beta-2M and elevated lactic dehydrogenase (LDH) were additional high-risk features for EFS. Time to CR, as a time-dependent covariate, was associated with longer EFS.

Distinguishing baseline features for long-term survivors were tandem AT performed within 12 months, absence of CA at baseline, and lower levels of C-reactive protein (CRP), anemia and normal LDH. The TT1 data both in the original publication and in the long-term update support the presence of distinct myeloma subgroups, which can be distinguished by metaphase cytogenetics. More recently, gene expression profiling has recognized several myeloma subentities at the molecular level which are predictive for outcome in Total

Therapy 2 and 3 and have differing clinical, cytogenetic, radiologic and biochemical features (see below).[2,15]

The successor Phase III trial, TT2 with 668 enrollees, delivered more intense treatment by intensifying remission induction, by adding consolidation chemotherapy post tandem AT, and by providing high-dose pulsed dexamethasone during maintenance with INF-α.[95] In addition, patients were randomized to receive thalidomide from the outset until disease progression or adverse events. The addition of thalidomide, the first new active drug since MEL and prednisone, was based on its ability to salvage patients with refractory and/or relapsed myeloma.[96] Overall, 65% of patients survived 5 years in both the thalidomide and non-thalidomide arms, and the median survival has not been reached at >8 years. The thalidomide group had significantly higher CR rates and 5-years EFS compared to the control group (62% vs 43%, and 56% vs 44%, respectively). However, the 5-year OS was approximately 65% in both arms of the study, which could be explained by worse postrelapse survival in the thalidomide arm, suggesting that continuous exposure to thalidomide may promote drug resistance. EFS and OS were adversely influenced by calcium (CA), elevated LDH and albumin <3.5 g/dl. Attainment of CR, analyzed as a time dependent co-variate variable, was a good prognostic feature.

The non-thalidomide arms in TT2 and TT1 were recently compared in order to examine the potential benefit conferred by dose-intensified induction chemotherapy and post-tandem AT consolidation chemotherapy applied in TT2 without having thalidomide as a confounding variable.[97] The CR rates in both trials were similar at 41% and 43%. However, the 5-year estimates of continuous CR (45% vs 32%), and 5-year EFS (43% vs 28%) were significantly superior in TT2, with a trend to improved OS (62% vs 57%). Patients who achieved CR in the first year and had tandem AT within 1 year also had superior OS. The treatment-related mortality was similar in both trials at approximately 7%. These data indicate that, overall, TT2 without thalidomide was superior to TT1. Since CA is an important prognostic factor, the outcome was examined in both trials in patients with good-risk (normal CA) and high-risk features (abnormal CA). TT2 especially benefited the two-thirds of good-risk patient who entered CR more frequently and had a longer duration of CR with superior EFS and OS. The influence of consolidation therapy was analyzed using a landmark set at 6 months post tandem AT. Post-transplant consolidation significantly improved survival in TT2 patients who had CA compared to similar patients in TT1. In fact, consolidation improved the outcome in the high-risk CA group in TT2 to the level obtained in the low-risk TT1 group. Despite the progress being made in TT2, it is clear that MM with abnormal CA remains a therapeutic challenge. It is, at present, not known whether the poor outcome in patients with abnormal CA is due to inherent drug resistance or whether it represents rapid regrowth in more proliferative myeloma, thus not allowing sustained tumor reduction.

Bortezomib alone has significant activity in advanced myeloma.[98] It has been suggested that bortezomib may overcome therapy resistance in myeloma with abnormal CA.[99] We observed synergistic activity of the combination of bortezomib, thalidomide and dexamethasone (VTD), which had profound activity in relapsed myeloma post AT, effecting a PR and CR of 60% and 15% respectively.[100] Therefore, in TT3 VTD was combined with the PACE portion of the highly cytoreductive DTPACE regimen allowing the reduction of remission induction to only two cycles of chemotherapy.[101] Post-tandem AT consolidation comprised two cycles of VDTPACE followed by 1 year maintenance with VTD and 2 years with dexamethasone and thalidomide alone. Treatment-free periods were covered by so-called 'bridging therapy', with thalidomide and dexamethasone, in order to reduce post-chemotherapy and AT release of cytokines which potentially protect any surviving myeloma cells by exerting antiapoptotic effects.[102] The initial results are very promising and show that EFS and OS track very closely at 86% and 84%, respectively, with an unprecedented 80% of patients remaining in CR at 2 years with a treatment-related mortality of only 5%. The 2-year rates of nCR (only immunofixation positive) and CR were significantly higher in TT3 compared to TT2 (83% vs 68%, and 56% vs 44%, respectively).

Randomized European studies

Several randomized European trials have studied the tandem AT concept, including the IFM94, the Dutch-Belgian HOVON and the Bologna 96 studies[103–106] (Table 8.3). All trials have confirmed that tandem AT does not confer excessive toxicity. The French Intergroup compared in the IFM 94 study a single transplant with MEL 140 with tandem transplants comprising conditioning with MEL 140 and MEL 140/TBI with the first and second transplant respectively.[103] A superior 7-year probability of EFS and OS in the tandem AT arm (20% vs 10% and 42% vs 21%, respectively) was observed. The EFS and OS curves separated after 3 years, and survival benefit only became statistically evident when the follow-up exceeded 5 years, indicating that it is important to obtain long-term follow-up data and not choose CR as a surrogate for an early outcome endpoint. In multivariate analysis, absence of CA, younger age, lower serum LDH and beta-2M levels, and assignment to tandem AT were associated with improved OS. The patients who benefited most from tandem AT were those who did not achieve at least a very good partial response at 3 months post first AT.

In the recently published Bologna 96 study, double AT significantly increased the probability to achieve (near) CR from 33% to 47% and

Table 8.3 Randomized trials of single versus double AT

Group	n	Age limit	Follow-up (months)	Regimen	CR% (single vs double)	Median EFS (mo) (single vs double)	Median OS (single vs double)	Conclusion
IFM 94[103]	399	≤60	75	MEL 140 + TBI → MEL 140	42 vs 50	25 vs 30	48 vs 58	OS/EFS better in double AT
HOVON24[253]	304	≤65	56	MEL 140 → Cy 120 + TBI	13 vs 28	20 vs 22	55 vs 50	EFS was better, but not OS with double AT
MAG 95[254]	227	≤55	53	MEL 140 + CCNU/ VP 16/Cy/TBI versus MEL 140 → MEL 140 + TBI	39 vs 37	31 vs 33	49 vs 73	No difference in EFS. OS is better with double AT
Bologna 96[255]	228	≤60	55	MEL 200 → MEL 120 + BU 12	35 vs 48	25 vs 35	59 vs 73	OS/EFS better in double AT
GMMG HD2[256]	261	≤65	NR	MEL 200→ MEL 200	Not available	23 vs 29	No difference	EFS better with double AT

extended the 5-year EFS from 29% to 17%.[104] Tandem AT prolonged EFS by approximately 1 year and was related to a higher CR rate. Twenty percent of patients who failed to achieve (n)CR post after the first transplant did so after the second transplant. Patients who were sensitive to conventional chemotherapy with VAD achieved a CR rate of 73% with double AT, versus 52% in the single AT group. Conversely, the CR rates in the single and tandem AT arms were similar in patients refractory to VAD, suggesting that resistance to conventional chemotherapy was difficult to overcome even by double AT. There was no benefit in terms of OS, which was similar after single and double AT (46% vs 43%). The 2-year OS from relapse in the single transplant arm was longer than in the second transplant arm (62% vs 51%), which can be explained by the sequential application of salvage therapies. Approximately one-third of the patients received a second, unplanned AT, obscuring the survival benefit conferred by a second planned procedure. In addition, half were treated with novel agents such as thalidomide and bortezomib, which may have the potential to reverse resistance to HDT.

The Dutch-Belgian HOVON24 study compared two cycles of 'intensified' chemotherapy with MEL 70 mg/m² in the standard arm with a high dose comprising two cycles of 'intensified' chemotherapy with MEL 70 mg/m² followed by cyclophosphamide/TBI with AT.[105] Patients were induced with VAD and randomization was performed after remission induction chemotherapy. Three hundred and seventy-nine patients were enrolled and only 261 were randomized. The CR was higher after myeloablative therapy (29% vs 13%), and time to progression (TTP) was longer (31 vs 25 months). However, EFS and OS were similar in both arms. In a subgroup of 120 patients with cytogenetic studies, abnormalities of chromosome 1p/q predicted inferior EFS, TTP and OS. The CR in the high-dose arm was relatively low and this study can be criticized for using cyclophosphamide and TBI as the myeloablative regimen. Cy/TBI is inferior to the more commonly used high-dose MEL with regard to myeloma cytoreduction, and it is perhaps not surprising that at least the EFS was not significantly better in the high-dose arm. The French MAG 95 used a two × two design in 230 patients younger than 56 years to study the effects of both tandem AT and purging of the autograft using CD34+ selection.[106] Tandem AT using unselected CD34+ cells resulted in improved OS compared to single AT. CD34+ cell selection did not confer survival benefit and was associated with an increased risk of infectious complications.

It is clear that tandem AT is well tolerated by younger patients with good organ function and has acceptable treatment-related morbidity and mortality. Most studies have demonstrated improved EFS with tandem AT, and MEL 200 mg/m² is currently considered to be the optimum conditioning regimen. Patients who appear to benefit most from a second AT procedure are those who are not in (n)CR after the first AT. Patients with aggressive disease, e.g. abnormal CA, do not seem to do better with tandem AT, although in TT3 the poor prognosis imparted by abnormal CA seems to be mitigated.

The best results have been reported when the two transplants are performed within 12 months of each other.[94,106] The early results of TT3 look very good and seem to support the incorporation of bortezomib or other novel drugs into transplant programs. Intuitively, it seems reasonable to assume that two planned transplants within a short time frame will achieve superior cytoreduction and outcome. However, tandem AT has never been formally compared in a randomized fashion to a single AT followed by a second, salvage AT in cases of relapse, and the optimal timing for a second transplant is therefore not known.[107–110] It should be noted that the frequency of both abnormal cytogenetics and a high-risk gene expression profile is increased at relapse, suggesting more evolved disease, which is likely to respond less well to a salvage procedure.

Maintenance

The absence of a plateau on survival curves post HDT and AT with ongoing relapses justifies the exploration of maintenance strategies with the prolongation of response duration as the goal. In addition, AT may result in a very low tumor burden, which may be susceptible to long-term suppression by drugs or immunomodulatory agents. A number of agents have been or are being explored for maintenance, including interferon-alpha (IFN-α), corticosteroids, bisphosphonates, thalidomide, lenalidomide, bortezomib, and combinations of these drugs.

IFN was one of the first drugs to be studied as maintenance post AT. It yielded a small benefit in a meta-analysis from the European Group for Blood and Marrow Transplantation (EBMT).[111] However, two randomized trials have not shown any significant survival benefit.[48,112] In the IFM99 studies, patients were randomized post AT to no maintenance, pamidronate or a combination of pamidronate and thalidomide.[113] The 3-year EFS landmarked from randomization were, respectively, 36%, 37% and 52%, indicating that thalidomide is an effective maintenance strategy. Patients who benefited were those who did not achieve a CR or very good partial response (VGPR) and who did not have deletion of chromosome 13. The Arkansas results suggest that thalidomide should perhaps be reserved for post AT to avoid the development of drug resistance. In TT2, thalidomide was used throughout the therapeutic program and prolonged EFS, but not OS, due to a shorter postrelapse survival caused by drug resistance. The shorter postrelapse survival was due to increased amplification of chromosome 1q21.[114] In both the French and Arkansas studies there was a considerable drop-out rate due to neuropathy. The median thalidomide dose used in the IFM study was 200 mg. Doses of up to 400 mg have been explored, but were not tolerated in up to 68% of patients, and required dose adjustment within 6 months, suggesting that maintenance therapy with thalidomide should not exceed 200 mg daily.[115,116] In fact, the exact therapeutic dose of thalidomide is not known and responses have been observed with as little as 50 mg per day.[117,118] Lenalidomide has been suggested as an alternative to thalidomide since it does not cause neuropathy. However, in the post-AT setting lenalidomide has to be used judiciously since it can cause significant myelosuppression, presumably due to unmasking of reduced post-AT marrow reserve.

Is it important to obtain a complete remission post AT?

In the context of AT trials for myeloma, disappearance of the M-protein is generally thought to play a pivotal role in predicting superior survival.[44,45,52,119–123] The premise that CR is a crucial step towards achieving a cure in myeloma is extrapolated from the experience in acute leukemia, where meaningful survival without early onset of CR is impossible. However, several observations have challenged the notion that a CR is an absolute requirement for prolongation of survival in myeloma.[124] The Mayo Clinic has reported that patients who underwent AT have similar PFS and OS irrespective of whether they achieved CR.[125] Patients with CA in TT2 had similar CR rates of 40% compared to those without CA, yet their median survival was significantly shorter post high-dose MEL therapy. A similar observation applied to the thalidomide arm in TT2 where a higher CR rate and EFS did not translate into superior survival.

Attainment of CR in myeloma is often a gradual and cumulative process. The median time to CR in TT2 was 12 months despite the application of an intensive therapeutic program.[95] In addition, the disappearance of MRI-defined focal lesions (FL), which are potential sites for surviving resistant myeloma cells, lags 2 years behind the disappearance of M-protein from blood and urine.[126] Paradoxically, more aggressive disease features such as CA, elevated LDH, and IgA isotype are predictors of CR.[97] We have recently reported that high serum free light chain levels at diagnosis are predictive for achieving CR.[127] These parameters reflect more proliferative myeloma which, on the one hand, is inherently more sensitive to combination chemotherapy, and on the other is linked to shorter EFS and OS due to rapid myeloma regrowth when tumor reduction is insufficiently radical.

Conversely, patients with myeloma evolving from monoclonal gammopathy of unknown significance (MGUS) or with smoldering myeloma have significantly lower CR rates, yet equal EFS and OS compared to patients with de novo myeloma. The lower CR rate in these patients is likely to be due to a lower proliferative rate, reflecting more indolent disease, which is less susceptible to eradication by both standard- and high-dose chemotherapy. Interestingly, these patients also have fewer MRI-defined FL. It is presently unknown whether all de novo myeloma initially arises from MGUS. We have recently defined an entity called MGUS-like myeloma through microarray analysis, which has a gene signature similar to patients with MGUS or myeloma evolved from MGUS.[4] Patients with MGUS-like myeloma have favorable clinical characteristics, with lower CR rates yet superior survival compared to patients with non-MGUS-like myeloma. Interestingly, an MGUS-like signature was found in most patients who are long-term survivors (>10 years) on the TT1 study.[94] Taken together, these considerations suggest that the correlation between CR and survival does not pertain to all myeloma patients.

We have recently defined a 70-gene model which identifies 13–14% of patients who are at very high risk of early disease-related death due to short durations of CR (see below).[7] The 70-gene model proved much more powerful in predicting outcome in TT2 patients when compared to standard prognostic variables, including metaphase cytogenetics. TT2 patients who had a high risk score and did not achieve CR had unprecedented high hazard ratios for OS and EFS (Fig. 8.1). Conversely, the absence of a CR in patients with a favorable 70-gene score was not detrimental. It appears, therefore, that achieving a CR is only critical for prolonging survival in a truly high-risk group of myeloma that thus far can only be captured by gene expression profiling.[128] These data also suggest that the use of CR as a surrogate marker for OS and EFS in clinical trials of novel agents cannot be applied without characterizing myeloma at the molecular level and should be used with extreme caution.

Outcome after AT can be predicted by cytogenetics and gene expression profiling

Therapy for myeloma has hitherto not been targeted at distinct myeloma subgroups. Several standard prognostic factors (SPF) have been identified which influence prognosis after AT. Elevated LDH, in analogy to aggressive lymphoma, reflects both the presence of a high tumor burden and is frequently associated with extramedullary disease.[129] The commonly used International Staging System (ISS) is based on serum levels of beta 2-microglobulin, associated with tumor burden, and albumin, indicative of elevated cytokine levels, but this staging system does not take into account the role of cytogenetics, since few patients were assessed for this variable.[130] Metaphase CA poses a greater hazard that exceeds the risk conferred by standard prognostic variables. Other prognostic variables which have been described include hypodiploidy, the proliferative potential of myeloma measured by plasma cell labeling index, circulating plasma cells and proteasomes.[131–133]

Myeloma displays an enormous genomic complexity, despite the common pathology reflected in an uncontrolled proliferation of plasma cells. Recent developments in cellular and molecular genetics have given unprecedented novel insights into the pathobiology and classification of myeloma.[5] A comprehensive understanding of genomic aberrations identified by cytogenetics and gene expression profiling (GEP) and their relation to response to therapy is of paramount importance for the development of risk-adopted strategies. Abnormal metaphase cytogenetics can be detected in approximately 30% of patients.[134] Metaphase cytogenetics are more powerful in predicting outcome compared to interphase fluorescence in situ hybridization (FISH) since they imply the presence of cells with autonomous proliferative capacity in the myeloma clone, which do not require the support of the bone marrow micro-environment (ME). Interphase FISH is not dependent on dividing cells and can capture genomic aberrations in non-cycling cells as well, thus increasing the detection of abnormal cells to 80–90%.[135] Interphase FISH can also detect important cytogenetically silent translocations such as t(4;14) and can be performed on stored material.[136,137]

The universal activation of one of the three cyclin D genes is consistent with the hypothesis that this is the initiating event in myelomagenesis.[138] Aneuploidy, as measured by flow cytometry, is present in a very high percentage of myeloma patients.[100,139] Myeloma can be divided into hyperdiploid and non-hyperdiploid types. Hyperdiploid

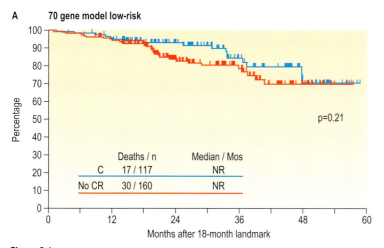

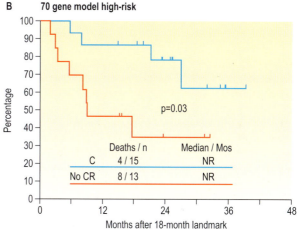

Figure 8.1
Achievement of CR for OS is only important in patients who have high-risk myeloma.

myeloma occurs in 60% of cases and is typified by trisomies of uneven chromosomes, including trisomy 1, 3,5,7,9,11,15,19 and 21, which is not associated with a poor prognosis.[140] Hyperdiploid myeloma is characterized by an increased incidence of bony lesions and is associated with increased expression of DKK1.[141,142] Myeloma cell lines are usually not hyperdiploid, suggesting that they can survive without the support of the ME. Both the increased incidence of bony lesions in myeloma and the lack of hyperdiploid cell lines suggest that hyperdiploid myeloma is more dependent on interaction with the ME.[138,142,143] A subgroup of hyperdiploid myeloma has gains of chromosome 1q and 7, del 13, and absence of trisomy 11 and has a more guarded prognosis.[144] The Groupe Français de Cytogénétique Hématologique demonstrated that the chromosome number pattern is an important prognostic factor in myeloma.[131] Hyperdiploid patients, with trisomies of uneven chromosomes, fared significantly better than the hypodiploid cases (median OS 34 vs 14 months).

The remaining 40% of cases consists of non-hyperdiploid myeloma, which is characterized by translocations at 14q32, the immunoglobulin heavy chain locus, resulting in the transcriptional activation of usually inactive proto-oncogenes. This results in recurrent IgH translocations which activate: *CCDN1* t (11;14), incidence 17%; the *FGFR3* and *MMSET* genes t(4;14), incidence 17%; *c-MAF* t(14;16), incidence 6%; *MAFB* t(14;20), incidence 6%; and *CCND3* t(6;14), incidence 3%.[5,135,145] Trisomy 11 or t(11;14) results in *Cyclin D1* overexpression, which is associated with a favorable response to STD and AT.[146–148] Translocations involving *MAF* and *FGFR3/MMSET* genes have a significantly worse outcome when compared to t(11;14).[131,146,149] Other poor cytogenetic features include deletion of chromosome 17p, hypodiploidy and deletion of chromosome 13q14, which is tightly associated with the aforementioned IgH-associated translocations, and a MM-MDS karyotype.[121,150–154]

The Arkansas group has systematically performed metaphase cytogenetics since 1989 and it was recognized early on that deletion of chromosome 13 and other cytogenetic abnormalities conferred a poor prognosis[52,134,137,155,156] (Fig. 8.2). Abnormal metaphase cytogenetics were independently associated with worse OS and EFS survival in all three TT trials, and were surpassed in predictive power only by data derived from gene expression profiling. The poor prognosis conferred by del 13 has been confirmed by other groups using both interphase FISH and metaphase cytogenetics.[140,157,158]

The presence of both hypoploidy and a high beta-2M identified a very poor-risk population.[131] A similar observation has been made for the combination of del 13 and high beta-2M in 110 patients treated with AT.[159] Keats et al reported that t (4 : 14) predicted for poor response to VAD induction chemotherapy and survival post AT in a series of 208 patients.[150] The presence of 17p13.1, the locus of the tumor suppressor gene p53, also imparts a poorer prognosis following AT.[160,161] In the Eastern Cooperative Oncology trial E9486/9487, Fonseca et al recognized three distinct prognostic groups in patients treated with conventional chemotherapy: a poor prognosis was typified by t(4;14) and/or t(14;16) and/or del 17p; an intermediate prognosis by del 13q but without t(4;14),t(14;16) and del 17p; and a good prognosis group who have t(11;14) or no abnormalities.[149] Similar observations have been reported for del 17p, t(4;14) and t(14;16) in the setting of AT.[147,153,161]

Avet-Loiseau et al recently published FISH data of nearly 1000 patients enrolled on the IFM99 therapeutic trials.[162] Del 13q, t(4;14) and del 17p all adversely influenced OS and EFS. On multivariate analysis, only del 17p and t(4;14) independently prognosticated for EFS and OS. The deleterious effect of del13q was dependent on its frequent association with the detection of t(4;14) and del 17p. The OS and EFS in patients who did not have t(4;14) and del 17p were similar, regardless of the presence of del 13q. Further, t(4;14) and del 17p separated distinct groups within each ISS stage. Patients who lacked

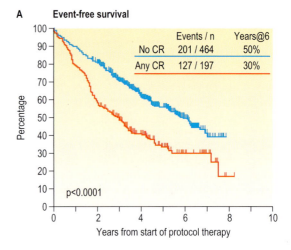

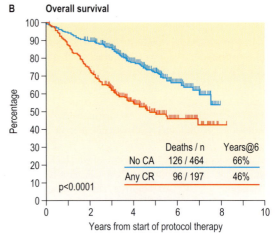

Figure 8.2
Importance of abnormal cytogenetics (CA): patients on TT2 with normal cytogenetics have superior EFS and OS.

t(4;14) and del 17p and who had a beta-2M of <4 mg/l had an excellent 4-year OS of 83% and clearly benefited from tandem AT. Conversely, patients who had either t(4;14) or del 17p combined with a beta-2M of <4 mg/l had a poor prognosis of OS of only 19 months after AT and it was considered that these patients should be considered for other treatment options.

It has been recognized that tandem duplications and jumping translocations of chromosome 1 are related to a more advanced myeloma phenotype.[163–166] Gain of 1q21 region has also been recognized as one of the most frequent recurrent abnormalities in human cancers.[167–170] In an analysis of 479 myeloma patients the incidence of amplification 1q21 (amp1q21) increased from diagnosis to relapse (72% vs 43%), suggesting that this genetic lesion plays a role in disease progression.[114] Both the proportion of cells with 1q21 and the copy number of 1q21 increased at relapse, indicating the existence of a gene dosage effect promoting drug resistance. Amp1q21 also shortened postrelapse survival. Newly diagnosed patients with amp1q21 treated on TT2 had inferior 5-year EFS and OS (38% vs 52%, and 62% vs 78%, respectively; both p < 0.001) (Fig. 8.3). Correlation with gene array data showed that 100% of cases with c-MAF, t(14;16), and 75% of cases with FGFR3/MMSET, (t4;14) spikes had amp1q21. This is analogous to the findings in the IFM99 tandem AT study where del 13 is strongly correlated to t(14;16) and (t4;14).[162] Interestingly, thalidomide only improved EFS in patients who lacked gain of 1q21, which suggests that amp1q21 may be an important determinant for assigning patients to AT regimens which incorporate thalidomide.[150] The gene *CKS1B*,

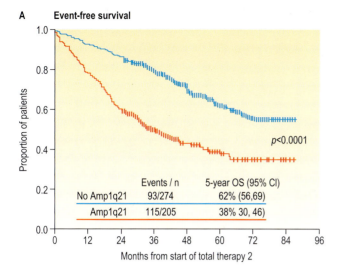

A Event-free survival

	Events / n	5-year OS (95% CI)
No Amp1q21	93/274	62% (56,69)
Amp1q21	115/205	38% 30, 46)

p<0.0001

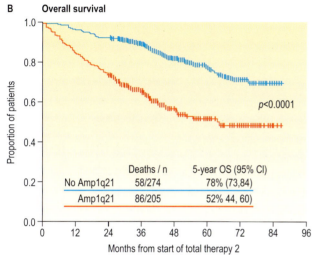

B Overall survival

	Deaths / n	5-year OS (95% CI)
No Amp1q21	58/274	78% (73,84)
Amp1q21	86/205	52% 44, 60)

p<0.0001

Figure 8.3
Patients without amp1q21 have superior EFS and OS on the TT2 protocol myeloma.

located at 1q21, has been linked to shorter progression-free survival post AT.[171] *CKS1-B* promotes the ubiquination and degradation of the cyclin-dependent kinase inhibitor p27(Kip1), which controls the G1 to S transition of the cell cycle.[172]

Taken together, these data support the notion that the systematic application of metaphase and FISH cytogenetic techniques can identify high-risk groups of patients who tend not to do well with AT approaches, including patients with high-level amp1q21, t(4;14), t(14;16), t(16;20) and MM-MDS karyotype.

The prognosis of individual patients remains highly variable, despite the progress being made in identifying high-risk patients by cytogenetics. This is underscored by a recent multivariate analysis of the TT2 data set, where standard prognostic factors and metaphase cytogenetics had limited ability to account for survival variability with hazard ratios not exceeding 2.0 in multivariate analyses.[128] Gene expression profiling in leukemias and lymphoma has assisted in delineating disease subclassifications, which are clinically relevant.[173–177] This suggests that for treatment advances to occur, outcome data have to be analyzed in the context of genetic data. Zhan et al described seven subgroups in myeloma, based on common gene expression signatures, with distinct clinical features and response to tandem AT.[5] Three high-risk entities were identified, one with overexpression of proliferation genes, the PROLIFERATION group, the second with overexpression of *MMSET* (t4;14), and the last one with spiked

expression of *c-MAF* or *MAFB*. A striking feature of these high-risk groups was the overexpression of genes on chromosome 1q. Shaughnessy et al hypothesized that gene expression extremes might be representative of gene copy number changes which are predictive of survival.[7] Genes located on chromosome 1 were overrepresented in 70 genes which were either highly overexpressed (chr.1q) or had marked reduced expression levels (chr.1p). Thirteen percent of patients had a high-risk score, as defined by the ratio of mean expression levels of upregulated to downregulated genes (Fig. 8. 4). This high-risk score was associated with shorter CR duration, OS and EFS in 532 patients treated on two separate tandem AT protocols. Unlike traditional SPF and CA with hazard ratios not exceeding 2, the 70-gene model captured a very high-risk group of patients with unprecedented high hazard ratios (>6 and >5, respectively, for OS and EFS) in those not attaining a CR, independent of SPF, ISS staging system and cytogenetics.[128] Interestingly the t(4;14) group could be divided into two groups with good and poor outcome based on the 70-gene risk score, which clearly indicates that not all patients with t(4;14) have a poor prognosis, as has previously been suggested.[178] At relapse, 76% of patients had a high-risk score, providing molecular evidence of clonal evolution that determines postrelapse outcome. Using a multivariate discriminant analysis 17 genes were identified, which had similar predictive power to detect high-risk myeloma.[7] The 2-year probabilities of OS and EFS in the high- and low-risk groups in TT3 were, respectively, 91% vs 88%, and 50% vs 54%. A 17-gene PCR kit is in development, which will provide a simple and very powerful molecular-based prognostic test, replacing SPF and cytogenetics and eliminating the need for testing of many prognostic variables with only limited prognostic implications.

Allogeneic stem cell transplantation for myeloma

Full myeloablative conditioning followed by allo-SCT has proven to be toxic in myeloma and is associated with a high TRM of 25–50%.[179–184] A report from the EBMT registry did report improvement in the TRM when comparing patients transplanted in the periods 1983–1993 (n = 334) and 1994–1998 (n = 356), presumably due to selection of less heavily pretreated patients and progress in supportive care. TRM reduced from 46% to 30%, but the regimen-related mortality rate remained unacceptably high.[185] In general, no more than 20% of patients remain in CR for more than 5 years post allo-SCT.[180,181,184] Two case–control studies by the EBMT and HOVON groups have, in fact, suggested longer survivals with AT rather than allo-SCT.[179,186] The high TRM essentially neutralizes the potential advantages of allografting over autografting, and full myeloablative allografts have therefore mostly been abandoned.

However, allo-SCT for myeloma remains a subject of continuing interest, because of the potential benefits attached to using allogeneic cells for transplantation. First, an allograft is not contaminated by myeloma cells. Relapse rates after syngeneic transplant were lower when compared to case-matched controls undergoing AT (36% vs 78% at 4 years), suggesting that some of the relapses in the AT setting may originate from a contaminated graft, although a graft-versus-myeloma (GvM) effect in the syngeneic setting cannot be ruled out.[187] Second, there is substantive evidence to suggest that there is a GvM effect mediated by allogeneic donor cells. Withdrawal of immunosuppression resulted in patients with relapse in GvM associated with GvHD.[188] A number of studies have documented an antimyeloma effect post donor leukocyte infusion (DLI) for relapse.[189,190] Although the initial results were very encouraging and presumably reflected reporting bias, more recent studies suggest that the CR rate after DLI may not be higher than 30%.[191–193] A single-center study of 27 patients reported

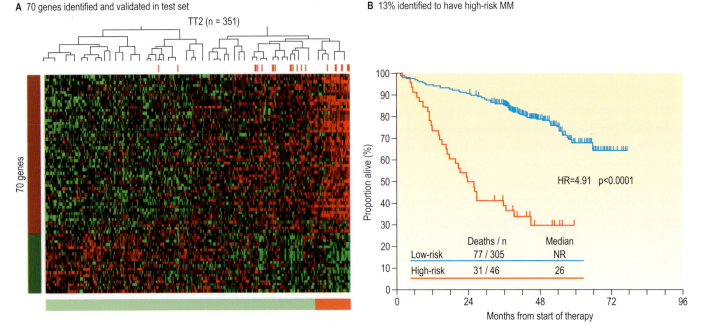

A 70 genes identified and validated in test set

B 13% identified to have high-risk MM

Figure 8.4
(a) Heat maps of the 70 genes show remarkable similarity in newly diagnosed myeloma. The 51 genes in rows indicated by the red bar are highly upregulated and the 19 genes designated by the green bar are highly downregulated in patients at risk of early death due to disease. Red bars above the columns indicate patients with disease-related death.
(b) OS is significantly worse in the 13% of patients who have high-risk myeloma (red curve).

only five with a response that lasted more than 30 months.[194] Further, the development of a GvM effect is very strongly linked to GvHD, which can be severe.[193]

A review of 29 patients reported a GvM effect in 82% of patients who developed GvHD compared to only 29% of patient without clinically evident GvHD.[195] The development of chronic GvHD post allo-SCT for myeloma is also associated with a reduction in relapse rate, underlining the close association between GvM and GvHD in myeloma.[196] Third, allo-SCT appears to be able to cytoreduce myeloma to a level undetectable by sensitive molecular techniques. Molecular remissions as defined by a negative PCR for immunoglobulin gene rearrangements are observed more frequently post allogeneic transplant rather than AT, and predict improved survival.[197,198] These findings were confirmed in 48 patients in hematologic remission post myeloablative SCT who had a cumulative risk of relapse at 5 years of 100% when PCR positive compared to 0% in patients who remained persistently PCR negative.[199] They suggest that allografting has the potential to achieve superior cytoreduction, which may, in some cases, translate into cure.

The high TRM rate with full myeloablative allografting has led to the introduction of reduced-intensity regimens for conditioning prior to allografting (RICT allografting). RICT allografting was initially developed in Seattle in canine models and subsequently introduced in humans.[200–206] The basic premise is that reduced-intensity conditioning (RIC) is associated with less regimen-related toxicity and principally provides immunosuppression, allowing establishment of the donor graft. Tumor eradication is subsequently achieved by immunocompetent donor cells contained in the graft, which recognize minor histocompatibility and other antigens. Several studies suggest that RICT is not a good salvage strategy for patients who have failed autografting or who have chemotherapy-resistant disease, although there was a substantial reduction in TRM.[207–209] In one study, relapse from a prior AT predicted for TRM, relapse and death.[210] When comparing the results of DLI for the therapy of relapse after allografting, it appears that the GvM effect is not as potent as the antitumor effects observed in relapsed chronic myeloid leukemia, chronic lymphocytic leukemias

and lymphomas. A natural step forwards was therefore to combine the cytoreductive effect of HDT with MEL 200 mg/m² with the GvM effect derived from a dose-reduced RICT allograft in a so-called tandem auto-'mini'-allograft procedure.[207,211,212]

There are, at present, no studies comparing tandem AT with tandem auto-'mini'-allografting in a randomized fashion. Published and ongoing studies (IFM9903, HOVON-50 and BMT-CTN0102) rely on 'genetic' randomization where patients with an HLA-identical sibling donor are assigned to tandem auto-'mini'-allografting. The IFM9903 study enrolled patients with high-risk myeloma as defined by beta-2M > 3 mg/l and FISH del 13, and compared the outcome of 219 patients allocated to the tandem AT arm with 65 patients assigned to the tandem auto-'mini'-allograft arm because of availability of an HLA-identical sibling donor.[213] The procedure was safe, with a 100-day mortality of 4.3% and TRM of 10.9%. However, on an intent-to-treat analysis there was no difference between the median OS (41 vs 35 months) and EFS (30 vs 25 months) in either arm. The estimated 5-year EFS was 0% with no plateau due to a high relapse rate, which can be explained by the fact that a poor-risk population was targeted. The results suggest that a tandem auto-'mini'-allograft does not offer any advantage over tandem AT in high-risk myeloma patients. This study has been criticized for the use of a relatively high dose of ATG (12.5 mg/kg) which may have attenuated the GvM effect in the tandem auto-'mini'-allograft arm.[214,215]

A multicenter Italian study used the same paradigm to assign 80 patients to a MEL 200 mg/m² AT followed by a mini-allograft after conditioning with 200 cGy TBI.[216] Nineteen percent of the patients actually receiving the mini-allograft were given DLI for relapse or progressive disease. In the comparator tandem AT arm, 82 patients received a first AT after MEL 200 mg/m² and a second AT after doses of MEL which varied from intermediate, at 100 mg/m², in some patients to ablative, at 140–200 mg/m², in the other group. The median and OS were superior in the tandem auto-'mini'-allograft arm (80 vs 54 months and 35 vs 29 months, respectively). The principal problem with this study, in contrast to the IFM study, is the absence of cytogenetic data, the most powerful predictor of outcome, in 64% of patients.

In addition, the 2-year incidence of extensive chronic GvHD was substantial at 32% at 2 years. In fact, the 5-year survival rate of 68% on TT2 in patients under the age of 65 (n = 532) is virtually identical to the reported outcome of the auto-allograft group without the unpredictable consequences of chronic GvHD.[217]

In general, it is difficult to interpret the many published RICT allograft studies since there is considerable variability in type of conditioning regimen, use of T-cell depletion, number of prior AT, pre-emptive or therapeutic use of DLI and lines and type of remission induction chemotherapy.[218] A number of factors have been reported which are predictors for a poor outcome, including use of an unrelated donor, use of alemtuzumab rather than ATG for T-cell depletion, lack of chronic GvHD, del 13q14, chemorefractory or relapsed myeloma and >1 prior AT.[207,219–226] In most of these studies, TRM has been considerably reduced to 15–30%. However, OS varies 30–40% and relapse rates vary from 40% to as high as 77%. Overall, the results are not clearly better than with tandem AT. One of the principal problems is the management of high-risk patients who seem to fare equally poorly with both tandem AT and tandem auto-'mini'-allografting. Conversely, good-risk patients have an excellent outcome with current AT approaches and it is not unreasonable to expect 10-year survivorships which exceed 50% in future studies, without the risk of early mortality and protracted GvHD incurred by allograft approaches.

The above interpretation of the RICT allograft data may leave the impression that allo-transplantation for myeloma is a 'dinosaur' destined to become extinct. This may not necessarily be the case. There are several ways in which RICT allografting for myeloma can be improved, and patients considered for allografting should be enrolled in clinical trials which explore novel therapeutic strategies. First, in many RICT allograft studies there may have been too much reliance on the GvM effect. Some of the myriad conditioning regimens used prior to RICT allografting are clearly inferior to MEL 200 mg/m^2 which remains the gold standard. Suboptimal regimens in terms of myeloma kill include fludarabine/low-dose TBI, MEL 100 mg/m^2, MEL 100 mg/m^2 fludarabine/low-dose TBI, and cyclophosphamide/low-dose TBI. These regimens could be easily supplanted by highly effective and equally well-tolerated regimens such as MEL 200 mg/m^2 or BEAM (carmustine, etoposide, cytarabine, melphalan). Incorporation of novel drugs into preparative regimens may potentially enhance cytoreduction. The addition of bortezomib and thalidomide to BEAM (VTD-BEAM) incurs little excess toxicity and is used by our group for 'salvage' AT (van Rhee et al, unpublished observations).

There also may be a role for the application of novel therapeutic agents post allografting. Thalidomide has been used for the therapy of chronic GvHD. One study has reported that the combination of low-dose thalidomide and DLI may improve response rates.[227] Murine studies have suggested that bortezomib may reduce GvHD yet retain a graft-versus-leukemia effect.[228] Bortezomib also selectively depletes allo-reactive T-cells and is currently being explored in clinical studies as an agent to prevent GvHD.[229] In the case of myeloma, it may confer additional antimyeloma activity. Lenalidomide may also find therapeutic application post allografting since it is a potent activator of NK cells and T-cells, although it could potentially activate GvHD.[230]

A major step forward in allografting for myeloma would be the dissociation of GvHD from GvM. Studies, pioneered by Barrett and Cavazzano-Calvi, have established platforms to separate GvHD from GvL.[231,232] However, of equal importance is to substantially enhance a specific GvM effect. Experimental studies have vaccinated healthy donors with idiotype or tumor lysate,[233,234] in order to allow transfer of antimyeloma immunity from donor to patients. We have recently demonstrated that immunization with the MAGE-A3 protein can produce potent cytotoxic, T-helper and humoral response in healthy donors and transfer this immunity post syngeneic transplant to a MAGE-A3 positive myeloma patient. In both patient and donor memory cytotoxic T-cells could be expanded more than 1 year after adoptive immune cell transfer.[235]

A number of other tumor-associated antigens have been described in myeloma which could be explored post allogeneic transplant. Selection for KIR mismatched donor and transfusion KIR mismatched DLI post allogeneic BMT could also specifically bolster the GvM effect.[226,232]

Finally, it is important to realize that allografting for myeloma will always have some limitations in application since myeloma is predominantly a disease of the elderly. When one takes into account the availability of matched donors, probably only ~10% of patients will be suitable candidates for allogeneic SCT.

Novel agents and risk-adopted treatment strategies

A number of novel agents including thalidomide, lenalidomide and bortezomib have proven activity for both relapsed/refractory and newly diagnosed myeloma.[96,98,236–240] Combinations of novel drugs including MPT, MPR, VTD, VMP, VMPT, PAD and ThaDD appear to be synergistic and in some trials high PR and n(CR) rates have been reported.[73–75,241–246] However, all these studies have a short median follow-up and it is presently not known whether these agents can achieve the benchmark of 30% survival at 10 years achieved with high-dose MEL-based AT. It is therefore too early to abandon high-dose MEL-based AT.

Several algorithms for the management of myeloma have been suggested. Most of these incorporate cytogenetics in addition to SPF.[6,247] Risk stratification models based on SPF alone have limited ability to account for variability in patient outcome and are therefore not likely to make a major contribution to improving outcome in myeloma.[123] Although cytogenetics are of importance, the state-of-art approach is to define high-risk disease by gene expression profiling. Disadvantages of GEP include sample attrition (especially in multi-center trials), expense, requirement for stringent quality control and sample turnaround time, which limits application outside so-called 'centers of excellence'.[248] The introduction of a 'myeloma PCR kit' may negate these issues and will in the very near future enable genetic stratification based on biologic disease risk. This will allow the separation of myeloma patients at diagnosis into standard and high risk, based on RT-PCR data of 17 genes. These 17 genes will provide a myeloma individualized risk-adopted therapy (MIRT) score. High-risk patients do poorly with all current approaches and should be entered into clinical trials exploring novel therapies and combination of novel drugs (Fig. 8.5). These patients are more likely to require 'genotoxic' therapy as part of a strategy designed to cure their disease since any surviving cells are likely to give rise to relapse. It is conceivable that standard- or low-risk patients, in the elderly population, would be amenable to therapeutic approaches aimed at providing long-term disease control. However, many unanswered questions remain in the standard-risk group, especially for younger patients. In future studies, these patients should be randomized prospectively to combinations of new drugs versus MEL-based HDT to study whether novel agents offer similar long-term survival. Other studies could address several unanswered questions in a randomized manner, including (a) which are the most efficacious and fastest induction regimens prior to AT, (b) the potential synergistic effect between new agents and high-dose MEL during AT and (c) the role of new drugs in sustaining remission post AT with maintenance. The latter is of particular importance since MEL-based AT does not seem to result in a plateau phase on the survival curve.

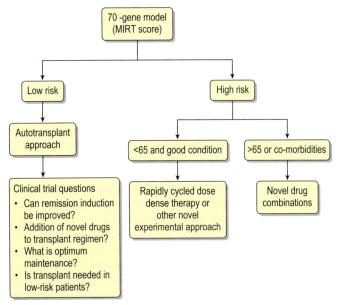

Figure 8.5
Risk-adopted approach based on gene expression defined risk (70-gene model) and potential clinical trials. The currently best available outcome data are from Total Therapy 3, which achieves unprecedented >90% (n)CR rates in good-risk patients with few relapses with a medial follow-up of 3 years. High-risk patients remain a formidable problem and should be entered into clinical trials exploring novel approaches.

Acknowledgements

We thank all the MIRT clinical, research, nursing and administrative staff for providing excellent care for our patients. Finally, we are grateful to our patients for participating in our research protocols and for continuing to put their confidence in MIRT.

References

1. SEER:http://seer.cancer.gov/csr/1975 2004/results merged/sect 18 myeloma.pdf)
2. Zhan F, Hardin J, Kordsmeier B et al. Global gene expression profiling of multiple myeloma, monoclonal gammopathy of undetermined significance and normal bone marrow plasma cells. Blood 2002;99:1745–1757
3. Bergsagel PL, Michael Kuehl WM et al. Molecular pathogenesis and a consequent classification of multiple myeloma. J Clin Oncol 2005;23:6333–6338
4. Zhan F, Barlogie B, Arzoumanian V et al. A gene expression signature of benign monoclonal gammopathy evident in multiple myeloma is linked to good prognosis. Blood 2007;109:1692–1700
5. Zhan F, Yongsheng H, Simona C et al. The molecular classification of multiple myeloma. Blood 2006;108:2020–2028
6. Dispenzieri A, Rajkumar V, Gertz MA et al. Treatment of newly diagnosed multiple myeloma based on Mayo stratification of myeloma and risk-adapted therapy (mSMART). Mayo Clin Proc 2007;82:323–341
7. Shaughnessy JD, Fenghuang JR, Burington BE et al. A validated gene expression model of high-risk multiple myeloma is defined by deregulated expression of genes mapping to chromosome 1. Blood 2007;109:2276–2284
8. Bergsagel DE, Sprague CC, Austin C, Griffith KM. Evaluation of new chemotherapeutic agents in the treatment of multiple myeloma: IV. L-Phenylalanine mustard (NC-8806). Cancer Chemother Rep 1962;21:87–89
9. Alexanian R, Haut A, Khan AU et al. Treatment for multiple myeloma. Combination chemotherapy with different melphalan dose regimens. JAMA 1969;208:1680–1685
10. Alexanian R, Dimopoulos M. The treatment of multiple myeloma. N Engl J Med 1994;330:484–489
11. Gregory WM, Richards MA, Malpas JS. Combination chemotherapy versus melphalan and prednisolone in the treatment of multiple myeloma: an overview of published poirtals. J Clin Oncol 1992;10:334–342
12. Group MTC. Combination chemotherapy versus melphalan plus prednisone as treatment for multiple myeloma: an overview of 6633 patients from 27 randomized trials. Myeloma Trialists' Collaborative Group. J Clin Oncol 1998;16:3832–3842
13. Fassas A, Tricot G. Result of high-dose treatment with autologous stem cell support in patients with multiple myeloma. Semin Hematol 2001;38:203–208
14. Lenhoff S, Hjorth M, Holmberg E et al. Impact on survival of high-dose therapy with autologous stem cell support in patients younger than 60 years with newly diagnosed multiple myeloma: a population-based study. Nordic Myeloma Study Group. Blood 2000;95:7–11
15. McElwain TJ, Powles RL. High-dose intravenous melphalan for plasma-cell leukaemia and myeloma. Lancet 1983;2:822–824
16. Selby PJ, McElwain TJ, Nandi A et al. Multiple myeloma treated with high dose intravenous melphalan. Br J Haematol 1987;66:55–62
17. Barlogie B, Hall R, Zander A et al. High-dose melphalan with autologous bone marrow transplantation for multiple myeloma. Blood 1986;67:1298–1301
18. Barlogie B, Alexanian R, Dicke KA et al. High-dose chemoradiotherapy and autologous bone marrow transplantation for resistant multiple myeloma. Blood 1987;70:869–872
19. Alexanian, R, Barlogie, B, Tucker S. VAD-based regimens as primary treatment for multiple myeloma. Am J Hematol 1990;33:86–89
20. Raje N, Powles R, Kulkarni S. A comparison of vincristine and doxorubicin infusional chemotherapy with methylprednisolone (VAMP) with the addition of weekly cyclophosphamide (C-VAMP) as induction treatment followed by autografting in previously untreated myeloma. Br J Haematol 1997;97(1):153–160
21. Ventura GJ, Barlogie B, Hester JP et al. High dose cyclophosphamide, BCNU and VP-16 with autologous blood stem cell support for refractory multiple myeloma. Bone Marrow Transplant 1990;5:265–268
22. Barlogie B, Gahrton G. Bone marrow transplantation in multiple myeloma. Bone Marrow Transplant 1991;7:71–79
23. Gore ME, Selby PJ, Viner C et al. Intensive treatment of multiple myeloma and criteria for complete remission. Lancet 1989;2:879–882
24. Jagannath S, Barlogie B, Dicke K et al. Autologous bone marrow transplantation in multiple myeloma: identification of prognostic factors. Blood 1990;76:1860–1866
25. Attal M, Huguet F, Schlaifer D et al. Intensive combined therapy for previously untreated aggressive myeloma. Blood 1992;79:1130–1136
26. Harousseau JL, Milpied N, Laporte JP et al. Double-intensive therapy in high-risk multiple myeloma. Blood 1992;79:2827–2833
27. Lokhorst HM, Meuwissen OJ, Verdonck LF, Dekker AW. High-risk multiple myeloma treated with high-dose melphalan. J Clin Oncol 1992;10:47–51
28. Anderson KC, Barut BA, Ritz J et al. Monoclonal antibody-purged autologous bone marrow transplantation therapy for multiple myeloma. Blood 1991;77:712–720
29. Reece DE, Barnett MJ, Connors JM et al. Treatment of multiple myeloma with intensive chemotherapy followed by autologous BMT using marrow purged with 4-hydroperoxycyclophosphamide. Bone Marrow Transplant 1993;11:139–146
30. Fermand JP, Chevret S, Ravaud P et al. High-dose chemoradiotherapy and autologous blood stem cell transplantation in multiple myeloma: results of a phase II trial involving 63 patients. Blood 1993;82:2005–2009
31. Reiffers J, Marit G, Boiron JM. Autologous blood stem cell transplantation in high-risk multiple myeloma. Br J Haematol 1989;72:296–297
32. Gianni AM, Tarella C, Bregni M et al. High-dose sequential chemoradiotherapy, a widely applicable regimen, confers survival benefit to patients with high-risk multiple myeloma. J Clin Oncol 1994;12:503–509
33. Cunningham D, Paz-Ares L, Gore ME et al. High-dose melphalan for multiple myeloma: long-term follow-up data. J Clin Oncol 1994;12:764–768
34. Cunningham D, Paz-Ares L, Milan S et al. High-dose melphalan and autologous bone marrow transplantation as consolidation in previously untreated myeloma. J Clin Oncol 1994;12:759–763
35. Vesole DH, Barlogie B, Jagannath S et al. High-dose therapy for refractory multiple myeloma: improved prognosis with better supportive care and double transplants. Blood 1994;84:950–956
36. Björkstrand B, Ljungman P, Bird JM et al. Double high-dose chemoradiotherapy with autologous stem cell transplantation can induce molecular remissions in multiple myeloma. Bone Marrow Transplant 1995;15:367–371
37. Dimopoulos MA, Alexanian R, Przepiorka D et al. Thiotepa, busulfan and cyclophosphamide: a new preparative regimen for autologous marrow or blood stem cell transplantation in high-risk multiple myeloma. Blood 1993;82:2324–2328
38. Bjorkstrand B, Ljungman P, Bird JM et al. Autologous stem cell transplantation in multiple myeloma: results of the European Group for Bone Marrow Transplantation. Stem Cells 1995;13(suppl 2):140–146
39. Alexanian R, Dimopoulous MA, Hester J et al. Early myeloablative therapy for multiple myeloma. Blood 1994;84:4278–4282
40. Harousseau JL, Attal M, Divine M et al. Autologous stem cell transplantation after first remission induction treatment in multiple myeloma: a report of the French Registry on autologous transplantation for myeloma. Blood 1995;85:3077–3085
41. Barlogie B, Jagannath S, Vesole D et al. Superiority of tandem autologous transplantation over standard therapy for previously untreated multiple myeloma. Blood 1997;89:789–793
42. Lenhoff S, Hjorth M, Holmberg E et al. Impact on survival of high-dose therapy with autologous stem cell support in patients younger than 60 years with newly diagnosed multiple myeloma: a population-based study. Blood 2000;95:7–11
43. Palumbo A, Triolo S, Argentino C et al. Dose-intensive melphalan with stem cell support (MEL100) is superior to standard treatment in elderly myeloma patients. Blood 1999;94:1248–1253
44. Attal M, Harousseau JL, Stoppa AM et al. A prospective, randomized trial of autologous bone marrow transplantation and chemotherapy in multiple myeloma. Intergroupe Français du Myélome. N Engl J Med 1996;335:91–97
45. Child JA, Morgan GJ, Davies FE et al. High-dose chemotherapy with hematopoietic stem-cell rescue for multiple myeloma. N Engl J Med 2003;348:1875–1883
46. Fermand JP, Katsahian S, Divine M et al. High-dose therapy and autologous blood stem-cell transplantation compared with conventional treatment in myeloma patients aged 55 to 65 years: long-term results of a randomized control trial from the Group Myeloma-Autogreffe. J Clin Oncol 2005;23:9227–9233
47. Bladé J, Rosinol L, Sureda A et al. High-dose therapy intensification compared with continued standard therapy in multiple myeloma patients responding to the initial chemotherapy: long-term results from a prospective randomized trial from the Spanish Cooperative Group PETHEMA. Blood 2005;106:3755–3759
48. Barlogie B, Kyle RA, Anderson KC et al. Standard chemotherapy compared with high-dose chemoradiotherapy for multiple myeloma: final results of phase III US Intergroup Trial S9321. J Clin Oncol 2006;24:929–936

49. Kyle RA, Rajkumar SV. Multiple myeloma. N Engl J Med 2004;351:1860–1873
50. Fassas A, Shaughnessy J, Barlogie B. Cure of myeloma: hype or reality? Bone Marrow Transplant 2005;35:215–224
51. Moreau P, Facon T, Attal M et al. Comparison of 200 mg/m^2 melphalan and 8 Gy total body irradiation plus 140 mg/m^2 melphalan as conditioning regimens for peripheral blood stem cell transplantation in patients with newly diagnosed multiple myeloma: final analysis of the Intergroupe Francophone du Myelome 9502 randomized trial. Blood 2002;99:731–735
52. Desikan KR, Tricot G, Dhodapkar M et al. Melphalan plus total body irradiation (MEL-TBI) or cyclophosphamide (MEL-CY) as a conditioning regimen with second auto-transplant in responding patients with myeloma is inferior compared to historical controls receiving tandem transplants with melphalan alone. Blood 2000;25:483–487
53. Goldschmidt U, Hegenbart M, Wallmeier M et al. High-dose therapy with peripheral blood progenitor cell transplantation in multiple myeloma. Ann Oncol 1997;8:243–246
54. Bladé J, Vesole DH, Gertz M. Transplantation for multiple myeloma: who, when, how often? Blood 2003;102:3469–3477
55. Buzaid AC, Durie BG. Management of refractory myeloma: a review. J Clin Oncol 1988;6:889–905
56. Barlogie B, Smith L, Alexanian R. Effective treatment of advanced multiple myeloma refractory to alkylating agents. N Engl J Med 1984;310:1353–1356
57. Alexanian R, Barlogie B, Dixon D. High-dose glucocorticoid treatment of resistant myeloma. Ann Intern Med 1986;105:8–11
58. Alexanian R, Dimopoulos MA, Hester J et al. Early myeloablative therapy for multiple myeloma. Blood 1994;84:4278–4282
59. Alexanian R, Dimopoulos MA, Smith T et al. Limited value of myeloablative therapy for late multiple myeloma. Blood 1994;83:512–516
60. Dimopoulos MA, Alexanian R, Przepiorka D et al. Thiotepa, busulfan, and cyclophosphamide: a new preparative regimen for autologous marrow or blood stem cell transplantation in high-risk multiple myeloma. Blood 1993;82:2324–2328
61. Vesole DH, Barlogie B, Jagannath S et al. High-dose therapy for refractory multiple myeloma: improved prognosis with better supportive care and double transplants. Blood 1994;84:950–956
62. Vesole DH, Tricot G, Jagannath S et al. Autotransplants in multiple myeloma: what have we learned? Blood 1996;88:838–847
63. Alexanian R, Weber D, Delasalle K et al. Clinical outcomes with intensive therapy for patients with primary resistant multiple myeloma. Bone Marrow Transplant 2004;34:229–234
64. Kumar S, Lacy MQ, Dispenzieri A et al. High-dose therapy and autologous stem cell transplantation for multiple myeloma poorly responsive to initial therapy. Bone Marrow Transplant 2004;34(2):161–167
65. Vesole DH, Crowley JJ, Catchatourian R et al. High-dose melphalan with autotransplantation for refractory multiple myeloma: results of a Southwest Oncology Group Phase II Trial. J Clin Oncol 1999;17:2173–2179
66. Singhal S, Powles R, Sirohi R et al. Response to induction chemotherapy is not essential to obtain survival benefit from high-dose melphalan and autotransplantation in myeloma. Bone Marrow Transplant 2002;30:273–279
67. Clavio M, Casciaro S, Gatti AM et al. Multiple myeloma in the elderly: clinical features and response to treatment in 113 Patients. Haematologica 1996;81:238–244
68. Bladé J, Munoz M, Fontanillas M et al. Treatment of multiple myeloma in elderly people: long-term results in 178 patients. Age Ageing 1996;25:357–361
69. Siegel DS, Desikan KR, Mehta J et al. Age is not a prognostic variable with autotransplants for multiple myeloma. Blood 1999;93:51–54
70. Badros A, Barlogie B, Siegel E et al. Autologous stem cell transplantation in elderly multiple myeloma patients over the age of 70 years. Br J Haematol 2001;114:600–607
71. Reece DE, Bredeson C, Perez WS et al. Autologous stem cell transplantation in multiple myeloma patients <60 vs >/= 60 years of age. Bone Marrow Transplant 2003;32: 1135–1143
72. Palumbo A, Bringhen S, Petrucci MT et al. Intermediate-dose melphalan improves survival of myeloma patients aged 50 to 70: results of a randomized controlled trial. Blood;2004:3052–3057
73. Palumbo A, Bringhen S, Caravita T et al. Oral melphalan and prednisone chemotherapy plus thalidomide compared with melphalan and prednisone alone in elderly patients with multiple myeloma: randomised controlled trial. Lancet 2006;367:825–831
74. Facon T, Mary JY, Hulin C et al. Major superiority of melphalan – prednisone (MP) + thalidomide (THAL) over MP and autologous stem cell transplantation in the treatment of newly diagnosed elderly patients with multiple myeloma. Blood 2005;106:780
75. Mateos M-V, Hernández J-M, Hernández M-T et al. Bortezomib plus melphalan and prednisone in elderly untreated patients with multiple myeloma: results of a multicenter phase 1/2 study. Blood 2006;108:2165–2172
76. Offidani M, Corvatta L, Piersantelli M-N et al. Thalidomide, dexamethasone, and pegylated liposomal doxorubicin (ThaDD) for patients older than 65 years with newly diagnosed multiple myeloma. Blood 2006;108:2159–2164
77. Knudsen LM, Hippe E, Hjorth M et al. Renal function in newly diagnosed multiple myeloma – a demographic study of 1353 patients. The Nordic Myeloma Study Group. Eur J Haematol 1994;53:207–212
78. Lee CK, Zangari M, Barlogie B et al. Dialysis-dependent renal failure in patients with myeloma can be reversed by high-dose myeloablative therapy and autotransplant. Bone Marrow Transplant 2004;33:823–828
79. Knudsen ML, Hjorth M, Hippe E, Nordic Myeloma Study Group. Renal failure in multiple myeloma: reversibility and impact on the prognosis. Eur J Haematol 2000;65:175–181
80. Bladé J, Fernandez-Llama P, Bosch F et al. Renal failure in multiple myeloma: presenting features and predictors of outcome in 94 patients from a single institution. Arch Intern Med 1998;158:1889–1893
81. Knudsen LM, Nielsen B, Gimsing P et al. Autologous stem cell transplantation in multiple myeloma: outcome in patients with renal failure. Eur J Haematol 2005;75:27–33
82. Bird JM, Rhian F, Sirohi B et al. The clinical outcome and toxicity of high-dose chemotherapy and autologous stem cell transplantation in patients with myeloma or amyloid and severe renal impairment: a British society of blood and marrow transplantation study. Br J Haematol 2006;134:385–390
83. Bardros A, Barlogie B, Siegel E et al. Results of autologous stem cell transplant in multiple myeloma patients with renal failure. Br J Haematol 2001;114:822–829
84. Tricot G, Alberts DS, Johnson C et al. Safety of autotransplants with high-dose melphalan in renal failure: a pharmacokinetic and toxicity study. Clin Cancer Res 1996;2:947–952
85. San Miguel JF, Lahuerta JJ, Garcia-Sanz R et al. Are myeloma patients with renal failure candidates for autologous stem cell transplantation? Hematol J 2000;1:28–36
86. Eleutherakis-Papaiakovou V, Bamias A, Gika D et al. Renal failure in multiple myeloma: Incidence, correlations, and prognostic significance. Leuk Lymph 2007;48:337–341
87. Raab MS, Breitkreutz I, Hundemer M et al. The outcome of autologous stem cell transplantation in patients with plasma cell disorders and dialysis-dependent renal failure. Haematologica 2006;91:1555–1558
88. Grazziutti M, Dong L, Miceli MH et al. Oral mucositis in myeloma patients undergoing melphalan-based autologous stem cell transplantation: incidence, risk factors and a severity predictive model. Bone Marrow Transplant 2006;38:501–506
89. Barlogie B, Jagannath S, Desikan KR et al. Total therapy with tandem transplants for newly diagnosed multiple myeloma. Blood 1999;93:55–65
90. Pui CH, Evans WE, Pharm D. Treatment of acute lymphoblastic leukemia. N Engl J Med 2006;354:166–178
91. Fermand JP, Levy Y, Benbunan JG et al. Treatment of aggressive multiple myeloma by high-dose chemotherapy and total body irradiation followed by blood stem cells autologous graft. Blood 1989;73:20–23
92. Cunningham D, Powles R, Malpas J et al. A randomized trial of maintenance interferon following high-dose chemotherapy in multiple myeloma: long-term follow-up results. Br J Haematol 1998;102:495–502
93. Ellison RR, Holland JF, Weil M. Arabinosyl cytosine: a useful agent in the treatment of acute leukemia in adults. Blood 1968;32:507–523
94. Barlogie B, Tricot G, van Rhee F et al. Long-term outcome results of the first tandem autotransplant trial for multiple myeloma.Br J Haematol 2006;135:158–164
95. Barlogie B, Tricot G, Anaissie E et al. Thalidomide and hematopoietic-cell transplantation for multiple myeloma. N Engl J Med 2006;354:1021–1030
96. Singhal S, Mehta J, Desikan R et al. Antitumor activity of thalidomide in refractory multiple myeloma. N Engl J Med 1999;341:1565–1571
97. Barlogie B, Tricot G, Rasmussen E et al. Total therapy 2 without thalidomide in comparison with total therapy 1: role of intensified induction and post transplantation consolidation therapies. Blood 2006;107:2633–2638
98. Richardson PG, Schenkein D, Anderson KC. Bortezomib or high-dose dexamethasone for relapsed multiple myeloma. N Engl J Med 2005;352:2487–2498
99. Jagannath S, Barlogie B, Berenson J.A phase 2 study of two doses of bortezomib in relapsed or refractory myeloma. Br J Haematol 2004;127:165–172
100. Barlogie B, Raber MN, Schumann J et al. Flow cytometry in clinical cancer research. Cancer Res 1983;43:3982–3997
101. Barlogie B, Shaughnessy J, Tricot G et al. Treatment of multiple myeloma. Blood 2006;103:20–32
102. Lee C-K, Barlogie B, Munshi N et al. DTPACE: an effective, novel combination chemotherapy with thalidomide for previously treated patients with myeloma. J Clin Oncol 2003;21:2732–2739
103. Attal M, Harousseau JL, Facon T et al. Single versus double autologous stem-cell transplantation for multiple myeloma. N Engl J Med 2003;349:2495–2502
104. Cavo M, Tosi P, Zamagni E et al. Prospective, randomized study of single compared with double autologous stem-cell transplantation for multiple myeloma: Bologna 96 clinical study. J Clin Oncol 2007;25:2434–2441
105. Segeren CM, Sonneveld P, van der Holt B et al. Overall and event-free survival are not improved by the use of myeloablative therapy following intensified chemotherapy in previously untreated patients with multiple myeloma: a prospective randomized phase 3 study. Blood 2003;101:2144–2151
106. Fermand JP, Alberti C, Morolleau JP. Single versus tandem high dose therapy (HDT) supported with autologous blood stem cell (ABSC) transplantation using unselected or CD34-enriched ABSC: results of a two by two designed randomized trial in 230 young patients with multiple myeloma (MM). Hematol J 2003;4:S59
107. Morris C, Iacobelli S, Brand R et al. Benefit and timing of second transplantations in multiple myeloma: clinical findings and methodological limitations in a European Group for Blood and Marrow Transplantation Registry study. J Clin Oncol 2004;22(9):1674–1681
108. Tricot G, Jagannath S, Vesole DH et al. Relapse of multiple myeloma after autologous transplantation: survival after salvage therapy. Bone Marrow Transplant 1995;16: 7–11
109. Mehta J, Tricot G, Jagannath S et al. Salvage autologous or allogeneic transplantation for multiple myeloma refractory to or relapsing after a first-line autograft? Bone Marrow Transplant 1998;21:887–892
110. Elice F, Raimondi R, Tosetto A et al. Prolonged overall survival with second on-demand autologous transplant in multiple myeloma. Am J Hematol 2006;81:426–431
111. Bjorkstrand B, Svensson H, Goldschmidt H et al. Alpha-interferon maintenance treatment is associated with improved survival after high-dose treatment and autologous stem cell transplantation in patients with multiple myeloma: a retrospective registry study from the EBMT. Bone Marrow Transplant 2001;27:511–515
112. Cunningham D, Powles R, Malpas J et al. A randomized trial of maintenance interferon following high-dose chemotherapy in multiple myeloma: long-term follow-up results. Br J Haematol 1999;102:495–502
113. Attal M, Harousseau JL, Leyvraz S et al. Maintenance therapy with thalidomide improves survival in patients with multiple myeloma. Blood 2006;108:3289–3294
114. Hanamura I, Stewart JP, Huang Y et al. Frequent gain of chromosome band 1q21 in plasma-cell dyscrasias detected by fluorescence in situ hybridization: incidence increases from MGUS to relapsed myeloma and is related to prognosis and disease progression following tandem stem-cell transplantation. Blood 2006;108:1724–1732

115. Stewart KA, Chen CI, Kang Howson-Jan K et al. Results of a multicenter randomized Phase II trial of thalidomide and prednisone maintenance therapy for multiple myeloma after autologous stem cell transplant. Clin Cancer Res 2004;24:8170–8176
116. Sahebi F, R Spielberger R, Kogut NM et al. Maintenance thalidomide following single cycle autologous peripheral blood stem cell transplant in patients with multiple myeloma. Bone Marrow Transplant 2006;37:825–829
117. Palumbo A, Bertola A, Falco P et al. Efficacy of low-dose thalidomide and dexamethasone as first salvage regimen in multiple myeloma. Haematol J 2004;5:318–324
118. Durie BG. Low-dose thalidomide in myeloma: efficacy and biologic significance. Semin Oncol 2002;29:34–38
119. Barlogie B, Jagannath S, Desikan KR et al. Total therapy with tandem transplants for newly diagnosed multiple myeloma. Blood 1999;93:55–65
120. Davies FE, Forsyth PD, Rawstron AC et al. The impact of attaining a minimal disease state after high-dose melphalan and autologous transplantation for multiple myeloma. Br J Haematol 2001;112:814–819
121. Shaughnessy J, Barlogie B, Sawyer J et al. Continuous absence of metaphase-defined cytogenetic abnormalities especially of chromosome 13 and hypodiploidy assures long-term survival in multiple myeloma treated with Total Therapy I: interpretation in the context of global gene expression. Blood 2003;101:3849–3856
122. Nadal E, Gine E, Blade J, Estevel J. High-dose therapy/autologous stem cell transplantation in patients with chemosensitive multiple myeloma: predictors of complete remission. Bone Marrow Transplant 2004;33(1):61–64
123. Alvares CL, Davies FE, Horton C et al. Long-term outcomes of previously untreated myeloma patients: responses to induction chemotherapy and high-dose melphalan incorporated within a risk stratification model can help to direct the use of novel treatments. Br J Haematol 2005;129:607–614
124. Barlogie B, Tricot G. Complete response in myeloma: a Trojan horse? Blood 2006;108:2134–2134
125. Rajkumar SV, Fonseca R, Dispenzieri A et al. Effect of complete response on outcome following autologous stem cell transplantation for myeloma. Bone Marrow Transplant 2000;26:979–983
126. Walker R, Barlogie B, Haessler J et al. Magnetic resonance imaging in multiple myeloma: diagnostic and clinical implications. J Clin Oncol 2007;25:1121–1128
127. van Rhee F, Bolejack V, Hollming K. High serum free-light chain levels and their rapid reduction in response to therapy define an aggressive multiple myeloma subtype with poor prognosis.Blood 2007;110(3):827–832
128. Haessler J, Shaughnessy JD Jr, Zhan F et al. Benefit of complete response in multiple myeloma limited to high-risk subgroup identified by gene expression profiling. Clin Cancer Res 2007;13(23):7073–7079
129. Barlogie B, Smallwood L, Smith T et al. High serum levels of lactic dehydrogenase identify a high-grade lymphoma-like myeloma. Ann Intern Med 1989;110:521–525
130. Greipp PR, San Miguel J, Durie BG et al. International Staging System for multiple myeloma. J Clin Oncol 2005;23:3412–3420
131. Smadja NV, Bastard C, Brigaudeau C et al. Hypodiploidy is a major prognostic factor in multiple myeloma. Blood 2001;98:2229–2238
132. Greipp PR, Lust JA, O'Fallon WM et al. Plasma cell labeling index and beta 2-microglobulin predict survival independent of thymidine kinase and C-reactive protein in multiple myeloma. Blood 1993;81:3382–3387
133. Jakob C, Egerer K, Liebisch P. Circulating proteasome levels are an independent prognostic factor for survival in multiple myeloma. Blood 2007;109:2100–2105
134. Sawyer JR, Waldron JA, Jagannath S, Barlogie B.Cytogenetic findings in 200 patients with multiple myeloma. Cancer Genet Cytogenet 1995;82:41–49
135. Fonseca R, Barlogie B, Bataille R et al. Genetics and cytogenetics of multiple myeloma: a workshop report. Cancer Res 2004;64:1546–1558
136. Tabernero D, San Miguel JF, Garcia-Sanz MD et al. Incidence of chromosome numerical changes in multiple myeloma: fluorescence in situ hybridization analysis using 15 chromosome-specific probes. Am J Pathol 1996;149:153–161
137. Shaughnessy J, Tian E, Sawyer J et al. High incidence of chromosome 13 deletion in multiple myeloma detected by multiprobe interphase FISH. Blood 2000;96:1505–1511
138. Bergsagel PL, Kuehl WM, Zhan F et al. Cyclin D dysregulation: an early and unifying pathogenic event in multiple myeloma. Blood 2005;106:296–303
139. Barlogie B, Alexanian R, Dixon D. Prognostic implications of tumor cell DNA and RNA content in multiple myeloma. Blood 1985;66:338–341
140. Pérez-Simón JA, García-Sanz R, Tabernero MD et al. Prognostic value of numerical chromosome aberrations in multiple myeloma: a FISH analysis of 15 different chromosomes. Blood 1998;91:3366–3371
141. Davide F, Robbiani MC, Bergsagel PL. Bone lesions in molecular subtypes of multiple myeloma. N Engl J Med 2004;351:197–198
142. Erming T, Fenghuang Z,Walker RD, Rasmussen E. The role of the Wnt-signaling antagonist DKK1 in the development of osteolytic lesions in multiple myeloma. N Engl J Med 2003;349:2483–2494
143. Robbiani DF, Chesi M, Bergsagel PL. Bone lesions in molecular subtypes of multiple myeloma. N Engl J Med 2004;351:197–198
144. Carrasco DR, Tonon G, Huang Y. High-resolution genomic profiles define distinct clinico-pathogenetic subgroups of multiple myeloma patients. Cancer Cell 2006;9:313–325
145. Shaughnessy J, Gabrea A, Qi Y et al. Cyclin D3 at 6p21 is dysregulated by recurrent Ig translocations in multiple myeloma. Blood 2001;98:217–223
146. Soverini S, Cavo M, Cellini C. Clinical observations, interventions, and therapeutic trials. Blood 2003;102:1588–1594
147. Moreau P, Facon T, Leleu X et al. Recurrent 14q32 translocations determine the prognosis of multiple myeloma, especially in patients receiving intensive chemotherapy. Blood 2002;100:1579–1583
148. Fonseca R, Emily A, Oken MM. Myeloma and the t(11;14)(q13; q32): evidence for a biologically defined unique subset of patients. Blood 2002;99:3735–3741
149. Fonseca R, Blood E, Rue M et al. Clinical and biologic implications of recurrent genomic aberrations in myeloma. Blood 2003;101:4569–4575
150. Keats JJ, Reiman T, Maxwell CA et al. In multiple myeloma, t(4;14)(p16;q32) is an adverse prognostic factor irrespective of FGFR3 expression. Blood 2003;101:1520–1529
151. Fassas A, Spencer T, Sawyer J et al. Both hypodiploidy and deletion of chromosome 13 independently confer poor prognosis in multiple myeloma. Br J Hematol 2002;118:1041–1047
152. Fonseca R, Harrington D, Oken MM et al. Biological and prognostic significance of interphase fluorescence in situ hybridization detection of chromosome 13 abnormalities (delta13) in multiple myeloma: an Eastern Cooperative Oncology Group study. Cancer Res 2002;62:715–720
153. Gertz MA, Lacy MQ, Dispenzieri A et al. Clinical implications of t(11;14)(q13; q32), t(4;14)(p16.3;q32), and −17p13 in myeloma patients treated with high-dose therapy. Blood 2005;106:2837–2840
154. Jacobson J, Barlogie B, Shaughnessy J et al. MDS-type abnormalities within myeloma signature karyotype (MM-MDS): only 13% 1-year survival despite tandem transplants. Br J Haematol 3003;123:430–440
155. Tricot G, Barlogie B, Jagannath S et al. Poor prognosis in multiple myeloma is associated only with partial or complete deletions of chromosome 13 or abnormalities involving 11q and not with other karyotype abnormalities. Blood 1995;86:4250–4256
156. Tricot G, Sawyer JR, Jagannath S et al. Unique role of cytogenetics in the prognosis of patients with myeloma receiving high-dose therapy and autotransplants. J Clin Oncol 1997;15:2659–2666
157. Zojer N, Königsberg K, Ackermann J. Deletion of 13q14 remains an independent adverse prognostic variable in multiple myeloma despite its frequent detection by interphase fluorescence in situ hybridization. Blood 2000;95:1925–1930
158. Seong C, Delasalle K, Hayes K et al. Prognostic value of cytogenetics in myeloma. Br J Haematol 1998;101:189–194
159. Facon T, Avet-Loiseau H, Guillerm G et al. Chromosome 13 abnormalities identified by FISH analysis and serum β2 microglobulin produce powerful myeloma staging system for patients receiving high-dose therapy. Blood 2001;97:1566–1571
160. Drach J, Ackermann J, Fritz E et al. Presence of a p53 gene deletion in patients with multiple myeloma predicts for short survival after conventional-dose chemotherapy. Blood 1998;92:802–809
161. Chang H, Qi-Long Q, Yi C, Reece K. *p53* gene deletion detected by fluorescence in situ hybridization is an adverse prognostic factor for patients with multiple myeloma following autologous stem cell transplantation. Blood 2005;105:358–360
162. Avet-Loiseau H, Attal M, Moreau P. Genetic abnormalities and survival in multiple myeloma: the experience of the Intergroupe Francophone du Myélome. Blood 2007;109:3489–3495
163. Sawyer JR, Tricot G, Mattox S et al. Jumping translocations of chromosome 1q in multiple myeloma: evidence for a mechanism involving decondensation of pericentromeric heterochromatin. Blood 1998;91:1732–1741
164. Le Baccon P, Leroux D, Dascalescu C et al. Novel evidence of a role for chromosome 1 pericentric heterochromatin in the pathogenesis of B-cell lymphoma and multiple myeloma. Genes Chrom Cancer 2001;32:250–264
165. Sawyer J, Tricot G, Lukacs J et al. Jumping segmental duplications: evidence for novel types of chromosome instability in myeloma. Genes Chrom Cancer 2005;42(1):95–106
166. Cremer FW, Bila J, Buck I et al. Delineation of distinct subgroups of multiple myeloma and a model for clonal evolution based on interphase cytogenetics. Genes Chromo Cancer 2005;44:194–203
167. Itoyama T, Nanjungud G, Chen W et al. Molecular cytogenetic analysis of genomic instability at the 1q12–22 chromosomal site in B-cell non-Hodgkin lymphoma. Genes Chrom Cancer 2002;35:318–328
168. Tarkkanen M, Elomaa I, Blomqvist C et al. DNA sequence copy number increase at 8q: A potential new prognostic marker in high-grade osteosarcoma. Int J Cancer 1999;84:114–121
169. Kudoh K, Takano M, Koshikawa T et al. Gains of 1q21-q22 and 13q12-q14 are potential indicators for resistance to cisplatin-based chemotherapy in ovarian cancer patients. Clin Cancer Res 1999;5:2526–2531
170. Petersen S, Aninat-Meyer M, Schluns K et al. Chromosomal alterations in the clonal evolution to the metastatic stage of squamous cell carcinomas of the lung. Br J Cancer 2000;82:65–73
171. Chang H, Qi X, Trieu Y et al. Multiple myeloma patients with CKS1B gene amplification have a shorter progression-free survival post-autologous stem cell transplanation. Br J Haematol 2006;135:486–491
172. Zhan F, Colla S, Wu X et al. *CKS1B*, over expressed in aggressive disease, regulates multiple myeloma growth and survival through SKP2- and p27(Kip1)-dependent and independent mechanisms. Blood 2007;109:4995–5001
173. Alizadeh AA, Eisen MB, Davis RE et al. Distinct types of diffuse large B-cell lymphoma identified by gene expression profiling. Nature 2000;43:868–874
174. Yeoh EJ, Ross ME, Shurtleff SA et al. Classification, subtype, discovery, and prediction of outcome in pediatric acute lymphoblastic leukemia by gene expression profiling. Cancer Cell 2002;1:133–143
175. Rosenwald A, Wright G, Leroy K. Molecular diagnosis of primary mediastinal B cell lymphoma identifies a clinically favorable subgroup of diffuse large B cell lymphoma related to Hodgkin lymphoma. J Exp Med 2003;198:851–862
176. Bullinger L, Dohner K, Bair E et al. Use of gene-expression profiling to identify prognostic subclasses in adult acute myeloid leukemia. N Engl J Med 2004;350:1605–1616
177. Lossos A, Czerwinski DK, Alizadeh AA et al. Prediction of survival in diffuse large-B-cell lymphoma based on the expression of six genes. N Engl J Med 2004;350:1605–1614
178. Cavo M, Terragna C, Renzulli M et al. Poor outcome with front-line autologous transplantation in t(4;14) multiple myeloma: low complete remission rate and short duration of remission. J Clin Oncol 2006;24: e4-e5
179. Bjorkstrand BB, Ljungman P, Svensson H et al. Allogeneic bone marrow transplantation versus autologous stem cell transplantation in multiple myeloma: a retrospective case-matched study from the European Group for Blood and Marrow Transplantation. Blood 1996;88:4711–4718

180. Gahrton G, Tura S, Ljungman P et al. Prognostic factors in allogeneic bone marrow transplantation for multiple myeloma. J Clin Oncol 1995;13:1312–1322
181. Bensinger W, Buckner CD, Anasetti C et al. Allogeneic marrow transplantation for multiple myeloma: an analysis of risk factors on outcome. Blood 1996;88:2787–2793
182. Reece D, Shepherd J, Klingemann H et al. Treatment of myeloma using intensive therapy and allogeneic bone marrow transplantation. Bone Marrow Transplant 1995;15:117–123
183. Cavo M, Bandini G, Benni M et al. High-dose busulfan and cyclophosphamide are an effective conditioning regimen for allogeneic bone marrow transplantation in chemosensitive multiple myeloma. Bone Marrow Transplant 1998;22:27–32
184. Mehta J, Tricot G, Jagannath S et al. Salvage autologous or allogeneic transplantation for multiple myeloma refractory to or relapsing after a first-line autograft? Bone Marrow Transplant 1998;21:887–982
185. Gahrton G, Svensson H, Cavo M et al. Progress in allogeneic bone marrow and peripheral blood stem cell transplantation for multiple myeloma: a comparison between transplants performed 1983–93 and 1994–8 at European Group for Blood and Marrow Transplantation centres. Br J Haematol 2001;113:209–216
186. Lokhorst HM, Segeren CM, Holt B et al. T-cell depleted allogeneic stem cell transplantation as part of first line treatment of multiple myeloma if inferior to intensive treatment alone. Results from a prospective donor versus no donor comparison in patients treated in the HOVON 24 study. Blood 2001;98:481a
187. Gahrton G, Svensson H, Bjorkstrand B et al. Syngeneic transplantation in multiple myeloma – a case-matched comparison with autologous and allogeneic transplantation. Bone Marrow Transplant 1999;24:741–745
188. Libura J, Hoffmann T, Passweg JR et al. Graft-versus-myeloma after withdrawal of immunosuppression following allogeneic peripheral stem cell transplantation. Bone Marrow Transplant 1999;24:925–927
189. Tricot G, Vesole DH, Jagannath S et al. Graft-versus-myeloma effect: proof of principle. Blood 1996;87:1196–1198
190. Verdonck LF, Lokhorst HM, Dekker AW et al. Graft-versus-myeloma effect in two cases. Lancet 1996;347:800–801
191. Collins RH, Shpilberg O, Drobyski WR et al. Donor leukocyte infusions in 140 patients with relapsed malignancy after allogeneic bone marrow transplantation. J Clin Oncol 1997;15:433–444
192. Aschan J, Lonnqvist B, Ringden O et al. Graft-versus-myeloma effect. Lancet 1996;348:346
193. Salama M, Nevill T, Marcellus D et al. Donor leukocyte infusions for multiple myeloma. Bone Marrow Transplant 2000;26:1179–1184
194. Lokhorst HM, Schattenberg A, Cornelissen JJ et al. Donor lymphocyte infusions for relapsed multiple myeloma after allogeneic stem-cell transplantation: predictive factors for response and long-term putcome. J Clin Oncol 2002;18:3031–3037
195. Mehta J, Singhal S. Graft-versus-myeloma. Bone Marrow Transplant 1998;22:835–843
196. Crawley C, Lalancette M, Szydlo R et al. Outcomes for reduced-intensity allogeneic transplantation for multiple myeloma: an analysis of prognostic factors from the Chronic Leukaemia Working Party of the EBMT. Blood 2005;105:4532–4539
197. Bird J, Russell N, Samson D. Minimal residual disease after bone marrow transplantation for multiple myeloma: evidence for cure in long-term survivors. Bone Marrow Transplant 1993;12:651–654
198. Corradini P, Voena C, Tarella C et al. Molecular and clinical remissions in multiple myeloma: role of autologous and allogeneic transplantation of hematopoietic cells. J Clin Oncol 1999;17:208–215
199. Corradini P, Cavo M, Lokhorst H et al. Molecular remission after myeloablative allogeneic stem cell transplantation predicts a better relapse-free survival in patients with multiple myeloma. Blood 2003;102:1927–1929
200. Yu C, Storb R, Mathey B et al. DLA-identical bone marrow grafts after low-dose total body irradiation: effects of high-dose corticosteroids and cyclosporine on engraftment. Blood 1995;86:4376–4381
201. Yu C, Seidel K, Nash RA et al. Synergism between mycophenolate mofetil and cyclosporine in preventing graft-versus-host disease among lethally irradiated dogs given DLA-nonidentical unrelated marrow grafts. Blood 1998;91:2581–2587
202. Storb R, Yu C, Wagner JL et al. Stable mixed hematopoietic chimerism in DLA-identical littermate dogs given sublethal total body irradiation before and pharmacological immunosuppression after marrow transplantation. Blood 1997;89:3048–3054
203. Georges GE, Storb R, Thompson JD et al. Adoptive immunotherapy in canine mixed chimeras after nonmyeloablative hematopoietic cell transplantation. Blood 2000;95:3262–3269
204. Giralt S, Estey E, Albitar M et al. Engraftment of allogeneic hematopoietic progenitor cells with purine analog-containing chemotherapy: harnessing graft-versus-leukemia without myeloablative therapy. Blood 1997;89:4531–4536
205. Slavin S, Nagler A, Naparstek E et al. Nonmyeloablative stem cell transplantation and cell therapy as an alternative to conventional bone marrow transplantation with lethal cytoreduction for the treatment of malignant and nonmalignant hematologic diseases. Blood 1998;91:756–763
206. Garban F, Attal M, Rossi JF et al. Immunotherapy by non-myeloablative allogeneic stem cell transplantation in multiple myeloma: results of a pilot study as salvage therapy after autologous transplantation. Leukemia 2001;15:642–646
207. Lee CK, Bensinger W, Goodman M et al. Prognostic factors in allogeneic transplantation for patients with high-risk multiple myeloma after reduced intensity conditioning. Exp Hematol 2003;31:73–80
208. Giralt S, Bensinger W, Goodman M et al. Ho-DOTMP plus melphalan followed by peripheral blood stem cell transplantation in patients with multiple myeloma: results of two phase 1/2 trials. Blood 2003;102:2684–2691
209. Einsele H, Schafer HJ, Hebart H et al. Follow-up of patients with progressive multiple myeloma undergoing allografts after reduced-intensity conditioning. Br J Haematol 2003;121:411–418
210. Kroger N, Perez-Simon JA, Myint H et al. Relapse to prior autograft and chronic graft-versus-host disease are the strongest prognostic factors for outcome of melphalan/fludarabine-based dose-reduced allogeneic stem cell transplantation in patients with multiple myeloma. Biol Blood Marrow Transplant 2004;10:698–708
211. Kroger N, Schwerdtfeger R, Kiehl M et al. Autologous stem cell transplantation followed by a dose-reduced allograft induces high complete remission rate in multiple myeloma. Blood 2002;100:755–760
212. Maloney DG, Molina AJ, Sahebi F et al. Allografting with non-myeloablative conditioning following cytoreductive autografts for the treatment of patients with multiple myeloma. Blood 2003;102:3447–3454
213. Garban F, Attal M, Michallet M et al. Prospective comparison of autologous stem cell transplantation followed by dose-reduced allograft (IFM99–03 trial) with tandem autologous stem cell transplantation (IFM99–04 trial) in high-risk de novo multiple myeloma. Blood 2006;107:3474–3480
214. Lokhorst HM. No RIC in high-risk myeloma? Blood 2006;107:3420–3421
215. Bensinger WI. The current status of reduced-intensity allogeneic hematopoietic stem cell transplantation for multiple myeloma. Leukemia 2006;20:1683–1689
216. Bruno B, Rotta M, Patriarca F. A comparison of allografting with autografting for newly diagnosed myeloma. N Engl J Med 2007;356:1110–1120
217. van Rhee F, Crowley J, Barlogie B. Allografting or autografting for myeloma (letter). N Engl J Med 2007;356:2647–2648
218. van Rhee F. Allografting for myeloma: con. Clin Adv Hematol Oncol 2006;4:4–7
219. Kröger N, Schwerdtfeger R, Kiehl M et al. Autologous stem cell transplantation followed by a dose-reduced allograft induces high complete remission rate in multiple myeloma. Blood 2002;100:755–760
220. Badros A, Barlogie B, Siegel E et al. Improved outcome of allogeneic transplantation in high-risk multiple myeloma patients after nonmyeloablative conditioning.[see comment]. J Clin Oncol 2002;20:1295–1303
221. Crawley C, Szydlo R, Lalancette M et al. Outcomes of reduced-intensity transplantation for chronic myeloid leukemia: an analysis of prognostic factors from the Chronic Leukemia Working Party of the EBMT. Blood 2005;106:2969–2976
222. Lee CK, Zangari M, Fassas A et al. Clonal cytogenetic changes and myeloma relapse after reduced intensity conditioning allogeneic transplantation. Bone Marrow Transplant 2006;37:511–515
223. Kroger N, Schilling G, Einsele H et al. Deletion of chromosome band 13q14 as detected by fluorescence in situ hybridization is a prognostic factor in patients with multiple myeloma who are receiving allogeneic dose-reduced stem cell transplantation. Blood 2004;103:4056–4061
224. Perez-Simon JA, Martino R, Alegre A et al. Chronic but not acute graft-versus-host disease improves outcome in multiple myeloma patients after non-myeloablative allogeneic transplantation. Br J Haematol 2003;121:104–108
225. Passweg JR, Meyer-Monard S, Gregor M et al. High stem cell dose will not compensate for T cell depletion in allogeneic non-myeloablative stem cell transplantation. [see comment]. Bone Marrow Transplant 2002;30:267–271
226. Kroger N, Shaw B, Iacobelli S et al. Comparison between antithymocyte globulin and alemtuzumab and the possible impact of KIR-ligand mismatch after dose-reduced conditioning and unrelated stem cell transplantation in patients with multiple myeloma. Br J Haematol 2005;129:631–643
227. Kroger N, Shimoni A, Zagrivnaja M et al. Low-dose thalidomide and donor lymphocyte infusion as adoptive immunotherapy after allogeneic stem cell transplantation in patients with multiple myeloma. Blood. 2004;104:3361–3363
228. Sun K, Wilkins DE, Anver MR et al. Differential effects of proteasome inhibition by bortezomib on murine acute graft-versus-host disease (GVHD): delayed administration of bortezomib results in increased GVHD-dependent gastrointestinal toxicity. Blood 2005;106:3293–3299
229. Blanco B, José A, Pérez-Simón JA et al. Bortezomib induces selective depletion of alloreactive T lymphocytes and decreases the production of Th1 cytokines Blood 2006;107:3575–3583
230. Chang DH, Liu N, Klimek V et al. Enhancement of ligand-dependent activation of human natural killer T cells by lenalidomide: therapeutic implications. Blood 2006;108:618–621
231. Solomon SR, Mielke S, Savani BN et al. Selective depletion of alloreactive donor lymphocytes: a novel method to reduce the severity of graft-versus-host disease in older patients undergoing matched sibling donor stem cell transplantation. Blood 2005;106:1123–1129
232. Cavazzano-Calvo M, Fromont C, Le DF et al. Specific elimination of alloreactive T cells by an anti-interleukin-2 receptor B chain-specific immunotoxin. Transplantation 1990;50:1–7
233. Kwak LW, Taub DD, Duffey PL et al. Transfer of myeloma idiotype-specific immunity from an actively immunized marrow donor. Lancet 1995;345:1016–1020
234. Neelapu SS, Munshi NC, Jagannath S et al. Tumor antigen immunization of sibling stem cell transplant donors in multiple myeloma. Bone Marrow Transplant 2005;36:315–323
235. Gnjatic S, Szmania S, Moreno A et al. Vaccination with MAGE-3 protein can induce a potent immune response in a healthy donor which can be adoptively transferred via stem cell transplant to a multiple myeloma patient. Blood 2005;106:620a
236. Richardson PG, Blood E, Mitsiades CS et al. A randomized phase 2 study of lenalidomide therapy for patients with relapsed or relapsed and refractory multiple myeloma. Blood 2006;108:3458–3464
237. Rajkumar SV, Hayman S, Gertz MA et al. Combination therapy with thalidomide plus dexamethasone for newly diagnosed myeloma. J Clin Oncol 2002;20:4319–4323
238. Rajkumar SV, Blood E, Vesole D et al. Phase III clinical trial of thalidomide plus dexamethasone compared with dexamethasone alone in newly diagnosed multiple myeloma: a clinical trial coordinated by the Eastern Cooperative Oncology Group. J Clin Oncol 2006;24:431–436
239. Rajkumar SV, Hayman SR, Martha QL et al. Combination therapy with lenalidomide plus dexamethasone (Rev/Dex) for newly diagnosed myeloma. Blood 2005;106:4050–4053

240. Jagannath S, Durie BGM, Wolf J et al. Bortezomib therapy alone and in combination with dexamethasone for previously untreated symptomatic multiple myeloma Br J Haematol 2005;129:776–783

241. Wang M, Delasalle K, Giralt S et al. Rapid control of previously untreated multiple myeloma with bortezomib-thalidomide-dexamethasone followed by early intensive therapy. Blood 2005;106:784

242. Richardson PG, Jagannath S, Avigan DE et al. Lenalidomide plus bortezomib (Rev-Vel) in relapsed and/or refractory multiple myeloma (MM): final results of a multicenter phase 1 trial. Blood 2006;108:405

243. Palumbo A, Falco P, Falcone A et al. Oral revlimid plus melphalan and prednisone (R-MP) for newly diagnosed multiple myeloma: results of a multicenter Phase I/II study. Blood 2006;108:800

244. Palumbo A, Ambrosini MT, Benevolo G et al. Bortezomib, melphalan, prednisone and thalidomide for relapsed multiple myeloma. Blood 2007;109:2767–2772

245. Orlowski R, Voorhees P, Garcia R et al. Phase 1 trial of the proteasome inhibitor bortezomib and pegylated liposomal doxorubicin in patients with advanced hematologic malignancies. Blood 2005;105:3058–3065

246. Oakervee HE, Popat R, Curry N et al. PAD combination therapy (PS-341/bortezomib, doxorubicin and dexamethasone) for previously untreated patients with multiple myeloma. Br J Haematol 2005;129:755–762

247. Hari P, Pasquini MC, Vesole DH. Cure of multiple myeloma – more hype, less reality. Bone Marrow Transplant 2006;37:1–18

248. Mulligan N, Mitsiades C, Bryant B et al. Gene expression profiling and correlation with outcome in clinical trials of the proteasome inhibitor bortezomib. Blood 2007;109:3177–3188

249. Dumontet C, Ketterer N, Espinouse D et al. Reduced progression-free survival in elderly patients receiving intensification with autologous peripheral blood stem cell reinfusion for multiple myeloma. Bone Marrow Transplant 1998;21:1037–1041

250. Sirohi B, Powles R, Treleaven J et al. The role of autologous transplantation in patients with multiple myeloma aged 65 years and over. Bone Marrow Transplant 2000;25: 533–539

251. Jantunen E, Kuittinen T, Penttila K et al. High-dose melphalan (200 mg/m2) supported by autologous stem cell transplantation is safe and effective in elderly (>or = 65 years) myeloma patients: comparison with younger patients treated on the same protocol. Bone Marrow Transplant 2006;37:917–922

252. Lenhoff S, Hjorth M, Westin J et al. Impact of age on survival after intensive therapy for multiple myeloma: a population-based study by the Nordic Myeloma Study Group. Br J Haematol 2006;133:389–396

253. Fermand JP. High dose therapy supported with autologous blood stem cell transplantation in multiple myeloma: long term follow up of prospective studies of the MAG group. Hematologica 2005;90(suppl 1):40

254. Sonneveld P, van der Holt B, Segeren CM. Intensive versus double intensive therapy in untreated multiple myeloma: update analysis of the randomized pahse III HOVON 24 study. Hematologica 2005;90:38

255. Goldschmidt H. Single vs double high dose therapy in multiple myeloma: second analysis of the GMMG-HD2 trial. Haematologica 2005;90:38

256. Cavo M, Cellini C, Zamagni E. Update on high dose therapy – Italian studies. Haematologica 2005;90:39

Hodgkin's disease and non-Hodgkin's lymphoma

Jürgen Finke

CHAPTER 9

Prognosis of the lymphomas depends on the type of histology as well as on disease-specific risk factors present at diagnosis. This chapter provides a brief overview of the classification and treatment of the lymphomas with special emphasis on those entities where stem cell transplantation is an established or an evolving treatment modality.

Prognostic index

The international prognosis index (IPI) was established in the early 1990s after multi-institutional analysis of patients with high-grade lymphomas. It is widely accepted today because of its good prognostic value regarding disease-free and overall survival in diffuse large B-cell, T-cell and, with slight modifications, follicular and mantle cell lymphomas.[1]

Five independent risk factors (RF) have been established:
1. advanced disease; Ann Arbor stage III or IV
2. lactic dehydrogenase (LDH) above upper normal limit
3. Karnofsky index less than 80%
4. more than one extranodal site involved
5. age greater than 60 years.

The age-adjusted index (aaIPI) only includes the first three variables (stage, LDH, Karnofsky score) and was originally intended to be applied to patients under 60 years of age. However, it is now also used in trials including older patients, especially when transplant strategies are involved, since the former upper age limit of 60 years for intensive therapies including autologous or allogeneic hematopoietic cell transplantation has been raised to include considerably older age groups.

Complete remission and 5-year overall survival (OS) rates differ between risk groups, ranging from 87% CR and 73% 5-year OS in low-risk patients – those with 0 or 1 risk factors according to IPI – to 44% CR and 26% 5-year OS in high-risk patients with four or five RF.

Using the age-adjusted IPI for patients less than 60 years of age, 5-year survival rates are 83%, 69%, 46%, and 32% for patients with no, one, two or three RF, respectively, according to the aaIPI.[1]

It is worth noting that these results were obtained in the pre-rituximab era. The addition of the anti-CD20 monoclonal antibody rituximab (R) to first-line anthracycline-based chemotherapy has improved remission rates and short-term outcomes in diffuse large B-cell lymphoma.

The World Health Organization classification

A unifying lymphoma classification has finally been established and accepted in the international scientific community. The WHO lymphoma classification was developed from the former REAL classifica-tion and depends on classic HE-stained light microscopy, as well as on immunophenotying and cytogenetic/molecular genetic analyses. These combined approaches make precise classification in the majority of lymphoma cases possible, which is a prerequisite when planning trials and analyzing and comparing published data. For example, case series of previously designated high-grade B-cell lymphomas contained lymphomas nowadays classified as mantle cell or follicular lymphoma. The WHO lymphoma classification comprises all entities of malignant diseases arising from lymphatic tissue.[2]

The precursor neoplasms contain B- or T-lymphoblastic leukemias and lymphomas with a particularly aggressive disease course. Conventional therapy is that of the intensive leukemia type, with repeated cycles of induction and consolidation, followed by transplantation, usually from an allogeneic donor, in patients with high-risk or relapsing disease.

The mature B-cell lymphomas cover a broad and heterogeneous spectrum, ranging from chronic lymphocytic leukemia (CLL) to Burkitt's lymphoma. Due to their growth pattern and clinical course, the lymphomas are categorized as indolent or aggressive, with Burkitt's lymphoma classified as highly aggressive. Mantle cell lymphoma (MCL) used to be classified as indolent or intermediate, but is now recognized as an aggressive type of lymphoma.

Mature T-cell and NK cell neoplasms include T-CLL and PLL, enteropathy-type T-cell lymphoma, mycosis fungoides and other cutaneous lymphomas, subcutaneous panniculitis-like T-cell lymphoma, peripheral T-cell and aggressive NK lymphomas, angio-immunoblastic (AILD) and anaplastic large cell lymphoma.

The histologies in Table 9.1 may be grouped as *indolent* lymphomas. Hodgkin's lymphoma, with six subgroups, is a B-cell lymphoma with a distinct clinical course and an excellent prognosis in the majority of cases after combination chemotherapy.

The major lymphoma entities are listed below.

Diffuse large B-cell lymphoma

Standard therapy: first-line treatment

Diffuse large B-cell lymphoma (DLBCL) is the most common type of lymphoma, with 31% of all cases occurring at a median age of 64 (14–98) years. Standard of care is anthracycline-containing combination chemotherapy plus rituximab (R). Present treatment strategies are risk stratified according to aaIPI, with more intensive therapies reserved for patients with two or three RF that have a dismal prognosis of less than 50% survival after 5 years. In low-risk patients with no or only one RF according to aaIPI, the combination of six cycles of CHOP (cyclophosphamide, adriamycin, vincristine, prednisone) plus

Table 9.1 Histology of indolent and aggressive forms of lymphoma

	B-cell types	T-cell types
Indolent		
	CLL	CLL
	Hairy cell leukemia (HCL)	T-cell large granular lymphocytic leukemia
	Waldenstrom's disease	Mycosis fungoides/Sezary syndrome
	Multiple myeloma	Primary cutaneous anaplastic large cell lymphoma
	Marginal zone lymphoma (MZL)	Lymphomatoid papulosis
	Mucosa-associated lymphoma tissue (MALT)	
	Follicular lymphoma (FL)	
Aggressive	B-prolymphocytic leukemia (B-PLL)	T-prolymphocytic leukemia (T-PLL)
	Diffuse large B-cell lymphoma (DLBCL)	Enteropathy-type T-cell lymphoma
	Mediastinal large B-cell lymphoma	Hepatosplenic lymphoma
	Mantle cell lymphoma (MCL) Intravascular lymphoma	Subcutaneous panniculitis-like T-cell lymphoma
	Primary effusion lymphoma	Peripheral T-cell and aggressive NK lymphomas
		Angio-immunoblastic (AILD)
		Anaplastic large cell lymphoma (ALCL)

rituximab resulted in a significantly improved 2-year survival of 95%, compared to 89% with CHOP alone.[3] Dose de-escalation with four versus six cycles of R-CHOP is being evaluated in low-risk patients with no RFs, as is the concept of dose density R-CHOP (14- versus 21-day cycles in patients with elevated LDH or bulky disease). Patients over 60 years undergo six cycles of R-CHOP plus two additional doses of R. The role of R as maintenance therapy is being assessed in several trials.

Hematopoietic cell transplantation as part of first-line treatment

The addition of rituximab, other cytotoxic agents such as etoposide or moderate-dose escalation have not significantly improved outcome in high-risk patients with two or three RF according to the aaIPI. The efficacy of high-dose chemotherapy and autologous stem cell transplantation within first-line treatment has been addressed in several trials, with varying results. Transplantation in first CR or PR after conventional chemotherapy resulted in 3-year survival rates of up to 84%.[4] Earlier trials were hampered by problems with feasibility due to early relapse while waiting for autologous marrow harvesting, treatment-related toxicities, or the inclusion of low-risk patients prior to the establishment of the IPI.[5–7]

The largest trials addressing the role of autologous stem cell transplantation in aggressive lymphoma have been performed by the French study group, GOELAMS. The data currently available show a lack of benefit in low-risk patients, who are best served with a combination of rituximab and CHOP-like chemotherapy. However, survival is significantly improved by auto-SCT in patients with two or three RF on aaIPI. For patients with two aaIPI RF, the study group reported a 5-year survival of 75% for patients treated with intensive CEEP (cyclo-

phosphamide, epirubicin, eldesin, prednisone) chemotherapy followed by high-dose BEAM (carmustine, etoposide, cytarabine, melphalan) and autologous SCT, compared to 45% in patients treated with repeated cycles of CHOP alone.[8] GOELAMS routinely uses high-dose chemotherapy and auto-SCT as part of first-line therapy for patients with three aaIPI RFs.[9,10]

The efficacy of additional rituximab during therapy and any potential as maintenance therapy remain to be demonstrated. There are reports of slower engraftment with R.[11] Improved response rates with repeated cycles of dose-escalated R-CHOP and autologous stem cell rescue in high-risk patients have been reported by the German HGNHL study group.[12] The optimum approach for high-risk patients may be a combination of early intensive chemotherapy combined with rituximab, followed by high-dose chemotherapy and autologous SCT. There have been no randomized trials comparing the different conditioning regimens available. Whereas total-body irradiation (TBI) (10–12 Gy) or high-dose busulfan (16 mg/kg)-containing regimens in combination with cyclophosphamide and/or VP16 were used until the late 1990s, most centers now favor the BEAM regimen due to its low regimen-related toxicity and high remission rates. The alkylating agents BCNU (carmustine) and melphalan effectively target resting (tumor) cells, contributing to the efficacy of this regimen.

Several strategies have been adopted to improve outcome in aggressive lymphoma. Sequential double autologous SCTs have been performed in patients with two or three aaIPI RF, consisting of a four-cycle induction with ACVBP (doxorubicin, cyclophosphamide, vindesine, bleomycin and prednisone). Peripheral blood stem cells (PBSC) of responding patients were collected after the fourth cycle of ACVBP (11 patients) or after an additional mobilization regimen (cyclophosphamide, VP16) (17 patients) followed by a first high-dose therapy (HDT) (mitoxantrone, cyclophosphamide, VP16 and carmustine) and autologous SCT. For a second HDT, busulfan, carboplatin and melphalan were given followed by SCT. The 3-year survival rate was 50% and the authors concluded that tandem transplantation did not improve the results of the LNH87–2 study, in which patients received a single consolidative HDT.[13]

In contrast, a single-center, prospective clinical trial was conducted evaluating two cycles of induction high-dose chemotherapy for adults under 65 years of age with aggressive non-Hodgkin's lymphoma (NHL) and 2–3 aaIPI RF. Patients received one cycle of standard CHOP, followed by one cycle of dose-intensive cyclophosphamide 5.25 g/m^2, etoposide 1.05 g/m^2, cisplatin 105 mg/m^2 (DICEP), and they then underwent autologous blood stem cell collection followed by one cycle of high-dose BEAM, and autologous SCT. Fifty five patients aged 20–63 years (median 44 years) were studied, 51 (92%) of whom had diffuse large B-cell NHL. Poor prognostic factors included stage 4 (n = 46), elevated LDH (n = 47), Eastern Cooperative Oncology Group (ECOG) performance status 2–4 (n = 43), bulky disease measuring more than 10 cm (n = 34), and marrow involvement (n = 16). Only one patient experienced non-relapse mortality. With a median follow-up of 49 months, the 4-year event-free survival (EFS) and overall survival (OS) rates for all 55 patients were 72% and 79%, respectively. This approach with CHOP-DICEP-BEAM has been regarded as encouraging for patients with poor-prognosis aggressive NHL.[14]

Aggressive lymphoma located exclusively in the brain, primary CNS lymphoma (PCNSL), presents a special clinical situation. PCNSL is histologically usually DLBCL, and, despite combined modality treatment with high-dose methotrexate followed by brain irradiation, the prognosis is dismal. High-dose busulfan, cyclophosphamide and thiotepa followed by autologous SCT in relapsed PCNSL resulted in a 53% 3-year EFS.[15] Several groups have recently published protocols involving high-dose alkylator-based chemotherapy and auto-SCT as part of first-line treatment.[16,17] A regimen including high-dose BCNU

400 mg/m^2 and thiotepa 20 mg/kg followed by auto-SCT and consolidating radiotherapy after induction chemotherapy with methotrexate and cytosine arabinoside resulted in 72% DFS at 5-year median follow-up.[18]

Relapsed, refractory disease

The prognosis of relapse after first remission is dismal, and less than 10% of patients with aggressive lymphoma survive beyond 5 years. The randomized Parma trial established the role of high-dose chemotherapy and autologous SCT for patients with chemosensitive relapse.[19] Patients in second remission after salvage DHAP (dexamethasone, cytarabine, cisplatin) received either high-dose BEAC (carmustine, etoposide, cytarabine, cyclophosphamide) followed by autologous marrow transplantation, or additional DHAP as consolidation. Patients in the transplant arm showed a significantly improved 5-year long-term survival of 46%, versus 12% in the non-transplant group.[19] Follow-up analysis revealed the prognostic value of the IPI. There was a strong correlation between the IPI at relapse and OS in patients treated in the DHAP arm (5-year OS: 48%, 21%, 33% and 0% for IPI 0, 1, 2 and 3, respectively; p = 0.006), but not in the BEAC arm (5-year OS: 51%, 47%, 50% and 50% for IPI 0, 1, 2 and 3, respectively; p = 0.90). OS was significantly superior in the BEAC arm in comparison with the DHAP arm in patients with an IPI > 0 (p < 0.05), but not in patients with an IPI of 0 (Fig. 9.1).[20]

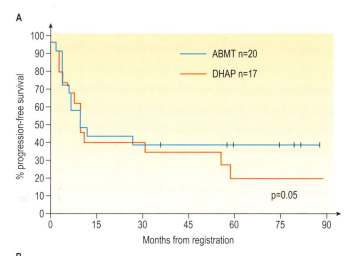

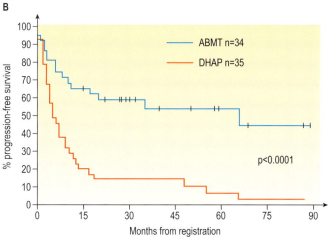

Figure 9.1
The International Prognostic Index correlates with survival in patients with aggressive lymphoma in relapse: analysis of the PARMA trial. Progression-free survival according to IPI at relapse. (a) Patients with IPI 0: autologous BMT versus DHAP. (b) Patients with IPI 1–3: autologous BMT versus DHAP. From Blay et al.[20]

Autologous SCT after high-dose BEAM conditioning can be given to patients beyond 60 years of age. Data from the Mayo Clinic showed equal success and treatment-related mortality (TRM) rates compared to younger adults for 93 patients older than 60 years with a median age of 66 (up to 76), with the age-adjusted IPI as the only prognostic factor.[21]

Thus, autologous SCT after intensive salvage therapy with DHAP or ICE (ifosfamide 5 g/m^2, carboplatinum AUC 5, etoposide3 × 100 mg/m^2),[22] usually combined nowadays with rituximab as RICE regimens, is the accepted standard treatment.[23] Worth noting is the presence of risk factors according to IPI at the time of salvage treatment, which are predictive for outcome and may result in the use of novel strategies including sequential autologous and allogeneic SCT.[24]

Patients not achieving complete remission after adequate full-dose first-line CHOP-like chemotherapy are regarded as having primary refractory disease, and their prognosis is poor. Several Phase II trials suggest a benefit for these patients of high-dose chemotherapy and autologous stem cell transplantation and show long-term progression-free survival (PFS) rates of 20–30%.[25,26] A multivariate analysis performed by the Autologous Blood and Marrow Registry on a study of 184 patients with aggressive lymphoma never achieving CR with conventional chemotherapy revealed certain adverse prognostic factors for overall survival.[27] These included chemotherapy resistance, Karnofsky performance score under 80 at transplantation, age 55 years or more at transplantation, three or more prior chemotherapy regimens, and no pre- or post-transplant involved-field irradiation therapy (Fig. 9.2).

The addition of rituximab, administered as two cycles of four standard doses, each starting 6 weeks post TBI, or BCNU, etoposide, cyclophosphamide high-dose conditioning and autologous B-cell depleted PBSCT, resulted in 2-year PFS of 81% in relapsed or refractory aggressive lymphoma, suggesting that R plays a beneficial role in this situation.[28]

The CORAL trial now being performed within the European Group for Blood and Bone Marrow Transplantation (EBMT) is randomly comparing three cycles each of R-DHAP with RICE in patients with relapsing or refractory CD20+ DLBCL, followed by BEAM and auto-SCT. For the post-transplant period, the role of six cycles of rituximab versus observation is being tested in a second randomization step.[29]

Radio-immunoconditioning with tositumomab, a radiolabeled iodine-131-anti-CD20 monoclonal antibody, in combination with high-dose etoposide and cyclophosphamide and autologous SCT, has been used for treating relapsing aggressive lymphoma, with a 2-year survival rate of 83%.[30]

FDG-PET positivity during induction or after completion of induction therapy implies an increased risk of relapse.[31] Whether these findings will ultimately indicate that different treatment strategies are appropriate, including early SCT, must be shown in prospective trials.

Follicular lymphoma

Follicular lymphoma (FL) is the second most common type of lymphoma, with a frequency of 22% among all lymphomas and a median age at onset of 59 years. FL is subdivided into three groups based on histology and number of blasts per high-power field; grade 3 (with more than 15 centroblasts) is treated like a DLCL.

Whereas limited stage I or II disease may be cured with radiation therapy, advanced stage III or IV FL, which is present in about two-thirds of patients at initial diagnosis, is regarded as incurable and only symptomatic patients are treated. In the pre-rituximab era, the median survival for all disease stages was in the range of 10 years. The IPI

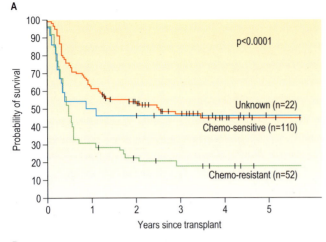

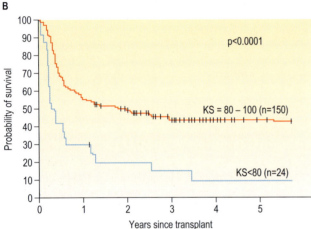

Figure 9.2
Autologous transplantation for diffuse aggressive non-Hodgkin's lymphoma in patients never achieving remission. (A) Probability of survival by sensitivity to chemotherapy. (B) Probability of survival by Karnofsky status at time of transplantation. From Vose et al with permission.[27]

has prognostic value, as in DLCL, sometimes modified by factors such as beta-2 microglobulin level or number of lymph node areas involved.

The addition of rituximab to CHOP or CVP (cyclophosphamide, vincristine, prednisolone)[33] has improved response rates and progression-free survivals. The combination of fludarabine and cyclophosphamide as first-line chemotherapy,[34] or as second-line treatment with additional R, are also very effective therapies for FL.

Autologous SCT

Several studies involving autologous SCT have been performed in patients with relapsed FL. These report high response rates, with median time-to-progression rates of 3–5 years.[35,36] Relapse rate after SCT was influenced by the number of different conventional therapy regimens given, as well as remission status and chemosensitivity prior to SCT. Although these trials compared favorably to historic controls involving similar patients treated with conventional therapy, there have been no randomized Phase III trials to date. During the 1990s, purging the autologous graft of disease-specific t(14;18) positive B-cells to PCR-undetectable levels resulted in better outcomes than were seen in patients with t(14;18) PCR-positive transplants. The ability to purge, however, may reflect disease burden in the patient. Which patients will benefit from high-dose chemotherapy and auto-SCT as second-line therapy remains speculative.[37]

Phase II trials have demonstrated feasibility and high CR rates for patients treated with high-dose radiation and chemotherapy and autologous SCT in first CR, resulting in an estimated 10-year survival of 86%.[38,39] A prospective, randomized Phase III German trial showed a benefit regarding CR rate, and a 5-year PFS of 65% for CHOP-sensitive patients receiving dexa-BEAM chemotherapy for stem cell mobilization, followed by TBI 12 Gy and cyclophosphamide 120 mg/kg followed by autologous SCT, compared to 33% in the IFN-α arm.[40] Acute toxicity was higher in the ASCT group, but early mortality was below 2.5% in both study arms. In that randomized, multicenter trial, high-dose radiochemotherapy followed by ASCT significantly improved PFS compared with IFN-α in patients with follicular lymphoma when given as consolidation in first remission. Longer follow-up is necessary to determine the effect of ASCT on overall survival.[40] Another randomized trial yielded similar data.[41]

A subsequent trial testing rituximab and CHOP in a randomized fashion against CHOP alone for induction therapy resulted in significantly improved CR and DFS rates for R-CHOP.[32] These results are equivalent to those seen after the earlier intensive radiochemotherapy and autologous SCT arm. A combination of both approaches is being tested in a prospective trial, including the possibility of using R as maintenance either post SCT or after R-CHOP.

Mantle cell lymphoma

Mantle cell lymphoma (MCL) occurs with a frequency of 6% of all lymphomas, at a median age of 63 years. It may behave indolently, but the median survival of most advanced-stage patients is under 2 years. The addition of R to first-line CHOP chemotherapy has significantly improved CR rates and PFS in MCL, as in DLBCL and FL.[42] Treatment of recurrent MCL is difficult and, although the combination of fludarabine, cyclophosphamide, mitoxantrone and rituximab is very effective in inducing remission, no survival plateau has been achieved.[43]

Autologous SCT

Autologous SCT in patients who have relapsed has not resulted in a long-term cure for the majority, although several reports show improved DFS and OS in patients with MCL transplanted in first remission.[44,45]

In a prospective Phase III trial, the European Mantle Cell Lymphoma Network showed that autologous SCT after high-dose TBI cyclophosphamide conditioning following CHOP-like induction therapy resulted in a CR rate of 81% and partial remission (PR) rate of 17%, compared to 37% CR and 62% PR in the interferon maintenance arm with no HD therapy and auto-SCT.[46] This approach is being evaluated within the EBMT in a 2-by-2 sequential randomized trial comparing R-CHOP with R-CHOP/R-DHAP induction and two different conditioning regimens: TBI 12 Gy, cyclophosphamide 120 mg/kg with TBI 10 Gy, AraC 2×2 g/m^2 and melphalan 140 mg/m^2 followed by autologous SCT. This trial will facilitate the optimization of transplant strategies within first-line therapy in MCL.

Burkitt's lymphoma

The very aggressive Burkitt's lymphoma (BL) is highly chemosensitive, and cure rates with a high-dose methotrexate-based combination chemotherapy regimen are in the order of 70%. However, patients who relapse rarely attain a second remission. The feasibility and efficacy of 'up-front' high-dose sequential chemotherapy followed by autologous SCT in previously untreated adults with BL, Burkitt-like lymphoma (BLL) or lymphoblastic lymphoma (LyLy) with no central nervous system or extensive bone marrow involvement were investigated in a multicenter Phase II study.[47] Treatment consisted of two sequential high-dose chemotherapy induction courses incorporating prednisone, cyclophosphamide, doxorubicin, etoposide and mitoxantrone, with no high-dose methotrexate or high-dose cytarabine. Patients who attained at least a PR continued with BEAM and ASCT. Treatment was completed by 85% of the BL/BLL and 87% of the LyLy patients. There were no toxic deaths, and response to treatment was 81% CR and 11% PR for patients with BL/BLL, and 73% CR and 20% PR for patients with LyLy. At a median follow-up of 61 months, six BL/BLL and eight LyLy patients had died. The actuarial 5-year overall and event-free survival estimates were 81% and 73% for BL/BLL, versus 46% and 40% for LyLy. Up-front high-dose sequential chemotherapy followed by ASCT was thus found to be highly effective in adults with BL/BLL with limited bone marrow involvement, but was less so in patients with LyLy.[47]

It remains unclear whether autologous SCT as consolidation in first CR offers further benefit to high-dose methotrexate-based chemotherapy, but this approach should be considered in high-risk disease.

Hodgkin's lymphoma

Modern combination chemotherapy results in 5-year survival rates of 97% in limited, low-risk Hodgkin's disease to 85% in advanced, high-risk disease. Late relapse after chemotherapy, defined as later than 1 year after the end of initial therapy, can be successfully salvaged with high-dose chemotherapy and autologous SCT. In a randomized trial which compared high-dose BEAM and autologous SCT after two cycles of dexa-BEAM with four cycles of dexa-BEAM without SCT, there was a 3-year PFS of 55%, significantly better than the dexa-BEAM arm with a PFS of 34%.[48] Early relapse and primary refractory disease both pose a difficult clinical situation and, despite autologous SCT, have higher relapse rates. The possibility of allogeneic SCT should be considered in such situations, perhaps with reduced-intensity conditioning.

A French study group used high-dose therapy with autologous SCT and combined-modality treatment as first-line therapy for Hodgkin's disease in patients who were clinical stage IV and/or had a mediastinal mass greater than or equal to 0.45 of the thoracic diameter at diagnosis, and who had had an incomplete response to first-line chemotherapy. Forty two patients who had been autografted were compared to 108 patients who had received combined-modality treatment from two protocols of the GOELAMS group. The 5-year freedom from progression and event-free survival rates were better for grafted patients (87% versus 55% for freedom from progression, and 81% versus 51% for event-free survival) whereas overall survival rates did not differ significantly at 85% for grafted patients versus 71% for those who had received combined modality treatment.[49]

On the Cologne high-dose sequential protocol, patients with primary progressive or relapsed Hodgkin's disease received two cycles of DHAP, followed by 4 g/m^2 cyclophosphamide and peripheral blood stem cell mobilization. They went on to receive one cycle each with methotrexate 8 g/m^2 and etoposide 2 g/m^2 and finally had a BEAM conditioned autologous SCT. Long-term DFS rates were between 62% and 39% for relapsed and refractory patients, respectively.[50] Similar results were obtained with a modified CBVP regimen containing cyclophosphamide 1.8 g/m^2, carmustine 0.5 g/m^2, etoposide 2.4 g/m^2 and cisplatin 150 mg/m^2.[51]

T-cell lymphomas

Six to eight percent of all lymphomas are histologically T-cell. These are highly divergent, as are the clinical manifestations. T-lymphoblastic lymphoma as a T-cell precursor neoplastic disease is treated with acute lymphoblastic leukemia-type protocols and shows promising 7-year DFS rates of 62%.[52] Transplantation, preferably allogeneic, is reserved for patients who respond inadequately or who relapse.

The majority of mature peripheral T-cell lymphomas (PTCL) have a dismal prognosis. A specific entity, namely anaplastic large cell lymphoma (ALCL) carrying the t(2;5) NPM/ALK translocation, shows better survival after anthracycline-based combination chemotherapy, with a 5-year survival rate close to 80% compared to NPM/ALK-negative ALCL peripheral T-cell lymphomas.

One thousand, eight hundred and eighty three patients with diffuse aggressive NHL included in the French LNH87 protocol were assessed for both morphology and immunophenotyping. Fifteen percent had PTCL and 85% had BCL. According to the Kiel classification, most PTCL were classified as angio-immunoblastic (AIL; 23%), pleomorphic medium and large T-cell (PML; 49%) or anaplastic large cell (ALCL; 20%) lymphomas. For BCL and PTCL, complete remission rates were 63% and 54%, respectively; the 5-year OS rates were 53% and 41%. The 5-year OS rate for T-ALCL (64%) was superior to those of other PTCL (35%) as well as diffuse large B-cell (53%) NHL. Using multivariate analysis with the IPI score as one factor, the study group found non-anaplastic PTCL to be an independent prognostic parameter.[54]

Autologous SCT

Autologous SCT was evaluated in patients with refractory or relapsing PTCL, chemosensitive to second-line chemotherapy, excluding patients with indolent histologies and those with anaplastic lymphoma kinase (ALK) expressing anaplastic large cell lymphoma. The results of 24 patients with PTCL were compared with those of 86 consecutive patients with chemosensitive relapsed or primary refractory diffuse large B-cell lymphoma (DLBCL). With a median follow-up time of 6 years for surviving patients with PTCL and DLBCL, the 5-year PFS rates for PTCL and DLBCL patients were 24% and 34%, respectively, and 33% and 39% overall survival rates were not significantly different. The age-adjusted IPI was the only variable prognostic for PFS and OS on multivariate analysis. The authors concluded that the outcome of SCT for patients with chemosensitive relapsed or primary refractory PTCL is similar to that seen in patients with DLBCL.[54]

Autologous SCT as part of first-line treatment was undertaken in 30 patients with T-cell lymphoma. Four to six courses of CHOP chemotherapy were followed by dexa-BEAM (dexamethasone, carmustine, melphalan, etoposide and cytarabine) or ESHAP (etoposide, methylprednisolone, cytarabine and cisplatin). Hyperfractionated TBI and high-dose cyclophosphamide with autologous peripheral blood stem cell transplant (APBSCT) were given to chemosensitive patients (21 of the 30 patients). Sixteen of the 21 patients transplanted remained in CR at a median follow-up of 15 months (range 6–32 months) from the beginning of treatment. Nine patients did not undergo APBSCT, mainly because of progressive disease.[56]

Success is frequently hampered by the fact that T-cell lymphomas may progress rapidly during chemotherapy and prior to planned autologous SCT. Of those patients treated in the French LNH87 and LNH93 trials, 330 under 60 years of age achieved complete remission after high-dose cyclophosphamide, doxorubicin, vincristine and prednisone, and received consolidative ASCT; 16% had T-cell NHL, with an IPI score of 2–3 in 66% of patients. At 5 years, OS and PFS were 75% and 67%, respectively. For T-cell lymphoma, the scores were 54% and 44%, respectively. On multivariate analysis, only the following parameters adversely affected OS and PFS: marrow involvement; more than one extranodal site involved; non-anaplastic T-cell histology versus other histologies; type of anthracycline used (mitoxantrone versus doxorubicin, for DFS only). These results suggest that ASCT can prevent relapse in patients with adverse IPI factors. A higher relapse risk is observed in patients presenting with a non-anaplastic T-cell phenotype, more than one extranodal site, or marrow involvement.[57]

The outcome for ALCL patients treated with high-dose chemotherapy and autologous SCT as part of their first-line therapy was analyzed in 202 intermediate or high-grade NHL patients in a prospective randomized trial. First-line chemotherapy comprised two alternating anthracycline-containing regimens. Responding patients were autografted after BEAM conditioning. Patients with bulky or residual masses received irradiation. Fifteen patients with ALCL had PFS and OS of 87% with a follow-up of over 5 years. These results are significantly better than those observed in the other 176 lymphoma patients in whom EFS was only 53% and OS reached 60%, demonstrating the efficacy of high-dose chemotherapy with autologous SCT in the treatment of ALCL.[58]

CHOP chemotherapy alone is insufficient for most patients and various approaches now combine high doses of Ara-C with CHOP-like chemotherapy and fludarabine, as well as monoclonal antibodies such as the anti-CD52, CAMPATH.

Allogeneic stem cell transplantation in treatment of lymphoma

In advanced lymphoma, novel therapeutic approaches using the monoclonal antibodies rituximab (anti-CD20) or CAMPATH (anti-CD52) and cytostatic drug combinations including purine analogs such as fludarabine may result in transient remission rates of 20–40% in relapsed low-grade lymphoma. However, although hematologic toxicities are manageable, increased rates of opportunistic infections, especially after CAMPATH therapy, are cause for concern. Allogeneic SCT was originally only used to treat end-stage disease and resulted in high TRM with significant relapse rates. Nevertheless, a graft-versus-lymphoma (GvL) effect was demonstrated for the majority of disease subgroups. Of interest, this GvL effect may result in disease eradication even in chemorefractory lymphoma, as has been demonstrated in vitro.[59] GvL frequently co-exists with GvHD and appears to be particularly effective in low-grade lymphoma, as has been demonstrated clinically after donor lymphocyte infusions (DLI) given for persistent disease or disease which has relapsed after allogeneic SCT.[60]

Allogeneic SCT from a related and unrelated donor offers the potential for rapid hematopoietic reconstitution after high-dose therapy as well as the establishment of a new, healthy immune system. Since the infused stem cells have not been exposed to prior chemotherapy, the 2–8% risk of secondary myelodysplastic syndrome after autologous SCT is not an issue after allogeneic SCT.[61]

The outcome of HLA-identical sibling bone marrow transplantation for advanced low-grade lymphoma was studied in an observational study of 113 patients conducted at 50 centers participating in the International Bone Marrow Transplant Registry (IBMTR).[62] The median patient age was 38 years (range, 15–61). Eighty percent had stage IV disease at the time of transplantation. The median number of prior chemotherapy regimens was two (range, 0–5). Thirty-eight percent had refractory disease and 29% a Karnofsky performance score (KPS) of less than 80%. Conditioning included TBI in 82% of patients and ciclosporin was used for GvHD prophylaxis in 74%. Three-year probabilities of recurrence, survival and PFS were 16%, 49% and 49%, respectively. Better survival was associated with a pretransplant KPS > 90%, chemotherapy-sensitive disease, use of a TBI-containing conditioning regimen, and age under 40 years.[62]

With novel reduced-intensity conditioning (RIC) regimens, combining the lymphoimmunotoxic effects of fludarabine with moderate doses of lymphomyelotoxic alkylating agents such as cyclophosphamide, melphalan, thiotepa or carmustine, TRM can be reduced considerably in this high-risk group.[63,64]

A different approach using only immunosuppressive conditioning with fludarabine and TBI 2 Gy has been successful in low-grade lymphoma in stable disease.[65-67] The Working Party on Lymphoma reported on the outcome of reduced-intensity allogeneic progenitor cell transplantation (allo-SCT) for 188 patients with lymphoma from the EBMT. The median patient age was 40 years, the median number of prior treatment courses was three, and 48% of patients had undergone a prior autologous transplant. Eighty-four percent of patients underwent conditioning with a fludarabine-based regimen, and 10% with BEAM. Full donor chimerism was confirmed in 71% of 100 patients assessed. A disease response to DLI was seen in 10 of 14 patients. With a median follow-up of 283 days, the overall survival rates at 1 and 2 years were 62% and 50%, respectively. The 100-day and 1-year transplantation-related mortality rates were 12.8% and 25.5%, respectively, and were significantly worse for older patients. The probabilities of disease progression at 1 year for patients with chemoresistant and chemosensitive disease were 75% and 25%, respectively. The PFS at 1 year was 46% and was significantly better for those with chemosensitive disease, Hodgkin's disease (HD), and low-grade NHL. Reduced-intensity progenitor cell transplantation is associated with reduced TRM and may control advanced HD and low-grade NHL. Results of DLI are promising (Fig. 9.3).[68]

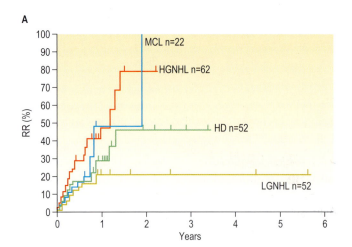

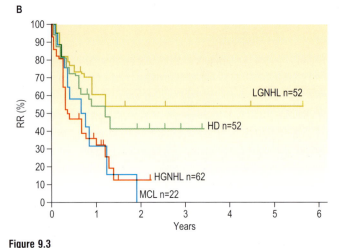

Figure 9.3

Chemoresistant or aggressive lymphoma predicts for a poor outcome following reduced-intensity alllogeneic SCT: an analysis from the Lymphoma Working Party of the EBMT. (A) Probability of progression according to disease category. (B) Probability of progression-free survival according to disease histology. From Robinson et al.[68]

Promising results have been reported for relapsed or refractory T-cell lymphomas. Seventeen patients with a median age of 41 years (range, 23–60 years) underwent salvage chemotherapy followed by RIC and allogeneic SCT. Conditioning was with thiotepa, fludarabine, and cyclophosphamide. GvHD prophylaxis was with ciclosporin and short-course methotrexate. Two patients had primary chemorefractory disease, and 15 had relapsed disease; eight patients (47%) had relapsed after an autologous transplant. After a median follow-up of 28 months from the day of study entry (range, 3–57 months), 14 of 17 patients were alive, two died from progressive disease, and one died from infection. The estimated 3-year overall and PFS rates were 81% and 64%, respectively. The estimated probability of non-relapse mortality at 2 years was 6%.[69]

Reduced-intensity conditioning regimens are currently predominantly used in the allogeneic setting for lymphoma. There are still no data available from randomized trials comparing these regimens with each other, or with 'standard' conditioning, i.e. TBI 12 Gy or busulfan 16 mg/kg plus cyclophosphamide. Therefore, any combined analyses performed under the heading RIC or 'non-myeloablative' should be considered with great caution. The focus is frequently solely on the conditioning regimen used, and the type of GvHD prophylaxis used is overlooked.

A widely used RIC regimen involving fludarabine and melphalan and GvHD prophylaxis with ciclosporin and CAMPATH resulted in promising early outcomes with little toxicity and almost no severe acute GvHD after matched sibling transplantation.[70,71] However, follow-up revealed an increased risk of late fatal infections and relapse. The optimum dose of the pan-specific antilymphocyte monoclonal antibody CAMPATH used for GvHD prophylaxis remains to be determined in dose-finding trials, and is likely to depend on the clinical and immunologic constellation, for example, sibling or unrelated donor, HLA matched or mismatched. Future strategies will examine the roles of earlier allogeneic SCT with reduced-intensity conditioning, optimized GvHD prophylaxis, and immunotherapy-based post-transplant strategies such as pre-emptive DLI, idiotype vaccination, and immunostimulation by cytokines to optimize any GvL effect.

Summary: optimizing transplantation in lymphoma patients

Autologous and, increasingly, allogeneic SCT play important roles in lymphoma therapy. The successful use of monoclonal antibodies as part of first-line chemotherapy may alter the indications from upfront autologous SCT in some situations, such as low-grade lymphomas, towards allogeneic SCT as a salvage procedure.

Monoclonal antibodies are also likely to improve outcome in patients with high-risk aggressive lymphomas, for example, a combination of rituximab with high-dose chemotherapy and SCT.

Table 9.2 Indications for SCT

Autologous
Chemosensitive relapse or failure to achieve first CR: DLBL, and other high-grade lymphomas, Hodgkin's disease
In first remission: high-risk aaIPI 2 or 3 high-grade NHL: DLCL, BL, peripheral T-cell lymphoma; advanced MCL as part of first-line therapy (trial); FL stage III–IV as part of first-line treatment (trial)

Allogeneic
Relapse after autologous SCT; progression after 2nd-line chemotherapy (including rituximab, fludarabine, anthracyclines); chemorefractory disease: MCL, FL, other low-grade histologies
Early relapse (<1 year) from 1st CR; relapse after autologous SCT, not in 1st CR, but with controllable disease: all high-grade lymphomas; in 1st CR: MRD-positive lymphoblastic lymphoma; high-risk aggressive T-cell lymphoma (e.g. marrow involvement)

References

1. International Non-Hodgkin's Lymphoma Prognostic Factors Project. A predictive model for aggressive non-Hodgkin's lymphoma. N Engl J Med 1993;329:987–994
2. Harris NL, Jaffe ES, Diebold J et al. World Health Organization classification of neoplastic diseases of the hematopoietic and lymphoid tissues: report of the Clinical Advisory Committee meeting-Airlie House, Virginia, November 1997. J Clin Oncol 1999;17:3835–3849
3. Pfreundschuh M, Trumper L, Osterborg A et al. CHOP-like chemotherapy plus rituximab versus CHOP-like chemotherapy alone in young patients with good-prognosis diffuse large-B-cell lymphoma: a randomized controlled trial by the MabThera International Trial (MInT) Group. Lancet Oncol 2006;7:379–391
4. Nademanee A, Molina A, O'Donnell MR et al. Results of high-dose therapy and autologous bone marrow/stem cell transplantation during remission in poor-risk intermediate- and high-grade lymphoma: international index high and high-intermediate risk group. Blood 1997;90:3844–3852
5. Kaiser U, Uebelacker I, Abel U et al. Randomized study to evaluate the use of high-dose therapy as part of primary treatment for 'aggressive' lymphoma. J Clin Oncol 2002;20:4413–4419
6. Vitolo U, Liberati AM, Cabras MG et al. High dose sequential chemotherapy with autologous transplantation versus dose-dense chemotherapy MegaCEOP as first line treatment in poor-prognosis diffuse large cell lymphoma: an 'Intergruppo Italiano Linfomi' randomized trial. Haematologica 2005;90:793–801
7. Olivieri A, Santini G, Patti C et al. Upfront high-dose sequential therapy (HDS) versus VACOP-B with or without HDS in aggressive non-Hodgkin's lymphoma: long-term results by the NHLCSG. Ann Oncol 2005;16:1941–1948
8. Milpied N, Deconinck E, Gaillard F et al. Initial treatment of aggressive lymphoma with high-dose chemotherapy and autologous stem-cell support. N Engl J Med 2004;350:1287–1295
9. Haioun C, Lepage E, Gisselbrecht C et al. Survival benefit of high-dose therapy in poor-risk aggressive non-Hodgkin's lymphoma: final analysis of the prospective LNH87–2 protocol – a groupe d'Etude des lymphomes de l'Adulte study. J Clin Oncol 2000;18:3025–3030
10. Haioun C, Lepage E, Gisselbrecht C et al. Benefit of autologous bone marrow transplantation over sequential chemotherapy in poor-risk aggressive non-Hodgkin's lymphoma: updated results of the prospective study LNH87–2. Groupe d'Etude des Lymphomes de l'Adulte. J Clin Oncol 1997;15:1131–1137
11. Khouri IF, Saliba RM, Hosing C et al. Concurrent administration of high-dose rituximab before and after autologous stem-cell transplantation for relapsed aggressive B-cell non-Hodgkin's lymphomas. J Clin Oncol 2005; 23; 2240–2247
12. Glass B, Kloess M, Bentz M et al. Dose-escalated CHOP plus etoposide (MegaCHOP) followed by repeated stem cell transplantation as primary treatment of aggressive high-risk non-Hodgkin lymphoma. Blood 2006;107:3058–3064
13. Haioun C, Mounier N, Quesnel B et al. Tandem autotransplant as first-line consolidative treatment in poor-risk aggressive lymphoma: a pilot study of 36 patients. Ann Oncol 2001;12:1749–1755
14. Stewart DA, Bahlis N, Valentine K et al. Upfront double high-dose chemotherapy with DICEP followed by BEAM and autologous stem cell transplantation for poor-prognosis aggressive non-Hodgkin lymphoma. Blood 2006;107:4623–4627
15. Soussain C, Suzan F, Hoang-Xuan K et al. Results of intensive chemotherapy followed by hematopoietic stem-cell rescue in 22 patients with refractory or recurrent primary CNS lymphoma or intraocular lymphoma. J Clin Oncol 2001;19:742–749
16. Cheng T, Forsyth P, Chaudhry A et al. High-dose thiotepa, busulfan, cyclophosphamide and ASCT without whole-brain radiotherapy for poor prognosis primary CNS lymphoma. Bone Marrow Transplant 2003;31:679–685
17. Abrey LE, Moskowitz CH, Mason WP et al. Intensive methotrexate and cytarabine followed by high-dose chemotherapy with autologous stem-cell rescue in patients with newly diagnosed primary CNS lymphoma: an intent-to-treat analysis. J Clin Oncol 2003;21:4151–4156
18. Illerhaus G, Marks R, Ihorst G et al. High-dose chemotherapy with autologous stem-cell transplantation and hyperfractionated radiotherapy as first-line treatment of primary CNS lymphoma. J Clin Oncol 2006;24:3865–3870
19. Philip T, Guglielmi C, Hagenbeek A et al. Autologous bone marrow transplantation as compared with salvage chemotherapy in relapses of chemotherapy-sensitive non-Hodgkin's lymphoma. N Engl J Med 1995;333:1540–1545
20. Blay J, Gomez F, Sebban C et al. The International Prognostic Index correlates to survival in patients with aggressive lymphoma in relapse: analysis of the PARMA trial. Parma Group. Blood 1998;92:3562–3568
21. Buadi FK, Micallef IN, Ansell SM et al. Autologous hematopoietic stem cell transplantation for older patients with relapsed non-Hodgkin's lymphoma. Bone Marrow Transplant 2006;37:1017–1022
22. Moskowitz CH, Bertino JR, Glassman JR et al. Ifosfamide, carboplatin, and etoposide: a highly effective cytoreduction and peripheral-blood progenitor-cell mobilization regimen for transplant-eligible patients with non-Hodgkin's lymphoma. J Clin Oncol 1999;17:3776–3785
23. Kewalramani T, Zelenetz AD, Nimer SD et al. Rituximab and ICE as second-line therapy before autologous stem cell transplantation for relapsed or primary refractory diffuse large B-cell lymphoma. Blood 2004;103:3684–3688
24. Hamlin PA, Zelenetz AD, Kewalramani T et al. Age-adjusted International Prognostic Index predicts autologous stem cell transplantation outcome for patients with relapsed or primary refractory diffuse large B-cell lymphoma. Blood 2003;102:1989–1996
25. Kewalramani T, Zelenetz AD, Hedrick EE et al. High-dose chemoradiotherapy and autologous stem cell transplantation for patients with primary refractory aggressive non-Hodgkin lymphoma: an intention-to-treat analysis. Blood 2000;96:2399–2404
26. Josting A, Sieniawski M, Glossmann JP et al. High-dose sequential chemotherapy followed by autologous stem cell transplantation in relapsed and refractory aggressive non-

Hodgkin's lymphoma: results of a multicenter phase II study. Ann Oncol 2005;16:1359–1365

27. Vose JM, Zhang MJ, Rowlings PA et al. Autologous transplantation for diffuse aggressive non-Hodgkin's lymphoma in patients never achieving remission: a report from the Autologous Blood and Marrow Transplant Registry. J Clin Oncol 2001;19:406–413

28. Horwitz SM, Negrin RS, Blume KG et al. Rituximab as adjuvant to high-dose therapy and autologous hematopoietic cell transplantation for aggressive non-Hodgkin lymphoma. Blood 2004;103:777–783

29. Hagberg H, Gisselbrecht C. Randomized phase III study of R-ICE versus R-DHAP in relapsed patients with CD20 diffuse large B-cell lymphoma (DLBCL) followed by high-dose therapy and a second randomization to maintenance treatment with rituximab or not: an update of the CORAL study. Ann Oncol 2006;17(suppl 4):iv31-iv32

30. Press OW, Eary JF, Gooley T et al. A phase I/II trial of iodine-131-tositumomab (anti-CD20), etoposide, cyclophosphamide, and autologous stem cell transplantation for relapsed B-cell lymphomas. Blood 2000;96:2934–2942

31. Haioun C, Itti E, Rahmouni A et al. PET scan in the therapeutic strategy. Hematol J. 2004;5(suppl 3):S149–S153

32. Hiddemann W, Kneba M, Dreyling M et al. Frontline therapy with rituximab added to the combination of cyclophosphamide, doxorubicin, vincristine, and prednisone (CHOP) significantly improves the outcome for patients with advanced-stage follicular lymphoma compared with therapy with CHOP alone: results of a prospective randomized study of the German Low-Grade Lymphoma Study Group. Blood 2005;106:3725–3732

33. Marcus R, Imrie K, Belch A et al. CVP chemotherapy plus rituximab compared with CVP as first-line treatment for advanced follicular lymphoma. Blood 2005;105:1417–1423

34. Flinn IW, Byrd JC, Morrison C et al. Fludarabine and cyclophosphamide with filgastrim support in patients with previously untreatedf indolent lymphoid malignancies. Blood 2000;96:71–75

35. Gribben JG, Freedman AS, Neuberg D et al. Immunologic purging of marrow assessed by PCR before autologous bone marrow transplantation for B-cell lymphoma. N Engl J Med 1991;325:1525–1533

36. Bastion Y, Brice P, Haioun C et al. Intensive therapy with peripheral blood progenitor cell transplantation in 60 patients with poor-prognosis follicular lymphoma. Blood 1995;86:3257–3262

37. Finke J. The role of stem cell transplantation in the treatment of follicular lymphoma. Semin Cancer Biol 2003;13:233–239

38. Horning SJ, Negrin RS, Hoppe RT et al. High-dose therapy and autologous bone marrow transplantation for follicular lymphoma in first complete or partial remission: results of a phase II clinical trial. Blood 2001;97:404–409

39. Ladetto M, Corradini P, Vallet S et al. High rate of clinical and molecular remissions in follicular lymphoma patients receiving high-dose sequential chemotherapy and autografting at diagnosis: a multicenter, prospective study by the Gruppo Italiano Trapianto Midollo Osseo (GITMO). Blood 2002;100:1559–1565

40. Lenz G, Dreyling M, Schiegnitz E et al. Myeloablative radiochemotherapy followed by autologous stem cell transplantation in first remission prolongs progression-free survival in follicular lymphoma: results of a prospective, randomized trial of the German Low-Grade Lymphoma Study Group. Blood 2004;104:2667–2674

41. Deconinck E, Foussard C, Milpied N et al. High-dose therapy followed by autologous purged stem-cell transplantation and doxorubicin-based chemotherapy in patients with advanced follicular lymphoma: a randomized multicenter study by GOELAMS. Blood 2005;105:3817–3823

42. Zelenetz AD. Mantle cell lymphoma: an update on management. Ann Oncol 2006;17(suppl 4):iv12-iv14

43. Forstpointner R, Dreyling M, Repp R et al. The addition of rituximab to a combination of fludarabine, cyclophosphamide, mitoxantrone (FCM) significantly increases the response rate and prolongs survival as compared with FCM alone in patients with relapsed and refractory follicular and mantle cell lymphomas: results of a prospective randomized study of the German Low-Grade Lymphoma Study Group. Blood 2004;104:3064–3071

44. de Guibert S, Jaccard A, Bernard M et al. Rituximab and DHAP followed by intensive therapy with autologous stem-cell transplantation as first-line therapy for mantle cell lymphoma. Haematologica 2006;91:425–426

45. Milpied N, Gaillard F, Moreau P et al. High-dose therapy with stem cell transplantation for mantle cell lymphoma: results and prognostic factors, a single center experience. Bone Marrow Transplant 1998;22:645–650

46. Dreyling M, Lenz G, Hoster E et al. Early consolidation by myeloablative radiochemotherapy followed by autologous stem cell transplantation in first remission significantly prolongs progression-free survival in mantle-cell lymphoma: results of a prospective randomized trial of the European MCL Network. Blood 2005;105:2677–2684

47. van Imhoff GW, van der Holt B, MacKenzie MA et al. Short intensive sequential therapy followed by autologous stem cell transplantation in adult Burkitt, Burkitt-like and lymphoblastic lymphoma. Leukemia 2005;19:945–952

48. Schmitz N, Pfistner B, Sextro M et al. Aggressive conventional chemotherapy compared with high-dose chemotherapy with autologous haemopoietic stem-cell transplantation for relapsed chemosensitive Hodgkin's disease: a randomized trial. Lancet 2002;359:2065–2071

49. Vigouroux S, Milpied N, Andrieu JM et al. Front-line high-dose therapy with autologous stem cell transplantation for high risk Hodgkin's disease: comparison with combined-modality therapy. Bone Marrow Transplant 2002;29:833–842

50. Josting A, Rudolph C, Mapara M et al. Cologne high-dose sequential chemotherapy in relapsed and refractory Hodgkin lymphoma: results of a large multicenter study of the German Hodgkin Lymphoma Study Group (GHSG). Ann Oncol 2005;16:116–123

51. Lavoie JC, Connors JM, Phillips GL et al. High-dose chemotherapy and autologous stem cell transplantation for primary refractory or relapsed Hodgkin lymphoma: long-term outcome in the first 100 patients treated in Vancouver. Blood 2005;106:1473–1478

52. Hoelzer D, Gokbuget N, Digel W et al. Outcome of adult patients with T-lymphoblastic lymphoma treated according to protocols for acute lymphoblastic leukemia. Blood 2002;99:4379–4385

53. Falini B, Pulford K, Pucciarini A et al. Lymphomas expressing ALK fusion protein(s) other than NPM-ALK. Blood 1999;94:3509–3515

54. Gisselbrecht C, Gaulard P, Lepage E et al. Prognostic significance of T-cell phenotype in aggressive non-Hodgkin's lymphomas. Groupe d'Etudes des Lymphomes de l'Adulte (GELA). Blood 1998;92:76–82

55. Kewalramani T, Zelenetz AD, Teruya-Feldstein J et al. Autologous transplantation for relapsed or primary refractory peripheral T-cell lymphoma. Br J Haematol 2006;134(2):202–207

56. Reimer P, Schertlin T, Rudiger T et al. Myeloablative radiochemotherapy followed by autologous peripheral blood stem cell transplantation as first-line therapy in peripheral T-cell lymphomas: first results of a prospective multicenter study. Hematol J 2004;5:304–311

57. Mounier N, Gisselbrecht C, Briere J et al. Prognostic factors in patients with aggressive non-Hodgkin's lymphoma treated by front-line autotransplantation after complete remission: a cohort study by the Groupe d'Etude des Lymphomes de l'Adulte. J Clin Oncol 2004;22:2826–2834

58. Deconinck E, Lamy T, Foussard C et al. Autologous stem cell transplantation for anaplastic large-cell lymphomas: results of a prospective trial. Br J Haematol 2000;109:736–742

59. Hoogendoorn M, Olde WJ, Smit WM et al. Primary allogeneic T-cell responses against mantle cell lymphoma antigen-presenting cells for adoptive immunotherapy after stem cell transplantation. Clin Cancer Res 2005;11:5310–5318

60. van Besien KW, de Lima M, Giralt SA et al. Management of lymphoma recurrence after allogeneic transplantation: the relevance of graft-versus-lymphoma effect. Bone Marrow Transplant 1997;19:977–982

61. Mach-Pascual S, Legare RD, Lu D et al. Predictive value of clonality assays in patients with non-Hodgkin's lymphoma undergoing autologous bone marrow transplant: a single institution study. Blood 1998;91:4496–4503

62. van Besien K, Sobocinski KA, Rowlings PA et al. Allogeneic bone marrow transplantation for low-grade lymphoma. Blood 1998;92:1832–1836

63. Bertz H, Illerhaus G, Veelken H, Finke J. Allogeneic hematopoetic stem-cell transplantation for patients with relapsed or refractory lymphomas: comparison of high-dose conventional conditioning versus fludarabine-based reduced-intensity regimens. Ann Oncol 2002;13:135–139

64. Khouri IF, Saliba RM, Giralt SA et al. Nonablative allogeneic hematopoietic transplantation as adoptive immunotherapy for indolent lymphoma: low incidence of toxicity, acute graft-versus-host disease, and treatment-related mortality. Blood 2001;98:3595–3599

65. Baron F, Maris MB, Sandmaier BM et al. Graft-versus-tumor effects after allogeneic hematopoietic cell transplantation with nonmyeloablative conditioning. J Clin Oncol 2005;23:1993–2003

66. Maris MB, Sandmaier BM, Storer BE et al. Allogeneic hematopoietic cell transplantation after fludarabine and 2 Gy total body irradiation for relapsed and refractory mantle cell lymphoma. Blood 2004;104:3535–3542

67. Sorror ML, Maris MB, Storer B et al. Comparing morbidity and mortality of HLA-matched unrelated donor hematopoietic cell transplantation after nonmyeloablative and myeloablative conditioning: influence of pretransplantation comorbidities. Blood 2004;104:961–968

68. Robinson SP, Goldstone AH, Mackinnon S et al. Chemoresistant or aggressive lymphoma predicts for a poor outcome following reduced-intensity allogeneic progenitor cell transplantation: an analysis from the Lymphoma Working Party of the European Group for Blood and Bone Marrow Transplantation. Blood 2002;100:4310–4316

69. Corradini P, Dodero A, Zallio F et al. Graft-versus-lymphoma effect in relapsed peripheral T-cell non-Hodgkin's lymphomas after reduced-intensity conditioning followed by allogeneic transplantation of hematopoietic cells. J Clin Oncol 2004;22:2172–2176

70. Kottaridis PD, Milligan DW, Chopra R et al. In vivo CAMPATH-1H prevents graft-versus-host disease following nonmyeloablative stem cell transplantation. Blood 2000;96:2419–2425

71. Morris E, Thomson K, Craddock C et al. Outcomes after alemtuzumab-containing reduced-intensity allogeneic transplantation regimen for relapsed and refractory non-Hodgkin lymphoma. Blood 2004;104:3865–3871

Chronic lymphocytic leukemia

Rifca Le Dieu and John G Gribben

CHAPTER 10

Introduction

There have been no randomized trials comparing the outcome of stem cell transplantation (SCT) with standard chemotherapy for patients with chronic lymphocytic leukemia (CLL), but both autologous and allogeneic SCT are being increasingly explored in this disease. Clinical trials have demonstrated that this approach is feasible, but that myeloablative SCT is associated with high mortality after allogeneic SCT and eventual relapse after autologous transplant. There is a clear demonstration of a graft-versus-leukemia (GvL) effect in CLL, with encouraging results seen after reduced-intensity conditioning (RIC) SCT. In the absence of any other treatment modalities currently capable of improving survival in this disease, the treatment of choice for younger patients with poor-risk CLL may well be SCT, but continued enrollment of appropriate patients into well-designed clinical trials is vital in the ongoing evaluation of the role of SCT in CLL, particularly in comparison with the improved responses seen with chemoimmunotherapy in this disease.

The major dilemma in CLL is to establish which patients have sufficiently high-risk disease to merit consideration for approaches such as SCT, with their attendant morbidity and treatment-related morality (TRM). Recently, there have been major advances in identifying prognostic factors in CLL which may help to select patients who are likely to have a sufficiently poor outcome using conventional therapy to merit this approach.

Prognostic and predictive factors

A number of prognostic factors have been identified in CLL. The Rai and Binet staging systems were based upon their prognostic significance and the stage of disease remains perhaps the most important prognostic factor in CLL, although there are increasing attempts to correlate prognosis with biologic markers. Although the majority of patients with high-risk disease (Rai stages III and IV and Binet stage C) have a rapidly progressive clinical course and short survival, the disease course is less uniform in the other groups, with some patients, particularly those with Rai stage 0, Binet stage A, following a benign or 'smoldering' course. Therefore, a number of other factors have been evaluated for their prognostic significance and have shown limited use in their ability to predict the course of disease.

Bone marrow (BM) biopsies are not needed to make the diagnosis of CLL, but the pattern of BM involvement (diffuse versus nodular or interstitial) has prognostic significance.[1] Atypical morphology with increased number of prolymphocytes is also an independent factor associated with an adverse prognosis.[2] A lymphocyte doubling time (LDT) of less than 12 months in untreated patients predicts a progres-

sive course.[3] Several other serum factors have been used to correlate tumor cell proliferation with clinical outcome, including beta-2 micro-globulin,[4] Ki67,[5] p27[6] and thymidine kinase.[7]

Cytogenetic and molecular analysis

Conventional cytogenetic analysis detects chromosome aberrations in only 40–50% of cases, but the introduction of fluorescent in situ hybridization (FISH) has greatly enhanced our ability to detect chromosomal abnormalities in CLL. Using FISH, chromosomal abnormalities are detected in more than 80% of CLL patients.[8] Genomic aberrations are important independent predictors of disease progression and survival. The most frequent changes observed are deletion in 13q, 11q and 17p, and trisomy 12q. Patients with deletion 17p and 11q have more advanced disease and shorter time to requirement for therapy and poorer prognosis than those without these deletions. The presence of 17p deletion predicts for treatment failure with alkylating agents and fludarabine and short survival times. In multivariate analysis, 11q and 17p deletions provided independent adverse prognostic information. These findings have implications for the design of risk-adapted treatment strategies, including selection of patients for SCT.[9]

Immunoglobulin gene mutation status, ZAP70 and CD38 expression

Patients with CLL who have unmutated immunoglobulin variable (IgV$_H$) region genes have poor prognoses compared to those whose immunoglobulin genes are mutated.[10,11] It has been suggested that higher levels of expression of CD38 are associated with unmutated IgV genes,[10] and on multivariate analysis, high levels of expression of CD38 on B-cell CLL cells were associated with more rapid disease progression and poor response to therapy.[12,13] In a multivariate analysis examining the prognostic significance of genetic abnormalities at presentation, clinical stage, lymphocyte morphology, CD38 expression, and IgV$_H$ gene status in 205 patients with CLL,[14] deletion of chromosome 11q23, absence of a deletion of chromosome 13q14, atypical lymphocyte morphology, and more than 30% CD38 expression were significantly associated with the presence of unmutated IgV$_H$ genes. Advanced stage, male sex, atypical morphology, more than 30% CD38 expression, trisomy 12, deletion of chromosome 11q23, loss or mutation of the p53 gene, and unmutated IgV$_H$ genes were all poor prognostic factors in the univariate analysis in this study. However, IgV$_H$ gene mutational status, loss or mutation of the p53 gene, and clinical stage retained prognostic significance in a multivariate analysis.[14] Expression of zeta-associated protein 70 (ZAP70) has been examined as a surrogate for IgV$_H$ mutational status and is also associated with poor prognosis in CLL.[15–17] Ongoing studies are addressing which combination of prognostic factors may be most predictive of poor response to chemoimmunotherapy approaches and might therefore be used to identify criteria more precisely for SCT in CLL.

Treatment of chronic lymphocytic leukemia

Evidence that current treatment can improve outcome is available only for patients with Rai III and IV or Binet B and C stages. Patients with earlier disease stages (Rai 0–II, Binet A) are generally not treated but monitored with a 'watch and wait' strategy. The decision to treat is guided by clinical staging, the presence of symptoms, and disease activity. Treatment is indicated in early stages only when disease-associated symptoms are present or there is evidence of disease progression, defined by a rapid increase in leukocyte count or size of lymph nodes.

Once treatment is indicated, the mainstay of treatment was previously with alkylator-based therapy, using chlorambucil, cyclophosphamide, doxorubicin, prednisone (CAP) or cyclophosphamide, doxorubicin, vincristine, prednisone (CHOP). Three large randomized trials have demonstrated that monotherapy with the purine analog fludarabine produces superior overall response rates and longer duration of responses compared with alkylating agent-based therapy including chlorambucil, CAP or CHOP.[18–20] However, this increased response rate has not translated into a survival advantage due to the relatively high response rates using salvage therapy with purine analogs for patients treated initially with alkylator-based approaches. The combination of fludarabine with cyclophosphamide (FC) has been shown in randomized trials to result in increased response rates and longer duration of response than has fludarabine alone.[21,22] As a single agent, the anti-CD20 monoclonal antibody rituximab has less activity in CLL than in follicular lymphoma. However, the addition of rituximab (R) to chemotherapy appears to improve response rates and duration of responses compared to fludarabine,[23] or fludarabine and cyclophosphamide using the FCR regimen.[24]

The management of relapsed CLL patients is dependent upon a number of factors, most importantly age, performance status, previous therapy administered, response and duration of response to such therapy, and time from last therapy. In addition, the goal of therapy, whether aggressive or palliative, must be factored in when deciding on the next line of treatment. The highest response rates seen occur in relapsed patients with the use of combination chemoimmunotherapy.[25] Nonetheless, there is no evidence to date that these treatments are curative and all patients invariably relapse and subsequently develop resistance to chemotherapy, often with the loss of function of p53.[26] In particular, once patients become refractory to purine analogs the prognosis is dismal, with a median survival of less than 1 year.[27]

The humanized anti-CD52 monoclonal antibody alemtuzumab is approved for CLL patients who are fludarabine refractory. In the pivotal study of alemtuzumab in 93 patients with fludarabine-refractory CLL, the overall response rate was 33%, although only 2% of patients achieved complete remission (CR).[28] The median time to progression for responders was 9.5 months and there was an improvement in survival in responding patients at 32 months, compared to 16 months for all patients. Of note, alemtuzumab appears to have activity against cases that are unresponsive to chemotherapy due to the presence of p53 mutations.[29,30] Alemtuzumab has poor activity against bulky lymphadenopathy, but demonstrates impressive efficacy in clearing the peripheral blood and bone marrow compartments of disease. Alemtuzumab has shown benefit when used in combination with fludarabine.[31,32] Studies are also examining the role of alemtuzumab treatment after chemotherapy to clear residual disease,[33] and

this may be an effective way to obtain autologous peripheral blood stem cells free of contamination with CLL.[34]

The role of transplantation in chronic lymphocytic leukemia

A number of studies have examined the role of SCT in patients with CLL to determine whether this has curative potential and can prevent or reverse the development of chemotherapy resistance. CLL is largely a disease of the elderly, with a median age of presentation between 65 and 70 years. Most patients with CLL are thus too elderly to consider such an approach, with its resulting morbidity and mortality in a disease perceived to be so indolent. However, 40% of patients with CLL are aged under 60 years of age, and 12% under 50 years at the time of diagnosis. Younger patients do not have a poorer prognosis than more elderly patients and have similar prognostic factors. Unlike older patients who often die of co-morbidities not associated with the CLL, more than 90% of younger patients die because of their CLL.[35] In addition, as described above, major advances in identification of prognostic factors in CLL may help to identify patients who are more unlikely to follow an indolent course or in whom chemoresistance will reduce the likelihood of durable responses to chemotherapy.

Indications for SCT in CLL

No clear guidelines have been defined for which patients are candidates for autologous SCT, but European Bone Marrow Transplant (EBMT) guidelines have now been established outlining indications for allogeneic SCT in CLL.[36] The guidelines conclude that there is an evidence base for the efficacy of allogeneic SCT in CLL and that this is indicated in high-risk CLL patents. Precisely what factors are defined as high risk is not defined clearly, but patients with p53 deletions or mutations are considered candidates in first remission, and ongoing studies are assessing the impact of biomarkers, including IgV_H mutational status and cytogenetic abnormalities, to identify patients at sufficiently high risk to merit consideration for transplant in first remission. The consensus of the EBMT working group was that allogeneic SCT was recommended early in the disease course for young patients with CLL who fail to achieve CR or who progress within 12 months after purine analogs, and those who relapse within 24 months after having achieved a response with purine analog-based combination therapy or autologous transplantation. It is clear that neither of these categories requires assessment of biologic risk factors, and ongoing prospective clinical studies will be required to determine the specific risk factors that identify patients at sufficiently high risk to merit use of allogeneic SCT in first CR. However, there is consensus that patients requiring treatment who have p53 abnormalities have a sufficiently poor prognosis to merit transplantation in first response.

Although SCT is not an option for many older patients who would not tolerate the approach or for those with indolent disease, younger patients with poor prognostic disease can be identified for whom SCT may offer a chance of cure. Questions remain regarding appropriate patient selection for consideration of SCT, timing of SCT in the clinical course of the disease, use of autologous versus allogeneic SCT, use of non-myeloablative regimens, and exploitation of the GvL effect, which are currently under investigation.

Autologous stem cell transplantation

The antitumor activity of autologous SCT is dependent upon a dose–response effect in CLL. There has been no prospective study directly comparing the outcome after conventional therapy compared to that obtained after autologous SCT, although a retrospective matched-pair analysis suggested a survival advantage for autologous SCT over

Table 10.1 Autologous transplantation for CLL

No. of patients	TRM	Ongoing CR	Median follow-up (months)	Reference
137	5 early 13 MDS/AML 15 other cancer	67	78	Gribben et al 2005[44]
77	0	50	28	Jantunen et al 2006[45]
65	1 early 5 MDS/AML	45	36	Milligan et al 2005[43]
16	2	5	37	Pavletic et al 1998[42]
13	0	12	19	Dreger et al 1998[41]
11	1	2	10	Khouri et al 1994[39]
8 20 enrolled 12 stem cells collected	0	5	36	Sutton et al 1998[81]
5	0	4	9	Itala et al 1997[40]

conventional therapy.[37] As induction regimens have evolved, it would now be useful to look at the new chemoimmunotherapeutic regimens in direct comparison with autologous SCT.

A number of Phase II studies have reported the outcome following autologous SCT for CLL (Table 10.1).[38–44] The approach is feasible in CLL with a peritransplant TRM of between 2% and 10%.[43,44] Encouraging early results were reported in patients with chemosensitive disease,[38] whereas patients transplanted in relapse or with chemoresistant disease had a poor outcome.[39] Poor results with a high relapse rate after autologous SCT in CLL were also observed in a study of 16 patients and, at a median follow-up of 41 months, eight had relapsed and six had died (three from progressive malignancy).[42] Other groups have observed better results. In 18 patients with CLL including early-stage disease, transplantation was performed in 13 patients, only one of whom had relapsed at the time of publication.[41] Eight heavily pretreated patients received auto-SCT with partially purged CD34+ peripheral blood stem cells, and although four patients remained in CR, the median follow-up was only 9 months.[40]

The experience in Finland has been updated recently for 72 patients autografted in five centers between 1995 and 2005.[45] Median patient age was 57 (range 38–69) with a median time from diagnosis of 32 months (range 6–181). The median number of prior therapies was one. The most commonly used conditioning regimen was total body irradiation (TBI) and cyclophosphamide (Cy) (n = 8, 53%). There were no early TRMs. Thirty-seven percent had relapsed or progressed after a median follow-up of 28 months. The projected median progression-free survival (PFS) and overall survival (OS) were 48 months and 95 months, respectively.

A pilot study from the Medical Research Council (MRC) in the UK enrolled previously untreated patients and followed them prospectively to assess the feasibility of performing autologous stem cell transplantation.[43] Only 65 of 115 patients (56%) entered into the study were able to proceed to autologous SCT. However, only one patient died of early transplant-related complications and the CR rate after transplantation was 74% (48 of 65). The 5-year OS was 77.5% and 5-year PFS was 51.5%. None of the variables examined at study entry was predictive of either OS or PFS. Sixteen of 20 evaluable patients achieved a molecular CR in the first 6 months following transplantation, and detectable molecular disease by PCR was highly predictive of disease recurrence. Of concern, five of 65 (8%) patients developed post-transplant acute myeloid leukemia/myelodysplastic syndrome.

Although the early TRM is low after auto-SCT, there is a high incidence of opportunistic infections in patients with CLL compared to other patient populations. Whether this is due to a greater degree of immune incompetence in patients with CLL or is secondary to the immunosuppressive effects of fludarabine and other therapy is unknown. Patients have a better outcome when they are treated early in the course of the disease and at a time when they have a small tumor burden. This suggests that selected patients should be transplanted as soon as treatment is indicated and perhaps even, for selected patients, as consolidation therapy of a first complete or partial remission. One difficulty in selecting high-risk patients is that these patients may also have an adverse outcome after transplant. The immunoglobulin gene mutation status maintains its poor prognostic significance after autologous transplantation[46] although it appears that this can be overcome using allogeneic transplant.[47,48] A randomized trial proposed by the European Bone Marrow Transplant Group should help to address this issue. The timing of the harvesting of the cells and whether they should be harvested in first remission and kept until later in the treatment course also needs to be further investigated. It is not always possible to collect enough CD34+ cells, especially in heavily pretreated patients,[49] and an interval of at least 3 months should be allowed between the last dose of fludarabine and stem cell collection.[50]

The major problem after autologous SCT remains disease relapse, and patients continue to relapse years later.[51] A number of methods including multiparameter flow cytometry analysis[52] and PCR[53] are being used to investigate whether persistence of minimal residual disease will predict which patients are likely to relapse following transplantation for CLL. Molecular remissions can be achieved in more than two-thirds of patients but these are not durable[43,53–55] and most patients who achieve CR post-autologous SCT will eventually relapse. Detectable molecular disease post transplant is, however, highly predictive of clinical recurrence.[43]

Of particular concern are recent reports of myelodysplasia and secondary acute myeloid leukemia (MDS/AML) post autograft. In the MRC CLL pilot study, among 65 newly diagnosed patients treated with fludarabine followed by autologous SCT, eight developed MDS/AML.[43] This equates to a 5-year actuarial risk of developing MDS/AML post autologous SCT of 12.4% (95% confidence interval (CI) 2.5–24%). No potential risk factor analyzed was predictive. The group postulates that potential causative factors may be fludarabine, low cell dose and use of TBI in the conditioning regimen. This finding has been supported by a long-term outcome report of a series from the Dana-Farber Cancer Institute, which reported an actuarial incidence of MDS/AML in CLL patients post autograft of 12% at 8 years.[44]

One of the major concerns in autologous transplantation is that reinfusion of tumor cells may theoretically contribute to the risk of relapse. Numerous groups have attempted to improve outcome by 'purging' the graft. The techniques most frequently employed utilize either negative selection using B-cell monoclonal antibodies to deplete tumor cells from the graft or positive selection of stem cells using CD34 antibodies. Unfortunately, these methods remain inefficient at removing CLL cells.[53] Purging also results in stem cell loss. If there has been difficulty in obtaining a sufficiently large harvest, as seen in 50% of cases in the MRC pilot study, purging cannot be performed. This problem could be bypassed by in vivo purging using alemtuzumab or rituximab pretransplant.

High-dose alemtuzumab was used for this purpose in the conditioning regimen for autologous transplants in one arm of the CLL3 trial from the German CLL Study Group, with unexpected consequences.[56] Sixteen patients were treated in this arm and received a median dose of alemtuzumab of 103 mg. A high incidence of initially unexplained skin rashes led to further analysis. Twelve of 16 patients (87%) developed a skin rash between 43 and 601 days post autologous SCT, in seven of whom a diagnosis of graft-versus-host disease (GvHD) could be made, compared with no cases in the TBI/Cy-only conditioned patients. Autologous GvHD is an autoimmune syndrome initiated by autologous effector T-cells that recognize self MHC Class II antigens and is usually self-limiting. In this case, however, all cases required immunosuppression and the median duration was 517 days (range 60–867). The trial was discontinued due to the high non-relapse mortality. However, of note, addition of alemtuzumab led to improved disease control at the molecular level. It is interesting that the use of alemtuzumab in combination with other immunosuppressants prior to allogeneic SCT results in effective prevention of GvHD. In this situation it was postulated that the markedly immunosuppressive regimen depleted regulatory CD4 and CD8 T-cells and NK cells, allowing subsequent development of autoimmune disease. The patients receiving alemtuzumab/TBI/Cy had a severe CD8 lymphopenia in the first year after SCT. The authors recommend that future trials investigating in vivo purging with alemtuzumab should use a less immunosuppressive conditioning regimen such as BEAM, and avoid the use of TBI.

The concept of using alemtuzumab for in vivo purging should perhaps not yet be discarded. When used at a modification from the standard doses (10 mg subcutaneously three times per week for 6 weeks) in 34 patients who had had a clinical response to a fludarabine-based regimen, the CR rate improved from 35% to 79.5%, with 56% achieving eradication of minimal residual disease (MRD).[57] Peripheral blood stem cell (PBSC) collection was subsequently successfully performed in 92%. Eighteen patients underwent autologous SCT, with 17 remaining in CR at a median follow-up of 14.5 months post SCT.

Myeloablative allogeneic stem cell transplantation

Allogeneic SCT extends the dose intensification effect of autologous transplantation by adding cellular immune therapy to generate a GvL effect. This results in better disease control but at the price of greater toxicity. The morbidity and mortality of allogeneic SCT relate to organ failure caused by the combination of the conditioning regimen, acute (a-GvHD) and chronic (c-GvHD) disease and infections. These risks are greater since many CLL patients are older.

The feasibility of allogeneic SCT in CLL was first demonstrated in 1988 in eight patients, five of whom were alive in CR after a median follow-up of 27 months post SCT.[58] The high TRM rate is apparent from registry data, with rates of 46–50% reported.[59] Despite the high TRM, patients who survive can have long-term disease control (Table 10.2).[38,59–62] Among 25 patients with CLL who underwent allogeneic SCT at the Fred Hutchinson Cancer Center,[62] 14 developed grades 2–4 a-GVHD and 10 clinical extensive c-GVHD. Non-relapse mortality at day 100 was unacceptably high at 57% for the seven patients conditioned with busulfan and cyclophosphamide, and 17% for the 18 patients conditioned with TBI-containing regimens. Actu-

Table 10.2 Myeloablative allogeneic transplantation for CLL

No.	TRM	Severe GvHD	Ongoing CR	Median follow-up (months)	Reference
54	25	18	24	27	Michallet et al 1996[59]
25	1 early 5 late	5	13 8 after DLI	78	Gribben et al 2005[44]
25	7	56	9	60	Doney et al 2002[62]
23	8	47	14	24	Pavletic et al 2000[61]
15	5	26	8	35	Khouri et al 1997[68]

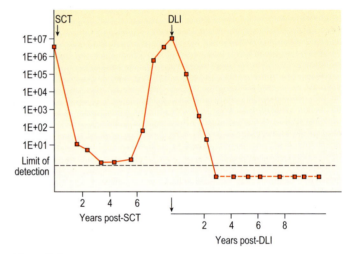

Figure 10.1
Response to donor lymphocyte infusion in CLL. Quantitive real-time PCR analysis of levels of disease following T-cell depleted allogeneic SCT. Donor lymphocyte infusion (DLI) administered as sole therapy after clinical evidence of relapse induced subsequent achievement of CR and eradication fo PCR detectable disease. Adapted with permission from Gribben et al.[44]

arial survival at 5 years for the 25 patients was 32%. All patients who received busulfan and cyclophosphamide died within 3 years of transplant. For the 14 patients transplanted since 1992 and who received TBI, the actuarial 5-year OS is 56%, suggesting that long-term disease-free survival (DFS) might be achieved in this disease.

The major advantage of allogeneic SCT appears to be the potential for a GvL effect. A strong GvL effect was noted, with those developing acute or chronic GvHD having near-complete protection from relapse.[63] This effect can be exploited by infusion of donor lymphocytes following allografting (Fig. 10.1)[44,64] or after cessation of immunosuppressive therapy.[65] Studies are under way addressing the issue of the number of lymphocytes required and the optimum timing of donor lymphocyte infusions (DLI) after allogeneic stem cell transplantation in this and other hematologic malignancies. Preclinical studies attempting to develop strategies to exploit maximal GvL effect without concomitant GvHD are also under way.

As HLA-matched sibling allogeneic transplants are only possible in a quarter of all potential recipients, the use of unrelated donor stem cells has been investigated. Among 38 heavily pretreated patients, 11 were alive and disease free at a median of 6 years post SCT.[66] The 5-year overall survival rate was 33%, TRM 38% and disease progression rate 32%. Of note, 45% developed grade 2–4 a-GvHD and 85% had c-GvHD. The authors concluded that lasting remissions could be achieved, but that the high TRM indicated that HLA-mismatched donors should be avoided.

Comparison of autologous and allogeneic SCT

Registry data have suggested that although durable responses were being achieved after allogeneic SCT, survival was worse than after autologous SCT, with the 3-year probability of survival reported as 45% for allogeneic SCT and 87% for autologous SCT.[67] Studies from the MD Anderson, however, have suggested improved outcome after allogeneic compared to autologous transplant.[39] In 14 patients with CLL refractory to or who had relapsed after chemotherapy with fludarabine, 13 (87%) achieved a complete remission post transplant. At the time of reporting, nine patients (53%) remained alive and in complete remission with a median follow-up of 36 months,[68] suggesting that allogeneic hematopoietic transplantation can induce durable remissions even in patients with CLL refractory to fludarabine. There are no studies directly comparing the outcome of autologous with allogeneic SCT. In a Phase II study at the Dana-Farber Cancer Institute (Fig. 10.2), 162 patients with high-risk CLL were enrolled in a study between 1989 and 1999, in which 25 patients with an HLA-matched sibling donor underwent T-cell depleted allogeneic transplantation and 137 with no sibling donor underwent B-cell purged autologous transplantation.[44] The 100-day mortality was 4% in both autologous and allogeneic SCT groups, although later TRM had a major impact on outcome. With a median follow-up of 6.5 years there was no difference in OS, with 58% after auto- and 55% after allogeneic SCT. PFS was significantly longer following autologous SCT than T-cell depleted allogeneic SCT, but no significant differences were observed in disease recurrence or deaths without recurrence according to type of transplant.

Reduced-intensity conditioning allogeneic stem cell transplantation

The rationale for the use of RIC allogeneic SCT is to capitalize on the GvL effect, avoiding the significant morbidity and mortality associated with myeloablative chemoradiotherapy. This approach is particularly applicable to the older age group of patients who develop CLL, and RIC regimens appear to be associated with a decreased mortality after allogeneic SCT, and then allow transplantation in older patients, making this approach more applicable to an increased number of CLL patients.[69–75] Patients in these studies were often heavily pretreated and refractory to therapy. Despite this, the majority demonstrated donor engraftment with a high CR rate. Survival is improved in patients

transplanted while they still have chemosensitive disease. These studies possibly provide the strongest direct evidence to date for a GvL effect that can be exploited in the management of CLL.

A major focus of ongoing research is the amount of pretransplant and post-transplant immunosuppression required to establish stable mixed chimerism and eventual full donor chimerism following non-myeloablative stem cell transplantation. It should be stressed that these procedures are currently investigational in nature and although the acute morbidity and mortality appear significantly lower compared to those seen after high-dose conditioning regimens with allogeneic transplantation, the longer term results with regard to morbidity of c-GvHD and disease control are currently lacking.

To examine whether RIC decreases TRM after allogeneic SCT for CLL, the outcome of 73 patients treated with RIC was compared with that of 82 matched patients from the European Bone Marrow Transplant Registry (EBMTR) database who had undergone standard myeloablative conditioning for CLL during the same time period.[76] Patients undergoing RIC had a significant reduction in TRM, but a higher incidence of relapse. There was no significant difference in OS or event-free survival (EFS) between the two groups.

The outcome has been reported after RIC allogeneic SCT for 64 patients with advanced CLL using the Fred Hutchinson Cancer Research Center multi-institutional protocol using related (n = 44) or unrelated (n = 20) donors (Fig. 10.3).[74] As shown in Table 10.3, the median age was 56 (range 44–69) years. The majority of patients were fludarabine refractory. TRM at 100 days was 11%, and 22% by 2

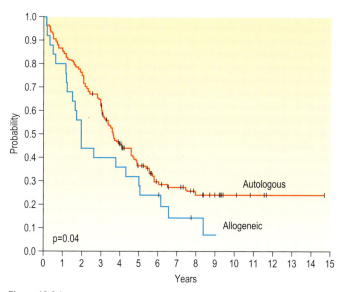

Figure 10.2
Progression-free survival after autologous and T-cell depleted allogeneic SCT. Adapted with permission from Gribben et al.[44]

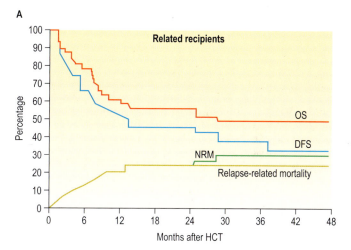

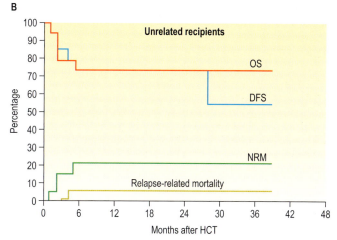

Figure 10.3
Outcome after RIC allo-SCT for CLL. Adapted with permission from Sorror et al.[74] OS, overall survival; DFS, disease-free survival; NRM, non-relapse mortality.

Table 10.3 RIC allogeneic SCT for CLL

n	Age, years (range)	Prior regimens (range)	Chemotherapy refractory	Donor (includes mismatch)	TRM	GvHD		Survival	Reference
						Acute grade 2–4	Chronic extensive		
30	50	3	47%	50% related	13% overall	56%	21%	OS 72% 2 yr	Schetelig et al 2002[69]
	(12–63)	(0–8)		50% unrelated				PFS 67%	
77	54	3	33%	81% related	18% 12m	34%	58%	OS 72% 2 yr	Dreger et al 2003[73]
	(30–66)	(0–8)	10 prior auto-SCT					PFS 56%	
64	56	4	53%	69% related	11% at 100 d	61%	50%	OS 60% 2 yr	Sorror et al 2005[74]
	(44–69)			31% unrelated	22% overall			PFS 52%	
39	57	3	Not stated	90% related	2% at 100 d	45%	58%	OS 48% 4 yr	Khouri et al 2006[82]
	(34–70)	(2–8)	*87% 'active' disease	10% unrelated				PFS 44%	
46	53	5	57%	33% related	17% overall	34%	43%	OS 54% 2 yr	Brown et al 2006[75]
	(35–67)	(1–10)	10 prior auto-SCT	67% unrelated				PFS 34%	
41	54	3	27%	58% related	5% at 100 d	10%	33%*	OS 51 2 yr	Delgado et al 2006[79]
	(37–67)	(1–8)	11 prior auto-SCT	42% unrelated	26% overall	(grade 3–4)		PFS 45%	

*after DLI.

years, with significant GvHD. At a median follow-up of 24 months, 39 patients were alive, 25 in complete remission. Two-year overall survival was 60% and disease-free survival was 52%. Although complications were more common in the patients with unrelated donors, there were higher CR and lower relapse rates than with related hematopoietic cell transplantation (HCT), suggesting more effective graft-versus-leukemia activity from the unrelated donors. A similar high rate of GvHD was seen in a smaller group of Australian patients.[77] Thus although RIC allogeneic SCTs are often termed 'mini-transplants', their morbidity, particularly in terms of GvHD, is still high.

The incidence of GvHD can be reduced by the use of alemtuzumab in the conditioning regimen, with consequent reduction in TRM. Unfortunately, it also delays post-SCT immune reconstitution, increases the risk of infective complications and potentially impairs the GvL effect. This impaired antitumor response may necessitate the early use of DLI post SCT.[78] A study by the British Society of Bone Marrow Transplantation (BSBMT) used alemtuzumab with fludarabine and melphalan as conditioning.[79] Forty-one consecutive patients were treated; 24 had HLA-matched sibling donors and 17 had unrelated volunteer donors (four mismatched). The conditioning regimen had significant antitumor effects, 100% of patients with chemosensitive disease and 86% with chemorefractory disease attaining CR or partial remission (PR). The TRM rate was 26%, overall survival 51% and relapse risk 29% at 2 years. GvHD rates were relatively low with a-GvHD occurring in 17 (41%) and c-GvHD in 13 (33%). The unexpectedly high TRM rate was due to a high incidence of fungal and viral infections. What emerged from this study was the clear adverse prognostic factor of fludarabine refractoriness. This group of patients had a 2-year overall survival of only 31%.

It has been demonstrated that patients with unmutated CLL who have undergone autologous SCT have a poor outcome.[37,46] This adverse event can be overcome with the use of allogeneic SCT.[48] Among 50 patients who underwent SCT, 34 had unmutated immunoglobulin variable heavy chain genes (IgV_H) (14 allogeneic SCT and 20 autologous SCT) and 16 had mutated IgV_H genes (nine allogeneic SCT and seven autologous SCT). There was no difference in CR rate between type of transplantation and IgV_H mutational status. After a median follow-up of 5 years, autologous SCT resulted in a significantly higher relapse rate than allogeneic SCT in both mutational groups. Thus the GvL effect of allogeneic SCT may overcome the negative impact of unmutated V_H gene status on outcome. Myeloablative conditioning may not

Table 10.4 The role of transplantation in CLL

Autologous SCT	No defined role
	Clinical trial only
Myeloablative allogeneic SCT	Chemorefractory disease in young patients
RIC allogeneic SCT	Incomplete response to first-line therapy
	Short duration of response after purine analog-containing regimens
	Richter's transformation
	p53 mutation at first treatment
	Other 'high-risk' in clinical trials

be required for this effect. In 30 patients with poor-prognosis CLL as defined by mutational status of V_H genes and cytogenetic abnormalities (11q-, 17p-) who had undergone RIC allogeneic SCT, OS and EFS for the poor-prognosis group were 90% and 92%, respectively, which was not significantly different to the rates seen in the good-prognosis group.[80]

Summary

High-dose therapy with autologous SCT is feasible in younger patients with poor-risk CLL. Myeloablative allogeneic SCT is associated with increased morbidity and mortality and should be restricted to patients with a very poor prognosis, and although no direct comparisons of myeloablative and RIC allogeneic SCT have been performed, given the older age of patients with CLL, it seems reasonable to consider RIC transplants as the approach of choice for CLL patients in whom allogeneic SCT is being considered. This should be undertaken early in the disease course to avoid development of refractory disease. The indications for these approaches are shown in Table 10.4. Autologous SCT offers a chance of lasting remission, with low TRM rates. However, it appears that this is not curative and all patients will eventually relapse. Whether this still results in improvement in survival, as has been observed in randomized trials in other diseases such as multiple myeloma, remains to be determined. Furthermore, it is currently unclear whether autologous SCT offers a superior survival advantage over the newer chemoimmunotherapeutic regimens.

Autologous transplantation will not overcome the poor prognosis conferred by unmutated V_H genes or poor risk cytogenetic abnormalities. Allogeneic SCT should be considered in these patients. Myeloablative regimens currently offer no survival advantage over autologous procedures, and a reduced-intensity conditioning regimen may therefore be the optimum approach to management. However, the high risk of GvHD needs to be taken into account. The optimum immunosuppressive conditioning regimen that minimizes GvHD while maximizing the GvL effect remains to be defined.

Despite encouraging initial results, we are still in the position where the follow-up of most clinical trials is too short to assess whether SCT can cure CLL. Future approaches to the management of this disease must take into account the balance between the increased morbidity and mortality of SCT in CLL and the curative potential that these approaches potentially offer. In the absence of any other treatment modalities currently capable of improving outcome in this disease, the treatment of choice for younger patients with poor-risk CLL may indeed be allogeneic or autologous SCT. Continued enrollment of appropriate patients into well-designed clinical trials is therefore vital for further progress.

References

1. Rozman C, Montserrat E, Rodriguez-Fernandez JM et al. Bone marrow histologic pattern – the best single prognostic parameter in chronic lymphocytic leukemia: a multivariate survival analysis of 329 cases. Blood 1984;64:642–648

2. Oscier DG, Matutes E, Copplestone A et al. Atypical lymphocyte morphology: an adverse prognostic factor for disease progression in stage A CLL independent of trisomy 12. Br J Haematol 1997;98:934–939

3. Montserrat E, Sanchez-Bisono J, Vinolas N, Rozman C. Lymphocyte doubling time in chronic lymphocytic leukemia: analysis of its prognostic significance. Br J Haematol 1986;62:567–575

4. Fayad L, Keating MJ, Reuben JM et al. Interleukin-6 and interleukin-10 levels in chronic lymphocytic leukemia: correlation with phenotypic characteristics and outcome. Blood 2001;97:256–263

5. Cordone I, Matutes E, Catovsky D. Monoclonal antibody Ki-67 identifies B and T cells in cycle in chronic lymphocytic leukemia: correlation with disease activity. Leukemia 1992;6:902–906

6. Vrhovac R, Delmer A, Tang R et al. Prognostic significance of the cell cycle inhibitor p27Kip1 in chronic B-cell lymphocytic leukemia. Blood 1998;91:4694–4700

7. Hallek M, Langenmayer I, Nerl C et al. Elevated serum thymidine kinase levels identify a subgroup at high risk of disease progression in early, nonsmoldering chronic lymphocytic leukemia. Blood 1999;93:1732–1737

8. Dohner H, Stilgenbauer S, Benner A et al. Genomic aberrations and survival in chronic lymphocytic leukemia. N Engl J Med 2000;343:1910–1916

9. Stilgenbauer S, Bullinger L, Lichter P, Dohner H. Genetics of chronic lymphocytic leukemia: genomic aberrations and V(H) gene mutation status in pathogenesis and clinical course. Leukemia. 2002;16:993–1007

10. Damle RN, Wasil T, Fais F et al. Ig V gene mutation status and CD38 expression as novel prognostic indicators in chronic lymphocytic leukemia. Blood 1999;94:1840–1847

11. Hamblin TJ, Davis Z, Gardiner A et al. Unmutated Ig V(H) genes are associated with a more aggressive form of chronic lymphocytic leukemia. Blood 1999;94:1848–1854

12. Tamburini A, Suppo G, Battaglia A et al. Clinical significance of CD38 expression in chronic lymphocytic leukemia. Blood 2001;98:2633–2639

13. Ibrahim S, Keating M, Do KA et al. CD38 expression as an important prognostic factor in B-cell chronic lymphocytic leukemia. Blood 2001;98:181–186

14. Oscier DG, Gardiner AC, Mould SJ et al. Multivariate analysis of prognostic factors in CLL: clinical stage, IGVH gene mutational status, and loss or mutation of the p53 gene are independent prognostic factors. Blood 2002;100:1177–1184

15. Crespo M, Bosch F, Villamor N et al. ZAP-70 expression as a surrogate for immunoglobulin-variable-region mutations in chronic lymphocytic leukemia. N Engl J Med 2003;348:1764–1775

16. Rassenti LZ, Huynh L, Toy TL et al. ZAP-70 compared with immunoglobulin heavy-chain gene mutation status as a predictor of disease progression in chronic lymphocytic leukemia. N Engl J Med 2004;351:893–901

17. Orchard JA, Ibbotson RE, Davis Z et al. ZAP-70 expression and prognosis in chronic lymphocytic leukemia. Lancet 2004;363:105–111

18. Johnson S, Smith AG, Loffler H et al. Multicentre prospective randomized trial of fludarabine versus cyclophosphamide, doxorubicin, and prednisone (CAP) for treatment of advanced-stage chronic lymphocytic leukemia. The French Cooperative Group on CLL. Lancet 1996;347:1432–1438

19. Rai KR, Peterson BL, Appelbaum FR et al. Fludarabine compared with chlorambucil as primary therapy for chronic lymphocytic leukemia. N Engl J Med 2000;343:1750–1757

20. Leporrier M, Chevret S, Cazin B et al. Randomized comparison of fludarabine, CAP, and ChOP in 938 previously untreated stage B and C chronic lymphocytic leukemia patients. Blood 2001;98:2319–2325

21. Eichhorst BF, Busch R, Hopfinger G et al. Fludarabine plus cyclophosphamide versus fludarabine alone in first-line therapy of younger patients with chronic lymphocytic leukemia. Blood 2006;107:885–891

22. Grever MR, Lucas DM, Dewald GW et al. Comprehensive assessment of genetic and molecular features predicting outcome in patients with chronic lymphocytic leukemia: results from the US Intergroup Phase III Trial E2997. J Clin Oncol 2007;25:799–804

23. Byrd JC, Rai K, Peterson BL et al. Addition of rituximab to fludarabine may prolong progression-free survival and overall survival in patients with previously untreated chronic lymphocytic leukemia: an updated retrospective comparative analysis of CALGB 9712 and CALGB 9011. Blood 2005;105:49–53

24. Keating MJ, O'Brien S, Albitar M et al. Early results of a chemoimmunotherapy regimen of fludarabine, cyclophosphamide, and rituximab as initial therapy for chronic lymphocytic leukemia. J Clin Oncol 2005;23:4079–4088

25. Wierda W, O'Brien S, Wen S et al. Chemoimmunotherapy with fludarabine, cyclophosphamide, and rituximab for relapsed and refractory chronic lymphocytic leukemia. J Clin Oncol 2005;23:4070–4078

26. Dohner H, Fischer K, Bentz M et al. p53 gene deletion predicts for poor survival and non-response to therapy with purine analogs in chronic B-cell leukemias. Blood 1995;85:1580–1589

27. Keating MJ, O'Brien S, Kontoyiannis D et al. Results of first salvage therapy for patients refractory to a fludarabine regimen in chronic lymphocytic leukemia. Leuk Lymphoma 2002;43:1755–1762

28. Keating MJ, Flinn I, Jain V et al. Therapeutic role of alemtuzumab (Campath-1H) in patients who have failed fludarabine: results of a large international study. Blood 2002;99:3554–3561

29. Stilgenbauer S, Dohner H. Campath-1H-induced complete remission of chronic lymphocytic leukemia despite p53 gene mutation and resistance to chemotherapy. N Engl J Med 2002;347:452–453

30. Lozanski G, Heerema NA, Flinn IW et al. Alemtuzumab is an effective therapy for chronic lymphocytic leukemia with p53 mutations and deletions. Blood 2004;103:3278–3281

31. Kennedy B, Rawstron A, Carter C et al. Campath-1H and fludarabine in combination are highly active in refractory chronic lymphocytic leukemia. Blood 2002;99:2245–2247

32. Elter T, Borchmann P, Schulz H et al. Fludarabine in combination with alemtuzumab is effective and feasible in patients with relapsed or refractory B-cell chronic lymphocytic leukemia: results of a phase II trial. J Clin Oncol 2005;23:7024–7031

33. Wendtner CM, Ritgen M, Schweighofer CD et al. Consolidation with alemtuzumab in patients with chronic lymphocytic leukemia (CLL) in first remission – experience on safety and efficacy within a randomized multicenter phase III trial of the German CLL Study Group (GCLLSG). Leukemia 2004;18:1093–1101

34. Montillo M, Tedeschi A, Rossi V et al. Successful CD34+ cell mobilization by intermediate-dose Ara-C in chronic lymphocytic leukemia patients treated with sequential fludarabine and Campath-1H. Leukemia 2004;18:57–62

35. Montserrat E, Gomis F, Vallespi T et al. Presenting features and prognosis of chronic lymphocytic leukemia in younger adults. Blood 1991;78:1545–1551

36. Dreger P, Corradini P, Kimby E et al. Indications for allogeneic stem cell transplantation in chronic lymphocytic leukemia: the EBMT transplant consensus. Leukemia 2007;21:12–17

37. Dreger P, Stilgenbauer S, Benner A et al. The prognostic impact of autologous stem cell transplantation in patients with chronic lymphocytic leukemia: a risk-matched analysis based on the VH gene mutational status. Blood 2004;103:2850–2858

38. Rabinowe SN, Soiffer RJ, Gribben JG et al. Autologous and allogeneic bone marrow transplantation for poor prognosis patients with B-cell chronic lymphocytic leukemia. Blood 1993;82:1366–1376

39. Khouri IF, Keating MJ, Vriesendorp HM et al. Autologous and allogeneic bone marrow transplantation for chronic lymphocytic leukemia: preliminary results. J Clin Oncol 1994;12:748–758

40. Itala M, Pelliniemi TT, Rajamaki A, Remes K. Autologous blood cell transplantation in B-CLL: response to chemotherapy prior to mobilization predicts the stem cell yield. Bone Marrow Transplant 1997;19:647–651

41. Dreger P, von Neuhoff N, Kuse R et al. Early stem cell transplantation for chronic lymphocytic leukemia: a chance for cure? Br J Cancer 1998;77:2291–2297

42. Pavletic ZS, Bierman PJ, Vose JM et al. High incidence of relapse after autologous stem-cell transplantation for B-cell chronic lymphocytic leukemia or small lymphocytic lymphoma. Ann Oncol 1998;9:1023–1026

43. Milligan DW, Fernandes S, Dasgupta R et al. Results of the MRC pilot study show autografting for younger patients with chronic lymphocytic leukemia is safe and achieves a high percentage of molecular responses. Blood 2005;105:397–404

44. Gribben JG, Zahrieh D, Stephans K et al. Autologous and allogeneic stem cell transplantation for poor risk chronic lymphocytic leukemia. Blood 2005;106:4389–4396

45. Jantunen E, Itala M, Siitonen T et al. Autologous stem cell transplantation in patients with chronic lymphocytic leukemia: the Finnish experience. Bone Marrow Transplant 2006;37:1093–1098

46. Ritgen M, Lange A, Stilgenbauer S et al. Unmutated immunoglobulin variable heavy-chain gene status remains an adverse prognostic factor after autologous stem cell transplantation for chronic lymphocytic leukemia. Blood 2003;101:2049–2053

47. Ritgen M, Stilgenbauer S, von Neuhoff N et al. Graft-versus-leukemia activity may overcome therapeutic resistance of chronic lymphocytic leukemia with unmutated immunoglobulin variable heavy-chain gene status: implications of minimal residual disease measurement with quantitative PCR. Blood 2004;104:2600–2602

48. Moreno C, Villamor N, Colomer D et al. Allogeneic stem-cell transplantation may overcome the adverse prognosis of unmutated VH gene in patients with chronic lymphocytic leukemia. J Clin Oncol 2005;23:3433–3438

49. Sala R, Mauro FR, Bellucci R et al. Evaluation of marrow and blood hemopoietic progenitors in chronic lymphocytic leukemia before and after chemotherapy. Eur J Hematol 1998;61:14–20

50. Michallet M, Thiebaut A, Dreger P et al. Peripheral blood stem cell (PBSC) mobilization and transplantation after fludarabine therapy in chronic lymphocytic leukemia (CLL):

a report of the European Blood and Marrow Transplantation (EBMT) CLL subcommittee on behalf of the EBMT Chronic Leukemias Working Party (CLWP). Br J Haematol 2000;108:595–601

51. Dreger P, Montserrat E. Autologous and allogeneic stem cell transplantation for chronic lymphocytic leukemia. Leukemia 2002;16:985–992

52. Rawstron AC, Kennedy B, Evans PA et al. Quantitation of minimal disease levels in chronic lymphocytic leukemia using a sensitive flow cytometric assay improves the prediction of outcome and can be used to optimize therapy. Blood 2001;98:29–35

53. Provan D, Bartlett-Pandite L, Zwicky C et al. Eradication of polymerase chain reaction-detectable chronic lymphocytic leukemia cells is associated with improved outcome after bone marrow transplantation. Blood 1996;88:2228–2235

54. Schey S, Ahsan G, Jones R. Dose intensification and molecular responses in patients with chronic lymphocytic leukemia: a phase II single centre study. Bone Marrow Transplant 1999;24:989–993

55. Schultze JL, Donovan JW, Gribben JG. Minimal residual disease detection after myeloablative chemotherapy in chronic lymphatic leukemia. J Mol Med 1999;77:259–265

56. Zenz T, Ritgen M, Dreger P et al. Autologous graft-versus-host disease-like syndrome after an alemtuzumab-containing conditioning regimen and autologous stem cell transplantation for chronic lymphocytic leukemia. Blood 2006;108:2127–2130

57. Montillo M, Tedeschi A, Miqueleiz S et al. Alemtuzumab as consolidation after a response to fludarabine is effective in purging residual disease in patients with chronic lymphocytic leukemia. J Clin Oncol 2006;24:2337–2342

58. Michallet M, Corront B, Hollard D et al. Allogeneic bone marrow transplantation in chronic lymphocytic leukemia: report from the European Cooperative Group for bone marrow transplantation (8 cases). Nouv Rev Fr Hematol 1988;30:467–470

59. Michallet M, Archimbaud E, Bandini G et al. HLA-identical sibling bone marrow transplantation in younger patients with chronic lymphocytic leukemia. European Group for blood and marrow transplantation and the International bone marrow transplant registry. Ann Intern Med 1996;124:311–315

60. Khouri I, Champlin R. Allogenic bone marrow transplantation in chronic lymphocytic leukemia. Ann Intern Med 1996;125:780–787

61. Pavletic ZS, Arrowsmith ER, Bierman PJ et al. Outcome of allogeneic stem cell transplantation for B cell chronic lymphocytic leukemia. Bone Marrow Transplant 2000;25:717–722

62. Doney KC, Chauncey T, Appelbaum FR. Allogeneic related donor hematopoietic stem cell transplantation for treatment of chronic lymphocytic leukemia. Bone Marrow Transplant 2002;29:817–823

63. Toze CL, Galal A, Barnett MJ et al. Myeloablative allografting for chronic lymphocytic leukemia: evidence for a potent graft-versus-leukemia effect associated with graft-versus-host disease. Bone Marrow Transplant 2005;36:825–830

64. Rondon G, Giralt S, Huh Y et al. Graft-versus-leukemia effect after allogeneic bone marrow transplantation for chronic lymphocytic leukemia. Bone Marrow Transplant 1996;18:669–672

65. deMagalhaes-Silverman M, Donnenberg A, Hammert L et al. Induction of graft-versus-leukemia effect in a patient with chronic lymphocytic leukemia. Bone Marrow Transplant 1997;20:175–177

66. Pavletic SZ, Khouri IF, Haagenson M et al. Unrelated donor marrow transplantation for B-cell chronic lymphocytic leukemia after using myeloablative conditioning: results from the Center for International Blood and Marrow Transplant research. J Clin Oncol 2005;23:5788–5794

67. Horowitz M, Montserrat E, Sobocinski K et al. Hemopoietic stem cell transplantation for chronic lymphocytic leukemia. Blood 2000;96(suppl 1):522a

68. Khouri IF, Przepiorka D, van Besien K et al. Allogeneic blood or marrow transplantation for chronic lymphocytic leukemia: timing of transplantation and potential effect of fludarabine on acute graft-versus-host disease. Br J Haematol 1997;97:466–473

69. Schetelig J, Thiede C, Bornhauser M et al. Reduced non-relapse mortality after reduced intensity conditioning in advanced chronic lymphocytic leukemia. Ann Hematol 2002;81(suppl 2):S47–48

70. Schetelig J, Thiede C, Bornhauser M et al. Evidence of a graft-versus-leukemia effect in chronic lymphocytic leukemia after reduced-intensity conditioning and allogeneic stem-cell transplantation: the Cooperative German Transplant Study Group. J Clin Oncol 2003;21:2747–2753

71. Khouri IF, Keating M, Korbling M et al. Transplant-lite: induction of graft-versus-malignancy using fludarabine-based nonablative chemotherapy and allogeneic blood progenitor cell transplantation as treatment for lymphoid malignancies. J Clin Oncol 1998;16:2817–2824

72. Khouri IF, Saliba RM, Giralt SA et al. Nonablative allogeneic hematopoietic transplantation as adoptive immunotherapy for indolent lymphoma: low incidence of toxicity, acute graft-versus-host disease, and treatment-related mortality. Blood 2001;98:3595–3599

73. Dreger P, Brand R, Hansz J et al. Treatment-related mortality and graft-versus-leukemia activity after allogeneic stem cell transplantation for chronic lymphocytic leukemia using intensity-reduced conditioning. Leukemia 2003;17:841–848

74. Sorror ML, Maris MB, Sandmaier BM et al. Hematopoietic cell transplantation after non-myeloablative conditioning for advanced chronic lymphocytic leukemia. J Clin Oncol 2005;23(16):3819–3829

75. Brown JR, Kim HT, Li S et al. Predictors of improved progression-free survival after non-myeloablative allogeneic stem cell transplantation for advanced chronic lymphocytic leukemia. Biol Blood Marrow Transplant 2006;12:1056–1064

76. Dreger P, Brand R, Milligan D et al. Reduced-intensity conditioning lowers treatment-related mortality of allogeneic stem cell transplantation for chronic lymphocytic leukemia: a population-matched analysis. Leukemia 2005;19:1029–1033

77. Hertzberg M, Grigg A, Gottlieb D et al. Reduced-intensity allogeneic hemopoietic stem cell transplantation induces durable responses in patients with chronic B-lymphoproliferative disorders. Bone Marrow Transplant 2006;37:923–928

78. Morris E, Thomson K, Craddock C et al. Outcomes after alemtuzumab-containing reduced-intensity allogeneic transplantation regimen for relapsed and refractory non-Hodgkin lymphoma. Blood 2004;104:3865–3871

79. Delgado J, Thomson K, Russell N et al. Results of alemtuzumab-based reduced-intensity allogeneic transplantation for chronic lymphocytic leukemia: a British Society of Blood and Marrow Transplantation Study. Blood 2006;107:1724–1730

80. Caballero D, Garcia-Marco JA, Martino R et al. Allogeneic transplant with reduced intensity conditioning regimens may overcome the poor prognosis of B-cell chronic lymphocytic leukemia with unmutated immunoglobulin variable heavy-chain gene and chromosomal abnormalities (11q- and 17p-). Clin Cancer Res 2005;11:7757–7763

81. Sutton L, Maloum K, Gonzalez H et al. Autologous hematopoietic stem cell transplantation as salvage treatment for advanced B cell chronic lymphocytic leukemia. Leukemia 1998;12:1699–1707

82. Khouri IF. Reduced-intensity regimens in allogeneic stem-cell transplantation for non-Hodgkin lymphoma and chronic lymphocytic leukemia. Hematology Am Soc Hematol Educ Program 2006:390–397

Solid tumors in children

Lochie Teague and Robin P Corbett

CHAPTER

11

Introduction

Over the last 40 years there have been dramatic improvements in the survival of children with most forms of cancer, but there are groups of childhood malignancy that remain difficult to cure with contemporary chemotherapy. Data from European and North American registries have helped to find a small group of children and young people for whom high-dose therapy (HDT) and stem cell transplant (SCT) can improve the chances of cure. While ongoing studies will continue to help optimize prognostic factors in patient selection, it is becoming clear that novel therapeutic approaches rather than HDT with SCT are required for the majority of patients with high-risk disease. Some of these new therapeutic approaches may be incorporated in combination with HDT and SCT.

This chapter will review the role of transplantation for each of the major solid tumors encountered in pediatric oncology.

Embryonal tumors

Neuroblastoma

Neuroblastoma is a malignancy originating from the embryonic neural crest cells that originally formed the adrenal medulla and peripheral sympathetic ganglia. Most tumors (approximately two-thirds) occur within the abdomen. Metastatic disease at time of diagnosis may be as high as 75%, and circulating tumor cells can also be detected in the blood in up to 50% of children with International Neuroblastoma Staging System (INSS – see below) stage 4 neuroblastoma at diagnosis.[1–3]

Neuroblastoma is the most common extracranial solid tumor in children, accounting for 8–10% of all childhood cancers with a median age at diagnosis of about 19 months. At diagnosis, 36% of patients are under 1 year, 89% under 5 years and 98% under 10 years. Neuroblastoma is clearly a diagnosis chiefly of infancy and early childhood.

Over time it has become clear that there is huge genetic heterogeneity. There is a propensity to differentiation either spontaneously or with various stimuli. Many genetic features in neuroblastoma have now been identified that correlate with clinical outcome. Widely accepted tumor characteristics at diagnosis are now incorporated into staging and risk classification used in the management of patients with neuroblastoma.

Most centers around the world use the surgical staging system, the International Neuroblastoma Staging System (INSS)[4] (Table 11.1).

The Children's Oncology Group and other co-operative groups have defined risk groups for suggested treatment assignment using the most widely validated and readily available markers (Table 11.2).[5]

The prognosis for low- and intermediate-risk patients is >90% and <80%, respectively, with current therapeutic approaches. Unfortunately, approximately 50% of patients over 1 year of age will be in the high-risk category. Until the last decade or so, the survival for this group was <15%. The most recent Phase III studies have now seen improvement in survival rates to 30–40% utilizing intensive induction chemotherapy, consolidation with high-dose chemotherapy and autologous stem cell transplant and therapy for minimal residual disease incorporating radiation therapy to tumor sites and non-cytotoxic agents (e.g. differentiating agents such as cis-retinoic acid).

Neuroblastoma is one of the few pediatric solid tumors in which there have been randomized studies to address the outcome of chemotherapy versus myeloablative therapy. The first randomized study performed by the European Neuroblastoma Study Group (ENSG)[6] between 1983 and 1985 in a relatively small number of patients (only 50% of 84 eligible stage IV patients randomized) demonstrated a moderate survival advantage to those who received the high-dose melphalan therapy. A larger Children's Cancer Group Phase III study[7] enrolling a total of 434 stage IV neuroblastoma patients between 1991 and 1996 showed a significantly better survival rate of 34% ± 4% 3-year event-free survival (EFS) in 189 patients who underwent a transplant, compared with 22% ± 4% EFS in those who received continuation chemotherapy. Importantly, a second randomization in the study, to test the value of 13 cis-retinoic acid, found this agent to improve EFS in both transplant and continued chemotherapy groups.

A successor study A3973 by the Children's Oncology Group opened in 2001 and recently closed to accrual. This was a randomized study of purged versus unpurged peripheral blood stem cell transplant following dose-intensive induction therapy for high-risk neuroblastoma. This study employed multiple monoclonal antibodies and magnetic beads to purify the stem cell graft ex vivo of neuroblastoma tumor cells. This manipulation was performed at only two centers during the study. The results of the study are still awaited. Another COG Phase III randomized study is comparing anti-GD2 antibody with cytokines plus 13 cis-retinoic acid with 13 cis-retinoic acid alone for patients in remission post stem cell transplant.

The rationale for purging the autologous product by either CD34+ stem cell selection or by monoclonal antibody or immunomagnetic beads has come from earlier evidence demonstrating that tumor cell contamination in the graft could contribute to relapse in children with neuroblastoma.[8,9] Even after 3 months of induction chemotherapy with marked reduction in circulating neuroblastoma tumor cells, contamination can be demonstrated in 25% of bone marrow samples and 7% of blood samples.[2] The efficacy of in vivo purging has been shown to correlate with EFS such that patients with >0.1 tumor cells in bone marrow at the end of induction have a poor outcome.

The optimal transplant conditioning regimen is yet to be determined. The European group of the International Society of Pediatric Oncology (SIOP) is comparing two different high-dose myeloablative regimens, based on preliminary data suggesting an advantage for busulfan/melphalan compared to the carboplatin, etoposide and melphalan regimen. The busulfan/melphalan approach (Table 11.3) may be less toxic and is also being used in the current Ewing's trials.

Further support for the role of megatherapy in autologous bone marrow transplant comes from a third randomized study[10] which enrolled 339 high-risk neuroblastoma patients in Germany and Switzerland between 1997 and 2002. This study compared myeloablative chemotherapy (melphalan, etoposide and carboplatin) with autologous stem cell transplant to oral maintenance chemotherapy with cyclophosphamide. The investigators showed, on an 'intention to treat' basis, that patients allocated megatherapy had an increased 3-year EFS compared with those on maintenance chemotherapy (47% (95% confidence interval (CI) 38–55) vs 31% (95% CI 23–39); hazard ratio (HR) 1.404 (95% CI 1.048–1.881), p =0.221), but did not have a significantly increased 3-year overall survival (OS) (62% (95% CI 54–70) vs 53% (95% CI 45–62); HR 1.329 (95% CI 0.958–1.843), p =0.0875).

Strategies utilizing the theoretical advantage of using non-cross resistant combinations of high-dose therapy with stem cell support have been tried and demonstrate the feasibility and safety of this approach in pilot and single institution studies.[11,12,13] However, randomized studies comparing single with double myeloablative regimens are awaited. Of concern has been the report of an increased incidence of the Epstein–Barr virus (EBV) lymphoproliferative disorder in children undergoing tandem transplants using autologous CD34 selected peripheral blood stem cells.[14]

Allogeneic bone marrow transplantation has also been utilized, although outcomes are not statistically different than with autologous bone marrow transplant.[15] This is presumably due to a relative lack of graft versus tumor effect in this disease (similarly for other pediatric solid tumors) and, due to greater morbidity and mortality of allograft bone marrow, this is not recommended.[16–22]

While the role of total-body irradiation (TBI) has not been well defined, as both TBI-containing and non-TBI containing regimens have been utilized in transplants for neuroblastoma, some TBI has been associated with many significant late effects in this age group of patients.[23–25] No current high-dose treatment regimens presently employ TBI in stem cell transplant for neuroblastoma.

In summary, high-dose therapy with autologous stem cell transplant support can certainly increase the proportion of patients surviving a high-risk neuroblastoma and is at present regarded as part of standard therapy for such patients. Long-term survival is still generally less than 40%, with less than 10% of those patients experiencing relapse

Table 11.1 International Neuroblastoma Staging System[4]

Stage	Definition
1	Localized tumor with complete gross excision, with or without microscopic residual disease; representative ipsilateral lymph nodes negative for tumor microscopically
2A	Localized tumor with incomplete gross excision; representative ipsilateral lymph nodes negative for tumor microscopically
2B	Localized tumor with or without complete gross excision, with ipsilateral lymph nodes positive for tumor. Enlarged contralateral lymph nodes must be negative microscopically
3	Unresectable unilateral tumor infiltrating across the midline, with or without regional lymph node involvement; or localized unilateral tumor with contralateral regional lymph node involvement; or midline tumor with bilateral extension by infiltration (unresectable) or by lymph node involvement
4	Any primary tumor with dissemination to distant lymph nodes, bone, bone marrow, liver and other organs (except as defined for stage 4S)
4S	Localized primary tumor (as defined as stage 1, 2A or 2B), in patient <1 year, with dissemination limited to skin, liver and/or bone marrow (marrow involvement should be minimal with malignant cells <10% of total nucleated cells)

Table 11.2 Neuroblastoma risk classification[5]

INSS	Age (days)	*MYCN*	Histology	Ploidy	Risk
1	Any	Any	Any	Any	Low
2A/2B	<365	Any	Any	Any	Low
	≥365	Non-amplified	Any	–	Low
	≥365	Amplified	FH	–	Low
	≥365	Amplified	UH	–	High
3	<365	Non-amplified	Any	Any	Intermediate
	<365	Amplified	Any	Any	High
	≥365	Non-amplified	FH	–	Intermediate
	≥365	Non-amplified	UH	–	High
	≥365	Non-amplified	Any	–	High
4	<365	Non-amplified	Any	Any	Intermediate
	<365	Amplified	Any	Any	High
	≥365	Any	Any	–	High
4S	<365	Non-amplified	FH	DI > 1	Low
	<365	Non-amplified	FH	DI = 1	Intermediate
	<365	Non-amplified	UH	Any	Intermediate
	<365	Amplified	Any	Any	High

Table 11.3 Busulfan-melphalan (Bu-Mel) regime

		D-7	D-6	D-5	D-4	D-3	D-2	D-1	D-0
Busulfan per os (po) 37.7 mg/m²/dose	0 h		X	X	X	X			
=150 mg/m²/d (4 divided doses per day)	6 h		X	X	X	X			
=600 mg/m² cumulative dose	12 h		X	X	X	X			
	18 h		X	X	X	X			
Melphalan iv 140 mg/m² iv infusion, 30 min							X		
Clonazepam po, iv 0.025–0.1 mg/kg/d		X	X	X	X	X	X	X	
Stem cell reinfusion min. 3 × 10⁶/kg CD34									X

NOTE: In patients ≥60 kg body weight, calculate dosage by kg BW, not m² BSA: cumulative dose 16 mg/kg, 16 divided doses, 1 mg/kg BW/dose, 4 daily doses over 4 days.
CONTRAINDICATIONS for Bu-Mel high-dose therapy: any patient who has received radiotherapy to central axial sites (e.g. chest, pelvis) is ineligible for busulfan high-dose therapy for reasons of anticipated toxicity.

or refractory disease being salvaged with any further therapy. Clearly, novel agents are required to treat this disease and a variety of different approaches, some incorporated with high-dose therapy, are presently in Phase I and II studies with the Neuroblastoma Therapy Consortium (NANT) and other co-operative groups. It is hoped that insights gained into the molecular pathogenesis of neuroblastoma will pave the way for more targeted molecular approaches that hold the promise not only of greater cure rates, but also less morbidity and mortality from both long- and short-term side-effects of current therapeutic approaches.

Wilms' tumor

Wilms' tumor has an incidence of approximately 6% of all childhood cancers and fortunately, due to a contemporary multimodality therapy either from SIOP or from NWTS approaches, dramatic improvements in survival rates have been demonstrated, which are now approaching 90%.[26,27] Approximately 15% of patients with favorable histology Wilms' tumor and 50% of patients with anaplastic Wilms' tumor experience relapse. Most recurrences occur within 2 years of diagnosis. However, survival for patients with recurrent disease is <30%,[28,29] particularly patients with heavy pretreatment, unfavorable histology and advanced stage at time of relapse or who have an early relapse (<12 months since diagnosis).

In the small numbers of patients treated with high-dose chemotherapy followed by stem cell transplant, the reported results have been sufficiently encouraging to promote consideration of this therapy in high-risk recurrent Wilms' tumor patients with chemoresponsive disease. Garaventa et al[30] for the European Bone Marrow Transplant Registry for Solid Tumors have published the reported outcomes on 25 resistant or relapsed Wilms' tumor patients who underwent therapy with high-dose chemotherapy followed by autologous bone marrow transplant (ABMT) between 1984 and 1991. Although seven different regimens were used, most included high-dose melphalan. Of 17 patients treated after achieving complete remission (CR) with salvage therapy, eight remained in continuous remission for a median of 34 months. However, only one of the eight patients treated with measurable disease at the time of transplant became a long-term survivor. Transplant-related mortality included three deaths due to *Pneumocystis*, which is generally higher than reported in more contemporary transplant studies.

Pein et al,[31] in the report for the French Society of Pediatric Oncology, reviewed 29 patients with high-risk recurrent Wilms' tumor who received treatment with high-dose chemotherapy followed by autologous stem cell rescue between 1994 and 1998. All patients had chemosensitive disease defined as having achieved complete or partial response with salvage chemotherapy, and 20 patients were entered into the study after their first recurrence. Consolidation chemotherapy consisted of melphalan, etoposide and carboplatin. Despite significant treatment-related toxicity, 12 patients remained in continuous CR at a median of 48.5 months.[36–96] The disease-free survival and overall survival at 3 years were 50% (±17%) and 60% (±18%), respectively. Patients treated after their first recurrence (second CR or partial remission (PR)) had a significantly better outcome than patients treated after their second recurrence, with a 3-year disease-free survival of 63.15% (±20%) versus 22.2% (±24%).

From April 1992 to December 1998, 23 patients with relapsed Wilms' tumor received high-dose chemotherapy followed by autologous stem cell rescue according to the German Co-operative Wilms' Tumor Study, as reported by Kremens et al.[32] Chemotherapy consisted of melphalan, etoposide and carboplatin, like the French study mentioned above. Ten of 13 patients transplanted in complete remission remain alive and free of disease, while only two of the 10 patients transplanted in partial response remain alive and free of disease. After

a median follow-up of 58 months[37–116] the EFS was 48.2% ±13.6% and the overall survival was 60.9% ±10.2%.

In both these studies it is important to note that most patients had chemosensitive disease involving only the lungs and were transplanted in complete remission. The patients with progressive disease did not receive high-dose stem cell therapy with transplant as part of consolidation therapy.

Tannous et al[33] have reported on the treatment of 66 patients with high-risk relapsed Wilms' tumor with chemotherapy consisting of two cycles of cyclophosphamide and etoposide (CE) followed by two cycles of carboplatin and etoposide (PE). Patients who achieved complete response of the tumor received maintenance therapy with five cycles of alternating CE and PE, while those with partial response or stable disease received ablative chemotherapy followed by ABMT. The 3-year EFS was 59% (±9%) and 40% (±14%) for the maintenance and ABMT subgroups, while 3-year OS was 64% (±8%) and 42% (±14%), respectively.

Most patients having a transplant for recurrent Wilms' tumor will only have a single remaining kidney and it is important to adjust the dosage of the nephrotoxic agents as appropriate. For example, carboplatin is typically adjusted to the individual glomerular filtration rate based on the formula defined by Calvert et al.[34]

High-dose chemotherapy (HDC) with stem cell transplantation has not been conclusively proven to be more effective or less toxic than second-line chemotherapy for patients with recurrent Wilms' tumor. However, the above studies suggest a possible improved survival with this therapeutic approach, with survival rates of between 36% and 73% for patients who achieve a good response to reinduction chemotherapy. The hypothesis that high-dose chemotherapy with stem cell transplant is superior is now the basis for a proposed Phase III randomized study within the Children's Oncology Group and this trial should help to clarify the role of high-dose chemotherapy with stem cell transplant for patients with relapsed Wilms' tumor.

Retinoblastoma

This rare pediatric malignancy occurs in about 1:18,000 live births; despite this, it is the most common eye cancer in childhood. The median age at diagnosis is 2 years. A significant proportion of patients harbor constitutional mutations or deletions in the RB1 and have hereditary retinoblastoma:

- 75% have unilateral disease – 15% of these have hereditary retinoblastoma
- 25% have bilateral disease – all have hereditary retinoblastoma.
Hereditary retinoblastoma is inherited in an autosomal recessive fashion with 90% penetrance.

Localized unilateral disease is usually treated with enucleation whereas localized bilateral disease is nowadays treated using combination chemotherapy and local ocular treatment such as laser therapy. The prognosis for such patients in terms of overall survival is excellent. A minority of children either present or relapse with extraocular metastatic disease involving one or more of bone marrow, bone, lymph nodes, liver or CNS. Studies have shown that such disease is often chemosensitive but survival is poor using conventional doses of chemotherapy.[35,36] However, relatively small studies consolidating treatment with HDC and autologous SCT (ASCT) have shown particularly promising results for that subgroup of children with metastatic disease *not* involving the CNS (Table 11.4).

Results of hematopoietic stem cell transplant (HSCT) in children with CNS metastases are not encouraging. In order to prospectively study the cohort of retinoblastoma patients with distant metastases, the United States Children's Oncology Group currently has an open trial in which high-dose carboplatin, thiotepa and etoposide with ASCT are delivered following courses of conventional chemotherapy.

Table 11.4 Results of studies reporting HDC with ASCT for metastatic retinoblastoma not involving the CNS[37,38]

Number of patients	Conditioning regimen	Number surviving (%)
11	Etoposide + carboplatin + cyclophosphamide	5 (45%) disease-free survival at 3 years
8	Carboplatin (C) + thiotepa (T) = 1 patient C + T + etoposide = 4 patients C + T + topotecan = 3 patients	7 (88%) event-free survival at 7 years
4	Carboplatin + etoposide = 1 Busulfan + cyclophosphamide + melphalan = 1 Cyclophosphamide + etoposide = 1 Cyclophosphamide + topotecan = 1	2 (50%) disease-free >6 years

Hepatoblastoma

This tumor comprises 1% of pediatric malignancies with onset usually between 6 months and 3 years of age.[40] Most cases present with disease localized to the liver; treatment comprises multiagent chemotherapy and surgery, and the prognosis is relatively optimistic. Approximately 20% present with disease metastatic to the lungs and/or lymph nodes, occasionally involving the CNS. In these cases, the outlook is extremely guarded. Data on HDC with ASCT in metastatic hepatoblastoma are scanty. However, Nishimura et al[41] treated three such patients using a variety of high-dose combinations (including etoposide, doxorubicin, platinum agents and 5-FU); all three remain alive without disease at the time of reporting. Hepatoblastoma is a chemosensitive embryonal tumor; further investigation of the role of HDC with ASCT may be warranted in high-risk disease.

Sarcoma

Ewing's sarcoma and primitive neuroectodermal tumors (PNET)

Ewing's sarcoma is the second most common indication for hematopoietic stem cell transplant after neuroblastoma. The Ewing's sarcoma and primitive neuroectodermal tumor (PNET) family are defined molecularly by the expression of the cell surface glycoprotein MIC-2 and the presence of a reciprocal translocation t(11;22)(q24;q12) that results in fusion of EWS with an *ets* family transcription factor, fli-I. Staging procedures as presently applied identify 20–25% of cases as metastatic at diagnosis. Survival with conventional chemotherapeutic approaches now results in 55–65% disease-free survival for localized disease, but patients with primary metastatic disease have only approximately 20% disease-free survival with few survivors if patients have bone and bone marrow metastases. Kushner[42] reported that patients with primary pulmonary metastases fared better than patients with primary bone marrow involvement. These findings are comparable to experience from earlier CESS and EICESS studies.[43–45] Most transplant preparative regimens have incorporated melphalan alone or busulfan/melphalan. More recent reported results, even with decreased transplant-related mortality incorporating tandem transplants, have failed to significantly improve results of earlier studies, with EFS rates ranging from 29% to 39%.[45–47]

Just as with neuroblastoma, tumor cells frequently contaminate stem cell harvests of Ewing's sarcoma patients and their presence following transplantation is associated with relapse.[48,49]

Updated results from the 1995 EBMT Solid Tumor Registry reported EFS at around 25% and 20% in patients who received an autologous or allogeneic stem cell transplant, respectively. There is little support for a graft-versus-Ewing's tumor effect being an effective

mechanism to further explore allogeneic stem cell transplantation in this disease.[50]

There have been small case series suggesting improved results for poor prognosis and recurrent disease[42–44,50–54] but results need to be interpreted with caution due to small numbers of patients and use of more intensive pretransplant therapy, and patients with bulky or aggressive disease during chemotherapy have been excluded from some of these analyses. 'Intention to treat' analyses are lacking.

A large Phase III Intergroup study of the European Ewing's Tumor Working Initiative of the National Group's Ewing's Tumor Studies 1999 (Euro-EWING99) is currently open and accruing patients with the objective of comparing, in a randomized trial, VAI (vincristine, dactinomycin, ifosphamide) consolidation chemotherapy with high-dose therapy (busulfan/melphalan) and peripheral blood stem cell rescue, (a) in patients with non-metastatic Ewing's sarcoma and poor physiologic response to standard induction VIDE (vincristine, ifosphamide, doxorubicin, etoposide) chemotherapy and (b) in patients with localized Ewing tumor ≥200 ml in volume. In a second objective, a randomized trial of VAI consolidation chemotherapy with whole lung irradiation is being compared to high-dose therapy (busulfan/melphalan) and peripheral blood progenitor cell (PBPC) rescue in patients with pulmonary or pleural metastases at diagnosis. The COG in 2003 began collaborating in the protocol for patients with isolated pulmonary metastases. The outcome of these trials is awaited with interest and should address the question of the role of high-dose therapy with stem cell support in Ewing's sarcoma.

Due to the inherent risks of high-dose chemotherapy and stem cell transplant, high-dose chemotherapy with stem cell transplant in the treatment of Ewing's sarcoma is presently only recommended in the context of a controlled clinical trial.

Novel therapeutic approaches are likely to be required to significantly improve outcomes for high-risk patients and even more so for those who experience relapse. Ewing's sarcoma patients for whom disease recurs usually have a fatal outcome even with high-dose therapy and stem cell transplant.[55,56]

Rhabdomyosarcoma

Rhabdomyosarcoma (RMS) is the most common soft tissue sarcoma in childhood, accounting for 8% of malignancies in this age group.[57] Multimodality treatment (chemotherapy, surgery and, in many cases, radiotherapy) has resulted in cure rates >75% for children with non-metastatic RMS. Unfortunately, for those who present with metastases or relapse, only 20–30% survive. The outlook for patients >10 years old with metastatic disease at diagnosis, or those of any age with involvement of the bones and/or bone marrow, is particularly poor. In an attempt to improve cure rates for this cohort, HDC with ASCT has been trialed following conventional chemotherapy. Weigel et al[58] analyzed the results of 22 published studies reporting on ASCT in RMS. The most commonly used conditioning agents were melphalan (44%), cyclophosphamide (40%) and thiotepa (24%); TBI was used in 28% of regimens. Results are shown in Table 11.5.

These results are not superior to those obtained using conventional chemotherapy. The largest single study published reported on 52 patients who received HDC and ASCT after six courses of conventional chemotherapy.[59] This cohort was compared with 44 patients who received 12 courses of conventional chemotherapy in place of HDC. The authors concluded that HDC may have prolonged progression-free survival but did not influence overall survival. It may be concluded that there is no convincing evidence in support of the role of HDC with ASCT in RMS. No randomized trial has been performed. Allogeneic transplantation is ineffective.[60] The major children's cancer study groups are currently investigating novel strategies to improve response rates in high-risk RMS.

Table 11.5 Outcome after HDC and ASCT in high-risk rhabdomyosarcoma[57]

Timing of HDC	Number of patients	EFS	OS
1st complete remission or 1st partial remission	161	24–29% at 3–6 years	20–40% at 2–6 years
2nd or 3rd remission	69	–	12–15% at 17months–3 years

Brain tumors

Tumors of the CNS constitute the second most common cancer in childhood. Advances in diagnosis, staging and treatment have improved outcome so that nowadays almost 70% of patients with brain tumors survive.[61] However, a significant proportion of survivors are troubled by the late sequelae of their tumors and treatment. Treatment for malignant brain tumors includes surgery and radiotherapy; in certain situations, for example, medulloblastoma and germ cell tumor, conventional chemotherapy is routinely added to the treatment regimen.

HDC has been trialed in pediatric CNS tumors in order to improve outcome and/or reduce the late sequelae of radiotherapy, particularly in young children. The relatively poor response of brain tumors to chemotherapy is usually explained by two factors:

- drug penetration into the CNS is obstructed by the blood–brain barrier
- brain tumors appear less responsive to chemotherapy compared with pediatric cancers arising outside the CNS.

HDC may 'swamp' the blood–brain barrier. Components of HDC are usually chosen for their ability to penetrate the CNS; the most commonly used agents include the alkylating agents (thiotepa, busulfan, cyclophosphamide and melphalan), etoposide and carboplatin.[62]

Medulloblastoma

Medulloblastoma is the most common malignant pediatric brain tumor; it arises in the posterior fossa. About 80% of patients with good surgical clearance and no metastases are long-term survivors after surgery, radiotherapy and conventional multiagent chemotherapy.[63] Those with metastases at diagnosis or who relapse are at greater risk. Dunkel & Finlay[64] summarized the treatment and results of HDC in relapsed medulloblastoma.

- HDC combinations included melphalan, thiotepa, busulfan, carboplatin and cyclophosphamide.
- Outcome ranged from 20% to 50% with 24–36 months follow-up.
- Disease-free survival was best for recurrence localized to the posterior fossa and worst for metastatic recurrence.

HDC certainly offers a realistic chance of cure for locally recurrent disease.

Supratentorial primitive neuroectodermal tumors

From a histologic perspective, medulloblastoma and supratentorial primitive neuroectodermal tumors (sPNET) are indistinguishable. A subset of sPNET arise in the pineal gland and are called pinealoblastoma. A significant proportion of children with sPNET are cured with a combination of surgery, radiotherapy and chemotherapy; however, the outcome for relapsed or progressive sPNET is grim when conventional chemotherapy is used.[65] Broniscer et al[66] have recently reported 17 patients with relapsed or refractory sPNET treated with high-dose thiotepa, etoposide ± carboplatin. Ten patients experienced relapse at

a median of 160 days after HDC; the 5-year EFS is 29%. All eight patients with pinealoblastoma died; statistical advantage was shown for surgery and radiotherapy in addition to HDC at the time of relapse. The authors analyzed six smaller, earlier studies of HDC in sPNET; eight of 19 patients are alive at the time of reporting. In conclusion, a subset of recurrent sPNET (excluding pinealoblastoma) can be salvaged using aggressive surgery, radiotherapy and HDC.

Germ cell tumors

CNS germ cell tumors (GCT) arise from the suprasellar or pineal regions and occur most frequently in the second and third decades of life. Germinomas respond extremely well to either radiotherapy alone or reduced-volume radiotherapy and chemotherapy; survival is excellent. In contrast, non-germinomatous GCTs (NGGCT) are less sensitive to radiotherapy and outcome is inferior compared with germinoma.[67] The French Society of Pediatric Oncology has reported on 13 patients with recurrent CNS GCT who received HDC (etoposide and thiotepa); 10 patients survived with a median follow-up of 16 months after HDC.[68] More recently, Modak et al[69] reported 21 patients with CNS GCTs with relapsed or progressive disease despite initial chemotherapy and/or radiotherapy. The HDC regimen was thiotepa based; overall and event-free survival at 4 years are 57% (±12%) and 52% (±14%), respectively. Seven of nine patients with germinoma survive disease free in contrast with only four of 12 with NGGCT. It appears that HDC is effective therapy for recurrent or progressive germinoma. In order to improve the prognosis of patients with NGGCT, the Children's Oncology Group is currently investigating HDC in a cohort of newly diagnosed patients with residual disease after initial chemotherapy and surgery.

High-grade glioma and diffuse intrinsic pontine tumors

Small studies reported in the early 1990s showed that a small proportion of children with recurrent high-grade glioma, arising outside the brainstem, were curable with HDC; prolonged survival appeared to be restricted to a cohort receiving HDC in the setting of minimal residual disease.[70] The Children's Cancer Group has run a number of studies of HDC in newly diagnosed high-grade glioma; approximately 25% of children survive progression free more than 5 years from treatment. Other studies have not demonstrated benefit from HDC.[71] In conclusion, the role of HDC in non-brainstem high-grade glioma remains inconclusive; there may be a role in patients with a good surgical clearance and the United States Children's Oncology Group is currently investigating this in a Phase III trial.[70] The situation regarding the role of any form of chemotherapy in brainstem (diffuse pontine) glioma remains dismal, and HDC cannot be justified on the basis of current evidence.

Infants with brain tumors

Infants with malignant brain tumors are regarded as a special group because radiation therapy at this age often results in major neurocognitive sequelae. Most children's cancer study groups have devised treatment regimens that rely upon surgery and chemotherapy, with radiotherapy reserved for poorly responding and relapsing disease. HDC has been trialed in recurrent disease, and then for upfront therapy. The Head Start I protocol was used to treat 62 infants with a variety of brain tumors; HDC consolidated therapy after 3 months of conventional chemotherapy treatment. Encouragingly, the 3-year overall and event-free survivals were 40% and 28%, respectively.[72] Best results were seen in children with medulloblastoma, sPNET and ependymoma while those with high-grade glioma fared poorly.

A high-dose thiotepa-based regimen has been used in 20 young children with brain tumors that recurred after chemotherapy (without initial radiotherapy); the 3-year EFS is 47% (±14%).[64] A recent summary of HDC in infants with brain tumors supports such treatment in medulloblastoma whilst cure in sPNET appears difficult to achieve using HDC without radiotherapy. Response of recurrent ependymoma to HDC is poor.[73] Co-operative children's cancer study groups are currently pursuing HDC in subsets of infant brain tumors.

Other brain tumors

Atypical teratoid/rhabdoid tumors (AT/RT) are rare, highly malignant embryonal tumors particularly affecting infants. There is increasing evidence for the role of aggressive chemotherapy in AT/RT, and prolonged disease-free survival is reported particularly in those where complete macroscopic excision of the tumor is achieved.[74] These authors reported 13 children who received HDC; six remained alive without disease 9.5–90 months from diagnosis. The Italian AIEOP group has similarly used HDC and a number of their patients remained disease free 5 years from treatment.[75] This group is currently investigating 'sarcoma-directed' conventional chemotherapy followed by HDC in AT/RT.[71]

Anaplastic oligodendrogliomas, particularly those with 1p and 19q genetic alterations, are chemosensitive.[76] A recent report documents the long-term follow-up of 39 adults who received high-dose thiotepa after conventional chemotherapy for newly diagnosed anaplastic or aggressive oligodendroglioma.[77] At the time of reporting the median progression-free survival was 78 months and the median overall survival had not yet been reached. Forty-six percent of patients have relapsed. These data are encouraging and justify further investigation of this strategy.

Choroid plexus tumors are uncommon CNS neoplasms that most frequently arise in the lateral or third ventricular system. A subset, choroid plexus carcinoma, appears to respond to chemotherapy and some investigators support the routine use of chemotherapy in this setting.[78] This is currently the subject of an International Society of Pediatric Oncology (SIOP) trial. There are anecdotal reports of HDC in relapsed choroid plexus carcinoma (J Finlay, personal communication, 2006). Two studies have reported on HDC in recurrent/refractory childhood ependymoma; neither showed particular benefit.[79,80]

Extracranial germ cell tumors

Germ cell tumors (GCT) comprise 3% of pediatric malignancies. This section deals with GCT arising outside the CNS; CNS GCTs are covered under Brain Tumors above. Conventional treatment for children with GCT consists of platinum drugs (either cisplatin or carboplatin) and surgery; this results in cure rates of more than 80%.[81] Given this, HDC with ASCT plays a very limited role. El-Helw & Coleman[82] reviewed the role of high-dose chemotherapy with ASCT in adults with GCT; single-arm studies have reported long-term disease-free survivals of:

- 13% for refractory/heavily pretreated disease
- 45% in first relapse
- 52% as first-line treatment in patients with poor-risk GCT.

However, a number of randomized trials in adults with initial poor risk disease, or those failing first-line chemotherapy, have failed to demonstrate benefit for HDC.[83] An analysis of the EBMT Registry revealed 23 children who received HDC with ASCT; 14 patients received treatment in second or third relapse while nine did so in first relapse. At the time of reporting, eight of 14 patients (57%) with extracranial GCT

remained disease free with a median follow-up of 66 months.[84] These results are encouraging, and HDC should be investigated in prospective clinical trials in relapsed GCT in childhood.

Lymphoma

Lymphoma is the third most common malignancy in childhood, accounting for about 12% of cancers. Two-thirds are non-Hodgkin's lymphoma and one-third Hodgkin's lymphoma. Most lymphoma in childhood is readily curable.

Hodgkin's lymphoma

Hodgkin's lymphoma (HL) is one of the most curable pediatric cancers with a 5-year overall survival close to 90%; this is usually achieved using a combined chemotherapy and radiotherapy approach. About 10–15% of children with HL either fail to achieve a complete remission or, more commonly, relapse. Children and adults with primarily refractory disease or who relapse after combined-modality treatment fare poorly with conventional salvage treatment. Fortunately, numerous reports attest to the efficacy of HDC in these high-risk settings (Table 11.6).[85–87]

In support of these data, studies in which adults with HL have been randomized to receive either HDC or conventional salvage treatment have shown significantly superior event-free survival in favor of the HDC arm.[88,89] In contrast, a recent retrospective, comparative study of relapsed childhood HL in 51 patients showed no benefit for relapsed disease, although there may have been a survival advantage for primarily refractory disease.[90]

Factors that negatively influence outcome after HDC in HL include extranodal disease at first relapse, the presence of a mediastinal mass at the time of HDC and primary induction failure.[85] Treatment-related mortality following HDC approaches 10%; particular risks include:

- prior mediastinal radiotherapy
- diffuse lung injury syndrome: this may complicate up to 40% of HDC procedures in HL. Risk factors for the development of pulmonary injury include prior mediastinal radiotherapy and bleomycin, and inclusion of BCNU in the HDC regimen.

Children with HL are at particular risk of developing second malignant neoplasms. Baker et al[91] studied the incidence of new malignancies following hematopoietic stem cell transplantation in adults and children; 14 of 124 (11%) with HL developed a post-transplantation malignancy. The most common new malignancies were myelodysplasia/acute myeloid leukemia. HDC has proven efficacy in high-risk HL; however, caution should be exercised regarding acute and long-term toxicities including second malignant neoplasms.

Non-Hodgkin's lymphoma

Non-Hodgkin's lymphomas (NHL) in children comprise the first group of malignant diseases originating from cells of the immune system that are not classified as Hodgkin's disease. Current WHO/REAL classification recognizes five distinct groups which comprise

Table 11.6 Outcome after HDC and ASCT in children with refractory or relapsed Hodgkin's lymphoma

Number of patients	Event-, progression-free or failure-free survival	OS	Reference
41	53% EFS at 5 years	68% at 5 years	Lieskovsky et al 2004[85]
53	31% FFS at 5 years	43% at 5 years	Baker et al 1999[86]
81	39% PFS at 3 years	64% at 3 years	Williams et al 1993[87]

the vast majority of subtypes of non-Hodgkin's lymphoma occurring in children. These are:

- Burkitt's lymphoma (40% of cases)
- diffuse large B-cell lymphoma (20% of cases)
- precursor B-cell lymphoblastic lymphoma (5% of cases)
- precursor T-cell lymphoblastic lymphoma (25% of cases)
- anaplastic large cell lymphoma (10% of cases).

Treatment of each of these has been shown to be most effective with leukemia-type chemotherapy protocols. Just as with standard and high-risk leukemia protocols in children, their best outcomes have been achieved without use of either autologous or allogeneic transplantation in first remission.

The role of transplantation in non-Hodgkin's lymphoma is confined, therefore, to relapsed patients.

Burkitt's lymphoma

Relapse of Burkitt's lymphoma tends to occur very early, often when the child is still receiving chemotherapy or shortly after ceasing primary therapy. Disease in this setting is aggressive and often resistant to chemotherapy. However, if future remission can be achieved with such agents as rituximab, then allogeneic or even autologous stem cell transplant results in the best chance of long-term survival.[92–94]

Relapsed precursor B- or T-cell lymphoma

Just as with relapse of acute lymphoblastic leukemia of precursor B- or T-cell lineage disease, allogeneic bone marrow transplant is favored due to the additional benefit of a graft-versus-lymphoma effect. However, Levine et al,[95] on behalf of the Lymphoma Study Writing Committee of the International Bone Marrow Transplant Registry and Autologous Blood and Marrow Transplant Registry, retrospectively analyzed the outcome of 128 patients undergoing autologous rescue and 76 patients receiving HLA-identical sibling allogeneic transplants. They observed that overall survival with autologous stem cell transplant was mildly improved over allogeneic transplant at 6 months post transplant, but in the longer term was not significantly superior, with overall survivals between the 2 groups at 1 and 5 years of 60% versus 45% (p =0.09) and 44% versus 39% (p =0.47), respectively. Independent of stem cell type, bone marrow involved at the time of transplantation and disease status more advanced than in complete remission were associated with inferior outcomes.

In summary, allogeneic stem cell transplantation for lymphoblastic lymphoma is associated with fewer relapses than autologous stem cell transplantation, but higher transplant-related mortality offsets any potential survival benefit. The transplant-related mortality reported in this series was 18% for allogeneic bone marrow transplant.

Anaplastic large cell lymphoma (ALCL)

ALCL was first described as a clinicopathologic entity by Stein and co-workers in 1985.[96] Morphologically, it is characterized by large, pleomorphic cells which express CD30, often together with epithelial membrane antigen (EMA) and the interleukin 2 (IL-2) receptor.[97,98] Lymphoid lineage specific antigens are of T-cell phenotype in the majority of cases. At the molecular level, almost 80% of pediatric and adolescent ALCL are characterized by a translocation involving the ALK receptor tyrosine kinase on chromosome 2.[98,99] Most often, the ALK gene gets fused to the NPM gene on chromosome 5, leading to an NPM-ALK fusion protein detectable by an ALK-1 monoclonal antibody.[98–102]

ALCL is a highly chemosensitive disease with complete remission rates ranging from 65% to over 90% with various multiagent chemotherapy protocols.[103–105] However, 25–40% of patients with ALCL relapse, usually during the first year after diagnosis.

Woessman,[106] on behalf of the BFM Group, recently published a retrospective review of 20 children and adolescents with high-risk relapse or refractory ALCL who underwent allogeneic hemopoietic stem cell transplant, and reported an EFS of 3 years after transplant of 75% (±10%). Eight patients received their transplants from matched sibling donors, eight from unrelated donors and four from haploidentical family donors. There was no influence of donor type or conditioning regimen on outcome. Two of six patients with progressive disease during frontline therapy survived, compared with 13 out of 14 patients with a first relapse after frontline therapy. The report concluded that allogeneic stem cell transplant is effective, with acceptable toxicity, as rescue therapy for high-risk ALCL relapse and even cured some patients with refractory disease, suggesting a graft versus ALCL effect.

Analysis of outcomes for patients with ALCL relapsing after BFM frontline therapy treated according to the non-Hodgkin's lymphoma BFM 1995 protocols in Germany, Australia and Switzerland has been used to define prognostic factors in developing a risk-adapted therapy for relapsed patients and forms the rationale for the current European Inter-Group Co-operation on Childhood non-Hodgkin's Lymphoma (EICNHL) international multicenter therapy study. This study opened in September 2005 and is projected to accrue patients through until 2011. The high-risk patients (relapsed during firstline therapy and/or those whose tumors are CD3+) will receive TBI/thiotepa/etoposide conditioning with an allogeneic stem cell transplant, matched sibling donor or 10/10 matched unrelated donor. Patients who have relapsed later and who are CD3– will receive a BEAM (carmustine, etoposide, cytarabine, melphalan) autologous stem cell transplant.[107]

Diffuse large B-cell lymphoma (DLBCL)

Children with DLBCL who relapse and other rare subtypes of relapsing lymphoma not already described are best treated with salvage chemotherapy protocols,[108] usually based on adult experience.[109–110] Just as with adult experience, best outcomes are obtained where relapsed disease is chemosensitive and the patient is in CR or very good partial response (VGPR) at time of subsequent allogeneic stem cell transplant.

The future direction in transplantation for lymphoma has been suggested by Cairo et al[111] to be with adoptive immunotherapy after reduced-intensity allogeneic stem cell transplant. This approach has the advantage of focusing the immunologic attack upon tumor cells and sparing the patient the toxicity of full myeloablative chemotherapy. Problems to overcome still include lack of efficacy in patients with progressive disease and/or high tumor burden, and a significant incidence of graft-versus-host disease. Graft failure has been noted to be a problem more particularly in non-malignant diseases utilizing reduced-intensity stem cell transplantation.

Histiocyte disorders

The histiocytoses are a group of conditions characterized by a pathologic increase of histiocytes within organs. Conditions under this umbrella include Langerhans cell histiocytosis (LCH), juvenile xanthogranuloma, hemophagocytic lymphohistiocytosis (HLH) and Rosai–Dorfman disease.[112] Although childhood histiocytic disorders are considered non-malignant, most HLH is extremely aggressive, necessitating treatment with chemotherapy and allogeneic HSCT. HSCT may be indicated in severe, multisystem LCH unresponsive to conventional therapy.[113]

Hemophagocytic lymphohistiocytosis

HLH is a rare condition. HLH may be familial (FLH) or secondary to a viral infection or malignancy (SHLH). However, it is important to

Table 11.7 Outcome after HSCT in HLH-94[117]

HSCT donor	Number	Percent surviving at 3 years (confidence interval)
Matched related	24	71 (±18)
Matched unrelated	33	70 (±16)
Family haploidentical	16	50 (±24)
Mismatched unrelated	13	54 (±27)
Total	86	64

note that the distinction between FLH and HLH is often blurred. The Histiocyte Society has developed guidelines for the diagnosis of HLH (HLH-2004 protocol).[114] HLH often results in rapid clinical deterioration; treatment may be indicated on the basis of strong clinical suspicion without fulfilment of the necessary criteria. Seven genetic mutations that result in FHL have been described; these generally oppose apoptosis of immune-regulating cells resulting in 'overactivity' of the immune system, histiocyte proliferation and activation. The most common mutation affects the perforin protein which is normally responsible for the introduction of cytotoxic effector molecules into target immune-regulating cells.[115]

Without treatment, HLH is invariably fatal; for FLH the median survival is 1–2 months.[116] In 1994, the Histiocyte Society developed a comprehensive treatment strategy (HLH-94) consisting of induction and continuation therapy; allogeneic HSCT was indicated for FLH, and HLH with persistent or relapsing disease. Overall survival is 55% (±9%) at 3 years.[117] Of 113 children entered into HLH-94, 86 received HSCT at a median age of 13 months.[118] The preparative regimen consisted of busulfan, cyclophosphamide and etoposide. Outcome related to donor selection is shown in Table 11.7.[118] Thirty-six percent died, 84% of these from transplant-related complications. Specific complications reported included:

- non-engraftment, a particular risk for those transplanted with active disease
- hepatic veno-occlusive disease (HVOD)
- 'hypercytokinemia syndrome' presenting with fever, capillary leak, vascular instability, respiratory distress and liver dysfunction – often mimicking HLH. This may be reversed with corticosteroids and/or antitumor necrosis factor agents.[118]

HLH-94 has resulted in a dramatic improvement in survival in HLH. The current Histiocyte Society HLH treatment strategy is HLH-2004. Clinicians are encouraged to actively search for genetic mutations responsible for FHL to more accurately identify those eligible for HSCT. Caution is advised when considering a matched related donor – a sibling may harbor a genetic mutation, as yet unexpressed clinically. A proportion of patients treated on HLH-94 have mixed chimerism, all with inactive disease a median time of 3 years after HSCT. With this in mind, reduced-intensity conditioning has been investigated in 12 patients.[119] Nine (75%) were alive and in remission a median of 30 months after HSCT. Reduced-intensity conditioning may be considered for HLH patients who are particularly ill at the time of transplant in an attempt to reduce the incidence of transplant-related mortality.

Langerhans cell histiocytosis

Langerhans cells are antigen-presenting histiocytes normally found in the skin. Langerhans cell histiocytosis (LCH) represents a clonal proliferation of these cells. LCH is an enigmatic disorder ranging from disease that spontaneously resolves to that which is unresponsive to multiagent therapy and associated with high mortality.[112] The latter group is characterized by children, usually between 1 and 3 years of age, with multisystem disease involving so-called 'risk organs' – bone marrow, spleen, liver and/or lung.

Studies conducted by the Histiocyte Society (LCH-I and II) and the German Co-operative Group (DAL HX-83 and 90) have shown that, for those with 'risk' disease, 50% have active LCH at week 12 of therapy and 75% of this subgroup die from progressive LCH. Allogeneic HSCT has been used for a small number of patients with unresponsive disease; 13 out of 22 children remained alive at the time of reporting. Toxicity-related mortality is high; a number were transplanted with active disease.[120,121] Four of five patients who received autologous HSCT had persistent active disease after transplantation. There may be an increased risk of second malignant neoplasm in survivors of allogeneic transplantation.[122] Allogeneic HSCT is not regarded as a standard therapeutic option for patients with refractory aggressive disease and should be considered investigational.[112]

References

1. Moss TJ, Cairo M, Santana VM et al. Clonogenicity of circulating neuroblastoma cells: implications regarding peripheral blood stem cell transplantation. Blood 1994;893: 3085–3089
2. Seeger RC, Reynolds CP, Gallego R et al. Quantitative tumor cell content of bone marrow and blood as a predictor of outcome in stage IV neuroblastoma: a Children's Cancer Group Study. J Clin Oncol 2000;18:4067–4076
3. Burchill SA, Lewis IJ, Abrams KR et al. Circulating neuroblastoma cells detected by reverse transcriptase-polymerase chain reaction for tyrosine hydroxylase mRNA are an independent poor prognostic indicator in stage 4 neuroblastoma in children over 1 year. J Clin Oncol 2001;19:1795–1801
4. Brodeur GM, Pritchard J, Berthold F et al. Revisions of the international criteria for neuroblastoma diagnosis, staging, and response to treatment. J Clin Oncol 1993;11: 1466–1477
5. Matthay KK, Castleberry RP. Treatment of advanced neuroblastoma: the US experience. In: Brodeur GM, Sawada T, Tsuchida Y, Voûte PA (eds) Neuroblastoma. Elsevier Science, Amsterdam, 2000:417–436
6. Pinkerton CR. ENSG 1-randomized study of high-dose melphalan in neuroblastoma. Bone Marrow Transplant 1991;7(suppl):112–113
7. Matthay KK, Villablanca JG, Seeger RC et al. Treatment of high-risk neuroblastoma with intensive chemotherapy, radiotherapy, autologous bone marrow transplantation, and 13-cis-retinoic acid: Children's Cancer Group. N Engl J Med 1999;341:1165–1173
8. Rill DR, Santana VM, Roberts WM et al. Direct demonstration that autologous bone marrow transplantation for solid tumors can return a multiplicity of tumorigenic cells. Blood 1994;84:380–383
9. Handgretinger R, Leung W, Ihm K et al. Tumor cell contamination of autologous stem cells grafts in high-risk neuroblastoma: the good news? Br J Cancer 2003;88:1874–1877
10. Berthold F, Boos J, Burdach S et al. Myeloablative megatherapy with autologous stem-cell rescue versus oral maintenance chemotherapy as consolidation treatment in patients with high-risk neuroblastoma: a randomized controlled trial. Lancet Oncol 2005;6: 649–658
11. Grupp SA, Stern JW, Bunin N et al. Tandem high-dose therapy in rapid sequence for children with high-risk neuroblastoma. J Clin Oncol 2000;18:2567–2575
12. Kletzel M, Katzenstein HM, Haut PR et al. Treatment of high-risk neuroblastoma with triple-tandem high-dose therapy and stem-cell rescue: results of the Chicago Pilot II Study. J Clin Oncol 2002;20:2284–2292
13. Marcus KJ, Shamberger R, Litman H et al. Primary tumor control in patients with stage 3/4 unfavorable neuroblastoma treated with tandem double autologous stem cell transplants. J Pediatr Hematol Oncol 2003;25:934–940
14. Powell JL, Bunin NJ, Callahan C et al. An unexpectedly high incidence of Epstein-Barr virus lymphoproliferative disease after CD34+ selected autologous peripheral blood stem cell transplant in neuroblastoma. Bone Marrow Transplant 2004;33:651–657
15. Ladenstein R, Lasset C, Hartmann O et al. Comparison of auto versus allografting as consolidation of primary treatments in advanced neuroblastoma over 1 year of age at diagnosis: report from the European Group for Bone Marrow Transplantation. Bone Marrow Transplant 1994;14:37–46
16. August CS, Serota FT, Koch PA et al. Treatment of advanced neuroblastoma with supralethal chemotherapy, radiation, and allogeneic or autologous marrow reconstitution. J Clin Oncol 1984;2:609–616
17. Pole JG, Casper J, Elfenbein G et al. High-dose chemoradiotherapy supported by marrow infusions for advanced neuroblastoma: a Pediatric Oncology Group study. J Clin Oncol 1991;9:152–158. [Published erratum appears in J Clin Oncol 1991;9:1094.]
18. Kamani N, August CS, Bunin N et al. A study of thiotepa, etoposide and fractionated total body irradiation as a preparative regimen prior to bone marrow transplantation for poor prognosis patients with neuroblastoma. Bone Marrow Transplant 1996;17:911–916
19. Evans AE, August CS, Kamani N et al. Bone marrow transplantation for high risk neuroblastoma at the Children's Hospital of Philadelphia: an update. Med Pediatr Oncol 1994;23:323–327
20. Kremens B, Klingebiel T, Herrmann F et al. High-dose consolidation with local radiation and bone marrow rescue in patients with advanced neuroblastoma. Med Pediatr Oncol 1994;23:470–475
21. Dopfer R, Berthold F, Einsele H et al. Bone marrow transplantation in children with neuroblastoma. Folia Hematol Int Mag Klin Morph Blutforsch 1989;116:427–436

22. Garaventa A, Rondelli R, Lanino E et al. Myeloablative therapy and bone marrow rescue in advanced neuroblastoma. Report from the Italian Bone Marrow Transplant Registry. Italian Association of Pediatric Hematology-Oncology. BMT Group. Bone Marrow Transplant 1996;18:125–130

23. Smedler AC, Bolme P. Neuropsychological deficits in very young bone marrow transplant recipients. Act Pediatr Japon 1995;84:429–433

24. Olshan JS, Willi SM, Gruccio D et al. Growth hormone function and treatment following bone marrow transplant for neuroblastoma. Bone Marrow Transplant 1993;12:381–385

25. Kolb HJ, Bender-Gotze CH. Late complications after allogeneic bone marrow transplantation for leukaemia. Bone Marrow Transplant 1990;6:61

26. D'Angio GJ, Evans AE, Breslow N et al. The treatment of Wilms' tumor. Results of the Second National Wilms' Tumor Study. Cancer 1981;47:2302–2311

27. Lemerle J, Voute PA, Tournade MF et al. Effectiveness of preoperative chemotherapy in Wilms' tumor: results of an International Society of Pediatric Oncology (SIOP) clinical trial. J Clin Oncol 1983;1:604–609

28. Grundy P, Breslow N, Green DM et al. Prognostic factors for children with recurrent Wilms' tumor: results from the Second and Third National Wilms' Tumor Study. J Clin Oncol 1989;7:638–647

29. Pinkerton CR, Groot-Loonen JJ, Morris-Jones PH et al. Response rates in relapsed Wilms' tumor. A need for new effective agents. Cancer 1991;67:567–571

30. Garaventa A, Hartmann O, Bernard H et al. Autologous bone marrow transplantation for pediatric Wilms' tumor: the experience of the European Bone Marrow Transplantation Solid Tumor Registry. Med Pediatr Oncol 1994;22:11–14

31. Pein F, Michon J, Valteau-Couanet D et al. High-dose melphalan, etoposide and carboplatin followed by autologous stem-cell rescue in pediatric high-risk recurrent Wilms' tumor: a French Society of Pediatric Oncology study. J Clin Oncol 1998;16:3295–3301

32. Kremens B, Gruhn B, Klingebiel T et al. High-dose chemotherapy with autologous stem cell rescue in children with nephroblastoma. Bone Marrow Transplant 2002;30:893–898

33. Tannous R, Giller R, Holmes E et al. Intensive therapy for high risk (HR) relapsed Wilms' tumor (WT). A CCG-4921/POG-9445 study report. Proc ASCO 2000;19:A2315

34. Calvert AH, Newell DR, Gumbrell LH et al. Carboplatin dosage: prospective evaluation of a simple formula based on renal function. J Clin Oncol 1989;7:1748–1756

35. Antoneli CBG, Steinhorst F, Ribiero KCB. Extraocular retinoblastoma: a 13 year experience. Cancer 2003;98:1292–1298

36. Chantada G, Fandino A, Casak S et al. Treatment of overt extraocular retinoblastoma. Med Pediatr Oncol 2003;40:158–161

37. Dunkel IJ, Aledo A, Finlay JL et al. Intensive multimodality therapy for metastatic retinoblastoma. Pediatr Blood Cancer 2004;43:378

38. Namouni F, Doz F, Tanguy ML et al. High-dose chemotherapy with carboplatin, etoposide and cyclophosphamide followed by hematopoietic stem cell rescue in patients with high-risk retinoblastoma: a SFOP and SFGM study. Eur J Cancer 1997;33:2368–2375

39. Rodriguez-Galindo C, Wilson MW, Haik BG et al. Treatment of metastatic retinoblastoma. Ophthalmology 2003;110:1237–1240

40. Schnater JM, Kohler SE, Lamers WH et al. Where do we stand with hepatoblastoma? Cancer 2003;98:668–678

41. Nishimura S-I, Sato T, Fujita N et al. High-dose chemotherapy in children with metastatic hepatoblastoma. Pediatr Int 2002;44:300–305

42. Kushner BH, Meyers PA, Gerald WL et al. Very-high-dose short-term chemotherapy for poor-risk peripheral primitive neuroectodermal tumors, including Ewing's sarcoma, in children and young adults. J Clin Oncol 1995;13:2796–2804

43. Cornbleet MA, Corringham RE, Prentice HG et al. Treatment of Ewing's sarcoma with high-dose melphalan and autologous bone marrow transplantation. Cancer Treat Rep 1981;65:241–244

44. Graham Pole J, Lazarus HM, Herzig RH et al. High-dose melphalan therapy for the treatment of children with refractory neuroblastoma and Ewing's sarcoma. Am J Pediatr Hematol Oncol 1984;6:17–26

45. Young MM, Kinsella TJ, Miser JS et al. Treatment of sarcomas of the chest wall using intensive combined modality therapy. Int J Radiat Oncol Biol Phys 1989;16:49–57

46. Burdach S, Meyer-Bahlburg A, Laws HJ et al. High-dose therapy for patients with primary multifocal and early relapsed Ewing's tumors: results of two consecutive regimens assessing the role of total-body irradiation. J Clin Oncol 2003;21:3072–3078

47. Hawkins DS, Felgenhauer J, Park J et al. Peripheral blood stem cell support reduces the toxicity of intensive chemotherapy for children and adolescents with metastatic sarcomas. Cancer 2002;95:1354–1365

48. Leung W, Chen AR, Klann RC et al. Frequent detection of tumor cells in hematopoietic grafts in neuroblastoma and Ewing's sarcoma. Bone Marrow Transplant 1998;22:971–979

49. Yaniv I, Cohen IJ, Stein J et al. Tumor cells are present in stem cell harvests of Ewing's sarcoma patients and their persistence following transplantation is associated with relapse. Pediatr Blood Cancer 2004;42:404–409

50. Burdach S, van Kaick B, Laws HJ et al. Allogeneic and autologous stem-cell transplantation in advanced Ewing tumors. An update after long-term follow-up from two centers of the European Intergroup study EICESS. Stem-Cell Transplant Programs at Dusseldorf University Medical Center, Germany and St. Anna Kinderspital, Vienna, Austria. Ann Oncol 2000;11:1451–1462

51. Hartmann O, Oberlin O, Beaujean F et al. [Role of high-dose chemotherapy followed by bone marrow autograft in the treatment of metastatic Ewing's sarcoma in children] Place de la chimiotherapie a hautes doses suivie d'autogreffe medullaire dans le traitement des sarcomes d'Ewing metastatiques de l'enfant. Bull Cancer Paris 1990;77:181–187

52. Burdach S, Jürgens H, Peters C et al. Myeloablative radiochemotherapy and hematopoietic stem-cell rescue in poor-prognosis Ewing's sarcoma and rhabdomyosarcoma. J Clin Oncol 1993;11:1482–1488

53. Horowitz ME, Kinsella TJ, Wexler LH et al. Total-body irradiation and autologous bone marrow transplant in the treatment of high-risk Ewing's sarcoma and rhabdomyosarcoma. J Clin Oncol 1993;11:1911–1918

54. Ladenstein R, Lasset C, Pinkerton R et al. Impact of megatherapy in children with high-risk Ewing's tumors in complete remission: a report from the EBMT Solid Tumor Registry. Bone Marrow Transplant 1995;15:697–705

55. Shankar AG, Ashley S, Craft AW et al. Outcome after relapse in an unselected cohort of children and adolescents with Ewing sarcoma. Med Pediatr Oncol 2003;40:141–147

56. Mackall C, Berzofsky J, Helman IJ. Targeting tumor specific translocations in sarcomas in pediatric patients for immunotherapy. Clin Orthop Relat Res 2000;373:25–31

57. McDowell HP. Update on childhood rhabdomyosarcoma. Arch Dis Child 2003;88:354–357

58. Weigel BJ, Breitfeld PP, Hawkins D et al. Role of high-dose chemotherapy with hematopoietic stem cell rescue in the treatment of metastatic or recurrent rhabdomyosarcoma. J Pediatr Hematol/Oncol 2001;23:272–276

59. Carli M, Colombatti R, Oberlin O et al. High-dose melphalan with autologous stem cell rescue in metastatic rhabdomyosarcoma. J Clin Oncol 1999;17:2796–2803

60. Doelken R, Weigel S, Schueler F et al. Poor outcome of two children with relapsed stage IV alveolar rhabdomyosarcoma after allogeneic stem cell transplantation. Pediatr Hematol Oncol 2005;22:699–703

61. Jemal A, Clegg LX, Ward E et al. Annual report to the nation on the status of cancer, 1975–2001, with a special feature regarding survival. Cancer 2004;101:3–27

62. Kalifa C, Valteau D, Pizer B et al. High-dose chemotherapy in childhood brain tumors. Child's Nerv Syst 1999;15:498–505

63. Packer RJ, Goldwein J, Nicholson HS et al. Treatment for children with medulloblastoma with reduced-dose craniospinal radiation therapy and adjuvant chemotherapy: a Children's Cancer Group study. J Clin Oncol 1999;17:2127–2136

64. Dunkel IJ, Finlay JL. High-dose chemotherapy with autologous stem cell rescue for brain tumors. Crit Rev Oncol/Hematol 2002;41:197–204

65. Van Eys J, Baram TZ, Cangir A et al. Salvage chemotherapy for recurrent primary brain tumors in children. J Pediatr 1988;113:601–606

66. Broniscer A, Nicolaides TP, Dunkel IJ et al. High-dose chemotherapy with autologous stem-cell rescue in the treatment of patients with recurrent non-cerebellar primitive neuroectodermal tumors. Pediatr Blood Cancer 2004;42:261–267

67. Matsutani M, Sano K, Takakura K et al. Primary intracranial germ cell tumors: a clinical analysis of 153 histologically verified cases. J Neurosurg 1997;86:446–455

68. Baranzelli MC, Pichon F, Patte C et al. High-dose etoposide and thiotepa for recurrent intracranial malignant germ cell tumors: experience of the SFOP. Child's Nerv Syst 1999;14:520

69. Modak S, Gardner S, Dunkel IJ et al. Thiotepa-based high-dose chemotherapy with autologous stem-cell rescue in patients with recurrent or progressive CNS germ cell tumors. J Clin Oncol 2004;22:1934–1943

70. Finlay JL, Zacharoulis S. The treatment of high grade gliomas and diffuse intrinsic pontine tumors of childhood and adolescence: a historical – and futuristic – perspective. J Neuro-Oncol 2005;75:253–266

71. Dallorso S, Dini G, Ladenstein R et al. Evolving role of myeloablative chemotherapy in the treatment of childhood brain tumors. Bone Marrow Transplant 2005;35:S31–S34

72. Mason WP, Grovas A, Halpern S et al. Intensive chemotherapy with bone marrow rescue for young children with newly diagnosed malignant brain tumors. J Clin Oncol 1998;16:210–221

73. Kalifa C, Grill J. The therapy of infantile malignant brain tumors: current status? J Neuro-Oncol 2005;75:279–285

74. Hilden JM, Meerbaum S, Burger P et al. Central nervous system atypical teratoid/rhabdoid tumor: results of therapy in children enrolled in a registry. J Clin Oncol 2004;22:2877–2884

75. Garré ML, Abate ME, Giangaspero F et al. Clinical features and treatment of CNS atypical teratoid/rhabdoid tumor. Med Pediatr Oncol 2002;39:275

76. Cairncross JG, Ueki K, Zlatescu MC et al. Specific predictors of chemotherapeutic response and survival in patients with anaplastic oligodendrogliomas. J Natl Cancer Inst 1998;90:1473–1479

77. Abrey LE, Childs BH, Paleologos N et al. High-dose chemotherapy with stem cell rescue as initial therapy for anaplastic oligodendroglioma: long-term follow-up. J Neuro-Oncol 2003;65:127–134

78. Greenberg ML. Chemotherapy of choroid plexus carcinoma. Child's Nerv Syst 1999;15:571–577

79. Grill J, Kalifa C, Doz F et al. A high-dose busulfan-thiotepa combination followed by autologous bone marrow transplantation in childhood recurrent ependymoma: a phase II study. Pediatr Neurosurg 1996;25:7–12

80. Mason WP, Goldman S, Yates AJ. Survival following intensive chemotherapy with bone marrow reconstitution for children with recurrent intracranial ependymoma – a report of the Children's Cancer Group. J Neuro-Oncol 1998;37:135–143

81. Mann JR, Raafat F, Robinson K et al. The United Kingdom Children's Cancer Study Group's second germ cell tumor study: carboplatin, etoposide and bleomycin are effective treatment for children with malignant extracranial germ cell tumors, with acceptable toxicity. J Clin Oncol 2000;18:3809–3818

82. El-Helw L, Coleman RE. Salvage, dose intense and high-dose chemotherapy for the treatment of poor prognosis or recurrent germ cell tumors. Cancer Treat Rev 2005;31:197–209

83. Shelley MD, Burgon K, Mason MD. Treatment of testicular germ-cell cancer: a Cochrane evidence-based systematic review. Cancer Treat Rev 2002;28:237–253

84. De Giorgi U, Rosti G, Slavin S et al. Salvage high-dose chemotherapy for children with extragonadal germ-cell tumors. Br J Cancer 2005;93:412–417

85. Lieskovsky YE, Donaldson SS, Torres MA et al. High-dose therapy and autologous hematopoietic stem-cell transplantation for recurrent or refractory pediatric Hodgkin's disease: results and prognostic indices. J Clin Oncol 2004;22:4532–4540

86. Baker KS, Gordon BG, Gross TG et al. Autologous hematopoietic stem-cell transplantation for relapsed or refractory Hodgkin's disease in children and adolescents. J Clin Oncol 1999;17:825–831

87. Williams CD, Goldstone AH, Pearce R et al. Autologous bone marrow transplantation for pediatric Hodgkin's disease: a case-matched comparison with adult patients by the Euro-

pean Bone Marrow Transplant Group Lymphoma Registry. J Clin Oncol 1993;11: 2243–2249

88. Linch DC, Winfield D, Goldstone AH et al. Dose intensification with autologous bone marrow transplantation in relapsed and resistant Hodgkin's disease: results of a BNLI randomized trial. Lancet 1993;341:1051–1054

89. Schmitz N, Pfistner B, Sextro M et al. Aggressive conventional chemotherapy compared with high-dose chemotherapy with autologous hemopoietic stem-cell transplantation for relapsed chemosensitive Hodgkin's disease: a randomized trial. Lancet 2002;359: 2065–2071

90. Stoneham S, Ashley S, Pinkerton CR et al. Outcome after autologous hemopoietic stem cell transplantation in relapsed or refractory childhood Hodgkin disease. J Pediatr Hematol/Oncol 2004;26:740–745

91. Baker KS, DeFor TE, Burns LJ et al. New malignancies after blood or marrow stem-cell transplantation in children and adults: incidence and risk factors. J Clin Oncol 2003;21: 1352–1358

92. Sandlung JT, Bowman L, Heslop HE et al. Intensive chemotherapy with hematopoietic stem-cell support for children with recurrent or refractory NHL. Cytotherapy 2002;4:253–258

93. Phillipe T, Hartmann O, Pinkerton R et al. Curability of relapsed childhood B-cell non-Hodgkins lymphoma after intensive first line therapy: report from the Societe Francaise d'Oncologie Pediatrique. Blood 1993;81:2003–2006

94. Ladenstein R, Pearce R, Hartmann O et al. High-dose chemotherapy with autologous bone marrow rescue in children with poor-risk Burkitt's lymphoma. A report from the European Lymphoma Bone Marrow Transplantation Registry. Blood 1997;90:2921–2930

95. Levine JE, Harris RE, Loberiza FR Jr et al. A comparison of allogeneic and autologous bone marrow transplant for lymphoblastic lymphoma. Blood 2003;101:2476–2482

96. Stein H, Mason DY, Gerdes J et al. The expression of the Hodgkin's disease associated antigen Ki-1 in reactive and neoplastic lymphoid tissue: evidence that Reed-Sternberg cells and histiocytic malignancies are derived from activated lymphoid cells. Blood 1985;66:848–858

97. Delsol G, Al Saati T, Gatter KC et al. Coexpression of epithelial membrane antigen (EMA), Ki-1, and interleukin-2 receptor by anaplastic large cell lymphomas. Diagnostic value in so-called malignant histiocytosis. Am J Pathol 1998;130:59–70

98. Stein H, Foss HD, Durkop H et al. CD30+ anaplastic large cell lymphoma: a review of its histopathologic, genetic, and clinical features. Blood 2000;96:3681–3695

99. Pulford K, Morris SW, Turturro F. Anaplastic lymphoma kinase proteins in growth control and cancer. J Cell Physiol 2004;199:330–358

100. Drexler HG, Gignac SM, von Wasielewski R et al. Pathobiology of NPM-ALK and variant fusion genes in anaplastic large cell lymphoma and other lymphomas. Leukemia 2000;14:1533–1559

101. Duyster J, Bai RY, Morris SW. Translocations involving anaplastic lymphoma kinase (ALK). Oncogene 2001;20:5623–5637

102. Falini B. Anaplastic large cell lymphoma: pathological, molecular and clinical features. Br J Haematol 2001;114:741–760

103. Brugieres L, Deley MC, Pacquement H et al. CD30+ anaplastic large-cell lymphoma in children: analysis of 82 patients enrolled in two consecutive studies of the French Society of Pediatric Oncology. Blood 1998;92:3591–3598

104. Seidemann K, Tiemann M, Schrappe M et al. Short-pulse B-non-Hodgkin lymphoma-type chemotherapy is efficacious treatment for pediatric anaplastic large cell lymphoma: a report of the Berlin-Frankfurt-Münster Group Trial NHL-BFM 90. Blood 2001;97:3699–3706

105. Reiter A, Schrappe M, Tiemann M et al. Successful treatment strategy for Ki-1 anaplastic large-cell lymphoma: a report of the Berlin-Frankfurt-Münster group studies. J Clin Oncol 1994;12:899–908

106. Woessman W, Peters C, Lenhard M et al. Allogeneic hematopoietic stem cell transplantation in relapsed or refractory anaplastic large cell lymphoma of children and adolescents – a Berlin-Frankfurt-Münster Group report. Br J Haematol 2006;133:176–182

107. Wojcik B, Kowalczyk JR, Chybicka A et al. Autologous stem-cell transplantations in children with non-Hodgkin lymphoma (article in Polish). Przegl Lek 2004;61(suppl 2):53–56

108. Imamura T, Yoshihara T, Morimoto A et al. Successful autologous peripheral blood stem cell transplantation with rituximab administration for pediatric diffuse large B-cell lymphoma. Pediatr Hematol Oncol 2006;23:19–24

109. Kobrinsky NL, Sposto R, Shah NR et al. Outcomes of treatment of children and adolescents with recurrent non-Hodgkin's lymphoma and Hodgkin's disease with dexamethasone, etoposide, cisplatin, cytarabine, and L-asparaginase, maintenance chemotherapy, and transplantation: Children's Cancer Group Study CCG-5912. J Clin Oncol 2001;19:2390–2396

110. Kung FH, Harris MB, Krischer IP. Ifosfamide/carboplatin/etoposide (ICE), an effective salvaging therapy for recurrent malignant non-Hodgkin lymphoma childhood: a Pediatric Oncology Group phase II study. Med Pediatr Oncol 1999;32:225–226

111. Cairo MS, Reiter AR. Second International Symposium on Childhood Adolescent and Adult non-Hodgkin's Lymphoma, May 2006. New York

112. Henter J-I, Tondini C, Pritchard J. Histiocyte disorders. Crit Rev Oncol/Hematol 2004;50:157–174

113. Kinugawa N, Imashuku S, Hirota Y et al. Hematopoietic stem cell transplantation (HSCT) for Langerhans cell histiocytosis (LCH) in Japan. Bone Marrow Transplant 1999;24:935–938

114. Henter J-I, Elinder G, Ost A. Diagnostic guidelines for hemophagocytic lymphohistiocytosis. Semin Oncol 1991;18:29–33

115. Verbsky JW, Grossman WJ. Hemophagocytic lymphohistiocytosis: diagnosis, pathophysiology, treatment and future perspectives. Ann Med 2006;38:20–31

116. Janka GE. Familial hemophagocytic lymphohistiocytosis. Eur J Pediatr 1983;140: 221–230

117. Henter J-I, Samuelsson-Horne A-C, Arico M et al. Treatment of hemophagocytic lymphohistiocytosis with HLH-94 immunochemotherapy and bone marrow transplantation. Blood 2002;100:2367–2373

118. Horne A-C, Janka G, Egeler RM et al. Hematopoietic stem cell transplantation in hemophagocytic lymphohistiocytosis. Br J Haematol 2005;129:622–630

119. Cooper N, Rao K, Gilmour K et al. Stem cell transplantation with reduced-intensity conditioning for hemophagocytic lymphohistiocytosis. Blood 2006;107:1233–1236

120. Akkari V, Donadieu J, Piguet C et al. Hematopoietic stem cell transplantation in patients with severe Langerhans cell histiocytosis and hematological dysfunction: experience of the French Langerhans Cell Study Group. Bone Marrow Transplant 2003;31:1097–1103

121. Hale GA, Bowman LC, Woodard JP et al. Allogeneic bone marrow transplantation for children with histiocytic disorders: use of TBI and omission of etoposide in the conditioning regimen. Bone Marrow Transplant 2003;31:981–986

122. Ringden O, Lonnqvist B, Holst M. 12-year follow-up of allogeneic transplantation for Langerhans cell histiocytosis. Lancet 1997;349:476

Breast cancer

Nancy M Hardy and Michael R Bishop

CHAPTER

12

Introduction: background and conventional treatment options

Breast cancer is the most common cancer in women and the leading cause of cancer deaths in women worldwide. More than 1.15 million cases of breast cancer are diagnosed annually, and in 2002 there were over 410,000 deaths due to this disease.[1,2] While breast cancer with limited spread is potentially curable, prognosis is heavily dependent on the degree of involvement of the axillary lymph nodes:[3] nearly 100% of women without lymph node involvement (stage I/IIA) are alive 10 years after diagnosis as compared to 45–59% of those with 4–9 involved lymph nodes (stage II/III), and 68–77% with 10 or more involved lymph nodes.[4] Locally advanced and inflammatory breast cancers are a heterogeneous group of tumors; as a consequence, prognosis is difficult to predict and is influenced largely by biologic characteristics of individual tumors.[5] Inflammatory breast cancers are an uncommon subtype characterized by dermal lymphatic invasion, often extensive local involvement, and aggressive behavior. Even with combined modality therapy, the 5-year disease-free survival (DFS) is approximately 30%.[6]

Fewer than 6% of women who are diagnosed with breast cancer present with distant metastases;[7] however, once there is metastatic spread, breast cancer is a chronic, virtually incurable disease, with 20% surviving 5 years, and a median survival of 2–3 years.[8] The high rate of recurrence after conventional therapy in patients with stage III disease, particularly in patients with 10 or more positive axillary nodes, and the poor prognosis after metastatic spread prompted evaluation of novel forms of therapy. High-dose chemotherapy (HDT) with autologous hematopoietic stem cell (AHSC) support and cellular immunotherapy using allogeneic lymphocyte-based or vaccine-based strategies have each been employed in the treatment of breast cancer.

Breast cancer presenting with locoregional spread is conventionally treated with combined-modality therapy aimed at eliminating the primary tumor (surgery) and preventing local (radiation therapy) and metastatic (systemic therapy) recurrence. Adjuvant polychemotherapy improves DFS and overall survival (OS) in women with early breast cancer, most demonstrably in women aged less than 50 years and with use of anthracycline-containing regimens.[9] Randomized, controlled trials suggest improved DFS and OS with both dose-escalated epirubicin[10] and combined anthracycline-taxane[10,11] regimens. Direct comparisons between these two approaches are limited, particularly for patients presenting with node-positive disease. However, an indirect comparison suggested that adjuvant therapy with six cycles of either docetaxel, doxorubicin and cyclophosphamide (TAC) or fluorouracil, epirubicin 100 mg/m^2 and cyclophosphamide (FEC100) may offer survival advantages over conventionally dosed anthracycline-based therapy to this subgroup of patients.[10] For patients whose tumors express estrogen and/or progesterone receptors or demonstrate increased expression of Her2/neu, therapy with estrogen antagonists[8] and the monoclonal antibody trastuzumab,[12,13] respectively, have shown DFS and OS benefits in the adjuvant setting. Conventional therapy for patients presenting with stage III breast cancer (including inflammatory breast cancer) involves aggressive treatment with neo-adjuvant chemotherapy, surgery and radiation therapy, and additional adjuvant systemic therapy.[14] Recurrence rates remain high, and the ideal choice of therapeutic agents, the sequence of treatment modalities and the number of chemotherapy cycles administered remain areas of investigation, hampered by heterogeneity of the biology of locally advanced tumors.

Chemotherapy, hormonal therapy, radiotherapy, biologic therapy and limited surgery are all used in the treatment of women with metastatic breast cancer (MBC). Almost all women with MBC will eventually become refractory to hormonal therapy, necessitating the use of systemic chemotherapy. The two most active classes of chemotherapy against MBC are anthracyclines and taxanes; however, both of these are more commonly being used together as part of adjuvant therapy, potentially limiting their usefulness in the metastatic setting.[15] A variety of second- and third-line chemotherapeutic agents is available, including vinorelbine, gemcitabine and capecitabine, either alone or in combination with biologic agents such as trastuzumab. Responses to these therapies are relatively consistent (15–30%), and median survival after their administration is generally less than 24 months.[16] While aggressive treatment strategies for local disease have resulted in reduced recurrence rates, particularly in tumors with histologic or genetic features suggestive of a poor prognosis, the prognosis for women with metastatic disease has changed comparatively little, in spite of a steady stream of new cytotoxic and biologic agents with breast cancer activity.[17] This failure has prompted continued search for alternative treatment paradigms to more effectively control advanced breast cancer.

High-dose chemotherapy for breast cancer

Observations of a dose–response relationship[18] and the importance of dose intensity[19] for efficacy of chemotherapy for breast cancer and ability to perform autologous hematopoietic stem cell transplantation led to the hypothesis that the use of HDT with AHSC support would improve outcomes in high-risk primary and metastatic breast cancer treatment. Early limitations in using this treatment modality for metastatic breast cancer included potential reinfusion of tumor cells with the stem cell product, and were minimized with the development of techniques for efficient peripheral blood stem cell mobilization and stem cell enrichment and sensitive assays for tumor contamination.[20,21]

HDT has been used extensively to treat both high-risk and metastatic breast cancer. Review of transplants registered with the Autologous Blood and Marrow Transplant Registry of North America (ABMTR) showed marked increases in use of this therapy in the late 1980s and early 1990s, and in 1993–1994, breast cancer was the most frequent indication for hematopoietic stem cell transplantation (HSCT) of all types.[22] Early enthusiasm based on promising non-randomized studies resulted in HDT becoming a standard treatment option for patients with poor prognoses, including those with extensive lymph node involvement or metastatic disease.[22,23] As a result, large, randomized trials accrued slowly; in the meantime, insurance company resistance, ensuing legislative battles[24,25] and reports of fraudulent data[26] added controversy to the field. When early reports of small, randomized trials failed to find significant benefit, enthusiasm for this approach waned rapidly. In recent years, however, results of larger randomized trials of AHSC-supported HDT have yielded provocative results that merit review here.

High-dose chemotherapy for high-risk primary breast cancer

As detailed above, patients with limited-stage breast cancer with extensive nodal involvement are at high risk of metastatic recurrence and death due to breast cancer. In high-risk primary breast cancer, including stage II or III disease with 4–9[27] and greater than 10[28–30] positive lymph nodes, non-randomized studies of HDT as consolidation after conventional adjuvant therapy found encouraging 5-year relapse-free survival rates of 73% and 50–70%, respectively. Sequential HDT instead of conventional adjuvant therapy yielded similarly promising results.[31] However, published randomized, controlled trial data have not shown consistent event-free survival (EFS) and OS benefits over conventional-dose adjuvant therapy or as consolidation after adjuvant therapy (Table 12.1). Results from 14 randomized studies using HDT in the treatment of high-risk primary breast cancer have been reported to date. Three studies reported significant differences favoring HDT, four suggested a possible benefit, six reported no difference in EFS or OS, and one study found that AHSC-supported HDT resulted in compromised outcomes.[32] However, this last study used consolidation with HDT (CTC: cyclophosphamide, thiotepa and carboplatin) as the control arm for the evaluation of adjuvant therapy with 'tailored' dosing of FEC (5-fluorouracil, epirubicin, and cyclophosphamide, dose adjusted to hematologic tolerance), and subjects in the study arm received significantly greater total doses of chemotherapy than those in the HDT arm.

In the largest of the studies finding a difference in favor of AHSC-supported HDT, the Dutch study reported by Rodenhuis et al[33] randomized 885 subjects with four or more involved lymph nodes treated with four cycles of FEC (fluorouracil 500 mg/m^2, epirubicin 90 mg/m^2 and cyclophosphamide 500 mg/m^2 every 3 weeks) to consolidation with HDT (CTC: cyclophosphamide 6000 mg/m^2, thiotepa 480 mg/m^2 and carboplatin 1600 mg/m^2) or a fifth cycle of conventionally dosed FEC. While differences in 5-year relapse-free survival (RFS) and OS were not statistically significant, HDT appeared to result in improved RFS at 5 years compared to conventional-dose therapy (CDT) in the subset of patients with 10 or more involved lymph nodes (61% vs 51%, p = 0.05).

In the West German Study Group trial reported by Nitz et al,[34] 403 subjects with primary breast cancer and 10 or more involved lymph nodes, after treatment with dose-dense EC (epirubicin 90 mg/m^2 and cyclophosphamide 600 mg/m^2 every 2 weeks), were randomized to

either two tandem cycles of AHSC-supported HDT (ECT: epirubicin 90 mg/m^2, cyclophosphamide 3000 mg/m^2 and thiotepa 400 mg/m^2) or three cycles of accelerated (14 day) iv CMF (cyclophosphamide 600 mg/m^2, methotrexate 40 mg/m^2 and fluorouracil 600 mg/m^2). This trial showed a statistically significant improvement in 4-year EFS (60% vs 44%, p = 0.00069) and OS (75% vs 70%, p = 0.02) favoring HDT.

The third study that demonstrated an advantage for HDT was the French PEGASE 01 trial.[35] In this study, 314 patients with seven or more involved lymph nodes were treated with four cycles of FEC100 (fluorouracil 500 mg/m^2, epirubicin 100 mg/m^2 and cyclophosphamide 500 mg/m^2 every 3 weeks) and randomized to receive AHSC-supported HDT (one cycle of CMA (cyclophosphamide 120 mg/kg, mitoxantrone 45 mg/m^2, and melphalan (Alkeran) 140 mg/m^2) or no further chemotherapy. The 3-year DFS was improved in the HDT arm (71% vs 55%, p = 0.002), as was EFS (68.5% vs 53.5%, p = 0.006). While OS was not different at 3 years, a subsequent report suggested improved OS in the HDT arm with longer follow-up.[36]

Four of the studies that did not find significant differences in outcomes after HDT suggested some evidence of superior activity. The International Breast Cancer Study Group (IBCSG) trial, reported by Basser et al,[37] randomized 344 patients with either 10 or more involved lymph nodes or five or more involved lymph nodes plus estrogen receptor-negative tumors or T3 tumors to three cycles of AHSC-supported high-dose EC (epirubicin 200 mg/m^2 and cyclophosphamide 4000 mg/m^2 every 21 days) or four cycles of AC (doxorubicin 60 mg/m^2 or epirubicin 90 mg/m,^{2} cyclophosphamide 600 mg/m,^{2} every 21 days) followed by three cycles of standard CMF (oral cyclophosphamide 100 mg/m^2 days 1–14, fluorouracil 600 mg/m^2 and methotrexate 40 mg/m,^{2} days 1 and 8, every 28 days). The HDT arm demonstrated a trend toward improved 5-year DFS (52% vs 43%, p = 0.07) but the difference in OS was not significantly significant (70% vs 61%, p = 0.17).

The second study was the German Adjuvant Breast-Cancer Group (GABG) trial reported by Zander et al,[38,39] in which 307 patients with 10 or more involved lymph nodes received four cycles of EC and were randomized to HDT with cyclophosphamide 6000 mg/m^2, thiotepa 600 mg/m^2 and mitoxantrone 40 mg/m^2 or three cycles of CMF (cyclophosphamide 500 mg/m^2, methotrexate 40 mg/m^2 and fluorouracil 600 mg/m^2 on days 1 and 8, every 28 days). While neither differences in EFS (hazard ratio (HR) 0.80, p = 0.15) nor OS (HR 0.84, p = 0.33) reached significance, patients with grade III tumors had a better outcome after HDT.

Third was the Cancer and Leukemia Group B (CALBG) trial, which randomized patients to consolidation after adjuvant CAF with high- versus intermediate-dose CBP (cyclophosphamide, cisplatin and carmustine), although in this last study an unplanned analysis suggested that patients age 50 years and older may have had better EFS following HDT.[115] The Italian study reported by Gianni et al[40] randomized 398 patients with four or more positive lymph nodes, and compared a conventional dosing regimen using three courses of epirubicin 120 mg/m^2 followed by six cycles of CMF with AHSC-supported HDT with cyclophosphamide 7000 mg/m^2, methotrexate 8000 mg/m^2 plus leucovorin, two courses of epirubicin 120 mg/m^2 and one cycle of thiotepa 600 mg/m^2 and melphalan 160–180 mg/m^2. At 52 months of follow-up, no differences were found in progression-free survival (PFS) or OS; however, younger patients (age less than 35) and those with 4–9 involved lymph nodes showed a trend for improved PFS HR 0.66 and 0.69, respectively, after HDT.

Three large, randomized trials in which HDT was evaluated in the setting of high-risk, primary breast cancer and there were 5 or more years of follow-up showed no difference in EFS or OS. The Eastern Co-operative Oncology Group (ECOG) trial,[41] which randomized 540

Table 12.1 Randomized, controlled trials comparing HDT with CDT in patients with high-risk primary breast cancer

Study	Eligibility	n	HDT	CDT/Control	EFS HDT vs CDT	OS HDT vs CDT	Median follow-up	Comments
Dutch Intergroup[33]	4 + LN	885 (10+: 317)	Induction: FEC × 4; HDT: CTC; XRT Tamoxifen	FEC × 5; XRT Tamoxifen	5-yr RFS: 65% vs 59% (p = 0.09); HR relapse: 0.83 (p = 0.09); 10+ nodes: 61% vs 51%, (p = 0.05)	p = 0.38	57 mo	HDT improved RFS for: Age < 40 (p = 0.05); Grade I (p = 0.002); Her-2-neg (p = 0.02); 2nd malig: HDT: 4.75% (21); (MDS/AML 0.2% (1)); CDT: 15 (MDS/AML: 0)
WSG[34]	10 + LN	403	Induction: EC × 2; HDT: ECT × 2; XRT Tamoxifen	EC × 2; EC × 4; XRT Tamoxifen	4-yr EFS: 60% vs 44% (p = 0.00069)	4-yr: 75% vs 70% (p = 0.02)	49 mo	TRM: None; AML: 1 patient in CDT arm after crossover to HDT
PEGASE 01[35,116]	7 + LN	314	FEC100 × 4; CMA × 1; XRT Tamoxifen	FEC100 × 4; XRT Tamoxifen	3-yr DFS: 71% vs 55% (p = 0.002); 3-yr EFS: 68.5 vs 53.5% (p = 0.006)	3-yr: 85% vs 84% (p = 0.33) *Reported significant at later follow-up[36]	39 mo	TRM 0.6%; 2nd malig: none
IBCSG[37,49]	10 + LN or 5 + LN & ER- or T3	344	HDT: EC × 3 Tamoxifen	AC or EC × 4; CMF × 3 Tamoxifen	5-yr DFS: 52% vs 43%; HR: 0.77 (p = 0.07)	5-yr: 70% vs 61%; HR: 0.79 (p = 0.17)	5.8 yr	TRM: 2.5%; 2nd malig: HDT/CDT: 5 vs 1, HDT 1 AML
JCOG 9208[48]	10 + LN	97	Induction: CAF × 6; C-T Tamoxifen	CAF × 6; Tamoxifen	RR 1.23 (0.85–1.79)	RR 1.01 (0.75–1.35)		TRM: None
GABG[38,39]	10 + LN	307	Induction: EC × 4; HDT: Cyclophosphamide Thiotepa Mitoxantrone Tamoxifen +/– XRT	EC × 4; CMF × 3 Tamoxifen +/– XRT	HR: 0.80 (p = 0.15)	HR: 0.84 (p = 0.33)	6.1 yr	TRM (HDT) 2%; Patients with tumor grade III had a better outcome with HDT (p = 0.049)
MDACC[44,45,110]	10 + LN or Stage III w/ 4 + LN	78	Induction: FAC × 8; HDT: CEC × 2; XRT Tamoxifen	FAC × 8; XRT Tamoxifen	10-yr RFS: 26% vs 40% (p = 0.11)	10-yr: 42% vs 47% (p = 0.13)	142.5 mo	TRM: 2.8%; MDS/AML: 2.8% (1 patient)
Dutch Pilot[46,47]	Level III nodes	81	Neoadj $FE_{120}C × 3$; 4th $FE_{120}C$; HDT: CTC; XRT Tamoxifen	Neoadj $FE_{120}C × 3$; 4th $FE_{120}C$; XRT Tamoxifen	5-yr DFS: 49% vs 47.5% (p = 0.37)	5-yr: 61 vs 62.5% (p = 0.85)	6.9 yr	MDS: 2.4%[117]; 2nd malig: HDT: 4.9%; CDT: 2.5%
ECOG[41]	10 + LN	540	Induction: CAF × 6; HDT: C-T	CAF × 6	6-yr DFS: 49 vs 47% (p = 0.55); Strict RFS: 55% vs 45% (p = 0.045)	6-yr: 58% vs 62% (p = 0.32)	6.1 yr	TRM: 3.3%; 2nd malig: CDT: 3.3%; HDT: Solid: 2.2%; MDS/AML: 3.3%

Table 12.1 Randomized, controlled trials comparing HDT with CDT in patients with high-risk primary breast cancer—cont'd

Study	Eligibility	n	HDT	CDT/Control	EFS HDT vs CDT	OS HDT vs CDT	Median follow-up	Comments
ACCOG[42]	4 + LN	605	Induction: Doxorubicin × 4 Cyclophosphamide × 1 HDT: C-T XRT Tamoxifen	Doxorubicin × 4 CMF × 8 XRT Tamoxifen	5-yr RFS: 57% vs 54% (p = 0.73)	5-yr: 62% vs 64% (p = 0.38)	6 yr	TRM (HDT): 1.6%
CALBG[78,115]	10 + LN	785	Induction: CAF × 4 HDT: 'TAMP I': CPB Tamoxifen	CAF × 4 Intermediatedose: Cyclophosphamide Cisplatin Carmustine Tamoxifen	5-yr EFS 61 vs 58% (NS)	5-yr 71% vs 71% (p = 0.75)	7.3 yr	TRM: 8.9% (3.8% 100-day) 2nd malig: HDT: 4.1% IDT: 5.1% MDS/AML: HDT: 1.8% vs IDT: 1.0% Age 50+ did better with HDT
ICCG[43]	4 + LN	281	Induction: FEC × 3 HDT: Cyclophosphamide Epirubicin Carboplatin XRT Tamoxifen	FEC × 3 CDT: 3 additional FEC XRT Tamoxifen	HR 1.06 (p = 0.76)	HR 1.18 (p = 0.40)	5.8 yr	TRM: HDT: 2.1% CDT: 3.6%
MCG[40,49]	4 + LN	398	Sequential Cyclophosphamide Methotrexate Epirubicin Thiotepa + Melphalan Tamoxifen	Epi 120 mg/m² CMF × 6 Tamoxifen	5-yr PFS: 65% vs 62% RR 1.05 (0.90–1.22)	5-yr 76% vs 77% RR 0.99 (0.88–1.10)	52 mo	TRM (HDT) 0.5% Trend toward improved PFS with HDT in patients: <36 yrs (n = 112, HR of 0.66), 4–9 LN+ (n = 147, HR of 0.69)
Scandinavian Breast Group 9401[32]	8 + LN or 5 + LN & poor prognostic feature	525	Induction: FEC HDT: CTC XRT Tamoxifen	'Tailored' FEC XRT Tamoxifen	3-yr RFS: 63% vs 72% (p = 0.013)	77% vs 83% (p = 0.12)	34.3 mo	FEC received higher dose intensity than HDT arm; 2nd malig: HDT: 2.2% FEC: 2.8% MDS/AML: 3.6% (8)

Abbreviations: AC, adriamycin and cyclophosphamide; CAF, cyclophosphamide, doxorubicin, 5-fluorouracil; CEC, cyclophosphamide, etoposide, cisplatin; CMA, cyclophosphamide, methotrexate and melphalan; CMF, cyclophosphamide, methotrexate and 5-fluorouracil; CPB, cyclophosphamide, cisplatin, carmustine; CTC, cyclophosphamide, thiotepa and carboplatin; EC, epirubicin and cyclophosphamide; ECT, epirubicin, cyclophosphamide and thiotepa; FAC, 5-fluorouracil, doxorubicin (adriamycin), cyclophosphamide; FEC, 5-fluorouracil, epirubicin, cyclophosphamide; XRT, radiation therapy patients with 10 or more involved lymph nodes and reported with a median follow-up of 6.1 years, found no difference in DFS or OS between observation and consolidation with HDT (cyclophosphamide 6000 mg/m² and thiotepa 800 mg/m²), following six 28-day cycles of adjuvant CAF (cyclophosphamide 100 mg/m² days 1–14, and adriamycin 30 mg/m² and fluorouracil 500 mg/m² on both days 1 and 8). However, when all protocol violations were excluded, the RFS was longer in the HDT arm (6-year RFS: 55% versus 45%, p = 0.045). The Anglo-Celtic Co-operative Oncology Group (ACCOG) trial, which randomized 605 patients with four or more involved lymph nodes and reported with a median follow-up of 60 months,[42] found no difference in RFS and OS between CDT (8 cycles of 21-day iv CMF: cyclophosphamide 600 mg/m², methotrexate 50 mg/m² and 5-fluorouracil 600 mg/m²) and HDT (cyclophosphamide mobilization 4000 mg/m², cyclophosphamide 6000 mg/m² and thiotepa 800 mg/m²) after adjuvant adriamycin (75 mg/m² × 4 cycles).

The International Collaborative Cancer Group (ICCG) trial[43] stopped accrual after 281 of the planned 300 patients were enrolled due to declining rates of accrual. The data reported were analyzed independently instead of as part of a planned meta-analysis with a parallel trial, so that sample size is significantly lower than anticipated. Patients with four or more involved lymph nodes (stratified by lymph node involvement of less than 10, or 10 or more) received three cycles of FEC (5-fluorouracil 600 mg/m², epirubicin 50 mg/m² and cyclophosphamide 600 mg/m²) and were randomized to receive three cycles of FEC (with 5-fluorouracil and cyclophosphamide repeated on day 8) followed by HDT with CTC (cyclophosphamide 6000 mg/m², thiotepa 500 mg/m² and carboplatin 800 mg/m²) or five additional monthly cycles of FEC (with 5-fluorouracil and cyclophosphamide repeated on day 8). At median follow-up of 5.82 years, there was no difference in RFS or OS. Planned subgroup analyses were not reported.

Three of the randomized trials reporting negative results were relatively small pilot studies with fewer than 100 subjects each, and all evaluated consolidation with HDT. The MD Anderson Cancer Center (MDACC) trial,[44,45] with a median follow-up of nearly 12 years, compared observation to consolidation with two tandem cycles of HDT using CEC (cyclophosphamide 5250 mg/m², etoposide 1200 mg/m² and cisplatin 165 mg/m²), following eight cycles of adjuvant standard-dose FAC (5-fluorouracil 500 mg/m², doxorubicin 50 mg/m² and cyclophosphamide 500 mg/m²). The Dutch Pilot Study,[46,47] with a median follow-up of nearly 7 years, compared observation to consolidation with one cycle of HDT with CTC (cyclophosphamide 6000 mg/m², thiotepa 480 mg/m² and carboplatin 1600 mg/m²), following neo-adjuvant FE₁₂₀C (5-fluorouracil 500 mg/m², epirubicin 120 mg/m², cyclophosphamide 500 mg/m²) and a fourth cycle of adjuvant FE₁₂₀C. And the Japan Clinical Oncology Group (JCOG) 9208 trial[48] compared observation to consolidation with one cycle of HDT (cyclophosphamide 6000 mg/m² and thiotepa 600 mg/m²), following six cycles of adjuvant standard CAF (cyclophosphamide 500 mg/m², adriamycin 40 mg/m² and fluorouracil 500 mg/m²). None of these trials showed any difference in EFS or OS.

The recent Cochrane meta-analysis of HDT for high-risk primary breast cancer[49] included 5064 patients, although much of the data were not mature at the time of the review. The meta-analysis identified statistically significant differences in TRM favoring CDT (relative risk (RR) 8.58, 95% confidence interval (CI) 4.13–17.70) and 3- and 4-year EFS favoring HDT (RR 1.12, 95% CI 1.06–1.19 and RR 1.30, 95% CI 1.16–1.45, respectively). There were no differences identified in 5- or 6-year EFS or in OS at 3, 4, 5 or 6 years. The authors pointed out that few of the data included in the meta-analysis were mature for the reported analyses, and that the late divergence in survival rates noted in some of the trials suggests that extended follow-up will be needed to determine the true value of HDT.

High-dose chemotherapy for inflammatory breast cancer

Prospective Phase II studies[50–52] as well as subset and retrospective analyses[53–56] suggest that women with stage IIIB inflammatory breast cancer may derive unique benefit from high-dose therapy in the adjuvant setting, with 5-year DFS of up to 54% reported,[6] and best results when used in conjunction with combined-modality treatment (Table 12.2). These results compare favorably with 5-year DFS of 30% observed after conventional combined-modality treatment strategies.[6] Investigations are continuing to further define the role of high-dose therapy in this subset of patients, and randomized, controlled trials are needed to confirm these promising results.

High-dose chemotherapy for metastatic breast cancer

High-dose chemotherapy has an extensive history in treating patients with metastatic disease. Again, results of Phase II studies were promising, with remarkable overall response rates of 73–100%, and up to 30% of patients maintaining complete remissions (CR) for well over a year, and occasionally for up to several years.[57–61] As a result of these preliminary data, HDT became a standard-care treatment option for MBC, with slow accrual to randomized, controlled clinical trials and frequent use of cross-over design hampering evaluation.[22] Unfortunately, the first reported randomized, controlled trial comparing HDT and CDT in the metastatic setting, which found a benefit with HDT,[62] was subsequently found to be based on fraudulent data.[26] Over the past few years, however, the results of several randomized, controlled trials have been reported[35,63–70] (Table 12.3). While time to progression (TTP) often reached statistical and in some cases clinical significance, only the French PEGASE 04 trial reported by Lotz et al[65] demonstrated improved OS with HDT.

In PEGASE 04, 61 patients without prior therapy for metastatic disease who had demonstration of chemoresponsive tumor were randomized to HDT with CMA (as in PEGASE 01, above) or maintenance/consolidation with the conventional chemotherapy regimen that had resulted in the response. The study enrolled only 61 of the planned 156 patients due to slow accrual. TTP was significantly longer in the HDT arm (12 vs 6 months, p < 0.0056), as was OS (44.1 vs 19.3 months, p < 0.0294).

However, other trials did not show OS benefit. The largest study was the National Cancer Institute of Canada trial reported by Crump et al,[71] in which patients without prior therapy for metastatic breast cancer were treated with four cycles of an anthracycline- or taxane-based regimen, and those with chemoresponsive tumor (224 patients) were randomized to receive up to two additional cycles of the same conventional therapy followed by HDT (cyclophosphamide 6000 mg/m², mitoxantrone 70 mg/m² and carboplatin 1800 mg/m²) or up to four additional cycles of CDT. With a median follow-up of 19 months, median TTP was longer in the HDT arm (12 vs 0.4 months, p = 0.014) although the difference in OS was not statistically significant (24 vs 27.6 months, p = 0.95).

The French PEGASE 03 trial randomized 180 patients with measurable metastatic disease who responded to FEC100 (5-fluorouracil 500 mg/m², epirubicin 100 mg/m², cyclophosphamide 500 mg/m²) to HDT ('CHUT': cyclophosphamide and thiotepa) or no further therapy.[72] After a median follow-up of 48 months, the HDT arm had improved TTP (11 vs 6.9 months, p = 0.0005) and 1-year DFS (46% vs 19%, p = 0.0001); the difference in OS had not reached significance (3-year: 38% vs 30%, p = 0.7).

In the Philadelphia Intergroup trial reported by Stadtmauer et al,[63] 199 (184 evaluable) of 553 chemoresponsive patients were random-

Table 12.2 HDT for inflammatory breast cancer

Study	n	HDT	CDT	EFS HDT vs CDT	OS	Median follow-up
PEGASE 02 and PEGASE 05[111–113]	223 (CDT) 95 (02) 54 (05)	(4 cycles) Neo-adjuvant Cyclophosphamide Doxorubicin 5-Fluorouracil or Cyclophosphamide Doxorubicin Docetaxel	Doxorubicin-based (historical)	3-yr DFS: 42% vs 52% vs 35%	3-yr: 65% vs 72% vs 50% Median OS: 60m vs NR vs 41 m	
Response Oncology[54]	56	15 Adjuvant 41 Neo-adjuvant Cyclophosphamide Thiotepa Carboplatin	n/a	3-yr EFS: 53%	3-yr: 75%	44 mo
Ottawa[118]	21 Randomized	(3 cycles) 5-Fluorouracil Doxorubicin Cyclophosphamide HDT: Adjuvant Tandem (2) Cyclophosphamide Etoposide Cisplatin	(9 cycles) 5-Fluorouracil Doxorubicin Cyclophosphamide	4-yr DFS: 39% vs 58%	4-yr: 64% vs 64%	
Ravenna[109]	21	Induction: Epirubicin × 4 HDT: Neo-adjuvant Tandem (2) Mitoxantrone Thiotepa Cyclophosphamide	n/a	DFS: 54 mo 5-yr DFS: 54%	53 mo 5-yr: 63%	48 mo
EBMTR[114]	921	Varied	n/a		Not reached	
Marseille[106]	74: 54 HDT	Cyclophosphamide Melphalan +/– Mitoxantrone or dose-intense CAF	Anthracycline-based	27 vs 13 mo 5-yr DFS: 28% vs 15%	5-yr: 50% vs 18%	48 mo (HDT:50 M vs CDT 13 mo)
City of Hope[52]	120	Doxorubicin-containing Neo-adj (73%)/ Adj (100%) CDT; 98% MRM; XRT: 93% Adjuvant HDT: Single or tandem doxorubicin-based (if eligible) or platinum-based +/– XRT	n/a	5-yr RFS: 44%	5-yr: 64%	61 mo (21–161)

Abbreviations: 02, PEGASE 02; 05, PEGASE 05; CAF, cyclophosphamide, doxorubicin, 5-fluorouracil; XRT, radiation therapy; NR, no response; MRM, modified radical mastectomy

ized to HDT with Solid Tumor Autologous Marrow Transplant Program regimen V (STAMP V: cyclophosphamide 6000 mg/m^2, thiotepa 500 mg/m^2 and carboplatin 800 mg/m^2) or CDT with up to 24 cycles of standard CMF.[63] The original study design called for randomization of 99 patients in complete response (CR) and 247 patients with PR. Due to slow accrual, the study was modified to 164 patients, without stratification by disease response. At a median follow-up of 69.5 months, there were no differences in TTP or OS between the two groups. However, subgroup analyses showed trends in favor of HDT for patients younger than 43 years, and in favor of conventional therapy for patients older than 42 years and patients with tumors expressing estrogen receptor.

Two studies did not require chemoresponsive disease for randomization. The International Randomized Breast Cancer Dose Intensity Study (IBDIS) reported by Crown et al[64,73,74] was unique in that it required stable disease rather than response to induction chemotherapy for randomization. The study randomized 110 patients without prior chemotherapy for MBC and no progression with three cycles of induction chemotherapy to tandem cycles of autograft-supported HDT or CDT. The regimens used were (1) induction: AT (doxorubicin 50 mg/ m^2 and docetaxel 75 mg/m^2); (2) the first HDT: ifosfamide 12000 mg/

m^2, carboplatin AUC18 and etoposide 12000 mg/m^2); (3) the second HDT: cyclophosphamide 6000 mg/m^2 and thiotepa 800 mg/m^2); and (4) CDT: a fourth cycle of AT followed by up to four cycles of IV CMF (cyclophosphamide 600 mg/m^2, methotrexate 40 mg/m^2 and 5-fluorouracil 600 mg/m^2 days 1, 8 of 28). The study was stopped with 110 of a planned 264 patients due to poor accrual. At median follow-up of 5 years, EFS was longer in the HDT arm (416 vs 312 days, p = 0.01) but the difference in OS had not reached statistical significance (949 vs 804 days, p = 0.145). Six patients in the HDT arm remained in CR at the 5-year follow-up compared with none of the patients on the CDT arm (p = 0.027).

The German trial reported by Schmid et al[66] enrolled 92 of the planned 440 patients before it, too, was terminated early due to poor accrual, so that planned determinations of superiority of CR rates (440 patients) or equivalence (additional 280 patients) between HDT and CDT could not be performed. Patients with measurable, untreated MBC were randomized at enrollment to tandem AHSC-supported (with cyclophosphamide mobilization) HDT (cyclophosphamide 2400 mg/m^2 (first), 4400 mg/m^2 (second), mitoxantrone 45 mg/m^2 and etoposide 2500 mg/m^2) or CDT (AT: doxorubicin 60 mg/m^2 and paclitaxel 200 mg/m^2 every 3 weeks for up to six courses); patients

Table 12.3 Randomized, controlled trials comparing HDT with CDT in patients with MBC

Study	Disease stage	n	HDT	Control	TTP HDT vs CDT (mo)	EFS HDT vs CDT	OS	Median follow-up (mo)	Comments
PEGASE 03[35,69]	iv, measurable disease, response to up to 4 cycles of induction FEC100	180	C-T	Observation	11 vs 6.9; (p = 0.0005)	1-yr DFS: 46% vs 19% (p = 0.0001)	3-yr: 38% vs 30% (p = 0.7)	48	TRM (HDT) 1.1%
PEGASE 04[35,65,69]	iv, response to up to 9 cycles of anthracycline-containing induction chemotherapy	61 (of 156 planned)	CMA	2–4 additional cycles of 'conventional treatment' (12/29 patients)	12 vs 6; (p < 0.0056)		44.1 vs 19.3; (p < 0.0294)	92 (HDT); 87 (CDT)	TRM: none
IBDIS[64]	iv, no prior chemotherapy for metastatic disease; adjuvant >1 yr; no progression with induction AT × 3	110 (of 264 planned)	Tandem HDT #1 HD ICE HDT #2 C-T	4th AT CMF × 4	14.4 vs 10.6; (p = 0.0033)	416 vs 312 (p = 0.01)	949 vs 804 days (p = 0.145)	60	TRM: 8.9% vs 3.7%
PBT-1[63,70]	iv, no prior chemotherapy for metastatic disease; no adjuvant within 6 months; no progression with induction CAF or CMF (4–6 cycles)	199 (of 346 planned, revised to 164)	CTC 'STAMP V'	Up to 24 cycles of CMF	9.6 vs 9.1; (p = 0.29)	5-yr: 4% vs 3%	25.8 vs 26.1 (p = 0.62) 5-yr: 14% vs 13%	67.5	TRM (HDT) 1% Longer TTP for estrogen receptor-positive patients with CDT (p = 0.05)
NCIC/Crump[69]	iv, no prior chemotherapy for metastatic disease; response with induction × 4 anthracycline or taxane based	224	+ 1–2 induction CMC ER+: Tam Solitary bone/soft tissue mets: XRT	+ 2 to 4 induction ER+: Tam Solitary bone/soft tissue mets: XRT	12 vs 8.4; (p = 0.014)		24 vs 27.6; (p = 0.95)	19	
Berlin[66]	iv, no cytotoxic therapy for metastatic disease Age < 60	92 (of planned 440 to 720)	Tandem (2) CME ER+: Tamoxifen	Up to 6 cycles: Doxorubicin Paclitaxel ER+: Tamoxifen	14.3 vs 10.3; (p = 0.0565)		26.9 vs 23.4; (p = 0.60)	14	TRM (HDT) 2.1% (1) 2o AML (HDT) 2.1% (1)
Duke University[67]	iv, bone-only metastases; no progression with 2–4 cycles of induction AFM	69	'STAMP-1': CPB Consolidation radiation therapy to soft tissue sites of disease	Consolidation radiation therapy to sites of disease		12 vs 4.3; (p < 0.0001)	35.6 vs 21.7; (p = 0.144)	97	TRM 9.7% MDS/AML: None Control arm treated with HDT at relapse
Duke University[68]	iv, hormone-insensitive; measurable disease, no prior chemotherapy for metastatic disease; CR with 2–4 cycles of induction AFM	100	'STAMP-1': CPB Consolidation radiation therapy to soft tissue sites of bulky disease	Consolidation radiation therapy to soft tissue sites of bulky disease		9.7 vs 3.8; (p = 0.006)	39.6 vs 25.2; (p = 0.20)	137	TRM: 8.6% Control arm treated with HDT at relapse

Abbreviations: AT, doxorubicin and docetaxel or paclitaxel; AFM, doxorubicin, 5-fluorouracil and methotrexate; C-T, cyclophosphamide and thiotepa; CMA, cyclophosphamide, mitoxantrone and melphalan; CMC, cyclophosphamide, mitoxantrone and carboplatin; CME, cyclophosphamide, mitoxantrone and etoposide; CMF, cyclophosphamide, methotrexate and 5-fluorouracil; CPB, cyclophosphamide, cisplatin and carmustine; FEC100, 5-fluorouracil, epirubicin, cyclophosphamide; HD-ICE, high-dose ifosfamide, carboplatin and etoposide; Tam, tamoxifen; XRT, radiation therapy

showing a partial response (PR) after six courses of AT could receive up to three courses of single-agent paclitaxel 200 mg/m². At a median follow-up of 14 months, TTP was marginally improved with HDT (14.3 vs 10.3 months, p = 0.0565) but there was no difference in OS (26.9 months vs 23.4 months, p = 0.60).

Long-term follow-up of two randomized trials from Duke University was recently reported by Vredenburgh et al.[67,68] These trials evaluated HDT as consolidation responses to intermediate-dose induction

chemotherapy. Both studies allowed crossover to HDT at the time of relapse in the observation arm, precluding evaluation of OS. One trial enrolled patients with measurable, hormone receptor-negative or hormone therapy-refractory MBC,[67] and a second enrolled patients with bone-only MBC.[68] The hormone-refractory study randomized those that achieved a CR with up to four cycles of intermediate-dose induction chemotherapy to AHST-supported HDT or observation (induction with AFM: 5-fluorouracil 750 mg/m²/day for days 1–5 and doxorubicin 25 mg/m²/day for days 3–5, and methotrexate 250 mg/m² on day 15 with leucovorin rescue, repeated every 3 weeks for up to four cycles; HDT with STAMP I: cyclophosphamide 5625 mg/m², cisplatin 165000 mg/m² and carmustine 600 mg/m²). In the hormone-refractory trial, there was a 27% CR rate to induction. At median follow-up of 11.4 years, the primary endpoint of EFS was significantly longer in the HDT arm (9.7 vs 3.8 months, p = 0.006); 11 patients in the HDT arm and five patients in the observation arm remained in CR. Forty-three patients in the observation arm underwent salvage HDT after relapse, with a 58% CR rate. Overall survival was not different between the two primary study arms (HDT: 39.6 months vs observation: 25.2 months, p = 0.20). The difference in OS between consolidation HDT and salvage HDT was not statistically significant (p = 0.69). In the bone-only metastases trial, 69 patients with stable disease after induction were randomized to the same HDT plus consolidation radiation therapy or consolidation radiation therapy alone. At median follow-up of 8.1 years, EFS was significantly longer in the HDT arm (12 months vs 4.3 months, p < 0.0001). All patients on the observation arm progressed, and 27 of 34 underwent salvage HDT with EFS of 5 months (compared with 12 months after immediate HDT, p = 0.0051). Differences in OS were not statistically significant (2.97 vs 1.81 years, p = 0.144). At the time of the report, four patients remained in CR after immediate HDT and two of the patients who achieved CR with salvage HDT remained free of progression.

An additional study randomized 187 patients with chemosensitive MBC to treatment with a single or tandem cycle of AHST-supported HDT using the STAMP-V regimen (cyclophosphamide, thiotepa and carboplatin). While the lack of a conventional treatment arm precludes conclusions regarding efficacy of HDT, the authors noted a trend toward improved PFS with tandem cycles over single cycle (11.2 vs 9.4 months, p = 0.06) and although not statistically significant, OS appeared worse with tandem cycles (23.5 vs 29 months, p = 0.4).

The recent Cochrane meta-analysis of HDT for metastatic breast cancer[69] included 438 patients, although much of the data were not mature at the time of the review. The meta-analysis identified statistically significant differences in TRM favoring CDT (RR 4.07, 95% CI 1.39–11.88) and 1- and 5-year EFS favoring HDT (RR 1.76, 95% CI 1.40–2.21 and RR 2.84, 95% CI 1.07–7.50 respectively). There were no differences identified in 3-year EFS or in OS at 1, 3 or 5 years. While the meta-analysis could not include TTP, the authors noted that four studies found statistically significant differences favoring HDT, an additional study observed a trend in favor of HDT, and only one study found no difference between the HDT and CDT arms in TTP.

Toxicities and long-term adverse events after high-dose chemotherapy

Treatment-related mortality (TRM) varied with the treatment regimens, but reached as high as 9.7%, and some centers within multicenter trials had much higher TRM.[68] The Cochrane meta-analyses of randomized trials of HDT found that the relative risk of treatment-related death among patients treated for high-risk primary breast cancer was 8.58, favoring CDT (95% CI 4.13–17.80)[49] and among patients treated for MBC, the relative risk of TRM with HDT was 4.07 (95% CI 1.39–11.88).[49]

Secondary malignancies, including myelodysplastic syndrome (MDS) and acute myelogenous leukemia (AML), are of concern following chemotherapy with alkylating agents and topoisomerase-II targeting drugs, including anthracyclines and anthracenediones. Given the frequent use of cyclophosphamide, anthracyclines and mitoxantrone in HDT regimens, the incidence of secondary MDS/AML was addressed in several trials and retrospective reviews. Rates of MDS and AML from trials that reported these are included in Tables 12.1

and 12.3. In general, rates of AML/MDS are 3% or less after HDT for high-risk primary breast cancer, although the length of follow-up likely underestimates the risk. In retrospective reviews, Laughlin et al[75] reported a 1.6% incidence of MDS/acute leukemia among 864 patients treated with cyclophosphamide, cisplatin and BCNU (STAMP I), and Kroger et al[76] found only one case of AML in their review of EBMT registry records among 364 patients with high-risk primary breast cancer treated with high-dose therapy. Kroger et al[77] reported three cases of secondary AML among 305 patients with high-risk primary breast cancer who received mitoxantrone-based HDT, which they noted could occur in up to 8% of patients receiving mitoxantrone as part of conventional adjuvant therapy. It appears that the risk of secondary MDS/AML may be somewhat lower after HDT than reported for conventional dosing of similar agents. This may be a reflection of younger age and absence of prior chemotherapy exposure in the majority of breast cancer patients treated with HDT.

If, in fact, HDT and CDT are equivalent with respect to disease outcome, it is reasonable to consider economic and quality-of-life (QOL) factors in clinical decision making. Comparative studies between HDT and intermediate-dose[78] and conventional therapy[79] in high-risk primary breast cancer found that QOL assessments at 3 months[78] or 6 months[79] favored conventional dosing, an effect that was lost by 12 months after starting treatment. The Cochrane review noted that most of the randomized, controlled trials of HDT in the adjuvant setting that reported QOL data found early, if any, differences favoring CDT, and only one study identified late detriment in QOL after HDT.[49]

It is plausible that the economic and QOL burdens of HDT are borne upfront, and that over the course of chronic MBC, these burdens would be reduced to below that sustained by patients undergoing ongoing treatment with CDT. However, the data do not support this. The Philadelphia Intergroup trial included a planned analysis of QOL. As in the adjuvant setting, QOL was negatively affected at 6 months after transplant, and later time points were not reported.[80] The Canadian NCIC trial also looked at QOL and found recipients of HDT scored significantly worse immediately after HDT, but by 6 and 9 months most scores had improved and were no longer significantly different from CDT recipients.[81] While cost-effectiveness data also favor conventional dosing in patients with MBC,[82] long-term economic data are lacking.

Implications for use of high-dose chemotherapy for breast cancer

Improved EFS and TTP with HDT were demonstrated in several randomized, controlled trials of HDT in the adjuvant setting as well as in the recent Cochrane meta-analysis of these trials. Although only one trial demonstrated an OS benefit, together these data suggest that this treatment modality may be of benefit to some patients, although the best timing and choice of agents are not clear. Patients who appeared to benefit were those with 10 or more involved lymph nodes, younger age, and her2-negative tumors. Major limitations on the interpretation of trial results for HDT in the adjuvant setting include heterogeneity among the regimens used and whether HDT was used as consolidation after conventional adjuvant therapy or instead of CDT, and, importantly, that the comparison arms of these trials used regimens that have been found inferior to currently used dose-dense chemotherapy as described above. The data in the metastatic setting are seriously compromised by early trial termination due to poor accrual, so the question of whether HDT benefits patients with MBC remains largely unanswered. Nonetheless, several trials showed improved EFS and TTP and reported durable CR after HDT and one trial demonstrated improved OS. The Cochrane meta-analysis of HDT in MBC[69] found significant improvement in EFS and TTP, and a non-significant trend toward improved OS, all favoring HDT. Together these reports suggest that longer follow-up and appropriate sample sizes might have identified patients with MBC who would benefit from HDT. While the data are not sufficient to change standard of care, it is reasonable to incorporate HDT into the design of trials evaluating targeted therapeutics, as a means of establishing a foundation of minimal residual disease.

Allogeneic cellular immunotherapy

Immunotherapy with allogeneic HSCT is an approach to treatment of MBC that is entirely distinct from AHSC-supported HDT. There have been a relatively small number of case reports, case series and Phase II trials describing allograft-versus-breast cancer effects (Table 12.4). The first case reports of breast cancer remissions after allogeneic HSCT were reported in the mid-1990s. In the first,[83] a patient treated with high-dose chemotherapy and matched sibling donor bone marrow

transplantation achieved a remission coincident with the development of acute graft-versus-host disease (GvHD). When GvHD was treated with steroids, the patient's breast cancer progressed. In vitro studies were suggestive of a graft-versus-tumor (GvT) effect, demonstrating host minor histocompatibility antigen-specific, major histocompatibility complex class I-restricted cytotoxic lymphocytes from the patient's peripheral blood at the time of the response that recognized a subset of breast cancer cell lines. A second report[84] described a woman diagnosed with simultaneous AML and chest wall recurrence of breast cancer. The chest wall tumor regressed completely over the 12 months following treatment with a matched-sibling donor HSCT.

Further support for graft-versus-breast cancer activity was reported by Ueno et al.[85] Ten women with MBC were treated with high-dose chemotherapy (CBP: cyclophosphamide 6000 mg/m², carmustine 450 mg/m² and thiotepa 720 mg/m²) and HLA matched-sibling donor peripheral HSCT transplantation. The overall response rate was 50%, with a median PFS of 238 days; at median follow-up of 408 days, the median OS had not been reached. After withdrawal of immune sup-

Table 12.4 Allogeneic HSCT for MBC

Study	n	Sites of metastatic disease	Conditioning	Late responses (GvT)	Associated GvHD (acute or chronic)	RR	EFS	OS	Median follow-up
Hadassah[84]	1	Chest wall, concurrent AML	Amsacrine/cytarabine etoposide/mitoxantrone Conditioning: n/s	1	Possible (rash c/w late-acute)	n/a	n/a	n/a	12 months
NCI[88,89]	16		Induction: Fludarabine Cyclophosphamide RIST: Fludarabine Cyclophosphamide	6	5/6 (acute (4) and chronic (1))	37.5%		10.3 months	23.4 months
Milan[107]	6 (updated to 9)[108]	Refractory MBC, evaluable disease	RIST: Thiotepa Fludarabine Cyclophosphamide	2	2/2 (late-acute/chronic)				Range: 109–1003 days
Genoa[90]	17	Any but brain	HDT/auto-SCT: Mitoxantrone Thiotepa RIST: Fludarabine Cyclophosphamide	4	4/4 (chronic)	24%			
Innsbruck[83]	1	Liver, bone	HDT: Thiotepa Carboplatin Cyclophosphamide	1 (day +27)	Y (acute)	n/a	n/a	n/a	d. Day +110
Hadassah[86]	6		HDT: Carboplatin Etoposide Thiotepa Melphalan Pre-donor cell therapy: cyclophosphamide 500–1000 mg/m² (D-1); non-mobilized donor PBL + IL-2; +/− IL-2 activation	4	0 (no engraftment)	n/a	7–12 months	n/a	11 months
MDACC[85]	10	Bone marrow and/or liver, stable or responding to standard-dose chemotherapy	Induction (CDT) HDT: Cyclophosphamide Carmustine Thiotepa	2	2/2 (acute)	50%	238	Median not reached	408 d
MDACC[87]	8	Any but brain, responding to standard-dose chemotherapy	RIST: Fludarabine Melphalan	4	3/4 (chronic)	37.5%	n/a	1-yr 75% median: 493 days	470.5 d

Abbreviations: AML, acute myelogenous leukemia; NCI, National Cancer Institute; RIST, reduced-intensity stem cell transplanatation; HDT, high-dose therapy; auto-SCT, autologous stem cell transplantation; Y, yes; d, death; PBL, peripheral blood lymphocytes; MDACC, University of Texas MD Anderson Cancer Center; CDT, conventional-dose therapy.

pression, two of four patients with progressive disease demonstrated regression of liver metastases in association with the development of acute GvHD of the skin. Both patients subsequently developed chronic GvHD and stabilization of their breast cancer through days 402 and 884 post transplant. Delayed responses achieved upon withdrawal of immunosuppression and coincident with clinical evidence of alloreactivity in the form of GvHD suggested an immune-mediated basis of these responses. In a second series reported by Or et al,[86] six patients with MBC were treated with HDT (carboplatin, etoposide, thiotepa and melphalan) with AHSC support followed by immune depletion, allogeneic lymphocyte infusions and exogenous interleukin-2. While none of the recipients demonstrated measurable donor engraftment, four patients had measurable disease responses to the allogeneic cell therapy. All patients achieved longer PFS after allogeneic cell therapy than after HDT alone, although the potential role of cyclophosphamide in maintaining disease control precluded definitive attribution to a GvT response.

Ueno et al[87] examined GvT effects in patients with metastatic or recurrent breast cancer and metastatic renal cell carcinoma treated with allogeneic HSCT following reduced-intensity conditioning (fludarabine and melphalan). In this study, immune suppression was tapered if patients had early (day 30) disease progression or persistent disease at day 100. This was followed by infusion of additional donor lymphocytes (DLI) in those without a response or GvHD. In the eight patients treated for MBC, there were two CR, one of which was late and associated with withdrawal of immune suppression, and one mixed response.

Bishop et al[88,89] reported results of a study designed to separate the effects of conditioning chemotherapy from potential GvT effects. Women with MBC and measurable disease received reduced-intensity conditioning (fludarabine/cyclophosphamide) followed by a T-cell depleted (1×10^5 T-cells/kg) PBSC allograft. In the absence of GvHD, immune suppression (ciclosporin) was rapidly tapered off from day 28 to day 42, and DLI were administered on days 42, 70 and 98. Six of 16 patients demonstrated tumor regression after day 28, including two patients with disease progression prior to DLI; these late responses were attributed to GvT effects of the allogeneic lymphocytes. The timing of these late tumor responses was highly suggestive of a graft-versus-breast cancer effect: regressions occurred at the time of or after the establishment of complete donor chimerism in the T-cell compartment and were strongly associated with the development of acute GvHD.

Most recently, Carella et al[90] reported on results of a study treating 17 women with measurable MBC with tandem autologous-allogeneic HSCT. HDT (mitoxantrone 45 mg/m² and thiotepa 600 mg/m²) with AHSC support was followed, upon recovery, with reduced-intensity conditioning (fludarabine and cyclophosphamide) and allogeneic HSCT. There was no TRM after autologous HDT or during the first 100 days after allogeneic HSCT. Following allogeneic HSCT, three patients converted partial response (PR) after HDT to CR, including one patient with persistent disease immediately after allogeneic HSCT who subsequently responded to DLI. A fourth patient achieved a partial response occurring 300 days after allogeneic HSCT, coincident with the development of chronic GvHD. Of note, all late responses, including stable disease, were associated with the development of chronic GvHD. The three patients who achieved late CR were alive and disease free at 1320, 1530 and 2160 days after allogeneic HSCT. From this trial, it appeared that GvT effects mediated by the allograft added to the response rates achieved with HDT.

In summary, there is a mounting body of evidence that an allo-mediated GvT effect may have clinical activity in controlling metastatic breast cancer. Combinations of HDT and allogeneic cell therapy, which take advantage of the significant disease response rates seen with HDT as well as of the improved toxicity profile of reduced-inten-

sity allogeneic HSCT, may be a feasible approach to minimize disease burden during the time a therapeutic response from immunotherapy is being established.

Future directions for stem cell therapies for breast cancer

Promising areas of ongoing investigation in transplantation and cellular immunotherapy for breast cancer often combine principles of HDT and/or allogeneic immunotherapy with novel approaches to improve efficacy. Ongoing trials evaluating novel immunologic approaches to breast cancer therapy are numerous and include therapeutic vaccine strategies, molecularly engineered cell therapies and allogeneic cell therapies. Vaccine approaches include modified cancer-cell vaccines (for example, the Dana Farber study, Vaccination with autologous breast cancer cells engineered to secrete granulocyte-macrophage colony-stimulating factor (GM-CSF) in metastatic breast cancer patients),[91] vaccines targeting breast cancer antigens such as CEA and MUC-1 (for example, the NCI study, Vaccine therapy before and after dose-intensive induction chemotherapy plus immune-depleting chemotherapy in treating patients with metastatic breast cancer),[92] Her2/neu (for example, the University of Washington study, HER-2/ Neu vaccine plus GM-CSF in treating patients with stage III or stage IV breast, ovarian, or non-small cell lung cancer),[93] tumor antigen- or RNA-loaded dendritic cell vaccines (such as the University of Pennsylvania's study, Vaccine therapy in treating patients who are undergoing surgery for ductal carcinoma in situ of the breast),[94] and the University of North Carolina's Vaccine therapy, trastuzumab, and vinorelbine in treating women with locally recurrent or metastatic breast cancer.[95] Engineered cell therapy trials include the NCI study of T-cells with genetically modified, tumor-specific T-cell receptors for treatment of patients with metastatic melanoma.[96,97]

Approaches building on the allogeneic HSCT platform are also being evaluated. Examples include adoptive transfer of mature allogeneic immune cells, including natural killer cell enrichment of the allograft (for example, the University of Minnesota study, Donor peripheral stem cell transplant after fludarabine and cyclophosphamide in treating patients with metastatic breast cancer),[98] after interleukin-2 activation (such as the Hadassah University study, Cell therapy of cancer with allogeneic blood lymphocytes activated with rIL-2 for metastatic solid tumors)[99] or using genetically modified donor lymphocytes (for example, the Hadassah University's Immunotherapy of cancer using donor lymphocytes labeled with in-vitro bispecific antibodies).[100]

Allogeneic cell therapy has the potential advantage of targeting multiple, often unknown tumor antigens, and the GvT effect appears to be less constrained by host regulatory cell populations than autologous cell vaccine strategies.[101] However, the GvT response to breast cancer, and perhaps to other tumors of epithelial origin, may be harder to separate from GvHD or have a narrower therapeutic index than more immunogenic and alloresponsive hematologic malignancies. Strategies to reduce GvHD while maintaining engraftment and GvT effects may broaden the therapeutic application of allogeneic cell therapy for patients with MBC.[102–105]

At present, the role of transplantation, including HSCT support for HDT and allogeneic cellular immunotherapy, remains investigational and limited to patients without proven curative treatment options. HDT and allogeneic immunotherapy offer their greatest promise as components of broader treatment strategies that build on progress in the development of molecularly targeted agents, therapeutic monoclonal antibodies, and clinical application of cellular immunology. As is nearly universal in the development of new therapeutic tools in the treatment of malignancy, while initial attempts are limited to patients with the poorest prognoses, with disease resistant to standard therapies, the greatest potential for improving the course of breast cancer lies in earlier treatment, when disease burden is lowest and tumor cells are most responsive to all forms of therapy. Given the demonstrated breast cancer activity of these aggressive investigational approaches, including allogeneic HSCT and combining allogeneic immunotherapy and/or HDT with emerging targeted therapeutics, they should be considered for young patients with good performance status who have metastatic disease that is not controlled by minimally toxic hormonal and/or Her2-directed therapies.

References

1. Bray F, McCarron P, Parkin DM. The changing global patterns of female breast cancer incidence and mortality. Breast Cancer Res 2004;6:229–239

2. Ferlay J, Bray F, Pisani P et al. GLOBOCAN 2002: cancer incidence, mortality and prevalence worldwide. CancerBase No. 5, version 2.0. IARC Press, Lyon, 2004

3. Fisher B, Bauer M, Wickerham DL et al. Relation of number of positive axillary nodes to the prognosis of patients with primary breast cancer. An NSABP update.Cancer 1983;52:1551–1557

4. Adjuvant! Online Database 2006. www.adjuvantonline.com

5. Walshe JM, Swain SM. Clinical aspects of inflammatory breast cancer. Breast Dis 2005;22:35–44

6. Yang CH, Cristofanilli M. Systemic treatments for inflammatory breast cancer. Breast Dis 2005;22:55–65

7. Surveillance, Epidemiology, and End Results (SEER) Program. SEER*Stat Database 2006. National Cancer Institute, DCCCPS, Surveillance Research Program, Cancer Statistics Branch, Bethesda, Maryland

8. Early Breast Cancer Trialists' Collaborative Group. Effects of chemotherapy and hormonal therapy for early breast cancer on recurrence and 15-year survival: an overview of the randomised trials. Lancet 2005;365:1687–1717

9. DeVita V, Hellman S, Rosenberg S et al. Cancer: principles and practice of oncology. Lippincott Williams and Wilkins, Philadelphia, 2005

10. Trudeau M, Charbonneau F, Gelmon K et al. Selection of adjuvant chemotherapy for treatment of node-positive breast cancer. Lancet Oncol 2005;6:886–898

11. Dang CT. Drug treatments for adjuvant chemotherapy in breast cancer: recent trials and future directions. Expert Rev Anticancer Ther 2006;6:427–436

12. Piccart-Gebhart MJ, Procter M, Leyland-Jones B et al. Trastuzumab after adjuvant chemotherapy in HER2-positive breast cancer. N Engl J Med 2005;353:1659–1672

13. Romond EH, Perez EA, Bryant J et al. Trastuzumab plus adjuvant chemotherapy for operable HER2-positive breast cancer. N Engl J Med 2005;353:1673–1684

14. Wood WC, Muss HB, Solin LJ, Olopade OI. Malignant tumors of the breast. In: DeVita V, Hellman S, Rosenberg S et al (eds) Cancer: principles and practice of oncology. Lippincott Williams and Wilkins, Philadelphia, 2005, 1415–1477

15. Perez EA. Adjuvant therapy approaches to breast cancer: should taxanes be incorporated? Curr Oncol Rep 2003;5:66–71

16. Crown J, Dieras V, Kaufmann M et al. Chemotherapy for metastatic breast cancer – report of a European expert panel. Lancet Oncol 2002;3:719–727

17. Gennari A, Conte P, Rosso R et al. Survival of metastatic breast carcinoma patients over a 20-year period: a retrospective analysis based on individual patient data from six consecutive studies. Cancer 2005;104:1742–1750

18. Frei E 3rd, Canellos GP. Dose: a critical factor in cancer chemotherapy. Am J Med 10980;69:585–594

19. Hryniuk W, Bush H. The importance of dose intensity in chemotherapy of metastatic breast cancer. J Clin Oncol 1984;2:1281–1288

20. Basser RL. New developments in high-dose chemotherapy for breast cancer. Recent Results Cancer Res 1998;152:355–367

21. Strobl FJ, Stadtmauer EA. Breast tumor cell contamination of hematopoietic stem cell collections. Breast Dis 2001;14:9–19

22. Antman KH, Rowlings PA, Vaughan WP et al. High-dose chemotherapy with autologous hematopoietic stem-cell support for breast cancer in North America. J Clin Oncol 1997;15:1870–1879

23. Crown J. Smart bombs versus blunderbusses: high-dose chemotherapy for breast cancer. Lancet 2004;364:1299–1300

24. Vogl DT, Stadtmauer EA. High-dose chemotherapy and autologous hematopoietic stem cell transplantation for metastatic breast cancer: a therapy whose time has passed. Bone Marrow Transplant 2006;37:985–987

25. Davidson NE. Out of the courtroom and into the clinic. J Clin Oncol 1992;10:517–519

26. Weiss RB, Rifkin RM, Stewart FM et al. High-dose chemotherapy for high-risk primary breast cancer: an on-site review of the Bezwoda study. Lancet 2000;355:999–1003

27. Stuart MJ, Peters WP, Broadwater G et al. High-dose chemotherapy and hematopoietic support for patients with high-risk primary breast cancer and involvement of 4 to 9 lymph nodes. Biol Blood Marrow Transplant 2002;8:666–673

28. Peters WP, Ross M, Vrendenburgh JJ et al. High-dose chemotherapy and autologous bone marrow support as consolidation after standard-dose adjuvant therapy for high-risk primary breast cancer. J Clin Oncol 1993;11:1132–1143

29. Somlo G, Doroshow JH, Forman SJ et al. High-dose chemotherapy and stem-cell rescue in the treatment of high-risk breast cancer: prognostic indicators of progression-free and overall survival. J Clin Oncol 1997;15:2882–2893

30. Cheng YC, Rondon G, Yang Y et al. The use of high-dose cyclophosphamide, carmustine, and thiotepa plus autologous hematopoietic stem cell transplantation as consolidation

31. Gianni AM, Siena S, Bregni M et al. Efficacy, toxicity, and applicability of high-dose sequential chemotherapy as adjuvant treatment in operable breast cancer with 10 or more involved axillary nodes: five-year results. J Clin Oncol 1997;15:2312–2321

32. Bergh J, Wiklund T, Erikstein B et al. Tailored fluorouracil, epirubicin, and cyclophosphamide compared with marrow-supported high-dose chemotherapy as adjuvant treatment for high-risk breast cancer: a randomised trial. Scandinavian Breast Group 9401 study. Lancet 2000;356:1384–1391

33. Rodenhuis S, Bontenbal M, Beex LV et al. High-dose chemotherapy with hematopoietic stem-cell rescue for high-risk breast cancer. N Engl J Med 2003;349:7–16

34. Nitz UA, Mohrmann S, Fischer J et al. Comparison of rapidly cycled tandem high-dose chemotherapy plus peripheral-blood stem-cell support versus dose-dense conventional chemotherapy for adjuvant treatment of high-risk breast cancer: results of a multicentre phase III trial. Lancet 2005;366:1935–1944

35. Roche H, Viens P, Biron P et al. High-dose chemotherapy for breast cancer: the French PEGASE experience. Cancer Control 2003;10:42–47

36. Zander AR, Kroger N. High-dose therapy for breast cancer – a case of suspended animation. Acta Haematol 2005;114:248–254

37. Basser RL, O'Neill A, Martinelli G et al. Multicycle dose-intensive chemotherapy for women with high-risk primary breast cancer: results of International Breast Cancer Study Group Trial 15–95. J Clin Oncol 2006;24:370–378

38. Zander AR, Kroger N, Schmoor C et al. High-dose chemotherapy with autologous hematopoietic stem-cell support compared with standard-dose chemotherapy in breast cancer patients with 10 or more positive lymph nodes: first results of a randomized trial. J Clin Oncol 2004;22:2273–2283

39. Zander AR, Kroeger N, Schmoor C et al. Randomized trial of high-dose chemotherapy with autologous haematopoietic stem cell support vs standard-dose chemotherapy in breast cancer patients with 10 or more positive lymph nodes: overall survival after 6 years of follow up. Proceedings of the ASCO Annual Meeting, 2006. J Clin Oncol 2006;24(18):672

40. Gianni AM, Bonadonna G. Five-year results of the randomized clinical trial comparing standard versus high-dose myeloablative chemotherapy in the adjuvant treatment of breast cancer with >3 positive nodes (LN+). Proceedings of the ASCO Annual Meeting 2001. ASCO, Alexandria, Virginia

41. Tallman MS, Gray R, Robert NJ et al. Conventional adjuvant chemotherapy with or without high-dose chemotherapy and autologous stem-cell transplantation in high-risk breast cancer. N Engl J Med 2003;349:17–26

42. Leonard R, Lind M, Twelves C et al. Conventional adjuvant chemotherapy versus single-cycle, autograft-supported, high-dose, late-intensification chemotherapy in high-risk breast cancer patients: a randomized trial. J Natl Cancer Inst 2004;96:1076–1083

43. Coombes RC, Howell A, Emson M et al. High dose chemotherapy and autologous stem cell transplantation as adjuvant therapy for primary breast cancer patients with four or more lymph nodes involved: long-term results of an international randomised trial. Ann Oncol 2005;16:726–734

44. Hortobagyi GN, Buzdar AU, Theriault RI et al. Randomized trial of high-dose chemotherapy and bone cell autografts for high-risk primary breast carcinoma. J Natl Cancer Inst 2000;92:225–233

45. Hanrahan EO, Broglio K, Frye D et al. Randomized trial of high-dose chemotherapy and autologous hematopoietic stem cell support for high-risk primary breast carcinoma: follow-up at 12 years. Cancer 2006;106:2327–2336

46. Rodenhuis S, Riche DJ, van der Wall E et al. Randomised trial of high-dose chemotherapy and haemopoietic progenitor-cell support in operable breast cancer with extensive axillary lymph-node involvement. Lancet 1998;352:515–521

47. Schrama JG, Faneyte IF, Schornagel JH et al. Randomized trial of high-dose chemotherapy and hematopoietic progenitor-cell support in operable breast cancer with extensive lymph node involvement: final analysis with 7 years of follow-up. Ann Oncol 2002;13:689–698

48. Tokuda Y, Tajima T, Narabayashi M et al. Randomized phase III study of high-dose chemotherapy (HDC) with autologous stem cell support as consolidation in high-risk postoperative breast cancer: Japan Clinical Oncology Group (JCOG9208). Proceedings of the ASCO Annual Meeting, 2001. ASCO, Alexandria, Virginia

49. Farquhar C, Marjoribanks J, Lethaby A et al. High dose chemotherapy and autologous bone marrow or stem cell transplantation versus conventional chemotherapy for women with early poor prognosis breast cancer. Cochrane Database Syst Rev 2005: CD003139

50. Ayash LJ, Elias A, Ibrahim J et al. High-dose multimodality therapy with autologous stem-cell support for stage IIIB breast carcinoma. J Clin Oncol 1998;16:1000–1007

51. Cagnoni PJ, Nieto Y, Shpall EJ et al. High-dose chemotherapy with autologous hematopoietic progenitor-cell support as part of combined modality therapy in patients with inflammatory breast cancer. J Clin Oncol 1998;16:1661–1668

52. Somlo G, Frankel P, Chow W et al. Prognostic indicators and survival in patients with stage IIIB inflammatory breast carcinoma after dose-intense chemotherapy. J Clin Oncol 2004;22:1839–1848

53. Adkins D, Brown R, Trinkaus K et al. Outcomes of high-dose chemotherapy and autologous stem-cell transplantation in stage IIIB inflammatory breast cancer. J Clin Oncol 1999;17:2006–2014

54. Schwartzberg L, Weaver C, Lewkow L et al. High-dose chemotherapy with peripheral blood stem cell support for stage IIIB inflammatory carcinoma of the breast. Bone Marrow Transplant 1999;24:981–987

55. Kasten-Sportes C, McCarthy NJ, Bishop MR et al. High-dose chemotherapy and autologous transplant for stage IIIB inflammatory breast cancer (abstract). Blood 2002;100:2447

56. Sportes C, McCarthy NJ, Hakim F et al. Establishing a platform for immunotherapy: clinical outcome and study of immune reconstitution after high-dose chemotherapy with progenitor cell support in breast cancer patients. Biol Blood Marrow Transplant 2005;11:472–483

57. Peters WP, Shpall EJ, Jones RB et al. High-dose combination alkylating agents with bone marrow support as initial treatment for metastatic breast cancer. J Clin Oncol 1988;6:1368–1376
58. Williams SF, Mick R, Desser R et al. High-dose consolidation therapy with autologous stem cell rescue in stage IV breast cancer. J Clin Oncol 1989;7:1824–1830
59. Kennedy MJ, Beveridge RA, Rowley SD et al. High-dose chemotherapy with reinfusion of purged autologous bone marrow following dose-intense induction as initial therapy for metastatic breast cancer. J Natl Cancer Inst 1991;83:920–926
60. Antman K, Ayash L, Elias A et al. A phase II study of high-dose cyclophosphamide, thiotepa, and carboplatin with autologous marrow support in women with measurable advanced breast cancer responding to standard-dose therapy. J Clin Oncol 1992;10:102–110
61. Williams SF, Gilewski T, Mick R et al. High-dose consolidation therapy with autologous stem-cell rescue in stage IV breast cancer: follow-up report. J Clin Oncol 1992;10:1743–1747
62. Bezwoda WR, Seymour L, Dansey RD et al. High-dose chemotherapy with hematopoietic rescue as primary treatment for metastatic breast cancer: a randomized trial. J Clin Oncol 1995;13:2483–2489
63. Stadtmauer EA, O'Neill A, Goldstein L et al. Conventional-dose chemotherapy compared with high-dose chemotherapy (HDC) plus autologous stem-cell transplantation (SCT) for metastatic breast cancer: 5-year update of the 'Philadelphia Trial' (PBT-1) (abstract 169). Proceedings of the ASCO Annual Meeting, 2002. ASCO, Alexandria, Virginia
64. Crown J, Leyvraz S, Verill M et al. High-dose chemotherapy (HDC) produces a superior rate of durable complete remission (DCR) compared to conventional chemotherapy in metastatic breast cancer (MBC): mature results of the International Breast Cancer Dose-Intensity Study. ESMO. Ann Oncol 2004;15(3):27
65. Lotz JP, Cure H, Janvier M et al. High-dose chemotherapy with haematopoietic stem cell transplantation for metastatic breast cancer patients: final results of the French multicentric randomised CMA/PEGASE 04 protocol. Eur J Cancer 2005;41:71–80
66. Schmid P, Schippinger W, Nitsch T et al. Up-front tandem high-dose chemotherapy compared with standard chemotherapy with doxorubicin and paclitaxel in metastatic breast cancer: results of a randomized trial. J Clin Oncol 2005;23:432–440
67. Vredenburgh JJ, Coniglio D, Broadwater G et al. Consolidation with high-dose combination alkylating agents with bone marrow transplantation significantly improves disease-free survival in hormone-insensitive metastatic breast cancer in complete remission compared with intensive standard-dose chemotherapy alone. Biol Blood Marrow Transplant 2006;12:195–203
68. Vredenburgh JJ, Madan B, Coniglio D et al. A randomized phase III comparative trial of immediate consolidation with high-dose chemotherapy and autologous peripheral blood progenitor cell support compared to observation with delayed consolidation in women with metastatic breast cancer and only bone metastases following intensive induction chemotherapy. Bone Marrow Transplant 2006;37:1009–1015
69. Farquhar C, Marjoribanks J, Basser R et al. High dose chemotherapy and autologous bone marrow or stem cell transplantation versus conventional chemotherapy for women with metastatic breast cancer. Cochrane Database Syst Rev 2005;CD003142
70. Stadtmauer EA, O'Neill A, Goldstein LJ et al. Conventional-dose chemotherapy compared with high-dose chemotherapy plus autologous hematopoietic stem-cell transplantation for metastatic breast cancer. Philadelphia Bone Marrow Transplant Group. N Engl J Med 2000;342:1069–1076
71. Crump M., Gluck S, Douglas Stewart D et al. A randomized trial of high-dose chemotherapy (HDC) with autologous peripheral blood stem cell support (ASCT) compared to standard therapy in women with metastatic breast cancer: a National Cancer Institute of Canada (NCIC) Clinical Trials Group Study (abstract 82). Proceedings of the ASCO Annual Meeting, 2001. ASCO, Alexandria, Virginia
72. Biron P, Durand M, Roche H et al. High dose thiotepa (TTP), cyclophosphamide (CPM) and stem cell transplantation after 4 FEC 100 compared with 4 FEC alone allowed a better disease free survival but the same overall survival in first line chemotherapy for metastatic breast cancer. Results of the PEGASE 03 French Protocole (abstract 167). Proceedings of the ASCO Annual Meeting, 2002. ASCO, Alexandria, Virginia
73. Crown J, Perey L, Lind M et al. Superiority of tandem high-dose chemotherapy (HDC) versus optimized conventionally-dosed chemotherapy (CDC) in patients (pts) with metastatic breast cancer (MBC): The International Randomized Breast Cancer Dose Intensity Study (IBDIS 1) (abstract 88). Proceedings of the ASCO Annual Meeting, 2003. ASCO, Alexandria, Virginia
74. Crown J, Leyvraz S, Verrill M et al. Effect of tandem high-dose chemotherapy (HDC) on long-term complete remissions (LTCR) in metastatic breast cancer (MBC), compared to conventional dose (CDC) in patients (pts) who were not selected on the basis of response to prior C: mature results of the IBDIS-I. Proceedings of the ASCO Annual Meeting, 2004. ASCO, Alexandria, Virginia
75. Laughlin MJ, McGaughey DS, Crews JR et al. Secondary myelodysplasia and acute leukemia in breast cancer patients after autologous bone marrow transplant. J Clin Oncol 1998;16:1008–1012
76. Kroger N, Zander AR, Martinelli G et al. Low incidence of secondary myelodysplasia and acute myeloid leukemia after high-dose chemotherapy as adjuvant therapy for breast cancer patients: a study by the Solid Tumors Working Party of the European Group for Blood and Marrow Transplantation. Ann Oncol 2003;14:554–558
77. Kroger N, Damon L, Zander AR et al. Secondary acute leukemia following mitoxantrone-based high-dose chemotherapy for primary breast cancer patients. Bone Marrow Transplant 2003;32:1153–1157
78. Peppercorn J, Herndon J 2nd, Kornblith AB et al. Quality of life among patients with Stage II and III breast carcinoma randomized to receive high-dose chemotherapy with autologous bone marrow support or intermediate-dose chemotherapy: results from Cancer and Leukemia Group B 9066. Cancer 2005;104:1580–1589
79. Malinovszky KM, Gould A, Foster E et al. Quality of life and sexual function after high-dose or conventional chemotherapy for high-risk breast cancer. Br J Cancer 2006;95:1626–1631
80. Daly M, Goldstein LJ, Topolsky D et al. Quality of life experience in women randomized to high-dose chemotherapy (HDC) and stem cell support (SCT) or standard dose chemotherapy for responding metastatic breast cancer in Philadelphia Intergroup Study (PBT-1) (abstract 327). Proceedings of the ASCO Annual Meeting, 2000. ASCO, Alexandria, Virginia
81. Dancey J, Crump M, Gluck S et al. Quality of life (QOL) analysis of a randomized trial of high-dose chemotherapy (HDCT) with peripheral stem cell transplant (PSCT) versus standard chemotherapy (SCT) in women with metastatic breast cancer (MBC): National Cancer Institute of Canada Clinical Trials Group study (NCIC CTG) MA-16 (abstract 301). Proceedings of the ASCO Annual Meeting, 2003. ASCO, Alexandria, Virginia
82. Schulman KA, Stadtmauer EA, Reed SD et al. Economic analysis of conventional-dose chemotherapy compared with high-dose chemotherapy plus autologous hematopoietic stem-cell transplantation for metastatic breast cancer. Bone Marrow Transplant 2003;31:205–210
83. Eibl B, Schwaighofer H, Nachbaur D et al. Evidence for a graft-versus-tumor effect in a patient treated with marrow ablative chemotherapy and allogeneic bone marrow transplantation for breast cancer. Blood 1996;88:1501–1508
84. Ben-Yosef R, Or R, Nagler A et al. Graft-versus-tumour and graft-versus-leukaemia effect in patients with concurrent breast cancer and acute myelocytic leukaemia. Lancet 1996;348:1242–1243
85. Ueno NT, Rondon G, Mirza NQ et al. Allogeneic peripheral-blood progenitor-cell transplantation for poor-risk patients with metastatic breast cancer. J Clin Oncol 1998;16:986–993
86. Or R, Ackerstein A, Nagler A et al. Allogeneic cell-mediated immunotherapy for breast cancer after autologous stem cell transplantation: a clinical pilot study. Cytokines Cell Mol Ther 1998;4:1–6
87. Ueno NT, Cheng YC, Rondon G et al. Rapid induction of complete donor chimerism by the use of a reduced-intensity conditioning regimen composed of fludarabine and melphalan in allogeneic stem cell transplantation for metastatic solid tumors. Blood 2003;102: 3829–3836
88. Bishop MR, Fowler DH, Marchigiani D et al. Allogeneic lymphocytes induce tumor regression of advanced metastatic breast cancer. J Clin Oncol 2004;22:3886–3892
89. Bishop MR, Steinberg SM, Gress RE et al. Targeted pretransplant host lymphocyte depletion prior to T-cell depleted reduced-intensity allogeneic stem cell transplantation. Br J Haematol 2004;126:837–843
90. Carella AM, Beltrami G, Corsetti MT et al. Reduced intensity conditioning for allograft after cytoreductive autograft in metastatic breast cancer. Lancet 2005;366: 318–320
91. Vaccination with autologous breast cancer cells engineered to secrete granulocyte-macrophage colony-stimulating factor (GM-CSF) in metastatic breast cancer. www.clinicaltrials.gov/ct/show/NCT00317603;jsessionid=5CBB223B14F69F918CE42FC5130962C3?order=50–17k-
92. Vaccine therapy before and after dose-intensive induction chemotherapy plus immune-depleting chemotherapy in treating patients with metastatic breast cancer. www.clinicaltrials.gov/ct/show /NCT00053170;
93. HER-2/Neu vaccine plus GM-CSF in treating patients with stage III or stage IV breast, ovarian, or non-small cell lung cancer. www.clinicaltrials.gov/ct/show/NCT00003002–17
94. Vaccine therapy in treating patients who are undergoing surgery for ductal carcinoma in situ of the breast. Protocol IDs: UPCC-08102. www.cancer411.org/clinicaltrials/ getTrialDetail.asp?Trial_Key=5340&PoliticalUnit=&City=-9k
95. Vaccine therapy, trastuzumab, and vinorelbine in treating women with locally recurrent or metastatic breast cancer. www.clinicaltrials.gov/ct/gui/show/ NCT00088985;jsessionid=AA3C32B2B3DF257FD750385AAD04B518?order=41–20k
96. Kershaw MH, Westwood JA, Parker LL et al. A phase I study on adoptive immunotherapy using gene-modified T cells for ovarian cancer. Clin Cancer Res 2006;12(20 Pt 1):6106–6115
97. Morgan RA, Dudley ME, Wunderlich JR et al. Cancer regression in patients after transfer of genetically engineered lymphocytes. Science 2006;314:126–129
98. Donor peripheral stem cell transplant after fludarabine and cyclophosphamide in treating patients with metastatic breast cancer. www.clinicaltrials.gov/ct/show/ NCT00376805?order=4
99. Cell therapy of cancer with allogeneic blood lymphocytes activated with rIL-2 for metastatic solid tumors. www.clinicaltrials.gov/ct/screen/BrowseAny;jsessionid=23688F63559D5716DF0F59B52D180486?
100. Immunotherapy of cancer using donor lymphocytes labelled with in-vitro bispecific antibodies. http://clinicaltrials.gov/ct/show/NCT00149019?order=1
101. Yang Y, Huang CT, Huang X et al. Persistent Toll-like receptor signals are required for reversal of regulatory T cell-mediated CD8 tolerance. Nat Immunol 2004;5:508–515
102. Fowler DH, Bishop MR, Gress RE et al. Immunoablative reduced-intensity stem cell transplantation: potential role of donor Th2 and Tc2 cells. Semin Oncol 2004;31:56–67
103. Fowler DH, Gress RE. CD8+ T cells of Tc2 phenotype mediate a GVL effect and prevent marrow rejection. Vox Sang 1998;74(suppl 2):331–340
104. Noonan K, Matsui W, Serafini P et al. Activated marrow-infiltrating lymphocytes effectively target plasma cells and their clonogenic precursors. Cancer Res 2005;65: 2026–2034
105. Hardy NM, Fowler DH, Bishop MR. Immunotherapy of metastatic breast cancer: phase I trail of reduced-intensity allogeneic hematopoietic stem cell transplantation with Th2/Tc2 T-cell exchange. Clin Breast Cancer 2006;7:87–89
106. Bertucci F, Tarpin C, Charafe-Jauffret E et al. Multivariate analysis of survival in inflammatory breast cancer: impact of intensity of chemotherapy in multimodality treatment. Bone Marrow Transplant 2004;33:913–920
107. Bregni M, Dodero A, Peccatori J et al. Nonmyeloablative conditioning followed by hematopoietic cell allografting and donor lymphocyte infusions for patients with metastatic renal and breast cancer. Blood 2002;99:4234–4236
108. Bregni M, Fleischhauer K, Bernardi M et al. Bone marrow mammaglobin expression as a marker of graft-versus-tumor effect after reduced-intensity allografting for advanced breast cancer. Bone Marrow Transplant 2006;37:311–315
109. Dazzi C, Cariello A, Rosti G et al. Neoadjuvant high dose chemotherapy plus peripheral blood progenitor cells in inflammatory breast cancer: a multicenter phase II pilot study. Haematologica 2001;86:523–529

110. Hortobagyi GN, Buzdar AU. RESPONSE: randomized trial of high-dose chemotherapy and blood cell autografts for high-risk primary breast carcinoma. J Natl Cancer Inst 2000;92:1273

111. Palangie T, Viens P, Roche H et al. Dose-intensified chemotherapy and additional Docetaxel may improve inflammatory breast cancer patients' outcome over two decades: results from Institut Curie protocols 1977–1987 and two consecutive French multicenter trials Pegase 02 (1995–96) and Pegase 05 (1997–99). J Clin Oncol 2004;22(14S): 848

112. Viens P, Palangie T, Janvier M et al. First-line high-dose sequential chemotherapy with rG-CSF and repeated blood stem cell transplantation in untreated inflammatory breast cancer: toxicity and response (PEGASE 02 trial). Br J Cancer 1999;81:449–456

113. Viens P, Penault-Llorca F, Jacquemier J et al. High-dose chemotherapy and haematopoietic stem cell transplantation for inflammatory breast cancer: pathologic response and outcome. Bone Marrow Transplant 1998;21:249–254

114. Pedrazzoli P, Ferrante P, Kulekci A et al. Autologous hematopoietic stem cell transplantation for breast cancer in Europe: critical evaluation of data from the European Group for Blood and Marrow Transplantation (EBMT) Registry 1990–1999. Bone Marrow Transplant 2003;32:489–494

115. Peters WP, Rosner GL, Vredenburgh JJ et al. Prospective, randomized comparison of high-dose chemotherapy with stem-cell support versus intermediate-dose chemotherapy after surgery and adjuvant chemotherapy in women with high-risk primary breast cancer: a report of CALGB 9082, SWOG 9114, and NCIC MA-13. J Clin Oncol 2005;23:2191–2200

116. Roche H, Pouillart P, Meyer N et al. Adjuvant high dose chemotherapy (HDC) improves early outcome for high risk (n > 7) breast cancer patients: the Pegase 01 Trial (abstract 102). Proceedings of the ASCO Annual Meeting, 2001. ASCO, Alexandria, Virginia

117. Schrama JG, Holtkamp MJ, Baars JW et al. Toxicity of the high-dose chemotherapy CTC regimen (cyclophosphamide, thiotepa, carboplatin): the Netherlands Cancer Institute experience. Br J Cancer 2003;88:1831–1838

118. Yau JC, Gertler SZ, Hanson J et al. A phase III study of high-dose intensification without hematopoietic progenitor cells support for patients with high-risk primary breast carcinoma. Am J Clin Oncol 2000;23:292–296

Solid tumors in adults

Andreas Lundqvist, Shivani Srivastava and Richard Childs

CHAPTER 13

Introduction

Hematopoietic cell transplantation (HCT) is an effective treatment for many life-threatening hematological, immunologic, metabolic and neoplastic diseases. HCT was first studied in animal models in the late 1940s as a method of rescuing marrow function in recipients exposed to myeloablative doses of cytotoxic drugs or total body irradiation. Today, the most common use of allogeneic and autologous HCT is for the treatment of hematologic malignancies. Over the past two decades, high-dose chemotherapy (HDC) with autologous stem cell transplantation (ASCT) has been explored for a variety of solid tumors in adults. Because only a small number of Phase III trials in solid tumors comparing HDC with ASCT versus conventional chemotherapy have been completed, the value of HDC for most solid tumors remains controversial and investigational. In myeloablative allogeneic HCT, the curative antitumor effects of the procedure occur as the consequence of both cytoreductive conditioning and immune-mediated antitumor effects generated by transplanted donor immune cells (i.e. the graft-versus-leukemia (GvL) or graft-versus-tumor (GvT) effect).

The curative potential of GvL/GvT against hematologic malignancies has recently attracted oncologists to explore the therapeutic potential of allogeneic HCT for solid tumors that have become refractory to conventional therapy. Preliminary data from small clinical trials have recently provided evidence that GvT effects can be generated against some chemotherapy-resistant solid tumors; reports of delayed tumor regression occurring in a subset of patients with metastatic renal cell, breast, ovarian, pancreatic and colon carcinoma have recently been published. However, relatively few complete responses have thus far been observed, perhaps due, in part, to the accrual of patients with extremely short survival expectation, advanced disease states and rapidly growing tumors.

This chapter discusses the results of autologous and allogeneic HCT for solid tumors and the development of allogeneic transplant strategies focused on optimizing the potential of the GvT effect.

Autologous hematopoietic stem cell transplantation

Autologous stem cell transplantation (ASCT), using either bone marrow (BM) or peripheral blood progenitor cells (PBPC), allows chemotherapeutic agents to be administered at a two- to tenfold increase in the drug dose. In vitro, HDC has substantially greater antitumor activity compared to standard-dose chemotherapy (SDC) for a number of tumors, an observation that led investigators to hypothesize that HDC would be associated with better outcome in

patients with advanced cancers. In ASCT, extramedullary organ toxicities are ultimately dose limiting. The widespread substitution of PBPC for BM as a source of hematopoietic progenitor cells and improvements in supportive care have increased the safety of HDC, resulting in current transplant-related mortality (TRM) rates of 5% or less.

Ovarian cancer

Less than 25% of patients with stage III ovarian carcinoma achieve long-term disease-free survival with conventional multimodal management including debulking surgery and combination chemotherapy. For patients with relapsed disease, salvage chemotherapy is palliative and not curative. Stage IV patients have an even worse prognosis, with a 5-year survival rate of less than 5%. In an attempt to improve outcome in poor-prognosis patients, high-dose chemotherapy and autologous stem cell transplantation have been investigated in the treatment of patients with relapsed disease, and as first-line consolidation after standard-dose chemotherapy and second-look surgery.

High-dose chemotherapy for recurrent ovarian cancer

Stiff et al reported a large, single-center experience in 100 heavily pretreated and predominantly platinum-refractory ovarian cancer patients treated with a carboplatin- or melphalan-based HDC regimen followed by autologous stem cell transplantation. Event-free survival (EFS) and overall survival (OS) were disappointingly low at 7 and 13 months, respectively. A subset analysis of patients with low tumor burden and platinum-sensitive disease appeared more encouraging, with a 1-year estimated progression-free survival (PFS) and OS survival rate of 76%.[1] An ABMTR retrospective analysis of 421 patients with relapsed ovarian cancer who received high-dose chemotherapy and autologous stem cell rescue from 1989 through 1996 reported similar results. In this poor-prognosis population, 2-year EFS and OS rates were 12% and 35% respectively. Patients who underwent transplantation who had good performance status and platinum-sensitive tumors had better EFS and OS rates of 22% and 55%, respectively.[2]

High-dose chemotherapy as front-line therapy for advanced ovarian cancer

Bertucci et al retrospectively analyzed 33 patients with advanced ovarian cancer sensitive to first-line chemotherapy who went on to receive high-dose melphalan conditioning followed by autologous stem cell rescue. Many of these patients had persistent disease after initial surgery. With a median follow-up of 5 years, EFS and OS rates were 29% and 45%, respectively. Patients with evidence of disease at second-look surgery had a dismal outcome. In contrast, patients who had a pathologic complete response (CR) at second-look surgery had a more encouraging outcome with 5-year EFS and OS rates of 43% and 75%, respectively.[3] A retrospective analysis of 254 patients from the EBMT registry evaluated the front-line use of high-dose chemotherapy followed by autologous stem cell rescue; about half of the patients in this analysis were transplanted with refractory residual disease, with 40% in first CR or near CR. Outcomes appeared to be improved for those transplanted in remission compared to those with resistant tumors, with a median EFS of 18 vs 9 months, and median OS of 33 vs 14 months.[4]

Cure et al conducted a randomized trial to address the efficacy of HDC in patients with low-burden, chemosensitive disease receiving first-line therapy. One hundred and ten patients were randomized to receive consolidation with high-dose carboplatin-cyclophosphamide with peripheral blood stem cell (PBSC) support or three maintenance cycles of conventional carboplatin-cyclophosphamide. No clear benefit of HDC was observed; at a median follow-up of 60 months, disease-free survival (DFS) and OS from randomization were 12.2 and 49.7 months, respectively, in the transplant arm which was not significantly different from that in the non-transplant conventional chemotherapy maintenance arm.[5]

More recently, Goncalves et al conducted a Phase II multicenter study evaluating HDC and autologous hematopoietic stem cell rescue postoperatively as front-line therapy in 34 patients with advanced ovarian cancer. Unfortunately, only 37% of transplanted patients achieved a pathologic CR, leading the authors to conclude that HDC with stem cell rescue offered no advantage over conventional chemotherapy.[6]

In conclusion, HDC with autologous stem cell support has largely failed to prove any beneficial role in the treatment of advanced ovarian cancer. At best, patients with platinum-sensitive disease at the time of remission might gain some benefit. The high level of toxicity encountered with such dose-intense strategies with questionable therapeutic benefit limits autologous transplants for ovarian cancer to the setting of a clinical trial.

Small cell lung cancer

Only 20–40% of patients with limited-stage small cell lung cancer (SCLC) and <5% of those with extensive-stage disease remain alive after 2 years with conventional therapies.[7–9] These discouraging outcomes prompted studies exploring HDC with ASCT in the early 1980s. Two different approaches were used: an early intensification approach offered the theoretical advantage that drug resistance would not have been induced by exposure to previous conventional doses of chemotherapy. In the late-intensification approach, it was hypothesized that minimal residual tumor cells, still responding to standard chemotherapy, may be more sensitive to intensified treatment. A summary of clinical trials exploring HDC with autologous stem cell rescue is shown in Table 13.1.

Humblet et al conducted the first randomized trial in small cell lung cancer in which 45 patients responding to induction chemotherapy were randomized to one additional chemotherapy cycle or to high-dose cyclophosphamide-BCNU-etoposide conditioning with ASCT and cranial radiation. Although the transplant arm showed an improved response rate and EFS, OS (68 weeks for the HDC group compared with 55 weeks for the conventional therapy group) was not different (p = 0.13) between the two arms, with an unacceptably high 17% incidence of TRM in the HDC cohort.[10]

A similar, dismal outcome was observed for SCLC in a larger multicenter Phase III EBMT trial conducted in 1996 comparing three cycles of sequential high-dose ICE (ifosfamide, carboplatin and etoposide) supported by PBPCs, versus six cycles of standard ICE; 145 patients were accrued, of whom 140 were evaluable (71 in the standard arm and 69 in the high-dose arm). CR rates were 32% and 37% for the standard and high-dose arms, respectively (p = 0.188). With a median follow-up of 4.9 years, median overall survival times were 15 months and 19.1 months (p = 0.659) for the standard and high-dose arms, respectively, with 19% of the patients alive at 3 years follow-up in both arms.[11]

In summary, the current literature (see Table 13.1) indicates that there is no evidence that the treatment of SCLC can be improved by increasing the dose intensity, the peak dose or the total dose of chemotherapy followed by ASCT and that such an intensification strategy should probably be abandoned. Moreover, bone marrow transplantation as initial therapy for SCLC patients is challenging in these patients as they frequently have an impaired performance status and pulmonary/cardiovascular dysfunction due to a prolonged smoking history that results in high mortality rates limiting the applicability of this treatment.

Melanoma

The prognosis of metastatic melanoma is dismal, with median survivals of less than 1 year. The vast majority of chemotherapeutic agents are inactive against this cancer. Further, the addition of IL-2 and IFN-alpha chemotherapy regimens has failed to significantly improve response rate, PFS or OS compared to chemotherapy alone.[12–15] Dose-intensive chemotherapy followed by autologous hematopoietic stem cell rescue was investigated as a strategy to overcome the resistance of melanoma to conventional chemotherapy. Response rates of 45–69% have been reported in trials investigating different HDC regimens followed by autologous bone marrow support. Early trials with high-dose single chemotherapeutic agents such as BCNU,[16] melphalan[17] or thiotepa[18] achieved higher than expected response rates compared to standard-dose chemotherapy although PFS was observed to be extremely short in the vast majority of responders.

Table 13.1 Clinical trials exploring HDC with autologous stem cell rescue for small cell lung cancer

Regimen + support	Patients (n)	CR (%)	MST (months)	2-year survival rate (%)	Reference
Ifo + Epi/Cb + Vp16 + PBPCs	35	66	24.6	51	119
ICE + PBPCs	140	37	19.1	19 (3 years)	11
Ctx + ABMT	36	33	20 (LD group)	NA	120
Ctx + Vp16 +/– A +/– Mtx X 2 + ABMT	32	28	NA	12.5	121
Ctx + BCNU + Vp16 + ABMT	23	60	NA	NA	10
Ctx + C + BCNU + ABMT +/– PBSCs	36	69	NA	57	27
Vp16 + Ifo + Cb + Epi + PBSC	30	23	8 (ED)	53 (LD)	122

Abbreviations: A, doxorubicin; ABMT, autologous bone marrow transplantation; BCNU, bischloroethylnitrosurea; C, cisplatin; Cb, carboplatin; CR, complete response; Ctx, cyclophosphamide; ED, extensive-stage disease; Epi, epirubicin; ICE, ifosfamide, carboplatin, etoposide; Ifo, ifosfamide; MST, median survival time; Mtx, methotrexate; PBSC, peripheral blood progenitor cell; Vp16, etoposide.

In high-risk non-metastatic melanoma, a small randomized trial compared HDC with cyclophosphamide-cisplatin-BCNU versus observation and HDC at relapse; 39 patients with five or more positive regional lymph nodes were enrolled, with no difference in outcome observed between cohorts.[19]

In summary, although HDC followed by ASCT in melanoma is associated with an improvement in response rate compared to conventional chemotherapy, progression-free survival is extremely short, negating any potential beneficial effect on OS. The use of HDC and ASCT as a means of cytoreducing the tumor before the administration of tumor-infiltrating lymphocytes and other types of immunotherapy to induce a more durable immune-mediated antitumor response is currently being explored in investigational trials.

Brain tumors

Most patients with malignant brain gliomas relapse after surgery and radiotherapy (RT) and die within 2 years of diagnosis. The addition of SDC offers a modest survival advantage, especially for younger patients with anaplastic astrocytoma.[20] Radiotherapy plus concomitant and adjuvant temozolomide has been shown to improve survival for glioblastoma. However, despite these maneuvers, the prognosis remains poor for the majority of patients with high-grade glioblastomas. High-dose chemotherapy with carmustine can improve response rates by increasing the overall chemotherapeutic dose delivered. The largest study to date of HDC in this setting was a retrospective analysis of 217 patients from the European Group for Blood and Marrow Transplantation analyzing outcomes in patients treated between 1988 and 2004. Ninety-six patients underwent complete surgical resection while 121 patients had partial resection or only biopsy. Carmustine was administered 1 month after neurosurgery followed 48–72 hours later by autologous stem cell infusion; cranial radiotherapy was started approximately 40 days after transplantation. Of the 121 patients evaluable, 53% had an objective response and 4.5% died from transplant-related causes. With a median follow-up of 8 years, survival and time to treatment failure were a median 20 months and 7 months, respectively. In glioblastoma multiforme (GM), age and surgery quality appeared to be prognostic factors.[21] These outcomes and outcomes of similar studies shown in Table 13.2 were similar to historical results in patients not receiving HDC, suggesting no benefit from high-dose BCNU with autologous stem cell rescue in patients with high-grade GM.

In summary, available results of HDC in adult patients with high-grade GM, largely employing high-dose single-agent BCNU, do not appear to improve outcome compared to conventional therapy. Further research may identify a role of HDC, in the setting of multimodal treatment, for young patients with atypical astrocytoma.

Adult bone and soft tissue sarcoma

Metastatic sarcomas represent a rare and heterogeneous disease. The prognosis of patients with unresectable or advanced metastatic bone and especially soft tissue sarcomas remains poor, with a disease-free survival of less than 10% at 5 years.[22] Few chemotherapeutic agents have been identified to be active, with response rates for single-agent doxorubicin, epirubicin and ifosfamide in the range of 20%.[23–25] A dose–response relationship of sarcomas to anthracyclines and ifosfamide has been shown to exist, leading to the investigation of high-dose chemotherapy with stem cell support by several investigators. Unfortunately, no randomized trials comparing HDC followed by ASCT with conventional therapy have yet been conducted, with all reported studies being relatively small, enrolling patients with heterogeneous subtypes of soft tissue sarcoma, in which outcome has been compared to historical controls.

Fagioli et al treated 32 patients with metastatic osteosarcoma with two cycles of high-dose chemotherapy consisting of carboplatin and etoposide followed by autologous stem cell support in a multimodality approach that included surgical debulking. The overall survival was 20% at 3 years, but the relapse rate was a disappointing 85%. Although this regimen was associated with high CR rates, the duration of remissions was very short.[26] Other studies with HDC followed by ASCT for the treatment of relapsed osteosarcoma, Ewing's sarcoma, and rhabdomyosarcoma failed to show any benefit over conventional chemotherapy.[23–26]

For soft tissue sarcomas, HDC followed by stem cell support when used upfront or as salvage therapy for refractory disease[27] did not result in a clear survival benefit. However, there is some suggestion that outcome may be improved when HDC followed by ASCT is used as consolidation after induction SDC, particularly for patients who are transplanted in CR. Blay et al treated 30 patients with responsive metastatic disease with high-dose ifosfamide, etoposide and cisplatin. At a median follow-up of 94 months, the EFS and OS rates were higher than expected at 21% and 23%, respectively. Patients in CR before HDC had superior outcome compared to those in partial response (PR) (5-year OS 75% vs 5%).[28] More recently, Engelhardt et al reported an analysis of 35 consecutive adult patients with poor-risk soft tissue sarcomas (n = 35) undergoing ASCT; with a median follow-up of 101 months following transplantation, median OS was 17.1 months and 11 patients were alive, including nine who remained in a sustained CR.[29]

Because randomized trials comparing conventional therapy with ASCT have not yet been published, the role of HDC for sarcomas remains unclear. One of the current challenges is to define those patients who are most likely to benefit from HDCT. The results of a

Table 13.2 Trials of adjuvant high-dose BCNU in malignant gliomas with autologous stem cell rescue

Patient characteristics	Patients (n)	Overall survival	Time to treatment failure	Reference
Malignant gliomas; adjuvant surgery (complete or partial resection)	217	20 months (survival rate at 5 years: 32%)	7 months	21
Malignant gliomas; adjuvant and recurrent surgery (complete or partial resection and biopsy)	36	NR	Adjuvant groups: 3 patients with progression-free survival at 70, 48 and 27 months	16
Malignant gliomas; unresectable grade 3 and 4	25	26 months	NR	123
Malignant gliomas; newly diagnosed and recurrent; surgery (complete or partial resection and biopsy)	98	12 months	NR	124
GM surgery (complete or partial resection and biopsy)	39	14 months (survival rate at 5 years: 25%)	NR	125
Malignant gliomas; adjuvant therapy; surgery (complete or partial resection and biopsy)	114	15 months (survival rate at 5 years: 32%)	9 months	126

Abbreviations: NR, not reported; GM, glioblastoma multiforme.

multicenter study currently being conducted in Europe and North America prospectively investigating HDC compared with maintenance therapy for sarcoma will hopefully better define what, if any, role dose-intensive chemotherapy plays in the treatment of this malignancy.[30]

Allogeneic tumor immunotherapy

Over the past two decades, immunotherapy has played an increasing role in the treatment of cancer. Advances in the field of immunology and in particular the discovery of major histocompatibility complex (MHC) restriction have accelerated the identification of several tumor-associated antigens (TAA). Most TAA identified to date are self-antigens expressed on both tumor cells and normal cells.[31] One of the primary goals of cancer vaccination therapies has been to target and break self-tolerance to these antigens to induce an effective T-cell mediated antitumor response. Many antigens shown to induce antitumor T-cell responses in preclinical mouse models are today being targeted in clinical cancer trials in humans.[32–36]

It has been established that vaccination against TAA can induce proliferation of antigen-specific T-cell populations that recognize and kill tumor cells, which in some cases can lead to tumor regression clinically.[37–40] Other immunotherapy strategies besides vaccination approaches include the adoptive infusion of ex vivo expanded tumor-reactive lymphocytes, which also induces regression of metastatic cancer in a subset of patients.[41–44] Although proof of the concept that the immune system can be harnessed to attack cancer cells has been established, only a minority of patients benefit from immunotherapeutic regimens designed to enhance the immune system of the cancer-bearing host. Increasing evidence exists that tumors possess a number of immune-evading mechanisms that may, in part, account for the marginal efficacy of conventional immunotherapeutic approaches; reduction in tumor cell antigen processing and presentation through downregulation of transporter associated with antigen processing and presentation (TAP), beta-2 microglobulin and MHC class I antigenic loss variants, upregulation of immunosuppressive cytokines (i.e. IL-10, IL-5), Fas-ligand upregulation leading to Fas-mediated T-cell apoptosis, and tumor evasion of death receptor signaling by upregulation of the serine protease inhibitor PI-9 rendering resistance to granzyme B-mediated killing have been reported.[45–51] More recently, the immunosuppressive effects of regulatory T-cells have been implicated in the spread of metastatic tumors and have been shown to hinder and potentially render ineffective adoptively transferred tumor-specific T-cells.[52–54]

In a quest to overcome at least some of these barriers, investigators in the mid-1990s began to explore the use of allogeneic hematopoietic cell transplantation (HCT) as an immunotherapeutic treatment alternative in patients with advanced solid tumors. For decades, allogeneic HCT had proven capable of curing patients with advanced hematologic malignancies.[55] Initially, myeloablative conditioning using dose-intensive chemotherapy with or without total body irradiation (TBI) was largely given credit for curing patients. Classic 'myeloablative' regimens were designed to ablate recipient hematopoiesis, the underlying malignancy, and the recipient's immune system to facilitate engraftment of the allogeneic transplant. The discovery that transplanted donor immune cells could eradicate residual or relapsed leukemia led to a paradigm shift in thinking regarding the relevance of the GvL/GvT effect. The ability of donor lymphocyte infusions (DLI) to cure relapsed CML was a seminal observation that provided the first definitive evidence that GvL was powerful enough to eradicate some cancers. Importantly, it led to the development of novel transplant approaches which utilized reduced-intensity conditioning or 'non-myeloablative' preparative regimens to reduce toxicity associated with

allogeneic HCT. This type of transplant was designed to provide immunosuppression at a level required to achieve engraftment of donor immune cells to allow for the induction of GvT effects.[56] The improved safety profile associated with reduced-intensity conditioning provided investigators in the late 1990s with a safer platform to test the potential of GvT to treat metastatic solid tumors.

The link between graft-versus-host disease and graft-versus-tumor effect

In order to harness the potential of GvT effect in patients with solid tumors, an understanding of the biology of allogeneic HCT is essential. Early HCT approaches utilizing high-dose conditioning regimens often resulted in direct organ toxicity leading to multisystem organ failure and a high risk of mortality.[57] Furthermore, the rapid and complete engraftment of donor immune cells and tissue destruction that occur as the consequence of dose-intensive conditioning predisposed recipients to developing severe GvHD.[57–59] In contrast, non-myeloablative transplants result in less conditioning-associated tissue injury and achieve a transient period where both donor and patient myeloid and lymphoid cells are detectable in the blood and bone marrow; a condition referred to as 'mixed chimerism'. Mixed chimerism appears to induce donor tolerance to recipient tissue, leading to a decreased risk of acute GvHD.[60,61] However, GvT effects are usually delayed after non-myeloablative conditioning and do not occur until mixed chimerism disappears, and full donor or an evolution towards increasing donor T-cell chimerism occurs.[62–64] Thus, non-myeloablative HCT regimens incorporate strategies to accelerate conversion from mixed to full donor chimerism by early discontinuation of GvHD prophylaxis and the infusion of donor lymphocytes.

Although significant advances have been made in both the prevention and treatment of GvHD, acute and chronic GvHD still remain a major obstacle to successful transplant outcome. However, patients who develop GvHD also are more likely to have beneficial GvT effects.[65–68] A retrospective analysis from the IBMTR of >2000 patients receiving allogeneic HCT was one of the first studies to provide overwhelming evidence that both acute and chronic GvHD were associated with a reduction in the risk of disease relapse.[69] In addition, attempts to reduce the incidence and severity of GvHD, including graft T-cell depletion, and use of additional immunosuppressive agents have repeatedly proven effective in reducing this complication at the expense of increasing the risk of leukemia relapse.[70–72]

Many solid tumors arise from epithelial tissues that are a target of alloreactive T-cells that cause GvHD. Since epithelial tissues such as gastrointestinal mucosal cells, hepatobiliary tissue, keratinocytes, and exocrine glands express alloantigens targeted by GvHD-inducing T-cells, it is likely that gastrointestinal malignancies, hepatomas, skin cancers, and glandular tumors would express the same alloantigens, leading alloreactive T-cells to mediate a GvT effect. Over the past decade, several small pilot trials have confirmed that GvT effects can extend beyond hematologic malignancies to a number of different solid tumors,[73–83] as depicted in Table 13.3.

Graft-versus-renal cell carcinoma (RCC)

Trials testing allogeneic HCT in solid tumors were first conducted against cancers that had a track record of sensitivity to autologous-based immunotherapy. Investigators first pursued reduced-intensity stem cell transplantation (RIST) or non-myeloablative HCT in patients with metastatic RCC in the late 1990s, shortly after the favorable results of non-myeloablative HCT in hematologic malignancies were published. Historically, myeloablative conditioning has been associated with considerable risk of morbidity and mortality and RCC has proven to be resistant to chemotherapy. Therefore, investigators uti-

Table 13.3 Clinical trials on RIST HCT against RCC

Number of patients	Conditioning regimen	GvHD prophylaxis	Regimen-related mortality	Response rate % (CR/PR/MR)	Response onset day (median)	Response to DLI reported	Reference
19	Flu + Cy	CSA	12%	53% (3/7/0)	129	Yes	77
7	Thio + Flu + Cy	CSA + MTX	14%	57% (0/4/0)	117	Yes	74
7	Flu + Cy	CSA + MTX	29%	0% (0/0/0)	NA	NA	80
12	Flu + Cy	Tac + MMF	33%	33% (0/4)	180	No	81
10	Flu + TBI	CSA + MMF	30%	30% (0/3)	NR	No	78
15	Flu + Mel	Tac + MTX	33%	47% (1/2/4)	NR	No	83

Abbreviations: Flu, fludarabine; Cy, cyclophosphamide; Thio, thiotepa; TBI, total-body irradiation; Bu, busulfan; GvHD, graft-versus-host disease; CSA, ciclosporin; MTX, methotrexate; NA, not applicable; MMF, mycophenolate mofetil; Tac, tacrolimus; Mel, melphalan; CR, complete response; PR, partial response; MR, minor response; NR, not reported.

lized a RIST approach to minimize regimen-related morbidity in an effort to evaluate the therapeutic potential of engrafting donor immune cells against this malignancy.

Over the past 8 years, graft-versus-solid tumor effects resulting in delayed regression of metastatic kidney cancer have been reported by investigators using a variety of different RIST approaches (see Table 13.3). Reported response rates have been extremely variable, ranging from 8% to 58%. An EBMT analysis of 124 patients with metastatic RCC undergoing RIST reported an overall response rate of 32%.[84] In general, regimens associated with more aggressive post-transplant immunosuppression withdrawal strategies have been associated with both a higher incidence of GvHD and tumor responses.

Most transplant regimens share the goal of maximizing the chances of inducing a GvT effect by utilizing highly immunosuppressive conditioning to knock out the recipient's immune system to facilitate donor T-cell engraftment while minimizing the time patients receive ciclosporin or tacrolimus for GvHD prophylaxis. In a pilot trial conducted at the National Heart, Lung and Blood Institute, 10 of the first 19 patients (54%) treated had tumor regression, including seven partial responses and three complete responses; the first patient treated remained without evidence of disease >8 years after transplantation.[77] In an updated series, 73/74 patients had sustained donor engraftment, with 38% of patients having either a partial (27%) or complete response (9%). Tumor responses were frequently preceded by tumor progression and were delayed a median 5 months (range, days 30–425) after transplantation, sometimes occurring after the administration of DLI or post-transplant IFN-α. Acute and chronic GvHD were observed in approximately 50% of the patients. Death from TRM occurred in 8% of the patients, half of whom died from complications related to GvHD.[85] GvT effects (determined radiographically) usually occurred following ciclosporin tapering and after T-cell chimerism had converted from mixed to predominantly full donor origin.

The observation that tumor regression can occur both in patients during GvHD and in those who never developed GvHD has provided indirect evidence that donor T-cells can be directed against minor histocompatibility antigens as well as antigens restricted to the tumor. Indeed, minor histocompatibility antigen-specific T-cell clones that recognize RCC cells in vitro have been isolated from patients with metastatic RCC undergoing non-myeloablative transplantation. More recently, T-cell clones that recognize a RCC antigen that is expressed in a significant percentage of kidney cancer cell lines have been identified from a patient who had a GvT effect after transplantation (Journal of Clinical Investigation 2008).

Advanced disease states, rapidly growing tumors, and accruals of patients with extremely short survivals are all factors that appear to limit the efficacy of this approach in patients with metastatic RCC. Because GvT effects are delayed by months after transplantation, patients with rapidly progressing disease frequently fail to benefit from a non-myeloablative transplant. Although published data are relatively limited, most responses reported to date have been partial, with complete responses occurring most often in patients with metastatic clear cell carcinoma with disease limited to the lungs. In general, patients with metastatic RCC appear to tolerate RIST well. Nevertheless, regimen-related mortality rates of 10–15% persist, largely as the consequence of severe acute GvHD. In addition, only 25% of patients have an HLA-matched sibling, limiting the procedure to a relatively small percentage of patients. Therefore, trials investigating the feasibility of using HLA-matched unrelated donors are currently being pursued.

As observed with hematologic malignancies, disease status at transplantation has a major impact on transplant outcome. Patients with slowly growing metastatic kidney cancer have the greatest chance of responding to an allogeneic HCT, while those with extensive, rapidly growing tumors are less likely to benefit. Efforts to cytoreduce the overall disease burden prior to transplantation, through surgical debulking or the use of newer agents that inhibit tumor angiogenesis such as sorafenib, sunitinib or bevacizumab, could potentially improve the chances of a GvT effect being induced after an allogeneic transplant.

GvT effects against solid tumors other than renal cell carcinoma

Analogous to RCC, melanoma appears to be susceptible to immune-mediated killing. However, the results of non-myeloablative HCT in patients with metastatic melanoma have, to date, been disappointing. A report on 25 patients undergoing RIST for metastatic melanoma from four different transplant centers reported a dismal outcome with a median survival of only 100 days; rapid disease progression was the major cause of death.[76] Although 24/25 patients had sustained donor engraftment and about half developed acute GvHD, only one patient had a delayed regression of subcutaneous melanoma lesions consistent with a GvT effect. These poor results may have been partly due to the inclusion of high-risk patients, in whom rapidly growing tumors precluded a delayed GvT effect. In another report, one out of two transplanted patients with metastatic melanoma showed regression of lymph node metastases; donor-derived tumor-specific CD8+ T-cells were subsequently expanded from this patient.[79] However, both patients died from disease progression within only 200 days of transplantation.

Evidence suggesting breast carcinoma, pancreatic, colon and metastatic ovarian carcinoma can be a target for a GVT effect has also recently been published.[78,86] Two of five patients with unresectable pancreatic carcinoma were reported to have a reduction in their tumor mass following a RIST. In one report, the observation that immunosuppressive therapy used to treat GvHD following a GvT effect was associated with disease progression again shows the strong association between GvT and GvHD.[82]

These trials have provided proof of the principle that allogeneic GvT effects can be generated against advanced solid tumors. Unfortunately, the inclusion of patients with extremely advanced disease, including treatment-refractory tumors, who proceed to transplantation as a final option after all other therapies have failed, has probably had a negative impact on the success of transplants for solid tumors. Preliminary data demonstrating disease-free survivals of greater than 3 years in some patients with metastatic breast cancer who were cytoreduced with an autologous transplant followed by an allogeneic RIST provide further evidence of the importance and need for achieving disease control to optimize transplant outcome.[87]

Improvements and future directions

Graft-versus-tumor effects in patients with solid tumors have most often been observed in those with a history of either acute or chronic GvHD, although disease regression has been observed in some patients without any apparent GvHD.[88,89] This observation provides indirect evidence that donor T-cells can be directed against both antigens restricted to normal tissue (i.e. minor histocompatibility antigens) as well as to the tumor (Fig. 13.1). Animal models of allogeneic HCT for cancer have demonstrated that donor T-cells can recognize minor histocompatibility antigens expressed on normal tissues as well as tumor cells, leading them to serve as targets for GvHD and GvT.[90–92] The list of known minor antigens is rapidly growing; to date, 17 minor histocompatibility antigens have been defined by CD8+ CTL recognition.[87] As observed with hematologic malignancies, minor histocompatibility antigen-specific T-cell clones that recognize tumor cells in vitro have been isolated from patients with metastatic renal cell carcinoma following allogeneic HCT.[88,89]

Although relatively few complete responses in patients with solid tumors undergoing allogeneic HCT have thus far been observed, the foundation has been laid for new transplant regimens that focus on methods to enhance the activity of donor immune cells mediating GvT effects. One of the major goals in allogeneic HCT for cancer is to separate beneficial GvT effects from the detrimental effects of GvHD. Methods of selectively depleting alloreactive T-cells that cause GvHD while preserving T-cells with antitumor effects are currently being investigated in clinical trials.[93,94] Preclinical transplantation murine models have provided evidence that host antigen-presenting cells (APC) play a major role in the induction of acute GvHD.[95,96] As a consequence, significant research is currently being devoted to pathways involved in host APC and donor T-cell interactions. Substantial evidence indicates that donor CD4+CD25+ regulatory T-cells can suppress GvHD lethality in animal models.[97,98] Edinger et al demonstrated that CD4+CD25+ regulatory T-cells suppress the early expansion of alloreactive donor T-cells and inhibit their capacity to induce GvHD without abrogating their beneficial GvT effector function.[99] Likewise, injection of 'regulatory APC' has been shown to induce regulatory T-cell differentiation leading to protection from acute GvHD while maintaining antileukemia effects.[100] Tumor antigen-primed memory CD4+ T-cells have also been shown to inhibit tumor growth in vivo without the induction of GvHD.[101] Based on these data, clinical trials investigating the impact of regulatory or memory T-cells on GvHD and GvT effects in humans will probably be undertaken.

Experimental animal models have demonstrated an increased GvT effect in recipients of allogeneic HCT receiving dendritic cell (DC)-based vaccinations.[102,103] Moreover, investigators have shown in pilot studies that adoptively transferred minor histocompatibility antigen or tumor antigen-specific T-cells can lead to enhanced antitumor effects in HCT recipients.[91,104]

Another area of investigation includes combining allogeneic immunotherapy with therapies specifically targeting molecular pathways critical to tumor growth. Molecular remissions following treatment with imatinib combined with DLI as salvage treatment for blast crisis Philadelphia chromosome-positive leukemias that have relapsed after non-myeloablative allogeneic HCT have recently been reported.[105] For RCC, the effects of combining sunitinib or sorafenib, two tyrosine kinase inhibitors recently approved by the FDA to treat metastatic RCC, with allogeneic immunotherapy are currently being investigated in animal models.[106–109]

Another strategy to potentiate GvT effects against solid tumors is to harness the enhanced antitumor effects of killer IgG-like receptor (KIR) ligand incompatible NK cells. In vitro, KIR incompatible NK cells have enhanced cytotoxicity against solid tumors such as RCC and melanoma compared to KIR matched or autologous NK cells.[110] Furthermore, recent literature suggests that KIR ligand incompatible ('alloreactive') NK cells reduce GvHD, possibly by elimination of host APC that survive transplant conditioning.[111–113] Over the past few years, a growing number of receptors involved in NK cell recognition of target cells have been identified. The largest group belongs to the immunoglobulin-like superfamily which binds to specific HLA subclasses.[114] Experimental animal models have demonstrated that infusion of alloreactive NK cells reduces the incidence and severity of GvHD.[112,115] Likewise, alloreactive NK cell infusion following allogeneic HCT in mice bearing murine RCC tumors was found to both decrease GvHD and mediate a GvT effect against murine RCC, resulting in a prolongation of survival.[116] Studies in humans evaluating the impact of KIR ligand incompatible allogeneic HCT have demonstrated a reduced incidence of AML leukemia relapse in recipients of haploidentical transplants and a reduction in the incidence of GvHD.[111,112,117] Based on the previously discussed in vitro data, a similar benefit of alloreactive NK cells for RCC might also exist. A recent retrospective analysis demonstrated significantly higher response rates and prolonged survival in RCC patients who lacked HLA-Bw4 (the KIR ligand for KIR3DL1) when they received a transplant from a donor who genotypically expressed KIR3DL1.[118] Whether adoptive infusions of alloreactive NK cells will improve transplant outcomes and enhance GvT effects (as observed in animal transplant models) for RCC will probably be evaluated in future clinical trials. If successful, such strategies could lead to a wider application of allogeneic immunotherapy for a number of different solid tumors.

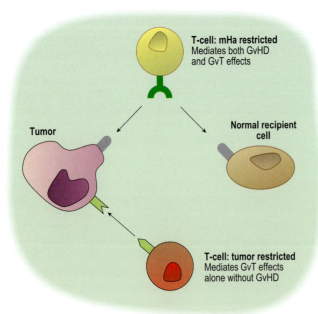

T-cell: mHa restricted
Mediates both GvHD and GvT effects

Normal recipient cell

Tumor

T-cell: tumor restricted
Mediates GvT effects alone without GvHD

Figure 13.1
Donor T-cells capable of killing solid tumors.

References

1. Stiff PJ, Bayer R, Kerger C et al. High-dose chemotherapy with autologous transplantation for persistent/relapsed ovarian cancer: a multivariate analysis of survival for 100 consecutively treated patients. J Clin Oncol 1997;15:1309–1317
2. Stiff P, Veum-Stone J, Lazarus H et al. High-dose chemotherapy and autologous stem-cell transplantation for ovarian cancer: an Autologous Blood and Marrow Transplant Registry report. Ann Intern Med 2000;133(7):504–515
3. Bertucci F, Viens P, Delpero JR et al. High-dose melphalan-based chemotherapy and autologous stem cell transplantation after second look laparotomy in patients with chemosensitive advanced ovarian carcinoma: long-term results. Bone Marrow Transplant 2000;26:61–67
4. Ledermann JA, Herd R, Maraninchi D et al. High-dose chemotherapy for ovarian carcinoma: long-term results from the Solid Tumour Registry of the European Group for Blood and Marrow Transplantation (EBMT). Ann Oncol 2001;12:693–699
5. Cure H, Guastalla. JP. Phase III randomized trial of high-dose chemotherapy (HDC) and peripheral blood stem cell (PBSC) support as consolidation in patients (pts) with advanced ovarian cancer (AOC): 5-year follow-up of a GINECO/FNCLCC/SFGM-TC study. J Clin Oncol 2004;229(suppl):14S
6. Goncalves A, Delva R, Fabbro M et al. Post-operative sequential high-dose chemotherapy with haematopoietic stem cell support as front-line treatment in advanced ovarian cancer: a phase II multicentre study. Bone Marrow Transplant 2006;37:651–659
7. Chrystal K, Cheong K, Harper P. Chemotherapy of small cell lung cancer: state of the art. Curr Opin Oncol 2004;16:136–140
8. Hoffman PC, Mauer AM, Vokes EE. Lung cancer. Lancet 2000;355:479–485
9. Zochbauer-Muller S, Pirker R, Huber H. Treatment of small cell lung cancer patients. Ann Oncol 1999;10(suppl 6):83–91
10. Humblet Y, Symann M, Bosly A et al. Late intensification chemotherapy with autologous bone marrow transplantation in selected small-cell carcinoma of the lung: a randomized study. J Clin Oncol 1987;5:1864–1873
11. Leyvraz S, Pampallona S, Martinelli G et al. Randomized phase III study of high dose sequential chemotherapy supported by peripheral blood progenitor cells for the treatment of small cell lung cancer: results of the EBMT Random-ICE trial. J Clin Oncol 2006;24(18S):7064
12. Eton O, Legha SS, Bedikian AY et al. Sequential biochemotherapy versus chemotherapy for metastatic melanoma: results from a phase III randomized trial. J Clin Oncol 2002;20:2045–2052
13. Flaherty LE, Atkins M, Sosman J et al. Outpatient biochemotherapy with interleukin-2 and interferon alfa-2b in patients with metastatic malignant melanoma: results of two phase II cytokine working group trials. J Clin Oncol 2001;19:3194–3202
14. McDermott DF, Mier JW, Lawrence DP et al. A phase II pilot trial of concurrent biochemotherapy with cisplatin, vinblastine, dacarbazine, interleukin 2, and interferon alpha-2B in patients with metastatic melanoma. Clin Cancer Res 2000;6:2201–2208
15. Rosenberg SA, Yang JC, Schwartzentruber DJ et al. Prospective randomized trial of the treatment of patients with metastatic melanoma using chemotherapy with cisplatin, dacarbazine, and tamoxifen alone or in combination with interleukin-2 and interferon alfa-2b. J Clin Oncol 1999;17:968–975
16. Phillips GL, Fay JW, Herzig GP et al. Intensive 1,3-bis(2-chloroethyl)-1-nitrosourea (BCNU), NSC #4366650 and cryopreserved autologous marrow transplantation for refractory cancer. A phase I-II study. Cancer 1983;52:1792–1802
17. Cornbleet MA, McElwain TJ, Kumar PJ et al. Treatment of advanced malignant melanoma with high-dose melphalan and autologous bone marrow transplantation. Br J Cancer 1983;48:329–334
18. Wolff SN, Herzig RH, Fay JW et al. High-dose thiotepa with autologous bone marrow transplantation for metastatic malignant melanoma: results of phase I and II studies of the North American Bone Marrow Transplantation Group. J Clin Oncol 1989;7:245–249
19. Meisenberg BR, Ross M, Vredenburgh JJ et al. Randomized trial of high-dose chemotherapy with autologous bone marrow support as adjuvant therapy for high-risk, multi-node-positive malignant melanoma. J Natl Cancer Inst 1993;85:1080–1085
20. Fine HA, Dear KB, Loeffler JS et al. Meta-analysis of radiation therapy with and without adjuvant chemotherapy for malignant gliomas in adults. Cancer 1993;71:2585–2597
21. Jacques-Olivier B, Claude L, Pierre B et al. Does high-dose carmustine increase overall survival in supratentorial high-grade malignant glioma? An EBMT retrospective study. Int J Cancer 2007;120:1782–1786
22. van Glabbeke M, van Oosterom AT, Oosterhuis JW et al. Prognostic factors for the outcome of chemotherapy in advanced soft tissue sarcoma: an analysis of 2,185 patients treated with anthracycline-containing first-line regimens – a European Organization for Research and Treatment of Cancer Soft Tissue and Bone Sarcoma Group Study. J Clin Oncol 1999;17:150–157
23. Antman K, Crowley J, Balcerzak SP et al. An intergroup phase III randomized study of doxorubicin and dacarbazine with or without ifosfamide and mesna in advanced soft tissue and bone sarcomas. J Clin Oncol 1993;11:1276–1785
24. Edmonson JH, Ryan LM, Blum RH et al. Randomized comparison of doxorubicin alone versus ifosfamide plus doxorubicin or mitomycin, doxorubicin, and cisplatin against advanced soft tissue sarcomas. J Clin Oncol 1993;11:1269–1275
25. Santoro A, Tursz T, Mouridsen H et al. Doxorubicin versus CYVADIC versus doxorubicin plus ifosfamide in first-line treatment of advanced soft tissue sarcomas: a randomized study of the European Organization for Research and Treatment of Cancer Soft Tissue and Bone Sarcoma Group. J Clin Oncol 1995;13:1537–1545
26. Fagioli F, Aglietta M, Tienghi A et al. High-dose chemotherapy in the treatment of relapsed osteosarcoma: an Italian sarcoma group study. J Clin Oncol 2002;20:2150–2156
27. Elias AD, Ayash LJ, Wheeler C et al. Phase I study of high-dose ifosfamide, carboplatin and etoposide with autologous hematopoietic stem cell support. Bone Marrow Transplant 1995;15:373–379
28. Blay JY, Bouhour D, Ray-Coquard I et al. High-dose chemotherapy with autologous hematopoietic stem-cell transplantation for advanced soft tissue sarcoma in adults. J Clin Oncol 2000;18:3643–3650
29. Engelhardt M, Zeiser R, Ihorst G et al. High-dose chemotherapy and autologous peripheral blood stem cell transplantation in adult patients with high-risk or advanced Ewing and soft tissue sarcoma. J Cancer Res Clin Oncol 2007;133:1–11
30. Clark MA, Fisher C, Judson I, Thomas JM. Soft-tissue sarcomas in adults. N Engl J Med 2005;353:701–711
31. van der Bruggen P, Stroobant V, van Pel A, van den Eynde B. T-cell defined tumor antigens. Cancer Immunity 2001; revised 2007. www.cancerimmunity.org/peptidedatabase/Tcellepitopes.htm#text
32. Eder JP, Kantoff PW, Roper K et al. A phase I trial of a recombinant vaccinia virus expressing prostate-specific antigen in advanced prostate cancer. Clin Cancer Res 2000;6:1632–1638
33. Panelli MC, Wunderlich J, Jeffries J et al. Phase 1 study in patients with metastatic melanoma of immunization with dendritic cells presenting epitopes derived from the melanoma-associated antigens MART-1 and gp100. J Immunother 2000;23:487–498
34. Phan GQ, Touloukian CE, Yang JC et al. Immunization of patients with metastatic melanoma using both class I- and class II-restricted peptides from melanoma-associated antigens. J Immunother 2003;26:349–356
35. Schwaab T, Lewis LD, Cole BF et al. Phase I pilot trial of the bispecific antibody MDXH210 (anti-Fc gamma RI X anti-HER-2/neu) in patients whose prostate cancer overexpresses HER-2/neu. J Immunother 2001;24:79–87
36. Thomas-Kaskel AK, Zeiser R, Jochim R et al. Vaccination of advanced prostate cancer patients with PSCA and PSA peptide-loaded dendritic cells induces DTH responses that correlate with superior overall survival. Int J Cancer 2006;119:2428–2434
37. Muderspach L, Wilczynski S, Roman L et al. A phase I trial of a human papillomavirus (HPV) peptide vaccine for women with high-grade cervical and vulvar intraepithelial neoplasia who are HPV 16 positive. Clin Cancer Res 2000;6:3406–3416
38. Nestle FO, Alijagic S, Gilliet M et al. Vaccination of melanoma patients with peptide- or tumor lysate-pulsed dendritic cells. Nat Med 1998;4:328–332
39. Peterson AC, Harlin H, Gajewski TF. Immunization with Melan-A peptide-pulsed peripheral blood mononuclear cells plus recombinant human interleukin-12 induces clinical activity and T-cell responses in advanced melanoma. J Clin Oncol 2003;21:2342–2348
40. Wierecky J, Muller MR, Wirths S et al. Immunologic and clinical responses after vaccinations with peptide-pulsed dendritic cells in metastatic renal cancer patients. Cancer Res 2006;66:5910–5918
41. Bukowski RM, Sharfman W, Murthy S et al. Clinical results and characterization of tumor-infiltrating lymphocytes with or without recombinant interleukin 2 in human metastatic renal cell carcinoma. Cancer Res 1991;51:4199–4205
42. Dudley ME, Wunderlich JR, Robbins PF et al. Cancer regression and autoimmunity in patients after clonal repopulation with antitumor lymphocytes. Science 2002;298:850–854
43. Morgan RA, Dudley ME, Wunderlich JR et al. Cancer regression in patients after transfer of genetically engineered lymphocytes. Science 2006;314:126–129
44. Savoldo B, Huls MH, Liu Z et al. Autologous Epstein-Barr virus (EBV)-specific cytotoxic T cells for the treatment of persistent active EBV infection. Blood 2002;100:4059–4066
45. Akdis CA, Blaser K. Mechanisms of interleukin-10-mediated immune suppression. Immunology 2001;103:131–136
46. Garcia-Lora A, Martinez M, Algarra I et al. MHC class I-deficient metastatic tumor variants immunoselected by T lymphocytes originate from the coordinated downregulation of APM components. Int J Cancer 2003;106:521–527
47. Hicklin DJ, Wang Z, Arienti F et al. beta2-Microglobulin mutations, HLA class I antigen loss, and tumor progression in melanoma. J Clin Invest 1998;101:2720–2729
48. Maeurer MJ, Gollin SM, Martin D et al. Tumor escape from immune recognition: lethal recurrent melanoma in a patient associated with downregulation of the peptide transporter protein TAP-1 and loss of expression of the immunodominant MART-1/Melan-A antigen. J Clin Invest 1996;98:1633–1641
49. Medema JP, de Jong J, Peltenburg LT et al. Blockade of the granzyme B/perforin pathway through overexpression of the serine protease inhibitor PI-9/SPI-6 constitutes a mechanism for immune escape by tumors. Proc Natl Acad Sci USA 2001;98:11515–11520
50. O'Connell J, Bennett MW, O'Sullivan GC et al. Fas counter-attack – the best form of tumor defense? Nat Med 1999;5:267–268
51. Seliger B, Hohne A, Jung D et al. Expression and function of the peptide transporters in escape variants of human renal cell carcinomas. Exp Hematol 1997;25:608–614
52. Antony PA, Piccirillo CA, Akpinarli A et al. CD8+ T cell immunity against a tumor/self-antigen is augmented by CD4+ T helper cells and hindered by naturally occurring T regulatory cells. J Immunol 2005;174:2591–2601
53. Curiel TJ, Coukos G, Zou L et al. Specific recruitment of regulatory T cells in ovarian carcinoma fosters immune privilege and predicts reduced survival. Nat Med 2004;10:942–949
54. Ormandy LA, Hillemann T, Wedemeyer H et al. Increased populations of regulatory T cells in peripheral blood of patients with hepatocellular carcinoma. Cancer Res 2005;65:2457–2464
55. Baron F, Storb R. Allogeneic hematopoietic cell transplantation as treatment for hematological malignancies: a review. Springer Semin Immunopathol 2004;26:71–94
56. Storb RF, Champlin R, Riddell SR et al. Non-myeloablative transplants for malignant disease. Hematology Am Soc Hematol Educ Program 2001:375–391
57. Parr MD, Messino MJ, McIntyre W. Allogeneic bone marrow transplantation: procedures and complications. Am J Hosp Pharm 1991;48:127–137
58. Majolino I, Saglio G, Scime R et al. High incidence of chronic GVHD after primary allogeneic peripheral blood stem cell transplantation in patients with hematologic malignancies. Bone Marrow Transplant 1996;17:555–560
59. Nash RA, Storb R. Graft-versus-host effect after allogeneic hematopoietic stem cell transplantation: GVHD and GVL. Curr Opin Immunol 1996;8:674–680

60. Mattsson J, Uzunel M, Remberger M, Ringden O. T cell mixed chimerism is significantly correlated to a decreased risk of acute graft-versus-host disease after allogeneic stem cell transplantation. Transplantation 2001;71:433–439

61. Trivedi HL, Vanikar AV, Modi PR et al. Allogeneic hematopoietic stem-cell transplantation, mixed chimerism, and tolerance in living related donor renal allograft recipients. Transplant Proc 2005;37:737–742

62. Childs R, Clave E, Contentin N et al. Engraftment kinetics after nonmyeloablative alloge-neic peripheral blood stem cell transplantation: full donor T-cell chimerism precedes allo-immune responses. Blood 1999;94:3234–3241

63. Imamura M, Tsutsumi Y, Miura Y et al. Immune reconstitution and tolerance after alloge-neic hematopoietic stem cell transplantation. Hematology 2003;8:19–26

64. Maris M, Sandmaier BM, Maloney DG et al. Non-myeloablative hematopoietic stem cell transplantation. Transfus Clin Biol 2001;8:231–234

65. Cross NC, Hughes TP, Feng L et al. Minimal residual disease after allogeneic bone marrow transplantation for chronic myeloid leukaemia in first chronic phase: correlations with acute graft-versus-host disease and relapse. Br J Haematol 1993;84:67–74

66. Enright H, Davies SM, DeFor T et al. Relapse after non-T-cell-depleted allogeneic bone marrow transplantation for chronic myelogenous leukemia: early transplantation, use of an unrelated donor, and chronic graft-versus-host disease are protective. Blood 1996;88:714–720

67. Sullivan KM, Fefer A, Witherspoon R et al. Graft-versus-leukemia in man: relationship of acute and chronic graft-versus-host disease to relapse of acute leukemia following alloge-neic bone marrow transplantation. Prog Clin Biol Res 1987;244:391–399

68. Zikos P, van Lint MT, Lamparelli T et al. Allogeneic hemopoietic stem cell transplantation for patients with high risk acute lymphoblastic leukemia: favorable impact of chronic graft-versus-host disease on survival and relapse. Haematologica 1998;83:896–903

69. Horowitz MM, Gale RP, Sondel PM et al. Graft-versus-leukemia reactions after bone marrow transplantation. Blood 1990;75:555–562

70. Apperley JF, Jones L, Hale G et al. Bone marrow transplantation for patients with chronic myeloid leukaemia: T-cell depletion with Campath-1 reduces the incidence of graft-versus-host disease but may increase the risk of leukaemic relapse. Bone Marrow Transplant 1986;1:53–66

71. Goldman JM, Gale RP, Horowitz MM et al. Bone marrow transplantation for chronic myelogenous leukemia in chronic phase. Increased risk for relapse associated with T-cell depletion. Ann Intern Med 1988;108:806–814

72. Martin PJ, Hansen JA, Buckner CD et al. Effects of in vitro depletion of T cells in HLA-identical allogeneic marrow grafts. Blood 1985;66:664–672

73. Bishop MR, Fowler DH, Marchigiani D et al. Allogeneic lymphocytes induce tumor regres-sion of advanced metastatic breast cancer. J Clin Oncol 2004;22:3886–3892

74. Bregni M, Dodero A, Peccatori J et al. Nonmyeloablative conditioning followed by hema-topoietic cell allografting and donor lymphocyte infusions for patients with metastatic renal and breast cancer. Blood 2002;99:4234–4236

75. Carella AM, Beltrami G, Corsetti MT et al. Reduced intensity conditioning for allograft after cytoreductive autograft in metastatic breast cancer. Lancet 2005;366:318–320

76. Childs R, Bradstock K. Non-myeloablative allogeneic stem cell transplantation (NST) for metastatic melanoma: nondurable chemotherapy responses without clinically meaningful graft-vs-tumor (GVT) effects. Society of Hematology Meeting, Philadelphia, USA, 2002 (abstracts)

77. Childs R, Chernoff A, Contentin N et al. Regression of metastatic renal-cell carcinoma after nonmyeloablative allogeneic peripheral-blood stem-cell transplantation. N Engl J Med 2000;343:750–758

78. Hentschke P, Barkholt L, Uzunel M et al. Low-intensity conditioning and hematopoietic stem cell transplantation in patients with renal and colon carcinoma. Bone Marrow Trans-plant 2003;31:253–261

79. Kurokawa T, Fischer K, Bertz H et al. In vitro and in vivo characterization of graft-versus-tumor responses in melanoma patients after allogeneic peripheral blood stem cell trans-plantation. Int J Cancer 2002;101:52–60

80. Pedrazzoli P, da Prada GA, Giorgiani G et al. Allogeneic blood stem cell transplantation after a reduced-intensity, preparative regimen: a pilot study in patients with refractory malignancies. Cancer 2002;94:2409–1245

81. Rini BI, Zimmerman T, Stadler WM et al. Allogeneic stem-cell transplantation of renal cell cancer after nonmyeloablative chemotherapy: feasibility, engraftment, and clinical results. J Clin Oncol 2002;20:2017–2024

82. Takahashi T, Omuro Y, Matsumoto G et al. Nonmyeloablative allogeneic stem cell trans-plantation for patients with unresectable pancreatic cancer. Pancreas 2004;28:e65–e69

83. Ueno NT, Cheng YC, Rondon G et al. Rapid induction of complete donor chimerism by the use of a reduced-intensity conditioning regimen composed of fludarabine and melphalan in allogeneic stem cell transplantation for metastatic solid tumors. Blood 2003;102:3829–3836

84. Barkholt L, Bregni M, Remberger M et al. Allogeneic haematopoietic stem cell transplanta-tion for metastatic renal carcinoma in Europe. Ann Oncol 2006;17:1134–1140

85. Bregni M, Ueno NT, Childs R. The second international meeting on allogeneic transplanta-tion in solid tumors. Bone Marrow Transplant 2006;38:527–537

86. Bay JO, Fleury J, Choufi B et al. Allogeneic hematopoietic stem cell transplantation in ovarian carcinoma: results of five patients. Bone Marrow Transplant 2002;30:95–102

87. Warren EH, Greenberg PD, Riddell SR. Cytotoxic T-lymphocyte-defined human minor histocompatibility antigens with a restricted tissue distribution. Blood 1998;91: 2197–2207

88. Tykodi SS, Warren EH, Thompson JA et al. Allogeneic hematopoietic cell transplantation for metastatic renal cell carcinoma after nonmyeloablative conditioning: toxicity, clinical response, and immunological response to minor histocompatibility antigens. Clin Cancer Res 2004;10:7799–7811

89. Warren EH, Tykodi SS, Murata M et al. T-cell therapy targeting minor histocompatibility Ags for the treatment of leukemia and renal-cell carcinoma. Cytotherapy 2002;4:441

90. Fontaine P, Roy-Proulx G, Knafo L et al. Adoptive transfer of minor histocompatibility antigen-specific T lymphocytes eradicates leukemia cells without causing graft-versus-host disease. Nat Med 2001;7:789–794

91. Mutis T. Targeting alloreactive donor T-cells to hematopoietic system-restricted minor histocompatibility antigens to dissect graft-versus-leukemia effects from graft-versus-host disease after allogeneic stem cell transplantation. Int J Hematol 2003;78: 208–212

92. Perreault C, Jutras J, Roy DC et al. Identification of an immunodominant mouse minor histocompatibility antigen (MiHA). T cell response to a single dominant MiHA causes graft-versus-host disease. J Clin Invest 1996;98:622–628

93. Amrolia PJ, Muccioli-Casadei G, Yvon E et al. Selective depletion of donor alloreactive T cells without loss of antiviral or antileukemic responses. Blood 2003;102:2292–2299

94. Solomon SR, Tran T, Carter CS et al. Optimized clinical-scale culture conditions for ex vivo selective depletion of host-reactive donor lymphocytes: a strategy for GvHD prophylaxis in allogeneic PBSC transplantation. Cytotherapy 2002;4:395–406

95. Matte CC, Liu J, Cormier J et al. Donor APCs are required for maximal GVHD but not for GVL. Nat Med 2004;10:987–992

96. Shlomchik WD, Couzens MS, Tang CB et al. Prevention of graft versus host disease by inactivation of host antigen-presenting cells. Science 1999;285:412–415

97. Cohen JL, Trenado A, Vasey D et al. CD4+D25+ immunoregulatory T Cells: new thera-peutics for graft-versus-host disease. J Exp Med 2002;196:401–406

98. Taylor PA, Lees CJ, Blazar BR. The infusion of ex vivo activated and expanded CD4+D25+ immune regulatory cells inhibits graft-versus-host disease lethality. Blood 2002;99: 3493–3499

99. Edinger M, Hoffmann P, Ermann J et al. CD4+CD25+ regulatory T cells preserve graft-versus-tumor activity while inhibiting graft-versus-host disease after bone marrow trans-plantation. Nat Med 2003;9:1144–1150

100. Sato K, Yamashita N, Baba M, Matsuyama T. Regulatory dendritic cells protect mice from murine acute graft-versus-host disease and leukemia relapse. Immunity 2003;18:367–379

101. Chen BJ, Cui X, Sempowski GD et al. Transfer of allogeneic CD62L- memory T cells without graft-versus-host disease. Blood 2004;103:1534–1541

102. Bendandi M, Rodriguez-Calvillo M, Inoges S et al. Combined vaccination with idiotype-pulsed allogeneic dendritic cells and soluble protein idiotype for multiple myeloma patients relapsing after reduced-intensity conditioning allogeneic stem cell transplantation. Leuk Lymphoma 2006;47:29–37

103. Zoller M. Tumor vaccination after allogeneic bone marrow cell reconstitution of the non-myeloablatively conditioned tumor-bearing murine host. J Immunol 2003;171:6941–6953

104. Ji YH, Weiss L, Zeira M et al. Allogeneic cell-mediated immunotherapy of leukemia with immune donor lymphocytes to upregulate antitumor effects and downregulate antihost responses. Bone Marrow Transplant 2003;32:495–504

105. Savani BN, Srinivasan R, Espinoza-Delgado I et al. Treatment of relapsed blast-phase Philadelphia-chromosome-positive leukaemia after non-myeloablative stem cell transplan-tation with donor lymphocytes and imatinib. Lancet Oncol 2005;6:809–812

106. Chalandon Y, Schwaller J. Targeting mutated protein tyrosine kinases and their signaling pathways in hematologic malignancies. Haematologica 2005;90:949–968

107. McInnes C, Fischer PM. Strategies for the design of potent and selective kinase inhibitors. Curr Pharm Des 2005;11:1845–1863

108. Murray N, Salgia R, Fossella FV. Targeted molecules in small cell lung cancer. Semin Oncol 2004;31(1 suppl 1):106–111

109. Wiedmann MW, Caca K. Molecularly targeted therapy for gastrointestinal cancer. Curr Cancer Drug Targets 2005;5:171–193

110. Igarashi T, Wynberg J, Srinivasan R et al. Enhanced cytotoxicity of allogeneic NK cells with killer immunoglobulin-like receptor ligand incompatibility against melanoma and renal cell carcinoma cells. Blood 2004;104:170–177

111. Ruggeri L, Capanni M, Casucci M et al. Role of natural killer cell alloreactivity in HLA-mismatched hematopoietic stem cell transplantation. Blood 1999;94:333–339

112. Ruggeri L, Capanni M, Urbani E et al. Effectiveness of donor natural killer cell alloreactiv-ity in mismatched hematopoietic transplants. Science 2002;295:2097–2100

113. Yu G, Xu X, Vu MD et al. NK cells promote transplant tolerance by killing donor antigen-presenting cells. J Exp Med 2006;203:1851–1858

114. Sentman CL, Barber MA, Barber A, Zhang T. NK cell receptors as tools in cancer immu-notherapy. Adv Cancer Res 2006;95:249–292

115. Asai O, Longo DL, Tian ZG et al. Suppression of graft-versus-host disease and amplifica-tion of graft-versus-tumor effects by activated natural killer cells after allogeneic bone marrow transplantation. J Clin Invest 1998;101:1835–1842

116. Lundqvist A, McCoy JP, Samsel L, Childs R. Reduction of GVHD and enhanced anti-tumor effects after adoptive infusion of alloreactive Ly49-mismatched NK-cells from MHC-matched donors. Blood 2007;109:3603–3606

117. Giebel S, Locatelli F, Lamparelli T et al. Survival advantage with KIR ligand incompatibil-ity in hematopoietic stem cell transplantation from unrelated donors. Blood 2003;102: 814–819

118. Srinivasan R, Carrington M, Suffredini D et al. Impact of KIR and HLA genotypes on outcome in nonmyeloablative hematopoietic cell transplantation (HCT) Using HLA matched related donors (ASH Annual Meeting Abstracts #323). Blood 2006; 108:11

119. van de Velde H, Bosquee L, Weynants P et al. Moderate dose-escalation of combination chemotherapy with concomitant thoracic radiotherapy in limited-disease small-cell lung cancer: prolonged intrathoracic tumor control and high central nervous system relapse rate. Groupe d'Oncologie-Pneumologie Clinique de l'Universite Catholique de Louvain, Brus-sels and Liege, Belgium. Ann Oncol 1999;10:1051–1057

120. Smith IE, Evans BD, Harland SJ et al. High-dose cyclophosphamide with autologous bone marrow rescue after conventional chemotherapy in the treatment of small cell lung carci-noma. Cancer Chemother Pharmacol 1985;14:120–124

121. Spitzer G, Farha P, Valdivieso M et al. High-dose intensification therapy with autologous bone marrow support for limited small-cell bronchogenic carcinoma. J Clin Oncol 1986;4:4–13

122. Fetscher S, Brugger W, Engelhardt R et al. Dose-intense therapy with etoposide, ifosfamide, cisplatin, and epirubicin (VIP-E) in 107 consecutive patients with limited- and extensive-stage non-small-cell lung cancer. Ann Oncol 1997;8:57–64

123. Johnson DB, Thompson JM, Corwin JA et al. Prolongation of survival for high-grade malignant gliomas with adjuvant high-dose BCNU and autologous bone marrow transplantation. J Clin Oncol 1987;5:783–789

124. Biron P, Vial C, Chauvin F. Strategy including surgery, high dose BCNU followed by ABMT and radiotherapy in supratentorial high grade astrocytomas: a report of 98 patients. In: Dicke KA, Armitage JO, Dicke-Evinger MJ (eds) Autologous bone marrow transplantation. Proceedings of the 5th International Symposium, University of Nebraska Medical Center, 1991, 637–645

125. Linassier C, Destrieux C, Benboubker L et al. [Role of high-dose chemotherapy with hemopoietic stem-cell support in the treatment of adult patients with high-grade glioma]. Bull Cancer 2001;88:871–876

126. Durando X, Lemaire JJ, Tortochaux J et al. High-dose BCNU followed by autologous hematopoietic stem cell transplantation in supratentorial high-grade malignant gliomas: a retrospective analysis of 114 patients. Bone Marrow Transplant 2003;31:559–564

Germ cell tumors

Alan Horwich and Duncan Gilbert

CHAPTER 14

Introduction

Germ cell tumors are the most common malignancies in young men (15–35 years) and are increasing in incidence for reasons as yet poorly understood. They include testicular and extragonadal areas of involvement such as retroperitoneal and mediastinal primary sites and are thought to derive from the primordial germ cell lineage. With the advent of cisplatin-containing combination chemotherapy, metastatic germ cell cancer has become a curable disease and increasingly efforts are focused on reducing the incidence of treatment-related toxicity. However, there is heterogeneity among patients and there exists a group with non-seminomatous germ cell tumors (NSGCT) whose prognosis remains poor despite standard chemotherapy regimens.

In 1997, the International Germ Cell Cancer Consensus Group (IGCCCG) published a prognostic index based on data from 5202 patients with NSGCT, based on multivariate risk factors identified from regression analysis, namely primary site, presence of non-pulmonary visceral metastasis and elevation of the tumor markers alpha-fetoprotein (AFP), beta-human chorionic gonadotrophin (HCG) and lactic dehydrogenase (LDH).[1] This divides patients into prognostic groups by expected survival rates, with good-prognosis patients expected to achieve 90% survival at 5 years, intermediate 80% survival but poor only 48% (Table 14.1). Poor-prognosis patients comprised 14% of those at presentation and were defined as those with high markers (beta-HCG >50,000 u/l, AFP >10,000 u/l or LDH >10x upper limit of normal), non-pulmonary visceral metastases, mediastinal primary or any combination thereof. Current standard treatment consists of 3–4 cycles of BEP (bleomycin, etoposide and cisplatin) chemotherapy. To date, no randomized trials have demonstrated a superior regimen, although a number of schedules have been reported as Phase II trials (Table 14.2). When considering non-randomized data, however, both the effect of the treating institution (larger centers achieve better results) and improving survival rates over time[2,3] must be considered, as well as case selection effects.

Surgery plays an important role in the management of residual disease after chemotherapy, and also in those who relapse after chemotherapy.[4] Retroperitoneal lymph node dissection and resection of other residual masses should be considered particularly in patients with persistently elevated tumor markers after chemotherapy or macroscopic disease. This aims to remove viable tumor, which is probably chemoresistant, and differentiated teratoma that may enlarge or undergo late malignant change.

Although around 85% of men presenting with metastatic cancer are cured, the outlook for patients experiencing relapse after chemotherapy is less good; 20–30% of patients with metastases will relapse and this confers a poor prognosis, though in some patients the disease remains sensitive to chemotherapy. Late relapse, i.e. more than 2 years after initial treatment, occurs in between 0.5–1% patients per year[5] and is relatively chemoresistant, requiring surgical resection wherever possible.

Thus, there are two groups of patients in whom the role for high-dose chemotherapy and stem cell transplant has been investigated: 'salvage' therapy in the setting of disease relapse, and 'first-line' therapy in those patients with a poor prognosis from the outset.

Non-myeloablative chemotherapy

First-line therapy

Recent studies seeking improved efficacy with conventional chemotherapy are summarized in Table 14.2. A variety of regimens has demonstrated efficacy in the poor-prognosis group broadly testing either increased dose intensity or new agents. Alternating chemotherapies is an attractive concept to allow dose escalation by avoiding specific cumulative toxicities, while minimizing the chances of drug resistance. The longest experience of this has been with POMB/ACE (cisplatin, vincristine, methotrexate, bleomycin alternating with actinomycin D, cyclophosphamide and etoposide), which in one study gave a 3-year survival of 75% (95% confidence interval (CI) 65–84%)[6] but has subsequently performed less well.[7,8] The Royal Marsden CBOP-BEP (carboplatin, bleomycin, vincristine and cisplatin, following by bleomycin, etoposide and cisplatin) schedule starts with 6 weeks of accelerated chemotherapy alternating carboplatin and cisplatin in combination with vincristine and bleomycin prior to three cycles of BEP (with the bleomycin dose reduced to remain within dose limits). In 54 men treated with this regime between 1989 and 2000, the 5-year overall survival was 87.6 % (95% CI 71.3–94.6%) and even primary mediastinal patients achieved 77.1% 3-year survival.[9] This schedule is currently being tested against standard BEP in an NCRI trial. At present, the only randomized data come from comparisons of BOP/VIP-B (bleomycin, vincristine, cisplatin (BOP)/etoposide, ifosfamide, cislatin and bleomycin (VIP-B))[10] or CISCA/VB (cisplatin, doxorubicin and cyclophosphamide alternated with vinblastine and bleomycin)[11] with BEP, and neither demonstrated any significant benefit. Substituting ifosfamide for bleomycin in BEP produced greater toxicity but was not more effective.[12] Paclitaxel has been added to BEP in a small study with encouraging response rates[13] and is currently the subject of an EORTC study in intermediate-prognosis patients. Oxaliplatin and gemcitabine are more recently developed agents with activity in GCTs,[14–17] and they have yet to be assessed in first-line chemotherapy.

Table 14.1 Prognostic groups within testicular GCT[1]

NSGCT	Seminoma
Good prognosis	
Testes/retroperitoneal primary and No non-pulmonary visceral metastases and Low serum markers 56% of NSGCT 5-year survival 92% 5-year PFS 89%	Any primary site and No non-pulmonary visceral metastases and Any marker (normal AFP) 90% of seminomas 5-year survival 86% 5-year PFS 82%
Intermediate prognosis	
Testes/retroperitoneal primary and No non-pulmonary visceral metastases and Intermediate markers 28% of NSGCT 5-year survival 80% 5-year PFS 75%	Any primary site and Non-pulmonary visceral metastases and Any marker 10% of seminomas 5-year survival 72% 5-year PFS 67%
Poor prognosis	
Mediastinal primary or Non-pulmonary visceral metastases or High markers 16% of NSGCT 5-year survival 48% 5-year PFS 41%	No patients classified as poor prognosis

Table 14.2 Outcomes in treating poor-prognosis disease at presentation (non-high dose)

Series	Drugs	Patients	Relapse-free survival (%)	Overall survival (%)
Bower (1997)[6]	POMB-ACE	92		75
Germa-Lluch (1999)[45]	POMB-EPI	22	58	
Decatris (2000)[46]	BEP-CEC	20		60
Fizazi (2002)[47]	BOP-CISCA POMB-ACE	38	65	
Schmoll (2003)[42]	HD VIP	182	69	
Christian (2003)[9]	CBOP-BEP	54	83	
Fossa (2005)[48]	CBOP-BEP	56	56	

Salvage regimens

In those failing after firstline chemotherapy, a worse outcome is predicted when the progression-free interval is less than 2 years, if there has been a less than complete response to induction treatment or there are markedly raised tumor markers.[18] Patients with all three risk factors fall into a poor prognostic group – in this data set none survived more than 3 years – whereas patients with at most two of these factors had a better outcome with a 5-year survival of 47%. These survivals were obtained with combination chemotherapy and subsequent consolidation with surgery or radiotherapy to residual disease. The Memorial Sloan Kettering Cancer Center (MSKCC) defines good prognosis at relapse as those patients with testicular primary tumors who achieve CR with first-line chemotherapy.

Chemotherapy schedules were typically ifosfamide, cisplatin and etoposide (IPE) or more recently paclitaxel, ifosfamide and cisplatin (TIP). This latter regime has been used in 46 MSKCC 'good prognosis relapse' patients, where 32 (70%) achieved a complete response to treatment and an overall progression-free survival (PFS) of 65% was seen.[19] In a Medical Research Council (MRC) Phase II trial of TIP[20] of 43 assessable patients, only eight complete responses (and 18

Table 14.3 Combination chemotherapy in relapsed/refractory GCT

Reference	Schedule	Number of patients	1-year PFS (%)
Pico (2005)[29]	Vinblastine/Etoposide Ifosfamide Cisplatin	128	35 (3 years)
Kondagunta (2005)[19]	Paclitaxel Ifosfamide Cisplatin	46 (selected MSKCC 'good prognosis')	65 (2 years)
Mead (2005)[20]	Paclitaxel Ifosfamide Cisplatin	43	36
Hinton (2002)[14]	Paclitaxel Gemcitabine	28	7
Pectasides (2004)[15]	Gemcitabine Oxaliplatin	29	10
Kollmannsberger (2004)[17]	Gemcitabine Oxaliplatin	35	11
Pectasides (2004)[16]	Irinotecan Oxaliplatin	18	11

partial responses with negative markers) were achieved with a subsequent 1-year failure-free survival of 36% (95% CI 22–50%). Results were much better in the MSKCC 'good prognosis relapse' group.

As previously discussed, late relapses (occurring more than 2 years after treatment) are associated with a higher degree of resistance to chemotherapy and subsequently do worse, although they may still respond to salvage treatment with TIP if they are not candidates for surgery.[21] Of the newer agents available, paclitaxel appears the most active drug in relapsed disease. Hence its use in first-line salvage combinations, but activity is also seen in combinations containing oxaliplatin or gemcitabine (Table 14.3), with response rates of around 30–40% (and durable responses seen in up to 10% patients).

Outcomes for high-dose chemotherapy

Salvage treatment

The rationale for considering high-dose chemotherapy in salvage of patients who have failed first-line chemotherapy for germ cell tumors is based on the chemosensitivity of this tumor type, the evidence for dose response to cisplatin at lower doses and the feasibility of significant dose escalation for a number of key drugs including carboplatin, etoposide and either cyclophosphamide or ifosfamide. When supported by hematopoietic precursor support, dose-limiting side-effects are mucositis for etoposide, renal toxicity for ifosfamide, especially in cisplatin-pretreated patients, and bowel toxicity for combinations of these drugs with carboplatin.

High-dose chemotherapy was first evaluated using support by autologous bone marrow transplantation. Trials of this approach began in Indiana University in 1986 using high-dose carboplatin and etoposide. In 32 patients registered for this study in the first 2 years chemotherapy comprised etoposide 1200 mg/m^2, together with carboplatin in an escalating dose schedule from 900 mg/m^2 to 2000 mg/m^2. Seven patients died of treatment-related problems and there were eight patients with complete remissions within a 42% overall response rate.[22] Further follow-up after the first 40 patients had been treated in the same study found that six patients (15%) were alive and continuously disease free at a minimum of 36 months follow-up. However, a further patient died of acute myelogenous leukemia while in remission 28 months after autologous bone marrow transplant (ABMT).[23] Data were recently reported in addition on 184 patients treated at Indiana

Table 14.4 Beyer prognostic groups[25]

Variable	Points
Platinum-refractory GCT	1
Primary mediastinal NSGCT	1
Progressive disease before HDCT	1
Absolute platinum refractory GCT	2
HCG >1000 u/ml	2
Cumulative point score	**Two-year PFS**
0	51%
1–2	27%
>2	5%

Abbreviations: GCT, germ cell tumor; HCG, human chorionic gonadotrophin; NSGCT, non-seminomatous germ cell tumor; HDCT, high-dose chemotherapy.

University with HDCE (high dose carboplatin + etoposide), of whom 63% remained disease free.[24]

Retrospective prognostic factor analysis of 310 patients treated with high-dose chemotherapy and autologous stem cell transplantation[25] identified a prognostic scoring system based on a number of factors (Table 14.4). Patients with none of these adverse features (score 0) had a failure-free survival rate at 2 years of 51%, as compared with intermediate scores (1 and 2) of 27% and poor-risk disease (>2) of 5%. The robustness of these features was demonstrated in a series of patients treated in Indiana between 1988 and 2001.[26]

The European experience with extragonadal tumors also shows significant long-term efficacy[27] with 30% disease-free survival at 58 months, but highlights the disparity between retroperitoneal (48% 3-year overall survival (OS)) and mediastinal (14% 3-year OS) disease. In this series there was a 5% toxic death rate.

Beyer's matched-pair analysis of 74 patients suggested an improvement in event-free survival of 9–11% in favor of high-dose chemotherapy at 2 years.[28] However, randomized trials have to date failed to demonstrate unequivocal benefit for a high-dose strategy over standard salvage chemotherapy. The largest of these, a multicenter European study,[29] randomized 280 patients with incomplete remission or relapse following first-line chemotherapy to either conventional dose salvage treatment (four cycles of cisplatin, ifosfamide and etoposide or vinblastine) or three such cycles followed by high-dose carboplatin, etoposide and cylophosphamide with stem cell support. There was no significant difference in 3-year event-free or overall survival, and 3% toxic deaths occurred with conventional treatment as opposed to 7% in the high-dose arm. A significant difference in relapse-free survival was observed in those achieving CR, in favor of high-dose treatment, but this did not translate to improved overall survival. It should be noted that given the numbers of patients enrolled, a difference of up to 15% in survival could not be excluded.

Despite the lack of evidence for the superiority of high-dose regimens, a German trial[30] randomized 216 patients with relapsed or refractory germ cell tumors to single or sequential high-dose chemotherapy (either 1 × VIP (etoposide, ifosfamide and cisplatin) and 3 × high-dose carboplatin and etoposide or 3 × VIP and 1 × high-dose carboplatin and etoposide (CE)), again powered to detect differences in excess of 15% between arms. However, the single high-dose treatment was associated with excess treatment-related mortality (15/105 patients) and the trial was prematurely closed with no significant difference between high-dose schedules (1-year PFS 55% vs 49%).

Paclitaxel has been introduced into salvage chemotherapy regimes and this is reflected in high-dose schedules such as TIP followed by high-dose carboplatin, etoposide and thiotepa which has demonstrated disease-free survival of 25% at 3 years.[31] Similar combinations (paclitaxel/ifosfamide induction and peripheral stem cell harvest followed by high-dose carboplatin/etoposide) yielded sustained responses in 15 of 37 patients (41%) at a median follow-up of 31 months.[32] Paclitaxel has

also been used with epirubicin as induction followed by three high-dose treatments (cyclophosphamide and thiotepa) then etoposide, ifosfamide and carboplatin.[33] This resulted in a 24% 3-year progression-free survival, although less than half of the 45 patients completed the course and there were five toxic deaths. Alternatively, paclitaxel can be given concurrently with the high-dose drugs etoposide, carboplatin and cyclophosphamide.[34] In this series of 36 patients, a 1-year event-free survival of 64% was seen in cisplatin-sensitive disease, falling to a 25% overall survival in cisplatin-refractory or absolute refractory disease. In addition, there were six treatment-related deaths.

Reported outcomes of the use of high-dose chemotherapy regimens in the salvage treatment of germ cell tumors are summarized in Table 14.5.

Primary treatment

High-dose chemotherapy has been investigated as an alternative approach to improve outcomes in patients identified as poor prognosis at presentation. Indications have been either as defined by the ICCCG criteria or using suboptimal marker decline to initial chemotherapy[35,36,37] and are summarized in Table 14.6.

Following encouraging results from a Phase II trial of 28 patients with poor-prognosis disease treated with two cycles of double-dose cisplatin, vinblastine, bleomycin and etoposide (modified PVeBV) and a single cycle of high-dose chemotherapy (double-dose cisplatin, etoposide and cyclophosphamide – PEC) followed by autologous bone marrow transplant,[38] this regime was tested in a randomized controlled trial.[39] However, this failed to demonstrate any therapeutic benefit of this approach. There is also evidence that the doses of cisplatin used (200 mg/m[2]) are no more effective than the standard dose of 100 mg/m[2].[40]

At the Memorial Sloan Kettering Cancer Center an analysis of tumor marker patterns following chemotherapy suggested that low or inadequate clearance of tumor markers was associated with a poor prognosis after conventional treatment and a protocol was introduced of switching patients to high-dose treatment if their marker clearance was slow. One problem with this approach is that the significance of tumor marker regression rates may depend upon the time when they are measured.[35] The results of this approach reported from MSKCC demonstrated that nine of 16 patients with slow marker response had a complete response to high-dose chemotherapy.[41]

A Phase I/II trial conducted in Germany investigated sequential high-dose etoposide, ifosfamide and cisplatin (VIP) with stem cell support, again with the aim of improving outcomes in the poor-prognostic group.[42] At 4 years median follow-up, 2- and 5-year PFS were 69% and 68%, respectively (n = 221) and this approach is being compared to standard 4 × BEP in a multicenter randomized EORTC trial.

Given the percieved superiority of first-line high-dose chemotherapy over historical controls, a recently completed US Intergroup trial randomized poor- and intermediate-prognosis patients to two cycles of BEP followed by two cycles of HDCT (cyclophosphamide, etoposide and carboplatin) against the standard 4 × BEP.[43] Two hundred and nineteen patients were enrolled, aiming to detect a 20% improvement in complete response at 1 year above a historical figure of 45%. However, 1-year complete responses were no different, being 52% for the high-dose arm and 48% for BEP alone.

Schema

High-dose chemotherapy with carboplatin and etoposide plus or minus an oxazaphosphorine followed by hematopoietic stem cell support therefore appears to be curative in 20–30% of patients with germ cell

Table 14.5 High-dose regimens as salvage for relapsed/progressive disease

Reference	High-dose regimen	Number of patients	Progression-free survival	Toxic deaths
Vaena (2003)[26]	Etoposide Carboplatin	80	32% (at 2 years)	6.3%
De Georgi (2005)[27]	Various	59	30% (at median 58 months)	5%
Pico (2005)[29]	Carboplatin Etoposide Cyclophosphamide	135	42% (at 3 years)	7%
Rick (2001)[31]	Carboplatin Etoposide Thiotepa	62	25% (at 3 years)	1.6%
Motzer (2000)[32]	Paclitaxel Ifosfamide Carboplatin Etoposide	37	41% (at median 30 months)	0%
Lotz (2005)[33]	Cyclophosphamide Thiotepa	45	23.5% (at 3 years)	11%
McNeish (2004)[34]	Carboplatin Etoposide Cyclophosphamide Paclitexel	36	48% (at 2 years)	17%
Lorch (2006)[30]	Carboplatin Etoposide Cyclophosphamide	216	55% at 1 year (1 × HDCT) 49% at 1 year (3 × HDCT)	14% 3.6%

Abbreviation: HDCT, high-dose chemotherapy.

Table 14.6 High-dose chemotherapy as primary treatment for poor-risk disease

Reference	High-dose regimen	Number of patients	Progression-free survival
Droz (1992)[38]	Cisplatin* Etoposide Cyclophosphamide	28	42% (at median 66 months)
Chevreau (1993)[39]	Cisplatin* Etoposide Cyclophosphamide	41	39% (at 2 years)
Flechon (1999)[49]	Variable	44	50% (at median 42 months)
Morris (1999)[41]	Carboplatin Etoposide Cyclophosphamide	220	50% (at median 30 months)
Schmoll (2003)[42]	Etoposide Ifosfamide Cisplatin	221	68% (at 5 years)
Bajorin (2006)[43]	Carboplatin Etoposide Cyclophosphamide	108	52% (at 1 year)

After El-Helw & Coleman.[44]
* Indicates double-dose cisplatin

Table 14.7 Royal Marsden Hospital high-dose chemotherapy regimen for GCT

Days -6 to -3 (i.e. 4 days)	Granisetron 1 mg iv Dexamethasone 8 mg iv Carboplatin AUC 6 (6 × (EDTA GFR +25)) iv Etoposide 150 mg/m² iv over 2 hours Etoposide 150 mg/m² iv over 2 hours Sodium chloride 0.9% 1 litre over 4 hours
Day 0	Stem cell return

tumors relapsing after cisplatin-based combination chemotherapy regimens. It is more effective in tumors that have retained some sensitivity to conventional-dose chemotherapy.

Given the toxicities involved and lack of randomized evidence in favor of high-dose treatment, multidisciplinary discussion to consider the relative merits of conventional dose salvage treatment paired with local therapy (surgery or radiotherapy) remains imperative. However, high-dose chemotherapy should be considered as second-line therapy with the possible exception of patients who relapse late with a limited extent of disease. Currently the use of high-dose chemotherapy in first-line treatment is not established.

Practically, the convenience of peripheral blood stem cell harvest has largely replaced bone marrow as the source of stem cells used for autografting. These can be readily mobilized despite pretreatment with

the first-line BEP regime, using conditioning chemotherapy followed by daily granulocyte colony-stimulating factor injection. Etoposide as a single agent, and in combination with ifosfamide and epirubicin (IVE), are both effective options for conditioning.

There are no reported data on the use of allografting in germ cell tumors.

An example of the high-dose regimen as used at the Royal Marsden Hospital for germ cell tumors is outlined in Table 14.7.

Future directions

As with the treatment of other cancers, a more comprehensive understanding of the molecular basis of germ cell tumors might improve treatments at both ends of the spectrum. Better identification of those patients who will not be cured with conventional chemotherapy might identify a subgroup who could benefit from dose intensification in the first instance and allow toxic treatments to be avoided when not necessary for cure. Equally, a better insight into mechanisms of chemoresistance should identify targets for rational drug design and treatments.

Conclusion

At present there is no clear evidence of benefit in either first-line or salvage settings from high-dose chemotherapy in the treatment of germ cell cancers. The Phase III trials have not been large enough, however, to exclude an improvement in disease control of up to 15%. This approach is therefore still likely to be used in selected patients.

Acknowledgements

This work was undertaken in the Royal Marsden NHS Trust, which received a proportion of its funding from the NHS Executive; the views expressed in this publication are those of the authors and not necessarily those of the NHS Executive. This work was supported by the Institute of Cancer Research, the Bob Champion Cancer Trust and Cancer Research UK Section of Radiotherapy [CUK] grant number C46/A2131.

References

1. International Germ Cell Cancer Collaborative Group. International Germ Cell Consensus Classification: a prognostic factor-based staging system for metastatic germ cell cancers. J Clin Oncol 1997;15:594–603

2. Collette L, Sylvester RJ, Stenning SP et al. Impact of the treating institution on survival of patients with 'poor prognosis' metastatic nonseminoma. J Natl Cancer Inst 1999;92:839–846

3. Sonneveld DJ, Hoekstra HJ, van der Graaf WT et al. Improved long term survival of patients with metastatic nonseminomatous testicular germ cell carcinoma in relation to prognostic classification systems during the cisplatin era. Cancer 2001;91:1304–1315

4. Horwich A, Huddart R. Retroperitoneal lymph-node dissection after chemotherapy for germ-cell cancer in patients with elevated levels of serum tumor markers. Nat Clin Pract Urol 2006;3:2–3

5. Shahidi M, Norman AR, Dearnaley DP et al. Late recurrence in 1263 men with testicular germ cell tumors: multivariate analysis of risk factors and implications for management. Cancer 2002;95:520–530

6. Bower M, Newlands ES, Holden L et al. Treatment of men with metastatic non-seminomatous germ cell tumors with cyclical POMB/ACE chemotherapy. Ann Oncol 1997;8:477–483

7. Bhala N, Coleman JM, Radstone CR et al. The management and survival of patients with advanced germ cell tumorous: improving outcome in intermediate and poor prognosis pateints. Clin Oncol 2004;16:40–47

8. Dorff TB, Rupani R, Wei DT et al. POMB-ACE therapy for patients with International Germ Cell Cancer Collaborative Group (IGCCCG) poor risk germ cell tumors (GCT): the USC experience. J Clin Oncol 2006;24(suppl):18

9. Christian JA, Huddart RA, Norman A et al. Intensive induction chemotherapy with CBOP/BEP in patients with poor prognosis germ cell tumors. J Clin Oncol 2003;21:871–877

10. Kaye SB, Mead GM, Fossa S et al. Intensive induction-sequential chemotherapy with BOP/VIP-B compared with treatment with BEP/EP for poor prognosis metastatic nonseminomatous germ cell tumor: a randomized Medical Research Council/European Organization for Research and Treatment of Cancer study. J Clin Oncol 1998;16:692–701

11. Droz JP, Pico JL, Ghosn M et al. Preliminary results of a randomized trial comparing bleomycin, etoposide, cisplatin (BEP) and cyclophosphamide, doxorubicin, cisplatin/vinblastin, bleomycin (CISCA/VB) for patients with intermediate and poor risk metastatic non seminomatous germ cell tumors (NSGCT) (abstract 690). Proceedings of the ASCO Annual Meeting, 2001. ASCO, Alexandria, Virginia

12. Nichols CR, Catalano PJ, Crawford ED et al. Randomized comparison of cisplatin and etoposide and either bleomycin or ifosfamide in treatment of advanced disseminated germ cell tumors: an Eastern Cooperative Oncology Group, Southwest Oncology Group, and Cancer and Leukemia Group B study. J Clin Oncol 1998;16:1287–1293

13. de Wit R, Louwerens M, de Mulder PH et al. Management of intermediate-prognosis germ-cell cancer: results of a phase I/II study of Taxol-BEP. Int J Cancer 1999;83:831–833

14. Hinton S, Catalano P, Einhorn LH et al. Phase II study of paclitaxel plus gemcitabine in refractory germ cell tumors (E9897): a trial of the Eastern Cooperative Oncology Group. J Clin Oncol 2002;20:1859–1863

15. Pectasides D, Pectasides M, Farmakis D et al. Gemcitabine and oxaliplatin (GEMOX) in patients with cisplatin-refractory germ cell tumors: a phase II study. Ann Oncol 2004;15:493–497

16. Pectasides D, Pectasides M, Farmakis D et al. Oxaliplatin and irinotecan plus granulocyte-colony stimulating factor as third-line treatment in relapsed or cisplatin-refractory germ-cell tumor patients: a phase II study. Eur Urol 2004;46:216–221

17. Kollmannsberger C, Beyer J, Liersch R et al. Combination chemotherapy with gemcitabine plus oxaliplatin in patients with intensively pretreated or refractory germ cell cancer: a study of the German Testicular Cancer Study Group. J Clin Oncol 2004;22:108–114

18. Fossa SD, Stenning SP, Gerl A et al. Prognostic factors in patients progressing after cisplatin-based chemotherapy for malignant non-seminomatous germ cell tumors. Br J Cancer 1999. 80:1392–1399

19. Kondagunta GV, Bacik J, Donadio A et al. Combination of paclitaxel, ifosfamide, and cisplatin is an effective second-line therapy for patients with relapsed testicular germ cell tumors. J Clin Oncol 2005;23:6549–6555

20. Mead GM, Cullen MH, Huddart R et al. MRC Testicular Tumor Working Party. A phase II trial of TIP (paclitaxel, ifosfamide and cisplatin) given as second-line (post-BEP) salvage chemotherapy for patients with metastatic germ cell cancer: a medical research council trial. Br J Cancer 2005;93:178–184

21. Ronnen EA, Kondagunta GV, Bacik J et al. Incidence of late-relapse germ cell tumor and outcome to salvage chemotherapy. J Clin Oncol 2005;23:6999–7004

22. Nichols CR, Tricot G, Williams SD et al. Dose-intensive chemotherapy in refractory germ cell cancer – a phase I/II trial of high-dose carboplatin and etoposide with autologous bone marrow transplantation. J Clin Oncol 1989;7:932–939

23. Broun ER, Nichols CR, Kneebone P et al. Long-term outcome of patients with relapsed and refractory germ cell tumors treated with high-dose chemotherapy and autologous bone marrow rescue. Ann Intern Med 1992;117:124–128

24. Einhorn LH, Williams S, Abonour RH. Salvage chemotherapy with high dose carboplatin + etoposide (HDCE) and peripheral blood stem cell transplant (PBSCT) in patients with germ cell tumors (GCT). J Clin Oncol 2006;24(suppl):4549

25. Beyer J, Stenning S, Gerl A et al. High-dose chemotherapy as salvage treatment in germ cell tumors: a multivariate analysis of prognostic variables. J Clin Oncol 1996;14:2638–2645

26. Vaena DA, Abonour R, Einhorn LH et al. Long-term survival after high-dose salvage chemotherapy for germ cell malignancies with adverse prognostic variables. J Clin Oncol 2003;21:4100–4104

27. De Giorgi U, Demirer T, Wandt H. Solid Tumor Working Party of the European Group for Blood and Marrow Transplantation 2005. Second-line high-dose chemotherapy in patients with mediastinal and retroperitoneal primary non-seminomatous germ cell tumors: the EBMT experience. Ann Oncol 2005;1:146–151

28. Beyer J, Stenning S, Gerl A et al. High-dose versus conventional-dose chemotherapy as first-salvage treatment in patients with non-seminomatous germ-cell tumors: a matched-pair analysis. Ann Oncol 2002;4:599–605

29. Pico JL, Rosti G, Kramar A, Genito-Urinary Group of the French Federation of Cancer Centers (GETUG-FNCLCC), France; European Group for Blood and Marrow Transplantation (EBMT) et al. A randomized trial of high-dose chemotherapy in the salvage treatment of patients failing first-line platinum chemotherapy for advanced germ cell tumors. Ann Oncol 2005;16:1152–1159

30. Lorch O, Rick JT, Hartmann C et al, for the German Testicular Cancer Study Group. Single versus sequential high-dose chemotherapy (HDCT) in patients with relapsed or refractory germ-cell tumors (GCT). J Clin Oncol 2006 2(suppl):4511

31. Rick O, Bokemeyer C, Beyer J et al. Salvage treatment with paclitaxel, ifosfamide, and cisplatin plus high-dose carboplatin, etoposide, and thiotepa followed by autologous stem-cell rescue in patients with relapsed or refractory germ cell cancer J Clin Oncol 2001;19:81–88

32. Motzer RJ, Sheinfeld J, Mazumdar M et al. Paclitaxel, ifosfamide, and cisplatin second-line therapy for patients with relapsed testicular germ cell cancer. J Clin Oncol 2000;18(12):2413–2418

33. Lotz JP, Bui B, Gomez F et al, on the behalf of the Groupe d'Etudes des Tumeurs Uro-Genitales (GETUG). Sequential high-dose chemotherapy protocol for relapsed poor prognosis germ cell tumors combining two mobilization and cytoreductive treatments followed by three high-dose chemotherapy regimens supported by autologous stem cell transplantation. Results of the phase II multicentric TAXIF trial. Ann Oncol 2005;16:411–418

34. McNeish IA, Kanfer EJ, Haynes R et al. Paclitaxel-containing high-dose chemotherapy for relapsed or refractory testicular germ cell tumors. Br J Cancer 2004;90:1169–1175

35. Stevens MJ, Norman AR, Dearnaley DP et al. Prognostic significance of early serum tumor marker half-life in metastatic testicular teratoma. J Clin Oncol 1995;13:87–92

36. Mazumdar M, Bajorin DF, Bacik J et al. Predicting outcome to chemotherapy in patients with germ cell tumors: the value of the rate of decline of human chorionic gonadotropin and alpha-fetoprotein during therapy. J Clin Oncol 2001;19:2534–2541

37. Fizazi K, Culine S, Kramar A et al. Early predicted time to normalization of tumor markers predicts outcome in poor-prognosis nonseminomatous germ cell tumors. J Clin Oncol 2004;22:3868–3876

38. Droz JP, Pico JL, Ghosn M et al. A phase II trial of early intensive chemotherapy with autologous bone marrow transplantation in the treatment of poor prognosis non seminomatous germ cell tumors. Bull Cancer 1992;79:497–507

39. Chevreau C, Droz, Pico JL et al. Early intensified chemotherapy with autologous bone marrow transplantation in first line treatment of poor risk non-seminomatous germ cell tumors. Preliminary results of a French randomized trial. Eur Urol 1993;23:213–217

40. Nichols CR, Williams SD, Loehrer PJ et al. Randomized study of cisplatin dose intensity in poor-risk germ cell tumors: a Southeastern Cancer Study Group and Southwest Oncology Group protocol. J Clin Oncol 1991;9:1163–1172

41. Morris MJ, Bosl GJ. High-dose chemotherapy as primary treatment for poor-risk germ-cell tumors: the Memorial Sloan-Kettering experience (1988–1999). Int J Cancer 1999;83:834–838

42. Schmoll HJ, Kollmannsberger C, Metzner B, German Testicular Cancer Study Group et al. Long-term results of first-line sequential high-dose etoposide, ifosfamide, and cisplatin chemotherapy plus autologous stem cell support for patients with advanced metastatic germ cell cancer: an extended phase I/II study of the German Testicular Cancer Study Group. J Clin Oncol 2003;21:4083–4091

43. Bajorin DF, Nichols CR, Margolin KA et al. Phase III trial of conventional-dose chemotherapy alone or with high-dose chemotherapy for metastatic germ cell tumors (GCT) patients (PTS): a cooperative group trial by Memorial Sloan-Kettering Cancer Center, ECOG, SWOG, and CALGB. J Clin Oncol 2006;24(suppl):4510

44. El-Helw L, Coleman RE. Salvage, dose intense and high-dose chemotherapy for the treatment of poor prognosis or recurrent germ cell tumors. Cancer Treat Rev 2005;3:197–209

45. Germa-Lluch JR, Garcia del Muro X, Tabernero JM et al. BOMP/EPI intensive alternating chemotherapy for IGCCC poor-prognosis germ-cell tumors: the Spanish Germ-Cell Cancer Group experience. Ann Oncol 1999;10:289–293

46. Decatris MP, Wilkinson PM, Welch RS et al. High-dose chemotherapy and autologous hemopoietic support in poor-risk seminomatous germ-cell tumors: an effective first-line therapy with minimal non-toxicity. Ann Oncol 2000;11:427–434

47. Fizazi K, Prow DM, Do KA et al. Alternating dose-dense chemotherapy in patients with high volume disseminated non-seminomatous germ cell tumors. Br J Cancer 2002;86:1555–1560

48. Fossa SD, Paluchowska B, Horwich A et al. Intensive induction chemotherapy with C-BOP/BEP for intermediate- and poor-risk metastatic germ cell tumors (EORTC trial 30948). Br J Cancer 2005;93:1209–1214

49. Flechon A, Biron P, Droz JP et al High-dose chemotherapy with hematopoietic stem-cell support in germ-cell tumor patient treatment: the French experience. Int J Cancer 1999;83:844–847

Primary immunodeficiency diseases

Paul Veys and H Bobby Gaspar

Introduction

Primary immunodeficiency (PID) diseases arise from intrinsic defects within lymphocytic or phagocytic cell lineages. Replacement of the defective lineage by hematopoietic stem cell transplantation (HSCT) remains the curative approach for most patients.

The first successful cases of transplantation for PID were reported in 1968: Gatti et al[1] described correction of severe combined immune deficiency (SCID), and Bach et al[2] described partial correction of Wiskott–Aldrich syndrome (WAS), using bone marrow from human leukocyte antigen (HLA)-matched sibling donors (MSD). Over three decades later, 30 different types of PID have now been corrected by SCT in more than 3500 patients.

Increased awareness of PID and availability of genetic testing have led to earlier diagnosis of PID, improving the clinical condition of patients approaching SCT. For those patients without matched family donors alternative HLA-identical donors have been obtained from molecular typing of volunteer unrelated donors (9 million worldwide) and cord blood banks (300,000 worldwide), while improved cell processing has facilitated the use of haploidentical-related donors in SCID. Reduced-intensity conditioning (RIC) has lowered transplant-related mortality (TRM) in patients with significant co-morbidities, and polymerase chain reaction (PCR)-based diagnostic tools coupled with improved antimicrobial therapies have reduced infectious complications in the peritransplant period. Taken together, these advances have led to dramatic improvements in the outcome of SCT for PID over recent years.

Newer therapies including enzyme replacement, gene transfer into autologous T-cells or stem cells, and transplantation of thymic tissue may provide an alternative approach to SCT in specific immune deficiencies; these latter approaches may be particularly advantageous when no closely matched allogeneic donor can be found.

Diseases

PID may be broadly divided into SCID and non-SCID immunodeficiencies. SCID can be further characterized by functional and genetic testing (Table 15.1); outcome of SCT in SCID may vary according to subtype, and alternative therapies are now available for certain SCID subtypes (see Alternative therapies, below). Non-SCID can be further subdivided into T-cell deficiencies, CD40 ligand deficiency, WAS, X-linked lymphoproliferative disorder (XLP), phagocytic cell disorders, hemophagocytic syndromes and autoimmune/immune dysregulatory disorders (Table 15.2).

Severe combined immune deficiency

The overall frequency of SCID is around 1 in 75,000 live births. The four main SCID syndromes are shown in Table 15.1 and represent inherited defects in T-cell ± B and NK cell differentiation leading to the absence or inactivity of the corresponding mature cells. Over the past two decades, striking progress has been made in defining the genetic mutations that cause the different forms of SCID, and the functional syndromes can now be further subdivided by their genetic basis (see Table 15.1).

Clinically, most patients present by age 3 months with unusually severe and frequent common infections or with opportunistic infections, often accompanied by one or more of diarrhea, dermatitis, and failure to thrive. SCID is an immunologic emergency because survival depends on expeditious stem cell reconstitution, and in the absence of successful SCT most children die in the first year or two of life from overwhelming infection.

It is recognized that as many of 50% of SCID patients are engrafted with maternal T-cells, but in most instances these cells do not initiate graft-versus-host disease (GvHD)[3] although on occasion they can lead to a severe disease distinguishable but pathologically similar to Omenn syndrome (see below). They may also contribute to graft rejection,[4] and it has therefore been suggested that in the setting of haploidentical SCT, the maternal donor is preferable if a conditioning cannot be used pretransplant. Transfusion-associated GvHD, on the other hand, is frequently lethal in SCID and any patient with a possible diagnosis of SCID should receive irradiated blood products.

Bacille Calmette–Guerin (BCG) vaccination can give rise to disseminated BCG-osis in SCID patients[5] and should be avoided at birth if there is any suspicion of immunodeficiency; frequently, symptoms and signs of BCG-osis appear for the first time or worsen with T-cell reconstitution, and temporary immunosuppression may be required alongside antituberculous therapy.

Matched sibling donor SCT for SCID

Since the first successful report of correction of SCID by MSD transplantation,[1] results have gradually improved such that, since 1985, the cure rate has exceeded 80%,[6] and is probably now in excess of 90%. Somewhat remarkably, sibling donor bone marrow (BM) may be infused into SCID recipients without the requirement for conditioning or GvHD prophylaxis. Severe GvHD occurs in less than 10% of cases,[7] presumably due to the young age of donor and recipient and the absence of tissue injury related to conditioning regimens. This would imply that the temporal improvements in outcome for SCID

Table 15.1 Classification of primary immunodeficiency: SCID

Functional	Genetic
T– B– NK–	ADA deficiency (AR) Reticular dysgenesis (XL or AR)
T– B– NK+	RAG deficiency (AR) SCID with Artemis (AR)
T– B+ NK–	γ deficiency (XL) Jak 3 kinase deficiency (AR)
T– B+ NK+	IL-7 Rα deficiency
Unspecified	
Other	

Table 15.2 Classification of primary immunodeficiency: non-SCID

T cell immunodeficiency/SCID variants
- CD4 lymphopenia
- Zap 70 kinase deficiency
- MHC class II deficiency
- PNP deficiency
- Omenn's syndrome
- Severe DiGeorge complex (22q 11del)
- CID with skeletal dysplasia
- Cartilage hair hypoplasia
- Other

C40 ligand deficiency (hyper-IGM syndrome)

WASP deficiency

XLP(Purtilo's syndrome)

Hemophagocytic syndromes
- Immunodeficiency with partial albinism
- Familial HLH
- Griscelli disease (partial albinism)
- Chediak–Higashi syndrome (CHS)

Phagocytic cell disorders
- Schwachman's syndrome
- Granule deficiency
- LAD
- X-linked CGD
- Kostmann disease
- AR-CGD
- IFN-γ receptor deficiency

Autoimmunune/immune dyregulatory disorders
- ALPS (fas deficiency)
- IPEX syndrome

probably reflect earlier diagnosis of SCID plus improved infection prophylaxis, surveillance, and treatment.

Infusion of sibling BM leads to the rapid development of T- and B-cell function post SCT, although usually only T-cells of donor origin develop, and myeloid and erythroid cells remain of recipient origin. While less than 50% of recipients become chimeric for donor B-cells, the donor-derived T-cells are able to co-operate with host-derived B-cells[8,9] and generate specific antibody production; some investigators have suggested that this co-operation might be facilitated by microchimerism of donor B-cells.[10] Only a minority (<10%) of SCID patients who undergo MSD SCT require supplementation with intravenous immunoglobulin in the long term.

Other matched family and unrelated donor SCT for SCID

Successes have also been reported with phenotypically matched related as well as unrelated donors.[6,11–13] In comparison to genotypically identical sibling donors, phenotypically matched related and unrelated transplants have a non-significant trend to reduced overall survival (81%, 72%, 63%, respectively)[6] (Fig. 15.1).

Unrelated donors have been variably defined as 'matched' using a combination of low- and/or high-resolution tissue typing techniques and measuring 6–10 HLA antigens; a single HLA antigen mismatch may be acceptable provided the marrow is T-cell depleted.[11] The risk of rejection/GvHD is considered too high for simple infusion of phenotypically matched marrow into SCID patients, so conditioning/GvHD prophylaxis is generally recommended. However, it may be that related/unrelated donors matched for extended haplotypes with up to 12 allelic loci (HLA, B, C, DRB1, DQB1, DPB1) could be treated in the same manner as sibling donors.

A significant issue with the use of unrelated donors in SCID is the necessary time involved in searching and acquiring the donor; this invariably prolongs the interval from diagnosis to SCT, although, in the current era of improved infection prophylaxis and treatment, it is not known whether this delay is detrimental to outcome. In a multivariate analysis, only age >12 months at the time of SCT and the lack of Septrin prophylaxis had a significant impact on survival of HLA-identical SCT.[6]

HLA-mismatched family donor for SCID

Prior to the development of unrelated donor banks, only approximately 20–30% of SCID patients had a healthy HLA-identical related donor available. Virtually all children have a haploidentical parental donor and as soon as T-cell depletion methods became available, HLA partially compatible SCT was proposed as an alternative to fetal liver transplantation which had only limited success.[14] In 1983 Reisner and co-workers successfully transplanted three patients with SCID with haplotype-disparate parental bone marrow depleted of T-cells by a combination of soyabean agglutination and sheep erythrocyte rosetting.[15] Durable lymphoid engraftment was achieved without pretransplant cytoreduction or post-transplant GvHD prophylaxis. With the introduction of peripheral blood progenitor cells (PBPCs) as a preferred stem cell source, most centers now employ CD34+ cell selection[16] or a large-scale CD3/CD19– depletion method[17] to achieve a 4–5 log T-cell depletion and a threshold of $1–5 \times 10^4$/kg CD3+ cells, below which GvHD prophylaxis is not required.[18] These improved depletion methods have, in turn, improved the outcome of haploidentical SCT in SCID, specifically by reducing the amount of GvHD, and in the largest cohort of patients treated by transplantation reported to date, survival rates which had been lower than with HLA-identical SCT (77% vs 54%; p = 0.02) were approaching 80% in the time cohort 1996–1999[6] (see Fig. 15.1).

In this European study, B– SCID had a poorer prognosis than B+ SCID, confirming a previous observation.[19] The reason for this appears to be multifactorial including lower engraftment rates in B– SCID, possibly caused by residual NK activity, a higher rate of severe post-SCT complications, and poorer long-term T- and B-cell reconstitution.[19,20] Within the B– SCID group, outcome may vary with genetic subtype. For instance, B– SCID characterized by increased cell sensitivity to radiation secondary to mutations of the DCLRE1C (Artemis) gene could carry a poorer prognosis because of defective repair of DNA breaks occurring in the peritransplant period from the damaging effects of chemotherapy, infection and GvHD.[20] For patients with ADA deficiency and reticular dysgenesis, survival rates were significantly worse with HLA-mismatched as compared to HLA-matched transplantation (29% vs 81%, and 29% vs 75%, respectively).

Use of conditioning

The use of myeloablative conditioning had a positive effect on survival in the B–SCID group, but not with the other SCID groups.[6]

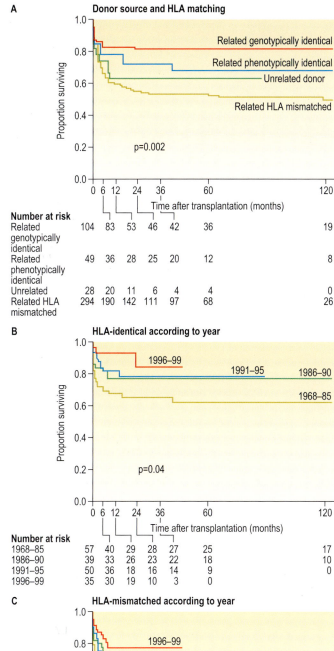

A   Donor source and HLA matching

Related genotypically identical
Related phenotypically identical
Unrelated donor
Related HLA mismatched

p=0.002

Time after transplantation (months)

Number at risk	0	6	12	24	36	42	60		120
Related genotypically identical	104	83	53	46	42		36		19
Related phenotypically identical	49	36	28	25	20		12		8
Unrelated	28	20	11	6	4		4		0
Related HLA mismatched	294	190	142	111	97		68		26

B   HLA-identical according to year

1996–99
1991–95
1986–90
1968–85

p=0.04

Time after transplantation (months)

Number at risk	0	6	12	24	36	60	120
1968–85	57	40	29	28	27	25	17
1986–90	39	33	26	23	22	18	10
1991–95	50	36	18	16	14	9	0
1996–99	35	30	19	10	3	0	

C   HLA-mismatched according to year

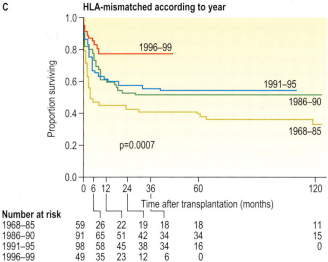

1996–99
1991–95
1986–90
1968–85

p=0.0007

Time after transplantation (months)

Number at risk	0	6	12	24	36	60	120
1968–85	59	26	22	19	18	18	11
1986–90	91	65	51	42	34	34	15
1991–95	98	58	45	38	34	16	0
1996–99	49	35	23	12	6	0	

Figure 15.1
Cumulative probability of survival in SCID patients, according to donor source (related or unrelated donor) and HLA-matching and year of transplantation. Reproduced with permission from Antoine et al 2003.[6]

However, the use of conditioning prior to haploidentical SCT in SCID remains controversial; Buckley[21] reported 81% survival among 89 patients with SCID who underwent haploidentical SCT without conditioning. SCID patients under 3 months of age had a likelihood of survival above 95%, probably as a combination of relative absence of infections prior to SCT and faster T-cell regeneration;[22] this group may be particularly suitable for unconditioned T-cell depleted haploidentical infusions. On the other hand, absence of conditioning may lead to delayed T-cell reconstitution and lack of B-cell (and myeloid) engraftment in up to 75% of cases, requiring ongoing intravenous immunoglobulin (IVIG) replacement.[20,21] Conversely, B-cell engraftment is secured in 75% of conditioned SCID patients.[23]

Immune reconstitution

The functional T-cells detected early after unmanipulated HLA-matched SCT are likely to have expanded from the mature T-cells transferred with the marrow inoculum. The kinetics of T- and B-lymphocyte function are much slower in recipients of T-depleted HLA-incompatible marrow.[24] Full T- and B-lymphocyte mediated responses were present only at day 505 compared to day 186 in recipients of HLA-identical transplants. This reflects the time taken for migration of donor lymphoid precursors to the thymus, maturation of thymic architecture and function, and subsequent differentiation of donor lymphocytes within the host environment. As evidence for thymic education, in patients with selective engraftment of donor T-cells (frequently seen after infusion of T-cell depleted haplotype-matched grafts), donor T-cells exhibit 'autoreativity' specific for donor MHC class II molecules.[25] This is probably caused by the lack of donor-derived MHC class II expressing dendritic cells in the host thymus, resulting in a lack of negative selection. The slow recovery of T-cell function after haploidentical SCT places patients at significant risk of viral, fungal and other opportunist infections;[26] the use of low-dose donor lymphocyte infusions (DLI) from haploidentical donors was not shown to improve immune reconstitution,[27] and is frequently associated with severe GvHD.[28]

Several groups have explored the possibility of returning DLI selectively depleted of alloreactive T-cells responsible for GvHD, by deleting T-cells that are activated in response to recipient antigen-presenting cells.[29,30] An alternative strategy might involve the use of genetically modified donor lymphocytes transduced with a herpes simplex virus thymidine kinase (HSV-TK) 'suicide' gene to allow their selective elimination by activating the prodrug ganciclovir, in the event of serious GvHD.[31,32]

T-cell output from the thymus declines with time in patients transplanted for SCID, with the number of recent thymic emigrants, as measured by T-cell receptor excision circles (TRECs), reducing to zero after 14 years.[33] Some of these patients require a second SCT procedure for problems related to recurrent immunodeficiency. The mechanism of this T-cell exhaustion is not fully understood but appears to be more common in those patients who do not have pluripotent hematopoietic stem cell engraftment as evidenced by lack of donor myeloid cells; premature thymus involution may therefore occur if the thymus is not provided with a supply of 'progenitor cells' from the bone marrow. Recent work has suggested that a 'plateau' of TRECs is reached within 2 years after haploidentical SCT. The onset of the plateau is determined by the age of the child, and the level of the plateau (which may determine the longevity of T-cell function) is increased by higher graft cell dose, and reduced by the occurrence of GvHD (P Schlegel, personal communication, 2006). It may be reasonable to consider SCID patients with poor T-cell recovery for a top-up procedure at this 2-year stage, before thymic involution and T cell exhaustion occur.

Table 15.3 Potential advantages and disadvantages of different types of stem cell donor

Donor	Availability	Access (re-access)	Cost	Rejection risk	Engraftment	GvHD risk	Immune reconstitution
Unrelated bone marrow	10/10 = 50% >9/10 = 80% ethnic minority =20%	Slow (possible)	High	Low	Moderate	Moderate	Moderate
Unrelated cord blood	>5/6Ags = 45% >4/6AgS = 90%	Fast (no)	Moderate	High	Slow	Low	Slow
Haploidentical family	>90%	Immediate (yes)	Low	Moderate	Fast	Low	Very slow

Unrelated cord blood transplantation for SCID

There are now in excess of 250,000 cord blood units stored worldwide.[34] There are some theoretical advantages for the use of cord blood stem cells for SCID: rapid availability (8 days to identify and request,[35] as with haplotype-matched parental donors, but no requirement for T-cell depletion; less risk of GvHD compared to adult unrelated donor;[36] no medical risk to the donor; and a greater proliferative lifespan which might be particularly important in such young recipients. There are also some specific disadvantages including: slower engraftment;[37] lack of viral specific cytotoxic T-cells; and lack of availability of the donor for a boost SCT. Of the 20 SCID patients who have undergone cord blood transplant (CBT) reported in the literature and reviewed recently,[38] three received cord blood cells from matched sibling donors, nine received cells from 6/6 HLA-matched unrelated cord blood donors, and four underwent 5/6, two 4/6, and two 3/6 HLA mismatched cord blood transplants. Four patients (20%) died, all of whom had pre-existing problems (one parainfluenza pneumonitis, one maternofetal engraftment, two chronic lung disease). One death was associated with significant GvHD. All surviving 16 patients (80%) had immune reconstitution including B-cell reconstitution.

CBT is in its relative infancy and outcomes are likely to improve with new techniques including expansion of cord blood progenitors[39] or the combination of multiple cords to increase cell dose[40] +/− the addition of mesenchymal stem cells to alleviate single-donor predominance,[41] co-transplantation of umbilical cord blood (UCB) and haploidentical family donors to shorten neutropenia,[42] and intraosseous infusion of cord blood to improve seeding efficiency.

Summary of SCT for SCID

In summary, in the absence of a matched sibling donor, and without the availability of gene therapy protocols for specific SCID types (see below), haplotype-mismatched and closely matched unrelated BM and CB may be appropriate alternative stem cell sources for SCID patients with equivalent outcomes. Choice will depend somewhat on preference and expertise of individual units as well as the clinical condition of the patient. Some of the advantages and disadvantages of each stem cell source are summarized in Table 15.3.

Non-severe combined immune deficiency

The major difference with non-SCID patients in comparison to SCID patients is the usual requirement for a conditioning regimen to achieve engraftment.[43] Omenn's syndrome may be an exception to this rule. There is now general consensus that the combination of busulfan 16–20 mg/kg with cyclophosphamide 200 mg/kg is the conditioning of choice for patients with non-SCID immunodeficiency treated by HLA-identical transplant.[44] There is large interpatient variability in busulfan exposure, particularly in young children receiving oral busulfan,[45] and therapeutic drug monitoring (TDM) may be required to target the

fairly narrow therapeutic index (AUC 900–1500 micromol/min). An alternative approach is to use iv busulfan on a bodyweight-based strategy which does not require TDM (G Vassal 2006, personal communication). A further option may be to replace busulfan with a structural analog of busulfan named treosulphan, which is similarly immuno- and myelosuppressive, but does not cause hepatic veno-occlusive disease (VOD).[46] Twenty-two children with genetic diseases, including six with non-SCID immunodeficiencies, have been transplanted with treosulphan 12–14 g/m² combined with fludarabine or cyclophosphamide. Despite significant co-morbidities, survival was as high as 90%.

Significant co-morbidities have been a frequent feature in non-SCID immunodeficiencies, which may then be exacerbated by myeloablative SCT. This is because the immunodeficiency is less pronounced than in SCID, and since these diseases are compatible with life for several years, ongoing infection with intracellular organisms gives rise to gradual but significant organ dysfunction. Early diagnosis of these disorders should permit allogeneic SCT as soon as possible and increase the chance of cure; indeed, in a European survey looking at all non-SCID immunodeficiencies, transplants performed before 2 years of age gave a 70% success rate versus 48% over 4 years of age.[47]

Among 444 non-SCID patients reported to the SCETIDE register in Europe,[6] survival was significantly better after HLA-matched than after HLA-mismatched SCT. Three-year survival after genotypically HLA-matched, phenotypically HLA-matched, HLA-mismatched related or unrelated donor transplantation was 71%, 42%, 42% and 59%, repectively (p = 0.0006) (Fig. 15.2). There was no difference in survival between genotypically HLA-identical and unrelated donor transplantation and so, unlike the situation in SCID patients, closely matched unrelated donors are preferable to HLA-mismatched related donors for non-SCID patients. Similarly, unrelated CB donors appear to give promising results in non-SCID immunodeficiency, with 29/32 (91%) patients surviving CBT matched for 4–6/6 HLA antigens.[38] By contrast with SCID, there has been no evidence of improvement in survival in non-SCID patients since 1985, whatever the donor origin or the HLA compatibility.[6] One approach to improving outcome in these patients, particularly those who have established organ dysfunction, may be to avoid myeloablative conditioning altogether by utilizing reduced-intensity conditioning prior to SCT.

Non-myeloablative SCT

Many children with PID have significant co-morbidities at the time of SCT, and conventional myeloablative preparation may be associated with significant treatment-related toxicity as well as long-term sequelae. Recent reports have suggested that non-myeloablative (NM) SCT may be a suitable alternative to achieve stable engraftment of immunocompetent donor cells with reduced procedure-related morbidity and mortality. Conventional SCT prevents rejection by the use of supralethal chemotherapy to remove host-versus-graft (HvG) reaction and create marrow space, often achieving full donor chimerism in the early months post SCT. NM-SCT prevents rejection by the use

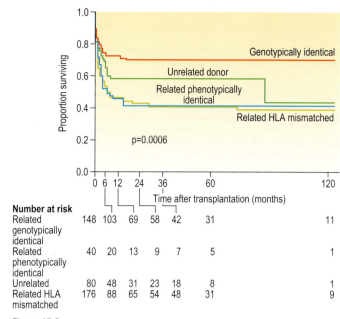

Figure 15.2
Cumulative probability of survival in non-SCID patients according to donor source (related or unrelated donor) and HLA matching. Reproduced with permission from Antoine et al 2003.[6]

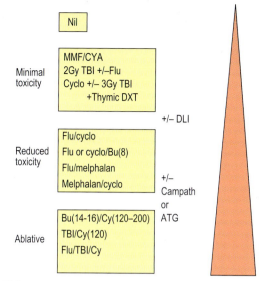

Figure 15.3
A hierarchy of conditioning intensity.

of pre ± post SCT immunosuppression to achieve tolerance, and a graft-versus-marrow (GvM) reaction to create space. In this setting, stable mixed chimerism is often achieved, which may be converted to full donor chimerism, if required, by tailing immunosuppression or DLI. Unlike the situation in malignant disease, stable mixed chimerism is usually sufficient to cure genetic disease.

Two general approaches have been used to develop NM-SCT regimens.[48] Regimens with 'reduced toxicity' (Fig. 15.3) have been developed by replacing myeloablative agents with more immunosuppressive and less myelosuppressive properties.[49,50] Such protocols have been used successfully in 7/8 patients with SCID/non-SCID immunodeficiencies surviving 8–17 months after transplant,[51] 7/10 patients with CGD surviving 16–26 months,[52] 9/12 patients with hemophagocytic lymphohistiocytosis (HLH)[53] surviving 5–61 months post SCT, and a variety of genetic diseases, including immunodeficiency, where patients achieved stable donor engraftment with low rates of regimen-related toxicity.[54]

There are no prospective studies comparing NM-SCT to conventional SCT in primary immunodeficiencies, although Rao[55] reported equivalent immune reconstitution and improved overall survival with RIC-SCT 31/33 (94%) compared to myeloablative SCT 10/19 (53%) in consecutive cohorts of patients. However, there were also problems associated with reduced-intensity SCT in immunodeficiency including high levels of viral reactivation,[56] particularly EBV,[57] and low-level donor chimerism following matched family donor SCT,[56] where the GvM effect may be reduced.

Secondly, regimens with 'minimal toxicity' (see Fig. 15.3) developed initially in animal models have used irradiation to induce a degree of immunosuppression pretransplant, followed by post-transplant immunosuppression given to control residual host, as well as newly infused donor, alloreactive T-cells.[58] By definition, the 'minimal toxicity' procedures have been associated with less toxicity than 'reduced toxicity' SCTs, but as the former rely solely on a GvH reaction to make marrow space, there is a suggestion that these procedures

are associated with an increased incidence of GvHD, particularly c-GvHD, especially with the use of unrelated donors. Four out of six patients with immunodeficiency survived with stable donor chimerism for 9–39 months after minimal toxicity SCT.[48] New minimal toxicity protocols are being developed where chemotherapeutic reagents are being replaced by monoclonal antibodies directed at hematopoietic cells such as anti-CD33 (Mylotarg), anti-CD45, anti-CD66 either naked or conjugated to toxins or radio-isotopes.

Studies to date indicate that NM-SCT may have an important role in treating primary immunodeficiency. Unlike more standard approaches, such regimens can be used without severe toxicity in patients with opportunist infections or severe pulmonary or hepatic disease. NM-SCT also offers the advantage that long-term sequelae such as infertility or growth retardation may be avoided or reduced. It is likely that NM-SCT will become the 'first step' towards establishing donor engraftment in children with immunodeficiency. Second infusions of donor stem cells, DLI or a second myeloablative transplant may be required in some patients with low-level donor chimerism or graft rejection.

Wiskott–Aldrich Syndrome (WAS)

WAS is an X-linked disorder with an incidence of 4 per million live male births, characterized by thrombocytopenia with small platelets, eczema, and progressive immunodeficiency.[59,60,61] The disorder is caused by mutations in the WASP gene at Xp11.22.[62] The gene encodes for a cytoplasmic protein, primarily expressed in hematopoietic cells, which is involved in the regulation of cytoskeletal reorganization.

Without SCT, WAS patients have a poor prognosis, with the major causes of death being infection, bleeding and lymphoproliferative disease (LPD). Splenectomy usually increases the platelet count and reduces the risk of significant hemorrhage, but the risk of death from sepsis is increased.[63] In 1968, Bach and associates[2] reported partial

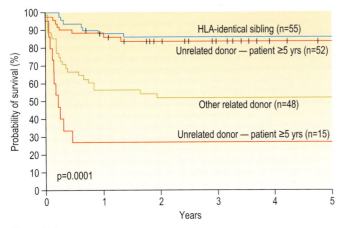

Figure 15.4
Probabilities of survival for 170 patients receiving bone marrow transplants for WAS by donor type and age. There was not a significant difference in the risk of mortality after HLA-matched sibling transplants and after unrelated donor transplants in children younger than 5 years. Significantly worse survival was associated with use of related donors other than HLA-identical siblings, regardless of recipient age, and with use of unrelated donors in patients over 5 years of age. Reproduced with permission from Filipovich et al 2001.[6]

Table 15.4 Three-year survival in non-SCID patients, according to primary disease and donor–recipient compatibility. Reproduced with permission from Antoine et al 2003[6]

Disorder	Genotypically identical		Related HLA-mismatched	
	n	% survival (95% CI)	n	% survival (95% CI)
Plagocytic cell disorders	23	70 (49–91)	14	69 (44–95)
Wiskott–Aldrich syndrome	32	81 (67–94)	43	45 (30–60)*
Hemophagocytic syndrome	32	68 (48–87)	28	49 (39–67)
T-cell deficiency	47	63 (50–77)	72	35 (24–46)

*p < 0.001 for difference between genotypically identical and related, mismatched transplants.

correction of WAS following high-dose cyclophosphamide and MSD BMT. Myeloid engraftment was not achieved and the patient remained thrombocytopenic. Full correction was achieved in 1978 by Parkman and colleagues[64] using myeloablative conditioning. A worldwide review from 1968 through to 1995 reported long-term survival in 57/65 (88%) children with WAS undergoing MSD BMT,[65] and HLA-matched sibling grafts administered after myeloablative conditioning remain the treatment of choice for this disorder. In the absence of a matched related donor, impressive results have been reported from the International Bone Marrow Transplant Registry, with 71% of patients surviving after matched unrelated donor (UD) SCT.[66] Prognosis appeared much better when SCT was performed below the age of 5 years (89% cure versus 30%), with significant problems from GvHD in older children (Fig. 15.4). Good results have also been reported with unrelated CBT, with 80% survival among 15 children with WAS.[67] For patients who lack an HLA-identical donor, therapeutic options are limited. Results from haplotyped-mismatched related donors are significantly poorer than from related identical donors (45% vs 81% survival;[6] 52% vs 87% survival[66]) with failures due to graft rejection, EBV-LPD and GvHD. Splenectomy, if appropriate, and supportive care may be the preferred approach until alternative therapies (for example, gene therapy) become available.

All aspects of WAS are corrected by SCT if the patient remains a full donor chimera. If only donor T-cell chimerism is achieved, then thrombocytopenia may persist or return in the absence of donor myeloid engraftment. Thrombocytopenia may then respond to splenectomy, but there is concern that autoimmune problems may return or persist in such patients.

T-cell immunodeficiency

In the SCETIDE European study,[6] there was a tendency to poorer outcome for T-cell deficiencies, after both matched and mismatched related donors (63% and 35%) (Table 15.4).

HLA class II (MHC II) deficiency

MHC II deficiency patients seem to carry a particularly poor prognosis; in a summary of 23 patients who underwent BMT for MHC II deficiency in Europe up to 1996, disease-free survival was 40% for HLA-matched transplants (n = 9), but only 20% from HLA-mis-

matched transplants (n = 14).[68–70] Of the eight patients who remained well post SCT, all had persistently low CD4+ T-lymphocytes consistent with impaired thymic maturation caused by defective HLA class II expression on thymic epithelia, making the patients particularly susceptible to ongoing opportunist infection. In a study from the United Kingdom,[71] only 2/10 children were still alive despite eight attempts at SCT in six patients. Overwhelming viral infection was the predominant cause of death. Alternative transplant strategies or novel therapies are required for these patients.

Omenn syndrome (OS)

OS is characterized by SCID typically associated with the triad of erythroderma, hepatosplenomegaly, and lymphadenopathy.[72] There is a marked eosinophilia and a variable number of autologous, activated, and oligoclonal T-lymphocytes that infiltrate target organs and are generally poorly responsive to mitogens.[73,74] Villa[75] showed that OS is usually caused by hypomorphic mutations in the recombination activating gene (RAG) that result in residual protein expression and function. Cavadini[76] then demonstrated that patients with OS have defective thymic expression of AIRE, a transcription factor that controls expression of tissue-specific peptides by thymic medullary epithelial cells. This defect is likely to result in defective negative selection of autoreactive T-cells in OS that can therefore expand in the periphery in response to autoantigens.

Experience with SCT in OS has been mixed. Gomez[77] reported a 66.7% overall survival in a single center using matched related donors; a lower success rate of 16.7% has been reported in another study using mainly mismatched related and matched unrelated donors.[78] A more recent study examining the use of alternative donor SCT in a single center reported 11 OS patients undergoing altogether 15 SCT procedures (haploidentical n = 7, MUD n = 4, related phenoidentical n = 3, related genoidentical n = 1).[79] Nine out of 11 were alive and immunoreconstituted 30–146 months after SCT. The overall mortality in this study was lower than previously reported; this was due to early recognition of OS and rapid initiation of adequate supportive treatment, with topical/systemic immune suppression with steroids and/or ciclosporin, to control immune dysreactivity before proceeding to SCT.

CD40 ligand deficiency (X-linked hyper-IgM syndrome)

CD40 ligand deficiency is a rare X-linked T-cell immunodeficiency caused by mutations in the gene encoding CD40 ligand glycoprotein (CD154) expressed on the surface of activated T-lymphocytes.[80,81] CD40 ligand interacts with CD40 on B-lymphocytes, monocyte/macrophages and epithelial cells.[82] This interaction is critical in initiating immunoglobulin isotype class switching from IgM to IgG, IgA and IgE in B-cells, and for monocyte/macrophage activation. Patients present with *Pneumocystis carinii* pneumonia or recurrent bacterial sinopulmonary infection leading to bronchiectasis. Particular susceptibility to gastrointestinal infection with protozoa such as *Cryptosporidium parvum* may lead to sclerosing cholangitis, cirrhosis, and cholangiocarcinoma.[83] Without SCT, about 50% of patients survive to the fourth decade.[84] The largest SCT series reported 38 patients from eight European countries between 1993 and 2000.[85] Donor stem cell source included 14 HLA-identical siblings, 22 unrelated donors, and two phenotypically matched parental donors. SCT cured 58% of the patients, 72% of those without hepatic disease; 32% died from infection-related complications, with severe cryptosporidiosis in six. Pre-existing lung damage was the most important adverse risk factor. In this study, three patients underwent elective orthotopic hepatic transplantation prior to SCT because of pre-existing cirrhosis and hepatic failure.

X-linked lymphoproliferative syndrome (XLP)

XLP is a rare immunodeficiency caused by mutations in the signaling lymphocyte activating molecule (SLAM)-associated protein (SAP)/SH2D1A gene[86] and characterized by a dysregulated immune response to EBV and other pathogens. The clinical presentation is heterogeneous and includes fulminant infectious mononucleosis, hemophagocytic lymphohistiocytosis, lymphoma, hypogammaglobulinemia and aplastic anemia.

Although heterogeneous in their initial presentation, XLP patients usually die before the age of 20 without intervention by allogeneic SCT.[87] Since the first report of SCT for XLP in 1986,[88] 14 cases have been published in the literature.[89] Stem cell donors included MSD (n = 7), matched sibling CB (n = 1), MUD (n = 4) and unrelated CB (n = 1). Overall survival was 71% (10/14), and was significantly better for chemotherapy-only conditioning regimens versus TBI-based regimens (8/9 vs 1/5), although this probably reflects older age of the TBI group (19.4 versus 4.7 yrs), who had therefore acquired more infections and organ toxicity. It is logical to use EBV-positive donors for these patients, and if T-cell depletion is required for the SCT procedure, careful monitoring of the EBV viral load by EBV-specific RQ-PCR is advisable. The generation and use of EBV-specific cytotoxic T-lymphocytes (CTLs) may be beneficial,[90] as well as depletion of donor/recipient B-lymphocytes by the administration of rituximab.[91]

Phagocytic cell disorders

Kostmann syndrome

Severe congenital neutropenia (CN) (Kostmann syndrome) is a hematologic disorder characterized by a maturation arrest of myelopoiesis at the promyelocyte/myelocyte stage of development.[92,93] This arrest results in severe neutropenia leading to absolute neutrophil counts (ANC) below 0.2×10^9/l associated with severe bacterial infections from early infancy. The availability of recombinant human granulocyte colony-stimulating factor (r-HuG-CSF) in 1987 dramatically changed the prognosis and quality of life of patients with CN[94] (see Alternative therapies, below). More than 90% of CN patients respond to r-HuG-CSF with an increase in ANC > 1.0×10^9/l, and require fewer antibiotics and reduced hospitalization.[95]

All CN patients, regardless of their treatment or response to granulocyte colony-stimulating factor (G-CSF), are at risk of developing myelodysplasia (MDS) or acute myeloid leukemia (AML), but the risks of malignant transformation and septic death appear higher in less responsive patients: after 10 years, 40% of the less responsive patients developed MDS/AML and 14% died of sepsis, compared with 11% and 4%, respectively, of more responsive patients. Consequently, in less responsive CN patients, early SCT may be a rational option.

Zeidler and colleagues[96] reported on 11 patients who underwent SCT for reasons other than malignant transformation. Eight were primary non-responders, one was prior to the availability of G-CSF, and two had a G-CSF receptor mutation which is thought to be one step in the pathway to leukemic transformation.[97] All eight patients who received BM from a MSD are alive, although one rejected the graft but developed r-HuG-CSF responsive neutropenia; only 1/3 undergoing mismatched SCT survive with ongoing extensive chronic GvHD. SCT from an HLA-identical donor is therefore beneficial for CN patients refractory to r-HuG-CSF. However, the results after UD SCT remain more disappointing.[96,98,99] Outcome of transplantation after the development of frank leukemia in CN is poor; in one study only 3/18 patients who underwent SCT as treatment for leukemia survived.[96]

Leukocyte adhesion deficiency (LAD)

LAD is an autosomal recessive disorder characterized by impaired migration of neutrophils from the intravascular space,[100] due to partial or complete absence of B2 leukocyte integrins (CD11/CD18). Complete absence of CD11/CD18 leads to a severe phenotype of LAD which predisposes to severe bacterial infections, often leading to death within the first 5 years of life.[101]

Conventional myeloablative conditioning may not be sufficient to result in complete donor chimerism,[102] and addition of agents such as etoposide may be required in addition to busulfan and cyclophosphamide. Nevertheless, similarly good results have been achieved with genotypically identical and related HLA-mismatched donors (70% vs 69%). This is in contradiction to most other non-SCID patients in whom HLA-mismatched transplants tend to do less well. More immunosuppressive regimens may also be suitable for LAD; 3/3 patients are alive and fully engrafted after a RIC regimen including CAMPATH, fludarabine and melphalan.[103]

Interferon-gamma receptor (IFNγR1) deficiency

IFNγR1 deficiency is an autosomal recessive disorder with a very poor prognosis.[104,105] Only 20% of patients survive until the age of 12 years due to severe organ damage from poorly virulent mycobacteria (e.g. *M. avium* complex subspecies). Mutations in the IFNγR1 gene lead to lack of expression or function of surface-expressed IFN-γ receptor, which results in lack of activation of macrophages upon exposure to IFN-γ secreted by antigen-specific T-cells. Consequently, symptoms are attributed to profound decrease in tumor necrosis factor alpha (TNF-α) production, intracellular killing of pathogens, and granuloma formation.[106]

Roesler[107] reported on eight patients with IFNγR1 deficiency who received altogether 11 SCTs from family donors, including 10 using HLA-identical sibling and non-sibling donors and one HLA-haploidentical transplant. Four patients died within 8 months of SCT, two deaths directly related to IFNγR1 deficiency. Among the survivors, donor cell engraftment was absent or very low in two, and only two patients were cured with full remission of mycobacterial illness, 5 years post SCT. The latter two cases were the only ones who were transplanted with a non-T-cell depleted graft from an HLA-identical sibling following a fully myeloablative regimen.

Shwachman–Diamond syndrome (SDS)

SDS is a rare autosomal recessive disease of infancy, first described by Shwachman et al[108] with an incidence of 1 : 70–80,000 children.[109] Clinically, SDS is characterized by exocrine pancreatic insufficiency, metaphyseal dysostosis, growth retardation and/or short stature and bone marrow dysfunction. Recently, the causative gene has been identified on chromosome 7 and its function, although still unclear, seems to be related to RNA processing and metabolism.[110]

In patients with SDS, the main causes of death are infection and hemorrhage associated with development of various hematologic abnormalities including neutropenia, aplasia, and MDS/AML.[111] Apart from supportive measures (transfusion, pancreatic enzymes, G-CSF, and antibiotics), SCT represents the only worthwhile treatment once severe marrow aplasia or MDS/AML has developed. Cesaro et al[112] reported the outcome of SCT in 26 patients with SDS and severe bone marrow abnormalities. Twenty (77%) had a graft from an unrelated or family mismatched donor. Nine patients died after a median time of 70 days post SCT. After a median follow-up of 1.1 years, the transplant-related mortality was 35.5%, while the overall survival was 64.5%. The bone marrow cells of SDS patients have shown an abnormal susceptibility to Fas-mediated apoptosis that may expose such patients to major organ toxicity and infections secondary to their conditioning.[109] In this study, most of the fatalities were due to organ toxicity and infection, while the impact of GvHD was limited. For this reason, SDS patients might be more suited to a reduced-intensity conditioning regimen, particularly those with aplasia without cytogenetic/clonal abnormalities.

Chronic granulomatous disease (CGD)

CGD is an inherited disorder of phagocyte function, characterized by recurrent, often life-threatening bacterial and fungal infections and by granuloma formation in vital organs. Neutrophils, monocytes/macrophages, and eosinophils cannot generate microbicidal oxygen metabolites owing to a defect in one of the four subunits of the NADPH oxidase of phagocytes. Despite prophylactic treatment with co-trimoxazole, itraconazole and/or interferon gamma, there is an annual mortality of between 2% (autosomal recessive CGD (AR-CGD)) and 5% (X-linked CGD (X-CGD)),[114] with one-quarter of the deaths due to invasive aspergillosis.

Uncomplicated CGD in not an indication for SCT, but SCT is generally considered for X-CGD or AR-CGD patients who have an HLA-genoidentical donor and one or more of the following complications: non-availability of specialist medical care; non-compliance with long-term antimicrobial prophylaxis; at least one life-threatening infection; severe granulomatous disease with progressive organ dysfunction (e.g. lung restriction); steroid-dependent granulomatous disease (e.g. colitis); ongoing therapy-refractory infection (e.g. aspergillosis) (R Seger, personal communication, 2005).

Between 1985 and 2000, 27 patients underwent SCT for CGD complicated as above, in 14 co-operating European centers.[115] Most transplants were children (n = 25) who received a myeloablative busulfan-based regimen (n = 23), and had unmodified marrow allografts (n = 23) from HLA-identical sibling donors. Twenty-three of 27 survived, with 22/23 cured of CGD. Survival was especially good in patients without infection at the time of SCT (18/18). SCT during active infection was sometimes complicated by severe inflammatory reactions at the infected site at the time of neutrophil engraftment, and severe skin GvHD resembling Lyell disease – the pathogenesis of both of these reactions was thought to be mediated by raised levels of TNF-α.

Horwitz et al[116] used non-myeloablative conditioning followed by T-cell depleted PBPCs from HLA-identical siblings in five children and five adults with CGD. All patients then received graduated donor lymphocyte infusions, and after a median follow-up of 17 months 8/10 patients had donor neutrophil engraftment ranging from 33% to 100%. Graft failure occurred in two patients, and three patients died of graft failure, pneumococcal pneumonia and GvHD respectively. Gungor and colleagues[117] reported a successful outcome in three high-risk

adults with CGD and severe disease-related complications, using HLA-identical related/unrelated donors and a reduced-intensity conditioning with fludarabine, busulfan 8 mg/kg and antithymocyte globulin (ATG).

In conclusion, myeloablative SCT, if performed at the first signs of a severe course of the disease, is a valid theraputic option for children with CGD having an HLA-genoidentical donor. The use of unrelated donors and reduced-intensity conditioning awaits further evaluation.

Hemophagocytic syndromes

Familial hemophagocytic lymphohistiocytosis (FHL)

FHL is a genetically determined autosomal recessive disorder characterized by the early onset of fever and hepatosplenomegaly, associated with pancytopenia, hypertriglyceridemia, and hypofibrinogenemia, and hemophagocytosis in the bone marrow.[118–120] In addition, central nervous system (CNS) involvement may be severe and cause permanent CNS dysfunction. The pathogenesis of FHL has been associated with the impairment of the cytotoxic pathway in lymphocytes, where uncontrolled activation of T-lymphocytes results in raised levels of inflammatory cytokines.[121] Mutations within the perforin (PRF1) gene[122] account for 30% of cases, while mutations of MUNC13–4[123] account for perhaps another 30%. The incidence is around 1:50,000 live births and is fatal without adequate treatment, including SCT.

Initial therapy consists of either cycles of etoposide, dexamethasone and ciclosporin A (CsA) (HLH94)[124] or ATG, steroids and CsA,[125] with intrathecal methotrexate for CNS disease, and followed by SCT from the best available donor. Horne[126] examined the outcome in 86 patients treated initially with HLH94 followed by SCT conditioned mostly with VP16, busulfan and cyclophosphamide between 1995 and 2000. The overall estimated 3-year survival post SCT was 64%: matched-related donor 71%; matched unrelated donor 70%; familial haploidentical donor 54%; and mismatched unrelated donor 54%. The odds ratios for mortality were 2.75 for those with active disease after 2 months of therapy compared with inactive disease, and 1.8 for children with active as opposed to inactive disease at the time of SCT. Veno-occlusive disease is the major toxicity associated with transplants in HLH[127] and because donor lymphocyte chimerism >20% is associated with sustained remission, reduced-intensity conditioning (RIC) may be an alternative approach for FHL, with one report showing 8/11 children surviving after largely unrelated/haploidentical SCT following RIC conditioning.[53]

Chediak–Higashi syndrome (CHS)

CHS is a rare autosomal recessive syndrome characterized by oculocutaneous albinism, recurrent infections, microscopic finding of large granules in hematopoietic and other cells, neurologic abnormalities and bleeding diathesis.[128–130] Pathologic mutations in the lysosomal trafficking regulator gene (LYST) localized to human chromosome 1q42-q43 are responsible for the development of CHS.[131] Neutropenia and defects in natural killer cell activity, T-cell cytotoxicity, chemotaxis and bactericidal killing by granulocytes and monocytes result in increased susceptibility to infection. In survivors of infectious complications, an accelerated phase, manifested by life-threatening hemophagocytosis, occurs within the first or second decade.

Thirty-four children with CHS underwent SCT and were reported to the IBMTR (C Delatt, personal communication). Twenty had a history of a life-threatening accelerated phase prior to SCT, nine were in accelerated phase at transplantation. 79%, 67% and 30% survived after HLA-identical, unrelated donor and mismatched related donor SCT respectively, suggesting that SCT is effective therapy for the accelerated phase of CHS. However, progressive neurologic dysfunction, similar to that described in non-transplanted adults with a mild clinical course, has been reported in long-term survivors of SCT for CHS who had neither recurrent infections nor manifestations of hemophagocytic syndrome after SCT.[132] This suggests a steady long-term progression, despite SCT, of the lysosomal defect in neurones and glial cells, and may question the appropriateness of SCT in non-accelerated CHS.

Griscelli's syndrome (GS)

GS is a rare autosomal recessive disorder that associates hypopigmentation, characterized by a striking silver-gray sheen of the hair and the presence of large clusters of pigment in the hair shaft on electron microscopy, and the occurrence of either a primary neurologic impairment or a severe immune disorder.[133] Patients who have mutations of the myosin Va gene (GS1) have severe primary neurologic impairment,[134] whereas those with RAB27A gene mutations (GS2) suffer from immunodeficiency and hemophagocytic lymphohistiocytosis.[135] SCT prevents relapse of HLH in GS2 patients, and, as in other HLH patients, mixed chimerism is sufficient to achieve disease control.[136]

Other non-SCID immunodeficiencies

SCT has been shown to correct the autoimmune syndromes associated with autoimmune lymphoproliferative syndrome (ALPS) due to Fas deficiency[137] and X-linked immune dysregulation, associated with polyendocrinopathy and enteropathy (IPEX)[138] due to a deficiency of regulatory T-cells.

Alternative therapies

Growth factors

Alternative treatments to SCT have been developed for specific immunodeficiency conditions over the last two decades. For instance, severe congenital neutropenia is effectively treated by regular subcutaneous injections of G-SCF but long-term use of G-CSF may be associated with an increased risk of developing myelodysplasia and AML in specific subgroups of patients.[139,140] The prognosis of CGD has also been profoundly altered by the prophylactic use of antibiotics and possibly by the use of interferon-gamma therapy, though the latter is associated with side-effects such as fever.[141,142]

Enzyme replacement

Enzyme replacement has been used in the treatment of adenosine deaminase (ADA) deficiency since 1987.[143] Purified bovine ADA is conjugated with polyethylene glycol to decrease clearance of the compound. PEG-ADA is administered weekly or twice weekly by intramuscular injection and leads to rapid metabolic correction with normalization of dATP levels and normalization of plasma ADA activity which is then followed by cellular and humoral immune reconstitution. The extent of immune recovery is variable and although many children recover full immunity in the short term, a significant number (~50%) remain on immunoglobulin replacement.[144] Over a longer time period, patients show a decline in T-cell numbers and remain lymphopenic.[145] Despite this, follow-up suggests that patients remain clinically well and free of infection with normal growth parameters.

Gene therapy

Possibly the greatest advance has been the development of stem cell gene therapy for the treatment of defined genetic defects. The first human condition for which gene therapy has shown unequivocal benefit is X-linked severe combined immunodeficiency. Using retroviral mediated transfer of the IL-2RG gene into autologous CD34+ cells, successful reconstitution of cellular and humoral immunity has been demonstrated in the majority of patients treated in two trials in Paris and London.[146,147] Since gene transduced cells have a significant survival advantage, this procedure can be undertaken without prior cytoreductive therapy, and thus the short-term morbidity of the procedure is low.

A number of gene therapy trials for ADA deficiency were initiated in the early 1990s. Trials in the US and Europe used retroviral mediated gene transfer of the ADA gene into different autologous cellular fractions (peripheral blood lymphocytes, umbilical cord blood, bone marrow and CD34+ selected stem cells).[148-151] In all of these studies, PEG-ADA was continued in addition to gene therapy and the effect of gene therapy alone on correction of the immune parameters is not proven. More recently, two studies have shown gene therapy to be efficacious in correcting ADA deficiency.[152,153] The process appears to be more successful if PEG-ADA is withdrawn prior to gene therapy to allow a selective advantage to gene-transduced cells. Furthermore, a mild non-myeloablative conditioning regimen was used to allow engraftment of a greater number of gene-modified cells. In two patients with X-CGD, a similar retroviral vector-based protocol using a non-myeloablative conditioning regimen prior to the return of gene-transduced autologous cells showed substantial gene transfer into neutrophils, leading to a large number of functionally corrected phagocytes and notable clinical improvement.[153]

These gene therapy studies show clearly that gene transfer into autologous stem cells can result in functional immune correction. However, side-effects related to insertion of the retroviral vector into a proto-oncogene (LMO2) have resulted in the development of T-cell leukemia in three of 10 patients treated in one X-SCID gene therapy study.[154] The exact reasons for oncogenesis are yet to be determined and may be related to the nature of retroviral vector insertion or expression of the IL-2RG transgene itself. Modifications to vector design are in progress and may overcome the problems associated with these initial trials. It is likely that gene therapy studies for other immunodeficiencies (e.g. WAS) will be initiated in the coming years.

Thymic transplant

In severe forms of congenital thymic hypoplasia (e.g. severe DiGeorge and CHARGE syndrome), the profound abnormalities of T-cell development can only be treated by allogeneic HSCT from a matched family donor. SCT from other donor sources does not successfully allow tolerized T-cell development from stem cells due to the lack of a thymus, and T-cell engraftment from mismatched post-thymic donor cells runs the risk of severe GvHD. For these individuals, the only option is transplantation of allogeneic thymic organ cultures, which has resulted in successful development of functional autologous T-cells.[155,156] In these studies, thymic organ culture generated from tissue removed from neonates undergoing congenital cardiac surgery is cultured and implanted into peripheral muscle where it forms a thymic organ capable of supporting function thymopoiesis.

In utero transplant

Availability of prenatal diagnosis for several primary immunodeficiencies offers the option of in utero treatment.[157,158] The reported experience is limited, but suggests that at least in B+ forms of SCID, transplantation of haploidentical CD34+ stem cells in utero can result in functional T-cell recovery.[159] Given the wide variety of successful options available for treatment postnatally, it is likely that in utero HSCT will be reserved for exceptional cases.

Summary

There have been significant advances in both SCT and non-transplant strategies for PID over the last decade. In some diseases there are now a number of curative approaches using different conditioning protocols, different types of stem cell donor and stem cell source, as well as gene therapy protocols. There are probably too few patients to perform prospective randomized studies, and although immediate outcomes appear to be equivalent, longer term follow-up may reveal differences in the quality and longevity of immune reconstitution as well as the occurrence of late effects.

References

1. Gatti RA, Meuwissen HJ, Allen HD et al. Immunological reconstitution of sex linked lymphogenic immunological deficiency. Lancet 1968;ii:1366–1369
2. Bach FH, Albertini RJ, Anderson JL et al. Bone marrow transplantation in a patient with the Wiskott-Aldrich syndrome. Lancet 1968;ii:1364–1366
3. Pollack MS, Kirkpartick D, Kapoor N et al. Identification by HLA typing of intrauterine-derived maternal T cells in four patients with severe combined immunodeficiency. N Engl J Med 1982;307:662–666
4. Haddad E, Le Deist F, Aucouturier P et al. Long term chimerism and B cell function after bone marrow transplantation in patients with severe combined immunodeficiency with B cells: a single-centre study of 22 patients. Blood 1999;94:2923–2930
5. Heydermann RS, Morgan G, Levinsky RJ et al. Successful bone marrow transplantation and treatment of BCG infection in two patients with severe combined immunodeficiency. Eur J Pediatr 1991;150:477–480
6. Antoine C, Muller S, Cant A et al. Long- term survival and hematopoietic stem cell transplantation for immunodeficiencies: a survey of the European experience 1968–1999. Lancet 2003;361:553–560
7. Fisher A, Landais P, Friedrich W et al. European experience of bone marrow transplantation for SCID. Lancet 1990;ii:850–854
8. Fisher A, Griscelli C, Friedrich W et al. Bone marrow transplantation for immunodeficiencies and osteoporosis. A European survey, 1968–1985. Lancet 1986;ii:2:1080–1084
9. Buckley RH, Schiff SE, Schiff RI et al. Haploidentical bone marrow stem cell transplantation in human severe combined immune deficiency. Semin Hematol 1993;30:92–104
10. White H, Thrasher A, Veys P et al. Intrinsic defects of B cell function in X-linked severe combined immunodeficiency. Eur J Immunol 2000;30:732–737
11. Ash RC, Casper JT, Chitambar CR et al. Successful allogenic transplantation of T cell depleted bone marrow from closely HLA matched unrelated donors. N Engl J Med 1990;322:485–495
12. Filipovich AH, Shapiro RS, Ramsay NK et al. Unrelated donor bone marrow transplantation for correction of lethal congenital immunodeficiencies. Blood 1992;80:270–276
13. Dalal I, Reid B, Doyle J et al. Matched unrelated bone marrow transplantation for combined immunodeficiency. Bone Marrow Transplant 2000;25:613–621
14. O' Reilly RJ, Pollock MS, Kapoor N et al. Fetal liver transplantation in man and animals. In: Gale RP (ed) Recent advances in bone marrow transplantation. Alan R Liss, New York, 1989, 789–830
15. Reisner Y, Kapoor N, Kirkpatrick D et al. Transplantation for severe combined immunodeficiency with HLA-A,B,D,DR incompatible parental marrow cells fractionated by soybean agglutinin and sheep red blood cells. Blood 1983;61:341–348
16. Schumm M, Lang P, Taylor G et al. Isolation of highly purified autologous and allogeneic peripheral CD34+ cells using the CliniMACS device. J Hematother 1999;8:209–218
17. Handgretinger R, Leimig T, Babarin-Dorner A et al. The potential role of graft engineering strategies in haploidentical stem cell transplantation. Bone Marrow Transplant 2002;30:S11
18. Reisner Y, Martelli MF. Tolerance induction by 'megadose' transplants of CD34+ stem cells: a new option for leukemia patients without an HLA-matched donor. Curr Opin Immunol 2000;12:536–541
19. Bertrand Y, Landais P, Friedrich W et al. Influence of severe combined immunodeficiency phenotype on the outcome of HLA non-identical, t cell depleted bone marrow transplantation: a retrospective European survey from the European group for bone marrow transplantation and the European Society for Immunodeficiency. J Pediatr 1999;134:740–748
20. Haddad E, Landais P, Friedrich W et al. Long term immunological reconstitution and outcome after HLA-non-identical T-cell depleted BMT for SCID: An European retrospective study of 116 patients. Blood 1998;91(10):3646–3653
21. Buckley RH, Schiff SE, Schiff RI et al. Hematopoietic stem-cell transplantation for the treatment of severe combined immunodeficiency. N Engl J Med 1999;18(340):508–516
22. Myers LA, Patel DD, Puck JM et al. Hematopoietic stem cell transplantation for severe combined immunodeficiency in the neonatal period leads to superior thymic output and improved survival. Blood 2002;99:878–878
23. Brady KA, Cowan MJ, Leavitt AD. Circulating red cells usually remain of host origin after bone marrow transplantation for severe combined immunodeficiency. Transfusion 1996;36:314–317
24. Wijnaendts L, Le Deist F, Griscelli C et al. Development of immunological functions after BMT in 33 patients with SCID. Blood 1989;74:2212–2219
25. De Villartay JP, Griscelli C, Fisher RA. Self tolerance to host and donor following HLA mismatched BMT. Eur J Immunol 1986;19:323–329
26. Kook H, Goldman F, Padley D et al. Reconstruction of the immune system after unrelated or partially matched T-cell-depleted bone marrow transplantation in children: immunophenotypic analysis and factors affecting the speed of recovery. Blood 1996;88:1089–1097
27. Eyrich M, Lang P, Lal S et al. A prospective analysis of the pattern of immune reconstitution in a paediatric cohort following transplantation of positively selected human leukocyte antigen-disparate hematopoietic stem cells from parental donors. Br J Haematol 2001;114:422–432
28. Aversa F, Tabilio A, Velardi A et al. Treatment of high-risk acute leukemia with T-cell-depleted stem cells from related donors with one fully mismatched HLA haplotype. N Engl J Med 1998;339:1186–1193
29. Andre-Schmutz I, Le Deist F, Hacein-Bey-Abina S et al. Immune reconstitution without graft-versus-host disease after hemopoietic stem-cell transplantation: a phase 1/2 study. Lancet 2002;360:130–137
30. Amrolia PJ, Muccioli-Casadei G, Huls H et al. Adoptive immunotherapy with allodepleted donor T-cells improves immune reconstitution after haploidentical stem cell transplant. Blood 2006;108(6):1797–1808
31. Bonini C, Ferrari G, Verzeletti S et al. HSV-RK gene transfer into donor lymphocytes for control of allogeneic graft-versus-leukemia. Science 1997;276:1719–1724
32. Tiberghien P, Ferrand C, Lioure B et al. Administration of herpes simplex-thymidine kinase-expressing donor T cells with a T-cell-depleted allogeneic marrow graft. Blood 2001;97:63–72
33. Patel DD, Gooding ME, Parrott RA et al. Thymic function after hematopoietic stem cell transplantation for the treatment of severe combined immunodeficiency. N Engl J Med 2000;342:1325–1332
34. Gluckman E, Koegler G, Rocha V. Human leukocyte antigen matching in cord blood transplantation. Semin Hematol 2005;42:85–90
35. Bhattacharya A, Slatter MA, Chapman CE et al. Single centre experience of umbilical cord stem cell transplantation for primary immunodeficiency. Bone Marrow Transplant 2005;36:1–5
36. Rocha V, John MD, Wagner JE Jr et al. Graft versus host disease in children who have received a cord blood or bone marrow transplant from an HLA identical sibling. N Engl J Med 2000;342:1846 -1854
37. Benito AI, Diaz MA, Gonzalez-Vicent M et al. Hematopoietic stem cell transplantation using umbilical cord blood progenitors: review of current clinical results.Bone Marrow Transplant 2004;33:675–690
38. Slatter MA, Gennery AR. Umbilical cord stem cell transplantation for primary immunodeficiencies. Expert Opin Biol Ther 2006;6:555–565
39. Shpall EJ, Quinones R, Giller R et al. Transplantation of ex vivo expanded cord blood. Biol. Blood Marrow Transplant 2002;8:368–376
40. Barker JN, Weisdorf DF, Defor TE et al. Transplantation of 2 partially HLA matched umbilical cord blood units to enhance engraftments in adults with hematologic malignancy. Blood 2005;105:1343–1347
41. Kim DW, Chung YJ, Kim TG et al. Cotransplantation of third party mesenchymal stromal cells can alleviate single donor predominance and increase engraftment from double cord transplantation. Blood 2004;103:1741–1948
42. Fernandez MN, Regidor C, Cabrera R et al. Unrelated umbilical cord blood transplants in adults: Early recovery of neutrophils by supportive co-transplantation of a low number of highly purified peripheral blood CD34+ cells from an HLA haploidentical donor. Exp Hematol 2003;31:535–544
43. O'Reilly RJ, Brochstein J, Dinsmore R et al. Marrow transplantation for congenital disorders. Semin Hematol 1989;21:188–225
44. Blazar DR, Ramsay MKC, Kersey JH et al. Pretransplant conditioning with Busulfan and Cyclophosphamide for non malignant diseases. Transplantation 1985;39:597–603
45. Vassal G, Fischer A, Challien D et al. Busulfan disposition below the age of 3: alteration in children with lysosomal storage disease. Blood 1993;82:1030–1034
46. Wachowiak J, Chybicka A, Kowalczyk J et al. Treosulphan based preparative regimen for allogeneic hematopoietic stem cell transplantation in children with increased risk of conventional regimen toxicity. Blood 2005;106:500a-501a
47. Fisher A, Landais P, Friedrich W et al. Bone marrow transplant (BMT) in Europe for primary immunodeficiencies other than severe combined immunodeficiency: a report from the European group for BMT and the European group for immunodeficiency. Blood 1994;83:1149–1154
48. Woolfrey A, Pulsipher MA, Storb R. Non-myeloablative hematopoietic cell transplant for treatment of immune deficiency. Curr Opin Pediatr 2001;13:539–545
49. Giralt S, Estey E, Albitar M et al. Engraftment of allogeneic hematopoietic progenitor cells with purine analog-containing chemotherapy: harnessing graft-versus-leukemia without myeloablative therapy. Blood 1997;89:4531–4536
50. Slavin S, Nagler A, Naparstek E et al. Nonmyeloablative stem cell transplantation and cell therapy as an alternative to conventional bone marrow transplantation with lethal cytoreduction for the treatment of malignant and nonmalignant hematologic diseases. Blood 1998;91:756–763
51. Amrolia P, Gaspar B, Hassan A et al. Non-myeloablative stem cell transplantation for congenital immunodeficiencies. Blood 2000;96:1239–1246
52. Horowitz ME, Barrett AJ, Brown MR et al Treatment of chronic granulomatous disease with nonmyeloablative conditioning and a T-cell-depleted hematopoietic allograft. N Engl J Med 2001;344:881–488
53. Cooper N, Rao K, Gilmour K et al. Stem cell transplantation with reduced intensity conditioning for hemophagocytic lymphohistiocytosis. Blood 2006;107:1233–1236
54. Resnick IB, Shapira MY, Slavin S. Nonmyeloablative stem cell transplantation and cell therapy for malignant and non-malignant diseases. Transplant Immunol 2005;14:207–219
55. Rao K, Amrolia PJ, Jones A et al. Improved survival after unrelated donor bone marrow transplant in children with primary immunodeficiency using a reduced intensity conditioning regimen. Blood 2005;105:879–885
56. Veys P, Rao K, Amrolia P. Stem cell transplantation for congenital immunodeficiencies using reduced-intensity conditioning. Bone Marrow Transplant 2005;35(suppl 1):S45–47
57. Cohen J, Rogers V, Gaspar HB et al. Increased incidence of EBV-related disease following paediatric stem cell transplantation with reduced-intensity conditioning. Br J Haematol 2005;129:229–239

58. Storb R, Yu C, Wagner JL et al. Stable mixed hematopoietic chimerism in DLA identical littermate dogs given sublethal total body irradiation before and pharmacological immunosuppression after marrow transplantation. Blood 1997;89:3048–3054

59. Wiskott A. Familiärer, angeborener Morbus Werlhoffi? Monatsschrift für Kinderheilkunde 1937;68:212–216

60. Aldrich RA, Steinberg AG, Campbell DC. Pedigree demonstrating a sex-linked recessive condition characterized by draining ears, eczematoid dermatitis and bloody diarrhoea. Pediatrics 1954;13:133–139

61. Peddy GS, Spector BD, Schuman LM et al. The Wiskott-Aldrich syndrome in the United States and Canada (1892–1979). J Pediatr 1980;97:72–78

62. Derry JM, Ochs HD, Franke U. Isolation of a novel gene mutated in Wiskott-Aldrich syndrome. Cell 1994;78:635–644

63. Lum LG, Tubergen DG, Corash L et al. Splenectomy in the management of the thrombocytopenia of the Wiskott-Aldrich Syndrome. N Engl J Med 1980;302:892–896

64. Parkman R, Rappeport J, Geha R et al. Complete correction of the Wiskott-Aldrich syndrome by allogeneic bone marrow transplantation. N Engl J Med 1978;208:921–927

65. Buckley RH. Bone marrow reconstitution in primary immunodeficiency. Clin Immunol Principles Pract 1995;2:1813–1830

66. Filipovich AH, Stone JV, Tomany SC et al. Impact on donor type on outcome of bone marrow transplantation for Wiskott-Aldrich syndrome: collaborative study of the International Bone Marrow Transplant Registry and National Marrow Donor Program. Blood 2001;97:1598–1603

67. Kobayashi R, Ariga T, Nonoyama S et al. Outcome in patients with Wiskott-Aldrich syndrome following stem cell transplantation: an analysis of 57 patients in Japan. Br J Haematol 2006;135(3):362–366

68. Elhasid R, Etzioni A. Major histocompatability complex class II deficiency: a clinical review. Blood Rev 1996;10:242–248

69. Griscelli C, Lisowska-Grospierre B, Mach B. Combined immunodeficiency with defective expression of MHC class II genes. Immunodef Rev 1989;1:135–153

70. Klieg C, Cavazzana-Calvo M, Le Deist F et al. Bone marrow transplantation in major histocompatability complex class II deficiency: a single centre study of 19 patients. Blood 1995;85:580–587

71. Saleem MA, Arkwright PD, Davies EG et al. Clinical course of patients with major histocompatibility complex class II deficiency. Arch Dis Child 2000;83:356–359

72. Omenn G. Familial reticuloendotheliosis with eosinophilia. N Engl J Med 1965;273:427–432

73. Villa A, Sobacchi C, Notarangelo LD et al. V(D)J recombination defects in lymphocytes due to RAG mutations: severe immunodeficiency with a spectrum of clinical presentations. Blood 2001;97:81–88

74. Rieux-Laucat F, Bahadoran P, Brousse N et al. Highly restricted human T cell repertoire in peripheral blood and tissue-infiltrating lymphocytes in Omenn's syndrome. J Clin Invest 1998;102:312–321

75. Villa A, Santagata S, Bozzi F et al. Partial V(D)J recombination activity leads to Omenn's syndrome. Cell 1998;93:885–896

76. Cavadini P, Vermi W, Facchetti F et al. AIRE deficiency in thymus of 2 patients with Omenn symdrome. J Clin Invest 2005;115:728–732

77. Gomez L, Le Deist F, Blanche S et al. Treatment of Omenn syndrome by bone marrow transplantation. J Pediatr 1995;127:76–81

78. Loechelt BJ, Shapiro RS, Jyonouchi H et al. Mismatched bone marrow transplantation for Omenn syndrome: a variant of severe combined immunodeficiency. Bone Marrow Transplant 1995;16:381–385

79. Mazzolari E, Moshous D, Forino C et al. Hematopoietic stem cell transplantation in Omenn syndrome: a single centre experience. Bone Marrow Transplant 2005;36:107–114

80. Korthauer U, Graf D, Mages HW et al. Defective expression of T cell CD 40 ligand caused x linked immunodeficiency with hyper IgM. Nature 1993;361:539–541

81. Disanto JP, Bonnefoy JY, Gauchat JF et al. CD40 Ligand mutations in x linked immunodeficiency with hyper-IgM. Nature 1993;361:541–543

82. Van Kooten C, Banchereau J. Functions of CD40 on B cells, dendritic cells and other cells. Current Opin Immunol 1997;9:330–337

83. Heyward AR, Levy J, Facchetti F et al. Cholangiopathy and tumours of the pancreas, liver and bilary tree in boys with x linked immunodeficiency with hyper-IgM. J Immunol 1997;158:977–983

84. Toniati P, Savoldi G, Jones AM et al. Report of the ESID collaborative study on clinical features and molecular analysis of x linked hyper IgM syndrome (abstract). Eur Soc Immunodeficiencies Newsletter 2002;(supplement):F9:40

85. Gennery AR, Khawaja K, Veys P et al. Treatment of CD40 ligand deficiency by hematopoietic stem cell transplantation: a survey of the European experience, 1993–2002. Blood 2004;103:1152–1157

86. Sayos J, Wu C, Morra M et al. The X linked lymphoproliferative disease gene product SAP regulates signals through the co-receptor SLAM. Nature 1998;395:462–469

87. Seemayer TA, Gross TG, Egeler RM et al. X linked lymphoproliferative disease: twenty five years after the discovery. Pediatric Res 1995;38:471–478

88. Filipovich AH, Blazar BR, Ramsay NK et al. Allogeneic bone marrow transplantation for X linked lymphoproliferative syndrome. Transplantation 1986;42:222–224

89. Lankester AC, Visser LFA, Hartwig NG et al. Allogeneic stem cell transplantation in X linked lymphoproliferative disease: two cases in one family and review of the literature. Bone Marrow Transplant 2005;36:99–105

90. Rooney CM, Smith CA, Ng CY et al. Infusion of cytotoxic T cells for the prevention and treatment of Epstein-Barr virus induced lymphoma in allogeneic transplant recipients. Blood 1998;92:1549–1555

91. Milone M, Tsai DE, Hodinka RL et al. Treatment of primary Epstein-Barr virus infection in patients with X linked lymphoproliferative disease using B cell directed therapy. Blood 2005;105:994–996

92. Kostmann R. Infantile genetic agranulocytosis. Acta Pediatr Scand 1956;5:1

93. Kostmann R. Infantile genetic agranulocytosis: a review with presentation of ten new cases. Acta Pediatr Scand 1975;64:362

94. Bonilla M, Gillio A, Ruggeiro M et al. Effects of recombinant human granulocyte colony-stimulating factor on neutropenia in patients with congenital agranulocytosis. N Engl J Med 1989;320:1574

95. Welte K, Gabrilove J, Bronchud MH et al. Filgrastim (r-metHuG-CSF): the first 10 years. Blood 1996;88:1907

96. Zeidler C, Welte K, Barak Y et al. Stem cell transplantation in patients with severe congenital neutropenia without evidence of leukemic transformation. Blood 2000;4:1195–1198

97. Welte K, Boxer L. Severe chronic neutropenia: pathophysiology and therapy. Semin Hematol 1997;34:267

98. Choi SW, Boxer LA, Pulsipher MA et al. Stem cell transplantation in patients with severe congenital neutropenia with evidence of leukemic transformation. Bone Marrow Transplant 2005;35:473–477

99. Ferry C, Quachee M, Leblanc T et al. Hematopoietic stem cell transplantation in severe congenital neutropenia: experience of the French SCN register. Bone Marrow Transplant 2005;35:40–50

100. Lekstrom-Himes JA, Gallin JI. Immunodeficiency diseases caused by defects in phagocytes. N Engl J Med 2000;343:1703–1714

101. Laksman R, Finn A. Neutrophil disorders and their management. J Clin Pathol 2001;54:7–19

102. Thomas C, Le Deist F, Cavazzana-Calvo M et al. Results of allogeneic bone marrow transplantation in patients with leukocyte adhesion deficiency. Blood 1995;86:1629–1635

103. Rao K, Amrolia PJ, Jones A et al. Improved survival after unrelated donor bone marrow transplantation in children with primary immunodeficiency using a reduced-intensity conditioning regimen. Blood 2005;105:879–885

104. Dupuis S, Doffinger R, Picard C et al. Human interferon-gamma-mediated immunity is a genetically controlled continuous trait that determines the outcome of mycobacterial invasion. Immunol Rev 2000;178:129–137

105. Jouanguy E, Altare F, Lamhamedi-Cherradi S et al. Infections in IFNGR-1-deficient children. J Interferon Cytokine Res 1997;17:583–587

106. Newport MK, Huxley CM, Huston S et al. A mutation in the interferon-gamma-receptor gene and susceptibility to mycobacterial infection. N Engl J Med 1996;335:1941–1949

107. Roesler J, Horwitz ME, Picard C et al. Hematopoietic stem cell transplantation for complete IFN-gamma receptor 1 deficiency: a multi-institutional survey. J Pediatr 2004;145:806–812

108. Shwachman H, Diamond LK, Oski FA et al. The syndrome of pancreatic insufficiency and bone marrow dysfunction. J Paediatr 1964;65:645–663

109. Dror Y, Freedman MH. Shwachman–Diamond syndrome. Br J Haematol 2002;118:701–703

110. Savchenko A, Krogan N, Cort JR et al. The Shwachman-Bodian-Diamond syndrome protein family is involved in RNA metabolism. J Biol Chem 2005;280:19213–19220

111. Smith OP, Hann IM, Chessells JM et al. Hematological abnormalities in Shwachman-Diamond syndrome. Br J Haematol 1996;94:279–284

112. Cesaro S, Oneto R, Messina C et al 2006. Hematopoietic stem cell transplantation for Shwachman-Diamond disease: a study from the European Group for blood and marrow transplantation. Br J Haematol 2005;131:231–236

113. Dror Y, Freedman MH. Shwachman-Diamond syndrome marrow cells show abnormally increased aptosis mediated through Fas pathway. Blood 2001;97:3011–3016

114. Winkelstein JA, Marino MC, Johnston RB et al. Chronic granulomatous disease: report on a national registry of 368 patients. Medicine 2000;79:155–169

115. Seger RA, Gungor T, Belohradsky BH et al. Treatment of chronic granulomatous disease with myeloablative conditioning and an unmodified hemopoietic allograft: a survey of the European experience, 1985–2000. Blood 2002;13:4344–4350

116. Horwitz ME, Barrett J, Brown MR et al. Treatment of chronic granulomatous disease with nonmyeloablative conditioning and a T-cell-depleted hematopoietic allograft. N Engl J Med 2001;344:881–888

117. Gungor T, Halter J, Klink A et al. Successful low toxicity hematopoietic stem cell transplantation for high-risk adult chronic granulomatous disease patients. Transplantation 2005;79:1596–1606

118. Loy TS, Diaz-Arias AA, Perry MC. Familial erythrophagocytic lymphohistiocytosis. Semin Oncol 1991;18:34–39

119. Henter J, Elinder G, Ost A. Diagnostic guidelines for hemophagocytic lymphohistiocytosis. The FHL study group of the Histiocyte Society. Semin Oncol 1991;18:29–33

120. Filipovich AH. Hemophagocytic lymphohistiocytosis: a lethal disorder of immune regulation. J Pediatr 1997;130:337–338

121. Arico M, Danesino C, Pende D, Moretta L. Pathogenesis of hemophagocytic lymphohistiocytosis. Br J Haematol 2001;114:761–769

122. Stepp SE, Dufourcq-Lagelouse R, Le Deist F et al. Perforin gene defects in familial hemophagocytic lymphohistiocytosis. Science 1999;286:1957–1959

123. Feldmann J, Callebaut I, Raposo G et al. Munc13–4 is essential for cytolytic granules fusion and is mutated in a form of familial hemophagocytic lymphohistiocytosis (FHL3). Cell 2003;115:461–473

124. Henter J, Samuelsson-Horne A, Arico A et al. Treament of hemophagocytic lymphohistiocytosis with HLH 94 immunochemotherapy and bone marrow transplantation. Blood 2002;100:2367–2373

125. Stefan JL, Donadieu J, Ledeist F et al. Treatment of familial hemophagocytic lymphohistiocytosis with antithymocyte globulins, steroids and cyclosporin A. Blood 1993;82:2319–2323

126. Horne AC, Janka G, Maarten Egeler R et al. Hematopoietic stem cell transplantation on hemophagocytic lymphohistiocytosis. Br J Haematol 2005;129:622–630

127. Ouachee-Chardin M, Elie C, de Saint Basile G et al. Hematopoietic stem cell transplantation in hemophagocytic lymphohistiocytosis: a single-center report of 48 patients. Pediatrics 2006;117:e743–750

128. Barak Y, Nir E. Chediak-Higashi syndrome. Am J Hematol/Oncol 1987;9:42–55

129. Pettit RE, Berdal KG. Chediak-Higashi syndrome. Neurologic appearance. Arch Neurol 1984;41:1001–1002

130. Grossi CE, Crist WM, Abo T et al. Expression of the Chediak-Higashi lysosomal abnormality in human peripheral blood lymphocytes subpopulations. Blood 1985;65:837–844

131. Certain S, Barrat F, Pastural E et al. Protein truncation test of LYST reveals heterogeneous mutations in patients with Chediak-Higashi Syndrome. Blood 2000;95:979–983

132. Tardieu M, Lacroix C, Navern B et al. Progressive neurologic dysfunctions 20 years after allogeneic bone marrow transplantation for Chediak-Higashi Syndrome. Blood 2005;106:40–42

133. Griscelli C, Durandy A, Guy-Grand D et al. A syndrome associating partial albinism and immunodeficiency. Am J Med 1978;65:691–702

134. Pastural E, Barrat FJ, Dufourcq-Lagelouse R et al. Griscelli disease maps to chromosome 15q21 and is associated with mutations in the myosin-Va gene. Nat Genet 1997;16:289–292

135. Ménasché G, Pastural E, Feldmann J et al. Mutations in RAB27A cause Griscelli syndrome associated with hemophagocytic syndrome. Nat Genet 2000;25:173–176

136. Trigg ME, Schugar R. Chediak-Higashi syndrome hematopoietic chimerism corrects genetic defect. Bone Marrow Transplant 2001;27:1211–1213

137. Benkerrou M, Le Deist F, de Villartay JP et al. Correction of Fas (CD95) deficiency by haploidentical bone marrow transplantation. Eur J Immunol 1997;8:2043–2047

138. Baud O, Goulet O, Canioni D et al. Treatment of the immune dysregulation, polyendocrinopathy, enteropathy, X linked syndrome (IPEX) by allogeneic bone marrow transplantation. N Engl J Med 2001;344:1758–1762

139. Dale DC, Bonilla MA., Davis MW et al. A randomized controlled phase III trial of recombinant human granulocyte colony-stimulating factor (filgrastim) for treatment of severe chronic neutropenia. Blood 1993;81:2496–2502

140. Rosenberg PS, Alter BP, Bolyard AA et al. The incidence of leukemia and mortality from sepsis in patients with severe congenital neutropenia receiving long-term G-CSF therapy. Blood 2006;107:4628–4635

141. Marciano BE, Wesley R, de Carlo ES et al. Long-term interferon-gamma therapy for patients with chronic granulomatous disease. Clin Infect Dis 2004;39:692–699

142. International Chronic Granulomatous Disease Cooperative Study Group. A controlled trial of interferon gamma to prevent infection in chronic granulomatous disease. N Engl J Med 1991;324:509–516

143. Hershfield MS, Buckley RH, Greenberg ML et al. Treatment of adenosine deaminase deficiency with polyethylene glycol-modified adenosine deaminase. N Engl J Med 1987;316:589–596

144. Hershfield MS. PEG-ADA replacement therapy for adenosine deaminase deficiency: an update after 8.5 years. Clin Immunol Immunopathol 1995;76:S228–232

145. Chan B, Wara D, Bastian J et al. Long-term efficacy of enzyme replacement therapy for adenosine deaminase (ADA)-deficient Severe Combined Immunodeficiency (SCID). Clin Immunol 2005;117:133–143

146. Hacein-Bey-Abina S, Le Deist F, Carlier F et al. Sustained correction of X-linked severe combined immunodeficiency by ex vivo gene therapy. N Engl J Med 2002;346:1185–1193

147. Gaspar HB, Parsley KL, Howe S et al.Gene therapy of X-linked severe combined immunodeficiency by use of a pseudotyped gammaretroviral vector. Lancet 2004;364:2181–2187

148. Blaese RM, Culver KW, Miller AD et al. T lymphocyte-directed gene therapy for ADA-SCID: initial trial results after 4 years. Science 1995;270:475–480

149. Bordignon C, Notarangelo LD, Nobili N et al. Gene therapy in peripheral blood lymphocytes and bone marrow for ADA-immunodeficient patients. Science 1995;270:470–475

150. Kohn DB, Weinberg KI, Nolta JA et al. Engraftment of gene-modified umbilical cord blood cells in neonates with adenosine deaminase deficiency. Nat Med 1995;1:1017–1023

151. Hoogerbrugge PM, van Beusechem VW, Fischer A et al. Bone marrow gene transfer in three patients with adenosine deaminase deficiency. Gene Ther 1996;3:179–183

152. Aiuti A, Slavin S, Aker M et al. Correction of ADA-SCID by stem cell gene therapy combined with nonmyeloablative conditioning. Science 2002;296:2410–2413

153. Ott MG, Schmidt M, Schwarzwaelder K et al. Correction of X-linked chronic granulomatous disease by gene therapy, augmented by insertional activation of MDS1-EVI1, PRDM16 or SETBP1. Nat Med 2006;12:401–409

154. Hacein-Bey-Abina S, von Kalle C, Schmidt M et al. LMO2-associated clonal T cell proliferation in two patients after gene therapy for SCID-X1. Science 2003;302:415–419

155. Markert .L, Boeck A, Hale LP et al. Transplantation of thymus tissue in complete DiGeorge syndrome. N Engl J Med 1999;341:1180–1189

156. Markert ML, Sarzotti M, Ozaki DA et al. Thymus transplantation in complete DiGeorge syndrome: immunologic and safety evaluations in 12 patients. Blood 2003;102:1121–1130

157. Flake AW, Roncarolo MG, Puck JM et al. Treatment of X-linked severe combined immunodeficiency by in utero transplantation of paternal bone marrow [see comments]. N Engl J Med 1996;335:1806–1810

158. Wengler GS, Lanfranchi A, Frusca T et al. In-utero transplantation of parental CD34 haematopoietic progenitor cells in a patient with X-linked severe combined immunodeficiency (SCIDXI). Lancet 1996;348:1484–1487

159. Pirovano S, Notarangelo LD, Malacarne F et al. Reconstitution of T-cell compartment after in utero stem cell transplantation: analysis of T-cell repertoire and thymic output. Haematologica 2004;89:450–461

Acquired aplastic anemia and Fanconi anemia

CHAPTER 16

Vikas Gupta and Judith Marsh

Introduction

Aplastic anemia (AA) has traditionally been defined as the presence of peripheral blood pancytopenia associated with a hypocellular bone marrow in the absence of (a) an abnormal infiltrate, (b) an increase in reticulin and (c) morphologic abnormalities in the remaining hemopoietic cells (apart from dyserythropoiesis which occurs commonly in AA). The term AA includes cases of acquired AA and a variety of inherited bone marrow failure syndromes as listed in Table 16.1.

Acquired aplastic anemia

Acquired AA is a rare disorder with an overall annual incidence of 1–2 cases per million population in the studies conducted in Europe and North America. In Asia, the incidence is 2–4 fold higher, which may be related to environmental and genetic factors.[1-3] Acquired AA shows a bimodal age distribution with most patients presenting between the ages of 15 to 25 years or after 60 years.[3,4] In most cases, AA is an immune-mediated disease and immune attack by activated T-cells leads to marrow failure (reviewed in ref 5).

Diagnosis

The complete diagnosis of acquired AA requires careful exclusion of other causes of pancytopenia and defining the disease in terms of (a) whether the disease is acquired or congenital, (b) etiology, (c) presence and size of co-existing abnormal clones, and (d) disease severity.

Confirming the diagnosis

The diagnosis of AA in most cases is straightforward, but other conditions can sometimes present with pancytopenia and a hypocellular bone marrow and mimic AA, particularly hypocellular myelodysplastic syndrome (MDS) (reviewed in ref 6). Good-quality blood and marrow slides, and a good length biopsy are essential. Repeat bone marrow examination and special investigations such as cytogenetics, clonogenic cell cultures and clonality studies may be helpful in some, but not in all cases.

Excluding inherited forms of AA

A high index of suspicion for inherited forms of AA should be maintained in pediatric patients and young adults. These include Fanconi anemia (FA), dyskeratosis congenita (DC) and, very rarely, Shwachman–Diamond syndrome. A detailed family history and a thorough physical examination may provide clues towards the congenital causes of AA. Genetic investigations may help in the correct diagnosis (see Table 16.1). The wider availability of genetic testing has helped in correct diagnosis of inherited bone marrow failure syndromes in an increasing number of patients, who by clinical criteria appear to have idiopathic AA and do not have any physical abnormalities on clinical examination.[7-11] A diagnosis of FA and DC not only avoids unnecessary treatment with immunosuppressive therapy and delay in bone marrow transplantation (BMT), but helps in selecting the appropriate conditioning regimen, should BMT be indicated. It also avoids using inappropriate conditioning which would otherwise lead to major morbidity or death.

Presence of associated abnormal clones

All patients should be screened for abnormal cytogenetic clones, which can be detected in approximately 10% of AA patients at the time of diagnosis, in the absence of morphologic features of MDS. It is a subject of controversy as to whether this represents AA or hypocellular MDS.[12] A study from the St George's Hospital demonstrated an abnormal clone in 12% of newly diagnosed adult patients with AA.[13] A trisomy (+6, +8 or +15) was the most common abnormality (60%) and the clone was usually small in size.[13] In patients with a trisomy as abnormal cytogenetic clone, response to immunosuppressive therapy (IST), durability of the response and risk of later clonal disorders were similar to those with a normal karyotype, whereas patients with non-numerical cytogenetic abnormalities responded poorly to IST. The presence of monosomy 7 should alert one to the likely diagnosis of MDS.

Larger multicenter studies are needed to clarify further the prognostic significance of individual cytogenetic abnormalities in the presence of AA. Current data suggest that patients with AA and a trisomy as the abnormal cytogenetic clone should be treated in a similar manner to AA patients with a normal karyotype. The presence of a trisomy in AA patients should not be an automatic indication for BMT, if the treatment algorithm suggests other treatment.

Flow cytometric screening for paroxysmal nocturnal hemoglobinuria (PNH) clones should be done in all patients at the time of diagnosis. With flow cytometry, at least one-third of newly diagnosed patients with AA show PNH clones of various sizes.[14,15] Presence of the PNH clone has been associated with a better response to IST in Japanese patients.[16]

Defining the disease severity

Disease severity is defined by the historical criteria of Camitta et al for severe AA (SAA) and those of Bacigalupo for very severe AA (Table 16.2).[17,18] All remaining patients have non-severe AA (NSAA).

Table 16.1 Etiology and confirmatory tests for aplastic anemia

Etiology	Diagnosis	Confirmation of diagnosis
Congenital	Fanconi anemia	Increased spontaneous and DEB- or MMC-induced chromosome breakages of cultured peripheral blood lymphocytes
	Dyskeratosis congenita (DC)	DKC1 gene mutated in X-linked DC, TERC (encodes the RNA component of telomerase) mutated in autosomal dominant DC, TERT and TERC (the reverse transcriptase of TERC) are mutated in about 5% of apparent acquired AA patients ('cryptic DC').
	Shwachman–Diamond syndrome	SBDS gene mutated in 80% of patients
Acquired	Idiopathic (75–80%)	–
	Drugs, e.g. NSAIDs, gold, chloramphenicol, sulphonamides, etc.	Careful drug history, but no tests available to prove association
	Chemicals: benzene, paints, organochlorine, pesticides	Careful exposure history, but no tests available to prove association
	Viruses: hepatitis A or B, non-A, non-B, non-C, hepatitis, EBV rarely	Liver function tests, viral studies (hepatitis A, B, C, G, but usually negative, EBV rarely)
	PNH	Flow cytometry of GPI-anchored proteins on red cells, neutrophils and monocytes.
	Pregnancy	
	Rarely: SLE, thymoma, eosinophilic fasciitis, anorexia nervosa	–
		Autoimmune screen

Abbreviations: DEB, diepoxybutane; MMC, mitomycin C; DC, dyskeratosis congenita; SBDS, Shwachman–Bodian Diamond syndrome; NSAID, non-steroidal anti-inflammatory drug; GPI, glycosylphosphatidyl inositol; EBV, Epstein–Barr virus; SLE, systemic lupus erythematosus; PNH, paroxysmal nocturnal hemoglobinuria.

Table 16.2 Severity of AA

Severe AA (Camitta)[18]	Criteria: BM cellularity <25% or 25–50% with <30% residual hematopoietic cells with 2 out of 3 of the following: neutrophils <0.5 × 10⁹/l, platelets <20 × 10⁹/l, reticulocytes <20 × 10⁹/l
Very severe AA (Bacigalupo)[17]	Same as for severe AA, except neutrophil count <0.2 × 10⁹/l

These simple clinical criteria provide an important framework for therapeutic decision making for AA.

Treatment options

Supportive care

One of the most important factors which can impact significantly upon the outcome of AA is the supportive care provided to the patient prior to the definitive treatment. The main aim of supportive care is to prevent the complications related to bone marrow failure, mainly infection and bleeding.

Blood product support

During the late 1970s and early 1980s, results of marrow transplantation for severe AA indicated that outcome of relatively undertransfused patients was significantly superior to that of multiply transfused patients.[19] Following these observations, a policy of not transfusing newly diagnosed patients unless absolutely necessary was advocated so as to avoid alloimmunization prior to BMT. Consequently, vital platelet and red cell transfusions were sometimes withheld in patients with severe anemia and thrombocytopenia, resulting in fatal or near-fatal hemorrhages before patients ever got to transplant. Prediction of bleeding is difficult in an individual patient. Support with red cell and platelet transfusions is essential for patients with AA to maintain a safe blood count. Fatal hemorrhages, usually cerebral, are more

common in patients who have <10 × 10⁹/l platelets, extensive retinal hemorrhages, buccal hemorrhages or rapidly spreading purpura. It is recommended that prophylactic platelet transfusions are given when the platelet count is <10 × 10⁹/l (or <20 × 10⁹/l in the presence of sepsis or fever), rather than giving platelet transfusions only in response to bleeding manifestations.[6] Additional measures such as use of tranexamic acid and prevention of menorrhagia by use of oral contraceptives may be considered on an individual case basis.

The majority of patients with severe AA require regular transfusion support, and therefore may develop alloimmunization to leukocytes present in red cell and platelet transfusions by generating antibodies to human leukocyte antigen (HLA) and non-HLA (minor histocompatability) antigens.[20] This can result in platelet refractoriness, which can impact upon the outcome of BMT, mainly due to a high rate of graft rejection.[21] In the work-up of platelet refractoriness, causes such as sepsis and drugs should be excluded and patients should be screened for HLA antibodies.

Prestorage leukodepletion of blood products appears to help reduce the risk of alloimmunization.[22,23] A retrospective study from the UK reported significant reduction in the risk of alloimmunization in patients with AA from 50% (prior to introduction of prestorage leukodepletion of blood products) to 12% in patients who received leukodepleted blood products only.[24] If a patient is sensitized to random donor platelets resulting in platelet refractoriness, then HLA-matched platelets should be used.

As for all transplant recipients, patients should be given irradiated red cell and platelet transfusions from the beginning of the pretransplant conditioning regimen. It is a matter of debate whether irradiated blood products should be used in supportive therapy for potential transplant candidates prior to the planned BMT.

If a patient is a potential candidate for early or later BMT, then the patient should be transfused with only cytomegalovirus (CMV)-negative blood products until the patient's CMV status is known. CMV-negative blood products should then be continued only if both the patient and donor are CMV negative.[25]

Prevention of infection

Patients with AA are usually at risk of bacterial and fungal infections. The risk of infection in a patient with AA is determined by severity of neutropenia and monocyte count. The risk may also be determined on an individual basis as some patients tend to have repeated infections while others have few. Patients with a neutrophil count <0.2 × 10⁹/l are at high risk of infections and should be given prophylactic antibiotics. The majority of centers use a quinoline antibiotic such as ciprofloxacin. However, there has been concern about the emergence of quinoline-resistant bacteria and more gram-positive infections. Centers should follow the local guidelines for prevention of infection in severely neutropenic patients.

For antifungal prophylaxis, fluconazole is used most commonly. Consideration should be given to the use of itraconazole if there is any previous history suggestive of aspergillus infection as fluconazole is ineffective against aspergillus. As itraconazole capsules have erratic absorption, itraconazole suspension should be used where necessary. The role of newer antifungal agents in the prophylactic setting is being studied at present.

Routine use of prophylaxis against *Pneumocystis carinii* pneumonia (PCP) and antiviral drugs is not necessary in untreated patients with AA. Antiviral prophylaxis with aciclovir for 6 months is essential for all patients undergoing BMT or IST. Prophylaxis against PCP is essential for patients undergoing BMT but not indicated following antithymocyte globulin (ATG) treatment. Length of prophylaxis after BMT may vary depending on type of conditioning and donor, as patients treated with T-cell depleted grafts and those transplanted from alternative donors may require longer prophylaxis.

Treatment of infections

All infections in the setting of severe neutropenia should be treated aggressively. Local guidelines should be followed for treatment of febrile neutropenia. Empirical use of antifungal agents may be indicated in patients where fever does not subside after 48–72 hours of adequate antibiotics coverage. To investigate the source of infection, chest and sinus imaging studies, even in the absence of symptoms, should be done in patients whose response to antibiotics is inadequate. Some patients with AA with residual marrow hemopoietic activity are able to mount a response to granulocyte colony-stimulating factors (G-CSF). Therefore, consideration should also be given to use of G-CSF in patients with severe systemic infections not responding adequately to intravenous antibiotics and antifungals. If there is no improvement in neutrophil count after 5–7 days' use of G-CSF, this can be discontinued.

Specific treatment

The standard specific treatment of a newly diagnosed patient with acquired AA is either allogeneic BMT from an HLA-identical matched sibling donor (MSD) or IST with ATG and ciclosporin (CSA). The outcome of patients treated with BMT from MSD or IST has improved and more than 80% patients survive after any of these treatments.[26,27] The selection of BMT or IST depends on the age of the patient, severity of AA and availability of a suitable donor. An EBMT study showed increased mortality in patients >40 years of age undergoing marrow transplantation and showed clear superiority of IST over BMT in this age group. Therefore, there is general recommendation to consider BMT as first-line therapy in patients ≤40 years with SAA.[27] For patients with NSAA who are red cell and/or platelet transfusion dependent, IST with ATG and CSA is recommended as first-line treatment. The broad treatment strategies for a newly diagnosed patient with SAA are outlined in Figure 16.1.

Bone marrow transplantation

There has been steady improvement in the results of BMT for acquired AA over the years. Transplantation for SAA from an HLA-identical sibling donor is now very successful, with a 75–90% chance of long-term cure in young patients.[21,28–31] More recently, promising results have also been observed for alternative donor transplants for AA patients failing IST.[32,33] To optimize the outcomes of BMT in AA, the importance of careful pre-BMT assessment cannot be overemphasized.

The purpose of pre-BMT assessment is not only to re-confirm the diagnosis and severity of the disease, but also to understand the need for any necessary modifications in conditioning regimen or supportive care. Additional tests necessary prior to planned BMT are discussed below.

Reassessment of bone marrow morphology, cytogenetics and PNH status and ensuring that a congenital form of aplasia has been excluded It is important to reassess the bone marrow morphology, cytogenetics and PNH status of the patient prior to BMT to rule out evolution to a premalignant or malignant condition, since this would influence the choice of transplant conditioning regimen. Patients with Fanconi anemia or DC do not tolerate conventional-intensity conditioning used for acquired AA.

HLA antibody screening Repeated exposure of patients with AA to blood and platelet transfusions increases the risk of HLA alloimmu-

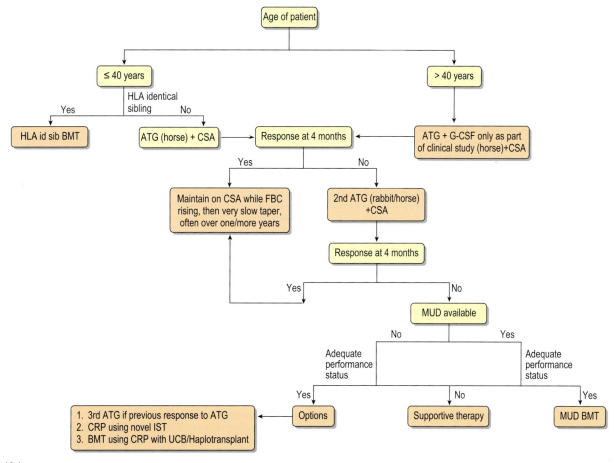

Figure 16.1

Treatment strategies for newly diagnosed patients with severe aplastic anemia. ATG, antithymocyte globulin; CSA, ciclosporin; MUD, matched unrelated donor; CRP, clinical research protocol; IST, immunosuppressive therapy; UCB, umbilical cord blood.

nization, resulting in resistance to random donor platelets. Earlier studies reported this risk to vary from 34% to 100%.[34,35] Leukocyte-depleted blood products are now routinely being used in many western European countries and North America and may help in decreasing the risk of alloimmunization. Poor incrementation to random platelet transfusions and the presence of HLA antibodies indicate the potential need for HLA-matched platelets and, ideally, these investigations should be completed before the start of conditioning therapy.

Co-morbidity assessment The adverse impact of pretransplant co-morbidities on non-relapse mortality has been reported in several studies in patients with hematologic malignancies.[36,37] Although this has not been formally studied in patients with AA, this may be an important factor determining transplant-related mortality, especially in older patients, in whom survival after marrow transplantation is significantly inferior to that seen in younger patients. Patients with high pretransplant co-morbidity scores may need modifications in the conditioning regimen, graft-versus-host disease (GvHD) prophylaxis or supportive care strategies.

Presence of active infections The presence of an active infection is an adverse factor for outcome after stem cell transplantation for AA.[38] Any active infection should be treated and the general condition stabilized before proceeding to BMT. However, it may sometimes be necessary to proceed with BMT in the presence of active infection, particularly fungal infection. Reduced- or minimal-intensity transplants are associated with a lower risk of complications in the immediate post-transplant period. Such a transplant offers the best chance of early neutrophil recovery and delaying the transplant may risk progression of the fungal infection.

Conditioning regimens for HLA-identical sibling donor transplantation

The optimum conditioning regimen for acquired AA has been a moving target. The transplant regimens commonly used for AA patients are usually non-myeloablative. The definition of intensity of conditioning regimens for patients with AA is a matter of controversy at present. For the discussion here, we will use the term 'conventional-intensity conditioning' for traditional high-dose cyclophosphamide-based protocols and 'minimal-intensity conditioning' for newer protocols using minimal doses of chemotherapy.

Conventional-intensity conditioning

Animal studies in the 1960s showed that cyclophosphamide was a powerful immunosuppressive agent that facilitated stable engraftment of transplanted allogeneic hematopoietic cells.[39–41] Since its initial introduction in the 1970s,[42,43] cyclophosphamide has been the major

component of conditioning regimens for patients with acquired AA. Initial studies showed a high rate of graft rejection in the range of 35–60% in AA patients.[42,44] Subsequently, ATG was introduced into this protocol as a measure to reduce graft rejection and significant improvement in graft rejection was observed.[28] Cyclophosphamide, given at a dose of 200 mg/kg (50 mg/kg × 4 (days −5 to −2)) in combination with equine ATG (total 90 mg/kg) is currently the conditioning regimen most commonly used for acquired AA.

The prognosis of the majority of newly diagnosed SAA patients undergoing BMT from MSD is good, and long-term survivals of 70–90% have been reported in various studies (Table 16.3).[21,29–31,38,45] The effect of age on HLA-identical sibling transplants was clearly demonstrated by a study from the EBMT.[27] In this study, actuarial survival of patients aged 16 years or less, 17–40, and greater than 40 years was 77%, 68% and 54%, respectively (p < 0.001). Other adverse prognostic factors are prior failed IST,[30] a long interval between diagnosis and BMT,[17,27,38,45] heavy transfusion burden,[17,21,27,38,45] platelet refractoriness and active infection before BMT.[21,38]

Minimal-intensity conditioning

The outcome of patients above the age of 40 years undergoing BMT with conventional-intensity protocols is significantly inferior when compared to the younger patients. The poor outcome in the older patients may be related to a combination of various factors such as prior failure of IST resulting in a heavy transfusion burden and late referral for BMT, increased regimen-related toxicities or an increased incidence of GvHD.

To improve outcomes in older patients with AA, various transplant groups have focused on using regimens which enhance immunosuppression but are minimally toxic to the marrow. The potential advantages of these protocols are to decrease the regimen-related toxicities such as hemorrhagic cystitis, cardiotoxicity, and late development of cancers of the urinary tract.[46,47] Various centers have reported encouraging preliminary results with good engraftment in heavily pretreated patients.[48–51] The doses of chemotherapy have varied between different studies. Usually, these protocols have used fludarabine (total dose 90–125 mg/m^2), low-dose cyclophosphamide (total dose 40–120 mg/kg) with or without ATG or alemtuzumab.

There are no data available at present comparing conventional-versus minimal-intensity conditioning in AA. Currently, it appears reasonable to offer these protocols to older patients or to patients with significant co-morbidities. Long-term and comparative data will be needed before these protocols can be offered to young patients with MSD, who usually do well with currently used conventional-intensity protocols.

Table 16.3 Recent studies of MSD stem cell transplantation for acquired AA

Reference/group	Year of transplants	n	Graft rejection	Acute GvHD II–IV	Chronic GvHD	Survival	Regimen
Passweg/IBMTR[38]	1988–1992	471	16%	19%	32%	66% at 5 years	Cy, 46%; Cy + TBI, 5%; Cy + LFR, 36%; Cy + ATG, 9%; others, 4%
Bacigalupo/EBMT[45]	1976–1998	1699	12%	13%	13% (limited) 10% (extensive)	66% at 4 years	Details not given, majority high-dose Cy-based protocol
Strob/Seattle[29]	1988–1999	94	4%	29%	32%	88% at 6 years	Cy + ATG
Kim/Seoul[31]	1995–2001	113	14%	11%	12%	89% at 6 years	Cy + procarbazine and ATG
Dulley/Sao Paolo	1993–2001	81	22%	37%	39%	56% at 6 years	Low-dose Bu (1 mg/kg) + Cy
Ades/Paris[30]	1978–2001	100 33	2% 6%	42% 0%	64% 42%	59% at 16 years 94% at 4.4 years	Cy + TAI Cy + ATG
Gupta/London[21]	1989–2003	33	24%	14%	4%	81% at 5 years	Cy + CAMPATH antibodies

Abbreviations: Cy, cyclophosphamide; TBI, total body irradiation; LFR, limited field radiation; ATG, antithymocyte globulin; NK, not known; Bu, busulfan; MSD, matched sibling donor.

GvHD prophylaxis

The introduction of CSA instead of methotrexate as GvHD prophylaxis helped in improving the survival of patients with SAA.[38,52] The patients who received a combination of CSA and short-term methotrexate (MTX) for GvHD prevention had better results compared to those receiving MTX alone.[53–55] A prospective randomized study from GITMO/EBMT compared the combination of CSA and short-term methotrexate with CSA alone in patients with SAA. This study showed improved survival in patients receiving CSA and MTX as GvHD prophylaxis.[56] Based on these data, a combination of CSA and short-term MTX is recommended GvHD prophylaxis for AA patients.

CAMPATH-1 antibodies or alemtuzumab have been used for the prevention of GvHD in AA. It is noteworthy that when CAMPATH antibodies are used in conditioning regimens for AA patients, CSA alone is sufficient for GvHD prevention.[21,57,58] As AA patients are at risk of late graft failure, GvHD prophylaxis is usually continued for 12 months, with slow tapering beginning at 9 months.[6]

Source and dose of hematopoietic progenitor cells

G-CSF mobilized peripheral blood stem cells (G-PBSC) have potential for earlier engraftment when compared to bone marrow stem cells. However, chronic GvHD is significantly higher after PBSC transplants. A recent retrospective study from the combined International and European Bone Marrow Transplant Registry (CIBMTR/EBMT) compared the outcomes after PBSC transplantation and BMT. Although engraftment was quicker with PBSC transplants, a significantly inferior outcome was noted after PBSC transplantation compared to BMT, mainly due to increased GvHD.[59] At present, routine use of PBSC transplants for AA is not recommended and this intervention should only be used as a part of a clinical research protocol.

Recently, there has been increasing interest in the use of G-CSF primed bone marrow (G-BM) as a source of hematopoietic cells.[60] A recent Phase III trial comparing G-BM and G-PBSC in matched sibling allograft recipients showed that G-BM produced similar hematologic recovery but a reduced incidence of extensive chronic GvHD.[61] This study mainly included patients with hematologic malignancies. No data are available on the utility of G-BM when compared to steady-state BM in patients with AA. A retrospective study is in progress at CIBMTR comparing the outcome of G-BM transplants with steady-state BM and PBSC transplants in patients with SAA. At present, the use of G-BM can only be recommended as a part of a well-designed clinical trial.

When using BM as a source of donor cells, it is important to give at least 3×10^8 nucleated marrow cells/kg because with lower doses, the risk of graft rejection is significantly higher.[62,63]

Post-transplant management

Once successful engraftment is achieved, the patient should be monitored closely for secondary graft failure. AA patients are at significant risk of secondary graft failure, which is most commonly associated with subtherapeutic CSA levels or early withdrawal of CSA. CSA trough levels should be maintained between 250 and 350 μg/l. It is important to monitor chimerism especially during CSA withdrawal. If there is any evidence of an increasing percentage of recipient cells, then CSA should not be reduced or withdrawn at that time.

Critical barriers for BMT in AA

Graft rejection

Compared to hematologic malignancies, AA patients have a higher rate of graft rejection. The cellular immunity in patients with hematologic malignancies is paralyzed due to the underlying disease and/or repeated cycles of chemotherapy. In comparison, the intact immunity in AA allows generation of a large rejection potential, further compounded by the underlying immune pathophysiology of the disease. Graft rejection rates following sibling BMT for AA vary from 5% to 20%.[64,65] Registry data from the EBMT indicate reduction of graft failure with time,[65] although this was not confirmed in an IBMTR study.[38]

Early graft rejection (no take) results in either no evidence of engraftment following transplantation with persistent pancytopenia or early engraftment with neutrophils and monocytes followed by pancytopenia. Late graft failure occurs after a period of established engraftment and may be associated with CMV infection, GvHD, drugs such as septrin or ganciclovir, and later, at 6–9 months, at the time of CSA withdrawal. The latter situation may respond to reintroduction of CSA therapy.

Factors affecting graft rejection

A heavy transfusion burden prior to BMT is one of the most important factors associated with graft rejection.[19,30,63,64] Although the definition of 'heavy transfusion burden' has varied from study to study, the majority of experts consider >50 transfusions prior to BMT as a 'heavy transfusion burden'. Multiple transfusions can result in alloimmunization to minor histocompatability antigens present on donor cells but lacking in recipients.[20] Use of CSA has led to a decrease in the incidence of graft rejection.[65,66] Interestingly, patients with posthepatitic AA have a low incidence of graft rejection, probably due to early referral and lower transfusion burden.[65] Use of irradiation as a means of extra immune suppression in conditioning resulted in a decreased incidence of graft rejection but was offset by increased regimen-related toxicities and GvHD, resulting in no improvement in survival.[52,64,65] A low dose of donor hemopoietic stem cells was associated with an increased incidence of graft failure in some studies,[62,63] but not confirmed by others.[64] T-cell depletion of donor marrow was associated with a high rate of graft rejection.[64] In studies from the UK using in vivo CAMPATH antibodies, the incidence of graft rejection was higher when CAMPATH was used, both before and after stem cell infusion.[21,57] Graft rejection decreased significantly when CAMPATH was used only prior to stem cell infusion, indicating that the timing of CAMPATH may be an important factor.[21]

Treatment strategies for graft rejection

If there is no evidence of engraftment by 4 weeks, it is reasonable to use growth factor support for 7–10 days. If there is no effect, then a second transplant should be planned. Good supportive care should be continued to prevent infection.

Patients who fail to engraft or develop graft failure after initial engraftment can benefit from a second transplant, provided they are in good physical condition and free of infection.[67] Various strategies have been used for second transplants such as using the same donor, another donor, cytokine mobilized peripheral blood stem cells and use of low-dose radiation in the conditioning regimen. It is difficult to make definitive recommendations in the absence of prospective studies. Such cases should be discussed with an experienced transplant center and the treatment strategy should be individualized according to the patient's circumstances.

To plan further management, it is important to ascertain whether the graft failure is due to failure to sustain donor hemopoiesis or recurrence of AA with re-establishment of recipient hemopoiesis. If the hemopoiesis is partly or completely of recipient origin, reconditioning of the recipient prior to second BMT is necessary. Graft rejection which is associated with inadequate donor hemopoiesis may benefit from 'booster' donor stem cells without the need for further immunosuppression. Late graft failure may respond to reintroduction of therapeutic doses of CSA if the rejection occurred after discontinuation or withdrawl of CSA.[66] Additional immunosuppression with methylpred-nisone may be considered. If these strategies fail, then a second transplant should be considered.

GvHD

GvHD (acute and chronic) is one of the most important complications, which can adversely impact upon performance status, quality of life and survival after marrow transplantation.[68,69] In a study from the Seattle group, among 209 patients who received marrow transplantation for acquired AA and survived 2 years, 86 (41%) had chronic GvHD.[68] A history of prior acute GvHD, infusion of viable donor buffy coat cells and older patient age were significant risk factors for chronic GvHD on univariate analysis, while use of ATG appeared to have a protective effect.

Chronic GvHD is a major risk factor for various long-term complications after transplantation. The adverse effects of chronic GvHD are related not only to the involvement of target organs, but also to the treatment of chronic GvHD. Long-term steroid use can result in significant morbidity due to infectious complications, skin problems, joint contractures, cataracts, restrictive or obstructive pulmonary disease, bone disease such as aseptic necrosis or osteoporosis, and psychiatric problems. With the high-dose Cy and ATG protocol, the risk of chronic GvHD is in the range of 30–40%.[29,30] The use of CAMPATH antibodies for marrow transplantation appears to have a favorable effect on acute and chronic GvHD.[21] In a study from St George's Hospital, the incidence of chronic GvHD was only 4% and none of the patients required steroids beyond 1 year after transplantation. Prevention of GvHD is one of the main goals of marrow transplantation in AA as there is no beneficial therapeutic effect of GvHD in this setting. The treatment strategies for acute and chronic GvHD in AA are similar to those with hematologic malignancies.

Long-term complications of BMT

Infertility

The chances of pregnancy or fathering a child are much higher in patients who receive a marrow transplant for AA compared to hematologic malignancies. Fertility is usually well preserved when irradiation is not used in the conditioning regimen.[70,71] Pregnancies in patients transplanted for AA usually have a successful outcome.[21] The presence of both acute and chronic GvHD appears to have an adverse impact on fertility.[68,72] With the current protocols using high-dose cyclophosphamide in combination with ATG or alemtuzumab, the chances of successful pregnancy or fathering a child are 35–45% after marrow transplantation for AA.[21,68] One major limitation of the reported literature is difficulty in determining precisely what proportion of patients attempted to have children. Fludarabine-based minimal intensity protocols use relatively lower doses of chemotherapy in the conditioning regimens and may have a theoretical advantage over conventional-intensity protocols in preserving fertility. However, data on gonadal function after fludarabine containing protocols are scanty at present.[73] Long-term data will be needed to evaluate the effect of fludarabine-based conditioning on fertility.

Secondary malignancies

After a long latency period, an increased frequency of solid tumor malignancies has been observed after marrow transplantation for AA.[30,68,74,75] The probability appears to be higher in patients with both acute and chronic GvHD when compared to patients with acute but no chronic GvHD (30% versus 0%).[68] A combined study from Seattle and Paris showed that treatment of chronic GvHD with azathioprine was a significant risk factor for post-transplant malignancies in AA.[76] Use of radiation in the conditioning regimens is associated with a higher incidence of malignancies compared to non-radiation based regimens.[76]

Immunosuppressive therapy

For patients who are not BMT candidates, the combination of ATG and CSA remains the current standard of immunosuppressive therapy for both SAA and transfusion-dependent NSAA. The response rate (as defined by transfusion independence) in severe AA is 60–70% at 6 months.[77,78] Long-term follow-up from the German prospective study, comparing ATG alone with ATG and CSA, reported an overall survival of 54–58% at 11.3 years and failure-free survival (defined as survival in the absence of relapse, no response, PNH, MDS, AML or solid tumors) of 39% at 11.3 years.[78]

Risk of relapse is 30–40%, but appears to be less with the more recent practice of prolonging CSA beyond 6 months. CSA dependency is observed in 26–62% of patients, necessitating long-term maintenance with the drug. The actuarial probability of developing hemolytic PNH, MDS/AML or a solid tumor after IST is 10%, 8% and 11% at 11 years, respectively, emphasizing the importance of long-term follow-up of all patients.[78]

Avascular necrosis may result in serious morbidity so the minimum dose of prednisolone should be given to prevent serum sickness.[79] The addition of G-CSF to ATG and CSA when administered daily for 3–4 months results in quicker neutrophil recovery but confers no benefit in terms of trilineage hematologic recovery or improved survival.[80] In children, the use of G-CSF in high dose, or for a more prolonged duration with IST, is a risk factor for MDS/AML with monosomy 7,[81] but not to date in adults.[80] A multicenter prospective randomized EBMT study is currently in progress to address the role of G-CSF in IST for SAA. The routine use of G-CSF in IST for SAA outside a research protocol is not recommended at present.

Quality of life (QOL) issues in AA

The outcomes of BMT and IST for AA have continued to improve so that differences in survival between the two treatment modalities have diminished. Therefore, differences in QOL issues become vitally important to inform decisions for clinicians and patients. There are no prospective studies that have compared the longitudinal QOL in AA patients undergoing BMT or IST. One retrospective study compared QOL outcomes between 52 transplanted patients and 155 patients receiving IST during the period 1976–1999 by using quality-adjusted time without symptoms and toxicity (Q-TWiST) methodology.[82] No differences in survival were observed. However, Q-TWiST analysis showed that IST-treated patients had longer periods of time with (a) symptoms from drug toxicity, (b) transfusion dependency, (c) partial remission and (d) secondary clonal disorders (Fig. 16.2). Transplanted patients spent more time in complete remission without drugs and had longer periods free from symptoms.

Patients who are refractory or who relapse after initial IST

About one-third of patients are refractory to ATG and CSA-based IST and approximately one-third of patients relapse after initial treatment with IST. If a matched sibling donor is available and the patient is in good physical condition, the option of BMT should be considered. For those without a MSD, it is now a common practice to offer a second course of ATG-containing IST. The response rate has varied from 30% to 60% in various studies.[83–86] While some studies did not report any difference in response rate between refractory or relapsed patients,[83–85] others reported a higher response rate in patients who relapsed after a previous course of ATG (68%) compared to refractory patients (33%).[86]

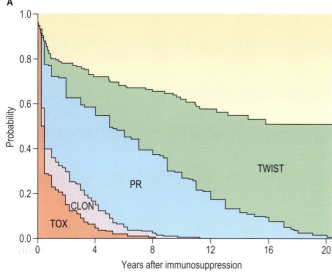

A

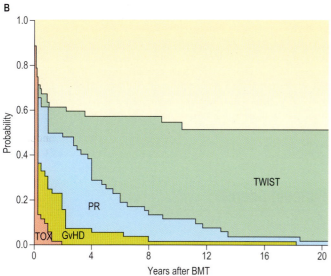

B

Figure 16.2
Quality-adjusted survival in patients with AA treated with immunosuppressive therapy or bone marrow transplantation. (a) Partitioning of survival time for patients treated with immunosuppressive therapy into the four clinically relevant states: TOX (time with toxicity and time with transfusion dependency), PR (including time in partial remission and time in complete remission but necessitating drugs), CLON (clonal complications) and TWiST (time without symptoms or toxicity). (b) Partitioning of survival time for patients treated with BMT into the four clinically relevant states: TOX (time with toxicity and time with transfusion dependency), PR (including time in partial remission and time in complete remission but necessitating drugs), GvHD (graft-versus-host disease and complications) and TWiST. Reproduced from Viollier et al,[82] with permission.

In the absence of any prospective study comparing rabbit with horse ATG, the choice of ATG preparation for a second course depends on whether a severe reaction occurred with the previous course, individual center preference and drug availability.

Marrow transplantation from alternative donors using a matched unrelated donor should be considered in patients who have failed two courses of IST (see Fig. 16.1). For patients who do not have a suitable donor, a third course of ATG-based treatment may be considered. A retrospective study from the UK showed that all of seven patients who had previously responded to a first or second course of ATG, but relapsed, responded again to a third course, whereas only two transient responses were observed among 11 patients refractory to the previous two courses.[87] Multiple courses of ATG are associated with an increasing risk of severe systemic reactions and anaphylaxis, so must be given

with great caution. Nevertheless, a third ATG course is often useful for relapsing patients, indicating that such patients may require some form of maintenance immunosuppression for presumed ongoing immune attack on hematopoiesis. For refractory patients, alternative experimental therapies should be considered.

Marrow transplantation from donors other than MSD

HLA phenotypically identical non-sibling BMT

In approximately 6% of patients, it is possible to find a phenotypically matched parent, or extended family testing may reveal a phenotypically matched family donor either by chance or due to consanguineous marriage. Limited available data indicate that outcomes similar to MSD transplants may be achievable in these patients.[88]

Syngeneic twin BMT

It was initially felt that conditioning therapy should not be necessary to prevent graft rejection in syngeneic BMT. Studies later showed high graft failure in patients who did not receive conditioning therapy. However, a large proportion of patients were rescued by second transplant.[89,90] There was no significant difference in survival noted in the IBMTR study in the patients who received syngeneic transplants with or without conditioning therapy.[90] Given the high rate of graft failure, it appears reasonable to give pretransplant conditioning to patients undergoing syngeneic transplant.

Matched unrelated donor (MUD) BMT

Compared to MSD transplants, the survival of patients transplanted from unrelated donors has only been in the range of 20–50%.[45,91,92] Main causes of transplantation failure in unrelated donor transplants have been a high incidence of graft failure, regimen-related toxicities and GvHD. The recent CIBMTR retrospective study of severe AA patients transplanted between 1988 and 1998 (see Table 16.4) highlighted the poor outcomes (39% survival at 5 years) and high rates of graft rejection, GvHD and infections after MUD BMT.[92] No improvement with time was noted in this study. A major limitation of this study was non-availability of high-resolution typing data.

The importance of better donor selection using high-resolution HLA typing in patients with SAA was demonstrated by a study from the Japan Marrow Donor Program (JMDP).[93] The 5-year overall survival of 154 patients transplanted for SAA was 56%. Of particular note, patients receiving a transplant from donors matched for A, B and DRB1 by high-resolution DNA typing had significantly superior survival, compared to those who had a mismatch at the A or B locus.

Recent attempts to reduce graft rejection and improve survival include the use of low-dose total-body irradiation (TBI) or a non-irradiation, fludarabine-based regimen (Table 16.4). In a prospective multicenter study, Deeg and colleagues reported a low graft rejection rate of 5% (2% for matched and 11% for mismatched donors) among 87 patients transplanted from unrelated donors, using a de-escalating dose of TBI in most patients. However, pulmonary toxicity was observed and GvHD remained a problem.[33] In contrast, a study from the EBMT using fludarabine, low-dose Cy (1200 mg/m^2) and ATG reported a higher graft rejection rate (18%), particularly among older patients, but a lower rate of acute and chronic GvHD with encouraging survival (Fig. 16.3).[32] Other approaches have been to use alemtuzumab instead of ATG in an otherwise similar regimen to that of the EBMT,[58] or G-CSF mobilized CD34+ selected PBSC.[94] However, both these latter approaches require further evaluation in larger studies.

Table 16.4 Recent studies of UD stem cell transplantation for acquired AA

Reference	Year of transplants	n	Graft rejection	Acute GvHD II–IV	Chronic GvHD All/extensive	Survival	Regimen
Kojima/Japan[93]	1993–2000	154 79 (MUD), 75 (M/M)	11%	29%	30%/15%	60% at 5 yr for A, B, DRB1 matches	Cy (120–200 mg/kg), irradiation ± ATG
Bacigalupo/EBMT[32]	1998–2004	38 28(MUD),10(M/M: 5 UD, 5 family)	18%	27%	27%/6%	73% at 5 yr	Fludarabine 120 mg/m², Cy 1200 mg/m², ATG
Passweg/CIBMTR[92]	1988–1998	181(MUD) 51 (M/M)	17% 51%	48% 37%	29%/NK 24%/NK	39% at 5 yr 36% at 5 yr	Cy ± irradiation ± antibodies
Deeg/North America[33]	1994–2004	62 (MUD) 25 (M/M)	2% (MUD) 11% (M/M)	69%(MUD) 77% (M/M)	52%/NK (MUD) 57%/NK (M/M)	61% at 5 yr (MUD) 40% (M/M)	Cy 200 mg/kg, ATG, low-dose TBI (2–6 Gy). If ATG intolerant, Cy 120 mg/kg, TBI 12 Gy

Abbreviations: UD, unrelated donor; MUD, matched unrelated donor; M/M, mismatched; UCB, umbilical cord blood; NK, not known.

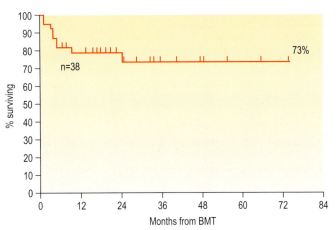

Figure 16.3
Survival of patients with SAA undergoing alternative donor transplants using a reduced-intensity approach (EBMT study). Actuarial survival of 38 patients with acquired SAA undergoing alternative donor (unrelated donors, 33; mismatched family donors, 5) transplants. Reproduced from Bacigalupo et al,[32] with permission.

Mismatched family donors

The outcome data of transplantation using mismatched family donors are scanty. There were no significant differences in outcomes of patients transplanted from a mismatched family donor compared to matched unrelated donors in a recent CIBMTR study.[92] Due to lack of high-resolution HLA typing data, this study was unable to discover whether a fully high-resolution matched unrelated donor is preferable to a mismatched family donor.

Cord blood transplantation

A potential advantage of using umbilical cord blood (UCB) as a source of stem cells for unrelated donor BMT in SAA is that HLA mismatching is better tolerated, so theoretically widely applicable. Published data for acquired AA UCB transplantation are limited. Furthermore, the low cell dose obtained from a UCB donation poses particular problems in AA where a good stem cell dose is important to help maximize engraftment. The recent use of double UCB transplants as a means of increasing the stem cell dose for adult recipients has been successful in achieving a high engraftment rate in high-risk MDS/AML.[95] For individual patients, only one of the two units engrafted long term. In acquired AA, a recent study from China demonstrated engraftment in seven of nine adults, with sustained mixed chimerism.[96] In four of the patients, two units of UCB were infused, one of which engrafted each patient.

Haploidentical transplantation

For patients who are refractory to two or more courses of IST and who do not have a suitable sibling or unrelated donor, the necessity of using alternative donors such as haploidentical family members is compelling. Nonetheless, haploidentical transplantation has rarely been performed in this context, probably because of the high risk of graft failure. Reported data are scanty at present and subject to publication bias.[97–100] These data show that some selected patients may benefit from this approach. Such transplants can only be recommended in experienced centers for young patients with a good performance status, who do not have alternative treatment options.

Fanconi anemia

Fanconi anemia (FA) is an autosomal recessive disorder (all complementation groups except FA-B group) or rarely an X-linked (FA-B group) recessive disorder.[101–103] FA can be divided into at least 12 complementation groups (A, B, C, D1, D2, E, F, G, I, J, L and M) defined by cell fusion studies, and 11 of the 12 genes have been identified.[102] FA patients show increased sensitivity to chromosome damage by DNA cross-linking agents because of a defect in DNA repair. FA proteins (including BRCA2/FANCD1) co-operate in the DNA repair process (the so called FA-BRCA pathway). Defects of FA genes have been found in many human cancers. The prevalence of FA is estimated to be 1–5 per million and the overall frequency of heterozygotes is 1 in 300, but higher in South African Africaans and Ashkenazi Jews. The disease is characterized by multiple congenital abnormalities, bone marrow failure, and predisposition to MDS, AML and solid tumors, especially head and neck squamous cell cancer, liver and gynecologic tumors. The risk of liver tumors is further increased in those patients treated with anabolic steroids. The common congenital defects seen in patients with FA include short stature (51%), abnormalities of the skin (55%), upper extremities (43%), head (26%), eyes (23%), kidneys (21%), and ears (11%), and developmental disability (11%).[104] Although the median age at diagnosis is 6.5 years for male patients and 8 years for female patients, atypical presentations are frequently reported with patients more than 20 years of age and with no morphologic abnormalities.[9,104]

The diagnosis is confirmed by increased chromosomal breakage in FA cells following exposure to DNA cross-linking agents such as mitomycin C and diepoxybutane.[105] FA subtyping (determination of the complementation group of each patient with FA) shows some correlation with phenotype, although there is pleotropic variation within a specific group.[106] FA patients have high levels of serum alpha-fetoprotein, and this test may be used as an initial preliminary screening investigation while waiting for confirmatory tests.[107]

The natural history of FA is to evolve toward progressive marrow failure, which is most often lethal before the end of the second decade of life without treatment. The actuarial risk of developing BM failure is above 90% by 40 years of age.[108,109] The risks of developing hematologic and non-hematologic neoplasms are 33% and 28%, respectively, by 40 years of age.[108]

Treatment of FA

Therapeutic interventions have focused on amelioration of the symptoms of bone marrow failure. Supportive care with red blood cell and platelet transfusions, antibiotic therapy, androgens and hematopoietic growth factors has helped to improve the survival of patients with FA. Oral oxymetholone induces a trilineage response in approximately 60% of patients. Most patients who respond later relapse, but it is a useful drug to help maintain blood counts while planning for SCT. The dose of oxymetholone is 2–5 mg/kg/day. Regular monitoring of liver function and liver ultrasound scan are important for early detection of liver complications while on androgen therapy. However, allogeneic stem cell transplantation is the only treatment option that can restore normal hemopoiesis in FA patients.

Outcome of marrow transplantation in FA

Stem cell transplantation is the treatment of choice for FA patients with severe hematologic manifestations. In the early 1980s, the Paris group made the observations of severe cyclophosphamide toxicity in patients with FA[110] and later on by in vitro studies demonstrated high sensitivity of FA patients to cyclophosphamide compared to parents of FA patients and healthy controls.[111] Subsequently, a lower dose of cyclophosphamide (20 mg/kg) and 5 Gy of thoracoabdominal irradiation (TAI) was used and good donor chimerism was observed in patients transplanted from matched sibling donors.[112]

In a study from the IBMTR, 151 patients receiving MSD transplants and 48 patients receiving alternative donor transplants were analyzed.[113] In this study, 2-year survival for MSD and alternative donor transplants was 66% and 29%, respectively. Younger age, high pretransplant platelet count, use of ATG, low-dose cyclophosphamide and limited field radiation and CSA for GvHD prophylaxis were associated with improved survival. In view of better survival in patients with higher platelet counts, earlier transplantation was recommended when a MSD was identified. Use of low-dose cyclophosphamide (20 mg/kg) and 4–6 Gy thoracoabdominal radiation helped to improve survival.[113,114] However, radiation also led to an increased risk of secondary malignancies, to which patients of FA are especially prone.[76,115–117] The risk of secondary malignancies was also higher in patients developing chronic GvHD.[76,116]

In a study from the EBMT, 69 FA patients transplanted from matched unrelated donors were reported and the 3-year survival was only 33%.[118] Extensive malformations, positive recipient cytomegalovirus serology, the use of androgens before transplant, and female donors were associated with a worse outcome.[118] Patients with extensive congenital malformations had a 3-year survival of 14%, compared to 44% for those with limited malformations. These patients had a higher rate of graft failure and GvHD. In particular, malformations of urogenital tract/kidneys and limbs were more frequently associated with GvHD.

In a study from Paris, the risk of acute and chronic GVHD was significantly higher in patients with FA compared to non-FA aplastic anemia.[117] Graft failure also appears higher in patients showing lymphocyte somatic mosaicism (i.e. the presence of diepoxybutane (DEB)-insensitive cells).[119]

More recently, fludarabine-based regimens have increasingly been used in patients with FA.[58,120–122] These small studies have reported an encouraging impact on engraftment and GvHD. However, follow-up is short at present and the impact on long-term complications, especially secondary malignancies, is not well known. These regimens have been used in related, unrelated donor and cord blood transplants and have also shown significant antileukemic activity.[120,123] In FA patients with MDS/AML at initial presentation, where possible, it seems preferable to proceed directly to stem cell transplantation rather than giving prior treatment with chemotherapy. Data from small studies indicate a favorable effect of ATG or alemtuzumab on GvHD;[58,120,121] however, larger well-designed prospective studies are needed. A small study of eight patients tested the feasibility of CD34-selected peripheral blood progenitor cells from alternative donors and showed a very low risk of GvHD in patients with FA.[124]

Compared to acquired AA, the incidence of malignancies in FA patients is very high. This is mainly due to genetic predisposition, in addition to other contributory factors such as chronic GvHD and use of radiation in the conditioning regimen. Also, these patients need to be monitored very closely for growth retardation, this being one of the classic features of the FA phenotype. After transplantation, additional factors may play a role in growth retardation.[116]

Stem cell transplantation for dyskeratosis congenita

Results of allogeneic BMT for dyskeratosis congenita (DC) have been poor, on account of early and late complications. These appear to be due to increased susceptibility to endothelial damage from conditioning therapy, causing a diffuse capillaritis of the gut and brain and contributing to pulmonary fibrosis. The capillaritis can cause fatal ulceration and hemorrhage from the gut. For this reason, a reduced-intensity conditioning regimen and avoidance of irradiation and busulfan have been recommended, although this does not necessarily remove this risk. Larger studies using reduced-intensity regimens in DC patients are required to evaluate this approach further.[125–127]

Prior to SCT, it is recommended that all new patients presenting with AA who are <35 years of age are screened for FAnemia. Increased awareness of other inherited forms of AA, such as DC and Shwachman–Diamond anemia, has led physicians to have a low threshold for additional genetic screening. For example, in the case of DC, screening for telomerase mutations should be considered in severe AA patients who fail to respond to IST, patients with a family history of AA or abnormal blood counts or macrocytosis, patients with unusual clinical features such as osteoporosis (and possibly avascular necrosis) or pulmonary symptoms, and adult patients who give a long history of low blood counts. For FA (and DC) patients, it is mandatory to also screen the potential family donor.

Summary

The outcome of marrow transplantation from MSD in younger patients with SAA has improved over the years. Better transfusion practices and supportive care facilities have played a major part in this improvement. Although there are no significant differences in survival after BMT or IST, time tends to favor BMT. In this group, the focus of clinical research is shifting to survivorship issues such as prevention of chronic GvHD, preservation of fertility and secondary malignancies to maximize quality of life. Older patients may benefit from newer minimal-intensity conditioning regimens. Better donor selection by high-resolution typing, decreasing the regimen-related toxicities by optimizing the intensity of conditioning regimens, and prevention of

GvHD by use of agents such as ATG or alemtuzumab have already shown promise for patients undergoing unrelated donor transplants, but require confirmation in larger studies. If the results of recent studies on unrelated donor transplantation can be reproduced in further larger studies, then the place of unrelated donor transplantation may need redefining in planning therapeutic strategies for SAA. Cord blood transplantation and haploidentical transplant approaches remain experimental at present and should only be attempted as part of clinical research protocols in patients with refractory disease.

For FA patients, the results of transplantation with fludarabine-based regimens appear encouraging at short term. Although the hematopoietic defect associated with FA may be cured by transplantation, careful monitoring and surveillance strategies are needed to monitor long-term complications.

References

1. Issaragrisil S, Kaufman DW, Anderson T et al. The epidemiology of aplastic anemia in Thailand. Blood 2006;107:1299–1307

2. Issaragrisil S, Leaverton PE, Chansung K et al. Regional patterns in the incidence of aplastic anemia in Thailand. The Aplastic Anemia Study Group. Am J Hematol 1999;61:164–168

3. Bottiger LE. Epidemiology and aetiology of aplastic anemia. Hematol Blood Transfus 1979;24:27–37

4. Davies SM, Walker DJ. Aplastic anemia in the Northern Region 1971–1978 and follow-up of long term survivors. Clin Lab Hematol 1986;8:307–313

5. Young NS, Calado RT, Scheinberg P. Current concepts in the pathophysiology and treatment of aplastic anemia. Blood 2006;108(8):2509–2519

6. Marsh JC, Ball SE, Darbyshire P et al. Guidelines for the diagnosis and management of acquired aplastic anemia. Br J Haematol 2003;123:782–801

7. Yamaguchi H, Calado RT, Ly H et al. Mutations in TERT, the gene for telomerase reverse transcriptase, in aplastic anemia. N Engl J Med 2005;352:1413–1424

8. Fogarty PF, Yamaguchi H, Wiestner A et al. Late presentation of dyskeratosis congenita as apparently acquired aplastic anemia due to mutations in telomerase RNA. Lancet 2003;362:1628–1630

9. Giampietro PF, Verlander PC, Davis JG, Auerbach AD. Diagnosis of Fanconi anemia in patients without congenital malformations: an international Fanconi Anemia Registry Study. Am J Med Genet 1997;68:58–61

10. Vulliamy TJ, Marrone A, Knight SW et al. Mutations in dyskeratosis congenita: their impact on telomere length and the diversity of clinical presentation. Blood 2006;107:2680–2685

11. Huck K, Hanenberg H, Gudowius S et al. Delayed diagnosis and complications of Fanconi anemia at advanced age–a paradigm. Br J Haematol 2006;133:188–197

12. Maciejewski JP, Selleri C. Evolution of clonal cytogenetic abnormalities in aplastic anemia. Leuk Lymphoma 2004;45:433–440

13. Gupta V, Brooker C, Tooze JA et al. Clinical relevance of cytogenetic abnormalities at diagnosis of acquired aplastic anemia in adults. Br J Haematol 2006;134:95–99

14. Maciejewski JP, Rivera C, Kook H et al. Relationship between bone marrow failure syndromes and the presence of glycophosphatidyl inositol-anchored protein-deficient clones. Br J Haematol 2001;115:1015–1022

15. Parker C, Omine M, Richards S et al. Diagnosis and management of paroxysmal nocturnal hemoglobinuria. Blood 2005;106:3699–3709

16. Sugimori C, Chuhjo T, Feng X et al. Minor population of CD55-CD59- blood cells predicts response to immunosuppressive therapy and prognosis in patients with aplastic anemia. Blood 2006;107:1308–1314

17. Bacigalupo A, Hows J, Gluckman E et al. Bone marrow transplantation (BMT) versus immunosuppression for the treatment of severe aplastic anemia (SAA): a report of the EBMT SAA working party. Br J Haematol 1988;70:177–182

18. Camitta BM, Thomas ED, Nathan DG et al. Severe aplastic anemia: a prospective study of the effect of early marrow transplantation on acute mortality. Blood 1976;48:63–70

19. Storb R, Thomas ED, Buckner CD et al. Marrow transplantation in thirty 'untransfused' patients with severe aplastic anemia. Ann Intern Med 1980;92:30–36

20. Kaminski ER, Hows JM, Goldman JM, Batchelor JR. Pretransfused patients with severe aplastic anemia exhibit high numbers of cytotoxic T lymphocyte precursors probably directed at non-HLA antigens. Br J Haematol 1990;76:401–405

21. Gupta V, Ball SE, Yi QL et al. Favorable effect on acute and chronic graft-versus-host disease with cyclophosphamide and in vivo anti-CD52 monoclonal antibodies for marrow transplantation from HLA-identical sibling donors for acquired aplastic anemia. Biol Blood Marrow Transplant 2004;10:867–876

22. Killick SB, Mufti G, Cavenagh JD et al. A pilot study of antithymocyte globulin (ATG) in the treatment of patients with 'low-risk' myelodysplasia. Br J Haematol 2003;120:679–684

23. Ljungman P. Supportive treatment of patients with severe aplastic anemia. In: Schrezenmeier H, Bacigalupo A (eds) Aplastic anemia, pathophysiology and treatment. Cambridge University Press, Cambridge, 2000:137–153

24. Killick SB, Win N, Marsh JC et al. Pilot study of HLA alloimmunization after transfusion with pre-storage leucodepleted blood products in aplastic anemia. Br J Haematol 1997;97:677–684

25. Pamphilon DH, Rider JR, Barbara JA, Williamson LM. Prevention of transfusion-transmitted cytomegalovirus infection. Transfus Med 1999;9:115–123

26. Doney K, Leisenring W, Storb R, Appelbaum FR. Primary treatment of acquired aplastic anemia: outcomes with bone marrow transplantation and immunosuppressive therapy. Seattle Bone Marrow Transplant Team. Ann Intern Med 1997;126:107–115

27. Bacigalupo A, Brand R, Oneto R et al. Treatment of acquired severe aplastic anemia: bone marrow transplantation compared with immunosuppressive therapy – The European Group for Blood and Marrow Transplantation experience. Semin Hematol 2000;37:69–80

28. Storb R, Etzioni R, Anasetti C et al. Cyclophosphamide combined with antithymocyte globulin in preparation for allogeneic marrow transplants in patients with aplastic anemia. Blood 1994;84:941–949

29. Storb R, Blume KG, O'Donnell MR et al. Cyclophosphamide and antithymocyte globulin to condition patients with aplastic anemia for allogeneic marrow transplantations: the experience in four centers. Biol Blood Marrow Transplant 2001;7:39–44

30. Ades L, Mary JY, Robin M et al. Long-term outcome after bone marrow transplantation for severe aplastic anemia. Blood 2004;103:2490–2497

31. Kim HJ, Park CY, Park YH et al. Successful allogeneic hematopoietic stem cell transplantation using triple agent immunosuppression in severe aplastic anemia patients. Bone Marrow Transplant 2003;31:79–86

32. Bacigalupo A, Locatelli F, Lanino E et al. Fludarabine, cyclophosphamide and antithymocyte globulin for alternative donor transplants in acquired severe aplastic anemia: a report from the EBMT-SAA Working Party. Bone Marrow Transplant 2005;36:947–950

33. Deeg HJ, O'Donnell M, Tolar J et al. Optimization of conditioning for marrow transplantation from unrelated donors for patients with aplastic anemia after failure of immunosuppressive therapy. Blood 2006;108(5):1485–1491

34. Klingemann HG, Self S, Banaji M et al. Refractoriness to random donor platelet transfusions in patients with aplastic anemia: a multivariate analysis of data from 264 cases. Br J Haematol 1987;66:115–121

35. Grumet FC, Yankee RA. Long-term platelet support of patients with aplastic anemia. Effect of splenectomy and steroid therapy. Ann Intern Med 1970;73:1–7

36. Sorror ML, Maris MB, Storb R et al. Hematopoietic cell transplantation (HCT)-specific comorbidity index: a new tool for risk assessment before allogeneic HCT. Blood 2005;106:2912–2919

37. Sorror ML, Maris MB, Storer B et al. Comparing morbidity and mortality of HLA-matched unrelated donor hematopoietic cell transplantation after nonmyeloablative and myeloablative conditioning: influence of pretransplantation comorbidities. Blood 2004;104:961–968

38. Passweg JR, Socie G, Hinterberger W et al. Bone marrow transplantation for severe aplastic anemia: has outcome improved? Blood 1997;90:858–864

39. Santos GW, Owens AH Jr. Allogeneic marrow transplants in cyclophosphamide treated mice. Transplant Proc 1969;1:44–46

40. Storb R, Epstein RB, Rudolph RH, Thomas ED. Allogeneic canine bone marrow transplantation following cyclophosphamide. Transplantation 1969;7:378–386

41. Storb R, Buckner CD, Dillingham LA, Thomas ED. Cyclophosphamide regimens in rhesus monkey with and without marrow infusion. Cancer Res 1970;30:2195–2203

42. Storb R, Thomas ED, Buckner CD et al. Allogeneic marrow grafting for treatment of aplastic anemia. Blood 1974;43:157–180

43. Thomas ED, Storb R, Fefer A et al. Aplastic anemia treated by marrow transplantation. Lancet 1972;1:284–289

44. Storb R, Thomas ED, Weiden PL et al. Aplastic anemia treated by allogeneic bone marrow transplantation: a report on 49 new cases from Seattle. Blood 1976;48:817–841

45. Bacigalupo A, Oneto R, Bruno B et al. Current results of bone marrow transplantation in patients with acquired severe aplastic anemia. Report of the European Group for Blood and Marrow transplantation. On behalf of the Working Party on Severe Aplastic Anemia of the European Group for Blood and Marrow Transplantation. Acta Hematol 2000;103:19–25

46. Haselberger MB, Schwinghammer TL. Efficacy of mesna for prevention of hemorrhagic cystitis after high-dose cyclophosphamide therapy. Ann Pharmacother 1995;29:918–921

47. Travis LB, Curtis RE, Glimelius B et al. Bladder and kidney cancer following cyclophosphamide therapy for non-Hodgkin's lymphoma. J Natl Cancer Inst 1995;87:524–530

48. Srinivasan R, Takahashi Y, McCoy JP et al. Overcoming graft rejection in heavily transfused and allo-immunised patients with bone marrow failure syndromes using fludarabine-based hematopoietic cell transplantation. Br J Haematol 2006;133:305–314

49. Rzepecki P, Sarosiek T, Szczylik C. Alemtuzumab, fludarabine and melphalan as a conditioning therapy in severe aplastic anemia and hypoplastic myelodysplastic syndrome – single center experience. Jpn J Clin Oncol 2006;36:46–49

50. Resnick IB, Aker M, Shapira MY et al. Allogeneic stem cell transplantation for severe acquired aplastic anemia using a fludarabine-based preparative regimen. Br J Haematol 2006;133:649–654

51. Kumar R, Prem S, Mahapatra M et al. Fludarabine, cyclophosphamide and horse antithymocyte globulin conditioning regimen for allogeneic peripheral blood stem cell transplantation performed in non-HEPA filter rooms for multiply transfused patients with severe aplastic anemia. Bone Marrow Transplant 2006;37:745–749

52. Gluckman E, Horowitz MM, Champlin RE et al. Bone marrow transplantation for severe aplastic anemia: influence of conditioning and graft-versus-host disease prophylaxis regimens on outcome. Blood 1992;79:269–275

53. Storb R, Deeg HJ, Farewell V et al. Marrow transplantation for severe aplastic anemia: methotrexate alone compared with a combination of methotrexate and cyclosporine for prevention of acute graft-versus-host disease. Blood 1986;68:119–125

54. Storb R, Sanders JE, Pepe M et al. Graft-versus-host disease prophylaxis with methotrexate/cyclosporine in children with severe aplastic anemia treated with cyclophosphamide and HLA-identical marrow grafts. Blood 1991;78:1144–1145

55. Storb R, Leisenring W, Deeg HJ et al. Long-term follow-up of a randomized trial of graft-versus-host disease prevention by methotrexate/cyclosporine versus methotrexate alone in patients given marrow grafts for severe aplastic anemia. Blood 1994;83:2749–2750

56. Locatelli F, Bruno B, Zecca M et al. Cyclosporin A and short-term methotrexate versus cyclosporin A as graft versus host disease prophylaxis in patients with severe aplastic anemia given allogeneic bone marrow transplantation from an HLA-identical sibling: results of a GITMO/EBMT randomized trial. Blood 2000;96:1690–1697

57. Hamblin M, Marsh JC, Lawler M et al. Campath-1G in vivo confers a low incidence of graft-versus-host disease associated with a high incidence of mixed chimerism after bone marrow transplantation for severe aplastic anemia using HLA-identical sibling donors. Bone Marrow Transplant 1996;17:819–824

58. Gupta V, Ball SE, Sage D et al. Marrow transplants from matched unrelated donors for aplastic anemia using alemtuzumab, fludarabine and cyclophosphamide based conditioning. Bone Marrow Transplant 2005;35:467–471

59. Schrezenmeier H, Bredeson C, Bruno B et al. Comparison of allogeneic bone marrow and peripheral blood stem cell transplantation for aplastic anemia: collaborative study of European Blood and Marrow Transplant Group (EBMT) and International Bone Marrow Transplant Registry (IBMTR). Blood 2003;102:79a (abstr)

60. Elfenbein GJ, Sackstein R. Primed marrow for autologous and allogeneic transplantation: a review comparing primed marrow to mobilized blood and steady-state marrow. Exp Hematol 2004;32:327–339

61. Morton J, Hutchins C, Durrant S. Granulocyte-colony-stimulating factor (G-CSF)-primed allogeneic bone marrow: significantly less graft-versus-host disease and comparable engraftment to G-CSF-mobilized peripheral blood stem cells. Blood 2001;98:3186–3191

62. Niederwieser D, Pepe M, Storb R et al. Improvement in rejection, engraftment rate and survival without increase in graft-versus-host disease by high marrow cell dose in patients transplanted for aplastic anemia. Br J Haematol 1988;69:23–28

63. Storb R, Prentice RL, Thomas ED. Marrow transplantation for treatment of aplastic anemia. An analysis of factors associated with graft rejection. N Engl J Med 1977;296:61–66

64. Champlin RE, Horowitz MM, van Bekkum DW et al. Graft failure following bone marrow transplantation for severe aplastic anemia: risk factors and treatment results. Blood 1989;73:606–613

65. McCann SR, Bacigalupo A, Gluckman E et al. Graft rejection and second bone marrow transplants for acquired aplastic anemia: a report from the Aplastic Anemia Working Party of the European Bone Marrow Transplant Group. Bone Marrow Transplant 1994;13:233–237

66. Hows JM, Palmer S, Gordon-Smith EC. Use of cyclosporin A in allogeneic bone marrow transplantation for severe aplastic anemia. Transplantation 1982;33:382–386

67. Stucki A, Leisenring W, Sandmaier BM et al. Decreased rejection and improved survival of first and second marrow transplants for severe aplastic anemia (a 26-year retrospective analysis). Blood 1998;92:2742–2749

68. Deeg HJ, Leisenring W, Storb R et al. Long-term outcome after marrow transplantation for severe aplastic anemia. Blood 1998;91:3637–3645

69. Syrjala KL, Langer SL, Abrams JR et al. Recovery and long-term function after hematopoietic cell transplantation for leukemia or lymphoma. JAMA 2004;291:2335–2343

70. Sanders JE, Hawley J, Levy W et al. Pregnancies following high-dose cyclophosphamide with or without high-dose busulfan or total-body irradiation and bone marrow transplantation. Blood 1996;87:3045–3052

71. Anserini P, Chiodi S, Spinelli S et al. Semen analysis following allogeneic bone marrow transplantation. Additional data for evidence-based counselling. Bone Marrow Transplant 2002;30:447–451

72. Rovo A, Tichelli A, Passweg JR et al. Spermatogenesis in long-term survivors after allogeneic hematopoietic stem cells transplantation is associated with age, time interval since transplantation and apparently with absence of chronic GvHD. Blood 2006;108(3):1100–1105

73. Kyriacou C, Kottaridis PD, Eliahoo J et al. Germ cell damage and Leydig cell insufficiency in recipients of nonmyeloablative transplantation for hematological malignancies. Bone Marrow Transplant 2003;31:45–50

74. Kojima S, Horibe K, Inaba J et al. Long-term outcome of acquired aplastic anemia in children: comparison between immunosuppressive therapy and bone marrow transplantation. Br J Haematol 2000;111:321–328

75. Socie G, Rosenfeld S, Frickhofen N et al. Late clonal diseases of treated aplastic anemia. Semin Hematol 2000;37:91–101

76. Deeg HJ, Socie G, Schoch G et al. Malignancies after marrow transplantation for aplastic anemia and fanconi anemia: a joint Seattle and Paris analysis of results in 700 patients. Blood 1996;87:386–392

77. Rosenfeld S, Follmann D, Nunez O, Young NS. Antithymocyte globulin and cyclosporine for severe aplastic anemia: association between hematologic response and long-term outcome. JAMA 2003;289:1130–1135

78. Frickhofen N, Heimpel H, Kaltwasser JP, Schrezenmeier H. Antithymocyte globulin with or without cyclosporin A: 11-year follow-up of a randomized trial comparing treatments of aplastic anemia. Blood 2003;101:1236–1242

79. Marsh JC, Zomas A, Hows JM et al. Avascular necrosis after treatment of aplastic anemia with antilymphocyte globulin and high-dose methylprednisolone. Br J Haematol 1993;84:731–735

80. Gluckman E, Rokicka-Milewska R, Hann I et al. Results and follow-up of a phase III randomized study of recombinant human-granulocyte stimulating factor as support for immunosuppressive therapy in patients with severe aplastic anemia. Br J Haematol 2002;119:1075–1082

81. Kojima S, Ohara A, Tsuchida M et al. Risk factors for evolution of acquired aplastic anemia into myelodysplastic syndrome and acute myeloid leukemia after immunosuppressive therapy in children. Blood 2002;100:786–790

82. Viollier R, Passweg J, Gregor M et al. Quality-adjusted survival analysis shows differences in outcome after immunosuppression or bone marrow transplantation in aplastic anemia. Ann Hematol 2005;84:47–55

83. Di Bona E, Rodeghiero F, Bruno B et al. Rabbit antithymocyte globulin (r-ATG) plus cyclosporine and granulocyte colony stimulating factor is an effective treatment for aplastic anemia patients unresponsive to a first course of intensive immunosuppressive therapy. Gruppo Italiano Trapianto di Midollo Osseo (GITMO). Br J Haematol 1999;107:330–334

84. Tichelli A, Passweg J, Nissen C et al. Repeated treatment with horse antilymphocyte globulin for severe aplastic anemia. Br J Haematol 1998;100:393–400

85. Schrezenmeier H, Marin P, Raghavachar A et al. Relapse of aplastic anemia after immunosuppressive treatment: a report from the European Bone Marrow Transplantation Group SAA Working Party. Br J Haematol 1993;85:371–377

86. Scheinberg P, Nunez O, Young NS. Retreatment with rabbit anti-thymocyte globulin and ciclosporin for patients with relapsed or refractory severe aplastic anemia. Br J Haematol 2006;133:622–627

87. Gupta V, Gordon-Smith EC, Cook G et al. A third course of anti-thymocyte globulin in aplastic anemia is only beneficial in previous responders. Br J Haematol 2005;129:110–117

88. Bacigalupo A, Hows J, Gordon-Smith EC et al. Bone marrow transplantation for severe aplastic anemia from donors other than HLA identical siblings: a report of the BMT Working Party. Bone Marrow Transplant 1988;3:531–535

89. Champlin RE, Feig SA, Sparkes RS, Galen RP. Bone marrow transplantation from identical twins in the treatment of aplastic anemia: implication for the pathogenesis of the disease. Br J Haematol 1984;56:455–463

90. Hinterberger W, Rowlings PA, Hinterberger-Fischer M et al. Results of transplanting bone marrow from genetically identical twins into patients with aplastic anemia. Ann Intern Med 1997;126:116–122

91. Hows J, Szydlo R, Anasetti C et al. Unrelated donor marrow transplants for severe acquired aplastic anemia. Bone Marrow Transplant 1992;10(suppl 1):102–106

92. Passweg JR, Perez WS, Eapen M et al. Bone marrow transplants from mismatched related and unrelated donors for severe aplastic anemia. Bone Marrow Transplant 2006;37:641–649

93. Kojima S, Matsuyama T, Kato S et al. Outcome of 154 patients with severe aplastic anemia who received transplants from unrelated donors: the Japan Marrow Donor Program. Blood 2002;100:799–803

94. Benesch M, Urban C, Sykora KW et al. Transplantation of highly purified CD34+ progenitor cells from alternative donors in children with refractory severe aplastic anemia. Br J Haematol 2004;125:58–63

95. Barker JN, Weisdorf DJ, Defor TE et al. Transplantation of 2 partially HLA-matched umbilical cord blood units to enhance engraftment in adults with hematologic malignancy. Blood 2005;105:1343–1347

96. Mao P, Zhu Z, Wang H et al. Sustained and stable hematopoietic donor-recipient mixed chimerism after unrelated cord blood transplantation for adult patients with severe aplastic anemia. Eur J Hematol 2005;75:430–435

97. Lacerda JF, Martins C, Carmo JA et al. Haploidentical stem cell transplantation with purified CD34+ cells after a chemotherapy-alone conditioning regimen in heavily transfused severe aplastic anemia. Biol Blood Marrow Transplant 2005;11:399–400

98. Tzeng CH, Chen PM, Fan S et al. CY/TBI-800 as a pretransplant regimen for allogeneic bone marrow transplantation for severe aplastic anemia using HLA-haploidentical family donors. Bone Marrow Transplant 1996;18:273–277

99. Woodard P, Cunningham JM, Benaim E et al. Effective donor lymphohematopoietic reconstitution after haploidentical CD34+-selected hematopoietic stem cell transplantation in children with refractory severe aplastic anemia. Bone Marrow Transplant 2004;33:411–418

100. Yabe H, Inoue H, Matsumoto M et al. Unmanipulated HLA-haploidentical bone marrow transplantation for the treatment of fatal, nonmalignant diseases in children and adolescents. Int J Hematol 2004;80:78–82

101. D'Andrea AD, Grompe M. Molecular biology of Fanconi anemia: implications for diagnosis and therapy. Blood 1997;90:1725–1736

102. Taniguchi T, D'Andrea AD. Molecular pathogenesis of Fanconi anemia: recent progress. Blood 2006;107:4223–4233

103. Meetei AR, Levitus M, Xue Y et al. X-linked inheritance of Fanconi anemia complementation group B. Nat Genet 2004;36:1219–1224

104. Alter B. Inherited bone marrow failure syndromes. In: Nathan and Oski's hematology of infancy and childhood, 6th edn. WB Saunders, Philadelphia, 2003;280–365

105. Joenje H, Patel KJ. The emerging genetic and molecular basis of Fanconi anemia. Nat Rev Genet 2001;2:446–457

106. Shimamura A, D'Andrea AD. Subtyping of Fanconi anemia patients: implications for clinical management. Blood 2003;102:3459

107. Cassinat B, Guardiola P, Chevret S et al. Constitutive elevation of serum alpha-fetoprotein in Fanconi anemia. Blood 2000;96:859–863

108. Kutler DI, Singh B, Satagopan J et al. A 20-year perspective on the International Fanconi Anemia Registry (IFAR). Blood 2003;101:1249–1256

109. Butturini A, Gale RP, Verlander PC et al. Hematologic abnormalities in Fanconi anemia: an International Fanconi Anemia Registry study. Blood 1994;84:1650–1655

110. Gluckman E, Devergie A, Schaison G et al. Bone marrow transplantation in Fanconi anemia. Br J Haematol 1980;45:557–564

111. Berger R, Bernheim A, Gluckman E, Gisselbrecht C. In vitro effect of cyclophosphamide metabolites on chromosomes of Fanconi anemia patients. Br J Haematol 1980;45:565–568

112. Socie G, Gluckman E, Raynal B et al. Bone marrow transplantation for Fanconi anemia using low-dose cyclophosphamide/thoracoabdominal irradiation as conditioning regimen: chimerism study by the polymerase chain reaction. Blood 1993;82:2249–2256

113. Gluckman E, Auerbach AD, Horowitz MM et al. Bone marrow transplantation for Fanconi anemia. Blood 1995;86:2856–2862

114. Kohli-Kumar M, Morris C, DeLaat C et al. Bone marrow transplantation in Fanconi anemia using matched sibling donors. Blood 1994;84:2050–2054

115. Guardiola P, Socie G, Pasquini R et al. Allogeneic stem cell transplantation for Fanconi anemia. Severe Aplastic Anemia Working Party of the EBMT and EUFAR. European Group for Blood and Marrow Transplantation. Bone Marrow Transplant 1998;21(suppl 2):S24–27

116. Socie G, Devergie A, Girinski T et al. Transplantation for Fanconi's anemia: long-term follow-up of fifty patients transplanted from a sibling donor after low-dose cyclophosphamide and thoraco-abdominal irradiation for conditioning. Br J Haematol 1998;103:249–255

117. Guardiola P, Socie G, Li X et al. Acute graft-versus-host disease in patients with Fanconi anemia or acquired aplastic anemia undergoing bone marrow transplantation from HLA-identical sibling donors: risk factors and influence on outcome. Blood 2004;103:73–77

118. Guardiola P, Pasquini R, Dokal I et al. Outcome of 69 allogeneic stem cell transplantations for Fanconi anemia using HLA-matched unrelated donors: a study on behalf of the European Group for Blood and Marrow Transplantation. Blood 2000;95:422–429

119. MacMillan ML, Auerbach AD, Davies SM et al. Hematopoietic cell transplantation in patients with Fanconi anemia using alternate donors: results of a total body irradiation dose escalation trial. Br J Haematol 2000;109:121–129

120. Bitan M, Or R, Shapira MY et al. Fludarabine-based reduced intensity conditioning for stem cell transplantation of fanconi anemia patients from fully matched related and unrelated donors. Biol Blood Marrow Transplant 2006;12:712–718

121. de la Fuente J, Reiss S, McCloy M et al. Non-TBI stem cell transplantation protocol for Fanconi anemia using HLA-compatible sibling and unrelated donors. Bone Marrow Transplant 2003;32:653–656

122. Tan PL, Wagner JE, Auerbach AD et al. Successful engraftment without radiation after fludarabine-based regimen in Fanconi anemia patients undergoing genotypically identical donor hematopoietic cell transplantation. Pediatr Blood Cancer 2006;46:630–636

123. Guardiola P, Kurre P, Vlad A et al. Effective graft-versus-leukaemia effect after allogeneic stem cell transplantation using reduced-intensity preparative regimens in Fanconi anaemia patients with myelodysplastic syndrome or acute myeloid leukaemia. Br J Haematol 2003;122:806–809

124. Boyer MW, Gross TG, Loechelt B et al. Low risk of graft-versus-host disease with transplantation of CD34 selected peripheral blood progenitor cells from alternative donors for Fanconi anemia. J Pediatr Hematol Oncol 2003;25:890–895

125. Nobili B, Rossi G, De Stefano P et al. Successful umbilical cord blood transplantation in a child with dyskeratosis congenita after a fludarabine-based reduced-intensity conditioning regimen. Br J Haematol 2002;119:573–574

126. Brazzola P, Duval M, Fournet JC et al. Fatal diffuse capillaritis after hematopoietic stem-cell transplantation for dyskeratosis congenita despite low-intensity conditioning regimen. Bone Marrow Transplant 2005;36:1103–1105; author reply 1105

127. Dror Y, Freedman MH, Leaker M et al. Low-intensity hematopoietic stem-cell transplantation across human leukocyte antigen barriers in dyskeratosis congenita. Bone Marrow Transplant 2003;31:847–850

Thalassemia and sickle cell disease

CHAPTER 17

Irene AG Roberts and Josu de la Fuente

Introduction

Advances in supportive care for patients with thalassemia and sickle cell disease have dramatically improved life expectancy. Nevertheless, patients continue to suffer disabling symptoms, particularly during their adult years, and most will die prematurely from complications of the disorders and/or their treatment. Stem cell transplantation (SCT) offers the only proven cure, effecting both resolution of the symptoms of disease and freedom from life-long emotionally and physically demanding treatment. For hemoglobinopathy patients and their physicians, the decision to undergo SCT, given the inherent risks involved, is difficult since these disorders are not usually immediately life-threatening. In this chapter we address the most important issues to consider in each case and summarize the evidence available to help patients and their healthcare teams decide whether or not to proceed.

Stem cell transplantation for thalassemia major

Clinical features and natural history of thalassemia

Recent estimates suggest that worldwide more than 120,000 children with thalassemia are born annually.[1] The highest prevalence is in families who live in or originate from the Indian subcontinent and Middle East. Virtually all those eligible for SCT have β-thalassemia major but occasional cases of β-thalassemia intermedia and HbE-β-thalassemia also benefit from SCT,[2] as do the rare children with α-thalassemia major who survive in good health after prenatal diagnosis and intrauterine transfusion.[3]

Thalassemia major presents with anemia and failure to thrive during the first year of life. Most children also have hepatosplenomegaly at presentation due to extramedullary hematopoiesis. Without red cell transfusion most children with thalassemia major die before the end of the first decade. Where red cell transfusion is available, most patients start regular transfusions before their first birthday and, in the absence of curative therapy, will remain dependent on 3–4 weekly red cell transfusions throughout life.[4] Transfusion ameliorates the symptoms of anemia, restores normal growth, reduces the increased iron absorption and prevents the adverse effects of extramedullary hematopoiesis in the chest, abdomen and skeleton.[5] Unfortunately, all patients develop transfusion-associated iron overload which leads to progressive multiorgan failure particularly affecting the heart, liver,

pancreas and pituitary. The resultant cardiac arrhythmias, cardiac failure, cirrhosis, diabetes and impaired growth and pubertal development contribute to the high mortality in the third decade unless effective iron chelation therapy is used, even in developed countries.[6] Compliance with iron chelation is the major predictor of life expectancy in transfused patients with thalassemia: for those who comply well with treatment, recent data indicate that up to 68–92% survive into their fourth decade albeit with considerable morbidity;[7,8] for those who do not comply well with iron chelation therapy, few survive beyond the age of 35 years.[6,7]

Treatment options for thalassemia

There are two broad treatment options for thalassemia major: regular red cell transfusions together with iron chelation, or SCT. SCT is the only proven curative option; gene therapy trials are beginning and offer promise for the future but are likely to face many modifications before they translate into clinical benefit for patients.[9,10] It is vital that transplant physicians remain up to date with advances in non-SCT options for therapy; changes in efficacy and tolerability of iron chelators or safety of blood transfusion must be included in decisions made about proceeding to SCT. In most developed countries, risks of blood transfusion have fallen due to patient vaccination, leukocyte depletion and donor testing to reduce transfusion-associated infections, and red cell phenotyping to minimize alloimmunization. However, risks of prion-associated or unknown pathogens remain a concern[11] and difficulties with vascular access and the complications of implanted venous access devices affect many patients for much of their lives.[12]

Iron chelation, like transfusion, is a life-long requirement. The most widely used and effective iron chelator in thalassemia is desferrioxamine; this is expensive and difficult to use since it is administered parenterally at least four times per week, usually by nightly subcutaneous infusions, and must be monitored closely to prevent toxicity.[12] Compliance has improved using well-designed needles (e.g. Thalaset™), local anesthetic cream, rotating injection sites, balloon infusers and support from clinical nurse specialists. Therefore, families should have access to full psychosocial support to achieve the best possible compliance with iron chelation before deciding that SCT is the best option for their child. The recent availability of two oral iron chelators, deferiprone and desferasirox, may alter long-term morbidity and mortality due to iron overload in thalassemia. Deferiprone has impressive ability to remove cardiac iron but must be taken three times daily and may cause fatal agranulocytosis.[13] Desferasirox appears to be less toxic and to effectively reduce hepatic and iron overload but has only recently been licenced and its long-term effects are unknown.[14–16]

For patients with HbE-β-thalassemia or thalassemia intermedia, treatment is more complex and must be individually tailored as these diseases are heterogeneous: at the more severe end of the spectrum patients are red cell transfusion dependent and may benefit from SCT;[2] those with milder disease may respond to HbF-modulating agents, splenectomy and/or intermittent red cell transfusion, and SCT is rarely considered.[17]

The role of SCT in the management of thalassemia

The most important role of SCT is the high chance of cure for individuals who otherwise face a lifetime of invasive, demanding treatment and a reduced lifespan. Improvements in medical treatment mean that survival in childhood is close to 100% where compliance with chelation is good.[8] For such children SCT offers an improved quality of life and there is no measurable impact of SCT on survival until transplanted children reach their fourth or even fifth decade, when mortality for non-transplanted patients starts to climb steeply.[6–8] On the other hand, where compliance with chelation is poor, few patients survive beyond 35 years; for these patients SCT does offer a survival advantage as well as improved quality of life.

Bone marrow transplant from HLA-identical family donors:

Most transplants for thalassemia use marrow from human leukocyte antigen (HLA)-identical sibling donors. Although fewer than half of families seeking SCT have a suitable sibling donor, many decide to extend their families, with or without prenatal diagnosis, hoping future children will be HLA identical and thalassemia free. In addition, couples are increasingly exploring preimplantation genetic diagnosis and HLA typing (PGD-H) to identify a thalassemia-free, HLA-matched sibling donor, although the success rate is currently very low.[19–21] Thalassemia trait in sibling donors is not a contraindication to SCT since it has no significant impact on outcome. To obtain sufficient stem cells the donor should usually be at least 2 years old; even where cord blood is the intended source of donor stem cells, we recommend waiting until the donor is 2 years old so 'back-up' cells are available if necessary. Where there is consanguinity, close relatives sometimes provide an HLA-identical match and it is worth obtaining an accurate family tree and carrying out extended donor testing if SCT is clearly indicated. Data from these transplants are limited but no significant difference in outcome has been reported.[22] In contrast, using mismatched relatives has a high rate of graft rejection and mortality; the only published series reported six successful outcomes with 10 transplant-related deaths and 13 graft failures.[22]

Cord blood transplantation

Cord blood stem cells from HLA-identical sibling donors for hemoglobinopathy SCT have some advantages over bone marrow: cord blood cells will often, but not always, avoid the need for a donor bone marrow harvest, they may be associated with a reduced incidence of graft-versus-host disease (GvHD) and the Eurocord data show a high survival rate (100% of 33 thalassemia patients).[23] However, these data also showed increased graft rejection (21%). This may reflect the importance of cell dose where conditioning is not consistently myeloablative[24] and although cell dose did not predict engraftment in this study, graft rejection declined when the intensity of conditioning was increased by adding thiotepa[23] or when methotrexate was not used as GvHD prophylaxis.

Peripheral blood stem cell transplantation

There are few published reports of peripheral blood stem cells (PBSC) for transplantation of hemoglobinopathy patients and no large or prospective studies.[25–28] PBSC have not generally been chosen for thalassemia SCT since most donors are young children and there has been reluctance to use granulocyte-colony stimulating factor (G-CSF) or central venous catheters. In addition, in the largest of the retrospective series, which compared 73 patients receiving PBSC and 109 patients receiving bone marrow, the risk of severe GvHD was higher in PBSC transplants (relative risk (RR) 1.94; $p = 0.036$),[28] suggesting that marrow should remain the preferred stem cell source for thalassemia SCT.

Unrelated donor SCT

Experience of unrelated donor SCT for thalassemia is limited to small numbers of patients with a variety of conditioning regimens, patient age groups and donor types and relatively short follow-up.[29–34] The largest series, an Italian multicenter collaboration, reported an overall survival of 79% and thalassemia-free survival of 66% in 32 consecutive patients with a median age of 14 years.[29] These data show the feasibility of unrelated donor SCT for thalassemia and were recently updated with similar results in a total of 68 patients.[30] However, the role of unrelated donor SCT in thalassemia remains to be established and is best investigated through carefully selected donors and well-designed, controlled clinical trials.[30,34]

The outcome of SCT for thalassemia

Survival and thalassemia-free survival

The largest series of patients treated in a single center comes from the Pesaro group who pioneered SCT for thalassemia.[35] Over a 22-year period from 1981 to 2003, 1003 consecutive patients (aged 1–35 years) were transplanted with a >20-year Kaplan Meier probability of thalassemia-free survival of 68%,[36] showing that SCT achieves long-term cure of the disease. These data include transplants from mismatched and unrelated donors as well as HLA-identical sibling donors, and adults as well as children. In current clinical practice, the vast majority of transplants are performed in children using marrow from HLA-identical siblings and for these patients most groups, including the Pesaro group, report considerably better results with an overall survival of around 90% and thalassemia-free survival of 80–90% except in those with the most severe iron overload.[18,26,36–43] The results using unrelated donors are generally poorer. The updated results from La Nasa and colleagues confirmed the earlier results of lower overall (79%) and thalassemia-free survival (66%) in their series of 68 patients compared to those obtained after HLA-identical family donor SCT, although this may reflect the relatively high median age (15 years) of the unrelated donor recipients.[30]

Prognostic factors for survival and cure after SCT

Most information about prognostic factors comes from the Pesaro group, which identified three factors which predicted outcome after SCT for thalassemia in children: hepatomegaly, liver biopsy evidence of portal fibrosis and poor compliance with chelation.[44] These three factors can be used to classify an individual as good, intermediate or poor risk (Class 1, 2 and 3, respectively). Table 17.1 shows how these risk groups predicted overall survival, thalassemia-free survival and graft rejection in the Pesaro patients.[45] These data show that even modest organ damage pre-SCT reduces the chance of a successful outcome; for example, the presence of a single risk factor confers Class 2 status and an increase in transplant-related mortality (TRM) from 6% to 15%. Early analyses of the data also showed that poor-risk

Table 17.1 Outcome of BMT for thalassemia according to the Pesaro risk classification*

	Class 1	Class 2	Class 3
Survival (%)	94	84	80
Thalassemia-free survival (%)	87	81	56
Transplant-related mortality (%)	6	15	18
Graft rejection (%)	7	4	33

* Patients were classified as Class 3 if they had all three of the following risk factors: hepatomegaly (>2 cm below costal margin); portal fibrosis on liver biopsy; and a history of irregular chelation (desferrioxamine initiated >18 months after the first transfusion or administered less than 8 hours continuously on at least 5 days per week). Patients were identified as Class 2 if they had any one or two of these risk factors and Class 1 if they had none of these risk factors (Lucarelli et al[44]). Note that changes to the conditioning regimen have subsequently improved the outcome for Class 3 patients (Sodani et al[46]).

(Class 3) patients fare extremely badly with standard conditioning regimens (TRM in the early Class 3 cohort was 47%). Initial attempts at reducing the toxicity of conditioning led to the high rate of graft rejection shown in Table 17.1 (33%).[44,45] A more recent protocol using complex conditioning starting 45 days prior to transplant has dramatically improved both overall (93%) and thalassemia-free survival (85%),[46] but it is important to see whether this approach can be replicated by others.

The Pesaro classification does not predict outcome in all centers, possibly because of smaller numbers of patients, different conditioning and/or the low TRM in many recent series: UK data on 57 consecutive patients transplanted since 1993 show 95% overall survival,[18] and in our own center only one child from the 65 thalassemic patients transplanted has died. Nevertheless, the Pesaro classification has played a crucial role in identifying patients at highest risk who may not benefit from SCT or who may need a modified protocol, and also in providing benchmarking data against which other centers can evaluate their own results.

Impact of age

In children less than 17 years old, age is not an independent predictor for outcome of SCT. However, data from studies in adults consistently show inferior overall and thalassemia-free survival. Nevertheless, using the protocol developed for poor-risk children (Pesaro Class 3), about two-thirds of young adults with thalassemia are cured: of 107 patients aged 17–35 transplanted from HLA-identical related donors, 69 survived (64%), of whom 66 are thalassemia free[47] and remain so with a median follow-up of 12 years.[48] The high TRM confirms that in older patients SCT should be reserved for highly motivated individuals, with limited organ damage, who are aware of the risks involved. This conclusion is supported by recent preliminary data on the outcome of 15 adults with thalassemia transplanted using a reduced-intensity conditioning regimen which improved TRM from 37% to 27%,[48] indicating that this should still be regarded as a high-risk procedure in adults.

TRM and complications of SCT for thalassemia

Acute GvHD and infections are the two most common causes of mortality, accounting for 32% and 24% of deaths, respectively, in the Pesaro cohort,[45] followed by chronic GvHD, hepatic and cardiac disease and marrow aplasia due to graft rejection. Severe chronic GvHD after sibling donor SCT is fairly uncommon (2–5% of patients), probably reflecting the young age of the patients and relatively non-toxic conditioning.[18,49] Abnormal liver function is a major predictor of TRM, as discussed above. In the Pesaro series this was due to iron overload and chronic viral hepatitis. Hepatitis B or C infection per se does not increase TRM or reduce thalassemia-free survival, but they are associated with hepatic fibrosis; similarly, SCT does not aggravate

pre-existing hepatitis-associated hepatic fibrosis.[50,51] An increased risk of cardiac tamponade was reported in 8/400 transplants from the Pesaro group, of which six were fatal.[52] Therefore, all patients must be evaluated for evidence of cardiac iron deposition and cardiac function abnormalities prior to SCT since neither serum ferritin nor liver iron is a reliable surrogate measure of iron-related cardiac dysfunction.[53]

Graft rejection and mixed chimerism

Graft rejection is more common after SCT for thalassemia than for most other disorders, particularly in poor-risk patients. In most studies, the overall risk of graft rejection is around 10% after both sibling donor SCT[18,42,43,45] and unrelated donor SCT.[34] Data from several studies and our own experience suggest that addition of pretransplant immune suppression with ATG or alemtuzumab appears to reduce graft rejection,[41] but there have been no controlled trials. Failure of primary engraftment with persistent aplasia is rare and has a poor outcome even with a second allogeneic transplant; overall survival in the largest series (32 patients) was 49%, with thalassemia-free survival of only 33%.[54] In this setting, autologous transplantation of previously cryopreserved cells may be a safer option than allogeneic SCT; for this reason it remains our practice to perform autologous marrow harvesting several months prior to allogeneic SCT in all thalassemic patients.

Most patients who develop graft rejection have no, or a very transient, aplastic phase, instead experiencing prompt recovery of autologous thalassemic hematopoiesis and recurrence of transfusion-dependent anemia. Graft rejection most often occurs in the first 6 months after SCT,[24,55] although late rejection after the first 2 years has been reported.[56,57] Autologous reconstitution can be difficult to diagnose in the early stages, since patients are usually well and the only clue is usually increasing or maintained red cell transfusion dependence. Therefore, monthly measurement of donor/host chimerism for the first 3–6 months is recommended; this can be easily performed on peripheral blood mononuclear cells.[24] All patients with residual detectable host cells should be monitored, since serially falling levels of donor cells usually predict secondary graft rejection.[24,56] In this setting, withdrawal of immune suppression may re-establish donor hemopoiesis.[58] Anecdotal experience suggests that donor lymphocyte infusion (DLI) rarely reverses established rejection, although occasional successful cases have been reported,[57] and it is likely that DLI needs to be given early in the rejection process.

Mixed hematopoietic chimerism is common, occurring in up to one-third of patients.[24,55] A review of 295 patients showed that in the first 2 months post transplant, 95 (32%) had mixed chimerism; by the second year 42 of these had become fully donor, 33 had progressed to rejection and 20 had persistent mixed chimerism of 30–90% donor cells.[55] Interestingly, all of these latter patients remained well, off transfusions, with a stable hemoglobin >8 g/dl 2–11 years post-SCT.[56] These findings imply that complete ablation of donor hemopoiesis is not necessary for long-term cure, supporting data from animal models[59] and anecdotal reports of cure of thalassemia after non-myeloablative conditioning (discussed below).[60–62]

Conditioning regimens

Most conditioning regimens employ a combination of chemotherapy, using busulfan and cyclophosphamide, and immunosuppression with ciclosporin and methotrexate.[18,35] Methotrexate is generally omitted in cord blood transplants because it is associated with a significantly increased risk of graft rejection,[23] and some groups, including our own, also use lower than conventional doses of methotrexate after bone marrow transplant (BMT) for the same reason (2 doses of 10 mg/

m²), although evidence is lacking to support this approach.[18,46] Several groups have added antithymocyte globulin (ATG) or alemtuzumab to reduce graft rejection, with apparent success,[18,46] although there are no controlled trials to support this. Others have used melphalan,[42] thiotepa[23,34] or fludarabine in addition to[34,46] or in place of cyclophosphamide,[63] without an increase in short-term toxicity and with good engraftment rates even in Class 3 patients.

The optimum dose of busulfan is difficult to ascertain as there is considerable interindividual variation in its metabolism.[64–67] Doses of more than 16 mg/kg are toxic but lower doses are associated with increased graft rejection.[44,68,69] The most widely used regimen, and the one we have used since 1992, is a total busulfan dose of 14 mg/kg given over 4 days followed by cyclophosphamide 200 mg/kg over the next 4 days.[18,35] This regimen is generally well tolerated. The low rates of mucositis mean that opiates and parenteral nutrition are usually unnecessary. Some groups measure blood busulfan levels to optimize the dose but there is no evidence that this has a significant impact on overall or thalassemia-free survival.[43,65,70] These problems with dosing are one of the reasons why it is generally not recommended to transplant children under the age of 18 months.

As previously mentioned, a reduced dose of cyclophosphamide is recommended for Pesaro Class 3 patients to avoid a high TRM[46,69] but must be combined with other measures to prevent graft rejection. The most recent Pesaro protocol showed a much improved rejection rate (8%) when hypertransfusion and hydroxyurea were used to suppress erythropoiesis for several weeks prior to SCT and fludarabine was added to the conditioning regimen.[46] Other approaches to reducing toxicity include new drugs, such as intravenous busulfan[71] or treosulfan,[72] which are being investigated in small trials and non-myeloablative conditioning regimens.

Long-term effects of SCT for thalassemia major

Long-term effects of SCT are influenced by age at SCT, conditioning regimen, peritransplant complications and pre-existing damage due to thalassemia and iron overload.

Iron overload

Iron overload improves slowly post transplant but can be accelerated by 'de-ironing' by regular phlebotomy or chelation with desferrioxamine.[73–75] 'De-ironing' usually begins 9–12 months after SCT and continues until the total iron burden is approaching normal (i.e. liver iron <7 mg/g dry liver weight or serum ferritin <300 ng/ml). Recent evidence confirms the importance of reducing iron overload post-SCT in patients infected with hepatitis B and/or C who otherwise have a high risk of progression to severe liver fibrosis.[76]

Growth and development

It is difficult to separate the effects of SCT from those of iron overload since up to two-thirds of non-transplanted thalassemics have growth or developmental delay.[4,7] For children transplanted early (<8 years old), growth after transplant is normal. However, older children and those in Pesaro Class 3 may have impaired growth.[77,78] Growth hormone is rarely required but may be effective in milder cases.[79] About 37% of boys and 60% of girls fail to enter puberty spontaneously if transplanted, a proportion similar to those treated medically.[80,81] The majority of girls transplanted after puberty develop secondary amenorrhea, whereas most boys transplanted after puberty have normal testosterone and gonadotrophin levels.[81] There are few data on fertility post-SCT for thalassemia. Three successful pregnancies from women who had undergone SCT for thalassemia have been reported,[35,82] and three men have had normal, spontaneous paterni-

ties.[83] However, comprehensive studies of fertility after busulfan/cyclophosphamide conditioning in other disorders suggest infertility is likely to be common.[84,85] Recent advances in cryopreservation of testicular and ovarian tissue show great promise even for prepubertal children, and it is important to discuss available options fully with parents and children prior to SCT as many units are now able to offer this service.[86–88]

Secondary malignancy

The largest series recently reported a total of eight malignancies in their cohort of patients transplanted for hemoglobinopathies, giving a prevalence of 0.8%.[83] Three patients developed post-transplant lymphomas and one a late non-Hodgkin's lymphoma. A further four patients developed solid tumors: one case each of spinocellular cancer, Kaposi's sarcoma, melanoma and colon cancer.

Indications for SCT in thalassemia major

General considerations

The most important question for patients, their families and their physician to consider when deciding whether or not to proceed to SCT is: will it improve the prospect of long-term survival and/or quality of life? There are no controlled trials of SCT versus transfusion and no adequate quality of life studies to help answer this question. However, some reasonably firm conclusions can be drawn. Recent data show that patients who comply well with iron chelation and have no evidence of cardiac or liver damage can expect to survive into the fifth decade of life and probably beyond,[7,8] although it is very difficult to select this group of patients in childhood. Since the TRM associated with SCT is 2–5% and the risk of graft failure is around 5%, such patients have a predicted survival of around 90–95% into their mid-thirties with either therapeutic approach, and the decision to proceed to SCT will be based on quality of life – the perceived benefit of being free from life-long transfusions, chelation therapy and their long-term complications. By contrast, for patients with a history of poor compliance, it is clear that few survive into their mid-thirties, and for these patients SCT offers not only an improved quality of life but also a much greater chance of long-term survival.[89]

Recommendations (Table 17.2)

We suggest that SCT should be offered to all families of children with thalassemia major where the child is less than 16 years of age and there is a suitable HLA-identical family donor. The risks, benefits and alternatives should be fully discussed, and the decision should not be hurried. Where compliance is poor despite optimal support to the family, SCT offers a survival advantage, and the majority of families will choose SCT because of the perceived improvement in quality of life and the removal of much of the uncertainty about future health once the first few months after SCT have passed.

The most difficult decisions are identifying the best option for children less than 16 years old who comply well with chelation, patients more than 16 years old for whom the risks of SCT are much higher, and poor compliers without HLA-identical family donors. For children without HLA-identical family donors, SCT using an unrelated donor may be an option in experienced centers if all approaches to medical treatment fail and SCT is undertaken as part of a controlled clinical trial. The role of SCT for thalassemia patients more than 16 years of age is unclear. For some highly motivated individuals 17–35 years of age, the benefits of SCT may just exceed the risks using current conditioning regimens, and it is reasonable for experienced centers to consider SCT if there is an HLA-identical sibling or extended haplotype-matched unrelated donor.

Table 17.2 Indications for SCT in thalassemia major

Definite indication for SCT
Transfusion-dependent thalassemia major
Age ≤16 years
HLA-identical sibling donor
Patients who meet all these criteria should be offered SCT in conjunction with detailed counseling about the risks, benefits and alternatives.
Candidates who may be considered for SCT in special circumstances

Transfusion-dependent thalassemia major
    Age 17–35 years *or*
    ≤16 years old, with an HLA-identical *non-sibling* family member

Thalassemia relapsing after previous SCT
Transfusion dependent Sβ^0 thalassemia
Factors affecting the decision to transplant a patient with thalassemia
Likelihood of cure and TRM
Risk of extensive chronic GvHD
Importance of fertility
Age of the patient
Availability of an HLA-identical donor
Predicted long-term survival without SCT based on compliance and iron overload

Table 17.3 Clinical features of sickle cell disease

All patients
Chronic hemolytic anemia
Increased susceptibility to infections
Recurrent painful vaso-occlusive crises
Reduced life expectancy (homozygous sickle cell disease)
Acute problems
Acute chest syndrome
Mesenteric crises
Splenic and hepatic sequestration
Aplastic crisis due to parvovirus B19
Priapism
Chronic organ damage
CNS damage, including overt stroke, seizures, occult damage
Chronic sickle lung disease
Chronic renal damage – renal failure, papillary necrosis, malignancy
Cardiomyopathy
Pulmonary hypertension

Prospects for improved management of thalassemia major in the future

Advances in medical treatment and in prevention of transplant-related complications over the next decade will influence the decisions of physicians and their patients about the role of SCT. The main advances in medical treatment are likely to come from 'tailored' chelation regimes based on magnetic resonance imaging (MRI) assessment of liver and heart,[90] greater knowledge about the long-term effects of the new oral iron chelators, improvements in red cell matching and safety and greater understanding of the impact of genotypic differences on the complications of thalassemia and treatment response.[91] In SCT, the main advances should focus on development of effective non-myeloablative conditioning to reduce transplant-related toxicity without the currently observed high risk of graft rejection. Finally, clinical trials of gene therapy have now begun bringing the prospect of cure to all those with thalassemia major and not just those with an HLA-identical donor.[9,10]

Stem cell transplant for sickle cell disease

Clinical features and natural history of sickle cell disease

Worldwide, approximately 250,000 children are born with sickle cell disease every year, the majority of them in underdeveloped countries where most die in the first few years of life.[1] Even in developed countries, the median survival for patients with the most severe and most common form of the disease (homozygous sickle cell disease) is 45 years, and more than 10% of children die before reaching adulthood.[92,93] In most centers, including our own, only patients with homozygous sickle cell disease and sickle-β^0 thalassemia, another severe sickling disorder, are considered for SCT. The frequency and severity of sickle-related complications are much lower in milder forms of the disease, such as hemoglobin SC disease and sickle-β$^+$ thalassemia, and SCT would only rarely be indicated in such patients. The remainder of this chapter will therefore focus entirely on the two severe forms and will refer to them collectively as sickle cell disease.

The clinical course of sickle cell disease is very variable, both between patients and in a single patient over time.[94] This unpredictability is one of the biggest problems for both families and physicians in managing the disease and in identifying the patients likely to benefit most from SCT. The main clinical features are shown in Table 17.3. Symptoms usually begin around the age of 2 years and persist throughout life. Many patients experience episodes of sickle-related acute chest syndrome with rapidly developing respiratory distress (life-long risk around 40%); this is recurrent in most patients and has a fatality rate of 1% per episode in children and almost 10% in adults.[95] Patients with sickle cell disease also have a life-long increased risk of stroke of around 25%.[96,97] Chronic damage increases with age and can affect almost any organ including the heart, lungs, liver, kidneys, bones and brain.[98–100] The most common causes of death are acute chest syndrome, infection and multiorgan failure.[95,98,101]

Treatment options for sickle cell disease

Treatment options depend on the nature and severity of the clinical problems. All patients require preventive measures and supportive treatment (penicillin, vaccination, folic acid and analgesia and psychosocial support for painful crises). For those with severe recurrent painful crises, the mainstay of treatment is hydroxyurea which reduces the frequency and severity of crises in the majority of adults and children.[102–104] Hydroxyurea is also the treatment of choice to prevent recurrent chest syndrome[104] and, used long-term, reduces mortality.[99] While hydroxyurea has improved the outlook for many severely affected patients, SCT offers the only available cure and should be considered where hydroxyurea has failed.[104,105]

Management of sickle cell disease patients with stroke requires a different approach. The risk of recurrent stroke after a first episode is at least 67%, particularly within the first 3 years.[97] This risk can be reduced to around 10% by monthly red cell transfusions.[97] Most patients develop transfusion-associated iron overload and require iron chelation after 12–18 months of transfusion. Duration of transfusion therapy is controversial, but for the majority of children, persistence

Table 17.4 Indications for BMT in sickle cell disease

Criteria for inclusion
1. Age <16 years and HLA-matched sibling donor
2. One or more of the following:
(a) Sickle cell disease related neurologic deficit, stroke or subarachnoid hemorrhage
(b) Recurrent acute sickle chest syndrome (>2 episodes) which has failed to respond to a trial of hydroxyurea of at least 6 months or where hydroxyurea is contraindicated
(c) Recurrent, severe debilitating pain due to vaso-occlusive crises which has failed to respond to a trial of hydroxyurea of at least 6 months or where hydroxyurea is contraindicated
(d) Problems relating to future medical care, e.g. unavailability of adequately screened blood products

Exclusions
1. Donor with major hemoglobinopathy
2. One or more of the following: (a) Karnofsky performance score <70%, (b) major intellectual impairment, (c) moderate/severe portal fibrosis, (d) glomerular filtration rate <30% predicted, (e) stage III and IV sickle lung disease, (f) cardiomyopathy and (g) HIV infection.

Modified from the British Paediatric Haematology Forum Criteria (Amrolia et al[105]).

of cerebral white matter changes on MRI or of angiopathy on MRA and Doppler studies will lead to transfusion programs being continued throughout childhood.[106–108] In this situation, SCT should be considered as the main alternative to prolonged transfusions with chelation; hydroxyurea at best ameliorates the disease and there is no good evidence yet that it can prevent stroke.[103,109–111]

Role of SCT in the management of sickle cell disease

Indications for SCT in sickle cell disease are summarized in Table 17.4. Although sickle cell disease is heterogeneous, the presence of specific clinical features (such as recurrent severe painful crises over a number of years, recurrent acute chest syndrome and stroke) helps to mark out a population of patients with a poor prognosis.[92,98,112,113]

SCT from HLA-identical family donors

The majority of SCT have been carried out using bone marrow from HLA-identical siblings. Unfortunately, only one in five children who fulfills the criteria for SCT has a suitable HLA-identical sibling donor.[114,115] It is unusual to find an HLA-matched family donor in the extended family given the low rate of consanguinity. PGD-H is increasingly sought by families with no HLA-identical sibling donors. Sickle cell trait in the donor is not a contraindication to transplantation.

Cord blood and unrelated donor transplantation

Data regarding cord blood transplantation are still limited. Related cord blood transplantation is feasible and effective,[23] and directed donation (collection of cord blood from unaffected siblings) is now common practice in sickle cell disease and thalassemia.[116] As with thalassemia, there may be an increased risk of graft rejection.[23] This can be minimized by adding thiotepa and omitting methotrexate from post-SCT GvHD prophylaxis, but we recommend autologous marrow harvesting prior to all hemoglobinopathy SCT because of this risk, and also deferring SCT until the cord blood donor is at least 2 years of age to allow a bone marrow 'top-up' infusion to be given if necessary. The use of volunteer unrelated donors might considerably expand the availability of SCT for patients with sickle cell disease. However, a recent study found that fewer than 5% of patients would have an HLA-matched cord blood unit available[117] and, to date, the experience of this approach is limited to case reports.[118,119]

Table 17.5 Results of major published series of myeloablative BMT for sickle cell disease

	Walters et al 2000[123] (n = 50)	Bernaudin et al 1997[121] (n = 26)	Vermylen et al 1998[122] (n = 50)
Overall survival	94% (6 yr)	92% (8 yr)	93% (11 yr)
Event-free survival	84% (6 yr)	75% (8 yr)	82% (11 yr)
Graft rejection*	10%	18%	10%
Acute GvHD ≥Grade 2	7.7%	23%	20%
Chronic GvHD – limited	Not available	7.7%	14%
Chronic GvHD – extensive	3.8%	7.7%	6%

* All had autologous reconstitution with relapse of sickle cell disease.

The outcome of SCT for sickle cell disease

Survival and disease-free survival

Approximately 250 patients with sickle cell disease have been transplanted worldwide, virtually all of them less than 16 years of age.[120] There are three major series from France, Belgium and an international group of 27 American and European centers.[121–123] These studies have all used myeloablative conditioning and their results are summarized in Table 17.5. Overall survival was just over 90% and disease-free survival 82–86%; TRM was 7–8% and graft rejection 8%.[120,124] There was no significant difference in outcome between the studies even though the French and international series included only symptomatic patients with severe disease, while the Belgian series included both symptomatic patients and very young patients with few symptoms. However, interestingly, the Belgian data showed that the children with more severe disease (n = 36) had less good overall survivals (88%) and disease-free survivals (75%) than did the small number of young children (n = 14) who had been transplanted early before overt sickle-related complications (overall survivals 100%, disease-free survivals 93%).[124] In all of the studies, no patients with stable engraftment any longer had clinical manifestations of sickle cell disease.

Prognostic factors

None of the studies to date is sufficiently large to allow identification of independent prognostic factors. However, it is worth noting that in contrast to the encouraging results in children less than 16 years of age, the results of SCT with full myeloablative conditioning in adults have been generally disappointing with as many deaths as survivors reported, although the numbers are very small,[120,125] supporting the investigation of reduced-intensity regimens (see below).

Transplant-related mortality and other complications

The most common causes of death are GvHD and infections. Acute GvHD occurs in 20–30% of transplants but is seldom severe.[120–122] Hemorrhagic cystitis, pneumococcal sepsis, veno-occlusive disease and aseptic necrosis have all been described, as with SCT for other disorders.[122] More important is the risk of neurologic problems. Patients with sickle cell disease have a markedly increased risk of neurologic complications in the peritransplant period, particularly seizures and intracranial hemorrhage. Initial results from the international study reported neurologic complications in a third of their 21 patients, particularly those with a prior history of stroke.[126] The introduction of prophylactic measures (including anticonvulsant therapy starting before SCT and continuing until at least 6 months post-SCT, maintaining the platelet count >50 × 10^9/l and hemoglobin levels between 9 and 11 g/dl, and rigorous control of levels of ciclosporin, magnesium and blood pressure) has reduced TRM, although a high risk of seizures (20%) remains.[123] Chronic GvHD occurs in 12% of patients, around 50% of whom have had extensive disease.[121–123]

Graft rejection and mixed hemopoietic chimerism

The incidence of graft failure is fairly high at 10–18%.[120,122] In the majority of cases, rejection is accompanied by autologous reconstitution and relapse of sickle cell disease[122,123] although the HbF may remain high for many months after relapse, obviating the need to reintroduce other therapy.[127] No clear risk factors for rejection have been identified, but Bernaudin and colleagues reported that addition of ATG to pretransplant conditioning decreased rejection from 25% to 7%,[121] and Bachet et al recently reported no episodes of graft rejection in a subgroup of patients given both ATG and hydroxyurea prior to SCT.[128]

Stable mixed chimerism, without evolution to rejection, occurs in around 25% of patients given the conventional myeloablative protocol discussed below.[129,130] Occasional cases with evolving chimerism and progressively reducing donor cells occur, and restoration to 100% donor hematopoiesis by donor lymphocyte infusions has been reported.[131] These observations suggest that non-myeloablative regimens with graft manipulation by immunosuppression and DLI may improve results, although early studies have to date been disappointing, with disease-free survivals of 9–50% in the 29 patients so far reported.[120,125,132–136] Further work is needed to understand mechanisms of engraftment and rejection of allogeneic cells in sickle cell disease, and the results of ongoing studies are awaited with interest.

Conditioning regimens

The most commonly used myeloablative regimens use oral busulfan (14–16 mg/kg) and intravenous cyclophosphamide (200 mg/kg) as for thalassemia; some studies have added thiotepa, fludarabine or melphalan with the aim of reducing graft rejection, but their role is not yet clear.[125,135] Other groups, including ours, have added ATG or alemtuzumab to pre-SCT conditioning to reduce graft rejection, with encouraging results, although it is important not to employ the high doses used by others to prevent GvHD.[121,123,135] Most studies use ciclosporin and methotrexate as GvHD prophylaxis; as for thalassemia, we use a low dose (2 doses of 10 mg/m²) to reduce the risk of graft rejection.

Long-term effects of SCT in sickle cell disease

Impact of SCT on pre-existing organ dysfunction

At least some of the organ damage associated with sickle cell disease can be stabilized and even reversed post transplant. Symptomatic CNS disease improves post-SCT in the majority of cases[123] but subtle MRI/MRA evidence of deterioration of existing neurologic damage occurs in a small proportion of patients.[137] Pulmonary function stabilizes[123] and improvement in splenic reticuloendothelial function post-SCT has been reported.[138]

Growth and development

Most patients with sickle cell disease demonstrate improved growth post-SCT unless they remain on immunosuppression for chronic GvHD or they undergo SCT at or near the adolescent growth spurt.[139] Unfortunately, gonadal failure and delayed sexual development appear fairly common, although there are too few patients to assess this properly. In the reported series, 11 of 13 girls had primary amenorrhea and most evaluable males have normal sexual development but follow-up remains short and many have not yet entered puberty.[122,123] Experience with busulfan and cyclophosphamide in other transplant settings suggests infertility is likely to be common.

Secondary malignancy

Although the number of SCT is small and the follow-up relatively short, one secondary malignancy was seen in the Belgian series – myelodysplasia evolving to acute myeloid leukemia 4 years post-SCT.[122]

Quality of life

There have been no detailed quality of life studies, although families' perception of the impact of SCT on quality of life is clearly an important issue in their choosing or refusing SCT.[140] In the international and Belgian series, more than 90% of engrafted patients had Karnofsky or Lansky scores of 100%.[122,123]

Indications for SCT in sickle cell disease

General considerations

Most transplants in sickle cell disease have been carried out for specific complications of sickle cell disease which predict for a poor prognosis (see Table 17.4).[124,141] Using these criteria, it is estimated that less than 10% of children with sickle cell disease fulfill the criteria for SCT, only one in five of whom will have an HLA-identical sibling donor.[115,142] An alternative approach is to offer SCT to all children with homozygous sickle cell disease who have an HLA-identical family donor, on the grounds that overall survival is superior to that with medical treatment, particularly when families wish to live in countries without reliable access to good-quality medical care.[124] This approach is supported by the excellent overall survival (100%) and disease-free survival (93%) in the young Belgian cohort transplanted using these criteria,[122] but is not generally recommended for those living in developed countries because of the long-term effects as well as the inevitability of some early TRM.

Once the decision to proceed to SCT in principle has been taken, a rigorous pretransplant work-up, including cranial MRI/MRA and neurocognitive assessment, is essential. It is important to make clear to families that the pre-SCT assessment may reveal severe organ damage, particularly neurologic or pulmonary damage, which may make SCT too hazardous. The final decision should be taken jointly by families, physicians and the SCT team. Involvement of parents and patients in the decision-making process is essential and has been shown to produce helpful insight into the different criteria which are used to identify treatment preferences by patients with severe sickle cell disease.[140,143,144]

Recommendations (Table 17.4)

The indications followed by our center and most centers in the UK are a modified version of the British Paediatric Haematology Forum criteria devised in 1993.[105] Guidelines from the international study are similar but include severe sickle nephropathy, retinopathy, osteonecrosis and red cell alloimmunization.[123] In the UK, SCT as a recommended option has been limited to patients with homozygous sickle cell disease or Sβ⁰ thalassemia. The most commn indications for transplant are CNS disease (stroke or recurrent transient ischemic attacks) and recurrent acute chest syndrome. Since hydroxyurea reduces the incidence and severity of acute chest syndrome and painful vaso-occlusive sickle crises, a trial of hydroxyurea is strongly recommended as a first step, and SCT considered only where hydroxyurea fails.[105] Patients identified by transcranial Doppler studies as being at increased risk of stroke, but who have not yet had a cerebrovascular accident, are not currently considered eligible for transplant, as blood transfusion has been shown to be protective in this setting.[97,145] However, the recent data from the STOP II trial suggesting that the protective effect of blood transfusion is lost unless this is continued for life brings into consideration the complications of this form of therapy, particularly iron accumulation and infective/immune complications which may lead to a further subgroup of children who would benefit from SCT.

Prospects for improved management of sickle cell disease in the future

Myeloablative SCT is likely to have an important role for several years as the only proven cure which is durable and has acceptable risks. Toxicity of myeloablative conditioning may be reduced by advances in fertility preservation, and promising results of restoration of ovarian function after orthotopic transplantation of cryopreserved ovarian tissue offer some hope.[146] Reduced-intensity conditioning regimens are being adapted to solve the high rejection rate, based on better understanding of engraftment and rejection through mouse models and detailed studies in patients.[130,147,148] Numerous clinical trials in the management of neurologic and pulmonary complications, new agents identified through animal models of sickle cell disease[107–109,149] and HbF induction are planned or underway.[150] Finally, after extensive work in vitro and in animal models, trials of gene therapy for patients with sickle cell disease are now under way.[9]

Summary

SCT remains the only cure for sickle cell disease and thalassemia. Cure appears to be life-long and associated with minimal long-term risks. When deciding whether or not to proceed with SCT, families and physicians must weigh up the risks of the procedure, including TRM and graft failure, against the expected survival and quality of life with medical treatment. For thalassemia the outcome of SCT is best in patients under 16 years old who comply well with chelation treatment and who have no evidence of liver dysfunction. They can expect long-term survival of 95% and thalassemia-free survival of 90%. Patients with poor-risk features have a reduced chance of cure (56–82%) and higher TRM (up to 20%), but still have a long-term survival advantage over conventional medical management.

Sickle cell disease is more heterogeneous and the patients predicted to benefit most from SCT are those with CNS disease or recurrent acute chest syndrome despite hydroxyurea. Long-term disease-free survival after SCT for sickle cell disease in childhood is 82–86%. Since this is almost identical to recent US data on survival of homozygous sickle cell disease with medical treatment, SCT is likely to remain a valuable option even with advances in pharmacologic disease modifiers.

References

1. Weatherall DJ, Clegg JB. Inherited hemoglobin disorders: an increasing global health problem. Bull WHO 2001;79:1–15
2. Pakakasama S, Hongeng S, Chaisiripoomkere W et al. Allogeneic peripheral blood stem cell transplantation in children with homozygous beta-thalassemia and severe beta-thalassemia/hemoglobin E disease. Pediatr Hematol Oncol 2004;26:248–252
3. Thornley I, Lehrmann L, Ferguson WS et al. Homozygous alpha-thalassemia treated with intrauterine transfusions and postnatal hematopoietic stem cell transplantation. Bone Marrow Transplant 2003;32:341–342
4. Rund D, Rachmilewitz E. β-thalassemia. N Engl J Med 2005;353:1135–1146
5. Cunningham MJ, Macklin EA, Neufeld EJ, Cohen AR. Complications of β-thalassemia major in North America. Blood 2004;104:34–39
6. Modell B, Khan M, Darlison M. Survival in beta-thalassemia major in the UK: data from the UK Thalassaemia Register. Lancet 2000;355:2051–2052
7. Borgna-Pignatti C, Rugolotto S, di Stefano P et al. Survival and complications in patients with thalassemia major treated with transfusion and deferoxamine. Hematologica 2004;89:1187–1193
8. Telfer P, Coen PG, Christou S et al. Survival of medically treated thalassemia patients in Cyprus. Trends and risk factors over the period 1980–2004. Hematologica 2006;91:1187–1192
9. Bank A, Dorazio R, Leboulch P. A phase I/II clinical trial of beta-globin gene therapy for beta-thalassemia. Ann NY Acad Sci 2005;1054:308–316
10. Sadelain M, Boulad F, Galanello R et al. Therapeutic options for patients with severe b-thalassemia: the need for globin gene therapy. Hum Gene Ther 2007;18:1–9
11. Wroe SJ, Pal S, Siddique D et al. Clinical presentation and pre-mortem diagnosis of variant Creutzfeldt-Jakob disease associated with blood transfuion: a case report. Lancet 2006;368:2061–2067
12. Davis BA, Porter JB. Long-term outcome of continuous 24-hour desferrioxamine infusion via indwelling intravenous catheters in high-risk beta-thalassemia. Blood 2000;95:1229–1236
13. Ceci A, Biairdi P, Feliisi M et al. The safety and effectiveness of deferiprone in a large-scale, 3-year study in Italian patients. Br J Haematol 2002;118:330–336
14. Galanello R, Piga A, Forni GL et al. Phase II clinical evaluation of deferasirox, a once-daily oral chelating agent, in pediatric patients with β-thalassemia major. Hematologica 2006;91:1343–1351
15. Capellini MD, Cohen A, Piga A et al. A phase 3 study of deferasirox (ICL670), a once-daily iron chelator, in patients with b-thalassemia. Blood 2006;107:3455–3462
16. Piga A, Galanello R, Forni GL et al. Randomized phase II trial of deferasirox (Exjade, ICL 670), a once-daily, orally-administered iron chelator, in comparison with deferoxamine in thalassemia patients with transfusional iron overload. Hematologica 2006;91:873–880
17. Singer ST, Kuypers FA, Olivieri NF et al. Fetal hemoglobin augmentation in E/beta⁰ thalassemia: clinical and hematological outcome. Br J Haematol 2005;131:378–388
18. Lawson S, Roberts IAG, Amrolia P et al. Bone marrow transplantation for β-thalassemia major: the UK experience in two paediatric centres. Br J Haematol 2003;120:289–295
19. van de Velde H, Georgiou I, de Rycke M et al. Novel universal approach for preimplantation genetic diagnosis of beta-thalassemia in combination with HLA matching of embryos. Hum Reprod 2004;19:700–708
20. Kuliev A, Rechitsky S, Verlinsky O et al. Preimplantation diagnosis and HLA typing for hemoglobin disorders. Reprod Biomed Online2005;11:362–370
21. Qureshi N, Foote D, Walters MC et al. Outcomes of preimplantation genetic diagnosis therapy in treatment of beta-thalassemia: a retrospective analysis. Ann NY Acad Sci 2005;1054:500–503
22. Gaziev D, Galimberti M, Lucarelli G et al. Bone marrow transplantation from alternative donors for thalassemia: HLA-phenotypically identical relative and HLA-nonidentical sibling or parent transplants. Bone Marrow Transplant. 2000;25:815–821
23. Locatelli F, Rocha V, Reed W et al. Related umbilical cord blood transplant in patients with thalassemia and sickle cell disease. Blood 2003;101:2137–2143
24. Amrolia P, Vulliamy T, Vassiliou G et al. Analysis of chimaerism in thalassaemic children undergoing stem cell transplantation. Br J Haematol 2001;114:219–225
25. Yesilpek MA, Hazar V, Kupesiz A et al. Peripheral blood stem cell transplantation in children with beta-thalassemia. Bone Marrow Transplant 2001;28:1037–1040
26. Fang J, Huang S, Chen C et al. Allogeneic peripheral blood stem cell transplantation in β-thalassemia. Pediatr Hematol Oncol 2002;19:453–458
27. Farzana T, Shamshi TS, Irfan M et al. Peripheral blood stem cell transplantation in children with beta-thalassemia major. Coll Physicians Surg Pak 2003;13:204–206
28. Mohyeddin Bonab M, Alimoghaddam K, Vatandoust S et al. Are HLA antigens a risk factor for acute GVHD in patients receiving HLA-identical stem cell transplantation? Transplant Proc 2004;36:3190–3193
29. La Nasa G, Giardini C, Argiolu F et al. Unrelated donor bone marrow transplantation for thalassemia: the effect of extended haplotypes. Blood 2002;99:4350–4356
30. La Nasa G, Argiolu F, Giardini C et al. Unrelated bone marrow transplantation for beta-thalassemia patients: the experience of the Italian Bone Marrow Transplant Group. Ann NY Acad Sci 2005;1054:186–195
31. Jaing T-H, Hung I-J, Yang C-P et al. Rapid and complete donor chimerism after unrelated mismatched cord blood transplantation in 5 children with b-thalassemia major. Biol Blood Marrow Transplant 2005;11:349–353
32. Feng Z, Sun E, Lan H et al. Unrelated donor bone marrow transplantation for beta-thalassemia major- an experience from China. Bone Marrow Transplant 2006;37:171–174
33. Hongeng S, Pakakasama S, Chuansumrit A et al. Outcomes of transplantation with related-and unrelated-donor stem cells in children with severe thalassemia. Biol Blood Marrow Transplant 2006;12:683–687
34. Fleischauer K, Locatelli F, Zecca M et al. Graft rejection after unrelated donor hematopoietic stem cell transplantation for thalassemia is associated with nonpermissive HLA-DPB1 disparity in host-versus-graft direction. Blood 2006;107:2984–2992
35. Lucarelli G, Andreani M, Angelucci E. The cure of thalassemia by bone marrow transplantation. Blood Rev 2002;16:81–85
36. Schrier S, Angelucci E. New strategies in the treatment of the thalassemias. Ann Rev Med 2005;56:157–171
37. Di Bartolomeo P, Di Girolamo G, Olioso P et al. The Pescara experience. Bone Marrow Transplant 1997;19(suppl 2):48–53
38. Ghavamzadeh A, Nasseri P, Eshraghian M et al. Prognostic factors in bone marrow transplantation for beta thalassemia major: experiences from Iran. Bone Marrow Transplant 1998;22:1167–1169
39. Mentzer W, Cowan M.Bone marrow transplantation for beta-thalassemia: the University of California San Francisco experience. J Pediatr Hematol Oncol 2000;22:598–601
40. Peristeri J, Kitra V, Goussetis E et al. Hematopoietic stem cell transplantation for the management of hemoglobinopathies in Greek patients. Transfus Sci 2000;23:263–264
41. Li CK, Shng MM, Chik KW et al. Hamatopoietic stem cell transplantation for thalassemia major in Hong Kong: prognostic factors and outcome. Bone Marrow Transplant 2002;29:101–105
42. Ball LM, Lankester AC, Giordano PC et al. Pediatric allogeneic bone marrow transplantation for homozygous beta-thalassemia, the Dutch experience. Bone Marrow Transplant 2003;31:1081–1087
43. Chandy M, Balasubramanian P, Ramachandran SV et al. Randomized trial of two different conditioning regimens for bone marrow transplantation in thalassemia- the role of busulfan pharmacokinetics in determining outcome. Bone Marrow Transplant 2005;36:839–845

44. Lucarelli G, Galimberti M, Polchi P et al. Bone marrow transplantation in patients with thalassemia. N Engl J Med 1990;322:417–421

45. Angelucci E, Lucarelli G. Bone marrow transplantation in beta thalassemia. In: Steinberg MH, Forget BG, Higgs DR, Nagel RL (eds) Disorders of hemoglobin: genetics, pathophysiology and clinical management. Cambridge University Press, Cambridge, 2001:1052–1072

46. Sodani P, Gaziev D, Polchi P et al. New approach for bone marrow transplantation in patients with class 3 thalassemia aged younger than 17 years. Blood 2004;104:1201–1203

47. Lucarelli G, Clift R Galimberti M et al. Bone marrow transplantation in adult thalassemic patients. Blood 1999;93:1164–1167

48. Gaziev J, Sodani P, Polchi P et al. Bone marrow transplantation in adults with thalassemia: treatment and long-term follow up. Ann NY Acad Sci 2005;1054:196–205

49. Gaziev D, Polchi P, Galimberti M et al. Graft-versus-host disease after bone marrow transplantation for thalassemia: an analysis of incidence and risk factors. Transplantation 1997;63:854–860

50. Giardini C, Galimberti M, Lucarelli G et al. Desferrioxamine therapy accelerates clearance of iron deposits after bone marrow transplantation for thalassemia. Br J Haematol 1995;89:868–873

51. Angelucci E, Muretto P, Nicolucci A et al. Effects of iron overload and hepatitis C virus positivity in determining progression of liver fibrosis in thalassemia following bone marrow transplantation. Blood 2002;100:17–21

52. Angelucci E, Mariotti E, Lucarelli G et al. Sudden cardiac tamponade after chemotherapy for marrow transplantation in thalassaemia. Lancet 1992;339:287–289

53. Anderson LJ, Wonke B, Prescott E et al. Comparative effects of oral deferiprone and subcutaneous desferrioxamine on myocardial iron concentrations and ventricular function in beta-thalassaemia. Lancet 2002;360:516–520

54. Gaziev D, Polchi P, Lucarelli G et al. Second bone marrow transplant for graft failure in patients with thalassemia. Bone Marrow Transplant 1999;24:1299–1306

55. Nesci S, Manna M, Lucarelli G et al. Mixed chimerism after bone marrow transplantation in thalassemia. Ann NY Acad Sci 1998;850:495–497

56. Andreani M, Nesci S, Lucarelli G et al. Long-term survival of ex-thalassemic patients with persistent mixed chimerism after bone marrow transplantation. Bone Marrow Transplant 2000;25:401–404

57. Aker M, Kapelushnik J, Pugatsch T et al. Donor lymphocyte infusions to displace residual host hematopoietic cells after allogeneic bone marrow transplantation for beta-thalassemia major. J. Pediatr Hematol Oncol 1998;20:145–148

58. Zakrzewski JL. Successful management of impending graft failure in a thalassemic bone marrow transplant recipient. Hematologica 2002;87:ECR32

59. Nishino T, Tubb J, Emery DW. Partial correction of murine beta-thalassemia with a gammaretrovirus vector for human gamma-globin. Blood Cells Mol Dis 2006;37:1–7

60. Hongeng S, Chuansumrit A, Chaisirpoomkere W et al. Full chimerism in nonmyeloablative stem cell transplantation in a β-thalassemia major patient (Class 3 Lucarelli). Bone Marrow Transplant 2002;30:299–314

61. Iannone R, Casella JF, Fuchs EJ et al. Results of minimally toxic nonmyeloablative transplantation in patients with sickle cell anemia and thalassemia. Biol Blood Marrow Transplant 2003;9:519–528

62. Horan JT, Liesveld JL, Fenton P et al. Hematopoietic stem cell transplantation for multiply transfused patients with sickle cell disease and thalassemia after low-dose total body irradiation, fludarabine and rabbit anti-thymocyte globulin. Bone Marrow Transplant 2005;35:171–177

63. Sauer M, Bettoni C, Lauten M et al. Complete substitution of cyclophosphamide by fludarabine and ATG in a busulfan-based preparative regimen for children and adolescents with beta-thalassemia. Bone Marrow Transplant 2005;36:383–387

64. Vassal G, Deroussent A, Challine D et al. Is 600 mg/m2 the appropriate dosage of busulfan in children undergoing bone marrow transplantation? Blood 1992;79:2475–2479

65. Yeager A, Wagner JE Jr, Graham M et al. Optimization of busulfan dosage in children undergoing bone marrow transplantation: a pharmacokinetic study of dose escalation. Blood 1992;80:2425–2428

66. Poonkuzhali B, Srivastava A, Quernin M et al. Pharmacokinetics of oral busulfan in children with beta thalassemia major undergoing allogeneic bone marrow transplantation. Bone Marrow Transplant 1999;24:5–11

67. Bostrom B, Enockson K, Johnson A et al. Plasma pharmacokinetics of high-dose oral busulfan in children and adults undergoing bone marrow transplantation. Pediatr Transplant 2003;7(suppl 3):12–18

68. Slattery J, Sanders J, Buckner C et al. Graft-rejection and toxicity following bone marrow transplantation in relation to busulfan pharmacokinetics. Bone Marrow Transplant 1995;16:31–42

69. Lucarelli G, Clift R, Galimberti M et al. Marrow transplantation for patients with thalassemia: results in class 3 patients. Blood 1996;87:2082–2088

70. Balasubramanian P, Chandy M, Krishnamoorthy R, Srivastava A. Evaluation of existing limited sampling models for busulfan kinetics in children with beta thalassemia major undergoing bone marrow transplantation. Bone Marrow Transplant 2001;28:821–825

71. Cremers S, Schoemaker R, Bredius R et al. Pharmacokinetics of intravenous busulfan in children prior to stem cell transplantation. Br J Clin Pharmacol 2002;53:386–389

72. Casper J, Knauf W, Blau I et al. Treosulfan/fludarabine: a new conditioning regimen in allogeneic transplantation. Ann Hematol 2004;83(suppl 1):S70–71

73. Giardini C, Galimberti M, Lucarelli G et al. Desferrioxamine therapy accelerates clearance of iron deposits after bone marrow transplantation for thalassaemia. Br J Haematol 1995;89:868–873

74. Angelucci E, Muretto P, Lucarelli G et al. Phlebotomy to reduce iron overload in patients cured of thalassemia by bone marrow transplantation. Italian Cooperative Group for Phlebotomy Treatment of Transplanted Thalassemia Patients. Blood 1997;90:994–998

75. Muretto P, Angelucci E, Lucarelli G. Reversibility of cirrhosis in patients cured of thalassemia by bone marrow transplantation. Ann Intern Med 2002;136:667–672

76. Angelucci E, Muretto P, Nicolucci A et al. Effects of iron overload and hepatitis C virus positivity in determining progression of liver fibrosis in thalassemia following bone marrow transplantation. Blood 2002;100:17–21

77. Gaziev D, Galimberti M, Giardini C et al. Growth in children after bone marrow transplantation for thalassemia. Bone Marrow Transplant 1993;19(suppl 2):100–101

78. de Sanctis V, Galimberti M, Lucarelli G et al. Growth and development in ex-thalassemic patients. Bone Marrow Transplant 1997;19(suppl 2):48–53

79. de Simone M, Olioso P, di Bartolomeo P et al. Growth and endocrine function following bone marrow transplantation for thalassemia. Bone Marrow Transplant 1995;15:227–233

80. de Sanctis V, Galimberti M, Lucarelli G et al. Gonadal function in long term survivors with b thalassemia major following bone marrow transplantation. Bone Marrow Transplant 1993;12(suppl 1):104

81. Vlachopapadopoulou E, Kitra V, Peristeri J et al. Gonadal function of young patients with beta-thalassemia following bone marrow transplantation. J Pediatr Endocrinol Metab 2005;18:477–483

82. Borgna-Pignatti C, Marradi P, Rugolotto S, Marcolongo A. successful pregnancy after bone marrow transplantation for thalassemia. Bone Marrow Transplant 1996;18:235–236

83. Gaziev J, Lucarelli G. Stem cell transplantation for hemoglobinopathies. Curr Opin Pediatr 2003;15:24–31

84. Sanders J, Hawley J, Levy W et al. Pregnancies following high-dose cyclophosphamide with or without high-dose busulfan or total-body irradiation and bone marrow transplantation. Blood 1996;87:3045–3052

85. Gulati S, van Poznak C. Pregnancy after bone marrow transplantation. J Clin Oncol 1998;16:1978–1985

86. Tournaye H, Goossens E, Verheyen G et al. Preserving the reproductive potential of men and boys with cancer: current concepts and future prospects. Hum Reprod Update 2004;10:525–532

87. Donnez J, Martinez-Madrid B, Jadoul P et al. Ovarian tissue cryopreservation and transplantation: a review. Hum Reprod Update 2006;12:519–535

88. Poirot CJ, Martelli H, Genestie C et al. Feasibility of ovarian tissue cryopreservation for prepubertal females with cancer. Pediatr Blood Cancer 2007;49(1):74–78

89. Vassiliou G, Amrolia P, Roberts IAG. Allogeneic transplantation for hemoglobinopathies. Best Pract Res Clin Hematol 2001;14:807–822

90. Voskaridou E, Douskou M, Terpos E et al. Magnetic resonance imaging in the evaluation of iron overload in patients with b-thalassaemia and sickle cell disease. Br J Haematol 2004;126:736–742

91. Weatherall DJ. Weak phenotype-genotype relationships in monogenic disease: lessons from the thalassemias. Nat Rev Genet 2001;2:245–255

92. Platt O, Brambilla D, Rosse W et al. Mortality in sickle cell disease. Life expectancy and risk factors for early death. N Engl J Med 1994;330:1639–1644

93. Quinn CT, Rogers ZR, Buchanan GR. Survival of children with sickle cell disease. Blood 2004;103:4023–4027

94. Buchanan GR, DeBaun M, Quinn CT, Steinberg MH. Sickle cell disease. Hematology (Am Soc Hematol Educ Program) 2004;35–47

95. Vichinsky E, Neumayr LD, Earles AN et al. Causes and outcome of the acute chest syndrome in sickle cell disease. N Engl J Med 2000;342:1855–1865

96. Ohene-Frempong K, Weiner SJ, Sleeper LA et al. Cerebrovascular accidents in sickle cell disease: rates and risk factors. Blood 1998;91:288–294

97. Kirkham FJ, DeBaun M. Stroke in children with sickle cell disease. Curr Treat Options Neurol 2004;6:357–375

98. Manci EA, Culberson DE, Yang YM et al. Causes of death in sickle cell disease: an autopsy study. Br J Haematol 2003;123:359–365

99. Steinberg MH, Barton F, Castro O et al. Effect of hydroxyurea on mortality and morbidity in adult sickle cell anemia: risks and benefits up to 9 years of treatment. JAMA 2003;289:1645–1651

100. Gladwin MT, Sachdev V, Jison ML et al. Pulmonary hypertension as a risk factor for death in patients with sickle cell disease. N Engl J Med 2004;350:886–895

101. Perrone V, Roberts-Harewood M, Bachir D et al. Patterns of mortality in sickle cell disease in adults in France and England. Hematol J 2002;3:56–60

102. Charache S, Terrin ML, Moore RD et al. Effect of hydroxyurea on the frequency of painful crises in sickle cell anemia. Investigators of the Multicenter Study of Hydroxyurea in Sickle Cell Anemia. N Engl J Med 1995;332:1317–1322

103. Ferster A, Tahriri P, Vermylen C et al. Five years of experience with hydroxyurea in children and young adults with sickle cell disease. Blood 2001;97:3628–3632

104. Halsey C, Roberts IAG. The role of hydroxyurea in sickle cell disease. Br J Haematol 2003;120:177–186

105. Amrolia PJ, Almeida A, Halsey C et al. Therapeutic challenges in childhood sickle cell disease. Part 1: current and future treatment options. Br J Haematol 2003;120:725–736

106. Adams RJ, Brambilla D, STOP Investigators. Discontinuing prophylactic transfusions used to prevent stroke in sickle cell disease. N Engl J Med 2005;353:2769–2778

107. Kirkham FJ, Lerner MB, Noetzel M et al. Trials in sickle cell disease. Pediatr Neurol 2006;34:450–458

108. Platt O. Prevention and management of stroke in sickle cell anemia. Hematology (Am Soc Hematol Educ Program) 2006:54–57

109. Ware RE, Zimmerman SA, Schultz WH. Hydroxyurea as an alternative to blood transfusions for the prevention of recurrent stroke in children with sickle cell disease. Blood 1999;94:3022–3026

110. Ware RE, Zimmerman SA, Sylvestre PB et al. Prevention of secondary stroke and resolution of transfusional iron overload in children with sickle cell anemia using hydroxyurea and phlebotomy. J Pediatr 2004;145:346–352

111. de Montalembert M, Brousse V, Elie C et al. Long-term hydroxyurea treatment in children with sickle cell disease: tolerance and clinical outcomes. Hematologica 2006;91:125–128

112. Houston-Yu P, Rana SR, Beyer B, Castro O. Frequent and prolonged hospitalizations: a risk factor for early mortality in sickle cell disease patients. Am J Hematol 2003;72:201–203

113. Prasad R, Hasan S, Castro O et al. Long-term outcomes in patients with sickle cell disease and frequent vaso-occlusive crises. Am J Med Sci 2003;325:107–109

114. Mentzer WC, Heller S, Pearle PR et al. Availability of related donors for bone marrow transplantation in sickle cell anemia. Am J Pediatr Hematol Oncol 1994;16:27–29

115. Walters M, Patience M, Leisenring W et al. Barriers to bone marrow transplantation for sickle cell anemia. Biol Blood Marrow Transplant 1996;2:100–104

116. Walters MC, Quirolo L, Trachtenberg ET et al. Sibling donor cord blood transplantation for thalassemia major: experience of the Sibling Donor Cord Blood Program. Ann NY Acad Sci 2005;1054:206–213

117. Adamkiewicz TV, Boyer MW, Bray R et al. Identification of unrelated cord blood units for hematopoietic stem cell transplantation in children with sickle cell disease. J Pediatr Hematol Oncol 2006;28:29–32

118. Adamkiewicz TV, Mehta PS, Boyer MW et al. Transplantation of unrelated placental blood cells in children with high-risk sickle cell disease. Bone Marrow Transplant 2004;34:405–411

119. Mazur M, Kurtzberg J, Halperin E et al. Transplantation of a child with sickle cell anemia with an unrelated cord blood unit after reduced intensity conditioning. J Pediatr Hematol Oncol 2006;28:840–844

120. Morris CR, Singer ST, Walters MC. Clinical hemoglobinopathies: iron, lungs and new blood. Curr Opin Hematol 2006;13:407–418

121. Bernaudin F, Souillet G, Vannier JP et al. Report of the French experience concerning 26 children transplanted for severe sickle cell disease. Bone Marrow Transplant 1997;19(suppl 2):112–115

122. Vermylen C, Cornu G, Ferster A et al. Hematopoietic stem cell transplantation for sickle cell anemia: the first 50 patients transplanted in Belgium. Bone Marrow Transplant 1998;22:1–6

123. Walters M, Storb R, Patience M et al. Impact of bone marrow transplantation for symptomatic sickle cell disease: an interim report. Multicenter investigation of bone marrow transplantation for sickle cell disease. Blood 2000;95:1918–1924

124. Vermylen C. Hematopoietic stem cell transplantation in sickle cell disease. Blood Rev 2003;17:163–166

125. van Besien K, Bartholomew A, Stock W et al. Fludarabine-based conditioning for allogeneic transplantation in adults with sickle cell disease. Bone Marrow Transplant 2000;26:445–449

126. Walters M, Sullivan K, Bernaudin F et al. Neurologic complications after allogeneic marrow transplantation for sickle cell anemia. Blood 1995;85:879–884

127. Ferster A, Corraza F, Vertongen F et al. Transplanted sickle-cell disease patients with autologous bone marrow recovery after graft failure develop increased levels of fetal haemoglobin which corrects disease severity. Br J Haematol 1995;90:804–808

128. Bachet C, Azzi N, Demulder A et al. Hydroxyurea treatment for sickle cell disease: impact on hematopoietic stem cell transplantation's outcome. Bone Marrow Transplant 2004;33:799–803

129. Walters M, Patience M, Leisenring W et al. Stable mixed hematopoietic chimerism after bone marrow transplantation for sickle cell anemia. Biol Blood Marrow Transplant 2001;7:665–673

130. Walters MC. Stem cell therapy for sickle cell disease: transplantation and gene therapy. Hematology (Am Soc Educ Program) 2005;66–73

131. Baron F, Dresse MF, Beguin Y. Donor lymphocyte infusion to eradicate recurrent host hematopoiesis after allogeneic BMT for sickle cell disease. Transfusion 2000;40:1071–1073

132. Krishnamurti L, Blazar BR, Wagner JE. Bone marrow transplantation without myeloablation for sickle cell disease. N Engl J Med 2001;344:68

133. Schleuning M, Stoezer O, Waterhouse C et al. Hematopoietic stem cell transplantation after reduced-intensity conditioning as treatment for sickle cell disease. Exp Hematol 2002;30:7–10

134. Iannone R, Luznik L, Engstrom LW et al. Effects of mixed hematopoietic chimerism in a mouse model of bone marrow transplantation for sickle cell anemia. Blood 2001;97:3960–3965

135. Horan JT, Liesveld JL, Fenton P et al. Hematopoietic stem cell transplantation for multiply transfused patients with sickle cell disease and thalassemia after low-dose total body irradiation, fludarabine and rabbit anti-thymocyte globulin. Bone Marrow Transplant 2005;35:171–177

136. Shenoy S, Grossman WJ, Di Persio J et al. A novel reduced-intensity stem cell transplant regimen for nonmalignant disorders. Bone Marrow Transplant 2005;35:345–352

137. Woodard P, Helton KJ, Khan RB et al. Brain parenchymal damage after haematopoietic stem cell transplantation for severe sickle cell disease. Br J Haematol 2005;129:550–552

138. Ferster A, Bujan W, Corazza F et al. Bone marrow transplantation corrects the splenic reticuloendothelial dysfunction in sickle cell anemia. Blood 1993;81:1102–1105

139. Eggleston B, Patience M, Edwards S et al. Effects of myeloablative bone marrow transplantation on growth of children with sickle cell anaemia: results of the multicentre study of sickle cell anaemia. Br J Haematol 2007;2007;136:673–676

140. Hankins J, Hinds P, Day S et al. Therapy preference and decision-making among patients with severe sickle cell anemia and their families. Pediatr Blood Cancer 2007;48:705–710

141. Amrolia P, Almeida A, Davies SC, Roberts IAG. Therapeutic challenges in childhood sickle cell disease. Part 2: a problem-orientated approach. Br J Haematol 2003;120:737–743

142. Davies SC, Roberts IAG. Bone marrow transplant for sickle cell disease – an update. Arch Dis Child 1996;75:3–6

143. Kodish E, Lantos J, Stocking C et al. Bone marrow transplantation for sickle cell disease. A study of parents' decisions. N Engl J Med 1991;325:1349–1353

144. van Besien K, Koshy M, Anderson-Shaw L et al. Allogeneic stem cell transplantation for sickle cell disease. A study of patients' decisions. Bone Marrow Transplant 2001;28:545–549

145. Nietert PJ, Abboud M, Silverstein M, Jackson SM. Bone marrow transplantation versus periodic prophylactic blood transfusion in sickle cell patients at high risk of ischemic stroke: a decision analysis. Blood 2000;95:3057–3064

146. Donnez J, Dolmans MM, Demylle D et al. Restoration of ovarian function after orthotopic (intraovarian and periovarian) transplantation of cryopreserved ovarian tissue in a woman treated by bone marrow transplantation for sickle cell anemia: case report. Hum Reprod 2006;21:183–188

147. Iannone R, Ohene-Frempong K, Fuchs EJ et al. Bone marrow transplantation for sickle cell anemia: progress and prospects. Pediatr Blood Cancer 2005;44:436–440

148. Kean LS, Durham MM, Adams AB et al. A cure for murine sickle cell disease through stable mixed chimerism and tolerance induction after nonmyeloablative conditioning and major histocompatibility complex-mismatched bone marrow transplantation. Blood 2002;99:1840–1849

149. Manci EA, Hillery CA, Bodian CA. Pathology of Berkeley sickle cell mice: similarities and differences with human sickle cell disease. Blood 2006;107:1651–1658

150. Fathallah H, Atweh GF. Induction of fetal hemoglobin in the treatment of sickle cell disease. Hematology (Am Soc Educ Program) 2006:58–62

Lysosomal storage disorders

Robert Wynn

CHAPTER 18

Introduction

Lysosomes are intracellular membrane-bound acidic organelles containing hydrolytic enzymes that mediate hydrolysis of macromolecules. A discussion of lysosomal physiology is necessary to understand the rationale for stem cell transplantation in disorders of lysosomal function and to better understand other therapies available.[1]

Lysosomal pH is maintained by lysosomal enzyme electron pumps. Lysosomal enzymes and the macromolecules that they digest are delivered separately to the lysosymes. Substrate is from three sources.

1. *Endocytosis*. This is the method by which endogenous, extracellular macromolecules are delivered to the lysosome for catabolism. Substrates for lysosomal catabolism that are delivered by this route are those that accumulate in lysosomal storage disorders (LSDs).
2. *Phagocytosis*. This is the route of entry onto the cell for catabolism of extracellular debris and micro-organsims.
3. *Autophagosomes*. Intracellular material requiring catabolism is delivered to lysosome in this way.

Fusion of vesicles containing substrate via the above routes with the primary lysosome results in a secondary lysosome.

Lysosomal enzyme trafficking and principles of cross-correction

Lysosomal enzymes are made in the rough endoplasmic reticulum and travel to the Golgi. In the Golgi they acquire a mannose 6 phosphate ligand. This is added by the sequential action of two Golgi enzymes, a phosphotransferase and a diesterase, and it is the addition of the mannose 6 phosphate that identifies the protein as destined for the lysosome (Fig. 18.1).[2] There are two reasons for the importance of this step.

- First, without the action of either of these two enzymes that add mannose 6 phosphate to the precursor enzyme then lysosomal dysfunction will occur as though there were primary enzyme deficiency. Mucolipidosis II and III (I-cell disease) arise from deficiency of these two enzymes.[3]
- The second reason for the importance of mannose 6 phosphate-directed lysosomal targeting of enzyme is of more concern to the clinician, including the transplant team. Some enzyme is tagged but leaves the cell and is taken up by neighboring cells and delivered to the lysosome of that cell – again via the mannose 6 phosphate moiety. This means that: (1) enzyme can be secreted from enzyme-competent cells – in our field by leukocytes of an unaffected (donor) individual (Fig. 18.2), and (2) enzyme can be uptaken by (deficient) host cells as long as the mannose 6 phosphate moiety is tagged to the secreted enzyme (Fig. 18.2).

This, therefore, is the principle behind bone marrow transplantation and LSDs. Engrafted donor leukocytes secrete enzyme and this donor enzyme is taken up by deficient recipient cells and their lysosomes via mannose 6 phosphate receptors and cross-corrects them. It was first shown in the laboratory co-culture of LSD with normal fibroblasts that the LSD was corrected. In the same seminal experiments it was shown that the supernatant alone (containing secreted enzyme) of the normal fibroblasts corrected the LSD fibroblasts.[4] In the daily practice of bone marrow transplantation (BMT) for mucopolysaccharidosis type IH (MPSIH) we see the clinical evidence of cross-correction of autologous cells by secreted donor enzyme. In enzyme replacement therapy, exogenous enzyme is tagged with the mannose 6 phosphate and delivered by therapeutic enzyme infusion to deficient host tissue.[5,6]

Lysosomal storage diseases

Lysosomal storage disorders arise from single gene mutations in one of the lysosomal enzymes or in one of the enzymes that add the mannose 6 phosphate ligand that directs the newly synthesized enzyme from the Golgi to the lysosome.[1] Most are autosomal recessive, the exceptions being Hunter (MPS II) and Fabry disease, that are X-linked dominantly inherited. For each disease there are well-characterized mutations, some of which are associated with little residual enzyme and which are consequently associated with a more severe phenotype than those associated mutations that allow some residual enzyme activity.

These are rare disorders and the gene frequency is low. A risk factor for such illness is parental consanguinity, although the consanguinity that brings disease also brings, to the transplant team, the possibility of donors beyond siblings within the wider family.

Patterns of disease

LSDs are multisystem diseases, although the extent of disease within any particular system in any particular disease is variable between different LSDs. The reason for this is poorly understood. Within a single LSD the extent and severity of disease are determined by residual enzyme activity. This is an important consideration when considering therapy associated with risk such as BMT; in general, milder deficiency without CNS involvement is not considered for transplant even where this is an accepted modality of therapy.

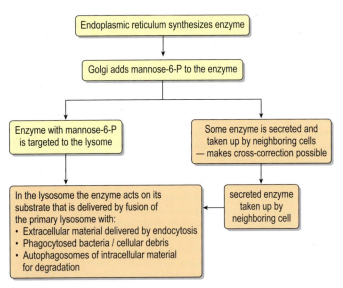

Figure 18.1
Lysosomal enzymes are made in the endoplasmic reticulum and trafficked via the Golgi to the lysosome. There they degrade specific macromolecules. Some lysosomal enzyme arrives from neighboring cells via specific receptors.

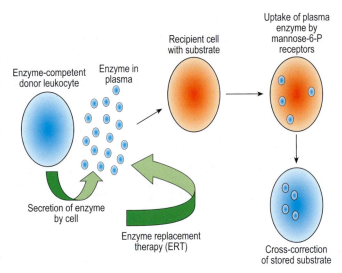

Figure 18.2
The principle of cross-correction that underlies ERT and stem cell therapy of LSDs. Enzyme is secreted into the plasma by donor, enzyme-competent leukocytes or is delivered there by intravenous infusion. Enzyme has the mannose 6 P tag that is taken up by enzyme-incompetent recipient cells. The enzyme is delivered to the lysosome and clears substrate accumulation after rendering the lysosome competent.

Briefly the effects may be seen in the following.

- *The CNS.* The extent of CNS involvement varies between diseases and within any disease is affected by the level of enzyme deficiency. In the severe forms there is early loss of skill acquisition and early intellectual decline
- *The skeleton.* This is involved in many of these illnesses and the characteristic change is dysostosis multiplex. There is widespread skeletal deformity with growth impairment and disordered bone growth leading to neurologic sequelae
- *The reticuloendothelial system.* Hepatosplenomegaly is a presenting feature of many of these diseases
- *The cardiac system.* Cardiomyopathy and cardiac valve abnormalities are frequently seen in these disorders
- *Dysmorphic appearances.* There are characteristic clinical appearances of affected individuals.

Pathophysiology of disease

Although failure of lysosomal function to catabolize a substrate leads to a particular lysosomal storage disorder, the etiologic relationship might not be clearcut. A consideration of the complexity of the pathophysiology of LSD is important for the transplant team as it aids understanding of why some diseases are better ameliorated than others by BMT and why some tissues within a particular condition are better corrected by exogenous enzyme delivery than others.

Lysosomal distension and cellular distortion are primary phenomena in LSD but trigger other events that contribute to the disease. Such events include macrophage activation so that aspects of the disease, in particular the bony disease, are inflammatory in nature.[7,8] Accumulation of extracellular matrix material appears to alter cytokine binding and cell signaling. Such alterations might explain the developmental abnormalities of the brain and other tissues.[9] These secondary events may be much less amenable to therapy with effective enzyme than the primary substrate accumulation itself.

CNS disease

The challenge of correcting the CNS in LSD is a formidable one. Not all LSDs have prominent CNS involvement, perhaps because the origins of substrate differ in the CNS than in the rest of the body. Thus in non-neuronopathic Gaucher disease residual enzyme activity is inadequate to deal with glucosylceramide (the substrate for the deficient enzyme) derived from red cell breakdown but adequate for breakdown of CNS ganglioside-derived substrate.[10] In neuronopathic forms the enzyme level is lower still, and inadequate to deal with systemic and CNS accumulation.[11]

The blood–brain barrier, formed by the close apposition of astrocytes to the capillary basement membrane, blocks the diffusion of soluble enzyme in the plasma. This acts as an impediment to the delivery of enzyme replacement therapy (ERT), given as intermittent therapeutic infusion in LSD with CNS involvement, and keeps the transplant unit involved in the care of such affected children even where a commercial enzyme is available.

Enzyme is delivered to the CNS after BMT by cells of the monocyte-macrophage system which cross this blood–brain barrier and become tissue macrophages, known in the CNS as microglial cells. These microglial cells are increasingly donor derived with increasing time after successful allogeneic BMT, and secrete enzyme for the CNS.[12,13]

Hemopoietic stem cell transplantation (HSCT) in LSD

Risk–benefit analysis of transplantation in the LSDs

The only common indication for BMT in the LSDs is MPSIH.[14] For this reason it is considered in more detail below. Necessarily much is inferred from this experience of Hurler BMT in the planning and practice of BMT in the other LSDs.

All transplants are performed after an assessment of the *risk* of transplant weighed against the possible *benefits* of donor cell engraftment. We specifically counsel families referred for transplantation in these terms. The risk of any transplant procedure is influenced by the closeness of the HLA match between donor and recipient and the well-being of the patient. Matching issues are generic to all transplants and choice of donor for Hurler patients is discussed below. The same discussion will apply to other patients with metabolic disease referred for BMT. In discussion of patient risk factors, patients with LSDs have significant pretransplant morbidity which will influence the pretransplant consent discussion. Once again, these factors are common to many LSDs referred for BMT and are discussed below in specific relation to Hurler BMT.

These risks, influenced by patient well-being and closeness of match, are weighed against the likelihood of patient benefit from the procedure. The untransplanted natural history of the underlying condition will also direct this discussion. Where the natural history without transplantation is adverse (early death, prominent CNS involvement) then the risks deemed acceptable will be higher than in situations where the disease natural history is less adverse. In some diseases too little is known, from the rarity of patients and paucity of transplants performed, for any firm conclusion on the exact influence of any therapy on disease outcome to be drawn. These uncertainties must, by necessity, be shared with the patient and their family. In these days of ERT the availability or impending availability of other treatments and their effect on the underlying disease and natural history must be considered.

Which LSDs should be considered for transplant?

For the reasons considered above there are few absolute indications in this field. Transplantation in Hurler disease is accepted practice but even there, individual patient factors, such as age at referral and co-morbidities, might influence transplant decision. The role of transplantation in other LSDs has been the topic of several reviews, and the current state of mainstream practice is summarized in Table 18.1.

Table 18.1 Summary of the current LSDs and their indications for transplant

	Disease
Standard indication	MPSIH (Hurler)
	MPS VII (Sly)
	α-Mannosidosis
	Presymptomatic Krabbe
	Late-onset globoid cell leukodystrophy
	Wolman
	MLD only late onset
Evidence for transplant efficacy but ERT increasingly first line	MPSIH/S, MPSIS (Hurler–Scheie, Scheie)
	MPS VI
	Gaucher disease
	Niemann-Pick type B
Insufficient data to draw definitive conclusions – transplant might be attempted	Fucosidosis
	Aspartylglucosaminuria
	Mucolipidosis type II (I-cell disease)
	Neuronal ceroid lipofucinosis (Batten's)
	Farber
No evidence for BMT	MPS II (Hunter syndrome)
	MPS III (San Filippo syndrome)
	MPS IV (Morquio)
	Fabry
	Tay–Sachs
	Sandhoff
	Glycogen storage type II (Pompe)
	Niemann-Pick types A and C

A fuller discussion of the individual diseases and the transplant experience is given in the text.

Mucopolysaccharidoses

While transplantation might be considered standard practice in MPSIH (Hurler syndrome),[15–21] it should not be considered routine, nor undertaken lightly. Any transplant has considerable risk and these risks are magnified in certain patients. Even with successful long-term donor cell engraftment there are long-term issues, and successful transplantation requires multidisciplinary long-term follow-up. This is discussed below. In milder forms where there is no CNS involvement (Hurler–Scheie and Scheie) the indication for transplantation is less clear. It is likely that ERT will be the mainstay of treatment[5] for these individuals although if transplant risk can be reduced, where an unaffected sibling donor is available or with continuing advances in BMT practice, then transplant might be considered.

There is no role for BMT in MPS II (Hunter syndrome) or MPS III (San Filippo syndrome).[22–26] There have been many reports of the failure of BMT to correct these illnesses, even where performed early in the disease and with a suitable donor. Whilst the consensus view is that there is no role for BMT in these diseases, cord blood transplant is routinely offered in certain American centers. The results of these experimental transplant programs *might* influence future transplant practice. In Manchester we have not been moved to change our opinion that transplant is not indicated in these conditions. It is interesting to speculate why transplant does not work in these conditions as the same principles of cross-correction of affected recipient tissue by secreted donor enzyme ought to apply as they do in MPSIH. Our best explanation is that the pace of the disease is such that there is insufficient time for donor enzyme to halt the CNS deterioration of this disorder.

In MPS IV (Morquio) the predominant manifestation of enzyme deficiency is skeletal and there is therefore little appetite for transplant as this is the manifestation of MPS disease that is least well corrected by BMT. In MPS VI (Maroteaux-Lamy) there are somatic effects of enzyme deficiency (cardiac disease, hepatosplenomegaly, corneal clouding) that have been reported to be corrected with successful donor cell engraftment.[26–28] However, in Manchester, with the advent of ERT for this condition, it has been our practice that these patients are no longer referred for BMT but managed with ERT.[28–30] MPS VII (Sly syndrome) patients are infrequent but transplants have been successful and the condition should be considered transplantable if the patient's neuropsychologic and clinical status is not adverse at the time of referral.[31]

Sphingolipidoses and other lipidoses

Globoid cell leukodystrophy exists in two forms. The early-onset form, known also as Krabbe disease, might be considered for BMT if diagnosed antenatally and the transplant performed in the neonatal period.[32–37] A recent study demonstrated that the state of disease at referral had an enormous influence on survival: all survived in the presymptomatic group compared to only 40% in the symptomatic group, in which disease progression was the most common cause of death.[35] Transplantation has a role in the later-onset forms, juvenile and adult, where it can stabilize the disease and the imaging abnormalities on MRI scan with appropriate timing.[28]

In metachromatic leukodystrophy (MLD) there are no large series of transplanted patients. However, the transplant experience of selected patients is such that it is generally recommended in presymptomatic patients or while neuropsychologic function and independence in activities of daily living remain good.[14,28,38,39] In Niemann-Pick (NP) disease, type A is not amenable to treatment because of its fulminant clinical course, and although there is some effect of donor cell engraftment in ameliorating NP type B, the advent of ERT will mean that most patients are referred for this therapy rather than stem cell transplantation.[40] Similarly, the clinical success and low morbidity associated with ERT have limited the role of transplantation for Gaucher disease, although this is clearly effective in alleviating most disease manifestations of this disorder. Transplantation is probably only indicated where there is neurologic deterioration or worsening pulmonary function in type III disease.[41]

There is only a single case report of SCT in Farber disease and that was complicated by graft loss.[42] Neurodevelopment continued to deteriorate, although the subcutaneous nodules improved. Definitive conclusions cannot be drawn.

Wolman's disease is characterized by massive hepatosplenomegaly which is a consequence of accumulation of cholesteryl esters and triglycerides in most body tissues. There is one report of an engrafted survivor, although in principle transplantation should be successful as there is no neurologic involvement. Transplant is limited by the rapid deterioration in early life and by liver disease so that four transplants have failed because of transplant-related mortality with probable veno-occlusive liver disease. Notwithstanding, we would transplant this disease if timely referral were made.[43,44]

In neuronal ceroid lipofucinosis (Batten's disease), transplant evidence from presymptomatic patients and animal models does not suggest benefit from transplant. However, more data are clearly needed before definitive conclusions can be drawn.[45,46]

In I-cell disease (mucolipidosis type II) few transplants have been performed and definitive data are therefore lacking. The rationale is present, and certainly donor cell engraftment can be accomplished. In patients transplanted in early life there is preservation of cardiopulmonary performance scores but affected children remain mildly to moderately delayed.[47]

Glycoproteinoses

Alpha-mannosidosis is clearly an indication for transplantation. Although few cases have been transplanted worldwide, the evidence from those cases suggests preservation of neurocognitive and cardiopulmonary function. In fucosidosis and aspartylglucosaminuria there are insufficient cases reported with long-term follow-up to allow an informed decision to be made about BMT. Certainly, there is a rationale for transplant and successful donor cell engraftment has been reported. Therefore, transplantation might be considered in an appropriate patient.[48,49]

Transplantation in MPSIH–Hurler syndrome

Natural history of Hurler syndrome

In Hurler syndrome there is a severe deficiency of the enzyme α-iduronidase. The genetics of the disease are becoming increasingly understood and there is a clear genotype-phenotype correlation. Most severe disease is caused by frameshift or premature stop mutations. Knowledge of the mutation in a particular patient will aid that family in antenatal diagnosis of subsequent pregnancies.[50]

Deficiency of this enzyme in the tissues leads to presentation in early life with a multisystem disorder. Without stem cell transplantation death occurs in childhood. Extent of the disease should be determined prior to transplantation in series of standardized tests. The number of general anesthetics should be kept to a minimum and children with MPSIH generally should not be sedated in an uncontrolled manner.

The importance of assessing the disease before transplantation is firstly so that morbidities that influence transplant can be identified and corrected. It further establishes a baseline for the post-transplant multidisciplinary follow-up of children. It also summarizes disease status for families before the transplant and serves as the basis for informed discussion about what successful donor cell engraftment can achieve and what it, unfortunately, will not achieve.

The features of the illness relevant to the BMT team are as follows.

- *Progressive neurocognitive decline.* Affected individuals gain skills early in life but are increasingly disabled as childhood progresses, with initial slowing and plateau in learning and subsequent dementia. Hydrocephalus may be a feature and needs specific intervention. Established neurocognitive problems are not reversed by transplantation. We do not usually transplant children over the age of 24 months but the earlier a child can be transplanted, the better neurodevelopmental outcome is likely to be. We aim to transplant children as soon as a donor is found and wherever possible within 3 months of referral to the transplant service. We use ERT where possible between referral and transplant (see below).

- There is *deposition of storage material* in the upper airways leading to anesthetic difficulties, obstructive sleep apnea, pulmonary hypertension, and conductive deafness. It is our routine practice to perform sleep studies in all pretransplant patients with MPS and to perform all surgical procedures on routine, as opposed to emergency, surgical lists with anesthetists experienced in the management of children with MPS. Our routine pretransplant assessment also includes an examination under anesthesia by the ENT surgical team. We aim to perform as many procedures as possible under the same general anesthetic to limit the risk that the anesthetic poses with a single procedure.

- *Cardiac disease.* There may be prominent cardiomyopathy and there will certainly be valvular heart disease. Untreated, the deposition of storage material in the coronary arteries means that early-onset ischemic heart disease is a feature of this condition. Recognition of cardiomyopathy is important, as ERT will improve fractional shortening and ejection fraction and should be given prior to transplant as conditioning usually involves cardiotoxic drugs such as cyclophosphamide.

- There is *hepatosplenomegaly.* There is little evidence in our experience that this increases the risk of hepatic complications during stem cell transplantation. Veno-occlusive disease might occur as a consequence of the use of busulfan and cyclophosphamide. The intra-abdominal organomegaly may further compromise respiratory performance and contribute to the development of umbilical and inguinal herniae. We might recommend the closure of these, especially inguinal herniae, before the transplant procedure and this should be carried out at the same time as other procedures requiring anesthesia pretransplant.

- There is *ophthalmic disease with corneal clouding.* This should be assessed by an ophthalmologist experienced in MPS but rarely requires intervention prior to transplant.

- There is *bony disease* which is severe and known as dysostosis multiplex. It may be severe from early life and may have led to suspicion and early diagnosis of MPS, through features such as congenital hip dislocation, prominent thoracolumbar gibbus and talipes. Instability at the atlantoaxial joint is relevant to the anesthetist but the presence of bony disease has little influence on transplant plans except in warning the family that bony disease is often least well corrected by successful donor cell engraftment after transplant.

Choice of donor

The principal factors influencing donor selection in the LSDs in general and MPSIH in particular are:
- HLA match
- speed of donor availability
- enzyme level of donor.

A family phenotypic match is still the donor of choice. Parental consanguinity creates disease but also creates a wider donor pool, and a genetics health visitor should construct a family tree of a consanguineous family to identify those individuals who might be HLA matched so that they can be tested. Using a donor within the family necessarily implies a risk of using a heterozygote donor – obligate heterozygote if parent, 50% risk if sibling donor. Because the enzyme level is reduced in heterozygote donors, and reduced again if there is mixed donor chimerism after the transplant, there is a *theoretical* possibility that these enzyme levels will less adequately cross over and correct recipient tissues than a fully engrafted non-heterozygote donor. There is a significant variable outcome in MPS transplantation, with some patients achieving a better long-term functional outcome than others. There are many possibilities for this (Table 18.2). Although use of a heterozygous donor might affect graft outcome, this should be the first-choice donor for transplant units unless it can be shown in ongoing retrospective and prospective multivariate analyses that it significantly adversely affects outcome. Even then, it would have to go into the risk-based decision of transplant planning, as unrelated donor transplantation is associated with increased risk during the transplant.

Where there is no HLA-matched family donor a recent EBMT working party has made donor recommendations, based on the UK pediatric BMT group (Table 18.3). Considerable weight should be given to the cell dose for the cord donors and matching is low resolution for class I (HLA-A and -B alone) and high resolution for class II. We would not use an adult donor matched at fewer than nine loci. Molecular matching is used for the adult marrow donors at HLA-A, B, Cw, DRB1 and DQB1.

There have been several impressive publications detailing cord blood transplantation in different diseases including Hurler disease. Duke University has reported a single series of cord blood-transplanted children with MPS.[16] In the EBMT registry data series there was no difference in the overall outcome of patients transplanted with cord cells but there was a higher level of full donor cell engraftment in the cord recipients.[51] Factors put forward to suggest this higher level of donor engraftment include a better graft-versus-marrow (GvM) effect because of the greater mismatch, the greater proliferative potential of cord blood stem cells and the presence of mesenchymal cells in the cord blood which favorably influences engraftment.

These impressive results are reflected in these guidelines for donor use, and indeed in the increasing use of cord blood transplants in this disease. Cell dose is important in cord blood transplantation and several lines of evidence suggest it is at least as important as HLA matching.[52,53] Most Hurler patients are less than 10 kg at transplant

and this clearly favorably influences cell dose. Cord blood is usually much more rapidly available than unrelated adult donor marrow or peripheral blood and this further influences the selection of cord blood as a donor source in a disease where there is some urgency to transplant once the diagnosis has been made. It is certainly now our practice to look for cord donors in newly referred patients with MPSIH and to select a cord unit first on the basis of matching and cell dose. We usually have other cord units identified in case of graft failure although we may also have adult donors identified as back-up.

Conditioning therapy

This has been the subject of a recent EBMT working party review and the key elements are as follows.

- *A full-intensity preparative regimen.* A recent EBMT retrospective study identified reduced-intensity preparative regimens in first transplants as a risk factor for treatment failure in multivariate analysis.[32,51]
- *Busulfan* should be given and monitored using pharmacokinetics. This is especially true when using an oral preparation. Use of busulfan pharmacokinetics in busulfan-based preparative regimens was associated with superior graft outcome in registry data of graft outcome of MPSIH.[32,51] Where the oral drug is used, the dose recommended is 40 mg/m² four times daily. We have recently been using intravenous busulfan, also given four times a day, in a weight-based manner, and have not been adjusting the drug as often as we used to when using the oral formulation. It should be noted that iv busulfan given four times daily in this way has considerable implications for the nursing staff. Some units have moved to twice-daily or even once-daily dosing but there is less evidence about efficacy using these dosing strategies.
- Usually busulfan is combined with *cyclophosphamide*, and there is no evidence that escalation of cyclophosphamide beyond the usual 200 mg/kg over 4 days is beneficial.
- There should be *no in vitro T-cell depletion* as this is associated with risks of graft failure.[32,51] The current EBMT recommendations are to use alemtuzumab or antithymocyte globulin (ATG) serotherapy in unrelated donor transplants and to use ATG in cord blood unrelated donor transplants. No serotherapy is utilized with HLA-matched related donor transplants.
- *Graft-versus-host disease(GvHD) prophylaxis* is ciclosporin and 'short' methotrexate in matched related donor transplantation. We use ciclosporin and prednisolone (1 mg/kg/day for 28 days, then tapered to zero over 2 weeks) in cord blood transplants, and ciclosporin/MMF (mycophenolate mofetil) (30 mgs /kg/day for 28 days) with unrelated donor transplants. Ciclosporin is continued for 6 months after cord blood transplantation but we taper it earlier, as early as starting to taper at 50 days, in unrelated donor transplants where there is no GvHD. This reflects our experience that GvHD is associated with superior graft survival and that if there is full donor chimerism at the point of stopping ciclosporin, then graft rejection will not happen later.

We have not performed many haploidentical transplants in MPSIH, preferring in recent years to undertake HLA-mismatched cord grafts. The conditioning protocol for such transplants is not therefore discussed in any detail here. The choice of conditioning therapy for second transplants is discussed below in the discussion of monitoring the graft in MPSIH.

Table 18.2 Factors influencing the variable long-term transplant outcome in Hurler disease transplantation

MPSIH genotype
Pretransplant disease severity, e.g. hydrocephalus
Age at transplant
Donor enzyme level
Level of donor chimerism
Transplant related complications, e.g. GvHD
Graft loss and need for second transplant
Intensity of post-transplant schooling, speech therapy, etc.

Table 18.3 Donor hierarchy in Hurler transplantation where no HLA-identical family donor is available

6/6 cord match = 10/10 adult donor
5/6 cord donor
9/10 adult donor
4/6 cord donor

Combining enzyme replacement therapy with bone marrow transplant

ERT has been available for treating iduronidase-deficient patients for several years. It is now probably the treatment of choice for patients without CNS involvement: Hurler–Scheie and Scheie patients.[5,54–56] We and others have been using it increasingly in combination with transplantation.[57] It is certainly safe and a recent analysis suggested that it did not influence transplant outcome in comparison with historical controls who received transplant without ERT.[58]

The two British centers performing transplant in Hurler patients have continued to use ERT between diagnosis and donor cell engraftment because it does not adversely influence outcome and because there is some evidence that the early exposure to enzyme is associated with a better long-term, functional outcome for the patient. We have found that patients are fitter and better able to tolerate the transplant procedure. Furthermore, there is an inevitable time interval in the real world of BMT between identification of a donor and identification of a space within the transplant schedule. We have felt that it is preferable for patients to be receiving enzyme in this interval. We have therefore interpreted the data indicating no difference in transplant outcome between ERT-treated and enzyme-naïve patients as an opportunity to improve patient fitness for transplant and influence long-term outcome without jeopardizing transplant outcome with sensitization to the deficient enzyme.

Monitoring graft function in Hurler transplants

All studies have recorded an increased rate of graft rejection in Hurler transplants.[15,17,18,20] Many factors have been put forward to explain this increased rate of graft rejection. The Hurler stroma is abnormal and we and others have described how this affects hemopoiesis in vitro.[59] This abnormal stroma might affect the engrafting normal donor cells and was part of the rationale for combined ERT and BMT. Certainly, graft rejection is increased by T-cell depletion and reduced-intensity conditioning, and reduced by busulfan pharmacokinetic monitoring and the use of cord blood as a donor cell source (see above).

Monitoring the graft is therefore important where there is such a high rate of graft failure. We monitor the graft using the following methods, at least monthly from white cell recovery after transplant until withdrawal of immune suppression and stabilization of graft. We continue to monitor graft function annually in the long-term follow-up clinic.

- Blood enzyme level: α-iduronidase
- Urinary substrate: glycosoaminoglycans (GAGs) expressed as total GAG and as the dermatan sulfate to chondroitin sulfate (DS/CS) ratio. This latter expresses more specifically the accumulating substrate in Hurler disease (Fig. 18.3)
- Molecular levels of engraftment using either short tandem repeat (STR) or variable number of tandem repeats (VNTR).

Using these methods we are able to distinguish five patterns of graft function.

1. Initial and continuing full donor cell engraftment. In this pattern of engraftment there is full donor engraftment with a good enzyme level, depending on donor source with lower levels in heterozygote donors, and declining GAG and DS/CS ratio. This engraftment pattern is shown in Figure 18.4.
2. Initial full donor cell engraftment but subsequent autologous reconstitution. Although there is an initial increase in the donor enzyme level it declines with loss of the donor cells. The GAGs and the DS/CS ratio fall with donor cell engraftment but subsequently rise again. It is important to recognize that the blood count remains the same during autologous reconstitution, and only specific monitoring of the graft as above will lead to an appreciation that the graft has actually been lost. This pattern of engraftment is shown in Figure 18.5.
3. Initial full donor cell engraftment but subsequent stabilization of donor chimerism. Whether this level of chimerism is adequate is an inexact science. We have tended to refer patients for retransplant where the chimerism does not support stable or falling GAGs levels. This pattern of engraftment is shown in Figure 18.6.
4. Primary graft failure. In this pattern there is never engraftment of donor cells. This is exceptionally rare, and in over 60 MPS transplants performed in Manchester we have only seen it once. Regrafting is indicated and if the patient is ill with aplastic complications we might return the autologous back-up marrow or obtain a second donation from the same or a different donor.
5. In cord blood transplants we have seen initial mixed chimeric engraftment but with continuing follow-up there is gradual progression to full donor cell engraftment. We have not seen such an engraftment pattern in grafts other than cords. In other donor cell

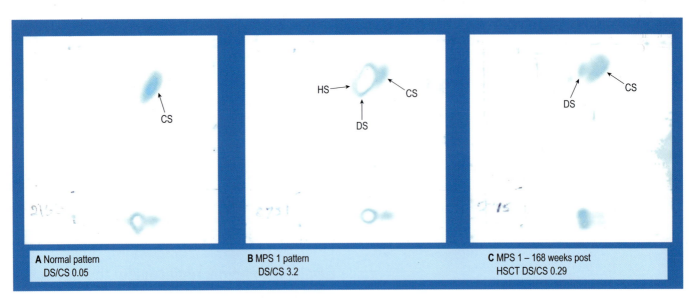

| A Normal pattern | B MPS 1 pattern | C MPS 1 – 168 weeks post |
| DS/CS 0.05 | DS/CS 3.2 | HSCT DS/CS 0.29 |

Figure 18.3
Children with MPS I show grossly elevated amounts of urinary dermatan sulfate (DS) and trace amounts of heparan sulfate (HS) (B) as compared with normal individuals (A) who show only chondroitin sulfate (CS). After HSCT the amount of DS detected in the urine decreases with time (C); this can be analyzed as a semi-quantitative technique and expressed as a DS/CS ratio.

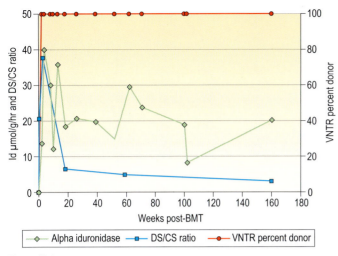

Figure 18.4
Patterns of graft function. Initial and continuing full donor cell engraftment. In this pattern of engraftment there is full donor engraftment with good enzyme level, depending on donor source, with lower levels in heterozygote donors, and declining GAG and DS/CS ratio.

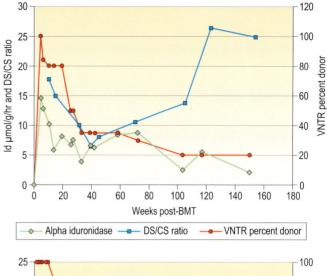

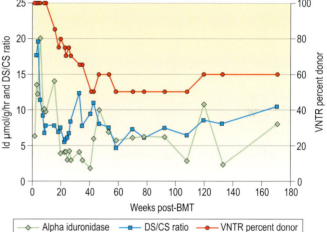

Figures 18.5 and 18.6
When autologous reconstitution occurs, there is early graft loss with recipient cells within the first 100 days after transplant.

sources, mixed chimerism is followed either by stabilization (pattern 3 above) or by inexorable graft loss (pattern 2 above). There are variable graft outcomes in individuals following the patterns of graft function above and using donors with different enzyme levels. In general terms, those with full donor engraftment and those with unaffected donors have higher enzyme levels than those with chimeric engraftment, especially where chimerism is with heterozygote levels. In Figure 18.7 it is demonstrated that engraftment can return GAG levels to baseline in the long term (Fig. 18.7a), that there is variation in engrafted enzyme levels according to donor used and chimerism obtained (Fig. 18.7b) and that this variation is closely correlated with substrate clearance (Fig. 18.7c). The relation between graft outcome and patient outcome is unknown and is affected by many factors (see Table 18.2, and discussion above).

Indications for and results of second transplants in Hurler disease

Graft failure is a common complication of Hurler SCT although we see it far less now that we use cord blood as our primary donor cell source. Graft failure usually occurs as late autologous reconstitution rather than primary graft failure. Where engraftment is complete and immune suppression is stopped we have not observed late graft failure. This is the rationale for early withdrawal of immune suppression in Hurler SCT – we commence ciclosporin withdrawal at day 50 in the absence of GvHD after unrelated donor transplantation. Where we see autologous reconstitution we see early graft loss with recipient cells within the first 100 days after transplant (see Figs 18.5 and 18.6).

We have not found any intervention measure (reduction or increase of ciclosporin) to influence the subsequent fate of the graft. We have avoided the use of donor lymphocyte infusion (DLI) in Hurler and other non-malignant conditions. Whilst DLI is a rational intervention and its use is supported by the observation that where GvHD occurs there is less graft loss, we have avoided its use as it is uncontrolled and likely to be associated with significant morbidity from GvHD. We have instead preferred to see if acceptable stabilization occurs, and if not, then perform a second transplant. We have preferred this route, as results of second BMT in our hands are good and treatment-related morbidity and mortality are low.

Our indication for a second transplant is inadequate graft function to clear substrate, and we are influenced by enzyme levels below the heterozygote range and by rising GAG levels. Others have reported prolonged good CNS correction with low-level donor chimerism, and it is difficult to make exact recommendations. We use the same donor in the second transplant and we use a reduced-intensity protocol with fludarabine (30 mg/m^2 for 5 days) with a single dose of melphalan 140 mg/m^2. We add alemtuzumab 0.2 mg/kg/day for 5 days if unrelated donor, and 0.1 mg/kg/day for 3 days if family donor. We use ciclosporin alone as GvHD prophylaxis and withdraw it early in the absence of GvHD and in the presence of full donor cell engraftment.

Recent EBMT registry data report similar results for myeloablative and non-myeloablative second transplants, with about 80% alive and engrafted. These figures are better than the alive and engrafted rates after a first transplant. Very few patients have received a third transplant but such a procedure is also likely to be associated with a good outcome, and we would recommend that a third transplant be performed if necessary in the case of continuing graft failure.[51]

Long-term follow-up of transplanted mucopolysaccharidosis type IH – what can bone marrow transplant achieve?

BMT in Hurler's disease has created a new clinical entity – the long-term engrafted transplant recipient. To some extent we are learning

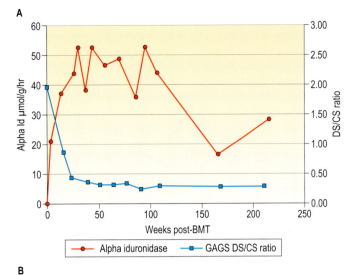

A

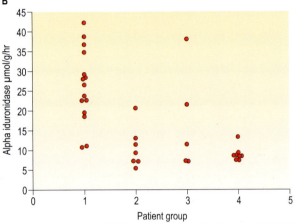

B

- 1. Normal donor, full engraftment
- 2. Heterozygous donor, full engraftment
- 3. Normal donor, chimeric graft
- 4. Heterozygous donor, chimeric graft

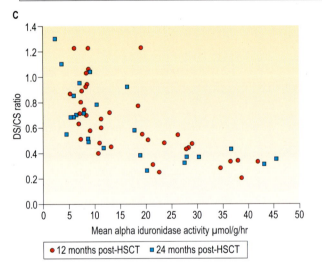

C

- 12 months post-HSCT
- 24 months post-HSCT

Figure 18.7

(a) This patient has undergone HSCT from a normal donor and has fully engrafted (100% donor). Iduronidase activity shows natural fluctuation within the normal range. Residual GAGs have fallen in the initial 6 months post transplant, reaching a plateau that shows a DS/CS ratio consistently <0.5. These data are typical of patients showing full engraftment from normal donors. (b) Individual mean iduronidase measurement for each patient over the initial 12 months post HSCT. Group 1 mean = 26.1, Group 2 mean = 10.2, Group 3 mean = 17.0, Group 4 mean = 7.1. (c) The relationship between mean iduronidase measurement for each patient over the initial 12 months and 12–24 months post HSCT, and the DS/CS ratio. Spearman's rank correlation coefficient (Rho) 12 months = −0.760, p < 0.0001. 12–24 months = −0.755, p < 0.0001. The greater the levels of circulating enzyme, the greater the reduction in urinary GAGs.

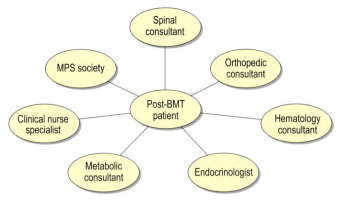

Figure 18.8
The post-transplant follow-up for the first months is carried out by the transplant team and thereafter by a multidisciplinary team.

about the natural history of these recipients as they survive into adulthood, the first successful transplants having been performed in the early 1980s.[60] Knowledge of how transplants affect patient outcome is, however, important for families referred for SCT. In general terms, the effects of transplant are as follows.

- There is correction of cardiac disease and lowering of risk of early cardiac ischemic death. Tachyarrhythmia is eliminated. Cardiac valvular problems may require surgical correction.[61–63]
- The airway corrects rapidly and the risk of anesthesia rapidly declines. Obstructive airway symptoms and hearing both improve.[64,65]
- Corneal clouding is stabilized.[66]
- There is rapid reduction in size of the enlarged liver and spleen to normal.
- We state that there is stabilization of the CNS disease from the point of transplant. Many factors affect outcome, and speech therapy appears to improve outcome.[67]
- Dysmorphic appearances resolve or are much less pronounced.

However, medical problems continue. These are more pronounced in some individuals than in others. It is difficult to accurately predict outcome in terms of ongoing medical problems. The particular organ least well corrected is the dysostosis multiplex of bony disease. This perhaps reflects poor penetration of the engrafted enzyme into bone and cartilage, or perhaps that the disease is inflammatory in nature and driven by cytokines rather than simple substrate accumulation. Many children require ongoing orthopedic procedures, although the enthusiasm with which the orthopedic team embarks on these is declining and varies from center to center.

In Manchester, the post-transplant follow-up for the first months is carried out by the transplant team and thereafter by a multidisciplinary team (Fig. 18.8). In a series of annual assessments and clinics, the patient is seen by all relevant specialists in the same day or during the same visit. Present at these clinics is the patients' organization that helps in areas not covered by the medical and nursing teams and it will advocate the patient's needs to the doctors where necessary. The proximity of other successfully transplanted Hurler children is a source of support and shared experience to families and these clinics are quite sociable occasions.

Summary

MPS transplantation is a rewarding experience. There are problems, and this chapter has discussed many of these. We see children on a daily basis whose life has been transformed by a stem cell transplant and their vitality and that of their families sustains us all in our work. This chapter is dedicated to those children and their families (see Fig. 18.9).

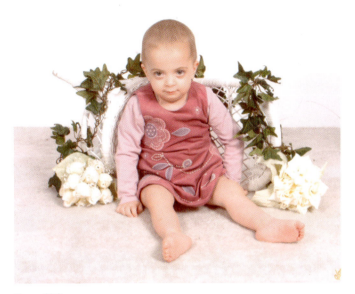

Figure 18.9
Rachel, months after a second transplant for Hurler syndrome.

References

1. Vellodi A. Lysosomal storage disorders. Br J Haematol 2005;128(4):413–431
2. Waheed A, Hasilik A, von Figura K. Processing of the phosphorylated recognition marker in lysosomal enzymes. Characterization and partial purification of a microsomal alpha-N-acetylglucosaminyl phosphodiesterase. J Biol Chem 1981;256(11):5717–5721
3. Hickman S, Neufeld EF. A hypothesis for I-cell disease: defective hydrolases that do not enter lysosomes. Biochem Biophys Res Commun 1972;49(4):992–999
4. O'Brien JS, Miller AL, Loverde AW et al. Sanfilippo disease type B: enzyme replacement and metabolic correction in cultured fibroblasts. Science 1973;181(101):753–755
5. Wraith JE, Clarke LA, Beck M et al. Enzyme replacement therapy for mucopolysaccharidosis I: a randomized, double-blinded, placebo-controlled, multinational study of recombinant human alpha-L-iduronidase (laronidase). J Pediatr 2004;144(5):581–588
6. Eng CM, Guffon N, Wilcox W et al. Safety and efficacy of recombinant human alpha-galactosidase A- replacement therapy in Fabry's disease. N Engl J Med 2001;345(1):9–16
7. Simonaro CM, Haskins ME, Schuchman EH. Articular chondrocytes from animals with a dermatan sulfate storage disease undergo a high rate of apoptosis and release nitric oxide and inflammatory cytokines: a possible mechanism underlying degenerative joint disease in the mucopolysaccharidoses. Lab Invest 2001;81(9):1319–1328
8. Simonaro CM, D'Angelo M, Haskins ME et al. Joint and bone disease in mucopolysaccharidoses VI and VII: identification of new therapeutic targets and biomarkers using animal models. Pediatr Res 2005;57(5 Pt 1):701–707
9. Futerman AH, van Meer G. The cell biology of lysosomal storage disorders. Nat Rev Mol Cell Biol 2004;5(7):554–565
10. Brady RO, Barton NW, Grabowski GA. The role of neurogenetics in Gaucher disease. Arch Neurol 1993;50(11):1212–1224
11. Zhao H, Bailey LA, Elsas LJ 2nd et al. Gaucher disease: in vivo evidence for allele dose leading to neuronopathic and nonneuronopathic phenotypes. Am J Med Genet A 2003;116(1):52–56
12. Ling EA, Wong WC. The origin and nature of ramified and amoeboid microglia: a historical review and current concepts. Glia 1993;7(1):9–18
13. Walkley SU, Thrall MA, Dobrenis K et al. Bone marrow transplantation corrects the enzyme defect in neurons of the central nervous system in a lysosomal storage disease. Proc Natl Acad Sci USA 1994;91(8):2970–2974
14. Peters C, Steward CG. Hematopoietic cell transplantation for inherited metabolic diseases: an overview of outcomes and practice guidelines. Bone Marrow Transplant 2003;31(4):229–239
15. Vellodi A, Young EP, Cooper A et al. Bone marrow transplantation for mucopolysaccharidosis type I: experience of two British centres. Arch Dis Child 1997;76(2):92–99
16. Staba SL, Escolar ML, Poe M et al. Cord-blood transplants from unrelated donors in patients with Hurler's syndrome. N Engl J Med 2004;350(19):1960–1969
17. Souillet G, Guffon N, Maire I et al. Outcome of 27 patients with Hurler's syndrome transplanted from either related or unrelated hematopoietic stem cell sources. Bone Marrow Transplant 2003;31(12):1105–1117
18. Peters C, Shapiro EG, Krivit W. Hurler syndrome: past, present, and future. J Pediatr 1998;133(1):7–9
19. Peters C, Shapiro EG, Krivit W. Neuropsychological development in children with Hurler syndrome following hematopoietic stem cell transplantation. Pediatr Transplant 1998;2(4):250–253
20. Peters C, Shapiro EG, Anderson J et al. Hurler syndrome: II. Outcome of HLA-genotypically identical sibling and HLA-haploidentical related donor bone marrow transplantation

in fifty-four children. The Storage Disease Collaborative Study Group. Blood 1998;91(7):2601–2608
21. Guffon N, Souillet G, Maire I et al. Follow-up of nine patients with Hurler syndrome after bone marrow transplantation. J Pediatr 1998;133(1):119–125
22. Vellodi A, Young E, New M et al. Bone marrow transplantation for Sanfilippo disease type B. J Inherit Metab Dis 1992;15(6):911–918
23. Vellodi A, Young E, Cooper A et al. Long-term follow-up following bone marrow transplantation for Hunter disease. J Inherit Metab Dis 1999;22(5):638–648
24. Sivakumur P, Wraith JE. Bone marrow transplantation in mucopolysaccharidosis type IIIA: a comparison of an early treated patient with his untreated sibling. J Inherit Metab Dis 1999;22(7):849–850
25. Bergstrom SK, Quinn JJ, Greenstein R et al. Long-term follow-up of a patient transplanted for Hunter's disease type IIB: a case report and literature review. Bone Marrow Transplant 1994;14(4):653–658
26. Krivit W, Pierpont ME, Ayaz K et al. Bone-marrow transplantation in the Maroteaux-Lamy syndrome (mucopolysaccharidosis type VI). Biochemical and clinical status 24 months after transplantation. N Engl J Med 1984;311(25):1606–1611
27. Herskhovitz E, Young E, Rainer J et al. Bone marrow transplantation for Maroteaux-Lamy syndrome (MPS VI): long-term follow-up. J Inherit Metab Dis 1999;22(1):50–62
28. Krivit W, Aubourg P, Shapiro E et al. Bone marrow transplantation for globoid cell leukodystrophy, adrenoleukodystrophy, metachromatic leukodystrophy, and Hurler syndrome. Curr Opin Hematol 1999;6(6):377–382
29. Hein LK, Meikle PJ, Dean CJ et al. Development of an assay for the detection of mucopolysaccharidosis type VI patients using dried blood-spots. Clin Chim Acta 2005;353(1–2):67–74
30. Desnick RJ. Enzyme replacement and enhancement therapies for lysosomal diseases. J Inherit Metab Dis 2004;27(3):385–410
31. Yamada Y, Kato K, Sukegawa K et al. Treatment of MPS VII (Sly disease) by allogeneic BMT in a female with homozygous A619V mutation. Bone Marrow Transplant 1998;21(6):629–634
32. Boelens JJ. Trends in hematopoietic cell transplantation for inborn errors of metabolism. J Inherit Metab Dis 2006;29(2–3):413–420
33. Martin PL, Carter SL, Kernan NA et al. Results of the cord blood transplantation study (COBLT): outcomes of unrelated donor umbilical cord blood transplantation in pediatric patients with lysosomal and peroxisomal storage diseases. Biol Blood Marrow Transplant 2006;12(2):184–194
34. McGraw P, Liang L, Escolar M et al. Krabbe disease treated with hematopoietic stem cell transplantation: serial assessment of anisotropy measurements – initial experience. Radiology 2005;236(1):221–230
35. Escolar ML, Poe MD, Provenzale JM et al. Transplantation of umbilical-cord blood in babies with infantile Krabbe's disease. N Engl J Med 2005;352(20):2069–2081
36. Wenger DA, Susuki K, Susuki Y. Galactosylceramide lipidosis: globoid cell leukodystrophy (Krabbe Disease). In: Scriver CR (ed) The metabolic and molecular basis of inherited disease, 8th edn. McGraw-Hill, New York, 2001:3669–3964
37. Krivit W. Allogeneic stem cell transplantation for the treatment of lysosomal and peroxisomal metabolic diseases. Springer Semin Immunopathol 2004;26(1–2):119–132
38. Malm G, Ringden O, Winiarski J et al. Clinical outcome in four children with metachromatic leukodystrophy treated by bone marrow transplantation. Bone Marrow Transplant 1996;17(6):1003–1008
39. Krivit W, Lipton ME, Lockman LA et al. Prevention of deterioration in metachromatic leukodystrophy by bone marrow transplantation. Am J Med Sci 1987;294(2):80–85
40. Vellodi A, Hobbs JR, O'Donnell NM et al. Treatment of Niemann-Pick disease type B by allogeneic bone marrow transplantation. BMJ (Clin Res Ed) 1987;295(6610):1375–1376
41. Schiffmann R, Brady RO. New prospects for the treatment of lysosomal storage diseases. Drugs 2002;62(5):733–742
42. Yeager AM, Uhas KA, Coles CD et al. Bone marrow transplantation for infantile ceramidase deficiency (Farber disease). Bone Marrow Transplant, 2000;26(3):357–363
43. Krivit W, Peters C, Dusenbery K et al. Wolman disease successfully treated by bone marrow transplantation. Bone Marrow Transplant 2000;26(5):567–570
44. Krivit W, Freese D, Chan KW et al. Wolman's disease: a review of treatment with bone marrow transplantation and considerations for the future. Bone Marrow Transplant 1992;10(suppl 1):97–101
45. Lake BD, Henderson DC, Oakhill A et al. Bone marrow transplantation in Batten disease (neuronal ceroid-lipofuscinosis). Will it work? Preliminary studies on coculture experiments and on bone marrow transplant in late infantile Batten disease. Am J Med Genet 1995;57(2):369–373
46. Deeg HJ, Shulman HM, Albrechtsen D et al. Batten's disease: failure of allogeneic bone marrow transplantation to arrest disease progression in a canine model. Clin Genet 1990;37(4):264–270
47. Yamaguchi K, Hayasaka S, Hara S et al. Improvement of tear lysosomal enzyme levels after treatment with bone marrow transplantation in a patient with I-cell disease. Ophthalmic Res 1989;21(3):226–229
48. Krivit WC, Peters C, Shapiro EG. Bone marrow transplantation as effective treatment of central nervous system disease in globoid cell leukodystrophy, metachromatic leukodystrophy, adrenoleukodystrophy, mannosidosis, fucosidosis, aspartylglucosaminuria, Hurler, Maroteaux-Lamy, and Sly syndromes, and Gaucher disease type III. Curr Opin Neurol 1999;12(2):167–176
49. Grewal SS, Shapiro EG, Krivit W et al. Effective treatment of alpha-mannosidosis by allogeneic hematopoietic stem cell transplantation. J Pediatr 2004;144(5):569–573
50. Neufeld EF, Muenzer J. The mucopolysaccharidoses. In: Scriver CR (ed) The metabolic and molecular basis of inherited disease, 8th edn. McGraw-Hill, New York, 2001:3421–3452
51. Boelens JJ, Wynn R, O'Mearra A et al. Results of hemopoietic stem cell transplantation for Hurler Syndrome: European experience 1994–2004 ASH 2005. Blood 2005;106(11):121a

52. Gluckman E, Rocha V, Arcese W et al. Factors associated with outcomes of unrelated cord blood transplant: guidelines for donor choice. Exp Hematol 2004;32(4):397–407

53. Kogler G, Enczmann J, Rocha V et al. High-resolution HLA typing by sequencing for HLA-A, -B, -C, -DR, -DQ in 122 unrelated cord blood/patient pair transplants hardly improves long-term clinical outcome. Bone Marrow Transplant 2005;36(12):1033–1041

54. Wraith JE. Limitations of enzyme replacement therapy: current and future. J Inherit Metab Dis 2006;29(2–3):442–447

55. Harmatz P, Giugliani R, Schwartz I. MPS VI Phase 3 Study Group. Enzyme replacement therapy for mucopolysaccharidosis VI: a phase 3, randomized, double-blind, placebo-controlled, multinational study of recombinant human N-acetylgalactosamine 4-sulfatase (recombinant human arylsulfatase B or rhASB) and follow-on, open-label extension study. J Pediatr 2006;148(4):533–539

56. Wraith JE. The first 5 years of clinical experience with laronidase enzyme replacement therapy for mucopolysaccharidosis I. Expert Opin Pharmacother 2005;6(3):489–506

57. Grewal SS, Wynn R, Abdenur JE et al. Safety and efficacy of enzyme replacement therapy in combination with hematopoietic stem cell transplantation in Hurler syndrome. Genet Med 2005;7(2):143–146

58. Cox-Brinkman J, Boelens JJ, Wraith JE et al. Hematopoietic cell transplantation (HCT) in combination with enzyme replacement therapy (ERT) in patients with Hurler syndrome. Bone Marrow Transplant 2006;38(1):17–21

59. Baxter MA, Wynn RF, Schyma L et al. Marrow stromal cells from patients affected by MPS I differentially support hematopoietic progenitor cell development. J Inherit Metab Dis 2005;28(6):1045–1053

60. Hobbs JR, Hugh-Jones K, Barrett AJ et al. Reversal of clinical features of Hurler's disease and biochemical improvement after treatment by bone-marrow transplantation. Lancet 1981;2(8249):709–712

61. Braunlin EA, Stauffer NR, Peters CH et al. Usefulness of bone marrow transplantation in the Hurler syndrome. Am J Cardiol 2003;92(7):882–886

62. Braunlin EA, Rose AG, Hopwood JJ et al. Coronary artery patency following long-term successful engraftment 14 years after bone marrow transplantation in the Hurler syndrome. Am J Cardiol 2001;88(9):1075–1077

63. Braunlin EA, Hunter DW, Krivit W et al. Evaluation of coronary artery disease in the Hurler syndrome by angiography. Am J Cardiol 1992;69(17):1487–1489

64. Whitley CB, Ramsay NK, Kersey JH et al. Bone marrow transplantation for Hurler syndrome: assessment of metabolic correction. Birth Defects Orig Artic Ser 1986;22(1):7–24

65. Malone BN, Whitley CB, Duvall AJ et al. Resolution of obstructive sleep apnea in Hurler syndrome after bone marrow transplantation. Int J Pediatr Otorhinolaryngol 1988;15(1):23–31

66. Summers CG, Purple RL, Krivit W et al. Ocular changes in the mucopolysaccharidoses after bone marrow transplantation. A preliminary report. Ophthalmology 1989;96(7):977–984; discussion 984–985

67. Shapiro EG, Lockman LA, Balthazor M et al. Neuropsychological outcomes of several storage diseases with and without bone marrow transplantation. J Inherit Metab Dis 1995;18(4):413–429

Autoimmune disorders

Paolo Muraro, Jaap van Laar, Gabor Illei
and Steven Pavletic

CHAPTER 19

Introduction

Autoimmune diseases comprise a relatively new field in hematopoietic stem cell transplantation (HSCT) and the first transplants undertaken specifically for these indications were initiated in the mid-1990s. Several developments set the stage, including the steadily improving safety of HSCT, promising results from animal models of autoimmune disease, case reports of cures of concomitant autoimmune disease after transplantation for another indication, and the steady need for better treatments for patients with therapy-refractory autoimmune disease.[1,2] The now historic consensus conferences held in Seattle in 1995 and Basel 1996 defined guidelines on how to proceed, and autologous HSCT was recommended as the modality of choice in early pilot trials.[3]

To date, more than 1000 patients with various severe autoimmune diseases have been treated worldwide by HSCT, most commonly for diagnoses of multiple sclerosis, systemic sclerosis, rheumatoid and juvenile arthritis and systemic lupus erythematosus.[4] In recent years, several randomized, prospective clinical trials have been initiated in the USA and Europe to address the role of autologous HSCT as compared to standard therapy in the treatment of severe systemic sclerosis, multiple sclerosis, systemic lupus erythematosus and Crohn's disease.[5]

Potential mechanisms of action of HSCT for autoimmune disease are presented in Table 19.1. In spite of 10 years of experience with HSCT for autoimmune disease, there is a profound lack of studies designed to explain the mechanisms of action and disease control in transplanted patients. The main question relating to autologous HSCT is whether HSCT qualitatively changes the diseased immune system or whether the observed effects are only due to dose-intensive lymphoablation. Studies have recently begun to demonstrate the regeneration of a new T-cell repertoire following autologous HSCT[6] and the restoration of impaired immunoregulatory circuits[7] in the context of the quantitatively fully recovered immune system. Today, it is evident that autologous HSCT can result in clinical disease control in about half of patients with a duration of several years. However, there is still room for significant improvements in safety and efficacy, and it still remains unclear whether autologous HSCT can cure patients or whether it only suppresses and delays disease progression.

The appeal of HSCT is its curative potential, avoiding cumulative toxicities, disability costs, impairment of quality of life and late mortality of patients receiving the life-long treatments that are needed for refractory autoimmune disease. Transplant-related mortality is, however, a limitation and is related to dose intensity, underlying disease and pre-existing organ damage.[8] On the other hand, disease control in autologous HSCT is better with higher intensity regimens,

which poses challenges when designing better HSCT strategies. Current efforts in the field are focused on three main aspects:
- pursuing well-planned prospective randomized trials to determine the role of autologous HSCT in selected disease
- pursuing innovative pilot studies of autologous HSCT to capitalize on current progress and explore better transplant regimens, including the role of cellular therapy[9]
- initiating carefully planned pilot trials of allogeneic HSCT.[10]

Optimum patient selection remains among the greatest ongoing challenges and there is an urgent need for studies and markers which will better define high-risk groups in patients who fail standard therapies. HSCT for severe autoimmune disease is an interdisciplinary effort in the true sense, and progress towards cure is only possible within integrated teams that include transplant specialists, disease specialists and basic scientists.

In the following sections we present the state of the art of clinical HSCT for the five most commonly transplanted autoimmune diseases: multiple sclerosis, systemic sclerosis, rheumatoid and juvenile arthritis, and systemic lupus erythematosus.

Results of transplantation

Multiple sclerosis

Background

Multiple sclerosis is the most common acquired demyelinating disease of the central nervous system (CNS), with prevalence rates ranging between 80 and 240 in 100,000 in Northern European and American countries.[11] The initial disease course, typically manifesting in young adulthood between age 20 and 40, is characterized by transient episodes of neurologic disturbances, developing over several hours and lasting a number of days, followed by remission (relapsing-remitting MS). The clinical symptoms may involve any component of neurologic function, and frequently affect vision, sensation or motion (including strength, co-ordination or both) in any combination. Later in the disease course, recovery from relapses may become less complete, resulting in an accumulation of residual neurologic disability. Many patients will eventually start progressing chronically between relapses, and even in the absence of relapses (secondary progressive MS).

Less commonly, the disease starts with chronically progressing symptoms (primary progressive). Clinical severity ranges from benign (no disability after 15 years of disease) to malignant MS, characterized by an aggressive course resulting in rapid accumulation of significant disability or death.[12] The majority of patients experience a disease course of intermediate severity between these two extremes. The most

Table 19.1 HSCT for autoimmune disease – potential mechanisms of action

	Auto	Allo
Dose intensity effect	++	+/-
Eradication of memory cells	+	++
Acquisition of self tolerance	+	+
Resetting immune system	+	+
Changing genetics	–	+/?
Graft-vs-host/autoimmunity	–	+

HSCT, hematopoietic stem cell transplantation; Auto, autologous; Allo, allogeneic.

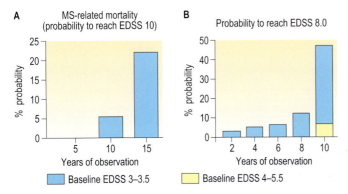

Figure 19.1
Probability of progression to death attributable to multiple sclerosis (a) or to advanced disability (defined as reaching an EDSS score of 8.0; equivalent to bed-ridden; (b) in an untreated MS population (n = 285). Source of data is the Silvia Lawry Center for Multiple Sclerosis Research (Daumer et al[14]).

commonly used rating scale to grade neurologic disability in patients with MS is the Expanded Disability Status Scale (EDSS), which ranges from 0 (normal neurologic status) to 10 (death due to MS), in non-linear 0.5-point intervals.[13]

MS has traditionally been seen as a disease that does not reduce life expectancy. This is true for the majority of patients with milder disease. Patients with severe or advanced disease, however, are at increased risk of developing life-threatening complications which may result from immobility and neurologic dysfunction, such as urinary tract infections and pneumonia. In a recent database survey of untreated MS patients who had started undergoing observation with intermediate grades of disability (EDSS 4.0 to 5.5), disease-related mortality was zero at five years, but 5.4% at 10 years and 22% at 15 years.[14] In the same patient subgroup, the risk of becoming bedridden (EDSS 8.0) was 12% after 5 years and rose to 40% after 10 years (Fig. 19.1). However, extrapolating these data to the general population of patients suffering from MS is problematic owing to disease heterogeneity and the risk of a selection bias. Unfavorable prognostic factors for progression to severe disability include male gender, older age at onset, polysymptomatic onset, and early high relapse rate.[15] Motor, cerebellar and sphincter involvement are also factors which were found to be associated with a poorer outcome.[15,16] Magnetic resonance imaging (MRI) has become an invaluable tool not only for diagnosis, but also for monitoring evolution and understanding the disease process in MS. In addition to conventional MRI measures which reveal disease activity (new or gadolinium-enhancing lesions) and progression (accumulation of lesions, atrophy),[17] new modalities such as magnetization transfer are likely to predict future extent of disability.[18]

Current knowledge suggests that MS is the result of an autoimmune inflammatory attack initiated by T- and B-cells and directed against components of CNS myelin. Relative sparing of axons is generally observed in relapsing-remitting MS, but axonal damage becomes prominent in secondary progressive disease and is thought to be a lead cause of clinical disability. It is generally felt that in these stages, axonal degeneration can progress independent of ongoing inflammation.

There is no therapy proven to be curative in MS. Treatment options can be grouped as treatment of acute relapse and maintenance therapy. Relapses are normally treated with intravenous steroids, with the objective of improving speed and extent of recovery. Realistic goals of maintenance treatment in MS are to prevent or reduce frequency and severity of the inflammatory attacks and development of new CNS white matter lesions. Current medications are only partially successful or have significant side-effects and risks that limit their long-term use. Approved immunomodulatory treatments such as interferon-β and glatiramer acetate typically achieve positive clinical responses in approximately one-third of patients. In the remaining subjects there is either no response, or an initial response is followed by breakthroughs of disease activity.

Natalizumab is a monoclonal antibody that inhibits lymphocyte migration into the CNS and it has proven effective in reducing disease activity in clinical trials. However, its high cost and associated risk of causing progressive multifocal encephalitis have delayed its introduction to routine MS care in most countries. Additional biologic agents such as daclizumab and fingolimod (FTY720) have resulted in promising reductions in disease activity such as relapse rates and numbers of gadolinium-enhancing lesions in proof-of-concept studies and await evaluation in larger and longer-term trials.[19,20] Study results and clinical practice, however, indicate that some patients, particularly those with more aggressive disease, derive very limited or no benefit from any of the available immunomodulatory drugs. In those patients, treatment with immune suppressants is often required to control disease activity. Immunosuppressive treatment options include oral azathioprine, monthly pulsed cyclophosphamide, and mitoxantrone (the only chemotherapy with regulatory approval for secondary progressive MS). Long-term use of the two latter agents is, however, limited by toxicities, and breakthroughs of disease activity are fairly common.

CAMPATH-1H (alemtuzumab) is highly immunosuppressive and trials in MS have resulted in protracted remissions from inflammatory disease activity although it did not prevent progression of chronic disability in patients with advanced, progressive disease.[21] Development of secondary autoimmune disorders including hyperthyroidism and idiopathic thrombocytopenias has been observed after CAMPATH-1H treatment.[22,23] High-dose cyclophosphamide (HDC) without stem cell support, pioneered by the Johns Hopkins group,[24] has shown no unexpected toxicities and has led to complete remissions lasting from 6 to 24 months of follow-up in a recent study of 12 patients with MS.[25] These encouraging results should stimulate further studies in larger series of patients, to assess durability of the clinical response after HDC.

Autologous hematopoietic stem cell transplantation

Rationale

Immune ablation followed by HSCT is being evaluated in MS as an experimental therapeutic approach aiming to induce complete, medication-free remission from new disease activity. The fundamental rationale of this therapy for MS is the same as for other autoimmune diseases, that is to purge the existing immune system that harbors disease-mediating cells and regenerate a new and healthy immune system.[26] Support for the rationale of testing HSCT as a therapy for MS came from data from an animal model of autoimmune demyelination, experimental allergic encephalomyelitis (EAE).[27] Studies in the EAE model showed that acute autoimmune demyelination could be prevented or blocked after clinical onset, although chronic neurologic damage could not be reversed.[27,28]

Clinical experience

To date, more than 300 patients with MS have undergone auto-HSCT worldwide. The Center for International Blood and Marrow Transplant Research (CIBMTR) registry includes 77 patients with MS who received an autologous transplant from 1996 to 2005 from centers in North and South America, and only one allogeneic transplant (Dr M C Pasquini, personal communication). In December 2006, the European Group for Blood and Marrow Transplantation (EBMT) registry included 264 patients who had received an autotransplant for MS (Dr R Saccardi, personal communication). To our knowledge, no similar registry data are available for the other continents.

Early reports of clinical trials included few patients and short follow-ups. They did not establish efficacy, but established proof of the principle that HSCT could induce disease remissions in patients with severe MS. A summary of the results of clinical trials and relevant retrospective surveys published since year 2000 is provided in Table 19.2. In spite of the limitations that include heterogeneous patient populations and transplantation regimens, small numbers of patients, and lack of a control arm, these studies provide important information.

Firstly, HSCT generally exerted profound beneficial effects on outcome, based on suppression of inflammatory disease activity such as acute clinical exacerbations, persistence of gadolinium-enhancing lesions on MRI of the brain or spinal cord post-transplantation, or both. Very few neurologic relapses were reported after treatment, other than those observed early post transplantation in association with fever related to antithymocyte globulin (ATG) administration or engraftment syndrome, which are attributable to release of soluble mediators, and have been shown to be preventable by corticosteroid administration.[29,30] Abrogation of inflammatory disease activity after HSCT has been most eloquently demonstrated in studies that undertook systematic contrast-enhanced MRI assessments such as those reported by Mancardi et al,[31] Saiz et al[32] and Saccardi et al[33] (Fig. 19.2).

Secondly, stabilization of the clinical disease course during follow-up post therapy was observed in major proportions of treated patients in all but one study.[34] Continued worsening of disability post therapy was frequently observed in patients who had a severe and chronically established degree of disability prior to HSCT (EDSS 6.0 and above), strongly suggesting that chronic deterioration in these patients was more likely to be related to axonal and oligodendroglial degenerative processes rather than to failure to suppress an active inflammatory process. This notion is supported by work showing ongoing CNS demyelination and axonal injury in association with activated microglia, in spite of suppressed inflammation post transplantation.[35]

Thirdly, it is conceivable that the most intensive conditioning regimens and graft lymphocyte depletion may present greater risks of toxicity and infectious complications; however, conclusive assessment is not possible due to diversity of the available data.

The high frequency at which continuous neurologic progression has been seen after treatment regimens that included total-body irradiation (TBI)[29,34,36] has raised awareness of the CNS-specific detrimental effects of radiation and cautioned against its use in future trials. A recent large-scale retrospective survey of the European registry provides an historical analysis of treatment-related mortality (TRM).[37] TRM was observed only until the end of year 2000 (overall TRM 5.3%) and no toxic deaths were recorded after that date, suggesting that increased experience with transplantation in MS, including more appropriate patient selection, has led to improved safety. Furthermore, no TRM was reported in the group of 53 patients who received a transplant regimen of BEAM (carmustine, etoposide, cytosine-arabinoside, melphalan) followed by ATG, without manipulation of the autologous graft, again lending support to the notion of differences in toxicities among various transplant regimens.

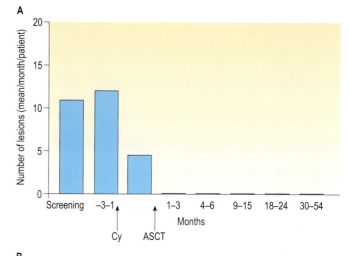

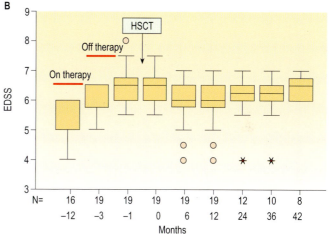

Figure 19.2

Effects of autologous transplantation on inflammatory disease activity and clinical disability in patients with severe multiple sclerosis. Reproduced with permission from Saccardi et al.[33] (a) MRI results. The mean numbers of lesions per month per patient are reported at baseline during the 3-month period before mobilization (-3–1) after mobilization (Cy), and after transplantation (AHSCT) to last follow-up. (b) EDSS outcome. Box plot of the changes in EDSS score over the entire study period and in the year before the enrollment. Error bars indicate the highest and lowest values, excluding outliers, which are cases with values between 1.5 and 3 box lengths from the upper or lower edge of the box. Extremes* are cases with values more than 3 box lengths from the upper or lower edge of the box; the box length is the interquartile range.

Ongoing and future clinical trials

Type of study, patient selection, treatment regimen, and outcome measures are some key issues to be considered in the planning stages of trials of HSCT to treat MS.

Type of study There is consensus among specialists in the field that whenever possible, patients with MS should receive hematopoietic transplantation in the context of a clinical trial rather than on an individual, compassionate basis. However, opinions are split on the design of the new studies to be conducted, with some specialists feeling that stronger evidence of safety and efficacy should be obtained from additional Phase II trials, and others being supportive of randomized, controlled studies. Two controlled clinical trials are currently recruiting patients: the Autologous Stem cell Transplantation International Multiple Sclerosis Trial (ASTIMS; www.astims.org) in which the transplantation arm consists of BEAM-ATG and no graft manipulation, and a study of non-myeloablative hematopoietic transplantation (principal investigator R Burt, Northwestern University, Chicago, IL). The control arms for the two studies are mitoxantrone and approved

Table 19.2 Recent trials of autologous HSCT in patients with multiple sclerosis

Reference (no.)	No. of patients treated	MS subtype[1]	EDSS at inclusion (range)	Graft manipulation[2]	Conditioning regimen[3]	Life-threatening toxicities[4]	Follow-up median (range)	Response on inflammatory activity (MRI or relapses)[5]	Response on neurologic disability (EDSS)[6]
Fassas et al 2000[43]	24	13 SPMS, 8 PPMS, 3 PRMS	4.5–8.0	CD34+ selection in 9 cases	BEAM+ATG	1 death from aspergillosis; 1 liver VOD, 1 TTP	40 mo (21–51)	No enhancing lesions in 21/23 (91%)	18/23 (78%) stabilized or improved
Kozak et al 2000[44]	8	SPMS	6.5–7.5	CD34+ selection+T depletion	BEAM (+ATG in 1 pt)	None	8.5 months (8–12)	No new or enhancing lesions in 6/7 (86%)[7]	7/8 (87%) stabilized or improved
Mancardi et al 2001[31]	10	SPMS	5.5–6.5	None	BEAM+ATG	None	15 months (4–30)	No new or enhancing lesions after 3 months post-TX in 10/10 (100%)	10/10 stabilized or improved
Fassas et al 2002[45]	85[8]	60 SPMS, 22 PPMS, 3 RRMS	4.5–8.5	Various	Various	7 deaths, from neurologic deterioration (2), cardiac toxicity (1), aspergillosis (1), septicemia (1), influenza pneumonitis (1), postoperative pneumococcal septicemia (1)	16 months (3–59)	No enhancing lesions in 56/61 (92%)	Confirmed progression-free survival 74% (±12%) at 3 years
Nash et al 2003[29]	26	17 SPMS, 8 PPMS, 1 RRMS	5.0–8.0	CD34+ selection	TBI+ATG	1 death from EBV-related post-transplantation lymphoproliferative disorder	24 months (3–36)	No new or enhancing lesions in 21/25 (84%); one neurologic deterioration associated with fever (engraftment syndrome)	19/25 (76%) stabilized or improved
Burt et al 2003[36]	21	14 SPMS, 6 PPMS, 1 RRMS	3.0–8.5	CD34+ selection	CY+TBI	2 deaths from complications of neurologic deterioration	24 months (5–60)	No new or enhancing lesions in 13/18 (72%); one confirmed relapse at 14 months	13/21 (62%) stabilized or improved. 9/9 patients with pre-Tx EDSS 3.0–6.0; and 4/12 patients with EDSS > 6.0
Saiz et al 2004[46]	15	9 SPMS, 6 RRMS	4.5–6.5	CD34+ selection	Carmustine+CY+ATG	None	36 months (19–55)	No enhancing lesions in 15/15 (100%); confirmed relapses in 2 patients	12/15 (80%) stabilized or improved
Saccardi et al 2005[33]	19	15 SPMS, 4 RRMS	5.0–6.5	None	BEAM+ATG	1 gastric ulcer bleeding requiring endoscopic intervention	36 months (12–72)	No enhancing lesions in 18/19 (95%)	18/19 (95%) improved or stabilized
Ni et al 2006[47]	21	16 SPMS, 2 PPMS, 2 PRMS, 1 malignant MS	5.0–9.5	CD34+ selection	BEAM (20 patients) or CY+TBI (1 pt)	2 deaths from pneumonia (1) and VZV hepatitis (1)	42 months (6–65)	No enhancing lesions in 18/21 (86%)	16/19 (84%) improved or stabilized
Samijn et al 2006[34]	14	SPMS	5.5–6.5	CD34+ selection	CY+TBI+ATG	EBV-related post-transplantation lymphoproliferative disorder (1), myelodysplastic syndrome (1). One death from respiratory infection 5 years from transplantation	36 months (7–36)	No enhancing lesions in 14/14 (100%)	5/14 (36%) improved or stabilized
Saccardi et al 2006[33]	178[8]	99 SPMS, 32 PPMS, 19 RPMS, 22 RRMS, 11 unknown	3.5–9.0	Various	Various	5.3% treatment-related mortality during 1995–2000; None 2000 onwards	41.7 months	Not available	90/142 (63%) improved or stabilized

1. SPMS, secondary progressive MS; PPMS, primary progressive MS; PRMS, progressive relapsing MS; RRMS relapsing-remitting MS.
2. Hematopoietic graft was peripheral blood stem cells for all studies except Samijn et al (bone marrow).
3. BEAM, carmustine, etoposide, cytosine-arabinoside, melphalan; CY, cyclophosphamide; BU, busulfan; ATG, antithymocyte globulin; TBI, total body irradiation.
4. VOD, veno-occlusive disease; TTP, thrombotic thrombocytopenic purpura.
5. With the exception of Mancardi et al 2001 no trial required presence of enhancing MRI lesions pretransplantation for patient inclusion.
6. The definition of stabilization differed among studies, with some requiring no EDSS change and others allowing an increase of 0.5 EDSS.
7. Corticosteroid treatment chronically administered post transplantation to all patients.
8. Retrospective multicenter observational analysis. The survey by Saccardi et al includes data from European studies that were previously reported independently as well as the earlier retrospective report by Fassas et al.

standard of care (i.e. interferon, copaxone, or mitoxantrone), respectively.

Patient selection Both the experience gained from clinical trials of HSCT and the improved understanding of the pathophysiologic evolution of MS should guide criteria for selecting the appropriate patients as candidates for HSCT. Since HSCT effectively stops CNS 'acute inflammation' in MS (focal blood–brain barrier disruption, peripheral immune cell infiltration and acute clinical relapses) in a remarkably high proportion of subjects, the best candidates for treatment are thought to be those patients who have an aggressive disease course but little disability and who experience high inflammatory activity (see Fig. 19.2). In contrast, subjects who are already in the advanced, progressive stages of disease are unlikely to benefit. The main challenge of the next round of clinical trials will be to select patients who have aggressive disease but who have not had it for long enough or sufficiently severely to have entered a phase of irreversible deterioration. These basic principles had already been identified in a consensus conference held in Milan in 1998.[38] Today's updated knowledge suggests further refinement of the inclusion criteria as follows.

- MS diagnosed according to McDonald's criteria[39]
- Relapsing–remitting, secondary progressive (only if with relapses), progressive relapsing courses
- Age 18–50
- Disease duration = 1 year but less than 10 years from diagnosis
- EDSS between 3.0 and 5.5
- Recent (in the last year) and significant (at least 1 point of EDSS) progression of disability, sustained for at least 3 months
- At least two relapses in the year preceding enrollment, or one relapse plus MRI evidence corroborating disease activity
- Presence of MRI-enhancing lesions on baseline scans
- Failure to respond to other available therapies

Ongoing or planned clinical trials utilize some or many of these criteria but assessment of what may be the optimum inclusion criteria is not unanimous. This uncertainty arises from the lack of an accepted definition of aggressive MS and the inability to accurately identify patients at high risk of a poor prognosis, either through clinical features or biomarkers.

Treatment regimens Two priorities concerning transplantation procedure in future clinical trials of autologous HSCT can be identified: (a) standardization; (b) dose de-escalation. It is imperative to standardize treatment regimens and reduce dispersal into a multitude of center- (or investigator-) specific procedures. The disappointing results of TBI-based immunoablative regimens and the remarkable efficacy and acceptable safety of BEAM-ATG will be likely to consolidate the role of the latter as the conventional transplantation regimen in MS. Accordingly, a National Institutes of Health-funded multicentric United States trial of HSCT in MS (R Nash, principal investigator) has adopted BEAM-ATG, with the addition of graft CD34+ selection. Two trials of autologous transplantation following reduced-intensity ('non-myeloablative') conditioning regimens are under way: the randomized trial at Northwestern University (mentioned above) and a pilot study initiated by G L Mancardi, University of Genoa, Italy and sponsored by the Italian Multiple Sclerosis Society. These studies will begin to address whether reduced-intensity regimens can achieve similar results with less toxicity than full-dose, myeloablative regimens. If development of these trials is positive, a less toxic, non-myeloablative conditioning regimen could be employed to treat patients during the appropriate window of opportunity, i.e. earlier in the course of disease than in the studies conducted to date (Fig. 19.3).

Outcome measures In addition to the established clinical measures based on neurologic disability and relapses, future trials should perform rigorous serial MRI analysis as the best available marker of subclinical disease activity. Quantitative assessment of brain atrophy

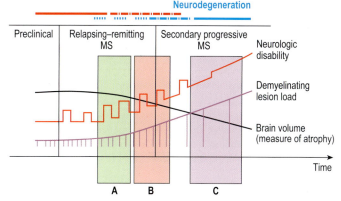

Figure 19.3
Pathogenetic components of MS and windows of opportunity for HSCT. Flares of inflammation characterize the early phases of relapsing-remitting MS, but repair and compensatory mechanisms allow good functional recuperation in the majority of patients. However, in patients who have aggressive disease, poor recovery or both conditions, accumulation of demyelinating lesions begins, resulting in initial neurologic disability (a). This may represent the ideal window of opportunity for therapies aiming to radically stop disease progression, including in theory HSCT. Practical considerations involving the availability of well-tolerated immunomodulatory drugs and the difficulty in predicting the evolution of disease in an individual patient typically lead to consideration of intensive treatments only later in the disease course, such as when the transition from relapsing-remitting to secondary progression approaches or occurs (b). At this stage glial and neuronal degeneration have already started as can be shown by measures of brain atrophy, and even though abrogation of CNS inflammation is less likely to completely stop clinical progression, HSCT could still beneficially affect the course of disease by reducing further inflammatory damage. Current trials of auto-HSCT are aiming to recruit patients at this stage. At more advanced stages the disease is characterized by reduced inflammatory activity and chronic progressive degenerative changes (c). The majority of patients who underwent HSCT to date were at a similar stage of disease; however, this late phase does not represent a suitable window of opportunity for immunotherapies unless these are combined with neural repair-promoting treatments.

should be included in trials as early as in initial screening visits, based on reported evidence of brain volume loss in the first year post transplantation,[32,40,41] but baseline information clinical metrics should include assessment of fatigue and quality of life in order to capture important components of the effects of treatment on the course of disease from the patient's perspective.

Allogeneic hematopoietic stem cell transplantation

Allogeneic HSCT is theoretically attractive as therapy for severe MS for two main reasons:

- it offers the prospect of correcting the genetic predisposition to autoimmunity by replacing the host's immune system with that of a healthy donor
- it may establish active control of autoimmune disease by the mechanism known as the graft-versus-autoimmunity effect. This effect has been demonstrated in experimental animal models but it is not known whether graft-versus-autoimmunity exists and can occur distinct from GvHD in humans.

Experience in allogeneic HSCT for MS is limited to anecdotal cases of patients treated for a malignancy who experienced prolonged remission of a concomitant autoimmune disease.[42] Currently, allogeneic HSCT remains an appealing notion but most neurologists do not feel that, for MS, the prospect of greater efficacy of allogeneic over autologous transplantation outweighs the increased morbidity and mortality risks. However, patients with aggressive MS who have failed autologous HSCT and who have a fully matched donor available could be seen as appropriate candidates for small exploratory clinical trials of allo-HSCT.[10]

Conclusions

- Results of clinical trials of autologous HSCT for MS have established its potential to induce long-term complete remissions or reduce the severity of aggressive forms of MS.
- Studies of the mechanism of action have confirmed the rationale that HSCT can regenerate a new, healthier immune system.
- Clinical results suggest that patients with early disease and high inflammatory disease activity are the most likely to benefit from treatment. Selection of the appropriate patient population is of fundamental importance since HSCT may not favorably modify the course of disease in patients with progressive forms and advanced disability.
- HSCT for MS (as for other immune diseases) remains an experimental therapy and should be performed whenever possible within clinical trials.

Systemic sclerosis

Background

Systemic sclerosis (SSc), also referred to as 'scleroderma', is a rare, heterogeneous condition of unknown etiology characterized by microvascular injury, inflammation, features of immune dysregulation such as the presence of autoantibodies, and the deposition of excess collagen in skin and internal organs.[48] A genetic predisposition is present, as illustrated by the finding that monozygotic twins clinically discordant for scleroderma showed concordance for fibroblast gene expression profiles.

There are two main clinical subsets of SSc as defined by criteria set up by the American Rheumatism Association. Limited cutaneous and diffuse cutaneous forms of the disease are distinguishable by the extent of skin involvement, their autoantibody profile, and the pattern of organ involvement. Limited SSc is characterized by skin involvement limited to hands, feet, face and/or forearms and is associated with a high incidence of anticentromere autoantibodies. Diffuse SSc is characterized by skin involvement on upper arms and trunk, is associated with an early incidence of interstitial lung disease, hypertensive crisis and renal failure, diffuse gastrointestinal disease and myocardial involvement, and presence of anti-Scl70 antibodies. Both forms of the disease are associated with vascular abnormalities clinically manifesting as Raynaud's phenomenon or as pulmonary artery hypertension.

Systemic sclerosis is the prototype fibrosing disease. Scleroderma skin and lung fibroblasts produce excessive amounts of type I collagen in vitro. It is thought that an autoimmune response precedes the development of fibrosis because lymphocytic infiltration is evident early in the disease in skin and lung, and autoantibodies are frequently present prior to the development of disease. Antibodies to the nuclear autoantigen topoisomerase I and the centromere proteins are rarely seen other than with this disease and are associated with particular HLA-D genotypes. A recent study found that the serum of SSc patients also contains stimulatory antibodies to the platelet-derived growth factor receptor, which selectively induced intracellular transcription factors and reactive oxygen species, and stimulated type I collagen-gene expression and myofibroblast phenotype conversion in normal human primary fibroblasts.[49] Despite this evidence, the relationship between autoimmune responses and vascular pathology is unclear and vascular abnormalities may be evident many years prior to the onset of disease. Similarly, the extent to which autoimmune responses and inflammation contribute to the maintenance of fibrosis remains unresolved, but it is thought that once established, the fibrotic process becomes independent of the immune drive and continues as an autonomous process.

Severe organ involvement occurs early in diffuse SSc, suggesting there is a window of opportunity to modify the disease course. Rapidly progressive diffuse SSc has the worst prognosis and is associated with a significant mortality (estimated to be 40–50% in 5 years) secondary to cardiac, renal and, particularly, pulmonary involvement.[49,50] Interstitial lung disease is now the leading cause of death in SSc patients. Pulmonary manifestations can be identified by pulmonary function testing in approximately half of SSc patients. The cumulative 10-year survival of SSc patients with a forced vital capacity (FVC) < 50% predicted is close to 50%. Diffusion capacity (DLCO), however, is the lung function parameter that best reflects the extent of alveolitis in SSc, and a DLCO < 70% is a predictor of early mortality, especially when accompanied by proteinuria and elevated erythrocyte sedimentation rate (ESR).

Autologous stem cell transplantation in systemic sclerosis

Until recently, there existed no proven effective therapy to prevent disease progression or to reverse fibrosis. D-Penicillamine, alpha-interferon, 5-fluorouracil, and chlorambucil were ineffective in controlled trials.[51] Methotrexate showed beneficial effects on skin thickening but not on organ dysfunction in a large multicenter, prospective, placebo-controlled, randomized trial.[52] There is no evidence for the efficacy of corticosteroids as monotherapy in SSc, and high-dose corticosteroid therapy, i.e. 15 mg/day prednisone or equivalent, is associated with the development of scleroderma renal crisis, which may lead to irreversible renal failure. Cyclophosphamide with or without corticosteroids has been shown to improve skin thickening, stabilize pulmonary function and increase survival in a number of non-randomized studies, particularly in early disease.

The beneficial effects of cyclophosphamide were recently confirmed in two prospective placebo-controlled multicenter clinical trials in SSc patients with alveolitis. In the North American Scleroderma Lung Study in 162 patients, cyclophosphamide had a statistically significant effect on FVC, dyspnea index, skin score, functional ability, and quality-of-life scores, compared to patients receiving placebo.[53] In the UK Fibrosing Alveolitis in Scleroderma Trial (FAST), involving 45 patients, there was also a statistically significant treatment difference in active treatment versus placebo in the FVC.[54] No differences were noted in the DLCO, computed tomography (CT) changes and dyspnea scores. The results of these studies convincingly demonstrated a disease-modifying effect of cyclophosphamide in SSc for the first time, albeit a modest one. Progress has also been made in the treatment of pulmonary hypertension associated with SSc with the advent of specific prostaglandins, endothelin-1 receptor antagonists, and phosphodiesterase inhibitors.[55]

The effectiveness of cyclophosphamide in SSc has prompted studies to investigate feasibility, safety and efficacy of dose intensification of cyclophosphamide with or without additional lymphoablative agents, followed by autologous HSCT in severe SSc. In view of the poor prognosis of SSc, the presumed autoimmune origin, and the lack of available therapies, this disease was considered particularly suitable for initial investigation of the tolerability and efficacy of autologous SCT.[56–59] The results collected by the Working Party on Autoimmune Diseases from the EBMT and European League Against Rheumatism (EULAR) on the first 41 SSc patients with at least 3 months follow-up suggested a significant impact on skin score with a trend to stabilization of lung function: 69% of the patients achieved an improvement of 25% or more in skin score[59] (Fig. 19.4).

In a recent analysis of 65 patients (which included the first cohort) the transplant-related mortality was 12.3% at 1 year, and 7.7% with exclusion of patients who did not meet the consensus guidelines on

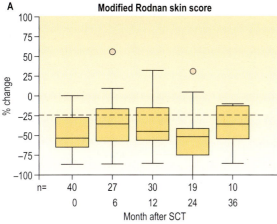

A Modified Rodnan skin score

p<0.001 at all times points versus baseline (Wilcoxon signed rank test)

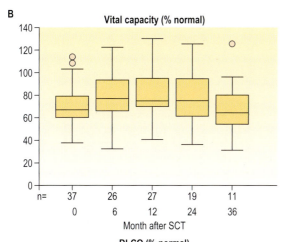

B Vital capacity (% normal)

DLCO (% normal)

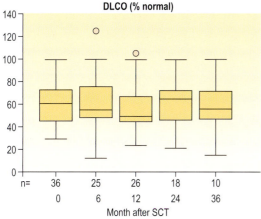

Figure 19.4
Results collected by EBMT and EULAR on the first 41 systemic sclerosis patients with at least 3 months follow-up suggest a significant impact on the Rodnan skin score (a skin thickness score assessment tool) with 69% of the patients achieving an improvement of 25% or more.

patient selection.[60] Detailed results were obtained from multicenter pilot studies conducted in the USA and France. The North American study involved 19 patients with poor-prognosis SSc, median age 40 years (range, 23–61 years), median modified Rodnan skin score (a measure of dermal sclerosis) of 31 (max. 51), and a median DLCO of 57%.[61] Conditioning therapy consisted of 800 cGy TBI (± lung shielding to approximately 200 cGy), 120 mg/kg cyclophosphamide, and 90 mg/kg equine ATG, followed by reinfusion of CD34-selected G-CSF mobilized autologous blood stem cells for hematopoietic

rescue. With a median follow-up of 14.7 months, the Kaplan–Meier estimated 2-year survival rate was 79%. Three patients died of treatment-related complications and one of disease progression. Two of the first eight patients had fatal regimen-related pulmonary injury, a complication not found among 11 subsequent patients who received lung shielding for TBI. Internal organ functions were stable to slightly worse after SCT, and four patients had progressive or non-responsive disease. As measured by skin scores and a disability index, significant disease responses occurred in 12 of 12 patients evaluated at 1 year.

In the French study, 12 patients were enrolled.[62] Peripheral blood stem cells were collected using cyclophosphamide (4 g/m²) and recombinant human G-CSF and enriched for CD34+ cells. Conditioning involved cyclophosphamide (200 mg/kg) or melphalan (140 mg/m²) according to cardiac function. One patient failed mobilization, one CD34+ selection and one intensification. Eleven patients received a transplant, one of these a bone marrow graft, the others peripheral blood stem cells. There was one procedure-related death. Hematologic recovery was uneventful. With a median follow-up of 18 months (range 1–26), eight out of 11 patients had a major or partial response.

Recent updates of the North American and French trials (the latter now including patients from The Netherlands treated with the same transplant protocol) confirmed the sustained clinical efficacy of high-dose immunosuppressive therapy and SCT.[63,64] In the former trial, skin thickening improved significantly by 73% and the disability index by 56% at 4 years in evaluable patients compared to baseline. Five-year estimated overall survival was 64%. In the latter study, the Kaplan–Meier estimated survival at 7 years was 57%, and 15 out of 16 patients with a follow-up of 5 years still had significant improvement of skin score and performance status.

The data obtained from the pilot studies formed the basis of the ongoing prospective Autologous Stem cell Transplantation International Scleroderma (ASTIS) and Scleroderma Cyclophosphamide Or Transplant (SCOT) trials in Europe and North America respectively, to test whether indeed this novel approach provides a survival advantage over conventional approaches in the long term. To combine safety and efficacy, medium-intensity regimens were chosen to achieve immunoablation. In the ASTIS protocol, hematopoietic stem cells are mobilized with cyclophosphamide (2 × 2 g/m²) plus G-CSF, and then enriched for CD34+ cells, while conditioning consists of high-dose cyclophosphamide (200 mg/kg), rabbit ATG (7.5 mg/kg), followed by SCT. The investigational arm in the SCOT trial comprises mobilization of peripheral blood stem cells with G-CSF plus subsequent enrichment of CD34+ cells, while the conditioning regimen consists of 8 Gy (fractionated) TBI with lung shielding, cyclophosphamide (120 mg/kg), and equine ATG (90 mg/kg). The control treatments in the trials are almost identical: a first intravenous pulse of 750 mg/m² or 500 mg/m² in ASTIS and SCOT respectively, followed by 11× monthly pulses at 750 mg/m². The trials target patients with early diffuse systemic sclerosis at risk of early mortality. These include patients with early disease, extensive skin thickening, and evidence of heart, lung or kidney disease. Exclusion criteria are end-stage organ failure, extensive pretreatment with cyclophosphamide, and other reasons that preclude participation in a trial. The primary endpoint is event-free survival, defined as the time in days since randomization until death or development of irreversible end-stage organ failure. The major secondary endpoints are progression-free survival, treatment-related mortality, and toxicity according to WHO criteria. It is postulated that SCT is a better treatment than pulse therapy because of its more profound perturbation of the immune system, although other mechanisms may also be involved. To date, in the ASTIS study, 87 patients have been randomized, with encouraging interim safety results, while the SCOT trial is now also open.[5]

Allogeneic stem cell transplantation in systemic sclerosis

Allogeneic SCT has not yet been systematically evaluated in SSc, but the experience in two cases is illustrative, showing both the curative potential and risks of allografting. Two SSc patients with diffuse SSc and lung involvement refractory to conventional immunosuppressive medication were treated with a myeloablative conditioning regimen which included busulfan, cyclophosphamide, and ATG.[65] Prophylaxis for graft-versus-host disease (GvHD) consisted of ciclosporin and methotrexate. Bone marrow was transplanted from HLA-identical siblings. In one patient, there were no complications related to the conditioning regimen, and GvHD did not develop after transplantation. At 5 years after SCT, there was nearly complete resolution of the scleroderma, improvement of lung function and marked improvement in physical functioning. On examination of serial skin biopsy samples, there was resolution of the dermal fibrosis. The other patient experienced skin toxicity from the conditioning regimen and a hypertensive crisis that was likely to have been related to high-dose corticosteroids given for treatment of GvHD. Although this patient experienced an improvement in scleroderma and overall functioning, he died from an opportunistic infection 17 months after SCT.

Summary and conclusions

- Immunoablative therapy and autologous HSCT is evolving as a promising therapy for patients with severe systemic sclerosis.
- Impressive improvements of skin thickening have been observed, not seen with conventional immunosuppressive therapy.
- Treatment-related toxicity and mortality have been reduced through improved patient selection and modifications in treatment regimens.
- Ongoing prospective randomized trials with long-term follow-up will determine whether the benefits of SCT outweigh the risks.
- Allogeneic HSCT is a treatment option for patients with severe SSc with a HLA-matched donor, but experience to date is limited.

Rheumatoid arthritis and juvenile idiopathic arthritis

Background

Rheumatoid arthritis (RA) and juvenile idiopathic arthritis (JIA) are the most common rheumatic diseases, with a prevalence of 1% and 0.1% in adults and children, respectively. RA is a systemic disease predominantly affecting synovial joints. JIA is a more heterogeneous disease entity, ranging from oligoarticular and polyarticular joint disease (the pediatric equivalent of RA) to so-called systemic JIA, characterized by fever, lymphadenopathy, serositis, hepatosplenomegaly, and secondary complications such as growth failure, osteoporosis, secondary amyloidosis, etc. Major clinical hallmarks of RA and JIA are chronicity and joint destruction. The disease course of both conditions is, however, variable. While most patients have relapsing-remitting disease, others experience progressive disease, resulting in joint destruction and severe disability, or even death. The severity of RA and JIA is not only determined by joint symptoms, but also by systemic and extra-articular symptoms. Epidemiologic studies have shown that overall mortality in RA and (systemic) JIA is increased in comparison to healthy individuals of the same age and sex.[66,67] Estimates of reduced life expectancy in RA vary from 3 to 18 years, although it is likely that better disease control with new therapies (see below) will translate into better survival.

In RA, several factors have been identified which predispose to severe progressive disease. These include particular HLA class II antigens, the presence in the serum of IgM rheumatoid factor and/or

IgG antibodies specific for citrullinated cyclic peptide (anti-CCP), all features suggestive of an autoimmune diathesis. The pathology of chronic synovitis in RA and JIA is characterized by complex interactions of cytokine-producing CD4+ Th1 lymphocytes, B-cells, macrophages and synoviocytes.[68] Being a prototype inflammatory disease, it is not surprising that immunosuppressive drugs including corticosteroids have been the principal component in the treatment of RA and JIA.

The search to optimize RA and JIA treatment has culminated in efforts to control the disease aggressively with disease-modifying antirheumatic drugs (DMARD) and biologics.[69] Methotrexate is probably the most common DMARD used, being effective as monotherapy, but more so in combination with other DMARDs, corticosteroids or biologics. Biologics constitute a novel therapeutic category, designed to specifically target a cellular subset or proinflammatory cytokine.

The introduction of monoclonal antibodies and soluble receptors directed against TNF-alpha (infliximab, adalimumab, etanercept), IL-6 (MRA), and B-cell depleting antibodies (rituximab) and shifting paradigms towards more aggressive treatment of early disease have had a significant impact on the disease course and outcome of RA and JIA patients in recent years. Nevertheless, even with the best of current conventional therapies, the majority of patients with newly diagnosed RA and a significant proportion of JIA patients do not enjoy a long-term, drug-free, complete remission, underscoring the need to further explore curative options such as stem cell transplantation.

The curative potential of HSCT in systemic autoimmune diseases was first investigated in experimental animal models.[1] The animal studies were paralleled by clinical observations of remissions in RA patients following immunoablation and *allogeneic* HSCT for concomitant hemato- or oncologic conditions. Two RA patients treated with *autologous* transplantation for non-Hodgkin's lymphoma[70,71] had a relapse of RA 5 weeks and 20 months after autologous HSCT. These relapses were attributed to the fact that the graft was not depleted of potentially autoreactive lymphocytes. Nevertheless, the mortality and morbidity of allografting using 'classic' conditioning regimens were felt not to be justified with a chronic disease such as RA in which prevention of morbidity instead of mortality is the major goal. Also, relapse has been seen in the setting of allogeneic HSCT.[72]

Autologous stem cell transplantation in RA and JIA

Based on the premise that immune abnormalities can be corrected by immunoablative therapy and that HSCT promotes recapitulation of a naïve, self-tolerant, immune system, this treatment modality seemed worth investigating in RA and JIA. Several protocols were developed along consensus guidelines issued by the EBMT in 1995.[3] At the time the first protocols were designed, it was, however, unknown whether mobilization of stem cells was possible in RA patients because intrinsic stem cell defects could hamper successful mobilization. In a larger, retrospective analysis of 187 cases, including 37 RA patients, it was shown that stem cells can be collected successfully in patients with autoimmune diseases, including rheumatoid arthritis.[73,74] In this study, the combination of G-CSF and cyclophosphamide caused fewer flares than G-CSF alone and resulted in a higher stem cell yield.

The pivotal role of T-cells in the pathogenesis of experimental arthritis and chronic human arthritis formed the rationale for T-cell depletion of the graft to prevent reinfusion of autoreactive T- and B-cells. Several methods have been employed to deplete T-cells from the marrow or blood cell graft, but most involved administration of anti-T-cell monoclonal antibodies (either with or without complement) or enrichment of CD34+ cells. A small randomized trial to compare T-cell depleted versus unmanipulated HSCT after high-dose chemotherapy (cyclophosphamide 200 mg/kg) in 31 RA patients failed to show significant differences with respect to length or quality of remissions between the two groups.[74] These findings argue against the importance of ex vivo T-cell depletion, at least in a setting of incomplete in vivo lymphoablation. Regarding conditioning regimens, most centers have used high-dose cyclophosphamide with or without ATG or TBIrradiation to achieve lymphoablation. Myeloablative regimens have been employed less frequently because of concerns of toxicity.[24,75–82]

Results from these heterogeneous studies are difficult to compare, but the treatment steps appeared feasible and safe in all patients. No unexpected major toxicity- or treatment-related mortality occurred, although infectious complications necessitated extra hospital admissions for parenteral antibiotic treatment in several patients. One patient, treated with a myeloablative regimen (busulfan-cyclophosphamide) died as a consequence of sepsis and concomitant lung cancer. Prompt, but transient improvement in disease activity was observed after mobilization with high-dose cyclophosphamide, while more durable responses were induced by subsequent intensification and HSCT. Single-center results of the 2-year follow-up of eight patients are depicted in Figure 19.5.[83]

A pooled analysis of this and other cases from the EBMT/EULAR database, in total 76 cases from 15 centers and a median follow-up of 16 months (range 3–55), confirmed the results from the pilot studies.[84] A good clinical response was seen in two-thirds of patients, defined by at least 50% improvement measured using the American College of Rheumatology criteria. Importantly, there was also a significant reduction in the level of functional disability measured by health assessment questionnaire (HAQ). The fact that these patients had previously failed a mean of five (range 2–9) DMARDs attests to the potential efficacy of HSCT. Nevertheless, recurrence of disease activity occurred in most patients, usually within 3 years, indicating immunoablative therapy and autologous HSCT are not curative. Of note, reinstitution of DMARDs for relapse resulted in substantial improvement of disease activity in the majority of patients who had been refractory to these drugs (even in higher doses) before transplantation, suggesting that some degree of sensitivity to conventional drugs had been regained. In a small series of 10 RA patients with recurrent disease following HSCT, rituximab was very effective in eight patients, again suggesting the disease had become more amenable to treatment.[85]

Relapse of RA after autologous HSCT could be due to persistence, or reinfusion and subsequent in vivo expansion of pathogenic T- or B-lymphocyte clones, emergence of newly formed pathogenic lymphocytes from stem cells as a result of exposure to novel autoantigens, and/or intrinsic stem cell defects. Also, the possibility that advanced disease persists because of autonomous growth of synoviocytes cannot be excluded.[80]

Although tempting to believe, there are no data in RA to show that further intensification, such as by in vivo T-cell depletion or by the use of myeloablation, would increase the likelihood and duration of remission. It remains to be shown that any superior efficacy of a more rigorous approach will compensate for increased toxicity in terms of quality-adjusted life expectancy.[86] This issue particularly applies to allogeneic HSCT which has not yet been systematically investigated as a primary treatment for patients with RA due to risks of transplant-related mortality and graft-versus-host disease.

In JIA, a recent retrospective analysis of follow-up data on 34 children with JIA who were treated with autologous HSCT (AHSCT) in nine different European transplant centers revealed a complete drug-free remission in 18 patients (53%) with a follow-up of 12–60 months.[87] Seven of these patients had previously failed treatment with anti-TNF. Six of the 34 patients (18%) showed a partial response (ranging from 30% to 70% improvement), and seven (21%) achieved no response to AHSCT. Infectious complications were common. There were three cases of transplant-related mortality (9%) and two of

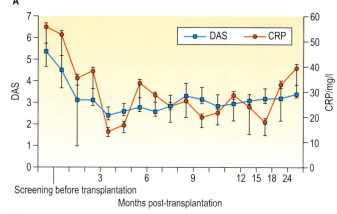

A

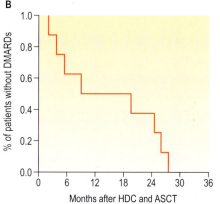

B

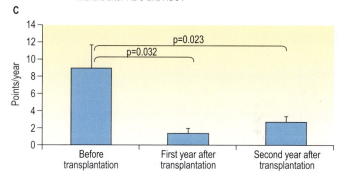

C

Figure 19.5

Single-center clinical results of eight patients with RA treated with high-dose chemotherapy (HDC) and CD34+ selected autologous blood stem cell transplantation (AHSCT). (a) Disease course as measured by mean (±SEM) disease activity scores (DAS, a validated composite score of tender and swollen joint counts, ESR, and patient assessment of disease activity by visual analog scale) and serum concentrations of C-reactive protein (mg/l). (b) Time after HDC and AHSCT until DMARDs were reinstituted. The mean time patients were off DMARDs was 14.8 months (95% CI 7.4–22.2). (c) Mean radiologic progression (in points per year) after HDC and AHSCT in the small joints of hands and feet.

disease-related mortality (6%). All cases of mortality and all partial and complete relapses of disease occurred in the first 18 months after AHSCT (Fig. 19.6). The three treatment-related deaths were precipitated by macrophage activation syndrome (MAS), which in two cases was infection related. A similar, non-fatal case of MAS after autologous BMT occurred in a young adult with systemic JIA in the US.[87] MAS is a serious and potentially lethal complication of rheumatic diseases in general, but particularly of systemic-onset JIA. It is characterized by fever, hepatosplenomegaly and lymphadenopathy, and also includes hematologic abnormalities, disseminated intravascular coagulation, and neurologic involvement. There is evidence of macrophage hemophagocytosis in the bone marrow, lymph nodes, liver

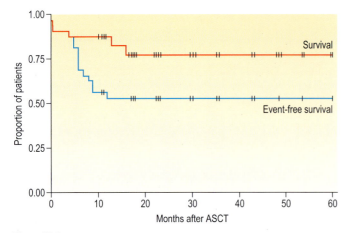

Figure 19.6
Kaplan-Meier curves showing the proportion of surviving patients with JIA and the proportion of event-free surviving JIA patients. An event is defined as either a partial or complete recurrence of disease. Each bar mark represents the maximum follow-up of a particular JIA patient.

and spleen. MAS frequently follows infections, but antirheumatic medications have also been implicated as triggering agents.

Allogeneic stem cell transplantation in RA

Allogeneic HSCT may be more effective than autologous HSCT if intrinsic stem cell abnormalities exist and if host hematopoiesis and abnormal immune cell populations can be eradicated via a graft-versus-autoimmunity effect. Recent advances in allografting have improved safety, thereby allowing its application in non-malignant conditions such as RA. Most non-myeloablative conditioning regimens currently used provide sufficient immunosuppression of the host to allow rapid engraftment of an allograft, in a relatively safe manner. Preliminary evidence of the excellent safety profile and potential efficacy of a reduced-intensity regimen and HLA-matched allogeneic HSCT was obtained in two RA patients.[88]

Summary and conclusions

- Immunoablative therapy and autologous HSCT have been shown to induce partial and complete remissions in the majority of RA and JIA patients, irrespective of the regimen employed.
- In RA, no major toxicities have been observed, and treatment-related mortality has been surprisingly low.
- In JIA, deaths due to macrophage activation syndrome have prompted modifications of treatment regimens including attenuation of the extent of T-cell depletion, prophylactic administration of antiviral drugs, and elimination of TBI from the conditioning regimen.
- With the adoption of more aggressive conventional treatment regimens and advent of highly effective biologics, however, the landscape of RA and JIA treatment has dramatically altered, and immunoablative therapy and autologous HSCT are unlikely to become routine therapy in these diseases.
- Allografting may, in the near future, become an attractive experimental treatment strategy if a suitable donor is available for patients with progressive (but not advanced) RA or JIA who have failed standard therapy.

Systemic lupus erythematosus

Background

Systemic lupus erythematosus (SLE) is the prototypic systemic autoimmune disorder with a heterogeneous clinical presentation and course. The prevalence of lupus in the US is estimated to range from 15 to 51 cases per 100,000 persons, with African-Americans, Hispanics, and Asians having a greater incidence and more severe course of SLE than Caucasians. SLE affects females nine times more frequently than males, and usually presents during child-bearing years. There is a 24% concordance of disease between monozygotic twins, compared to only 2% between dizygotic twins,[89] suggesting an important effect of the genetic background but at the same time implying an important role for environmental or stochastic factors.

The severity of SLE is determined by the pattern of major organ involvement. Clinically significant renal involvement is present in 50–60% of patients. CNS involvement, such as behavioral changes and cognitive deficits, is common in SLE. Acute inflammatory involvement of the brain and spine (cerebral vasculitis, cerebritis, transverse myelitis) is rare but presents as a real medical emergency. Other, acutely life-threatening manifestations include lupus pneumonitis, pulmonary embolism, pulmonary hemorrhage or alveolitis and catastrophic antiphospholipid syndrome. A minority of patients can also develop severe treatment-resistant autoimmune hemolytic anemia or autoimmune thrombocytopenia.

Determinants of mortality in SLE

Overall 10-year survival rates in SLE range from 64% to 93%. The standardized mortality rate (SMR), which compares mortality to the general population, is increased fourfold[90] and is highest in younger patients. Regarding the clinical and laboratory features of SLE, major organ involvement and persistent overall disease activity are by far the most important predictors of poor outcome (reviewed in references 91 and 92).

The majority of fatalities among patients with SLE are attributable to major organ failure due to active disease, followed by infections and cardiovascular disease.[92] Active SLE most commonly causes death due to nephritis, multiorgan failure or CNS disease. Infections most commonly occur in the setting of active SLE in patients receiving high-dose corticosteroids and/or immunosuppressive therapy.[93] Comorbid conditions and other complications of therapy account for the remainder of deaths.

Treatment of major organ involvement

Lupus nephritis is the only major organ manifestation for which effective treatment has been established in controlled clinical trials.[94–98] The treatment of other major organ manifestations is empirical and based on the experience with lupus nephritis and/or similar manifestations in non-lupus patients combined with organ-specific supportive therapy.[99,100]

The cornerstone of treatment of major organ manifestations is high-dose corticosteroid therapy used as daily treatment (prednisone 0.5–1.0 mg/kg/d) or as bolus intravenous therapy (methylprednisolone 0.5–1.0 g for 1–3 days). For most major organ manifestations another immunosuppressive agent is started at the same time. Based on the experience of treating severe lupus nephritis, cyclophosphamide is the traditional choice for the most severe manifestations; it can be given daily or as monthly intravenous pulse therapy. Cyclophosphamide-induced infertility, the risk of which increases with the cumulative dose and patient age, is common and of major concern, since the majority of patients are women in their child-bearing years.[101] Recently, several studies have suggested that mycophenolate mofetil, which has no effect on fertility, may be an alternative to cyclophosphamide in treating lupus nephritis.[95,96] Immune-mediated hemolytic anemia and thrombocytopenia in SLE are treated as their idiopathic counterparts, autoimmune hemolytic anemia (AIHA) and idiopathic thrombocytopenic purpura (ITP). Protracted immunosuppressive therapy decreases flare rate and improves long-term outcomes but is associated with significant treatment-related morbidities.[102] However, the ultimate long-term goal of treatment-free remission or cure has been elusive to date. Up to one-third of patients do not achieve a complete response, and another third may experience a flare after achieving a response.[103] There are several clinical studies under way evaluating new biologics, such as B-cell depleting agents (rituximab, epratuzumab), anti-CTLA4-Ig and anti-Blys for SLE; however, none of these is considered potentially curative.

Autologous hematopoetic stem cell transplantation
Rationale in SLE

A general model of the complex pathogenesis of SLE is that in a genetically susceptible individual, an initial breakdown in tolerance creates primary autoreactive effectors, which then propagate the autoimmune response by a variety of mechanisms.[104,105] Production of autoantibodies targeted against conserved nuclear antigens, such as DNA, complement activation, immune complex deposition, and leukocyte infiltration of target organs are key immunopathogenic events. The primary event in the initiation of autoimmunity is unknown, but by the time SLE is clinically evident there is an ongoing activation of autoreactive B- and T-cells in the lymphoid organs in a self-perpetuating process. Both activated B-cells and T-cells produce inflammatory cytokines that contribute to organ damage and provide an inflammatory milieu for abnormal presentation of autoantigen by antigen-presenting cells. Deleting B-cells in established disease may lead to a decrease in autoantigen presentation in the lymphoid organs that in turn may decrease the number of autoreactive T-cells and decrease both autoantibody production and activation of other effector cells. Deleting activated T-cells at the same time may be necessary to prevent activation of remaining precursors of autoreactive B-cells, and to prevent T-cell help to naturally occurring low-affinity autoreactive cells that may develop during regeneration of the immune system.

Clinical experience

To date, over 100 patients have been enrolled in early studies of autologous HSCT for the primary indication of severe SLE.[106] The two largest series come from the registry data of the EBMT/EULAR, and the largest single center experience from Northwestern University, Chicago (Table 19.3).

EBMT and EULAR registry experience Data from 53 patients (reported by 23 teams from 12 countries) who underwent autologous HSCT for SLE were analyzed.[107] The mean duration of follow-up after transplant was 26 months. In 41/53 cases the stem cell source was peripheral blood rather than bone marrow, and the most common method of stem cell mobilization was a combination of cyclophosphamide and G-CSF. Conditioning regimens were typically non-myeloablative, most commonly high-dose cyclophosphamide with ATG, without (n = 25) or with (n = 11) total-lymphoid irradiation. Positive selection of CD34+ hematopoietic stem cells for T-cell depletion was used in 41%. There were 12 deaths post transplant; six died related to the procedure within the first 100 days (gastrointestinal bleeding 1, infection 3, thrombotic thrombocytopenic purpura (TTP) 1, unknown 1), one late death was due to suicide at 6 months and one at 4 years from secondary acute myelogenous leukemia. Four patients died due to progressive SLE at 1, 24, 32, and 40 months. Lupus activity decreased significantly; average SLEDAI (Systemic Lupus Erythematosus Disease Activity Index) scores fell from 33.2 pretransplant to a mean of 2.6–3.8 after transplant. Remission of SLE, defined as SLEDAI score <3 and prednisone dose <10 mg/d, occurred in 33 (66%) cases. Remission was not associated with any pretransplant variables. Of those achieving remission, 32% relapsed. CD34+ cell selection did not show any association with relapse. Decrease in auto-

Table 19.3 Autologous HSCT in patients with systemic lupus erythematosus

Study	No. of patients treated	Major organ manifestation (%)[1]	Graft manipulation	Conditioning regimen[2]	Life-threatening complications[3]	Follow-up	Response[4]	Estimated long-term benefit (at 5 years)[5]
Jayne 2004[107]	53	Renal: 65 CNS: 46 Lung: 35 Vasculitis: 34	None: 28/51 CD34+ selection: 21/51 CD34+ selection with neg. T-cell selection: 2/51	CY+ATG: 25 (48%) TLI ± CY+ATG 11 (22%) Other 14 (27%)	12 deaths TRM: 7 SLE: 4 Suicide: 1 Serious AEs Infections: 22 Autoimmune events: 5 EBV-PTLD: 1 AML: 1	Median 23 months (range 0–78)	50 evaluable pts at 6 months NR: 1 (2%) PR: 7 (14%) R: 33 (66%) Relapse: 10/31 (32%)	Probability of survival: 62% Disease-free survival: 50%
Burt 2006[5]	50	Renal: 50 CNS: 64 Lung: 48 Vasculitis: 18 APS: 44	CD34+ selection	CY+ATG	8 deaths 2 preconditioning: SLE: 1 (premobilization) Infection; 1 (postmobilization) 6 post-transplant SLE: 4 Unintentional injury: 1 Infection: 1 Serious AEs Infections Early: 27 Late: 9 Lung toxicity: 6 Cytokine release: 19 Immune events: 3 Renal: 2	Mean 29 months (range 6 months–7 years)	48 evaluable pts NR: 4 (8%) PR: NS R: S Relapse: NS	Probability of survival: 84% Disease-free survival: 50%

1. Patients may have had more than one major organ involvement.
2. CY, cyclophosphamide; ATG, antithymocyte globulin; TLI, total lymphoid irradiation.[3]
3. TRM, transplant-related mortality; PTLD, post-transplant lymphoproliferative disease; AML, acute myeloid leukemia.
4. NR, no response; PR, partial response; R, remission. The definition of remission differed among studies. NS, not specified.
5. Survival probability as determined by Kaplan-Meier estimates.

antibody levels was seen in most patients but was only temporary in many. At the time of last follow-up, steroids were successfully withdrawn in only 8/22 (36%) evaluable patients and additional individuals remained on other post-transplant immunosuppression for disease control, most commonly mycophenolate mofetil (13/30).

Northwestern University experience In the largest single center study at Northwestern University in Chicago, 50 patients with severe and treatment-refractory SLE underwent autologous HSCT.[108] Stem cells were mobilized with cyclophosphamide (2.0 g/m^2) and G-CSF (5 µg/kg/day). Lymphocytes were depleted from the graft by selection of CD34+ stem cells. The conditioning regimen used was cyclophosphamide (200 mg/kg), horse ATG (90 mg/kg), and methylprednisolone (3 g). The primary endpoints were overall and disease-free survival. Mean follow-up was 29 months (6 months–7.5 years). Two patients died (one from mucormycosis and one from lupus) after mobilization but before conditioning. No treatment-related deaths were reported among the 48 patients who underwent HSCT. Six patients died from non-treatment related events; four of these had complications of active lupus or its treatment. The probability of 5-year survival was 84%, whereas the probability of disease-free survival defined as no evidence of active disease and no immunosuppressive therapy except <10 mg of prednisone, and hydroxychloroquine was 50% at 5 years.

Future clinical trials of HSCT for SLE

Patient selection

Until reliable estimates of the actual risks and long-term outcomes of autologous HSCT are available, it is imperative to select patients who may benefit the most and at the same time have a reasonable chance of survival. Since the risk of TRM is strongly associated with the general medical condition of subjects at the time of transplant, the optimal timing of stem cell transplant in SLE may be early in the diseases course before the development of any significant organ damage. Until we have reliable markers that identify patients early who have an adverse prognosis, we should only consider patients for stem cell transplant if they have failed a reasonable length of conventional therapy, but we should not wait until they fail all available treatment options. The general goal is to select patients who are in an acceptable general medical condition and who have therapy-resistant, active severe lupus with the potential of long-term response.

The lupus-specific eligibility criteria can be defined along three principles. Subjects must have a severe major organ manifestation associated with increased mortality or the risk of severe disability, such as diffuse proliferative glomerulonephritis or pulmonary vasculitis. At the time of enrollment, patients must have manifestations of active disease known to respond to immunosuppressive therapy. Active disease must be distinguished from permanent damage. Treatment-refractory disease is defined as objective worsening of disease despite adequate immunosuppressive therapy, or the inability to taper prednisone due to flare in the target organ. The minimum length of prior immunosuppressive therapy can be defined specifically for each organ involved (for example, 6 months of cyclophosphamide for lupus nephritis).

Treatment regimens

An important consideration in choosing the optimal conditioning regimen is to define the ultimate goal of HSCT in SLE where HSCT can be used either as salvage therapy or a potentially curative intervention. If used as a salvage treatment for patients who have failed conventional therapy, the primary goal is to arrest an active process and turn it into a more manageable condition. Therefore, it is less important if the benefit is due to the high-intensity immunosuppressive therapy or to a fundamental change in the disease. This can be viewed as a relatively short- to medium-term goal, and only a small increase in short-term mortality would be acceptable. The Northwestern data demonstrate that a high-dose cyclophosphamide-based lymphoablative regimen can be used relatively safely in experienced centers and leads to clinical response in most patients.

The second strategy implies that the long-term goals of HSCT in lupus should be achievement of durable immunologic tolerance and cure rather than just a delay of disease progression or attenuation of symptoms. However, if the goal of HSCT is to achieve long-lasting immunologic tolerance or cure of SLE, a more aggressive approach may be needed. Data about the important role of innate immunity and other non-immunologically mediated mechanisms in the initiation and maintenance of autoimmunity are rapidly accumulating. The impact of these 'secondary', non-lymphocyte depleting effects of conditioning regimens on the underlying pathology of autoimmune disease is largely unknown today but suggests that purely lymphodepleting approaches may not be sufficient to avoid recurrence of the disease if the innate immune system remains abnormal. This notion is supported by the fact that in both the EBMT registry and in the Northwestern experience the 5-year disease-free survival after autologous HSCT in SLE is 50%. The potential curative effect of more aggressive conditioning regimens should initially be addressed in carefully designed pilot studies.

Response criteria

One of the most concerning limitations of the available data is the uncertain quality of reported remissions post transplant, the pattern of relapses, and the large number of patients not being able to discontinue prednisone. All these raise doubts about the overall curative potential of current autologous HSCT for SLE. Thus, it is essential to have predefined criteria of both response and failure. The response criteria should reflect major favorable responses of the underlying autoimmune process in the target organ with a concomitant improvement in general disease activity measured by disease activity indices. Since concomitant corticosteroid therapy is a significant confounder of outcome, successful tapering of corticosteroids according to a predetermined regimen is a necessary criterion of response. Different grades of responses (complete, partial or no response) should be defined for every target organ and the bar for success should be set high.

Allogeneic hematopoietic stem cell transplantation

The fact that about half of the patients with SLE who undergo autologous HSCT do not achieve sustained disease-free remission raises a fundamental and still unanswered question of whether the underlying pathology is due to an inherent genetic or acquired abnormality of hematopoietic stem cells. In either case, allogeneic transplant would provide a rational alternative due to the potential for a much more profound and sustained eradication of the host immune system which is replaced by a new healthy donor-derived immune system.[109] Besides supportive evidence from animal experiments[110,111] there is also some anecdotal clinical evidence in SLE that allogeneic stem cell transplantation may be effective in curing lupus.[112–115] The major limiting factor of using allogeneic HSCT for lupus is the higher expected mortality rate and the risk of graft-versus-host disease.

Summary and conclusions

- High-dose immunosuppression followed by autologous hematopoietic stem cell therapy is effective in inducing short- to medium-term responses in patients with treatment-resistant systemic lupus erythematosus. In some of these patients such responses are durable for at least several years.

- Procedure-related mortality varies among studies between 4% and 12% and is lower in relatively larger single-center studies. However, the curative potential of this procedure in severe SLE is still unknown.
- Allogeneic hematopoietic stem cell therapy holds a potential promise for cure but is as yet untested in humans.
- To accomplish the best therapeutic and scientific results, it is necessary to treat all patients with carefully planned protocols by specialized teams of lupus specialists and transplanters. All protocols should incorporate studies of immune reconstitution to understand the mechanisms of cure or failure.

References

1. van Bekkum DW. Experimental basis for the treatment of autoimmune diseases with autologous hematopoietic stem cell transplantation. Bone Marrow Transplant 2003;32(suppl 1):S37–39
2. Snowden JA, Patton WN, O'Donnell JL et al. Prolonged remission of longstanding systemic lupus erythematosus after autologous bone marrow transplant for non-Hodgkin's lymphoma. Bone Marrow Transplant 1997;19:1247–1250
3. Tyndall A, Gratwohl A. Blood and marrow stem cell transplants in auto-immune disease: a consensus report written on behalf of the European League against Rheumatism (EULAR) and the European Group for Blood and Marrow Transplantation (EBMT). Bone Marrow Transplant 1997;19:643–645
4. van Laar JM, Tyndall A. Adult stem cells in the treatment of autoimmune diseases. Rheumatology (Oxford) 2006;45:1187–1193
5. Burt RK, Marmont A, Oyama Y et al. Randomized controlled trials of autologous hematopoietic stem cell transplantation for autoimmune diseases: the evolution from myeloablative to lymphoablative transplant regimens. Arthritis Rheum 2006;54:3750–3760
6. Muraro PA, Douek DC, Packer A et al. Thymic output generates a new and diverse TCR repertoire after autologous stem cell transplantation in multiple sclerosis patients. J Exp Med 2005;201:805–816
7. de Kleer I, Vastert B, Klein M et al. Autologous stem cell transplantation for autoimmunity induces immunologic self-tolerance by reprogramming autoreactive T-cells and restoring the CD4+CD25+ immune regulatory network. Blood 2005;1:1
8. Gratwohl A, Passweg J, Bocelli-Tyndall C et al. Autologous hematopoietic stem cell transplantation for autoimmune diseases. Bone Marrow Transplant 2005;35:869–879
9. Dazzi F, van Laar JM, Cope A, Tyndall A. Cell therapy for autoimmune diseases. Arthritis Res Ther 2007;9:206
10. Griffith LM, Pavletic SZ et al. Feasibility of allogeneic hematopoietic stem cell transplantation for autoimmune disease: position statement from a National Institute of Allergy and Infectious Diseases and National Cancer Institute-Sponsored International Workshop, Bethesda, MD, March 12 and 13, 2005. Biol Blood Marrow Transplant 2005;11:862–870
11. The atlas of MS. Multiple Sclerosis International Federation;2006. www.atlasofms.org/index.aspx
12. Lublin FD, Reingold SC. Defining the clinical course of multiple sclerosis: results of an international survey. National Multiple Sclerosis Society (USA) Advisory Committee on Clinical Trials of New Agents in Multiple Sclerosis. Neurology 1996;46:907–911
13. Kurtzke JF. Rating neurologic impairment in multiple sclerosis: an expanded disability status scale (EDSS). Neurology 1983;33:1444–1452
14. Daumer M, Griffith LM, Meister W et al. Survival, and time to an advanced disease state or progression, of untreated patients with moderately severe multiple sclerosis in a multicenter observational database: relevance for design of a clinical trial for high dose immunosuppressive therapy with autologous hematopoietic stem cell transplantation. Mult Scler 2006;12:174–179
15. Bergamaschi R. Prognosis of multiple sclerosis: clinical factors predicting the late evolution for an early treatment decision. Expert Rev Neurother 2006;6:357–364
16. Weinshenker BG, Bass B, Rice GP et al. The natural history of multiple sclerosis: a geographically based study. 2. Predictive value of the early clinical course. Brain 1989;112(Pt 6):1419–1428
17. Brex PA, Ciccarelli O, O'Riordan JI et al. A longitudinal study of abnormalities on MRI and disability from multiple sclerosis. N Engl J Med 2002;346:158–164
18. Agosta F, Rovaris M, Pagani E et al. Magnetization transfer MRI metrics predict the accumulation of disability 8 years later in patients with multiple sclerosis. Brain 2006;129(Pt 10):2620–2627
19. Bielekova B, Richert N, Howard T et al. Humanized anti-CD25 (daclizumab) inhibits disease activity in multiple sclerosis patients failing to respond to interferon beta. Proc Natl Acad Sci USA 2004;101:8705–8708
20. Kappos L, Antel J, Comi G et al. Oral fingolimod (FTY720) for relapsing multiple sclerosis. N Engl J Med 2006;355:1124–1140
21. Coles AJ, Cox A, Le Page E et al. The window of therapeutic opportunity in multiple sclerosis. Evidence from monoclonal antibody therapy. J Neurol 2005;27:27
22. Coles AJ, Wing M, Smith S et al. Pulsed monoclonal antibody treatment and autoimmune thyroid disease in multiple sclerosis. Lancet 1999;354:1691–1695
23. Loh Y, Oyama Y, Statkute L et al. Development of a secondary autoimmune disorder after hematopoietic stem cell transplantation for autoimmune diseases: role of conditioning regimen used? Blood 2007;109:2643–2648
24. Brodsky RA, Petri M, Smith BD et al. Immunoablative high-dose cyclophosphamide without stem-cell rescue for refractory, severe autoimmune disease. Ann Intern Med 1998;129:1031–1035
25. Gladstone DE, Zamkoff KW, Krupp L et al. High-dose cyclophosphamide for moderate to severe refractory multiple sclerosis. Arch Neurol 2006;63:1388–1393

26. Muraro PA, Douek DC. Renewing the T cell repertoire to arrest autoimmune aggression. Trends Immunol 2006;27:61–67
27. Karussis DM, Vourka-Karussis U, Lehmann D et al. Prevention and reversal of adoptively transferred, chronic relapsing experimental autoimmune encephalomyelitis with a single high dose cytoreductive treatment followed by syngeneic bone marrow transplantation. J Clin Invest 1993;92:765–772
28. Burt RK, Padilla J, Begolka WS et al. Effect of disease stage on clinical outcome after syngeneic bone marrow transplantation for relapsing experimental autoimmune encephalomyelitis. Blood 1998;91:2609–2616.
29. Nash RA, Bowen JD, McSweeney PA et al. High-dose immunosuppressive therapy and autologous peripheral blood stem cell transplantation for severe multiple sclerosis. Blood 2003;102:2364–2372
30. Oyama Y, Cohen B, Traynor A et al, Burt RK. Engraftment syndrome: a common cause for rash and fever following autologous hematopoietic stem cell transplantation for multiple sclerosis. Bone Marrow Transplant 2002;29:81–85
31. Mancardi GL, Saccardi R, Filippi M et al. Autologous hematopoietic stem cell transplantation suppresses Gd-enhanced MRI activity in MS. Neurology 2001;57:62–68
32. Saiz A, Carreras E, Berenguer J et al. MRI and CSF oligoclonal bands after autologous hematopoietic stem cell transplantation in MS. Neurology 2001;56:1084–1089
33. Saccardi R, Mancardi GL, Solari A et al. Autologous HSCT for severe progressive multiple sclerosis in a multicenter trial: impact on disease activity and quality of life. Blood 2005;105:2601–2607
34. Samijn JP, te Boekhorst PA, Mondria T et al. Intense T cell depletion followed by autologous bone marrow transplantation for severe multiple sclerosis. J Neurol Neurosurg Psychiatry 2006;77:46–50
35. Metz I, Lucchinetti CF, Openshaw H et al. Multiple sclerosis pathology after autologous stem cell transplantation: ongoing demyelination and neurodegeneration despite suppressed inflammation. Mult Scler 2006;12:S9
36. Burt RK, Cohen BA, Russell E et al. Hematopoietic stem cell transplantation for progressive multiple sclerosis: failure of a total body irradiation-based conditioning regimen to prevent disease progression in patients with high disability scores. Blood 2003;102: 2373–2378
37. Saccardi R, Kozak T, Bocelli-Tyndall C et al. Autologous stem cell transplantation for progressive multiple sclerosis: update of the European group for blood and marrow transplantation auto immune diseases working party database. Mult Scler 2006;12:1–10
38. Comi G, Kappos L, Clanet M et al. Guidelines for autologous blood and marrow stem cell transplantation in multiple sclerosis: a consensus report written on behalf of the European Group for Blood and Marrow Transplantation and the European Charcot Foundation. BMT-MS Study Group. J Neurol 2000;247:376–382
39. McDonald WI, Compston A, Edan G et al. Recommended diagnostic criteria for multiple sclerosis: guidelines from the International Panel on the diagnosis of multiple sclerosis. Ann Neurol 2001;50:121–127
40. Inglese M, Mancardi GL, Pagani E et al. Brain tissue loss occurs after suppression of enhancement in patients with multiple sclerosis treated with autologous haematopoietic stem cell transplantation. J Neurol Neurosurg Psychiatry 2004;75:643–644
41. Chen JT, Collins DL, Atkins HL et al. Brain atrophy after immunoablation and stem cell transplantation in multiple sclerosis. Neurology 2006;66:1935–1937
42. McAllister LD, Beatty PG, Rose J. Allogeneic bone marrow transplant for chronic myelogenous leukemia in a patient with multiple sclerosis. Bone Marrow Transplant 1997;19:395–397
43. Fassas A, Anagnostopoulos A, Kazis A et al. Autologous stem cell transplantation in progressive multiple sclerosis – an interim analysis of efficacy. J Clin Immunol 2000;20:24–30
44. Kozak T, Havrdova E, Pit'ha J et al. High-dose immunosuppressive therapy with PBPC support in the treatment of poor risk multiple sclerosis. Bone Marrow Transplant 2000;25:525–531
45. Fassas A, Passweg JR, Anagnostopoulos A et al. Hematopoietic stem cell transplantation for multiple sclerosis. A retrospective multicenter study. J Neurol 2002;249:1088–1097
46. Saiz A, Blanco Y, Carreras E et al. Clinical and MRI outcome after autologous hematopoietic stem cell transplantation in MS. Neurology 2004;62:282–284
47. Ni XS, Ouyang J, Zhu WH et al. Autologous hematopoietic stem cell transplantation for progressive multiple sclerosis: report of efficacy and safety at three years of follow up in 21 patients. Clin Transplant 2006;20:485–489
48. Charles C, Clements P, Furst DE. Systemic sclerosis: hypothesis-driven treatment strategies. Lancet 2006;367:1683–1691
49. Baroni SS, Santillo M, Bevilacqua F et al. Stimulatory autoantibodies to the PDGF receptor in systemic sclerosis. N Engl J Med 2006;354:2667–2676
50. Trad S, Amoura Z, Beigelman C et al. Pulmonary arterial hypertension is a major mortality factor in diffuse systemic sclerosis, independent of interstitial lung disease. Arthritis Rheum 2006;54:184–191
51. Furst DE, Clements PJ. D-penicillamine is not an effective treatment in systemic sclerosis. Scand J Rheumatol 2001;30:189–191
52. Pope JE, Bellamy N, Seibold JR et al. A randomized, controlled trial of methotrexate versus placebo in early diffuse scleroderma. Arthritis Rheum 2001;44:1351–1358
53. Tashkin DP, Elashoff R, Clements PJ et al. Cyclophosphamide versus placebo in scleroderma lung disease. N Engl J Med 2006;354:2655–2666
54. Hoyles RK, Ellis RW, Wellsbury J et al. A multicenter, prospective, randomized, double-blind, placebo-controlled trial of corticosteroids and intravenous cyclophosphamide followed by oral azathioprine for the treatment of pulmonary fibrosis in scleroderma. Arthritis Rheum 2006;54:3962–3970
55. Williams MH, Das C, Handler CE et al. Systemic sclerosis associated pulmonary hypertension: improved survival in the current era. Heart 2006;92:926–932
56. Tyndall A, Black C, Finke J et al. Treatment of systemic sclerosis with autologous haemopoietic stem cell transplantation. Lancet 1997;349:254
57. Komatsuda A, Kawabata Y, Horiuchi T et al. Successful autologous peripheral blood stem cell transplantation using thiotepa in a patient with systemic sclerosis and cardiac involvement. Tohoku J Exp Med 2006;209:61–67

58. Miniati I, Saccardi R, Pagliai F et al. [The treatment of diffuse cutaneous systemic sclerosis with autologous hemopoietic stem cells transplantation (HSCT): our experience on 2 cases.] Reumatismo 2005;57:277–282

59. Tsukamoto H, Nagafuji K, Horiuchi T et al. A phase I-II trial of autologous peripheral blood stem cell transplantation in the treatment of refractory autoimmune disease. Ann Rheum Dis 2006;65:508–514

60. Farge D, Passweg J, van Laar JM et al. Autologous stem cell transplantation in the treatment of systemic sclerosis: report from the EBMT/EULAR Registry. Ann Rheum Dis 2004;63:974–981

61. McSweeney PA, Nash RA, Sullivan KM et al. High-dose immunosuppressive therapy for severe systemic sclerosis: initial outcomes. Blood 2002;100:1602–1610

62. Farge D, Marolleau JP, Zohar S et al. Autologous bone marrow transplantation in the treatment of refractory systemic sclerosis: early results from a French multicentre phase I-II study. Br J Haematol 2002;119:726–739

63. van Laar JM, McSweeney PA. High-dose immunosuppressive therapy and autologous progenitor cell transplantation for systemic sclerosis. Best Pract Res Clin Haematol 2004;17:233–245

64. van Laar JM, Farge D, Tyndall A. Autologous Stem cell Transplantation International Scleroderma (ASTIS) trial: hope on the horizon for patients with severe systemic sclerosis. Ann Rheum Dis 2005;64:1515

65. Nash RA, McSweeney PA, Nelson JL et al. Allogeneic marrow transplantation in patients with severe systemic sclerosis: resolution of dermal fibrosis. Arthritis Rheum 2006;54: 1982–1986

66. Myllykangas-Luosujarvi RA, Aho K, Isomaki HA. Mortality in rheumatoid arthritis. Semin Arthritis Rheum 1995;25:193–202

67. Borchers AT, Selmi C, Cheema G et al. Juvenile idiopathic arthritis. Autoimmun Rev 2006;5:279–298

68. Choy EH, Panayi GS. Cytokine pathways and joint inflammation in rheumatoid arthritis. N Engl J Med 2001;344:907–916

69. Savage C, St Clair EW. New therapeutics in rheumatoid arthritis. Rheum Dis Clin North Am 2006;32:57–74

70. Euler HH, Marmont AM, Bacigalupo A et al. Early recurrence or persistence of autoimmune diseases after unmanipulated autologous stem cell transplantation. Blood 1996;88:3621–3625

71. Cooley HM, Snowden JA, Grigg AP, Wicks IP. Outcome of rheumatoid arthritis and psoriasis following autologous stem cell transplantation for hematologic malignancy. Arthritis Rheum 1997;40:1712–1715

72. McKendry RJ, Huebsch L, Leclair B. Progression of rheumatoid arthritis following bone marrow transplantation. A case report with a 13-year followup. Arthritis Rheum 1996;39:1246–1253

73. Burt RK, Fassas A, Snowden J et al. Collection of hematopoietic stem cells from patients with autoimmune diseases. Bone Marrow Transplant 2001;28:1–12

74. Moore J, Brooks P, Milliken S et al. A pilot randomized trial comparing CD34-selected versus unmanipulated hemopoietic stem cell transplantation for severe, refractory rheumatoid arthritis. Arthritis Rheum 2002;46:2301–2309

75. Joske DJ, Ma DT, Langlands DR, Owen ET. Autologous bone-marrow transplantation for rheumatoid arthritis. Lancet 1997;350:337–338

76. Durez P, Toungouz M, Schandene L et al. Remission and immune reconstitution after T-cell-depleted stem-cell transplantation for rheumatoid arthritis. Lancet 1998;352: 881

77. Burt RK, Traynor AE, Pope R et al. Treatment of autoimmune disease by intense immunosuppressive conditioning and autologous hematopoietic stem cell transplantation. Blood 1998;92:3505–3514

78. Snowden JA, Biggs JC, Milliken ST et al. A phase I/II dose escalation study of intensified cyclophosphamide and autologous blood stem cell rescue in severe, active rheumatoid arthritis. Arthritis Rheum 1999;42:2286–2292

79. Lowenthal RM, Graham SR. Does hemopoietic stem cell transplantation have a role in treatment of severe rheumatoid arthritis? J Clin Immunol 2000;20:17–23

80. Verburg RJ, Toes RE, Fibbe WE et al. High dose chemotherapy and autologous hematopoietic stem cell transplantation for rheumatoid arthritis: a review. Hum Immunol 2002;63:627–637

81. Bingham SJ, Snowden J, McGonagle D et al. Autologous stem cell transplantation for rheumatoid arthritis – interim report of 6 patients. J Rheumatol 2001;64(suppl):21–24

82. Pavletic SZ, Odell JR, Pirruccello SJ et al. Intensive immunoablation and autologous blood stem cell transplantation in patients with refractory rheumatoid arthritis: the University of Nebraska experience. J Rheumatol 2001;64(suppl):13–20

83. Verburg RJ, Sont JK, van Laar JM. Reduction of joint damage in severe rheumatoid arthritis by high-dose chemotherapy and autologous stem cell transplantation. Arthritis Rheum 2005;52:421–424

84. Snowden JA, Passweg J, Moore JJ et al. Autologous hemopoietic stem cell transplantation in severe rheumatoid arthritis: a report from the EBMT and ABMTR. J Rheumatol 2004;31:482–488

85. Moore J, Ma D, Will R et al. A phase II study of Rituximab in rheumatoid arthritis patients with recurrent disease following haematopoietic stem cell transplantation. Bone Marrow Transplant 2004;34:241–247

86. Verburg RJ, Sont JK, Vliet Vlieland TP et al. High dose chemotherapy followed by autologous peripheral blood stem cell transplantation or conventional pharmacologic treatment for refractory rheumatoid arthritis? A Markov decision analysis. J Rheumatol 2001;28:719–727

87. De Kleer IM, Brinkman DM, Ferster A et al. Autologous stem cell transplantation for refractory juvenile idiopathic arthritis: analysis of clinical effects, mortality, and transplant related morbidity. Ann Rheum Dis 2004;63:1318–1326

88. Burt RK, Oyama Y, Verda L et al. Induction of remission of severe and refractory rheumatoid arthritis by allogeneic mixed chimerism. Arthritis Rheum 2004;50:2466–2470

89. Deapen D, Escalante A, Weinrib L et al. A revised estimate of twin concordance in systemic lupus erythematosus. Arthritis Rheum 1992;35:311–318

90. Urowitz MB, Gladman DD, Abu-Shakra M, Farewell VT. Mortality studies in systemic lupus erythematosus. Results from a single center. III. Improved survival over 24 years. J Rheumatol 1997;24:1061–1065

91. Rus V, Hochberg.MC. The epidemiology of systemic lupus erythematosus. In: Wallace DJ, Hahn BH (eds) Dubois' lupus erythematosus, 6th edn. Lippincott Williams and Wilkins, Philadelphia, 2002:65–86

92. Trager J, Ward MM. Mortality and causes of death in systemic lupus erythematosus. Curr Opin Rheumatol 2001;13:345–351

93. Pryor BD, Bologna SG, Kahl LE. Risk factors for serious infection during treatment with cyclophosphamide and high-dose corticosteroids for systemic lupus erythematosus. Arthritis Rheum 1996;39:1475–1482

94. Boumpas DT, Austin HA, Vaughn EM et al. Controlled trial of pulse methylprednisolone versus two regimens of pulse cyclophosphamide in severe lupus nephritis. Lancet 1992;340:741–745

95. Contreras G, Pardo V, Leclercq B et al. Sequential therapies for proliferative lupus nephritis. 2004;350:971–980

96. Ginzler EM, Dooley MA, Aranow C et al. Mycophenolate mofetil or intravenous cyclophosphamide for lupus nephritis. N Engl J Med 2005;353:2219–2228

97. Gourley MF, Austin HA, III, Scott D et al. Methylprednisolone and cyclophosphamide, alone or in combination, in patients with lupus nephritis. A randomized, controlled trial. Ann Intern Med 1996;125:549–557

98. Houssiau FA, Vasconcelos C, D'Cruz D et al. Immunosuppressive therapy in lupus nephritis: the Euro-Lupus Nephritis Trial, a randomized trial of low-dose versus high-dose intravenous cyclophosphamide. Arthritis Rheum 2002;46:2121–2131

99. Boumpas DT, Austin HA, Fessler BJ et al. Systemic lupus erythematosus: emerging concepts. Part 1: Renal, neuropsychiatric, cardiovascular, pulmonary, and hematologic disease. Ann Intern Med 1995;122:940–950

100. Boumpas DT, Austin HA, Fessler BJ et al. Systemic lupus erythematosus: emerging concepts. Part 1: Renal, neuropsychiatric, cardiovascular, pulmonary, and hematologic disease. Ann Intern Med 1995;122:940–950

101. Boumpas DT, Austin HA, Vaughan EM et al. Risk for sustained amenorrhea in patients with systemic lupus erythematosus receiving intermittent pulse cyclophosphamide therapy. Ann Intern Med 1993;119:366–369

102. Illei GG, Austin HA, Crane M et al. Combination therapy with pulse cyclophosphamide plus pulse methylprednisolone improves long-term renal outcome without adding toxicity in patients with lupus nephritis. Ann Intern Med 2001;135:248–257

103. Illei GG, Takada K, Parkin D et al. Renal flares are common in patients with severe proliferative lupus nephritis treated with pulse immunosuppressive therapy: long-term followup of a cohort of 145 patients participating in randomized controlled studies. Arthritis Rheum 2002;46:995–1002

104. Lipsky PE. Systemic lupus erythematosus: an autoimmune disease of B cell hyperactivity. Nat Immunol 2001;2:764–766

105. Shlomchik MJ, Craft JE, Mamula MJ. From T to B and back again: positive feedback in systemic autoimmune disease. Nat Rev Immunol 2001;1:147–153

106. Pavletic SZ, Illei GG. The role of immune ablation and stem cell transplantation in severe SLE. Best Pract Res Clin Rheumatol 2005;19:839–858

107. Jayne D, Passweg J, Marmont A et al. Autologous stem cell transplantation for systemic lupus erythematosus. Lupus 2004;13:168–176

108. Burt RK, Traynor A, Statkute L et al. Nonmyeloablative hematopoietic stem cell transplantation for systemic lupus erythematosus. JAMA 2006;295:527–535

109. Pavletic SZ. Nonmyeloablative allogeneic hematopoietic stem cell transplantation for autoimmune disease. Arthritis Rheum 2004;50:2387–2390

110. Ikehara S, Good RA, Nakamura T et al. Rationale for bone marrow transplantation in the treatment of autoimmune diseases. Proc Natl Acad Sci USA 1985;82:2483–2487

111. Jones OY, Steele A, Jones JM et al. Nonmyeloablative bone marrow transplantation of BXSB lupus mice using fully matched allogeneic donor cells from green fluorescent protein transgenic mice. J Immunol 2004;172:5415–5419

112. Gur-Lavi M. Long-term remission with allogeneic bone marrow transplantation in systemic lupus erythematosus. Arthritis Rheum 1999;42:1777

113. Khorshid O, Hosing C, Bibawi S et al. Nonmyeloablative stem cell transplant in a patient with advanced systemic sclerosis and systemic lupus erythematosus. J Rheumatol 2004;31:2513–2516

114. Olalla JI, Ortin M, Hermida G et al. Disappearance of lupus anticoagulant after allogeneic bone marrow transplantation. Bone Marrow Transplant 1999;23:83–85

115. Lu Q, Lu L, Niu X et al. Non-myeloablative allogeneic stem cell transplant in a patient with refractory systemic lupus erythematosus. Bone Marrow Transplant 2006;37: 979–981

PART 3

PREPARATION FOR TRANSPLANT

Patient selection: preliminary interview, screening of patient and donor

Samar Kulkarni and Jennifer Treleaven

Introduction

The field of hematopoietic stem cell transplantation (HSCT) has evolved rapidly over the last three decades. From the initial unsuccessful attempts at performing transplants in high-risk, end-stage malignant conditions, these treatments are now routinely offered to patients early in the course of their disease, with the aim of achieving cure. As described in earlier chapters, stem cell transplantation procedures are also being used with increasing frequency as therapy for nonmalignant conditions, albeit those which would cause severe morbidity and even mortality if left untreated. Refinements in the transplant procedures themselves, with better understanding of the problems associated with high-dose chemoradiotherapy as well as improvements in supportive care, have led to a reduction in transplant-related problems. Many of these can now be effectively treated because of the availability of better antibiotics, antifungal and antiviral agents, the availability of more agents to control graft-versus-host disease (GvHD), and improved blood product support.

However, in spite of all these improvements allogeneic transplantation remains associated with a significant risk of treatment-related morbidity and mortality, and the principal causes of treatment failure remain essentially the same as when they were initially described by Thomas et al in the 1970s and 1980s – disease relapse, GvHD and its complications, and pneumonitis.[1,2] Significant numbers of patients may die from transplant-related complications in the allograft setting depending on their individual risk factors, which include increased recipient age, degree of human leukocyte antigen (HLA) disparity between donor and recipient, amount of prior treatment and disease stage, which are all well recognized as being associated with outcome.[3–5] It is important that patients being considered for all transplant procedures are given a realistic but positive breakdown of the wide range of possible complications without being rendered too fearful to accept a potentially life-saving treatment.

In the autograft setting, procedure-associated mortality has dropped to around 5%, again depending on factors such as the patient's performance status, but it should not be overlooked that even a relatively fit patient who has not been heavily pretreated could fall prey to overwhelming sepsis while neutropenic, in spite of the improvements in antibiotic therapy, and again, patients should be apprised of possible complications.

Traditionally, full-intensity conditioned allogeneic transplants are not usually recommended beyond the age of 55 years because of the increased incidence of complications above this age. This led to a major discrepancy between the number of patients who could be offered a transplant and the number of those who need one. Earlier on, an autograft procedure would have been the only possible treatment option for some patients, but more recently non-myeloablative

and reduced-intensity conditioned (RIC) allogeneic transplants have become commonplace. This has resulted in many older patients and patients with high-risk disease being able to receive an allograft and possibly to benefit from a graft-versus-tumor effect which does not exist in the autograft setting.

Blood and marrow transplants are medically so invasive that a good outcome can never be guaranteed even in what are perceived to be the best-risk patients. They are also very expensive. It is therefore important that the appropriateness of the intended procedure is very carefully evaluated for each individual patient, taking into consideration all of his/her individual risk factors so that a realistic estimate can be given of the chances of a successful outcome.

This chapter summarizes our current understanding of appropriate patient selection for autologous and allogeneic hematopoietic stem cell transplantation, and donor selection in the allogeneic setting. It also discusses the issues which should be covered during a consultation with the patient and his donor if an allograft procedure is to be undertaken. Investigations for donor and recipient which must be undertaken prior to transplantation are also listed. Table 20.1 summarizes the general approach to a patient who is being considered for a blood or marrow transplant and lists the most important considerations

Patient selection

Type of transplant

Patients deemed to be appropriate recipients of a stem cell transplant procedure by virtue of their disease status can be broadly divided in three groups:

1. those eligible for a full-intensity conditioned transplant
2. those eligible for a non-myeloablative or RIC transplant
3. those suited to an autograft.

Overall, an allograft procedure is usually considered preferable when the disease being treated is known to be susceptible to a graft-versus-tumor effect, but such transplants are associated with much more significant morbidity and mortality than are autograft procedures, although in survivors of an allograft procedure disease relapse is much less likely. An allograft is also the only transplant treatment option for bone marrow failure syndromes such as aplastic anemia and for the immunodeficiency disorders and inborn errors of metabolism such as Hurler's syndrome.

If an allogeneic transplant is intended, it is, of course, imperative that a suitable allogeneic donor be identified, either an HLA-matched sibling or an unrelated donor. In the event that no such donor can be identified, the patient may instead be referred for an autograft if there

Table 20.1 General approach to a patient who is being considered for a blood or marrow transplant

1. Is transplantation the best therapy under the circumstances?
2. Are there any obvious contraindications to transplantation (age, performance status, complicating medical problems, etc.)?
3. Autograft or allograft preferable?
4. If allograft preferable, is there a suitable HLA-compatible donor available?
5. If no information is available on donors:
   a. has typing on family members been arranged?
   b. has a preliminary search for unrelated donors been started?
5. If autograft preferable or no allogeneic donor available:
   a. have cells already been harvested?
   b. when to harvest?
   c. peripheral blood stem cells or marrow?
   d. how to mobilize peripheral blood stem cells?
   e. purged/selected or unmanipulated?
6. If allograft preferable and a donor is available:
   a. peripheral blood stem cells or marrow?
   b. RIC or full-intensity conditioning?
   c. what type of GvHD prophylaxis?
7. When to transplant?
8. What conditioning regimen to use?

From Mehta & Singhal.[90]

are data available to suggest an advantage for this treatment approach with the underlying disease. Indeed, for some diseases an autograft may be the preferred transplant approach. For example, patients with multiple myeloma tend to be older at presentation, and results of autografting following conditioning with high-dose melphalan are favorable.[6,7] With myeloma, an allograft should probably be reserved for the younger patients when a suitable donor can be identified.

Another important question that remains unanswered is whether the results of RIC or non-myeloablative transplants (NMT) are similar to or better than those seen after full-intensity allografting, if RIC transplantation is performed in patients who are eligible for full-intensity transplantation. Theoretically, by reducing the treatment-related mortality in this group of patients, the overall results should be better provided that the graft evokes a strong graft-versus-tumor influence. However, there are currently few data available to answer this question.

Patient age

As mentioned earlier, full-intensity conditioned transplants are generally not recommended above the age of 55 years. Treatment-related mortality in the patient groups above this age cut-off is significantly higher than in the younger age groups, and transplant-related morbidity and mortality (TRM) increase overall with increasing age, as has been clearly shown by figures from the International Bone Marrow Transplant Registry (IBMTR).[8,9] Hence, patients above the age of 55 are candidates for RIC transplantation, and such transplants have been successfully undertaken in patients up to the age of 70. It should, however, be appreciated that although RIC and NMT have expanded the number of patients and the age group which can receive transplantation, they may still be associated with considerable toxicity, and no randomized studies are available to date to clarify their role in the management of specific malignant conditions.

Type of disease

The spectrum of diseases that has been treated with transplantation requires constant evaluation and refining in the light of developments in other areas of therapy. For example, with the advent of tyrosine kinase inhibitors (TKIs),[10] it is much less common for patients with chronic myeloid leukemia to require allografting, this normally arising

only if a patient has ceased to respond to imatinib and the newer related TKIs or if the mutational status of their disease has changed so that they are resistant to all the currently available TKIs. The European Organization for Research and Treatment of Cancer (EORTC) and the European Bone Marrow Transplant Registry (EBMT) have reviewed the published data on allografting which they have used as a basis for defining the current valid indications.[11–13] This is a useful starting point but, as already mentioned, the decisions must be specific for an individual patient, taking into account all the factors that influence the likelihood of success. Indications for transplantation in the various hematologic and immunologic conditions are discussed in detail in Chapters 3–19.

Stage of disease

The results of full-intensity transplants are better if they are performed when patients are in complete remission.[14,15] It is also well established that the results in first complete remission (CR) are better than in subsequent remissions. This is likely to be due to more previous treatment and the presence of drug-resistant cell populations.

Co-morbidities and performance status

Optimal organ function pretransplant is an important requisite to minimize post-transplant complications and mortality. Older patients undergoing RIC transplantation are more likely to have various age-related illnesses that could influence the transplant procedure. In view of this it would be beneficial to have an assessment tool that can predict post-transplant outcomes. Various scales have been devised to assess co-morbidities in transplant patients.[4] It is also interesting to know that the prediction potential is not influenced by the choice of donor, i.e. related or unrelated.

The co-morbidity index seems to be a significant predictor in specific malignancies,[4] and also in high-risk patients such as those who have received NMT/RIC after having failed prior myeloablative transplant.[16] Another simple measure widely employed is the performance status. In the preliminary studies by Artz et al[3] it was shown that combining performance status with co-morbidity scale increases the power of prediction over co-morbidity index alone. However, most of the data were retrospective and the perfect scale remains to be defined. In addition to identifying the risk to an individual patient, co-morbidity scales are likely to help in tailoring the therapy for particular situations. It is also helpful to compare the data from various studies, and hence prospective studies in this field are warranted.

Organ assessment

Liver

Development of liver dysfunction following HSCT has significant impact on mortality. Early consequences of liver dysfunction include development of edema/ascites, low albumin levels, deranged clotting, risk of bleeding, abnormal drug metabolism and development of veno-occlusive disease, while later sequelae are liver fibrosis, cirrhosis and hepatocellular carcinoma. All patients planned for HSCT should be questioned regarding factors which could influence hepatic function, including previous viral hepatitis, alcohol intake, medications, symptoms suggestive of portal hypertension or any familial history of liver diseases. Physical examination to seek evidence of hepatosplenomegaly and signs of liver dysfunction such as icterus, ascites, edema, spider nevi and gynecomastia should be undertaken in every patient.

Liver function tests that are commonly used in evaluation are serum bilirubin, serum albumin, clotting studies, alkaline phosphatase, lactate dehydrogenase, alanine and aspartate transaminase, and gamma glutamyl transpeptidase. Abnormalities prior to transplantation have been shown to correlate with subsequent hepatic dysfunction.[17,18] Elevated serum ferritin levels have also been shown to correlate adversely with transplant outcome.[19,20] In certain cases, studies such as CT scanning, Doppler ultrasound and even liver biopsy may be needed if the results of liver function tests suggest significant liver impairment. For more details about this subject, the reader is referred to the recent excellent review by Carreras.[21]

Heart

Mortality directly attributable to a cardiac event is uncommon in HSCT patients,[22,23] probably because, in general, transplants are performed in relatively young patients. However, now that NMT/RIC transplants are being offered to older patients, it is more likely that there will be an underlying cardiac disorder. HSCT induces cardiac stress through various mechanisms including anemia, fluid overload, chemotherapy, sepsis and arrhythmias.[24–26] Patients likely to be at particular risk of cardiac problems include those with previous exposure to anthracyclines, and those with amyloidosis, systemic sclerosis, autoimmune disorders, hemoglobinopathies, a storage disorder, or previous myocardial infarction. There is no standardized, universally accepted protocol for cardiac evaluation pre-HSCT and traditionally, patients with an ejection fraction above 40% have been considered to have adequate reserve for HSCT.[27] In recent years, biochemical markers of cardiac damage including troponins and N-terminal pro-brain natriuretic peptide have become available and have shown correlation with increased risk post HSCT.[28,29] A more detailed discussion of pretransplant cardiac evaluation is to be found in a recent review.[30]

Lungs

Evaluation of lung function using standard pulmonary function testing (PFT) and diffusing capacity (DLCO) is routinely performed before HSCT. Patients with poor PFT or DLCO are traditionally considered unsuitable for myeloablative transplant. There are few studies evaluating the influence of pre-HSCT PFT/DLCO on mortality. Crawford & Fisher[31] found that abnormal DLCO (>80% predicted) and a P(A-a) O_2 gradient more than 20 mmHg were independently associated with TRM. Similar results have been reported by others.[32] Unfortunately, it is still not established what minimum level of lung function is required below which HSCT becomes untenable, and so patients should be assessed for SCT in the context of other co-morbidities.

Kidneys

Renal impairment develops in 30–40% patients post HSCT. The predominant causes include drug toxicity, sepsis and radiation nephritis. Another important, although less common cause for nephrotoxicity is hemolytic uremic syndrome. Multivariate analyses of renal dysfunction after SCT indicate that degree of renal impairment is strongly associated with TRM.[33,34]

Chronic renal impairment is not very common after HSCT in contrast to solid organ transplantation, mostly due to the fact that ciclosporin is generally stopped at 6 months post HSCT. In children, Grönroos et al[35] found that glomerular filtration rate (GFR) and effective renal plasma flow (ERPF) were significantly reduced at 1 year post HSCT. Renal impairment was found in 41% of patients at 1 year, 31% at 3 years and 11% at 7 years. There was slight recovery of GFR at 3 years but ERPF was unchanged. Similar results have been reported by Miralbell et al.[36]

A high serum creatinine pre-HSCT has been shown to be associated with chronic renal failure,[37] and serum creatinine along with renal creatinine clearance estimated by ethylenediaminetetra-acetic acid (EDTA) clearance are most commonly used to assess renal function pretransplant. This also helps to decide the doses of conditioning chemotherapy agents, especially fludarabine, used for RIC/NMT. It also helps to identify patients who may benefit from dose reductions, avoidance of potentially nephrotoxic agents and having pre-emptive measures like volume replacement and alkalinization of urine.

Viral status

Evaluation of ongoing or previous exposure to viral pathogens is important for both patient and potential donor. Over the years there have been significant developments in the management of viral infections, especially cytomegalovirus (CMV) reactivation. The aim of pre-HSCT testing is to avoid donors who have been exposed to certain viruses, identify the best combination of donor/patient viral status and identify patients who are at higher risk of viral reactivation post HSCT. For most viruses, serologic methods are used to identify previous exposure. Type of antibody, whether IgG or IgM, will help to define previous or recent infection. Chapter 42 gives a fuller account of the current situation with regard to viruses in the stem cell transplantation setting.

Human immunodeficiency virus (HIV)

Positivity for HIV is a contraindication for HSCT for the patient although to date few case reports have been published, with only short follow-ups.[38–41] The situation is probably better for HIV-positive patients in the autograft setting owing to the less profound immunosuppression necessary.[40] It is contraindicated to use an HIV-positive donor.

Human T-lymphoma virus (HTLV-1 and HTLV-2)

HTLV-1 is associated with adult T-cell leukemia and lymphoma (ATLL). Reduced-intensity allogeneic HSCT has been used successfully to treat this condition.[42–44] HTLV-1 positive donors should be avoided, and it is contraindicated to use HTLV-2 positive donors.[45]

Cytomegalovirus

For a seronegative patient, it is ideal to have a seronegative donor, since use of a seropositive donor in a seronegative patient increases the risk of CMV reactivation. In CMV-seropositive patients the data are controversial. One large study has shown a beneficial effect of using seropositive donors,[46] especially in unrelated donor transplants, but others have found no survival advantage using CMV-positive donors.[47,48]

Herpes simplex virus (HSV)

Reactivation of HSV is very common after HSCT, but the availability of aciclovir since the 1980s[49] means that this does not usually become a significant problem, particularly as most centers use aciclovir or valaciclovir prophylaxis.[50] For the same reason, HSV status of the donor is not critical as patients can be easily treated should they develop signs of infection.

Epstein–Barr virus (EBV)

EBV is known to be associated with post-transplant lymphoproliferative disorder (PTLD).[51,52] The risk in HSCT is much smaller than in solid organ transplants (1% compared to >10%)[53] and risk in HSCT is higher with unrelated and mismatched donors or use of T-depletion.[54] EBV serology is recommended in both HSCT patients and donors.

Varicella zoster virus (VZV)

VZV serology of patients is useful in certain situations. If the seronegative patient is exposed to VZV in the community, prophylactic human immunoglobulin and extended antiviral prophylaxis may be useful, and as the antibody titer may decrease over time it is useful to know VZV serostatus even in long-term survivors.[55,56]

Hepatitis viruses

Transfusion-transmitted viral hepatitis is very rare now, but in certain parts of the world hepatitis B positivity has been reported to be as high as 30%.[57] Similar figures are quoted in the literature for hepatitis C viruses.[17,58,59]

Hepatitis B virus (HBV)

For evaluation of HBV status, tests include HBsAg, HbeAg, anti-HBc (IgM/IgG), anti-HBs, anti-HBe and HBV-DNA. The patient's viral status can be determined by the pattern of antigens and antibodies detected. The status of the patient not only predicts if there is increased risk of hepatic complications, but also what group of patients should receive prophylactic antiviral therapy.[60–62] If the patient has active hepatitis (abnormal liver function tests (LFTs)), it is safer to delay the transplant.

Prophylactic antivirals are indicated in patients who are HBV-DNA positive and those who have pre-core mutant (HBeAg-, anti-HBe+, HBV-DNA+). There is no contraindication to HSCT in HBsAg-positive patients who do not have abnormal liver function. In patients who are HBsAg negative but who are anti-HBc+ and anti-HBs+, testing for HBV-DNA is recommended and antivirals should be started if the test becomes positive.[63,64] Vaccination of the donor is also recommended.[59]

As HBsAg+ donors transmit the virus in a significant number of cases, an alternative donor should be used if possible. If only a donor positive for HBV-DNA is available, either treatment of the donor with antivirals before donation should be undertaken, or the patient's HBV-DNA should be monitored after HSCT with a view to starting antivirals if it becomes positive.[60] Patients who are anti-HBc+ or anti-HBs+ and negative for HbeAg and HBV-DNA are unlikely to transmit infection.

Hepatitis C virus (HCV)

Conventional serologic testing is not always adequate to rule out HCV infection and hence assessment of viremia using polymerase chain reaction (PCR) is used for testing. In patients who are HCV-DNA positive, have abnormal liver function and have significant fibrosis on liver biopsy, myeloablative transplants are likely to result in high TRM.[61,62] Hence, other treatment approaches should be explored. Since 25% of long-term survivors with HCV infection will develop cirrhosis after SCT, long-term follow-up is required.[65] Transplant is not contraindicated in patients who are HCV-DNA positive but have normal liver function tests. However, it is contraindicated to use HCV-DNA+ donors as transmission of HCV occurs in almost all cases.[66]

Other viruses

In patients or donors who are symptomatic, testing for other viruses including respiratory syncytial virus (RSV),[67] adenovirus[68] or West Nile virus may be indicated. However, routine testing is not recommended.

Table 20.2 Routine screening procedures to be performed in HSCT recipients

Tissue typing
ABO group and Rhesus typing with antibody screen
Full blood count
Coagulation studies
Urea and electrolytes
Creatinine clearance
Liver function tests
Blood sugar
Chest X-ray
Electrocardiogram and MUGA scan
Bone marrow aspirate and trephine
Screening for MRSA, *C.diff* and VRE
Viral screens for: Cytomegalovirus Epstein–Barr virus Hepatitis B (HBsAg) Hepatitis C HIV Herpes simplex virus Varicella zoster virus
Screening for syphilis (VDRL, TPHA)
Toxoplasma screen
Cardiac evaluation
Renal function evaluation
Pulmonary function tests
Dental check
Complete disease restaging

Tables 20.2 and 20.3 depict the routine screening test to be undertaken on patients and prospective donors prior to SCT.

The initial interview, information to be given and consenting process

It is very important that the patient planned to receive a transplant should be adequately prepared. Using various risk classifications for individual malignancies, it is possible to identify the potential candidates for transplantation early on during treatment. This should enable the transplant team to start giving information to the patient and hence allow adequate time for the individual to assimilate and assess the information with the view of making an informed decision. It also gives time for the patient to identify his/her individual concerns, and any special issues can be addressed.

A detailed history is very important. This should include smoking, alcohol intake, recreational drug use, long-term medications, previous illnesses, infections and allergies, since all of these factors can impact upon transplant outcome.[69] The interview should be conducted in a comfortable and non-threatening environment and it should be remembered that patients being referred for a transplant procedure from elsewhere are likely to be even more nervous and unable to fully assimilate information given to them than are 'in-house' patients who have had all their initial treatment at the hospital where the transplant will be undertaken. A nurse transplant co-ordinator should be present when possible, who can provide additional information and support to the patient, particularly regarding matters such as dietary restrictions and visiting. The 'transplant talk' should then cover the topics covered below.

Table 20.3 Pretransplant investigations for the donor

Blood group and antibody screening
Coagulation studies
Complete blood count
Full tissue typing
Liver function tests
Pregnancy test
Urea and creatinine
VDRL
Viral serology Cytomegalovirus Epstein–Barr virus Hepatitis B (HBsAg) Hepatitis C HIV Herpes simplex virus Varicella zoster virus
Chest X-ray
Electrocardiogram
Under certain circumstances
Cytogenetic studies (chromosome fragility)
Bone marrow examination
Echocardiogram and/or MUGA scan
Hemoglobin electrophoresis
Lung function tests
Sickle test
Toxoplasma titer

Nature of the intended treatment

HSCT is an intensive modality of treatment and is likely to be associated with fatal outcome in 20–50% patients. Patients who are planned for HSCT should know the rationale behind choosing the particular modality and what outcomes are expected, and alternative options. Using the statistics and data from literature may not help to make decisions about an individual person but it certainly helps to make the decision process a little easier for the patient.

The most important part of the initial interview is to explain the exact nature of the transplant procedure. As most of the patients are likely to have limited knowledge of the medical terminology, it is always helpful to simplify the discussion in layman's terms. Various websites are available that can be used to obtain appropriate information, and most institutions have written documents and leaflets informing the patient about transplant issues. They may also have their own, individualized written information. It is helpful for the patient to know what is going to happen in chronologic order. The discussion should include mention of the drugs to be used for conditioning, the dose and fractionation schedule of total body irradiation, a description of pre- and post-transplant immunosuppression and any additional measures to be used such as alemtuzumab.

Side-effects

Discussion of the acute side-effects should include the temporal pattern, severity and expected duration for each. It is helpful for the patient to know what measures will be taken to prevent and treat the side-effects. Most patients will have experienced common early side-effects such as nausea, vomiting and diarrhea during the previous induction therapy. Similarly, myelosuppression and infections will

have occurred during previous treatments. Viral infections, especially CMV reactivation, can occur late after myeloid recovery and hence patients may need treatment well after the initial discharge from hospital.

Patients should be aware that severe mucositis is likely to prevent adequate oral intake and hence there may be a need for enteral or parenteral nutrition. The discussion about GvHD should include an explanation of the clinical manifestations, scoring of severity and treatment options. It is essential for patients to know that the initial development of GvHD may occur beyond the first month and that prompt medical help should be sought on development of signs and symptoms. Treatment options and side-effects of these should be explained.

Patients should be informed about the clinical symptoms, investigations and management options for veno-occlusive disease, and they should be made aware of the need for compliance with the prophylactic antibiotics and *Pneumocystis* prophylaxis. It should be possible to give an estimate of the chances of vital organ dysfunction overall in each individual situation.

Long-term complications

It is also important to discuss the chances of late and long-term complications, as covered in Chapter 46. Patients should be aware that they are likely to be immune deficient for a long period of time, and hyposplenic for the rest of their lives, especially after myeloablative transplant. Infertility is almost inevitable after myeloablative transplantation. Data regarding NMT/RIC are not available.

Time to be spent in hospital

Patients should realize that their initial hospitalization could be in excess of 6 weeks, and that many will need 2–3 readmissions after the first discharge. If the patient is to be nursed in isolation, the exact nature of the isolation, visiting policy and restrictions implemented during this phase should be explained. Physical recovery may not be substantial for as long as 6 months and in some cases it could be longer than 1 year. During this period patients are unlikely to be able to work and this can have serious financial implications for the family. Patients should be offered information about the institutions they can contact to seek help.

Donor selection

HLA match

The most important factor determining the overall success and risk of mortality after HSCT is the degree of HLA match between the recipient and donor. HLA typing and matching are discussed in Chapter 23. The EBMT and Bone Marrow Donors Worldwide (BMDW) have published guidelines about selection of unrelated donors.[70]

CMV status

As discussed above, for a CMV-seronegative patient the best option is a CMV-negative donor. For a CMV-seropositive patient, CMV status of the donor is less important but there is some old evidence to suggest that a CMV-seropositive donor is preferable for a CMV-positive patient receiving a T-cell depleted allograft, as a CMV-immune donor may be able to protect the recipient from CMV infection.[46,48,71] Prior donor CMV exposure may place seronegative recipients at increased risk of CMV conversion. However, multivariable analysis indicated that prior donor CMV exposure significantly reduced the risk of CMV reactivation in seropositive recipients. It seems that the CMV serology status of the recipient, rather than the donor, is the primary determinant of risk for CMV conversion, and immunity against CMV seems to be transferred with the donor graft and protects seropositive HSCT recipients from CMV reactivation.[72]

Blood group and Rh status

Blood group and/or Rh mismatch are not a contraindication for transplant. With bone marrow donation, major blood group mismatch requires manipulation of the stem cell product to remove red cells so that the risk of intravascular hemolysis is reduced.[73,74] There are conflicting data regarding the role of blood group mismatch and the risk of relapse post transplant[75,76] but a number of publications suggest that ABO and Rh mismatch do not influence transplant outcome.[75,77,78]

Sex match

Donor–recipient sex match is an important predictor of transplant-related mortality, and the combination of male recipient with a female donor is known to be associated with increased risk of chronic GvHD and higher TRM,[79] but this does not result in a reduction in relapse risk in all diseases,[80] although in multiple myeloma relapse risk does appear to be reduced.[81] Female patients with male donors show an increased risk of graft rejection in aplastic anemia.[82]

Parity

Parous females are exposed to fetal antigens in utero and there is a high incidence of HLA-specific antibodies in these women.[83] It is well known that parous female stem cell donation to male or female recipients is associated with a higher risk of chronic GvHD.[47] Hence, it is recommended that whenever possible, parous female donors are avoided.

Age

Younger donor age at the time of donation has a favorable effect on outcome after HSCT. The risks of acute GvHD (grade III or more) and chronic GvHD are higher and the overall survival is lower with increasing donor age.[47,48,84]

Special considerations for screening of elderly donors

More than 25% of HSCTs are performed for elderly patients,[85] and thus the chances of using a donor above the age of 55 are also higher in the matched sibling situation. As this group of donors is more likely to have medical problems, it has been recommended recently that additional tests should be conducted in donors more than 55 years of age so as to reduce the risk of transmission of donor-derived disease to the patient and also to ensure the safety of the donor. The additional tests aim to reduce the risk of transmission of malignant and congenital disorders. They include prostate-specific antigen (PSA) in males, occult blood in stools, bone marrow aspiration if medical history or tests are abnormal, protein electrophoresis, lactate dehydrogenase (LDH), and computed tomography (CT) scanning of the chest if there is history of smoking.[86]

Stem cell source and blood loss

Peripheral blood stem cells (PBSC) are now the most usual source of stem cells, whereas until about 10 years ago bone marrow was virtually always used. There are advantages and disadvantages to each method of donation which, in one study, were examined in a group of normal donors who donated both blood- and marrow-derived stem cells so that a comparison could be made.[87] Blood loss is not significant with PBSC harvesting. However, good venous access is a prerequisite and it is necessary to administer G-CSF to mobilize the stem cells into the peripheral blood, which causes significant bone pain.

During the period when bone marrow was used as a stem cell source, one or two units of autologous units of blood were often collected over the 2–4 weeks preceding the marrow harvest for intra- or postoperative transfusion, and folic acid and iron supplementation were prescribed. Erythropoietin has also been administered with good effect to both normal donors and patients to minimize transfusion requirements.[88,89]

Consent

Written consent from the patient should be obtained at the end of the pretransplant evaluation, when all the investigations have been completed. The transplant consent form should ideally specify the exact nature of the transplant, the conditioning regimen, the source of cells, and the GvHD prophylaxis to be used. The consent form may be an institution-specific document, accompanied by an information sheet describing the proposed procedure. Alternatively, it may be deemed appropriate to combine the information sheet with a generic consent form to produce a detailed, procedure-specific consent form.

For peripheral blood stem cell harvests, consent for administration of growth factors should be included for both normal donors and patients, along with consent for insertion of a central venous access device, should this be needed. A summary of possible side-effects should also be given.

References

1. Thomas ED, Buckner CD, Banaji M et al. One hundred patients with acute leukemia treated by chemotherapy, total body irradiation, and allogeneic marrow transplantation. Blood 1977;49:511–533
2. Thomas ED. Bone-marrow transplantation in acute leukaemia. Lancet 1978;1:876
3. Artz AS, Pollyea DA, Kocherginsky M et al. Performance status and comorbidity predict transplant-related mortality after allogeneic hematopoietic cell transplantation. Biol Blood Marrow Transplant 2006;12:954–964
4. Sorror ML, Sandmaier BM, Storer BE et al. Comorbidity and disease status based risk stratification of outcomes among patients with acute myeloid leukemia or myelodysplasia receiving allogeneic hematopoietic cell transplantation. J Clin Oncol 2007;25:4246–4254
5. Sorror ML, Maris MB, Storb RF et al. Hematopoietic cell transplantation (HCT)-specific comorbidity index: a new tool for risk assessment before allogeneic HCT. Blood 2005;106:2912–2919
6. McElwain TJ, Gore ME, Meldrum M et al. VAMP followed by high dose melphalan and autologous bone marrow transplantation for multiple myeloma. Bone Marrow Transplant 1989;4(suppl 4):109–112
7. Gore ME, Selby PJ, Viner C et al. Intensive treatment of multiple myeloma and criteria for complete remission. Lancet 1989;2:879–882
8. Ringden O, Horowitz MM, Gale RP et al. Outcome after allogeneic bone marrow transplant for leukemia in older adults. JAMA 1993;270:57–60
9. Horowitz MM, Loberiza FR, Bredeson CN et al. Transplant registries: guiding clinical decisions and improving outcomes. Oncology (Williston Park) 2001;15:649–659
10. Goldman JM, Melo JV. Editorial: targeting the BCR-ABL tyrosine kinase in chronic myeloid leukemia. N Engl J Med 2001;344:1084–1086
11. Gratwohl A, Passweg J, Baldomero H, Hermans J. Blood and marrow transplantation activity in Europe 1997. European Group for Blood and Marrow Transplantation (EBMT). Bone Marrow Transplant 1999;24:231–245
12. Gratwohl A, Baldomero H, Passweg J et al. Accreditation Committee of the European Group for Blood and Marrow Transplantation (EBMT); Working Parties Acute (ALWP) Chronic Leukemias (CLWP); Lymphoma Working Party. Hematopoietic stem cell transplantation for hematological malignancies in Europe. Leukemia 2003;17:941–959
13. Ljungman P, Urbano-Ispizua A, Cavazzana-Calvo M et al. Allogeneic and autologous transplantation for haematological diseases, solid tumours and immune disorders: definitions and current practice in Europe. Bone Marrow Transplant 2006;37:439–449
14. Hunault M, Harousseau JL, Delain M et al. Better outcome of adult acute lymphoblastic leukemia after early genoidentical allogeneic bone marrow transplantation (BMT) than after late high-dose therapy and autologous BMT: a GOELAMS trial. Blood 2004;104:3028–3037
15. Runde V, de Witte T, Arnold R et al. Bone marrow transplantation from HLA-identical siblings as first-line treatment in patients with myelodysplastic syndromes: early transplantation is associated with improved outcome. Chronic Leukemia Working Party of the European Group for Blood and Marrow Transplantation. Bone Marrow Transplant 1998;21:255–261

16. Baron F, Storb R, Storer BE et al. Factors associated with outcomes in allogeneic hematopoietic cell transplantation with nonmyeloablative conditioning after failed myeloablative hematopoietic cell transplantation. J Clin Oncol 2006;24:4150–4157

17. Locasciulli A, Alberti A, de Bock R et al. Impact of liver disease and hepatitis infections on allogeneic bone marrow transplantation in Europe: a survey from the European Bone Marrow Transplantation (EBMT) Group – Infectious Diseases Working Party. Bone Marrow Transplant 1994;14:833–837

18. Carreras E, Bertz H, Arcese W et al. Incidence and outcome of hepatic veno-occlusive disease after blood or marrow transplantation: a prospective cohort study of the European Group for Blood and Marrow Transplantation. European Group for Blood and Marrow Transplantation Chronic Leukemia Working Party. Blood 1998;92:3599–3604

19. Angelucci E, Muretto P, Nicolucci A et al. Effects of iron overload and hepatitis C virus positivity in determining progression of liver fibrosis in thalassemia following bone marrow transplantation, Blood 2002;100:17–21

20. Armand P, Kim HT, Cutler CS et al. Prognostic impact of elevated pretransplantation serum ferritin in patients undergoing myeloablative stem cell transplantation. Blood 2007;109:4586–4588

21. Carreras E. Risk assessment in hematopoietic stem cell transplantation: the liver as a risk factor. Best Pract Res Clin Hematol 2007;20:231–246

22. Cazin B, Gorin NC, Laporte JP et al. Cardiac complications after bone marrow transplantation. A report on a series of 63 consecutive transplantations. Cancer 1986;57:2061–2069

23. Murdych T, Weisdorf DJ. Serious cardiac complications during bone marrow transplantation at the University of Minnesota, 1977–1997. Bone Marrow Transplant 2001;28:283–287

24. von Bernuth G, Adam D, Hofstetter R et al. Cyclophosphamide cardiotoxicity. Eur J Pediatr 1980;134:87–90

25. Artucio H, Digenio A, Pereyra M. Left ventricular function during sepsis. Crit Care Med 1989;17:323–327

26. Mackenzie I. The hemodynamics of human septic shock. Anaesthesia 2001;56:130–144

27. Bearman SI, Petersen FB, Schor RA et al. Radionuclide ejection fractions in the evaluation of patients being considered for bone marrow transplantation: risk for cardiac toxicity. Bone Marrow Transplant 1990;5:173–177

28. Dispenzieri A, Gertz M, Kyle R et al. Prognostication of survival using cardiac troponins and N-terminal pro-brain natriuretic peptide in patients with primary systemic amyloidosis undergoing peripheral blood stem cell transplantation. Blood 2004;104:1181–1887

29. Horacek JM, Pudil R, Tichy M et al. The use of biochemical markers in cardiotoxicity monitoring in patients treated for leukemia, Neoplasma 2005;52:430–434

30. Coghlan JG, Handler CE, Kottaridis PD. Cardiac assessment of patients for hematopoietic stem cell transplantation. Best Pract Res Clin Hematol 2007;20:247–263

31. Crawford SW, Fisher L. Predictive value of pulmonary function tests before marrow transplantation. Chest 1992;101:1257–1264

32. Goldberg SL, Klumpp TR, Magdalinski AJ, Mangan KF. Value of the pretransplant evaluation in predicting toxic day-100 mortality among blood stem-cell and bone marrow transplant recipients J Clin Oncol 1998;16:3796–3802

33. Parikh CR, Coca SG. Acute renal failure in hematopoietic cell transplantation. Kidney Int 2006;69:430–435

34. Parimon T, Au DH, Martin PJ, Chien JW. A risk score for mortality after allogeneic hematopoietic cell transplantation. Ann Intern Med 2006;144:407–414

35. Grönroos MH, Bolme P, Winiarski J, Berg UB. Long-term renal function following bone marrow transplantation. Bone Marrow Transplant 2007;39:717–723

36. Miralbell R, Sancho G, Bieri S et al. Renal insufficiency in patients with hematologic malignancies undergoing total body irradiation and bone marrow transplantation: a prospective assessment. Int J Radiat Oncol Biol Phys 2004;58:809–816

37. Kist-van Holthe JE, Bresters D, Ahmed-Ousenkova Y-M et al. Long-term renal function after hemopoietic stem cell transplantation in children Bone Marrow Transplant 2005;36:605–610

38. Molina A, Zaia J, Krishnan A.Treatment of human immunodeficiency virus-related lymphoma with hematopoietic stem cell transplantation. Blood Rev 2003;17:249–258

39. Sorà F, Antinori A, Piccirillo N et al. Highly active antiretroviral therapy and allogeneic CD34+ peripheral blood progenitor cells transplantation in an HIV/HCV coinfected patient with acute myeloid leukemia. Exp Hematol 2002;30:279–284

40. Wolf T, Rickerts V, Staszewski S et al. First case of successful allogeneic stem cell transplantation in an HIV-patient who acquired severe aplastic anemia. Haematologica 2007;92:56–58

41. Kang EM, de Witte M, Malech H et al. Nonmyeloablative conditioning followed by transplantation of genetically modified HLA-matched peripheral blood progenitor cells for hematologic malignancies in patients with acquired immunodeficiency syndrome. Blood 2002;99:698–701

42. Fukushima T, Miyazaki Y, Honda S et al. Allogeneic hematopoietic stem cell transplantation provides sustained long-term survival for patients with adult T-cell leukemia/lymphoma. Leukemia 2005;19:829–834

43. Kami M, Hamaki T, Miyakoshi S et al. Allogeneic haematopoietic stem cell transplantation for the treatment of adult T-cell leukaemia/lymphoma. Br J Haematol 2003;120:304–309

44. Okamura J, Utsunomiya A, Tanosaki R et al. Allogeneic stem-cell transplantation with reduced conditioning intensity as a novel immunotherapy and antiviral therapy for adult T-cell leukemia/lymphoma. Blood 2005;105:4143–4145

45. CDC, Infectious Disease Society of America, American Society of Blood and Marrow Transplantation. Guidelines for preventing opportunistic infections among hematopoietic stem cell transplant recipients. Recommendations of CDC, the Infectious Disease Society of America, and the American Society of Blood and Marrow Transplantation 2000/49(RR10). www.cdc.gov/mmwr/preview/mmwrhtml/rr4910al.htm

46. Ljungman P, Brand R, Einsele H et al. Donor CMV serologic status and outcome of CMV-seropositive recipients after unrelated donor stem cell transplantation: an EBMT megafile analysis. Blood 2003;102:4255–4260

47. Kollman C, Howe CW, Anasetti C et al. Donor characteristics as risk factors in recipients after transplantation of bone marrow from unrelated donors: the effect of donor age. Blood 2001;98:2043–2051

48. Boeckh M, Nichols WG. The impact of cytomegalovirus serostatus of donor and recipient before hematopoietic stem cell transplantation in the era of antiviral prophylaxis and pre-emptive therapy. Blood 2004;103:2003–2008

49. Gluckman E, Lotsberg J, Devergie A et al. Prophylaxis of herpes infections after bone-marrow transplantation by oral acyclovir. Lancet 1983;2:706–708

50. Dignani MC, Mykietiuk A, Michelet M et al. Valacyclovir prophylaxis for the prevention of Herpes simplex virus reactivation in recipients of progenitor cells transplantation. Bone Marrow Transplant 2002;29:263–267

51. Paya CV, Fung JJ, Nalesnik MA et al. Epstein–Barr virus-induced posttransplant lymphoproliferative disorders. ASTS/ASTP EBV-PTLD Task Force and The Mayo Clinic Organized International Consensus Development Meeting. Transplantation 1999;68:1517–1525

52. Sundin M, LeBlanc K, Ringdén O et al. The role of HLA mismatch, splenectomy and recipient Epstein-Barr virus seronegativity as risk factors in post-transplant lymphoproliferative disorder following allogeneic hematopoietic stem cell transplantation. Haematologica 2006;91:1059–1068

53. Everly MJ, Bloom RD, Tsai DE, Trofe J. Posttransplant lymphoproliferative disorder. Ann Pharmacother 2007;41:1850–1858

54. Juvonen E, Aalto S, Tarkkanen J et al. Retrospective evaluation of serum Epstein Barr virus DNA levels in 406 allogeneic stem cell transplant patients. Haematologica 2007;92:819–825

55. Boeckh M, Kim HW, Flowers ME et al. Long-term acyclovir for prevention of varicella zoster virus disease after allogeneic hematopoietic cell transplantation – a randomized double-blind placebo-controlled study. Blood 2006;107:1800–1805

56. Steer CB, Szer J, Sasadeusz J et al. Varicella-zoster infection after allogeneic bone marrow transplantation: incidence, risk factors and prevention with low-dose aciclovir and ganciclovir. Bone Marrow Transplant 2000;25:657–664

57. Yim HJ, Lok AS. Natural history of chronic hepatitis B virus infection: what we knew in 1981 and what we know in 2005. Hepatology 2006;43(suppl 1):S173–S181

58. Locasciulli A, Testa M, Valsecchi MG et al. The role of hepatitis C and B virus infections as risk factors for severe liver complications following allogeneic BMT: a prospective study by the Infectious Disease Working Party of the European Blood and Marrow Transplantation Group. Transplantation 1999;68:1486–1491

59. Idilman R, Ustün C, Karayalçin S et al. Hepatitis B virus vaccination of recipients and donors of allogeneic peripheral blood stem cell transplantation. Clin Transplant 2003;17:438–443

60. Lau GK, Lie AK, Kwong YL et al. A case-controlled study on the use of HBsAg-positive donors for allogeneic hematopoietic cell transplantation. Blood 2000;96:452–458

61. Strasser SI, McDonald GB. Hepatitis viruses and hematopoietic cell transplantation: a guide to patient and donor management. Blood 1999;93:1127–1136

62. Locasciulli A, Bruno B, Alessandrino EP et al. Hepatitis reactivation and liver failure in hemopoietic stem cell transplants for hepatitis B virus (HBV)/hepatitis C virus (HCV) positive recipients: a retrospective study by the Italian group for blood and marrow transplantation. Bone Marrow Transplant 2003;31:295–300

63. Hsiao LT, Chiou TJ, Liu JH et al. Extended lamivudine therapy against hepatitis B virus infection in hematopoietic stem cell transplant recipients. Biol Blood Marrow Transplant 2006;12:84–94

64. Hui CK, Lie A, Au WY et al. Effectiveness of prophylactic Anti-HBV therapy in allogeneic hematopoietic stem cell transplantation with HBsAg positive donors. Am J Transplant 2005;5:1437–1445

65. Peffault R, de Latour R, Levy V et al. Long-term outcome of hepatitis C infection after bone marrow transplantation. Blood 2004;103:1618–1624

66. Shuhart MC, Myerson D, Childs BH et al. Marrow transplantation from hepatitis C virus seropositive donors: transmission rate and clinical course. Blood 1994;84:3229–3235

67. Peck AJ, Corey L, Boeckh M. Pretransplantation respiratory syncytial virus infection: impact of a strategy to delay transplantation. Clin Infect Dis 2004;39:673–680

68. Runde V, Ross S, Trenschel R et al. Adenoviral infection after allogeneic stem cell transplantation (SCT): report on 130 patients from a single SCT unit involved in a prospective multi center surveillance study. Bone Marrow Transplant 2001;28:51–57

69. Hoodin F, Kalbfleisch KR, Thornton J, Ratanatharathorn V. Psychosocial influences on 305 adults' survival after bone marrow transplantation: depression, smoking, and behavioral self-regulation. J Psychosom Res 2004;57:145–154

70. Wiegand T, Raffoux C, Hurley CK et al. World Marrow Donor Association Quality Assurance Work Group, WMDA Donor Registries Working Group. A special report: suggested procedures for international unrelated donor search from the donor registries and quality assurance working groups of the World Marrow Donor Association (WMDA). Bone Marrow Transplant 2004;34:97–101

71. Grob JP, Grundy JE, Prentice HG et al. Immune donors can protect marrow-transplant recipients from severe cytomegalovirus infections. Lancet 1987;1:774–776

72. Lin TS, Zahrieh D, Weller E et al. Risk factors for cytomegalovirus reactivation after CD6+ T-cell-depleted allogeneic bone marrow transplantation. Transplantation 2002;74:49–54

73. Guttridge MG, Sidders C, Booth-Davey E et al. Factors affecting volume reduction and red blood cell depletion of bone marrow on the COBE Spectra cell separator before hematopoietic stem cell transplantation. Bone Marrow Transplant 2006;38:175–181

74. Larghero J, Rea D, Esperou H et al. ABO-mismatched marrow processing for transplantation: results of 114 procedures and analysis of immediate adverse events and hematopoietic recovery. Transfusion 2006;46:398–402

75. Seebach JD, Stussi G, Passweg JR et al. GVHD Working Committee of Center for International Blood and Marrow Transplant Research. ABO blood group barrier in allogeneic bone marrow transplantation revisited. Biol Blood Marrow Transplant 2005;11:1006–1013

76. Mehta J, Powles R, Sirohi B et al. Does donor-recipient ABO incompatibility protect against relapse after allogeneic bone marrow transplantation in first remission acute myeloid leukemia? Bone Marrow Transplant 2002;29:853–859

77. Klumpp TR, Herman JH, Ulicny J et al. Lack of effect of donor-recipient ABO mismatching on outcome following allogeneic hematopoietic stem cell transplantation. Bone Marrow Transplant 2006;38:615–620

78. Wirk B, Klumpp TR, Ulicny J et al. Lack of effect of donor-recipient Rh mismatch on outcomes after allogeneic hematopoietic stem cell transplantation. Transfusion 2007; Sept 27 (epub ahead of print)

79. Gratwohl AH, Niederwieser D, van Biezen A et al. Female donors influence transplant-related mortality and relapse incidence in male recipients of sibling blood and marrow transplants. Hematol J 2001;2:363–370

80. Loren AW, Bunin GR, Boudreau C et al. Impact of donor and recipient sex and parity on outcomes of HLA-identical sibling allogeneic hematopoietic stem cell transplantation. Biol Blood Marrow Transplant 2006;12:758–769

81. Gahrton G, Iacobelli S, Apperley J et al. The impact of donor gender on outcome of allogeneic hematopoietic stem cell transplantation for multiple myeloma: reduced relapse risk in female to male transplants. Bone Marrow Transplant 2005;35:609–617

82. Stern M, Passweg J, Locasciulli A et al. Influence of donor/recipient sex matching on outcome of allogeneic hematopoietic stem cell transplantation for aplastic anemia. Transplantation 2006;82:218–226

83. James E, Chai JG, Dewchand H et al. Multiparity induces priming to male-specific minor histocompatibility antigen, HY, in mice and humans. Blood 2003;102:388–393

84. Carreras E, Jiménez M, Gómez-García V et al. Donor age and degree of HLA matching have a major impact on the outcome of unrelated donor hematopoietic cell transplantation for chronic myeloid leukemia. Bone Marrow Transplant 2006;37:33–40

85. McSweeney PA, Niederwieser D, Shizuru JA et al. Hematopoietic cell transplantation in older patients with hematologic malignancies: replacing high-dose cytotoxic therapy with graft-versus-tumor effects. Blood 2001;97:3390–3400

86. Niederwieser D, Gentilini C, Hegenbart U et al. Transmission of donor illness by stem cell transplantation: should screening be different in older donors? Bone Marrow Transplant 2004;34:657–665

87. Powles R, Mehta J, Kulkarni S et al. Allogeneic blood and bone-marrow stem cell transplantation in haematological malignant disease: a randomised trial. Lancet 2000;335:1231–1237

88. Mitus AJ, Antin JH, Rutherford CJ et al. Use of recombinant human erythropoietin in allogeneic bone marrow transplant donor/recipient pairs. Blood 1994;83:1952–1957

89. Martínez AM, Sastre A, Muñoz A et al. Recombinant human erythropoietin (rh-Epo) administration to normal child bone marrow donors. Bone Marrow Transplant 1998;22:137–138

90. Mehta J, Singhal S. Pre-transplant evaluation of the patient and the donor. In: Barrett AJ, Treleaven JG (eds) The clinical practice of stem cell transplantation. Isis Medical Media, Oxford, 1998

Stem cell donor registries

Susan Cleaver

CHAPTER 21

Introduction

'10 million bone marrow donors – 10 million chances of life.' So stated the global press release on November 16 2005, celebrating the addition of the 10 millionth donor to the Bone Marrow Donors Worldwide (BMDW) database.[1] This represented the successful collaborative effort of 57 stem cell donor registries and 38 cord blood banks in 42 countries working together for the common good of patients requiring treatment by hematopoietic stem cell transplantation (HSCT) from unrelated donors. The BMDW, as an initiative, dates back to1988, when Professor JJ van Rood, on behalf of the Immunology Working Party of the European Group for Blood and Marrow Transplantation (EBMT), undertook to collect all the HLA phenotypes of all the unrelated volunteer donors in the world and collate them into one file in Leiden, The Netherlands. In this format they would be readily available for patient searches.

Since February 1989 when the first edition was distributed with data from 155,000 volunteer donors from eight bone marrow registers, their HLA types recorded on paper, some remarkable progress has been made in terms of donor numbers and the information technology necessary to produce the present sophisticated matching programs. To quote Professor van Rood in his official statement to the world in November 2005, 'BMDW is a symbol of hope and a testimony of the goodwill of people in our world, united in their effort to provide life-saving help to those who need it'. Over the intervening years, since its inception, the importance of such a collaborative effort has become more evident. The advent of molecular typing techniques has demonstrated the scale of the polymorphism of the human major histocompatibility complex, so that as recently as 2005 more than a third (39%) of unrelated HSC transplants that took place used foreign donors, and in 64% of the countries performing unrelated donor transplants, foreign donors had to be used for at least half of the patients.[2] The crossing of international borders is essential if lives are to be saved.

Number and location of stem cell donor registries

The BMDW is an indispensable tool in the search for an unrelated donor. A visit to the website www.bmdw.org provides a variety of useful information which includes the names and contact details of all the contributing registries and cord blood banks, as well as the current number of donors or cord units of each participant. (Those few registries and cord blood banks not yet participating are also listed.) The donor or cord unit numbers are totalled per registry and the percentage which are HLA-A, B, DR typed, and number that are class I and class II typed by molecular techniques is given. These figures are updated monthly.

The main feature is the online match programs that give a rapid overview of the worldwide unrelated donor situation for a patient. They can be accessed with appropriate authorization, details of which are given on the website. Authorization is primarily obtained through the national hub, this being the Anthony Nolan Trust in the UK, and is available for transplant physicians and search co-ordinators. People who are not professional members of the bone marrow transplant (BMT) community will not be authorized.

The majority of donors in the world are of north-west European origin due to the number and size of registers located in Europe and North America. Almost half of the donors (46%) reside in North America, 42% in Europe and the remaining 12% originate from other countries (Fig. 21.1). Historically, the first dedicated unrelated bone marrow donor register was that of the Anthony Nolan Trust, set up in the UK in 1974 (www.anthonynolan.org.uk). The founder, Shirley Nolan, was awarded the OBE in the Millennium Honors List, 2000, in recognition of her vision and determination in setting up a bone marrow register. This endeavor has helped over 4600 patients in the intervening 30-plus years, although sadly her son, Anthony, died without receiving a transplant. The present largest register in the world, the National Marrow Donor Program (NMDP), USA, was formed in July 1986 when, after enthusiastic campaigning by concerned individuals, Congress directed the US Navy to establish a national registry (www.marrow.org). By the early 1990s most European countries had formed their own register and some Asian countries too, such as the Japan Marrow Donor Program, Tokyo, Japan, and the Buddhist Tzu Chi Stem Cells Center, Taiwan.

Although new registers are generally modeled on existing registers, organizational features do differ. Donors are recruited and managed by 'donor centers' which either have an in-house HLA typing laboratory or contract out for typing services. The 'registry' is a national organization whose responsibility is to process requests for HSCs from donors originating within the country and from abroad. The registry is where the HLA typing information on donors is stored and made available in an anonymous fashion for patient searches, through computer-based matching programs. The registry may serve one in-house donor center, as at the Anthony Nolan Trust, or many donor centers in various locations within the country, such as the German register, Zentrales Knochenmarkspender-Register Deutschland (ZKRD), which manages data from 2.7 million donors from 35 donor centers, the largest of which is Deutsche Knockenmarkspenderdatei (DKMS) in Tübingen, with 1.4 million donors. The registry acts as the intermediary between the donor center(s) of that country and transplant centers within the country. For international activity, the registry liaises with similar registries in other countries and

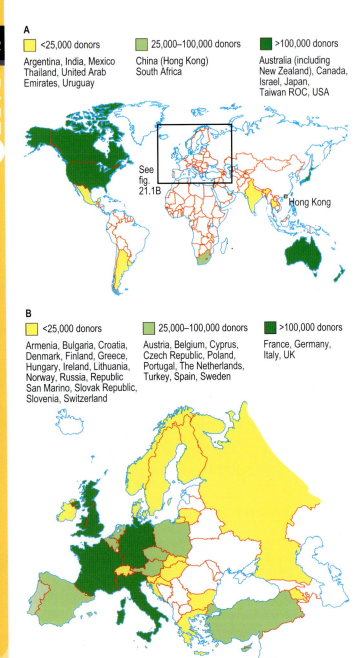

A

- <25,000 donors
  Argentina, India, Mexico Thailand, United Arab Emirates, Uruguay
- 25,000–100,000 donors
  China (Hong Kong) South Africa
- >100,000 donors
  Australia (including New Zealand), Canada, Israel, Japan, Taiwan ROC, USA

See fig. 21.1B

Hong Kong

B

- <25,000 donors
  Armenia, Bulgaria, Croatia, Denmark, Finland, Greece, Hungary, Ireland, Lithuania, Norway, Russia, Republic San Marino, Slovak Republic, Slovenia, Switzerland
- 25,000–100,000 donors
  Austria, Belgium, Cyprus, Czech Republic, Poland, Portugal, The Netherlands, Turkey, Spain, Sweden
- >100,000 donors
  France, Germany, Italy, UK

Figure 21.1
(A) Distribution of stem cell donors in the world from Bone Marrow Donors Worldwide Annual Report 2005. (B) Distribution of stem cell donors in Europe from Bone Marrow Donors Worldwide Annual Report 2005.

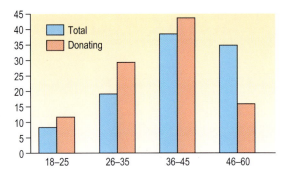

Figure 21.2
Percentage of total volunteers on the Anthony Nolan Trust Register and those donating in 2005, by age range.

becomes designated as the 'hub' as its interactions radiate out to donor centers and transplant centers within its own country and to those in other countries via the foreign hub. This arrangement concentrates a body of expertise within the hub that can facilitate searches and HSC procurement, both nationally and internationally, and streamline all the associated administrative and financial processes. The hub concept has been developed by the World Marrow Donor Association.[3]

New donor recruitment strategies and targets

Despite 10 million donors worldwide, there are still many patients who do not find matches. In 2005, of the 1080 new patients referred for searches from UK transplant centers, 76 (7%) had no matching donor worldwide. This may be because they had an uncommon cau-

casoid HLA type or because they were of a racial or ethnic group whose HLA phenotypes are underrepresented amongst the world's donors. Although other transplant options such as cord blood or haploidentical donors may be available for these patients, the recruitment of new donors continues, in order to help future patients in their donor search. Some of these donors are being added in parts of the world previously without large registers, such as Armenia and Mexico, but the majority are being recruited to existing registers. The Anthony Nolan Trust succeeded in recruiting 20,000 new donors in 2006. Key factors have been identified as being of importance in new donor recruitment.

Aging of registers, aging of donors

As many registers have existed for 15 or more years, aging of donors is a recognized problem. Worldwide in 2005, 101,274 donors were retired from registers due to their reaching the upper age limit, necessitating new donor recruitment to offset this loss.[2] The German donor center DKMS, which has 1.4 million donors, has found that the average age of registered DKMS donors has increased from 33.5 years in 1991 to 40.4 years in 2005. In the same period the average age of newly recruited donors remained nearly constant at 33.5 years in 1991 versus 34.1 years in 2005 (Schmidt A, Rutt C, unpublished work, 2006). The experience of the Anthony Nolan Trust is similar, with the median age of donors on the register in 1993 being 35 years, increasing to 41 years in 2006. Younger donors are successfully targeted for recruitment, with 46% of those added to the Anthony Nolan Register in 2005 being in the age group 18–25.

Evidence shows that the use of younger donors may lower the incidence of graft-versus-host disease and improve survival after bone marrow transplantation.[4] A preference for younger donors is borne out by the donor choices made by transplant centers. Bearing in mind that HLA match is of the utmost importance, there are proportionally a larger number of younger donors used in transplants than donors in the older age ranges (Fig. 21.2). This is compounded by the fact that younger donors are more likely to be CMV negative, a desirable donor attribute for a CMV-negative recipient. From the point of view of the registry, younger donors are a better financial investment because theoretically there is a longer period in which they could donate. Additionally, if newly recruited donors are young they are more likely to be fit, and thereby to meet the stringent health criteria for donating.

Although donors can remain on registers to be available to donate up to a maximum age of 60 years (or younger, according to national regulations), most registers set a much lower age limit for joining the register. The Italian Bone Marrow Donor Register, for example, has an age limit of 18–35 years to join their register, and at the Anthony Nolan Trust this is 18–40 years. Strategies to recruit at the lower end of these age ranges include targeting high schools, universities and colleges.

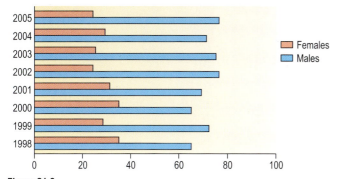

Figure 21.3
Percentage of HSC donations annually from Anthony Nolan Trust donors, by gender.

Gender of donors

Although transplants with successful outcome are achieved with both male and female donors, experience shows that male donors are preferred (Fig. 21.3). There is some scientific evidence to suggest a higher incidence of graft-versus-host disease with multiparous female donor to male recipient,[5] and from the practical point of view the perception is that men, being generally of a heavier build, can provide a higher stem cell count. Females of child-bearing age are made temporarily unavailable to donate for up to 2 years during pregnancy, childbirth and breastfeeding.

Of the 53 registers worldwide contributing data on donor gender, 76% have more female than male potential donors. This results in a figure of 1.4 million more female than male volunteer donors.[2] For many years, the policy at the Anthony Nolan Trust has been to target recruitment of male donors, without excluding interested females, and this has led to a gradual increase in the percentage of male donors on the register, from 39% at the end of 1995 to 41.7% at the end of 2005.

Donor typing strategies

Guidelines for new donor typing suggest that, at a minimum, HLA-A, B and DR should be tested at low-resolution/split antigen level.[6] DNA-based typing is generally commissioned by registries, in preference to serology, for all loci tested. Ideally, every new donor would be typed by molecular technology to a high resolution at all the HLA loci deemed to have significance in transplantation, thus speeding up the search for a patient. In reality, however, a balance has to be struck so that limited resources are used in the most effective way. Generally this results in a two-stage testing scheme, whereby newly recruited donors are low/intermediate resolution typed for HLA-A, B, DRB1 (in preference) or for HLA-A, B, followed by selected donors being typed at a higher resolution and for additional HLA loci. This further typing may occur prospectively, as a planned registry typing improvement program, or it may be directed to benefit specific patients, as and when donors are potential matches and are called for tests.

Ethnicity and human leukocyte antigen diversity of donors

Whereas caucasoid, northern European patients referred from the UK have approximately a 70% chance of a matching donor on the preliminary search of the Anthony Nolan Trust Register, this figure drops to 20–30% for patients from racial or ethnic minorities. Recruitment of new donors should aim to increase the diversity of tissue types on

registers and one way to achieve this is by targeting ethnic minorities within a country. The Anthony Nolan Trust has nine donor recruitment officers, two of whom are Black Minority Ethnic (BME) Officers, one to work specifically with the African/African-Caribbean community and one with the Asian community in the UK, primarily to raise awareness of the need for donors. This type of recruitment is often associated with a patient in need of a transplant, who agrees to be the focus of an appeal.

Considerable HLA diversity also occurs amongst the indigenous population of a country. This has been illustrated in studies from the Anthony Nolan Research Institute with the development of a software package, Cactus, that allows patterns of diversity to be calculated using allele, haplotype and phenotype frequencies. Using this approach, it has been possible to map the variation in HLA allele and haplotype frequencies on the Anthony Nolan Trust Register amongst the endemic North European caucasoid population across the UK, determining regions with high and low HLA phenotypic diversity (Marsh SGE, personal communication, 2006). Such analyses can help target future recruitment to improve the efficiency with which further diversity can be added to the register.

As many of the world's populations are underrepresented on HSC registers, it is incumbent upon well-established registries to assist the development of new registries in varying countries of the world. In this respect, the Anthony Nolan Trust has always welcomed visitors to its offices and/or laboratories, for short or extended periods of training. Several registries, including the Anthony Nolan Trust, have offered practical support through the sharing of software for matching programs and donor management.

Contribution of the World Marrow Donor Association

World Marrow Donor Association (WMDA) aims and initiatives

The importance of international collaboration and sharing of experience was recognized early on in the development of donor registries with the formation of the Co-operative Marrow Donor Program as an informal group in 1988, renamed the World Marrow Donor Association (WMDA) in 1994 and established as a foundation with an office in Leiden, The Netherlands. As stated in the WMDA mission statement:

The World Marrow Donor Association (WMDA) strives to improve and simplify stem cell donation for donors and patients worldwide. Founded in 1994 to address the obstacles faced when transplantation involved donors and recipients in different countries, today the WMDA establishes international guidelines for the collection and transfer of hematopoietic stem cells. Members include donor registries, cord blood registries and numerous individuals working together to advance hematopoietic stem cell transplantation.

The WMDA initiatives are:
- publishing annual reports that summarize global activity in unrelated hematopoietic stem cell transplantation. These reports are a valuable resource for assessing trends in the field, current growth obstacles and optimal strategies for donor recruitment and selection
- providing forums to discuss issues related to the international facilitation of HSCT. This includes forums at the annual meetings of the EBMT, at meetings of the US National Marrow Donor Program and at the biennial International Donor Registry conferences

- developing consensus about uniform HLA testing and terminology to facilitate communication among registries
- developing template forms for all aspects of donor registry operations
- analyzing and publicizing issues related to donor safety, ethics and confidentiality
- providing data and expertise to national and international bodies addressing regulatory issues in HSCT. The WMDA works to harmonize regulations among member countries and minimize impediments to global exchange of hematopoietic stem cells
- development of a WMDA accreditation program for hematopoietic stem cell registries. WMDA accreditation is an indication that a registry has committed to follow WMDA standards. These standards promote the quality and timeliness of the procedure to obtain hematopoietic stem cells from the most suitable unrelated volunteer donor while protecting the donor's anonymity, health and well-being.

The standards cover:

- general organization of registry
- donor recruitment
- donor characterization
- information technology
- facilitation of search requests
- second/subsequent donations
- collection/processing/transport of stem cells.

Details of these initiatives can be found on the website (www.world-marrow.org), together with information about membership, meetings, publications, ongoing activities of the working groups and subcommittees, and the WMDA standards. To comply with WMDA standards, it is necessary that a registry has a quality management system and has in place service level agreements with its donor centers, collection centers and transplant centers, through which vehicle these bodies also agree to respect WMDA standards.

Stem cell regulatory issues

Unlike the majority of blood and organ donations, HSC are directed donations for a particular patient, the donor being, at times, the only donor in the world who can best fulfill that patient's transplant need. In an era of heightened regulatory activity in the field, the WMDA represents registries and the interests of patients, in both campaigning to harmonize regulations in different parts of the world and to catalog those regulations that do exist, in order to streamline the movement of products across international boundaries. In Europe, the EU Tissues and Cells Directive 2004/23/EC came into force throughout the EU in April 2006 to set standards of quality and safety for the donation, procurement, testing, processing, preservation, storage and distribution of human tissues and cells. In the USA the Food and Drug Administration (FDA) requires imported cells to comply with its own specific requirements for donor eligibility and donor testing (particularly with reference to infectious disease markers (IDM)) and also requires collection centers in the country of origin to be registered with the FDA. The Regulatory Issues subcommittee of the WMDA Donor Registries Working Group has gathered data from many countries concerning regulations associated with IDM testing, product labeling, product packaging, diagnostic specimen shipment, product customs requirements and documentation, to ease import and export of HSC and other associated blood products.

The WMDA works with other international organizations that implement their own standards, such as the FACT-JACIE standards and accreditation system for HSC transplant facilities, and the FACT-Netcord standards and accreditation system for cord blood banks, to compare and harmonize standards to cover all aspects of unrelated HSC procurement and donation.

Donor identification

HLA typing the patient and assessing the likelihood of a match

Given the polymorphism of the HLA system and the number of donors and registers in the world, the task of identifying a suitable unrelated donor for a given patient could seem daunting. The first essential step in the search for an unrelated donor is to ensure that the patient is HLA typed accurately and to a high resolution. The policy at the Anthony Nolan Trust dictates the following.

- HLA typing of the patient must be undertaken in a laboratory accredited by the European Federation for Immunogenetics (EFI) or by an agency with similar standards and accreditation process.
- HLA typing of the patient must be undertaken on two occasions using samples drawn at different times, so that the typing and identity are confirmed.
- HLA typing of the patient must be by DNA methods, but may be supplemented by serology to ascertain protein expression (the presence or absence of null alleles).
- HLA loci A, B, C and DRB1 must be typed at a minimum. Additionally, HLA-DRB3, DRB4, DRB5 and DQB1 typing are considered desirable, and DPB1 optional.
- The resolution of typing should ideally be high resolution for HLA-A, B and DRB1, resolving polymorphisms within exons 2 and 3 for HLA-A and B, and polymorphisms within exon 2 for HLA-DRB1, at a minimum. All serologically defined antigens should be discriminated.

With the advent of molecular HLA typing techniques, many donors are typed to intermediate/high resolution, with the possibility of identifying a good molecular match on the preliminary search of the registers. This reinforces the main reasons for high-resolution typing the patient at the start of the search.

- Many sophisticated matching programs, such as those of the Anthony Nolan Trust, BMDW and the NMDP, will match at the allelic level on HLA class I (A and B, or A, B and C), and class II (DRB1, or DRB1, and DQB1), sorting the best matching donors to the top of the list. Without patient high-resolution typing at the outset, long donor lists may be curtailed, removing from view what are actually the best matches.
- Restricting the donor list to the most appropriate donors on whom to request further tests, by high-resolution typing the patient, enables time and money to be saved, both valuable commodities in an unrelated donor search.
- If there are no fully matching donors and a one-antigen mismatch donor is to be considered, it will be important to be able to ascertain the degree of match at the other 'matched' HLA loci.

The importance must be stressed of using an HLA expert to review the patient's HLA type and assess the likelihood of a match at the number of loci and level of resolution desired by the transplant center. The following factors will affect the probability of identifying a matching donor.

- *Racial/ethnic match between patient and donor pool.* As haplotypes have different distributions in different populations and may be population specific, the HLA specialist will use allele and haplotype frequencies and racial/ethnic information to determine the most appropriate registries in which to search.
- *Accuracy of patient and donor typing.* The HLA expert can assess the probability of a missed or wrongly assigned antigen/allele, particularly those that may have occurred in donor HLA types

dating back in time and performed by serology rather than a molecular technique.

- *Resolution of donor types and number of loci tested.* The HLA expert can deduce probable types from incomplete information, based on knowledge of common haplotypes, thus focusing on the best donors for further testing.

- *Level of match required.* Some centers require patients and donors for transplant to be matched at HLA-A, B, DRB1 (6/6), others require HLA-A, B, C, DRB1 (8/8) or HLA-A, B, C, DRB1, DQB1 (10/10). The HLA specialist can recommend that in certain cases which are difficult to match, a larger than usual number of donors should be typed, to increase the possibility of identifying a matching donor. Alternatively, the transplant physician can be given the opportunity to reconsider the match requirements so that the patient can be transplanted in a timeframe compatible with the disease stage, or an alternative, non-transplant, strategy can be pursued.

The search process

The person conducting a search and selecting donors (the search co-ordinator) must be familiar with the complexity of the HLA nomenclature[7] and with the use of the shorthand alphabetical codes, devised by the NMDP, to represent allele strings. This NMDP coding system is widely used and was introduced to accommodate the sometimes very long allele strings resulting from intermediate-resolution molecular typing. They can be viewed on the NMDP website (www.marrow. org) in the bioinformatics section. Additionally, due to the varying techniques that have been used over the years for donor typing, giving results at various levels of resolution, these diverse assignments are converted to 'search determinants' before being included in a matching algorithm.[8] The search co-ordinator must be familiar with the variety of matching programs used by registers, with their varying search determinants, if potential matches are not to be missed. The NMDP took a major step forward in 2005 to support this search process, by introducing their enhanced matching algorithm known as Haplogic. This makes use of primary data on the DNA polymorphism of volunteer donors, collected over the years, and an analysis of allele-level HLA haplotype frequencies of donors on the NMDP Register, to predict the most likely high-resolution results prior to the actual typing, and giving a probability of a match to a patient.[9] The benefit of this program to patients is immeasurable, given the great size and ethnic diversity of the NMDP register.

The search procedure and matching program in operation at the Anthony Nolan Trust is described in the *Laboratories and operations department user guide* which is available to download from the website (www.anthonynolan.org). The matching program developed at the Anthony Nolan Trust includes the HLA-A, B and DRB1 molecular typing data in the sorting algorithm. Where ambiguities exist, resulting in intermediate-resolution results, the allele codes developed by the NMDP (USA) are utilized to enter data onto the computer. Searches will be extended to look for donors with a single mismatch at the HLA-A, B or DR locus if deemed appropriate. The standard sort format for donor listings is male donors before female (based on transplant center preference) and younger before older, within degree of HLA match. Additional information provided on matching donors, if known, includes blood group, cytomegalovirus (CMV) status, ethnic group, and weight. Most of these factors may be applied as optional filters to reduce a long list of matching donors. For example, a list of only the CMV-negative matching donors may be requested. Donors who are known to be temporarily unavailable are marked 'Unavailable' with a release date, and those in test for another patient are marked 'In Test'. Advice on selecting donors for patients can be provided by the Anthony Nolan Trust, either on an individual case basis

or via such a meeting as was hosted in London, in 2005.[10] However, the final decision on donor suitability is always the responsibility of the transplant center.

Although searches for acceptable unrelated HSC donors for northwest European patients have become more successful over time, further improvements could be made to the timespan of the search process.[11] A search for an unrelated donor should be commenced in a timely fashion. Although it will be usual to HLA type any siblings, and/or other close relatives before embarking on an unrelated donor search, there may be occasions, if siblings are temporarily unavailable, undecided or difficult to trace, when the unrelated donor search should commence as soon as the patient's HLA type is available. The preliminary search will involve ascertaining the likelihood of identifying a suitable donor and need not incur any expense.

The Anthony Nolan Trust accepts search requests from UK transplant centers that are maintaining accreditation by the Joint Accreditation Committee EBMT-ISCT Europe (JACIE), or working towards such accreditation (www. jacie.org). In addition to the name and contact details of the referring physician and transplant center affiliation, the patient information required for an unrelated donor search includes:[12]

- HLA type
- name
- date of birth
- diagnosis
- status of search (standard or urgent).

Additional useful patient information that will speed the search if available:

- date of diagnosis
- disease status and number of remissions (where applicable)
- gender
- race or ethnic group
- CMV status
- blood group (ABO/Rh)
- weight (particularly for a cord unit search)
- familial HLA haplotypes.

Search requests intended for the UK registers must be sent to each UK register independently, with the exception of those originating from a UK transplant center, where a co-operative agreement exists to exchange these requests on the day of receipt. Each UK register, the Anthony Nolan Trust, the British Bone Marrow Register (BBMR) and the Welsh Bone Marrow Donor Register (WBMDR), will produce its own separate donor list. The Anthony Nolan Trust will run all search requests originating from the UK against its own register, producing an Anthony Nolan Trust donor list, and also against the BMDW, to give the requesting physician the worldwide picture of the likelihood of a matching donor being identified.

International searching

At the request of the transplant center physician, after reviewing the search report, the search can be extended to any international registers that have potential matches. The role of the national registry, or hub, is to guide the transplant center through this process, by providing administrative information, co-ordinating sample requests/shipments, and advising on ways to expedite the search, or any foreseeable impediments to its smooth progress. The percentage of patients referred for international searches from the UK has steadily increased from 32% of patients in 2000 to 55% in 2005. The Anthony Nolan Trust has always encouraged transplant centers to seek the 'best' donor for their patients, so that whenever there is a choice of HLA-matched donors, other donor factors may be taken into account:

- age
- gender

- CMV status
- blood group
- weight
- parity (females)
- transfusion status
- likelihood of obtaining preferred product (usually PBSC)
- availability of donors
- reliability of donor HLA typing
- registry administrative factors (e.g. costs, speed of donor provision, restrictions on donor release).

International search reports are obtained by the registry either by fax or through the European Marrow Donor Information System (EMDIS) (www.zkrd.de/emdis.html?&L=1). EMDIS is an open communication system involving the exchange of a standard set of messages between the local databases of the national registries of many countries, both within Europe and more recently extending outside, to the USA. It covers all steps of the unrelated donor search, from preliminary search requests, repeat searches for updated donor lists, the exchange of requests and results, and finally the bone marrow prescription. This streamlining and automation of the communication process between national registries improves the speed and efficiency and, ultimately, the success of the search. The donor lists thus obtained are forwarded to the transplant center concerned, so that they may proceed with donor selection.

Donor testing

The vast majority of patients, 99%, who reach transplant with an Anthony Nolan Trust donor have that matching donor identified on the preliminary search of the register. Similarly, when foreign donors are selected, they are usually present on the preliminary international search report. If there is not a match amongst the over 7 million donors in the world who are already HLA-A, B and DR typed, there is rarely time to identify a matching donor by DR typing those donors who are only class I, HLA-A, B typed. The exception may be for a very rare class I type where, by definition, there will be few donors; in such cases additional testing for the DR locus may add the desired DR type due to linkage disequilibrium between these HLA genes.

Before donors can proceed to donation, it is mandatory that they be HLA typed by the same laboratory that typed the patient. This should use the same techniques for both, and be within a similar timeframe. This testing, known as confirmatory typing (CT), will usually be performed on a number of donors for a particular patient to ascertain the best matching donor before final selection. Infectious disease marker testing is also undertaken at this stage, usually by the donor center.

Donor availability

Many registries/donor centers have strategies for keeping in contact with donors so that they are available when needed. As most registries have been in operation for longer than 10 years, maintenance becomes a major part of a donor center's work. This may take the form of proactive communications with donors, such as newsletters, greetings cards or strategies to contact donors when they are actually needed as a potential match for a particular patient. Usually both ploys are necessary. Statistics from the WMDA 2005 Annual Report show that 32% of donor blood samples requested at CT stage are not shipped due to donor-related reasons, suggesting the advisability of requesting a larger number of donor samples, where possible, at the outset.

Worldwide, in 2005, the median percentage of national donors deferred at work-up, resulting in harvest cancellation, was 4.4%.[2] It is

likely that the majority of these were medical deferrals, due to conditions previously unidentified until the predonation physical examination and associated laboratory tests. At the Anthony Nolan Trust, donors are required to complete a comprehensive medical questionnaire when they join the register and on each subsequent occasion that they are called to give a blood sample as a potential match. This medical questionnaire is reviewed and updated periodically by the Trust's Medical Advisory Committee, and the Medical Officer will adjudicate on individual queries, eliciting further information from the donor where necessary. In this way, medical deferrals at work-up can be kept to a minimum.

It is advisable when possible, however, to continue testing donors until a back-up donor is identified. In The Netherlands, data on 502 unrelated donor work-up procedures performed for 425 Dutch patients between 1987 and 2002 showed one of 11 work-ups ending in the primary requested donor failing to donate. Of all donor-related cancellations (n = 46), 78% of the procedures were deferred for medical reasons and 22% due to non-medical reasons. In 50% of the cases for which a back-up donor was already identified, the patients were transplanted with a delay of less than 2 weeks; when no back-up donor was available, the median delay increased to 18 weeks.[13]

Donor commitment

Information and education are the key to donor commitment. Informed consent must be obtained at various stages of the search process – at recruitment; when giving further blood samples for confirmatory typing; and when actually requested to donate.[14] It must be understood by transplant physicians, and ultimately by the patient, that the nature of the consent is such that the donor is permitted to withdraw at any time, including the period while the patient is being conditioned.[15] In the light of this, all efforts are made by donor centers/ registries to exclude those potential donors who are within a predefined risk group, who appear physically or mentally unfit, or who show undue hesitation, perhaps due to fear of the procedure or lack of support from family or workplace. At the Anthony Nolan Trust, donors are provided with written information at each stage of the procedure and have the opportunity to discuss any aspect of the process with staff at the Trust and at the harvest/collection center. After donation, donors are requested to provide feedback through a questionnaire and in person to the Donor Welfare Officer assigned to them by the Anthony Nolan Trust. In this way the process is continually monitored and adjusted as necessary. The Donor Welfare Officers maintain contact with donors after donation during their recovery period and will be responsible for approaching a donor should a second donation request for the same patient be received. If at any time donors indicate that they would not be agreeable to being approached to consider a second donation, this information is relayed to the transplant center without delay.

Choice of peripheral blood stem cells or bone marrow-derived stem cells

Requests from transplant centers show a general preference for peripheral blood stem cells (PBSC) rather than bone marrow, although this is often dependent upon the patient's disease. Of the 400 requests received at the Anthony Nolan Trust in 2005 for first donations, 77% expressed a preference for PBSC, although in most cases bone marrow, as a second choice, would have been accepted.

The Anthony Nolan Trust began providing PBSCs on a regular basis in 2001. It was decided that, as many donors had joined the register prior to the PBSC donation era, the choice of which product

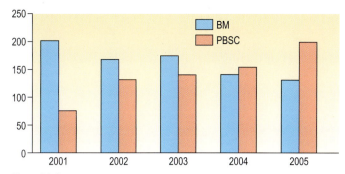

Figure 21.4
Donations from Anthony Nolan Trust donors by year, according to stem cell source, BM vs PBSC.

to donate should be that of the donor, following provision of sufficient information detailing the procedures and short- and long-term risks of both methods. Generally, donors are interested in providing the product most desired for a successful outcome to the transplant, and the preference of the transplant center is relayed to the donor if the donor queries this point. Since 2001, an increasing percentage of the donations provided by Anthony Nolan donors have been PBSC, in preference to bone marrow (Fig. 21.4). Registers in other countries have varying policies regarding availability of PBSCs from their donors, such information being available through the BMDW website or through national hubs.

Donor and recipient anonymity

It is essential for the success of unrelated HSC programs that strict anonymity for donor and patient is maintained, certainly prior to donation. This ensures that there is no coercion of an unrelated donor and no inducements offered of any kind. The right of the patient to privacy is also respected. Patient information given to donors who request it on the Anthony Nolan Register is limited to broad age range (i.e. child, young adult, adult) and patient gender. The geographical location of the patient and donor is strictly confidential and is rarely disclosed. Patient diagnosis is not generally given unless specifically requested, but is sometimes referred to in donor counseling, when estimating the likelihood of further product requests after the primary donation. Steps

are taken to ensure anonymity of the donor by coded labeling of blood samples sent to transplant centers and of the final HSC product itself. HSC label design ensures that the identity of the originating registry can be removed before it can become visible to the patient while being infused. If foreign donors are being provided for national patients, it is important that transplant center staff do not inadvertently reveal donor details to which they may be privy, such as donor nationality, and similarly, HSC couriers when delivering the product must respect confidentiality of donor origin.

References

1. Bone Marrow Donors Worldwide 2006. www.bmdw.org/
2. WMDA. Unrelated Stem Cell Donor Registries Annual Report 2005. www.worldmarrow.org
3. Goldman JM. A special report: bone marrow transplants using volunteer donors – recommendations and requirements for a standardized practice throughout the world – 1994 update. Blood 1994;84:2833–2839
4. Kollman C, Howe CWS, Anasetti C et al. Donor characteristics as risk factors in recipients after transplantation of bone marrow from unrelated donors: the effect of donor age. Blood 2001;98:2043–2051
5. Weisdorf D, Hakke R, Blazar B et al. Risk factors for acute graft-versus-host disease in histocompatible donor bone marrow transplantation. Transplantation 1991;51:1197–1203
6. Hurley CK, Wade JA, Oudshoorn M et al. A special report: histocompatibility testing guidelines for hematopoietic stem cell transplantation using volunteer donors. Tissue Antigens 1999;53:394–406
7. Marsh SGE, Albert ED, Bodmer WF et al. Nomenclature for factors of the HLA system, 2004. Tissue Antigens 2005;65:301–369
8. Hurley CK, Setterholm M, Lau M et al. Hematopoietic stem cell donor registry strategies for assigning search determinants and matching relationships. Bone Marrow Transplant 2004;33:443–450
9. Hurley CK, Wagner JE, Setterholm MI et al. Advances in HLA: practical implications for selecting adult donors and cord blood units. Biol Blood Marrow Transplant 2006;12(suppl 1):28–33
10. Duarte RF, Pamphilon D, Cornish J et al. Topical issues in unrelated haematopoietic stem cell transplants: a report from a workshop convened by the Anthony Nolan Trust in London – 2005. Bone Marrow Transplant 2006;37:901–908
11. Heemskerk MB, van Walraven SM, Cornelissen JJ et al. How to improve the search for an unrelated haematopoietic stem cell donor. Faster is better than more! Bone Marrow Transplant 2005;35:645–652
12. Wiegand T, Raffoux C, Hurley CK et al. A special report: suggested procedures for international unrelated donor search from the donor registries and quality assurance working groups of the World Marrow Donor Association (WMDA). Bone Marrow Transplant 2004;34:97–101
13. van Walraven SM, Heemskerk MB, Lie JL et al. Donor identification. The importance of identifying a back-up donor for unrelated stem cell transplantation. Bone Marrow Transplant 2005;35:437–440
14. Rosenmayr A, Hartwell L, Egeland T. Stem cell donation. Informed consent – suggested procedures for informed consent at various stages of recruitment, donor evaluation, and donor workup. Bone Marrow Transplant 2003;31:539–545
15. Bakken R, van Walraven A-M, Egeland T. Normal donors. Donor commitment and patient needs. Bone Marrow Transplant 2004;33:225–230

Cord blood banks and umbilical cord blood transplantation in children and adults

CHAPTER 22

Vanderson Rocha and Eliane Gluckman

Introduction

Umbilical cord blood transplantation (UCBT) has extended the availability of allogeneic hematopoietic stem cell transplantation (HSCT) to patients who would otherwise not be eligible for this curative approach. Since the first successful UCBT from an HLA-identical sibling in a child with severe Fanconi's anemia reported by Gluckman et al in 1989,[1] the number of UCB transplants from related and unrelated donors has increased dramatically, and we estimate that more than 8000 patients to date have undergone UCBT from unrelated donors for a variety of genetic, hematologic, immunologic, metabolic and oncologic disorders. A survey of the International Bone Marrow Transplant Registry (IBMTR) estimates that since 1998, 20% of stem cell transplants performed in young patients (<20 years old) have been cord blood transplants (IBMTR Newsletter). In Japan, approximately 50% of HSCT from unrelated donors are being performed with cord blood cells nowadays (T. Takahashi, Tokyo Cord Blood Bank, personal communication).

In comparison to other sources of allogeneic HSCT, UCB offers substantial logistic and clinical advantages including:
- significantly faster availability of banked cryopreserved UCB units, with patients receiving UCB transplantation in a median of 25–36 days earlier than those receiving bone marrow (BM)[2,3]
- extension of the donor pool due to tolerance of 1–2 HLA mismatches out of 6 (higher HLA mismatch is associated with lower probability of engraftment)
- lower incidence and severity of acute graft-versus-host disease (GvHD)
- lower risk of transmitting infections by latent viruses such as cytomegalovirus (CMV) and Epstein–Barr virus (EBV)
- lack of donor attrition
- lack of risk to the donor
- higher frequency of rare haplotypes compared to bone marrow registries, since it is easier to target ethnic minorities.[4]

The disadvantages of UCBT are:
- the low number of hematopoietic progenitor cells and HSCs in UCB compared with BM or mobilized peripheral blood stem cells (PBSC) which translates into increased risk of graft failure and delayed hematopoietic engraftment
- lack of possibility of using donor lymphocyte transfusion for immunotherapy.

Progress in the field of umbilical cord blood transplantation parallels the huge interest in establishing and developing cord blood banks worldwide. Today, more than 300,000 cord blood grafts are available in more than 40 cord blood banks. These banks play an important role in the process of cord blood transplantation. The Netcord group was created on behalf of Eurocord to establish good practices in umbilical cord blood storage, facilitate donor search, improve the quality of the grafts, standardize excellence criteria on an international scale and, importantly, to establish procedures for bank accreditation in collaboration with FACT (Foundation on Accreditation in Cell Therapy). The inventory of Netcord, the co-operative network of large, experienced UCB banks, currently has more than 130,000 cryopreserved UCB units ready for clinical use for unrelated recipients, and more than 5000 grafts have been shipped.[5] Recently, the National Marrow Donor Program (NMDP) has established a similar cord blood bank network in the USA with the financial support of the American Congress. Collaborations between Netcord-Eurocord and NMDP have been established with the goal of providing the most appropriate and high-quality cord blood unit for a specific patient. Other types of cord blood banks have been established such as sibling donor cord blood banks or autologous (or commercial family CB banking) where there is no existing transplant recipient.

This chapter reports the outcomes and risk factors of using related and unrelated cord blood cells for HSCT in children and adults for various hematologic diseases, the comparative results of transplants using other sources of hematopoietic stem cells, mainly bone marrow, and the development of different types of cord blood banks.

Clinical experience with related and unrelated umbilical cord blood transplantation

Eurocord registry

In order to develop research in the different biologic aspects of cord blood cells and evaluate cord blood transplants, the European Blood and Marrow Transplantation group (EBMT) with the support of the European Union organized the Eurocord group in 1995. One of the most important achievements of the Eurocord group was the establishment of the Eurocord registry. It works in close collaboration with Netcord banks, collecting and validating clinical data of patients transplanted with Netcord cord blood units. Thanks to this collaboration, from 1988 to February 2007, 3372 cord blood transplants have been reported to the Eurocord registry from 186 European transplant centers from 43 European countries (64% of cases), and 187 transplant centers (36% of cases) from other countries. Three hundred and fifty nine UCBT transplants have been reported using related donors (the majority HLA-identical sibling donors) mainly for children with malignant and non-malignant disorders, and 2965 have been performed in the unrelated transplant setting for children and adults. During the last 3 years, the number of unrelated UCBT reported to Eurocord has increased to more than 300 transplants/year, and since 2004 the number of adults transplanted with cord blood cells has overtaken the number of UCBT performed in children (Eurocord registry data).

Cord blood transplantation has been used to treat a variety of genetic, hematologic, immunologic, metabolic and oncologic disorders. Table 22.1 lists the patients reported to Eurocord, transplanted with an unrelated cord blood graft, according to age and diagnosis.

Umbilical cord blood transplantation from related donors

Related UCBT has been performed almost exclusively in children.[6] In an update of the Eurocord experience with a median follow-up of 41 months after related UCBT in children, the survival estimate at 3 years was 47 ± 5% in patients with malignancies (n = 96), 82 ± 7% in patients with bone marrow failure (n = 33), 100% (90% disease-free survival) in patients with hemoglobinopathies (n = 52), and 70 ± 15% (n = 10) in patients with inborn errors of metabolism or primary immunodeficiencies (Eurocord unpublished data). For children with malignancies, the 3-year overall survival was 71 ± 12% for early-phase disease (first complete remission of leukemia), 45 ± 7% for those in intermediate-phase disease (second complete remission), and 24 ± 7% for those with advanced phase disease.

A specific analysis has been performed and published for 44 children with thalassemia (Thal) and sickle cell disease (SCD) given a related UCBT.[7] We have updated this analysis and confirmed that all 63 patients are alive, and the 5-year disease-free survival (DFS) is 78% in the 44 Thal patients, and 94% for the 19 SCD patients. The absence of methotrexate in the graft-versus-host disease prophylaxis and the use of fludarabine in the conditioning regimen were the most important factors associated with increased DFS.

A joint study by the Eurocord and International Bone Marrow Transplant Registry[8] has compared the outcomes of 113 children who received UCB from HLA-identical siblings with those of 2052 children who underwent HLA-identical sibling BM transplantation (BMT). UCB transplant recipients had slower recovery of neutrophils and platelets, and a lower risk of acute and chronic GvHD. Interestingly, relapse-related deaths, mortality rate at 100 days after transplantation and overall survival were not significantly different between the two groups.[8] These findings suggest that, in children in the HLA-identical sibling setting, UCBT is as useful as BMT.

Based on these results, we recommend collecting and freezing cord blood units in families where a sibling child is suffering from a genetic or hematologic disease. In order to have high-quality familiar cord blood units, sibling cord blood bank programs have been established.[9]

Umbilical cord blood transplantation from unrelated donors in children with malignant and non-malignant disorders

Multicenter,[6,10,11] single institution[3,12,13] and consortium[14,15] studies have shown that unrelated donor UCBT in children is able to reconstitute hematopoiesis and achieve sustained engraftment in most cases, is associated with a low incidence of GvHD, and does not result in a higher relapse risk. Almost all pediatric series concerning UCBT from unrelated donors have demonstrated the profound impact of cell dose, measured as total nucleated cells, colony-forming cells, and CD34+ cells, on engraftment, adverse transplant-related events and survival.[6,10–12,16] Although the prognostic importance of HLA disparity was not clearly recognized in earlier series, it has become apparent in recent updates.[11,12,16]

Results of unrelated UCBT in children with specific diseases have been published in AML,[10] Hurler syndrome[14] and Krabbe disease.[15] The Eurocord group has recently conducted three studies (unpublished data): outcome of unrelated UCBT in childhood acute lymphoid leukemia (ALL), primary immunodeficiencies and Fanconi's anemia.

We have analyzed a total of 361 children with ALL receiving an UCBT, from 1994 to 2005, in 24 countries, mostly in Europe. Eighty seven children were transplanted in first complete remission (CR) with unfavorable cytogenetics (89% had t(9;22) or t(4;11)); 152 children were transplanted in second CR and 122 with more advanced disease. Median age was 6.5 years, median cell dose infused was 4.1×10^7/kg and the median follow time was 22 months (3–96). The graft was HLA disparate in 80% of cases, with one or two incompatibilities (HLA-A and B low-resolution typing or HLA-DRB1 by high-resolution typing). Overall, 3-year leukemia-free survival (LFS) was 33 ± 7% for patients in CR1; 35 ± 4% for patients in CR2 and 21 ± 4% for patients transplanted with advanced disease. On multivariate analysis, only CR1 and CR2 were associated with superior LFS (p < 0.0001). In the group of children tranplanted in CR2 (n = 151) the main risk factor associated with improved 2-year LFS on multivariate analysis was previous relapse before UCBT, either on or off therapy (p = 0.02). In fact, 3-year LFS was 26% if the patients relapsed while still receiving therapy compared to 45% for those relapsing off therapy. Other patient groups, diseases and graft characteristics were not associated with outcome on multivariate analysis (Eurocord; unpublished data).

Outcomes of 93 unrelated UCBT in children with severe primary immunodeficiencies (SPID) reported to Eurocord by 40 centres were analyzed (J. Ortega on behalf of Eurocord; unpublished data). Median age was 0.9 years (range 0–26), and median weight 8 kg (3–39). Diagnoses included severe combined immunodeficiency (n = 61), Wiskott–Aldrich syndrome (n = 20), and other (n = 12). Fifty-six patients were matched or had one HLA difference with the CB unit. The median number of nucleated cells (NC) infused was 8.3×10^7/kg (0.1–94) and the median CD34+ cell number 3.4×10^5/kg (0.4–33). Forty-four patients received busulfan/cyclophosphamide, 11 received no conditioning, and 74 patients received ciclosporin(CsA)/steroids as

Table 22.1 Number of unrelated CBT reported to Eurocord registry according to diagnosis and recipient age

Diagnosis	Children (≤ 16 years, n = 1602)	Adults (>16 years, n = 1136)
Acute lymphoblastic leukemia	579 (36.1%)	269 (23.7%)
Acute myeloid leukemia	257 (16%)	356 (31.3%)
Secondary acute leukemia	38 (2.4%)	63 (5.5%)
Myelodysplastic syndrome	120 (7.5%)	97 (8.5%)
Chronic myeloid leukemia	40 (2.5%)	119 (10.5%)
Chronic lymphocytic leukemia	–	16 (1.4%)
Hodgkin's/non-Hodgkin's lymphomas	31/- (1.9%)	97/32 (11.4%)
Myeloma	–	20 (1.8%)
Solid tumors	9 (0.6%)	5 (0.4%)
Histiocytosis	60 (3.7%)	1 (0.1%)
Congenital and acquired bone marrow failure syndromes	157 (9.8%)	50 (4.4%)
Hemoglobinopathies	4 (0.2%)	–
Primary immunodeficiencies	170 (10.6%)	1 (0.1%)
Metabolic diseases	126 (7.9%)	5 (0.4%)
Other disease	11 (0.7%)	5 (0.4%)

GvHD prophylaxis. Cumulative incidences (CIs) for neutrophil and platelet recoveries were 85% and 77%, respectively. CIs for acute grades II–IV and chronic GvHD were 41% and 23%, respectively. Transplant-related mortality at 2 years was 31%. Survival at 2 years was 68% overall, 78% if patient/CB unit were matched or had one HLA disparity, and 58% with 2–3 HLA differences (multivariate analysis, p = 0.04).

We also analyzed the results of unrelated UCBT in 93 Fanconi's anemia (FA) patients. Median age at transplantation was 8.6 years (1–45). The units transplanted were HLA-A, B, DRB1 identical in 12 cases, one HLA difference in 35 cases and two or three HLA differences in 45 cases. The median number of nucleated cells (NC) and CD34+ cells infused by recipient weight was 4.9×10^7/kg and 1.9×10^5/kg, respectively. Participating centers selected the preparative regimen of their choice; in 57 patients (61%), it included fludarabine. CI of neutrophil recovery was 60 ± 5% at day +60. On multivariate analysis, a fludarabine-containing preparative regimen and NC number infused 4.9×10^7/kg were associated with a higher probability of neutrophil recovery. CIs of grade II–IV acute and of chronic GvHD were 32 ± 5% and 16 ± 4%, respectively. Overall survival was 40 ± 5%. On multivariate analysis, factors associated with a favorable outcome were use of fludarabine in the conditioning regimen, number of NC infused > 4.9×10^7/kg and negative recipient CMV serology (unpublished data).

In summary, these results showed that unrelated UCBT can be considered as a source of allogeneic stem cells for transplantation for those children with genetic and metabolic diseases, or with malignant disorders who need a HSCT and who lack an HLA-identical sibling donor. Outcomes are associated with patient, disease and transplant characteristics. Therefore, better patient selection and factors easily modifiable such as cord blood unit selection and changes in conditioning regimens or GvHD prophylaxis can improve outcome.

Umbilical cord blood transplantation in children compared to bone marrow from unrelated donors

Comparison of the results of UCBT and BMT from unrelated donors in children is of paramount relevance, because for many patients the search process will identify both UCB units and UBM donors. Three published studies, two single center studies and a Eurocord registry series, have reported retrospective analyses comparing outcomes after UCBT and UBMT in children.[3,17,18] Briefly, in these three studies, recipients of UCBT were transplanted sooner compared to children given an UBMT; neutrophil and platelet recovery were delayed, acute GvHD was less and overall survival was not significant different after UCBT compared to UBMT. The Eurocord group has reported higher early TRM, probably due to infections related to delayed engraftment. It is important to note that all patients in the Eurocord series were transplanted before 1998, when UCBT was still considered to be a last option for leukemia treatment.

Recently, a meta-analysis combining these comparative studies was published.[19] A total of 161 children undergoing UCBT (mostly one or two antigen mismatched) and 316 children undergoing UBMT (almost entirely fully matched with the recipient) were analyzed. Pooled comparisons of studies of UCBT and UBMT in children found that the incidence of chronic GvHD was lower with UCBT, but the incidence of grade III–IV acute GvHD did not differ. There was no difference in 2-year overall survival (OS) between children given an unrelated UCBT or UBMT.

All these previous comparative studies have analyzed HLA-matched BMT using the definition of low-resolution HLA-A and B typing, and high-resolution HLA-DRB1 typing. In a preliminary analysis, Eapen

et al,[20] on behalf of the Center of the International Bone Marrow Transplant Registry (CIBMTR) and the New York Cord Blood Program, have recently compared results observed in 503 recipients of CB with those in 116 recipients of allele-matched BM (HLA-A, B, C and DRB1). Of the CB recipients, 35 were matched at the HLA A, B (antigen-level) and DRB1 (allele-level), 201 were mismatched at one locus and 267 were mismatched at two loci. All patients (aged <16 years) had acute leukemia and were transplanted between 1995 and 2003. Median follow-up was 45 and 59 months for CB and BM recipients, respectively. LFS was superior in recipients of HLA-matched CB (p = 0.040). Notably, LFS and OS at 5 years were comparable between those receiving allele-matched BM and one or two loci-mismatched CB. These results in LFS and OS are, in part, explained by differences in risks of transplant-related mortality (TRM) and relapse between patient populations. Compared to allele-matched BM transplants, TRM was similar in recipients of matched and one locus-mismatched/high cell dose (>0.3 × 10⁸/kg) CB and higher in recipients of one locus-mismatched/low cell dose (<0.3 × 10⁸/kg) and two loci-mismatched CB (any cell dose) (p = 0.005, p < 0.001, respectively). Conversely, relapse rates were lower in recipients of CB mismatched at one and two loci (p = 0.037, p = 0.003, respectively). As previously observed, probability of neutrophil recovery (>500/μl) at day 42 depended on graft type, HLA match and cell dose (98% with BM; 85% with matched CB; 79% with one or two loci-mismatched CB/high cell dose; 64% with one and two loci-mismatched CB/low cell dose). Compared to allele-matched BM, risks of grade 2–4 and grade 3–4 acute GvHD were lower after matched CB (relative risk (RR) 0.45, p = 0.035, RR 0.51, p = 0.035, respectively) and similar after mismatched CB. Risk of chronic GvHD was lower after matched or mismatched CB transplantation (RR 0.66, p = 0.036).

These data strongly suggest that UCB is an acceptable alternative to matched unrelated BM in children, and support starting a simultaneous search for BM and UCB unrelated donors. The final selection of unrelated donor BM versus UCB should be based on the urgency of the transplant, and characteristics of the BM and UCB unrelated donor such as cell dose and HLA compatibility. For those children requiring an urgent transplant, generally in less than 3 months, UCB seems advantageous. Moreover, cord blood banks should increase their inventories, with the aim of finding more closely matched CB grafts.

Umbilical cord blood transplantation from unrelated donors in adults

Progress in the field of cord blood transplantation has been largely restricted to children, mainly because of the impact of cell dose on engraftment and the risk of TRM. However, in recent years, due to improved cord blood unit selection, more clearly defined indications for transplantation and more experience of outcome, UCBTs in adults have improved (Fig. 22.1). Reviews focusing on the clinical results of unrelated donor UCBT in adults have been published.[21–23] To date, more than 2000 UCBTs have been performed in adults with a unit coming from the Netcord organization.[5] However, the information available in this setting is still limited. Six studies have reported outcomes and risk factors of single unit unrelated UCBT in adults.[24–29] As expected from retrospective and multicenter studies, the series were heterogeneous in terms of recipients and disease-related characteristics, such as type and status of the disease at transplant.[24,29] However, single centers report more homogeneous series of patients and diseases with standard conditioning regimens and GvHD prophylaxis.[25–27] For example, in the Japanese series,[26,27] the analyses are from a single center, reporting patients with myelodysplastic syndrome (MDS) or acute myeloid leukemia (AML), with a uniform conditioning regimen (without antithymocyte globulin (ATG)) and using

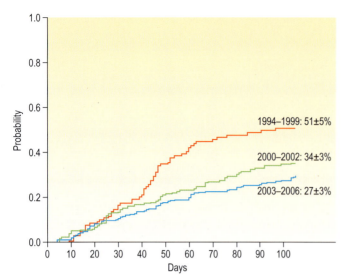

Figure 22.1
Probability of early transplant-related mortality in 557 adults with hematologic malignancies given a single cord blood transplant, according to the period of transplant.

methotrexate in combination with ciclosporin as GvHD prophylaxis. Another important difference is that in four of the six series, the median number of nucleated cells infused per kilogram recipient weight was below 2×10^7/kg, and several patients received less than 1.5×10^7 nucleated cells/kg, figures that are below recent recommendations.[12,16] However, in the Japanese series very few patients received a cord blood cell dose of less than 2×10^7/kg. GCSF was commonly used after UCBT in all series. The myeloid engraftment rate at 60 days ranged from 80% to 100% and the probability of platelet engraftment at 180 days was 65–90%. Median time to achieve a neutrophil count above 0.5×10^9/l varied from 22 to 32 days. The incidence of acute and chronic GvHD has differed widely in adults undergoing unrelated UCBT, as has TRM at 100 days (0–54%) and disease-free survival, which has varied from 15% to 76%. It is difficult to explain the reason for such differences, since factors such as patient and cord blood graft selection, disease and disease status, center effect and period of transplant may be involved.

Recently, the Eurocord group has published the outcomes and risk factors after UCBT in adults with hematologic malignancies given a single cord blood unit after a myeloablative conditioning regimen.[29] One hundred and seventy-one patients were transplanted after 1997. Their median age was 29 years (15–55) and the median follow-up time was 18 months (1–71). Most patients had acute or chronic leukemia (n = 142, 83%), Ninety-one (53%) were transplanted with advanced disease and an autologous transplant had failed in 32 (19%). Most patients (87%) received an HLA-mismatched cord blood unit with 1–2 HLA disparities. At infusion, the median number of NC and CD34+ cells was 2.1×10^7/kg and 1×10^5/kg, respectively. The cumulative incidence of neutrophil recovery at day 60 was 72 ± 3%, with a median of 28 days (11–57). A higher NC cell dose (>2.0×10^7/kg) and use of hematopoietic growth factors were independently associated with faster neutrophil recovery. The cumulative incidence of grade II–IV acute GvHD was 32 ± 4% and this complication was not associated with the number of HLA mismatches. The 2-year cumulative incidence of chronic GvHD, transplant related-mortality and relapse was 36 ± 10%, 51 ± 4% and 22 ± 4%, respectively. At 2 years, disease-free survival for patients transplanted in early, intermediate and advanced phases of their disease was 41 ± 9%, 34 ± 10% and 18 ± 4%, respectively. On multivariate analysis, advanced disease status was an adverse factor for relapse and disease-free survival.

Therefore, unrelated HLA-mismatched cord blood graft containing a higher cell dose should be considered as an alternative source of stem cells in adults with hematologic malignancies lacking an HLA-matched donor. In order to circumvent the problem of cell dose and transplant-related mortality, new approaches in adult UCB transplantation such as the use of double cord blood units and reduced-intensity conditioning have led to an increased use of cord blood cells in adults. These approaches are discussed later in this chapter.

Results of unrelated cord blood transplants compared to unrelated or related bone marrow transplants in adults with hematologic malignancies

Three retrospective studies comparing results of UCBT with UBMT in adults[30–32] have been published. Investigators from a single center in Japan compared the outcomes of 113 adult patients with hematologic malignancies who received unrelated UBMT (n = 45) or unrelated UCBT (n = 68). In this single-center analysis, time from donor search to transplantation was significantly shorter among UCBT recipients (median 2 months) compared to 11 months in UBMT. Neutrophil and platelet recovery were delayed in UCBT recipients. UCBT recipients experienced a faster tapering of immunosuppressant after transplantation, and treatment of acute GvHD with steroids was less frequent. Moreover, no UCBT recipient died of GvHD, in spite of the high HLA mismatching. TRM was decreased and DFS superior after UCBT when compared to UBMT. In this study, all but four patients received a cord blood cell dose of more than 2×10^7/kg.[30]

The Eurocord and Acute Leukemia Working Party of the EBMT has performed a retrospective registry-based comparative study of 98 UCBT with 584 UBMT from unrelated donors in adults with acute leukemia.[31] Transplants were performed between 1998 and 2002. Recipients of cord blood were younger (median 24.5 versus 32 years; p < 0.001), weighed less (median 58 versus 68 kg; p < 0.001), and had more advanced disease at the time of transplant (52% versus 33%, p < 0.001). All marrow transplants were HLA matched, whereas 94% of cord blood grafts were HLA incompatible (p < 0.001). The median number of nucleated cells infused was 2.3×10^7/kg for cord blood, and 2.9×10^8/kg for bone marrow; (p < 0.001). Multivariate analysis demonstrated a lower risk of grade II–IV acute GvHD after UCBT (RR 0.57; 95% confidence interval (CI) 0.37–0.87; p = 0.01), but neutrophil recovery was significantly delayed (RR 0.49; 95% CI 0.41–0.58, p < 0.001). Transplant-related mortality, relapse rate, chronic GvHD, and LFS were not significantly different in the two groups.

In another registry-based analysis, Laughlin et al, on behalf of the IBMTR, found inferior outcomes for patients with leukemia given an UCBT compared to an HLA-matched UBMT. However, similar outcomes were found when UCBT was compared to one HLA-mismatched UBMT.[32]

A meta-analysis pooling these studies has been published: 316 adults undergoing UCBT (mostly one or two antigen mismatched) were compared to 996 adults undergoing UBMT (almost entirely fully matched with the recipient) and, as expected, transplant-related mortality and disease-free survival were not statistically different between the groups, in spite of delayed neutrophil recovery in cord blood recipients.[19]

Interestingly, the same Japanese team which found that unrelated UCBT has better outcomes than UBMT compared results of HLA-genoidentical BM or peripheral blood stem cell (PBSC) transplants (n = 71) with HLA-mismatched cord blood transplants (n = 100) for adults with hematologic diseases. All patients received myeloablative regimens. Multivariate analysis demonstrated no statistically significant differences in TRM (9% in CBT and 13% in BMT/PBSCT recipients), relapse (17% in CBT and 26% in BMT/PBSCT recipients), and DFS (70% in CBT and 60% in BMT/PBSCT recipients) between groups.[33]

The results of these four comparative studies together with the meta-analysis showed that:

- UCBT is feasible in adults when a cord blood unit contains a high number of cells and should be considered an option as an allogeneic stem cell source for patients lacking an HLA-matched bone marrow donor
- despite increased HLA disparity, UCB from unrelated donors offers results as promising as those of matched UBM in adults with hematologic malignancies.

Therefore, the conclusion is that, as in children, the donor search process for BM and UCB from an unrelated donor should be started simultaneously, especially in patients with acute leukemia where the time factor is crucial.

Strategies to improve outcome after cord blood transplantation

Many approaches have been suggested to improve the results of unrelated cord blood transplantation. These have focused on accelerating hematopoietic recovery and reducing transplant-related toxicity. The following strategies are currently being explored.

Accelerating engraftment by increasing cell dose and homing of umbilical cord blood cells

Optimization of the process of UCB collection

Establishment of high-quality UCB banks, and expansion of the pool of donors, which is particularly relevant for ethnic and racial minorities, will prove most valuable.

Ex vivo expansion of cord blood cells

Two Phase I clinical trials using expanded cord blood cells have been reported.[34,35] Both studies have demonstrated the feasibility of ex vivo expansion but there is a need for more efficient expansion protocols and gene marking of expanded cells to evaluate their capacity for engraftment. New pharmacologic agents such as linear polyamine copper chelators that expand cord blood stem cells are currently being used in Phase I clinical trials in USA and Europe.

Transplantation of two partially HLA-matched UCB

Results with double cord blood transplantation with or without reduced-intensity conditioning, although preliminary, support the safety of the procedure which is used to overcome the cell dose barrier in adolescents and adults.[36–42] Chimerism data from these studies reveal that typically only one CB engrafts. In addition, preliminary data suggest that double UCBT is associated with a greater graft-versus-leukemia effect,[41] probably due to a higher incidence of acute GvHD, when recipients of single (n = 210) versus double (n = 169) UCBT have been compared.[42] Despite the increased risk of acute GvHD, TRM at 1 year was significantly lower in recipients of double UCBT (17%, 95% CI 5–29%), as compared to that seen in recipients of a single UCBT (47%, 95% CI 26–68%; p = 0.02) among those who developed grade III–IV acute GvHD. Survival at 1 year among those with grade III–IV acute GvHD was significantly higher after double UCBT (67%, 95% CI 51–83%) than after single UCBT (41%, 95% CI 21–61%; p = 0.04). These results may have important scientific implications in terms of understanding, immunology, nature of the hematopoietic stem cell niche and how modulation of this niche may impact upon transplant outcome.

Co-transplantation of an UCB unit with highly purified CD34+ cells from haploidentical family donors

Phase I–II clinical trials have already been published, with interesting results.[43]

Intrabone infusion of cord blood cells

In mice, it has been suggested that intrabone infusion of CD34+ CB cells confers an engraftment advantage 15 times greater than after intravenous infusion, probably because cell loss during circulation before homing is decreased.[44] This approach seems attractive. Recently, the group which described these findings has started a Phase I clinical trial. Ten adult patients were transplanted in advanced phase of leukemia with a median cell dose of 2.7×10^7/kg infused into the posterior iliac crest under a short anesthetic. All patients engrafted (100% donor cells), with a median of 20 (14–33) days of sustained neutrophil recovery. Follow-up is still short (3–11 months), but seven patients are alive and in remission.[45] These encouraging results require confirmation in larger series of patients.

Choosing the 'best' umbilical cord blood unit according to cell dose, HLA and diagnosis

It has been suggested that cell dose and number of HLA mismatches interact mutually on engraftment and on other outcomes. Thus, a higher cell dose in the graft could partially overcome the negative impact of HLA for each level of HLA disparity, but this hypothesis has not been yet been fully demonstrated. However, based on previous data[11,12] and Eurocord data,[16] we recommend cord blood grafts with no more than two HLA disparities and with more than 3×10^7/kg nucleated cells at cryopreservation. Other factors such as diagnosis have an important role in rate of engraftment. This is due to the fact that most patients have a full marrow and have not received chemotherapy or immunosuppression before conditioning or, in the cases of aplastic anemia, they have often received multiple transfusions previously or had a severe infection at the time of transplantation, thus increasing the risk of non-engraftment.

Recently, in the light of the observation that requirements regarding cell dose and HLA matching may differ in malignant and non-malignant diseases, we attempted to construct an algorithm to guide clinicians in choosing the 'best' cord blood unit, taking into account the impact of diagnosis, cell dose and HLA incompatibilities, in patients receiving a single UCBT. If the cell dose with a single unit is not achieved, a double cord blood transplant should be possible. With this objective, two different cohorts of patients who had received a single UCBT between 1994 and 2005 were analyzed: 925 patients had a malignant disease and 279 had a non-malignant disease (Eurocord; unpublished data). Donor–recipient histocompatibility was determined by serology or antigen typing for HLA-A and HLA-B and by DNA typing for HLA-DRB1.

Patients with malignant diseases

In patients with malignant diseases, the median age was 11 years (range 1 month–56 years). Diagnoses included acute myeloid leukemia in 24.6%, acute lymphoid leukemia in 44.3%, chronic leukemia in 9.1% and myelodysplastic syndrome in 10% of cases. Only 9% were classified as having class I antigens and class II alleles identical to their donor; 42% had one HLA difference, 40% had two HLA differences and the remainder had three or four HLA differences. For patients who had one HLA mismatch, 67% had a class I difference and 33% had a class II difference. For patients with two HLA differences, 38% had two class I differences, 7% had two class II differences, and 55% had one class I and one class II difference. The median number of NCs infused was 3.1×10^7 NC/kg (range 2–5 × 10^7 NC/kg). At day 100, the cumulative incidence (CI) of neutrophil recovery (the first day the neutrophil count reached >500 neutrophils/μl) was 77.4%

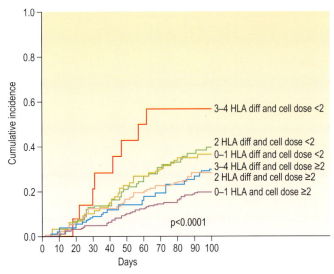

Figure 22.2
Transplant-related mortality in 925 UCBT recipients with malignant diseases according to number of nucleated cells infused (×10⁷/kg) and number of HLA disparities.

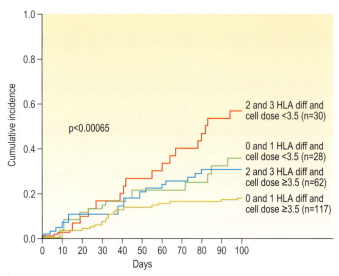

Figure 22.3
Transplant-related mortality in 268 patients with non-malignant disorders according to cell dose infused (×10⁷/kg) and HLA differences.

and the CI of platelet recovery (the first day the platelet count reached >20,000 platelets/μl) was 54.7%. This related to the number of cells infused (p < 0.0001). HLA was a second factor that affected neutrophil engraftment, with a difference between 0–1 (81%), 2 (75%) and 3–4 (63%) HLA incompatibilities (p = 0.037). The role of HLA mismatching was abrogated by an increase in cell dose, except in the group of patients who received a 3–4 HLA-mismatched transplant.

In the malignant disease group, we found that cell dose was the most important factor influencing outcome; a minimum cell dose of 3 × 10⁷ NC/kg at collection, and of 2 × 10⁷ NC/kg at infusion needed to be targeted. We also showed that the number of HLA mismatches increased the risk of delayed engraftment and led to a higher incidence of TRM and chronic GvHD (Fig. 22.2); however, it decreased the risk of relapse, resulting overall in a lack of influence of HLA mismatching on OS and DFS. Type of HLA mismatch did not influence outcome, but matching for HLA-DRB1 appeared better for patients receiving a graft that had two HLA incompatibilities. As stated earlier, increasing cell dose abrogated the effect of HLA mismatching, but not for grafts with three or four HLA incompatibilities.

Patients with non-malignant diseases

The median age of patients studied who had non-malignant diseases was 3 years (range 3 months–10 years). The diagnosis was bone marrow failure syndrome in 40%, primary immunodeficiency in 36% and a hereditary metabolic disorder in 24% of patients.

Only 18% were classified as identical for HLA class I antigens and class II allelic typing, whereas 43% had one HLA difference, 35% had two HLA differences and the remainder had three HLA differences. For patients with one HLA mismatch, 69% had a class I difference and 31% a class II difference. For patients with two HLA differences, 43% had two class I differences, 3% had two class II differences, and 54% one class I and one class II difference. The median number of NCs infused was 6.4 × 10⁷ NC/kg (range 0.8–66 × 10⁷ NC/kg).

At day 100, the CI of neutrophil recovery was 69.3% and CI of platelet recovery was 50%. Both outcomes were associated with the median number of cells infused (p < 0.000055). HLA was also an important factor associated with neutrophil recovery, with a statistical difference between 0–1 and ≥2 HLA mismatches (p = 0.046). The role of HLA mismatching was abrogated by increasing cell dose, except in the group of patients who received a 3–4 HLA-mismatched transplant. There was no correlation between neutrophil

recovery and class of HLA mismatching (class I or class II, or HLA-A, B or DRB1).

The CI of acute GvHD grade II–IV was 31.8% and grade III–IV 18%, and was only associated with the number of HLA incompatibilities (p = 0.0029). The CI of chronic GvHD was 24% and was also associated with the number of HLA incompatibilities (p = 0.01). The CI of OS at 100 months was 49%. It was influenced by cell dose and by the number of HLA mismatches. The group who received an UCBT with < 3.5 × 10⁷ NC/kg at infusion and a 2–3 HLA-mismatched transplant had <10% survival. Increasing cell dose partially abrogated the effect of HLA mismatches; there was no statistical difference between the groups who received a cell dose of >3.5 × 10⁷ NC/kg with a 0, 1-, 2- or 3-HLA-mismatched UCBT.

Thus, patients with a non-malignant disease must receive a higher cell dose to obtain engraftment than patients with a malignant disease; this should not be below 4.9 × 10⁷ NC/kg at collection and 3.5 × 10⁷ NC/kg at infusion. In non-malignant disorders, HLA mismatching played a major role in engraftment, GvHD, TRM (Fig. 22.3) and survival, which was partially abrogated by increasing cell dose. A CB graft containing two or more HLA disparities with a cell dose inferior to 3.5 × 10⁷ NC/kg should be avoided. Experience of double cord blood transplantation in non-malignant disorders is still too limited to allow routine recommendation of this type of transplant.

Reducing conditioning-related mortality

Encouraging results regarding engraftment and TRM have recently been reported with the use of reduced-intensity conditioning regimens.[37,46–48] Investigators from the University of Minnesota have reported the preliminary results of UCBT from mismatched unrelated donors after non-myeloablative (NMA) conditioning in 43 adult patients (median age 49.5 years) with advanced or high-risk hematologic malignancies.[46] In this series, some patients received two cord blood units, and two types of non-myeloablative conditioning: fludarabine 200 mg/m², busulfan 8 mg/kg and total-body irradiation (TBI) 200 cGY (Flu/Bu/TBI) for the 21 patients and fludarabine 200 mg/m², cyclophosphamide 50 mg/kg and TBI 200 cGY (Flu/Cy/TBI) for the remaining cases. All patients received CsA and mycophenolate mofetil (MMF) as GvHD prophylaxis. The median time to neutrophil recovery was 26 days (range 12–30 days), with the cumulative incidence of 76% for the Flu/Bu/TBI recipients and only 9.5 days (range 5–28 days) with a cumulative incidence of 94% for the Flu/Cy/TBI recipients. The cumulative incidence of acute GvHD grade II–IV and III–IV was 44% and 9%, respectively. TRM at day 100 was 48% for Bu/Flu/TBI recipients, and 28% for Flu/Cy/TBI. Causes of death during the first 100 days were predominantly organ failure and infection. DFS at 1 year in these high-risk patients was 24% for Flu/Bu/TBI recipients and 41% for Flu/Cy/TBI recipients. The same group of investigators have updated these results to include 95 patients given a single or double cord blood transplant after RIC. They have found an association between the use of ATG and a higher incidence of EBV reactivation and disease.[47] Other series of double UCBT using reduced-intensity conditioning regimens have been reported.[37]

We analyzed 65 patients with advanced hematologic malignancies (49% had advanced-phase disease and 39% had received a previous autologous transplant), mostly leukemias transplanted from 1999 to 2005 and reported to Eurocord.[48] The median follow-up was only 8 months (3–26) and the median age was 47 years (16–76). Conditioning varied according to disease and center: fludarabine(Flu)+endoxan (End)+TBI (2 Gy) was given to 33 patients, Flu+End or melphalan to 11, Flu+BU (<8 mg/kg) with or without other drugs in 13, and other regimens in eight patients. ATG/antilymphocyte globulin (ALG) was added in 26% of the cases. The median nucleated cell dose infused was 2.4×10^7/kg. The graft was HLA identical (6/6) in three cases, 5/6 in 15, 4/6 in 37 and 3/6 in 10. Median time to neutrophil recovery (>500/mm^3) was 20 days (0–56) and 35 days for platelets recovery (>20,000/mm^3). At day 60, probability of neutrophil recovery was 87 ± 7% for the 33 patients who received the Flu+End+TBI conditioning regimen and 65 ± 10% for patients receiving other regimens (p < 0.01). Grade II a-GvHD was observed in 13%, grade III in 7% and grade IV in 7%. TRM was 45 ± 7% overall; 50 ± 15% in acute leukemia, 30 ± 15% in lymphomas and 27 ± 16% for other diagnoses. TRM at 1 year for those receiving <2.4×10^7 TNC/kg was 53 ± 9%, and for those receiving >2.4×10^7 NC/kg 39 ± 10% (p = 0.07). For patients receiving Flu+End+TBI, TRM at 1 year was 24 ± 10%, and for those receiving other conditioning regimens 60 ± 9% (p = 0.001). DFS at 1 year for lymphomas was 50 ± 9%, for leukemias 27 ± 7% and for other diagnoses zero. When HLA compatibility was 6/6 or 5/6, DFS at 1 year was 42 ± 12%, for 4/6 disparities DFS was 27 ± 9% and for 3/6 disparities it was zero. DFS was 43 ± 11% for those receiving Flu+End+TBI, and 16 ± 7% for patients receiving other conditioning regimens (p = 0.005). For patients receiving > 2.4×10^7 NC/kg the DFS was 31 ± 12% and for patients receiving < 2.4×10^7 NC/kg it was 14 ± 8% (p = 0.05).

In conclusion, cell dose and HLA remain important factors in the RIC setting as well. Type of conditioning (Flu+End+TBI) seems to be associated with decreased TRM and better DFS, and other factors may also influence outcome after RIC-UCBT. More data are needed to establish criteria for the use of single and double cord blood transplants in the RIC setting.

Improving immune reconstitution

Immune recovery after UCBT is an area of great interest and concern owing to the low number and immaturity of UCB lymphocytes as well as the degree of HLA mismatching. Despite these factors, several studies have shown that immune reconstitution in children undergoing UCBT is not delayed compared to BMT in terms of numbers of T-, B- and NK lymphocyte subsets,[49] T-cell repertoire diversity and thymic function,[50] and recovery of specific immune responses toward viruses and fungi.[51] In contrast, central T-cell and lymphocyte recovery are delayed after UCBT in adults compared to children, especially in the presence of GvHD.[52] Whether or not infection is related to delayed neutrophil engraftment, GvHD or immune disturbances, it remains the major cause of death after UCBT.[11] Recently, pediatric recipients of UCBT who had undergone transplantation for acute leukemia were sequentially evaluated for their development of antigen-specific T-lymphocyte immunity to herpes viruses. The presence of an antigen-specific response resulted in a relapse-free survival advantage (p = 0.0001) primarily due to a decrease in leukemia relapse (p = 0.003). On multivariate analysis, negative antigen-specific T-lymphocyte proliferation was associated with an increased risk of relapse among other factors, Notably, neither acute nor chronic GvHD had any effect on the incidence of leukemia relapse.[53]

Cord blood banks

Cord blood transplantation has been made possible largely by the creation of worldwide umbilical cord blood banks (CBBs). The CBB consists of an integrated team, under a single CBB director, responsible for the collection, processing, testing, banking, selection and release of cord blood units. In accordance with the Netcord-FACT (Foundation for the Accreditation of Cellular Therapy) standards, the CBB, each collection facility and each processing facility is required to operate in compliance with local law and current national licensing and registration requirements.

There are two types of CBB: public and private, according to their economic interest and financial support, and three types of CBB according to type of donation and its use: unrelated donor, sibling donor or autologous CBB. Unrelated donor transplantation programs employ public banks as their source of donor cord blood units (CBU). These CBUs are donated on a volunteer basis by women delivering healthy babies at term. Private banks, which are for-profit entities, store 'directed donations' collected by obstetricians from babies born into families who intend to use the cord blood for the baby from whom it came (autologous donation) or for another family member in need of future transplantation therapy. Sibling donor cord blood banks (SDCBB) programs have been established publicly or privately for families within which there is an indication for hematopoietic stem cell transplant. The differences between these three types of banks are shown in Table 22.2.[54]

Unrelated cord blood banks

The number of unrelated cord blood banks, and in consequence, the number of available cord blood units for unrelated use is increasing worldwide. We estimate that more than 300,000 cord blood units are available for transplantation in more than 40 cord blood banks in many countries (www.bmdw.org, accessed in February 2007). The price of a cord blood unit varies between 15,000 and 22,000 euros.

Currently, there is an increasing number of international exchange cord blood units. For example, in France, from 1994 to 2005, 63% of UCBT were performed using a CBU coming from abroad. Therefore, many national regulatory agencies and transplant centers are aware of the need for international standards for cord blood collection, processing, testing, banking, selection and release. In 2006, Netcord-FACT published the third edition of the International standards for cord blood. Founded in 1998, Netcord is the international cord blood banking arm of Eurocord. The mission of Netcord is to promote high-quality cord blood banking and clinical use of umbilical cord blood for allogeneic stem cell transplantation. Through its online virtual office (www.netcord.org), cord blood units from member banks are made available for unrelated donor transplantation. Approximately 20 CBBs, mostly European, are Netcord members, accounting for almost 50% of worldwide available units. To be an active Netcord member, a Netcord-FACT accreditation is required, among other criteria. Some of Netcord CBBs have already been accredited and others are in the process of gaining accreditation. The major objective of these stan-

Table 22.2 Comparative features among three models for cord blood banking[54]

	Autologous	Unrelated	Sibling
Operating model			
Financial status	For-profit	Non-profit	Non-profit
Donation	Business transaction	Voluntary act	Motivated act
Donor's status	Payer	Neutral	Non-fiduciary benefit
Product ownership	Contingent upon payment?	Public	Family
Operating location	Remote sites	Few specified sites	Remote sites
Potential size/market	Very large	Large	Small
Safety and QA			
Eligibility	All who can pay	Medical and lab deferrals	Few absolute deferrals
ID testing	Unpublished	Full blood donor ± nat	Donor retested ± nat
Genetic disease testing	Unpublished	Yes, expanded testing under consideration	Established, often specific to family's mutation
Deliberate maneuvers to facilitate CB collection volume	No	No	Not excluded
Donor–recipient linkage	Defining property	Under debate	Intrinsic
Trained collectors	No	Yes	Limited training at the time of collection
Quality assurance	Unpublished	Established	Under development using blood center model
Disposition of units			
Likelihood of complete histocompatibility	100%	Low	~25%
Likelihood of use for transplant	Low to nil	Moderate	Relatively high
Research potential	Low to nil	High	Moderate to high
Crossed over for public use	No	N/a	Under discussion

dards is to promote quality medical and laboratory practices throughout all phases of cord blood banking, with the goal of achieving consistent production of high-quality placental and umbilical cord blood units for transplantation. These standards cover:

- collection of cord blood cells, regardless of the methodology or site of collection
- screening, testing, and eligibility determination of the maternal and infant donor according to local law
- all phases of processing and storage, including quarantine, testing, and characterization of the unit
- making the CB unit available for transplantation, either directly or through listing it with a search registry
- the search process for selection of specific cord blood units
- all transport or shipment of cord blood units, whether fresh or cryopreserved.

To be compliant with standards, CBBs must use validated methods, supplies, reagents, and equipment. They must maintain a comprehensive, properly documented quality management program, and track the clinical outcomes of patients who receive cord blood units from that bank. The accreditation process includes submission of written documentation and on-site inspection of collection, processing, and storage facilities. Netcord-FACT accredited CBBs are reinspected routinely every 3 years.

All the practical aspects of cord blood banking, such as need to obtain the mother's informed consent, collection techniques, labeling and identification, infectious disease and genetic disease testing, HLA typing, methodology of cell processing, cryopreservation, transportation and release, have been extensively published.[4,55] All these issues are detailed in the last version of the Netcord-FACT standards (www.factwebsite.org).

Sibling donor cord blood banks

Sibling donor cord blood bank (SDCBB) programs have been established for families in whom there is an indication for hematopoietic stem cell transplant.[9,54] Because there is a 25% probability that a new sibling will be HLA identical to the existing full sibling, a family and their child's physician often agree that it is prudent to collect and cryopreserve the new sibling's CB in the event that a clinical indication for CB transplantation arises. Currently, most of the cord blood units coming from a sibling cord blood donor are collected and frozen in hospitals where the family recipient is being treated. In order to unify and homogenize collection and cord blood unit processing following regulatory procedures, sibling donor cord blood banks have been established. Because these relatively few families give birth at a variety of smaller hospitals, it is a considerable logistical challenge to provide access to specialized high-quality SDCB banking services for them. An example of this type of national banking program is the SDCBB at The Children's Hospital, Oakland, USA.[9,54] Many of the operational procedures and medical policies have been developed for the national, comprehensive SDCB banking program.

Although far smaller than unrelated donor CB programs, the scope of need for SDCB banking services is considerable. Approximately 5000 children in the US aged 0–14 are newly diagnosed each year with a malignant process, and approximately 40% of these represent hematopoietic malignancies.[56] Enrollment in Oakland's SDCB program is consistent with this epidemiology; nearly half of the enrollments are from families caring for a child with a hematopoietic malignancy.

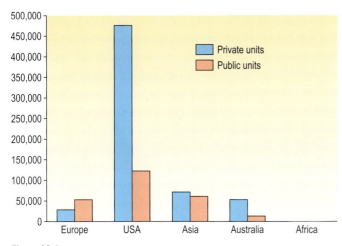

Figure 22.4
Number of cord blood units available in public and private banks worldwide.[57] (Source: BMDW, ESSEC 2005.)

Autologous cord blood banks

Public banks collect UCB intended for recipients suffering from hematologic diseases (related or unrelated allogeneic transplantation), and private banks store newborn blood in order to keep it for that same individual's possible future use (autotransplantation). In April 2006, there were 134 private banks worldwide, accounting for some 780,000 units[57] (Fig. 22.4). The 54 public banks owned a stock that was approximately one-third that size: 227,000 units (source: www.bmdw.org, April 2006).

The growth of public banks is constrained by the public funding on which it depends. In economic terms, the stock of private banks represents the demand of parents who are willing to pay for a service, whereas the public bank stock represents the supply of care services available to its national citizens. Since 75% of the umbilical cords stored worldwide are held by private banks, the imbalance between supply and demand could lead public banks to become dependent on the grafts kept by private banks. While private banks are prohibited in some European countries such as France and Italy, they are developing quickly in Belgium, Great Britain and Germany. They are growing extremely rapidly in Asia, Australia and the United States.[57] Since the year 2000, the three main American private banks have increased their graft stock by roughly 40% each year (www.parentsguidecordblood.org).

Many ethical issues have been raised concerning the scientific value of commercial CBBs for autologous CBT and their competition with the public CBBs.[57,58] In spite of the huge number of private units frozen for autologous use, only one case of autologous use has been recently reported concerning a child with acute leukemia.[59]

Acknowledgments

We would like to thank Dr G Sanz, from Valencia in Spain, for his suggestions and comments, and all Eurocord-Netcord members and data managers for providing data for the registry.

References

1. Gluckman E, Broxmeyer HE, Auerbach AD et al. Hematopoietic reconstitution in a patient with Fanconi's anemia by means of umbilical-cord blood from an HLA-identical sibling. N Engl J Med 1989;321:1174–1178
2. Barker JN, Krepski TP, DeFor T et al. Searching for unrelated donor hematopoietic stem cell grafts: availability and speed of umbilical cord blood versus bone marrow. Biol Blood Marrow Transplant 2002;8:257–260
3. Dalle JH, Duval M, Moghrabi A et al. Results of an unrelated transplant search strategy using partially HLA-mismatched cord blood as an immediate alternative to HLA-matched bone marrow. Bone Marrow Transplant 2004;33:605–611
4. Davey S, Armitage S, Rocha V et al. The London Cord Blood Bank: analysis of banking and transplantation outcome. Br J Haematol 2004;125:358–365
5. Wernet P. The Netcord inventory and use (Netcord website). Available at: https://office.de.netcord.org/inventory.gif. Accessed March 2007
6. Gluckman E, Rocha V, Boyer-Chammard A et al. Outcome of cord blood transplantation from related and unrelated donors. Eurocord Transplant Group and the European Blood and Marrow Transplantation Group. N Engl J Med 1997;337:373–381
7. Locatelli F, Rocha V, Reed W et al. Related umbilical cord blood transplant in patients with thalassemia and sickle cell disease. Blood 2003;101:2137–2143
8. Rocha V, Wagner JE, Sobocinski KA et al. Graft-versus-host disease in children who have received a cord blood or bone marrow transplant from an HLA-identical sibling. N Engl J Med 2000;342:1846–1854
9. Reed W, Smith R, Dekovic F et al. Comprehensive banking of sibling donor cord blood for children with malignant and nonmalignant disease. Blood 2003;101:351–357
10. Michel G, Rocha V, Chevret S et al. Unrelated cord blood transplantation for childhood acute myeloid leukemia: a Eurocord Group analysis. Blood 2003;102:4290–4297
11. Rubinstein P, Carrier C, Scaradavou A et al. Outcomes among 562 recipients of placental-blood transplants from unrelated donors. N Engl J Med 1998;339:1565–1577
12. Wagner JE, Barker JN, DeFor TE et al. Transplantation of unrelated donor umbilical cord blood in 102 patients with malignant and nonmalignant diseases: influence of CD34 cell dose and HLA disparity on treatment-related mortality and survival. Blood 2002;100:1611–1618
13. Styczynski J, Cheung YK, Garvin J et al. Outcomes of unrelated cord blood transplantation in pediatric recipients. Bone Marrow Transplant 2004;34:129–136
14. Staba SL, Escolar ML, Poe M et al. Cord-blood transplants from unrelated donors in patients with Hurler's syndrome. N Engl J Med 2004;350:1960–1969
15. Escolar ML, Poe MD, Provenzale JM et al. Transplantation of umbilical-cord blood in babies with infantile Krabbe's disease. N Engl J Med 2005;352:2069–2081
16. Gluckman E, Rocha V, Arcese W et al. Eurocord Group. Factors associated with outcomes of unrelated cord blood transplant: guidelines for donor choice. Exp Hematol 2004;32:397–407
17. Rocha V, Cornish J, Sievers E et al. Comparison of outcomes of unrelated bone marrow and umbilical cord blood transplants in children with acute leukemia. Blood 2001;97:2962–2971
18. Barker JN, Davies SM, DeFor T et al. Survival after transplantation of unrelated donor umbilical cord blood is comparable to that of human leukocyte antigen-matched unrelated donor bone marrow: results of a matched-pair analysis. Blood 2001;97:2957–2961
19. Hwang WY, Samuel M, Tan D et al. A meta-analysis of unrelated donor umbilical cord blood transplantation versus unrelated donor bone marrow transplantation in adult and pediatric patients. Biol Blood Marrow Transplant 2007;13:444–453
20. Eapen M, Rubinstein P, Zhang MJ et al. Unrelated donor hematopoietic stem cell transplantation (HSCT) in children with acute leukemia: risks and benefits of umbilical cord blood (CB) versus HLA A, B, C, DRB1 allele-matched bone marrow (BM). Blood 2006;108:434
21. Rocha V, Sanz G, Gluckman E, Eurocord and European Blood and Marrow Transplant Group. Umbilical cord blood transplantation. Curr Opin Hematol 2004;11:375–385
22. Brunstein CG, Setubal DC, Wagner JE. Expanding the role of umbilical cord blood transplantation. Br J Haematol 2007;137:20–35
23. Schoemans H, Theunissen K, Maertens J et al. Adult umbilical cord blood transplantation: a comprehensive review. Bone Marrow Transplant 2006;38:83–93
24. Laughlin MJ, Barker J, Bambach B et al. Hematopoietic engraftment and survival in adult recipients of umbilical-cord blood from unrelated donors. N Engl J Med 2001;344:1815–1822
25. Sanz GF, Saavedra S, Planelles D et al. Standardized, unrelated donor cord blood transplantation in adults with hematological malignancies. Blood 2001;98:2332–2338
26. Ooi J, Iseki T, Takahashi S et al. Unrelated cord blood transplantation for adult patients with de novo acute myeloid leukemia. Blood 2004;103:489–491
27. Ooi J, Iseki T, Takahashi S et al. Unrelated cord blood transplantation for adult patients with advanced myelodysplastic syndrome. Blood 2003;101:4711–4713
28. Long GD, Laughlin M, Madan B et al. Unrelated umbilical cord blood transplantation in adult patients. Biol Blood Marrow Transplant 2003;9:772–780
29. Arcese W, Rocha V, Labopin M et al, Eurocord-Netcord Transplant Group. Unrelated cord blood transplants in adults with hematologic malignancies. Haematologica 2006;91:223–230
30. Takahashi S, Iseki T, Ooi J et al. Single-institute comparative analysis of unrelated bone marrow transplantation and cord blood transplantation for adult patients with hematological malignancies. Blood 2004;104:3813–3820
31. Rocha V, Labopin M, Sanz G et al. Acute Leukemia Working Party of European Blood and Marrow Transplant Group; Eurocord-Netcord Registry. Transplants of umbilical-cord blood or bone marrow from unrelated donors in adults with acute leukemia. N Engl J Med 2004;351:2276–2285
32. Laughlin MJ, Eapen M, Rubinstein P et al. Outcomes after transplantation of cord blood or bone marrow from unrelated donors in adults with leukemia. N Engl J Med 2004;351:2265–2275
33. Takahashi S, Ooi J, Tomonari A et al. Comparative single-institute analysis of cord blood transplantation from unrelated donors with bone marrow or peripheral blood stem-cell transplants from related donors in adult patients with hematologic malignancies after myeloablative conditioning regimen. Blood 2007;109:1322–1330
34. Shpall EJ, Quinones R, Giller R et al. Transplantation of ex vivo expanded cord blood. Biol Blood Marrow Transplant 2002;8:368–376
35. Jaroscak J, Goltry K, Smith A et al. Augmentation of umbilical cord blood (UCB) transplantation with ex vivo-expanded UCB cells: results of a phase 1 trial using the Aastrom-Replicell System. Blood 2003;101:5061–5067

36. Barker JN, Weisdorf DJ, DeFor TE et al. Transplantation of 2 partially HLA-matched umbilical cord blood units to enhance engraftment in adults with hematologic malignancy. Blood 2005;105:1343–1347

37. Ballen KK, Spitzer TR, Yeap BY et al. Double unrelated reduced-intensity umbilical cordblood transplantation in adults. Biol Blood Marrow Transplant 2007;13:82–89

38. Fernandes J, Rocha V, Robin M et al. Second transplant with two unrelated cord blood units for early graft failure after haematopoietic stem cell transplantation. Br J Haematol 2007;137:248–251

39. Majhail NS, Brunstein CG, Wagner JE. Double umbilical cord blood transplantation. Curr Opin Immunol 2006;18:571–575

40. Rocha V, Madureira A, Robin M et al. Double cord blood transplantation for patients with high risk hematological diseases: delayed immune recovery and high incidence of infections. Blood 2006;108:2923

41. Verneris MR, Brunstein C, DeFor TE et al. Risk of relapse (REL) after umbilical cord blood transplantation (UCBT) in patients with acute leukemia: marked reduction in recipients of two units. Blood (ASH Annual Meeting Abstracts) 2005;106:305

42. MacMillan ML, Brunstein C, DeFor TE et al. Single versus double umbilical cord blood transplantation (UCBT): higher risk of acute graft-versus-host disease (GVHD) but lower transplant related mortality (TRM) in recipients of double UCBT. Blood (ASH Annual Meeting Abstracts) 2006;108:435

43. Magro E, Regidor C, Cabrera R et al. Early hematopoietic recovery after single unit unrelated cord blood transplantation in adults supported by co-infusion of mobilized stem cells from a third party donor. Haematologica 2006;91:640–648

44. Castello S, Podesta M, Menditto VG et al. Intra-bone marrow injection of bone marrow and cord blood cells: an alternative way of transplantation associated with a higher seeding efficiency. Exp Hematol 2004;32:782–787

45. Raiola A.M, Ibatici A, Gualandi F et al. Direct intra-bone marrow transplant of cord blood cells: a way to overcome delayed engraftment in adult patients. Bone Marrow Transplant 2007;39(suppl 1):S31

46. Barker JN, Weisdorf DJ, DeFor TE et al. Rapid and complete donor chimerism in adult recipients of unrelated donor umbilical cord blood transplantation after reduced-intensity conditioning. Blood 2003;102:1915–1919

47. Brunstein CG, Weisdorf DJ, DeFor T et al. Markedly increased risk of Epstein-Barr virus-related complications with the addition of antithymocyte globulin to a nonmyeloablative conditioning prior to unrelated umbilical cord blood transplantation. Blood 2006;108: 2874–2880

48. Rocha V, Rio B, Brunstein C et al. Unrelated cord blood transplantation after reduced intensity conditioning (RIC) in adults with hematological malignancy. An EBMT-Eurocord-Netcord, Société Française de Greffe de Moelle et de Thérapie cellulaire and University of Minnesota collaborative study. Blood 2007;110:603a

49. Niehues T, Rocha V, Filipovich A et al. Factors affecting lymphocyte subset reconstitution after either related or unrelated cord blood transplantation in children – a Eurocord analysis. Br J Haematol 2001;114:42–48

50. Talvensaari K, Clave E, Douay C et al. A broad T-cell repertoire diversity and an efficient thymic function indicate a favorable long-term immune reconstitution after cord blood stem cell transplantation. Blood 2002;99:1458–1464

51. Montagna D, Locatelli F, Moretta A et al. T lymphocytes of recipient origin may contribute to the recovery of specific immune response toward viruses and fungi in children undergoing cord blood transplantation. Blood 2004;103:4322–4329

52. Hamza NS, Lisgaris M, Yadavalli G et al. Kinetics of myeloid and lymphocyte recovery and infectious complications after unrelated umbilical cord blood versus HLA-matched unrelated donor allogeneic transplantation in adults. Br J Haematol 2004;124:488–498

53. Parkman R, Cohen G, Carter SL et al. Successful immune reconstitution decreases leukemic relapse and improves survival in recipients of unrelated cord blood transplantation. Biol Blood Marrow Transplant 200612:919–927

54. Lubin B, Trachtenberg E, Saba J et al. Banking of sibling donor cord blood for children with malignant and non-malignant disease. In: McCurdy P (ed) Cord blood banking. Marcel Dekker, New York, 2003

55. Rubinstein P. Why cord blood? Hum Immunol 2006;67:398–404

56. Nathan DG, Orkin SH (eds). Nathan and Oski's hematology of infancy and childhood, vol 2, 5th edn. WB Saunders, Philadelphia, 1998

57. Katz-Benichou G. Umbilical cord blood banking: economic and therapeutic challenges. Int J Healthcare Technol Management 2007;8:464–477

58. American Academy of Pediatrics Section on Hematology/Oncology, American Academy of Pediatrics Section on Allergy/Immunology, Lubin BH, Shearer WT. Cord blood banking for potential future transplantation. Pediatrics 2007;119:165–170

59. Hayani A, Lampeter E, Viswanatha D et al. First report of autologous cord blood transplantation in the treatment of a child with leukemia. Pediatrics 2007;119:296–300

Human leukocyte antigen matching, compatibility testing and donor selection

Bronwen E Shaw

Introduction

One of the major factors which has contributed to improving the outcomes of stem cell transplantation is the progress which has been made in the field of human leukocyte antigens (HLA). This is evident not only in the progress made in developing techniques for rapid and accurate tissue typing, but also in the greatly improved understanding of the HLA system, its function and the impact of HLA matching on transplant complications.

The aim of this chapter is first to outline the background of the major histocompatibility complex (MHC)/HLA and provide the reader with a vocabulary for further discussion. Second, to discuss the current methods used for tissue typing of samples and the relative pros and cons of each. Third, to provide guidance, based on current studies in the literature, for the selection of the most appropriate (unrelated, UD) donor.

Numerous studies considering the impact of HLA matching on the outcome of UD transplantation have been published. An excellent review by Petersdorf et al is recommended.[1] This chapter does not aim to report these in an exhaustive fashion, but rather to select data from the most recent and comprehensive studies and present this in a manner that it is hoped will prove helpful to transplant physicians in donor selection.

The major histocompatibility complex and human leukocyte antigens

Introduction

The major histocompatibility complex (MHC) was discovered during studies in mice by Peter Gorer and George Snell.[2,3] These studies uncovered an antigen (antigen II) which they found to be involved in the rejection of tumors between different strains of mice. They subsequently showed the presence of antigens related to antigen II in other strains of mice and recognized that these were probable alleles of the same 'tumor resistance' gene. This first major histocompatibility locus they named H (later renamed H-2).

The identification of similar antigens in humans followed the description of antileukocyte antisera, detectable by agglutination assays, in the sera of patients who had received multiple blood transfusions.[4] Unlike the situation in mice, the human population is completely outbred, increasing the complexity of identification of human histocompatibility antigens enormously.

The HLA are molecules of the immune system that are essential to T-cell mediated adaptive immunity, in the context of particular peptides bound to the HLA molecule. Whilst each allele can bind and present hundreds or thousands of different peptides, the T-cell receptor recognizes the peptide sequence only if it is presented by the same MHC molecule as encountered during priming, a concept known as MHC restriction.[5] This primary role of presenting peptide to T-cells enables them to recognize and eliminate 'foreign' particles present in an individual, as well as to prevent the recognition of 'self' as foreign. These natural functions need to be overcome (or manipulated) in order to allow grafts between allogeneic individuals to be accepted.

Genetic organization

The MHC contains more than 200 genes, many of which have functions related to immunity, and is contained within 4.2 Mbp on the short arm of chromosome 6 at 6p21.3.[6] It is divided into three main regions: at the telomeric end, the HLA Class I region, at the centromeric end, the HLA Class II region and lying between these, the Class III region. A comprehensive map of the HLA region has been published and is periodically updated.[7] Of principal interest in transplantation are the six 'classic' HLA genes which encode the highly polymorphic loci: HLA-A, B and C (in the Class I region) and HLA-DR, DQ and DP (in the Class II region).

A number of other important molecules are present within these two clusters, such as the MHC Class I chain related (MIC) family of genes and the genes for both subunits of the transporter associated with antigen processing (TAP). The Class III region is densely packed with genes including those encoding complement factors and tumor necrosis factor (TNF).

Polymorphism

The HLA region is the most polymorphic (with HLA-B the most polymorphic gene) currently known in the human genome (www.sanger.ac.uk/HGP/Chr6/).[6] The overall structure of the Class I and Class II molecules is similar, with most of the polymorphism located in the peptide-binding groove (PBG), i.e. concentrated in the areas which influence PBG conformation, and the sites of interaction with the T-cell receptor.[8] This extensive polymorphism is thought to be a result of balancing selection due to the need for the immune system to keep up with and control infectious pathogens (evolutionary pressure).[6,9,10]

The HLA Class I loci consist of an α-chain which is highly polymorphic. The second polypeptide chain contributing to Class I molecular structure is the non-polymorphic B_2m encoded outwith the MHC on chromosome 15. The Class II molecules consist of both an α- and a β-chain, encoded by separate genes. The β-chain of each locus is highly polymorphic, in contrast to the limited polymorphism exhibited in the α-chains. In July 2006 there were 2437 named HLA alleles (Table 23.1) (www.ebi.ac.uk/imgt/hla).

Table 23.1 The number of HLA alleles currently named at each locus

HLA locus	Number of Class I alleles	HLA locus	Number of Class II alleles
HLA–A	479	HLA–DRB1	460
HLA–B	805	HLA–DRB3, 4, 5	74
HLA–C	257	HLA–DQA1	34
		HLA–DQB1	73
		HLA–DPA1	23
		HLA–DPB1	125

Table 23.2 An example of HLA nomenclature and its relation to tissue typing techniques

Typing method	Nomenclature
Serologic	A1
DNA-based: low resolution	A*01
DNA-based: medium resolution	A*0101/0102/0104N/0106/0109
DNA-based: high resolution	A*0101/0104N
DNA-based: allele level	A*0101

HLA nomenclature

The nomenclature for the HLA system has changed over the years, reflecting not only the changing techniques for defining HLA types (serologic tests versus DNA methodologies), but also the importance of a precise nomenclature: that is, defining HLA alleles at nucleotide level. The need for continuity was recognized at an early stage in the history of HLA, and a series of international conferences (and workshops) were initiated in order to standardize HLA nomenclature. At the 10th International Histocompatibility Workshop (IHW) the naming of HLA alleles based on nucleotide sequencing was addressed, with the gene name being followed by an asterisk (which acts as a separator) and then a four-digit allele name. The first two digits indicate the serologic group to which the allele belongs and the second two indicate the number of the allele within the group.[11] Since that time, the complexity of the HLA system has required that the original four-digit allele name be extended. In the current nomenclature the allele name can extend to eight digits, with the fifth and sixth digits representing synonymous mutations, the seventh and eighth representing intronic (or other non-coding) variants and the addition of an optional letter at the end of a sequence to indicate a major alteration in its expression (e.g. an 'N' for a null allele) (Table 23.2).

The National Marrow Donor Program (NMDP) has created allele codes to facilitate the reporting of HLA alleles, which are used extensively by most tissue typing laboratories and donor registries. These codes, describing a 'string' of alleles, allow typing laboratories to provide the maximum amount of information to transplant centers within the design constraints of search reports by narrowing the number of alleles which need to be considered. For example, a report of DRB1*01AD means that the typing is either DRB1*0101 or DRB1*0104, but not DRB1*0102 or DRB1*0103 (further information on how to use these codes is at: http://bioinformatics.nmdp.org/HLA/allele_code_lists.html).

Haplotypes and linkage disequilibrium

A haplotype is defined as a chromosomal combination of genes.[12] Certain combinations of alleles occur on HLA haplotypes within the population at a higher frequency than expected. This is due to the phenomenon of non-random gametic association (genetic linkage disequilibrium). The linkage disequilibrium (LD) between alleles at different loci is dependent on the magnitude of the recombination fraction observed between loci.[13] In the human MHC LD is more frequently observed between loci that are in close proximity, although in many cases it may extend across the entire Class I, II and III regions.

Thus, very strong LD is displayed between the α- and β-subunit of each of the HLA Class II molecules.[14–17] Likewise, HLA-B and HLA-C display strong LD, as do HLA-DRB1 and HLA-DQB1. The fact that the HLA-C and DQB1 type could be inferred from the HLA-B and DRB1 types, respectively, explains why tissue typing at these loci lagged behind that for HLA-A, B and DRB1. However, as knowledge of the polymorphism seen in HLA increased, it became clear that there were numerous circumstances in which LD was not completely predictive. It has been shown that a number of HLA-C alleles may associate with certain HLA-B alleles and that HLA-C mismatches are common in HLA-A and B serologically matched pairs,[18] as well as in pairs matched at HLA-A, B, DRB and DQB1.[19,20] For example, while over 95% of caucasoid individuals who have HLA-B*0702 will have HLA-Cw*0702, those who express B*1801 may express Cw*0701 (38%), Cw*1203 (38%) or Cw*0501 (34%).[21] Likewise, DRB1*0401 may be seen in association with either DQB1*0301 or DQB1*0302 in roughly similar proportions.[22]

This phenomenon is present for a large proportion of the common HLA-B, C and HLA-DRB1, DQB1 alleles, making it essential to perform accurate high-resolution tissue typing at both loci, especially in certain circumstance (such as those mentioned above). When developing a high-resolution typing strategy, it may be reasonable (particularly where funding is an issue) to accept a medium resolution (or string) for those alleles where strong LD exists, but have a policy for always achieving four-digit unambiguous types for those alleles with multiple possible associations, e.g. B44, B18. A basic familiarity with these concepts and associations will also aid the transplant physician in selecting the most appropriate donors identified at the search on whom to request confirmatory typing.

In view of the evidence for LD extending, in many cases, across the Class III region to incorporate alleles in the Class I and Class II regions (for example, the common caucasoid haplotype: A*0101, Cw*0701, B*0801, DRB1*0301, DQB1*0201[23]), the question arises as to whether this predicts for complete identity in the intervening region, such that an unrelated donor may be as well matched as a sibling donor for the entire MHC region. This is not the case, as recombination events are known to occur with increased frequency at certain points within the MHC,[24] such as between the HLA-DP loci and the other Class II loci[25] and around the TNF-α gene.[23]

Typing methods

Introduction

It is no longer appropriate to perform low-resolution/serologic typing alone for unrelated donors prior to selection for transplantation, as typing at DNA level is essential to uncover all allelic differences which exist between recipient and donor. The current gold standard is four-digit (allele level) typing for both of the alleles at the five major transplantation loci (HLA-A, B, C, DRB1, DQB1). In practice this may not always be achievable due to financial, technologic and other constraints. However, an appropriate strategy should be agreed between physician and typing laboratory to identify possible areas where compromise may be accepted and others where this may not. The technologies now available focus on cost-effectiveness, as well as rapid, high-throughput techniques. Many donor registries are rapidly accruing new donors and the strategy now is to perform medium-/high-resolution tissue typing at the time of joining the register in order to facilitate rapid and appropriate donor searches when necessary (see Chapter 21). In the current era, transplanters should not have to accept mistakes or inadequate typing.

An example of a contemporary typing strategy, employed by the Anthony Nolan Trust (ANT) typing laboratories, is as follows (www.anthonynolan.org.uk).

- Siblings and unrelated donors undergo the same initial typing strategy as each other and the patient.
- A serologic type is performed for HLA-A and B. This quickly ensures that the correct samples are being typed and excludes the presence of null alleles.
- Simultaneously medium-/high-resolution typing is done, using Luminex technology (see below) for HLA-A, B, C, DRB1, DQB1, as well as DRB3, 4, 5.
- Further discrimination of DRB1 to allele level is always performed (using PCR-SSP, see below).
- For patients receiving unrelated donor transplants, both patient and donor are further typed by high-/allele-level resolution (PCR-SSP or direct sequencing) for HLA-A, B, C and DPB1.

High-throughput laboratories such as this benefit greatly from the availability of commercial platforms and kits, which are validated and standardized, and for 'big users' the cost is kept low.

Resolution

Techniques can result in low-, medium-, high- or allele-level resolution typing. Low resolution provides a serologic (antigenic) type. Medium-resolution typing implies that the result obtained is more specific than a serologic type, but not discriminatory enough to provide a precise allele assignment, i.e. it can define specific allele groups (often as a 'string' of possible alleles); for example, an HLA-A*0201 allele may be typed as an HLA- A*0201/0207/0209/0215N/0218/0220/0224/0229, etc. with the test unable to discriminate further between these. High-resolution typing methods resolve the tissue type further, e.g. A*0201/0209 whereas allele-level typing results in there being no ambiguities, e.g. A*0201.

DNA-based techniques

All of the medium- to high-resolution techniques currently employed are PCR based. For PCR, only small amounts of DNA are required and this is most commonly acquired from peripheral blood or buccal swabs. As no viable cells are required there is less urgency in the transport and processing of samples. Commercial DNA extraction kits can be employed, and in many laboratories this procedure is automated/semi-robotic in an attempt to eradicate labeling errors. Samples of DNA can be stored in small aliquots, reducing the space needed and cost of storing huge numbers of samples.

Due to the sensitivity of PCR, this technique is prone to contamination. Therefore, laboratories must ensure scrupulous techniques as well as separation into 'pre-PCR' and 'post-PCR' areas.

Sequence-specific oligonucleotide probing (SSOP)

This technique is medium to high resolution, depending on the number of probes used. SSOP (dot blot) 26 involves the immobilization of the product amplified by PCR onto a nylon membrane. The polymorphisms present in the amplified product are then detected using a number of short oligonucleotide probes which have been labeled, designed to react with these sequences. This technique can also be 'reversed' (the reverse dot blot),[27] where the sequence-specific probes are immobilized and the labeled sample DNA hybridized to these.

The Luminex xMAP system is an SSO-based technique, which is available in kit form for HLA DNA typing (for loci HLA-A, B, C, DRB1, DRB3, 4, 5, DQB1 and DPB1). This is a multiplexed microsphere-based suspension array platform.[28] Up to 100 different reactions can be analyzed and reported in a single reaction vessel. Each microsphere has a different oligonucleotide attached to its surface. The PCR product, which is biotinylated, is then hybridized to the beads. Analysis of results is by flow cytometric technology using the Luminex FlowMetrix system. This system allows high-volume, rapid-throughput typing and is appropriate for laboratories typing large numbers of samples. Further benefits of this technology are that additional typing systems are available, such as KIR haplotype typing. The benefits of SSOP are that it is reliable, requires only one PCR reaction per locus and is relatively cheap. However, due to the hybridization step it is slower than SSP.

Sequence-specific priming (SSP)

SSP is a medium- to high-resolution technique dependent on the number of PCR amplification primers used.[29,30] Sequence-specific primers (a panel of primers designed to detect all known polymorphisms for the locus being typed) are used for the PCR reaction. The products are then run on agarose gels and the HLA type is inferred from the presence or absence of specific bands from the various PCRs.

SSP is more rapid then SSOP and suited to typing small numbers of samples simultaneously. Fewer ambiguities are obtained using this method. The use of subtyping kits (i.e. the primers included are specific for a particular allele group at one locus) provides results at allele-level resolution.

Reference strand-mediated conformation analysis (RSCA)

RSCA is a method which provides medium- or high-resolution typing, depending on the locus/allele of interest.[31] A PCR reaction for a particular locus is performed. The product is then hybridized to a specific fluorescent-labeled reference DNA fragment. The sample is then separated, by mobility, by non-denaturing polyacrylamide gel electrophoresis (PAGE) in an automated DNA sequencer. These results are compared to a reference from which the alleles can be inferred. New alleles can also be identified by this technique.

Sequence-based typing (SBT)

This is a high-resolution technique, which employs a direct approach by determining the nucleotide sequence of the polymorphic exons of the alleles.[32,33] A PCR is performed, aimed at amplifying both alleles at a given locus. The two alleles are then sequenced as a mixture on a polyacrylamide gel, after the addition of fluorescent probes. The results are then analyzed using computer programs which identify the areas of heterozygosity. From comparisons of the patterns obtained with those expected for all combinations of alleles, the possible types in the sample can be inferred by the program. Allele-level typing may also be achieved by locus-specific sequencing. However, as the number of HLA polymorphisms has increased, it may be necessary to perform a second round of allele group-specific sequencing in order to achieve a single allele result.

SBT is slower than SSP, and an up-to-date database of all HLA alleles is required to efficiently resolve all ambiguities.

Serologic typing

This technique uses antibodies to detect antigens on the cell surface. A major limitation to this technique is that only a minority of the HLA

Class I and II alleles have a serologic equivalent, and are thus not recognized. This technique should only be used in combination with others.

Functional assays

Although initially the mixed lymphocyte culture (MLC) and cytotoxic T-lymphocyte precursor assay (CTLp) were widely employed by tissue typing laboratories as a form of cellular cross-match before transplantation, to predict for HLA Class II and Class I incompatibility respectively, this has largely been superseded by DNA typing methods. This is due to the speed and accuracy which DNA methodologies offer over functional assays, as well as the fact that the MLC or CTLp was not found to reliably predict for transplant complications.[20]

Although these assays are now not routinely used in most typing laboratories, a place for them in the future should not be excluded. Ideally, an appropriate functional assay should be rapid and reliable. It should provide predictive information prior to transplantation, including reactions due to non-HLA genetic factors and also identifying permissive versus non-permissive mismatches. Such methods would require validation before typing laboratories could use them with confidence.

Selecting the appropriate (unrelated) donor

HLA factors

The 'perfect' donor

Unfortunately the 'perfect donor' does not yet exist – at least, no formal algorithm may be applied to donor selection, which will always predict for a favorable outcome. In current transplantation practice the 'perfect' donor, at least with regards to HLA matching, is thought to be one who is matched at the allele level for HLA-A, B, C, DRB1, DQB1, i.e. a 10/10 match. There is also, however, evidence that some degree of mismatch may be tolerated in certain circumstances.

A 10/10 match?

The largest international and collaborative study to date is that performed by the International Histocompatibility Working Group (IHWG) in Hematopoietic Cell Transplantation, which has reported on outcomes in 4796 UD transplant pairs, receiving myeloablative conditioning regimens.[34] The pairs have been submitted from over 30 transplant centers/registers all over the world, and thus are demographically and clinically heterogeneous. Of those in the study, 61% were 10/10 matched and 39% were mismatched for a single allele or antigen. In this cohort, there was a significant survival detriment to having an HLA mismatch, with the hazard of mortality (adjusted for disease stage, age, and ethnicity) conferred by a single HLA mismatch being 1.20 (95% confidence interval (CI) 1.12–1.30; p = <0.0001). An important question asked by the investigators was whether the impact of a single mismatch differed dependent on the disease stage of the recipient. Interestingly, the impact of a single mismatch was found to be most marked in those with low-risk disease (hazard ratio (HR) 1.50; 95% CI 1.28–1.76, p = < 0.0001), less marked in those with intermediate-risk disease (HR 1.15: 95% CI 1.0–1.29, p = 0.02) and not statistically significantly different in those with high-risk disease (HR 1.06; 95% CI 0.92–1.22, p = 0.43). This phenomenon has previously been reported in a study of 948 UD transplant pairs,[35] which showed a significantly increased mortality in those with low-risk disease and a single HLA mismatch (HR 2.27), while a single HLA mismatch had no significant effect on mortality in those with either intermediate- (HR 1.0) or high-risk (HR 1.19) disease. The increase in mortality in

this study was attributable to an increase in transplant-related mortality (TRM) (HR 2.13).

Further support for the permissibility of selecting a donor with a single mismatch comes from the experience in reduced-intensity conditioned/non-myeloablative transplants. In a study of 144 recipients of T-cell depleted reduced-intensity conditioned UD transplants,[36] there was no significant difference in overall survival (OS) between matched or one antigen mismatched grafts, compared to those with two or more mismatches (p = 0.005). The only deleterious effect in this cohort due to a single HLA mismatch (equal risk to those with multiple mismatches) was an increase in the rate of primary graft failure (6/47,13% versus 1/93, 1%, p = 0.006).

These data are reiterated in an analysis of the impact of HLA matching on outcome in 423 UD pairs undertaken by the Anthony Nolan Research Institute (ANRI).[37] These were transplants which took place at multiple centers within the UK. As is the practice in the UK, the majority of patients had conditioning protocols including T-cell depleting agents, most commonly CAMPATH. Of the pairs, 67% were matched for 10/10 alleles, while 24% had a single mismatch and 9% had multiple mismatches. Those matched for their HLA loci had a significantly better OS at 3 years than mismatched pairs (47% versus 40%, p = 0.040). However, in patients with a single HLA mismatch the OS was 43%, while this was 30% in those with multiple mismatches (Fig. 23.1), i.e. there was a significantly worse OS in those with multiple mismatches, but not in those pairs with a single mismatch. This suggests that single HLA mismatches may be tolerated in the setting of T-cell depletion. However, despite the similar OS, the early TRM (at 1 year) was 40% in pairs with a single mismatch compared to 31% in matched pairs (Fig. 23.2). This may partially be explained by an increase in the incidence of acute graft-versus-host disease (a-GvHD) in the single antigen-mismatched group (59%) compared to the HLA-matched group (48%).

A study including 114 chronic myeloid leukemia (CML) patients who underwent myeloablative transplants (1/3 of whom received antithymocyte globulin (ATG)) showed a significant 5-year survival detriment (HR 2.43, p = 0.0019), and increase in TRM (HR 2.58, p = 0.0027), in patients with a 9 or less/10 match.[38] The authors found that the influence of HLA incompatibilities was 'scarcely evident' in patients receiving a T-cell depleted graft.

A large study of 1874 transplant pairs reported by the NMDP[39] considered the overall survival in 8/8 matched transplants (having

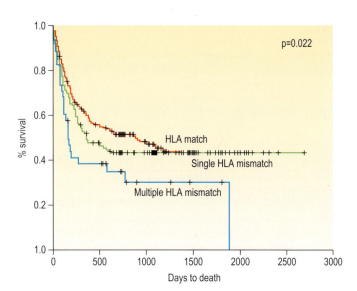

Figure 23.1

In a cohort of 423 patients transplanted in the UK from an UD, a single HLA mismatch is tolerated with regards to overall survival, while multiple mismatches are not.

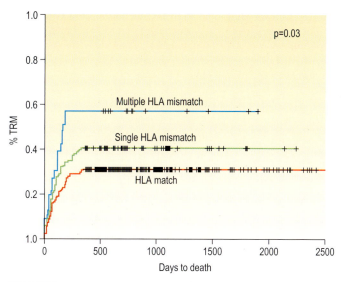

Figure 23.2
In a cohort of 423 patients transplanted in the UK from an UD, while TRM at 1 year is increased in those with a graft with a single HLA mismatch, it is significantly higher in those receiving grafts mismatched for multiple HLA alleles.

shown no deleterious effect due to DQB1 mismatches, this locus was excluded from this part of the analysis). In a multivariate analysis, the authors report a highly significant survival advantage for 8/8 matched pairs compared to those with one (RR 1.32) or two (RR 1.53) mismatches (p = 0.0003). This is mirrored by a significant rise in the relative risk of grades III–IV GvHD, with one (RR 1.53) or two (RR 1.78) mismatches (p = 0.001).

Thus, although the outcome using a 10/10 matched donor is best, using a 9/10 matched donor has been associated with an equally favorable outcome, in terms of overall survival, in those patients with later disease stage, or where T-cell depletion and/or reduced-intensity conditioning (RIC) transplant protocols have been used. These data together suggest that the choice of donor in individual circumstances may differ. In some circumstances it may be reasonable to select a donor with a single HLA mismatch, rather than delaying the procedure in order to find a 10/10 matched donor, without expecting a deleterious outcome (see Chapter 21 for discussion on waiting times).

A 9/10 match (or choice between mismatched donors)

A dilemma then, which often faces transplant physicians, is how to select between mismatched donors when no 10/10 matched donor is available. Does the locus at which the donor is mismatched matter? Is there evidence for 'permissive' mismatches at certain loci? Is an allelic mismatch 'better' than an antigenic mismatch?

In the early years of transplantation, when employing only serologic (or even medium-resolution) typing techniques pretransplantation, many mismatches remained 'hidden', thus making the interpretation of transplant outcomes, based on HLA matching status, confusing and inaccurate. The first strong data to support allele-level typing were presented by the Fred Hutchinson Cancer Research Center (FHCRC) in 1995.[40] In this analysis, the presence of an allele-level mismatch for DRB1 was significantly correlated with increased a-GvHD, increased TRM and a worse overall survival, in pairs serologically matched for HLA-A, B and DRB1. Based on these data, the selection of a donor matched at allele level for DRB1 became the gold standard in UD transplants, a situation which still exists today. It was some years before studies using equally precise methods of tissue typing for other HLA alleles were reported, and the interpretation of these studies may be influenced by the selection bias for DRB1 matching. A more recent study by the same group, reporting the results in

467 pairs transplanted from UD for CML,[1] showed a single Class II allele mismatch (DRB1 or DQB1) to be well tolerated with regard to OS (HR 1.1), although associated with an increase in a-GvHD (45% compared to 32% in 10/10 matched). In the same study a single Class I allele mismatch was well tolerated with regard to a-GvHD, but resulted in a greater HR for mortality (1.4).

The IHWG has addressed this question.[34] Single mismatches for HLA-A, B and C were significantly associated with a worse OS. In contrast, mismatches for a single HLA-DRB1 or DQB1 allele did not confer a significant survival detriment. A possible explanation for the lack of impact of a DRB1 mismatch is that there were relatively fewer DRB1-mismatched pairs in the analysis (111, compared to 414 at HLA-A, 179 at HLA-B, 744 at HLA-C and 239 at HLA-DQB1). Alternatively, it may be that the transplant procedure was modified in some way in these recipients in view of the knowledge of the mismatch.

HLA-DQB1 emerges in these data as a locus which may potentially be mismatched without significant harmful effect. This is supported by the data from the NMDP.[39] HLA-DQB1 was the only classic locus where mismatching was not shown to result in a significantly detrimental effect on overall survival. There was also no significant impact on acute or chronic GvHD or engraftment, leading the authors to suggest that this locus may be mismatched without deleterious effects. There are, however, data to suggest that in multiply mismatched patients, those with a DQB1 mismatch do worse than those without a DQB1 mismatch.[35]

In contrast, they have shown that mismatches for HLA-A, B, C or DRB1 result in a significant survival detriment. Interestingly, only HLA-A mismatches were associated with an increase in GvHD, in both the acute (RR 1.41, p = 0.005) and chronic (RR 1.35, p = 0.006) forms.

The analysis from the ANRI in 423 pairs also found no significant differences in outcome associated with mismatches for HLA-DRB1 or DQB1 (although the number of mismatches at these loci was small). In addition, there was no significant impact of mismatching for HLA-A. In contrast, there was a highly significant survival disadvantage to an HLA-B mismatch (log rank, p = 0.0005). This was contributed to by an increase in TRM at 1 year in the mismatched pairs (p = 0.072), as well as an increased rate of grade III–IV a-GvHD (11% versus 4%), although these were not statistically significant findings. Although HLA-C mismatched pairs were not shown to have a statistically different rate of OS, the incidence of a-GvHD was increased in the mismatched group compared to the matched group (57% versus 48%). The impact of this locus on chronic GvHD was even more striking. Mismatched pairs had a significantly greater risk of developing c-GvHD than did matched pairs (p = 0.002). This was reflected by an increased in limited (43% versus 28%) as well as extensive disease (21% versus 15%). In this study the presence of limited c-GvHD was significantly associated with a lower mortality, most likely explaining the lack of negative impact of mismatching at this locus on OS.[37] A survival detriment due to mismatching for HLA-B has also been reported in a study of 100 patients receiving T-cell depleted myeloablative transplants.[41]

Data reported by the Japanese Marrow Donor Program (JMDP) on 1298 pairs[42] found the worst 3-year survival to be in pairs mismatched for either HLA-A or B (39.9% compared to 65.4% in 10/10 matched pairs) (unfortunately they do not differentiate between these loci in the text, but there appear to be a roughly equal number of mismatches for either). This was true in both standard and high-risk disease. This survival detriment was due to an increase in 3-year TRM (54.6% in HLA-A or B mismatches compared to 27.7% in matched), associated with an increase in the incidence of severe acute GvHD as well as in the incidence and extent of chronic GvHD. Although HLA-C and DRB1 were both associated with a significant increase in a-GvHD, neither impacted significantly on OS or TRM. HLA-DQB1 mismatches were not found to be associated significantly with any adverse outcome. Any combination of two or more mismatches resulted in a worse overall survival.

An interesting aspect highlighted by the IHWG report is the possibility of 'permissive' mismatches, i.e. that certain mismatches within one locus may be tolerated, whilst others are not. They found that a single HLA-A mismatch was poorly tolerated in JMDP transplants (HR 2.27, 95% CI 1.14–4.53) while being less detrimental in the non-JMDP population (HR 1.24, 95% CI 0.92–1.67). In contrast, mismatches at HLA-C were well tolerated among the JMDP pairs (HR 1.05, 95% CI 0.50–2.23) but poorly tolerated among non-JMDP transplants (HR 1.68, 95%CI 1.36–2.08). On closer analysis, this effect is seen to be due to the differences in the actual allele mismatches in these separate populations.[43] The predominant HLA-A allele mismatch in the JMDP population was A*0201/A*0206, a mismatch which was less common in the non-JMDP population. When the effects of this mismatch on mortality were analyzed (compared to those with matched HLA-A alleles), there was a significant survival disadvantage (HR 1.58, p = < 0.001) irrespective of the ethnic background. No other particular HLA-A allele mismatch gave significant effects, although many were at a much lower number. Thus, this particular mismatch can be referred to as a 'non-permissive' mismatch, and explains why the effect of an HLA-A mismatch in the JMDP cohort was greater. Preliminary results show the presence of similarly non-permissive mismatches at other loci, and further study of these will greatly aid our ability to best choose between mismatched donors. Of course, as can be appreciated, a comprehensive analysis of permissive mismatches at all loci will require the study of large numbers of ethnically diverse transplant populations, who have been HLA typed at high resolution, and for whom complete clinical data are available.

Allelic versus antigenic mismatches

As a general rule, the difference between HLA allele and antigen mismatches lies in the fact that antigen mismatches are characterized by amino acid substitutions important in both peptide binding and T-cell recognition, whereas allelic mismatches are characterized by amino acid substitution only in the peptide-binding regions.[44] Allelic mismatches are usually not recognized by serologic typing techniques, leading to the question of whether these mismatches are likely to be as allogeneic as antigenic mismatches. In fact, there is an argument that the opposite situation is true. A report describing rejection of transplanted bone marrow induced by a single amino acid variant demonstrates that small differences are sufficient for development of in vivo alloreactivity.[45] Additionally, it has been suggested that limited differences may induce stronger alloresponses than numerous differences[46,47] because the foreign MHC molecule closely resembles self-MHC and is therefore more likely to cross-react with self-educated T-cells. Indeed, recent data from Heemskerk et al[48] showed that, in a substantial number of cases, Class I MHC molecules with numerous sequence differences did not elicit an allogeneic cytotoxic T-lymphocyte response.

An attempt to address this question was made in the large cohort reported by the NMDP.[39] This study found that the deleterious effects associated with low-resolution mismatches at HLA-A, B, C or DRB1 were more evident than the effects seen with high-resolution mismatches, implying that the alloreactive effects of an antigenic mismatch are greater than an allelic mismatch (however, they do remark that the number of patients within each of these subgroups may be too small to formally prove a true difference in outcome).

In a different study,[49] it was shown that while a single HLA Class I antigen mismatch significantly increased the risk of graft rejection, a single allele mismatch was tolerated. This risk was exacerbated if the recipient was HLA homozygous at the mismatched HLA locus. A later study reported by the same group[35] found no difference in the impact of allele or antigen mismatches on mortality. The study from the ANRI showed no difference on survival dependent on whether mismatches were allelic or antigenic.

Scoring (predictive) matching systems

Attempts have been made to create scoring systems which will electronically predict the likelihood of allogenicity between two mismatched pairs. An example of this is the HistoCheck software,[50] which aims to provide a score which takes into account both the functional and the structural difference between two HLA alleles at one locus. The predictive value of HistoCheck is based on the presumption that transplant success is improved by selecting a donor with an HLA type most similar to the patient, but as discussed above, this may not always be the case. In fact, a study performed by the ANRI considering 26 HLA-A mismatched pairs found that the score generated by the program was not correlated with complications or transplant outcomes.[51] Nevertheless, in the future, as larger studies on which these data can be based are performed and functional tests become more sophisticated, the applicability and appropriateness of such scoring systems are likely to increase. Certainly, a validated and efficient system would be of great benefit to transplant physicians.

Other HLA alleles

Thus far, most transplant analyses have concentrated on the effects of the five 'classic' HLA loci. However, we know that polymorphism is found at the other HLA loci (classic and non-classic molecules) as well as other non-HLA genetic determinants within the MHC region (e.g. TAP, MIC A and B). The most polymorphic of these loci is DPB1 (discussed below), which in fact displays more polymorphism than DQB1. In contrast, the degree of polymorphism at other loci is low and/or the LD is very strong between these and their neighboring loci (see above, Linkage disequilibrium). Thus most clinical studies have not concentrated on mismatching for these loci and the available data are minimal.[52–54] Nevertheless, as polymorphism does exist in these molecules, the possibility of an impact of mismatching on outcome, as suggested by some studies, cannot be discounted.

HLA-DPB1

Although HLA-DPB1 is highly polymorphic, the analysis of its impact on transplantation lagged behind that of the other classic transplantation loci. A number of reasons for this exist, the most compelling being the weak LD between HLA-DP and the rest of the HLA Class II molecules,[25] reducing the probability of finding a donor who is matched at DP in addition to the other five HLA loci. Studies investigating the mismatch frequency of this locus have reported figures of between 5.31% and 10.9% in sibling donors[55,56] and between 75% and 89% in UD.[16,57,58]

Despite this, there is now strong evidence supporting the allogenicity of this molecule and firmly establishing an impact due to matching status on transplantation outcome.[57–64] In addition, convincing evidence for the existence of 'permissive mismatches' has been reported for this locus.[63–65]

A number of studies have shown a significant increase in acute GvHD in pairs mismatched for one or two DPB1 alleles, with some of these demonstrating a 'threshold effect', i.e. the effect of two DPB1 mismatches being significantly greater than one.[57–62,66] In one study this resulted in an increased TRM and a consequently worse overall survival.[66] However, the majority of studies have shown no effect on overall survival despite an increase in a-GvHD. The largest of these studies to date is from the DPB1 working group of the IHWC[61] which found a significantly higher risk of both grade II–IV a-GvHD (HR 1.33, p < 0.0001) and grade III–IV a-GvHD (HR 1.26, p = 0.0007) in those pairs that were mismatched for DPB1 compared to those that were matched, without showing a threshold effect. TRM has not thus far been analyzed by this group.

A study of 423 patients, performed by the ANRI, examined the outcome of UK (largely T-cell depleted) transplants with respect to DPB1 matching status.[62] A trend was seen towards an increased incidence of a-GvHD in those pairs who were incompatible for DPB1 (93/180, 52%) compared to pairs with DPB1 compatibility (27/71, 38%) (chi-squared test, p = 0.051). Much more compelling was the highly significant increase in relapse in DPB1-matched pairs, whether in those matched for 10/10 alleles (74% as compared to 56%, log rank, p = 0.001) (Fig. 23.3) or in those with any additional HLA mismatches (i.e. 9 or less/10) (Fig. 23.4). Although the survival in the group overall was not significantly different dependent on DPB1 status, in acute lymphoblastic leukemia (ALL), DPB1-matched pairs had a significantly worse overall survival (log rank, p = 0.025).

These findings have now been repeated in the IHWC study[61] of 5930 patient–donor pairs. There was a significantly protective effect

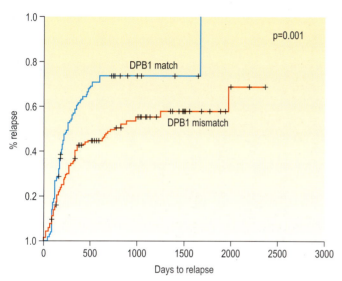

Figure 23.3
In a cohort of 282 patients (matched for 10/10 HLA alleles with their UD) a DPB1 mismatch is significantly associated with a reduced relapse rate.

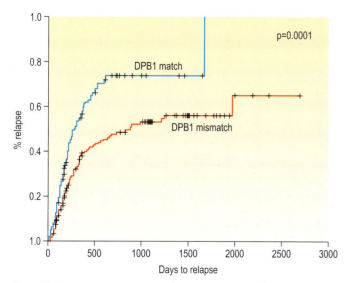

Figure 23.4
In a cohort of 423 patients the presence of a DPB1 mismatch is significantly associated with a reduced relapse rate.

on disease relapse in those pairs that were mismatched for DPB1 (HR 0.82, p = 0.01) compared to the pairs that were matched. Interestingly, this effect was marked in 10/10 matched pairs but, unlike the earlier study, not significant in pairs with mismatches for any other HLA alleles. A possible explanation for these discrepant results is the degree to which the different cohort included T-cell depletion as part of the conditioning protocol.

As mentioned above, recent data provide evidence for 'permissive' mismatches at the DPB1 locus.[63–65] Zino et al performed a functional 'epitope-based' analysis, in which they classified different DPB1 mismatches into those of lesser or greater immunogenicity, based on a shared T-cell epitope.[64] These data are based on a DPB1*0901 specific T-cell clone which they identified in a patient who rejected their graft (from a two allele-mismatched family member).[67] This T-cell clone has been shown, in the subsequent work, to cross-react strongly with certain alleles (termed group 1: DPB1*1001 and 1701), less strongly with other alleles (termed group 2: DPB1*0301, *1401 and *4501) and not at all with a large number of other alleles (termed group 3: including DPB1*0401, *0402, *0201, *1901 and *4601). Using their scoring system, transplant pairs could have a permissive or a non-permissive match. They analyzed 118 transplant pairs using this system and reported a significant increase in a-GvHD (grades II–IV) and 3-year TRM in pairs with a non-permissive mismatch (in a GvH or HvG direction), compared to those with a permissive mismatch. They did not see a significant impact on relapse or overall survival in their analysis. More recently, the same group have shown, in 72 patients receiving UD-HSCT for thalassemia, that a non-permissive mismatch in the HvG direction is associated with a significantly increased risk of rejection and consequent decreased thalassemia-free survival.[63]

Non-HLA factors

It is well recognized that even when the MHC loci are identical between the donor and the recipient (and in sibling transplants), complications may still occur. Thus, it is likely that other genetic factors exist, which may be mismatched between recipient and donor and can be implicated in outcome. The majority of these are far less well studied than HLA, and a discussion of these studies is beyond the scope of this chapter. However, many have been shown to impact significantly on outcome, including minor histocompatibility antigens,[68–71] cytokine gene polymorphisms,[72,73] and KIR haplotypes[74–77] among others.

In addition, it is important to remember the impact of other donor-related factors, such as donor age, CMV status and gender,[15,78–87] as well as donation-related factors, including route of donation and CD34 cell dose,[88–93] on transplant outcome.

Conclusion

There is no doubt that one of the factors implicated in the dramatic improvements in the outcome of UD transplantation over the years is the advances in HLA testing and matching and the understanding of donor selection issues. Nevertheless, as yet there is still no 'perfect' donor and much work remains to be done. Additional ways of analyzing HLA are in development, such as determining matching for haplotypes, rather than just for alleles. Not only are issues related to HLA important, but there is also growing interest and evidence that non-HLA genetic factors (e.g. KIR, minor histocompatibility antigens, NOD2 and cytokine polymorphisms) play an increasingly important role. In addition, non-HLA factors such as gender, cell dose, CMV status and stem cell source certainly influence outcome.

Ultimately, an algorithm for selecting the best donor should include all available genetic information as well as taking into account specific donor characteristics. In addition, this should be 'targeted' to the individual patient, taking into account factors such as disease type and stage.

The importance of international collaborations and data sharing cannot be overstated given the huge numbers of pairs that will need to be studied in order to dissect out the relative importance of all the factors discussed.

Summary of donor selection strategy (human leukocyte antigen matching)

1. Most data available suggest that a 10/10 matched donor is the best choice. Consideration should be given to typing the HLA-DPB1 locus in certain patients/circumstances. If more than one donor is available, the most appropriate DPB1 type could be chosen. If only one donor is available, modifications to conditioning/immunosuppression protocols could be considered.

2. In many circumstances the use of a 9/10 match has been associated with an outcome equally as good as a 10/10 match. However, the individual allele at which the donor is mismatched is likely to be important.

   • Most studies suggest that an HLA-DQB1 mismatch is the least likely to cause an adverse outcome.

   • Many recent analyses do not show a worse outcome due to DRB1 mismatches. This should be interpreted with some caution, given that donor selection strategies were likely to actively avoid DRB1 mismatches over the time that most of these studies were performed, thus potentially skewing the data.

   • Most studies report a worse outcome with Class I mismatches, but the locus-specific effects are conflicting. This is likely to reflect the allelic variation within certain populations. There is evidence that this may reflect the existence of 'permissive' mismatches. Advice in choosing between an HLA-A, B or C mismatched donor should be based on local studies and experience.

3. Two or more mismatches for the classic HLA alleles are usually associated with a poorer outcome.

4. There are no strong data currently available to suggest that allelic or antigenic mismatches are superior and should always be chosen out of preference.

References

1. Petersdorf EW, Anasetti C, Martin PJ, Hansen JA. Tissue typing in support of unrelated hematopoietic cell transplantation. Tissue Antigens 2003;61:1–11

2. Gorer P. The genetic and antigenic basis of tumour transplantation. J Pathol Bacteriol 1937;44:691–697

3. Gorer P, Lyman S, Snell G. Studies on the genetic and antigenic basis of tumour transplantation. Linkage between a histocompatibility gene and 'fused' in mice. Proc R Soc London Ser B 1948;135:499–505

4. Dausset J. Leuko-agglutinins IV. Leuko-agglutinins and blood transfusion. Vox Sang 1954;4:190–198

5. Zinkernagel RM, Doherty PC. Restriction of in vitro T-cell-mediated cytotoxicity in lymphocytic choriomeningitis within a syngeneic or semiallogeneic system. Nature 1974;248:701–702

6. MHC Sequencing Consortium. Complete sequence and gene map of a human major histocompatibility complex. Nature 1999;401:921–923

7. Campbell RD, Trowsdale J. A map of the human major histocompatibility complex. Immunol Today 1993;14:349–352

8. Parham P, Lawlor DA, Lomen CE, Ennis PD. Diversity and diversification of HLA-A,B,C alleles. J Immunol 1989;142:3937–3950

9. Hughes AL, Nei M. Pattern of nucleotide substitution at major histocompatibility complex class I loci reveals overdominant selection. Nature 1988;335:167–170

10. Parham P, Ohta T. Population biology of antigen presentation by MHC class I molecules. Science 1996;272:67–74

11. WHO Nomenclature Committee. Nomenclature for factors of the HLA system, 1987. Tissue Antigens 1988;32:177–187

12. Ceppellini R, Curtoni ES, Mattiuz PL et al. Genetics of leukocyte antigens: a family study of segregation and linkage. In: Curtoni ES, Mattiuz PL, Tosi RM (eds) Histocompatibility testing, vol. 1. Munksgaard, Copenhagen, 1967:149–187

13. Cavalli-Sforza LL, Bodmer WF. The genetics of human populations. Dover Publications, New York, 1999

14. Bodmer JG, Marsh SGE, Albert ED et al. Nomenclature for factors of the HLA system, 1991. WHO Nomenclature Committee for factors of the HLA system. Tissue Antigens 1992;39:161–173

15. Petersdorf EW, Longton GM, Anasetti C et al. Definition of HLA-DQ as a transplantation antigen. Proc Natl Acad Sci USA 1996;93:15358–15363

16. Hurley CK, Baxter-Lowe LA, Begovich AB et al. The extent of HLA class II allele level disparity in unrelated bone marrow transplantation: analysis of 1259 National Marrow Donor Program donor-recipient pairs. Bone Marrow Transplant 2000;25: 385–393

17. Sage DA, Evans PR, Howell WM. HLA DPA1-DPB1 linkage disequilibrium in the British caucasoid population. Tissue Antigens 1994;44:335–338

18. Scott I, O'Shea J, Bunce M et al. Molecular typing shows a high level of HLA class I incompatibility in serologically well matched donor/patient pairs: implications for unrelated bone marrow donor selection. Blood 1998;92:4864–4871

19. Petersdorf EW, Stanley JF, Martin PJ, Hansen JA. Molecular diversity of the HLA-C locus in unrelated marrow transplantation. Tissue Antigens 1994;44:93–99

20. El Kassar N, Legouvello S, Joseph CM et al. High resolution HLA class I and II typing and CTLp frequency in unrelated donor transplantation: a single-institution retrospective study of 69 BMTs. Bone Marrow Transplant 2001;27:35–43

21. Bunce M, Barnardo MC, Procter J et al. High resolution HLA-C typing by PCR-SSP: identification of allelic frequencies and linkage disequilibria in 604 unrelated random UK Caucasoids and a comparison with serology. Tissue Antigens 1996;48:680–691

22. Stastny P, Carcassi C, Mehra NK et al. HLA-DR4, DR53. In: Charron D (ed) HLA. Genetic diversity of HLA. Functional and medical implications, vol. 1. EDK, Paris, 1997:100–102

23. Vorechovsky I, Kralovicova J, Laycock MD et al. Short tandem repeat (STR) haplotypes in HLA: an integrated 50-kb STR/linkage disequilibrium/gene map between the RING3 and HLA-B genes and identification of STR haplotype diversification in the class III region. Eur J Hum Genet 2001;9:590–598

24. Foissac A, Salhi M, Cambon-Thomsen A. Microsatellites in the HLA region: 1999 update. Tissue Antigens 2000;55:477–509

25. Begovich AB, McClure GR, Suraj VC et al. Polymorphism, recombination, and linkage disequilibrium within the HLA class II region. J Immunol 1992;148:249–258

26. Tiercy JM, Morel C, Freidel AC et al. Selection of unrelated donors for bone marrow transplantation is improved by HLA class II genotyping with oligonucleotide hybridization. Proc Natl Acad Sci USA 1991;88:7121–7125

27. Trachtenberg EA, Erlich HA. DNA-based HLA typing for cord blood stem cell transplantation. J Hematother 1996;5:295–300

28. Dunbar SA. Applications of Luminex xMAP technology for rapid, high-throughput multiplexed nucleic acid detection. Clin Chim Acta 2006;363:71–82

29. Bunce M, Welsh KI. Rapid DNA typing for HLA-C using sequence-specific primers (PCR-SSP): identification of serological and non-serologically defined HLA-C alleles including several new alleles. Tissue Antigens 1994;43:7–17

30. Krausa P, Bodmer JG, Browning MJ. Defining the common subtypes of HLA A9, A10, A28 and A19 by use of ARMS/PCR. Tissue Antigens 1993;42:91–99

31. Arguello R, Pay AL, McDermott A et al. Complementary strand analysis: a new approach for allelic separation in complex polyallelic genetic systems. Nucleic Acids Res 1997;25:2236–2238

32. Rozemuller EH, Bouwens AG, van Oort E et al. Sequencing-based typing reveals new insight in HLA-DPA1 polymorphism. Tissue Antigens 1995;45:57–62

33. Scheltinga SA, Johnston-Dow LA, White CB et al. A generic sequencing based typing approach for the identification of HLA-A diversity. Hum Immunol 1997;57:120–128

34. Petersdorf EW, Gooley T, Malkki M et al, for the International Histocompatibility Working Group in Hematopoietic Cell Transplantation. Clinical significance of donor-recipient HLA matching on survival after myeloablative hematopoietic cell transplantation from unrelated donors. Tissue Antigens 2007;69(suppl 1):25–30

35. Petersdorf EW, Anasetti C, Martin PJ et al. Limits of HLA mismatching in unrelated hematopoietic cell transplantation. Blood 2004;104:2976–2980

36. Shaw BE, Russell NH, Devereux S et al. The impact of donor factors on primary non-engraftment in recipients of reduced intensity conditioned transplants from unrelated donors. Haematologica 2005;90:1562–1569

37. Shaw BE. Understanding the immunogenetic and clinical factors which influence the outcome of haematopoietic stem cell transplantation using unrelated donors. Anthony Nolan Research Institute. University of London, London, 2004:315

38. Tiercy JM, Passweg J, van Biezen A et al. Isolated HLA-C mismatches in unrelated donor transplantation for CML. Bone Marrow Transplant 2004;34:249–255

39. Flomenberg N, Baxter-Lowe LA, Confer D et al. Impact of HLA class I and class II high-resolution matching on outcomes of unrelated donor bone marrow transplantation: HLA-C mismatching is associated with a strong adverse effect on transplantation outcome. Blood 2004;104:1923–1930

40. Petersdorf EW, Longton GM, Anasetti C et al. The significance of HLA-DRB1 matching on clinical outcome after HLA-A, B, DR identical unrelated donor marrow transplantation. Blood 1995;86:1606–1613

41. Perz JB, Sergeant R, Szydlo R et al. Impact of HLA Class I and Class II DNA high-resolution HLA typing on outcome in adult unrelated stem cell transplantation after in vivo T-cell depletion with CAMPATH 1H: a single centre experience in 100 patients (abstract). Blood 2005;106:1804

42. Morishima Y, Sasazuki T, Inoko H et al. The clinical significance of human leukocyte antigen (HLA) allele compatibility in patients receiving a marrow transplant from serologically HLA-A, HLA-B, and HLA-DR matched unrelated donors. Blood 2002;99: 4200–4206

43. Morishima Y, Kawase T, Malkki M, Petersdorf EW. Effect of HLA-A2 allele disparity on clinical outcome in hematopoietic cell transplantation from unrelated donors. Tissue Antigens 2007;69(suppl 1):31–35

44. Bjorkman PJ, Saper MA, Samraoui B et al. Structure of the human class I histocompatibility antigen, HLA-A2. Nature 1987;329:506–512

45. Fleischhauer K, Kernan NA, O'Reilly RJ et al. Bone marrow-allograft rejection by T lymphocytes recognizing a single amino acid difference in HLA-B44. N Engl J Med 1990;323:1818–1822

46. Lechler RI, Lombardi G, Batchelor JR et al. The molecular basis of alloreactivity. Immunol Today 1990;11:83–88

47. Housset D, Malissen B. What do TCR-pMHC crystal structures teach us about MHC restriction and alloreactivity? Trends Immunol 2003;24:429–437

48. Heemskerk MB, Roelen DL, Dankers MK et al. Allogeneic MHC class I molecules with numerous sequence differences do not elicit a CTL response. Hum Immunol 2005;66:969–976

49. Petersdorf EW, Hansen JA, Martin PJ et al. Major-histocompatibility-complex class I alleles and antigens in hematopoietic-cell transplantation. N Engl J Med 2001;345:1794–1800

50. Elsner HA, DeLuca D, Strub J, Blasczyk R. HistoCheck: rating of HLA class I and II mismatches by an internet-based software tool. Bone Marrow Transplant 2004;33:165–169

51. Shaw BE, Barber LD, Madrigal JA et al. Scoring for HLA matching? A clinical test of HistoCheck. Bone Marrow Transplant 2004;33:165–169

52. Schaffer M, Aldener-Cannava A, Remberger M et al. Roles of HLA-B, HLA-C and HLA-DPA1 incompatibilities in the outcome of unrelated stem-cell transplantation. Tissue Antigens 2003;62:243–250

53. Tamouza R, Rocha V, Busson M et al. Association of HLA-E polymorphism with severe bacterial infection and early transplant-related mortality in matched unrelated bone marrow transplantation. Transplantation 2005;80:140–144

54. Kitcharoen K, Witt CS, Romphruk AV et al. MICA, MICB, and MHC beta block matching in bone marrow transplantation: relevance to transplantation outcome. Hum Immunol 2006;67:238–246

55. Buchler T, Gallardo D, Rodriguez-Luaces M et al. Frequency of HLA-DPB1 disparities detected by reference strand-mediated conformation analysis in HLA-A, -B, and -DRB1 matched siblings. Hum Immunol 2002;63:139–142

56. Nomura N, Ota M, Kato S et al. Severe acute graft-versus-host disease by HLA-DPB1 disparity in recombinant family of bone marrow transplantation between serologically HLA-identical siblings: an application of the polymerase chain reaction-restriction fragment length polymorphism method. Hum Immunol 1991;32:261–268

57. Varney MD, Lester S, McCluskey J et al. Matching for HLA DPA1 and DPB1 alleles in unrelated bone marrow transplantation. Hum Immunol 1999;60:532–538

58. Petersdorf EW, Gooley T, Malkki M et al. The biological significance of HLA-DP gene variation in haematopoietic cell transplantation. Br J Haematol 2001;112:988–994

59. Loiseau P, Esperou H, Busson M et al. DPB1 disparities contribute to severe GVHD and reduced patient survival after unrelated donor bone marrow transplantation. Bone Marrow Transplant 2002;30:497–502

60. Shaw BE, Potter MN, Mayor NP et al. The degree of matching at HLA-DPB1 predicts for acute graft-versus-host disease and disease relapse following haematopoietic stem cell transplantation. Bone Marrow Transplant 2003;31:1001–1008

61. Shaw BE, Gooley T, Madrigal JA et al. Clinical importance of HLA-DPB1 in haematopoietic cell transplantation: Joint Report from the IHWG in HCT. Tissue Antigens 2007;69(suppl 1):36–41

62. Shaw BE, Marsh SG, Mayor NP et al. HLA-DPB1 matching status has significant implications for recipients of unrelated donor stem cell transplants. Blood 2006;107:1220–1226

63. Fleischhauer K, Locatelli F, Zecca M et al. Graft rejection after unrelated donor hematopoietic stem cell transplantation for thalassemia is associated with nonpermissive HLA-DPB1 disparity in host-versus-graft direction. Blood 2006;107:2984–2992

64. Zino E, Frumento G, Marktel S et al. A T-cell epitope encoded by a subset of HLA-DPB1 alleles determines nonpermissive mismatches for hematologic stem cell transplantation. Blood 2004;103:1417–1424

64. Shaw BE, Marsh SGE, Mayor NP, Madrigal JA. Matching status at amino acid positions 57 and 65 of the HLA-DPB1 beta chain determines outcome in recipients of unrelated donor haematopoietic stem cell transplants (abstract). Blood 2004;104:827

66. Filion A, Loiseau P, Rocha V et al. Decreased transplant related mortality and better survival in HLA matched (12/12 A, B, C, DRB1, DQB1, DPB1) unrelated bone marrow transplants. Bone Marrow Transplantation 2004;33:S55

67. Fleischhauer K, Zino E, Mazzi B et al. Peripheral blood stem cell allograft rejection mediated by CD4(+) T lymphocytes recognizing a single mismatch at HLA-DP beta 1*0901. Blood 2001;98:1122–1126

68. Dickinson AM, Charron D. Non-HLA immunogenetics in hematopoietic stem cell transplantation. Curr Opin Immunol 2005;17:517–525

69. Goulmy E, Schipper R, Pool J et al. Mismatches of minor histocompatibility antigens between HLA-identical donors and recipients and the development of graft-versus-host disease after bone marrow transplantation. N Engl J Med 1996;334:281–285

70. Mutis T, Gillespie G, Schrama E et al. Tetrameric HLA class I-minor histocompatibility antigen peptide complexes demonstrate minor histocompatibility antigen-specific cytotoxic T lymphocytes in patients with graft-versus-host disease. Nat Med 1999;5:839–842

71. Hambach L, Goulmy E. Immunotherapy of cancer through targeting of minor histocompatibility antigens. Curr Opin Immunol 2005;17:202–210

72. Dickinson AM, Middleton PG. Beyond the HLA typing age: genetic polymorphisms predicting transplant outcome. Blood Rev 2005;19:333–340

73. Zeiser R, Marks R, Bertz H, Finke J. Immunopathogenesis of acute graft-versus-host disease: implications for novel preventive and therapeutic strategies. Ann Hematol 2004;83:551–565

74. Bignon JD, Gagne K. KIR matching in hematopoietic stem cell transplantation. Curr Opin Immunol 2005;17:553–559

75. Ruggeri L, Capanni M, Mancusi A et al. The impact of donor natural killer cell alloreactivity on allogeneic hematopoietic transplantation. Transpl Immunol 2005;14:203–206

76. Parham P. MHC class I molecules and KIRs in human history, health and survival. Nat Rev Immunol 2005;5:201–214

77. Hsu KC, Pinto-Agnello C, Gooley T et al. Hematopoietic stem cell transplantation: killer immunoglobulin receptor component. Tissue Antigens 2007;69(suppl 1):42–45

78. Buckner CD, Clift RA, Sanders JE et al. Marrow harvesting from normal donors. Blood 1984;64:630–634

79. Kollman C, Howe CW, Anasetti C et al. Donor characteristics as risk factors in recipients after transplantation of bone marrow from unrelated donors: the effect of donor age. Blood 2001;98:2043–2051

80. Hansen JA, Gooley TA, Martin PJ et al. Bone marrow transplants from unrelated donors for patients with chronic myeloid leukemia. N Engl J Med 1998;338:962–968

81. Davies SM, Kollman C, Anasetti C et al. Engraftment and survival after unrelated-donor bone marrow transplantation: a report from the national marrow donor program. Blood 2000;96:4096–4102

82. Meyers JD, Flournoy N, Thomas ED. Risk factors for cytomegalovirus infection after human marrow transplantation. J Infect Dis 1986;153:478–488

83. Ljungman P, Brand R, Einsele H et al. Donor CMV serologic status and outcome of CMV-seropositive recipients after unrelated donor stem cell transplantation: an EBMT megafile analysis. Blood 2003;102:4255–4260

84. Grob JP, Grundy JE, Prentice HG et al. Immune donors can protect marrow-transplant recipients from severe cytomegalovirus infections. Lancet 1987;1:774–776

85. Nichols WG, Corey L, Gooley T et al. High risk of death due to bacterial and fungal infection among cytomegalovirus (CMV)-seronegative recipients of stem cell transplants from seropositive donors: evidence for indirect effects of primary CMV infection. J Infect Dis 2002;185:273–282

86. Craddock C, Szydlo RM, Dazzi F et al. Cytomegalovirus seropositivity adversely influences outcome after T-depleted unrelated donor transplant in patients with chronic myeloid leukaemia: the case for tailored graft-versus-host disease prophylaxis. Br J Haematol 2001;112:228–236

87. Kroger N, Zabelina T, Kruger W et al. Patient cytomegalovirus seropositivity with or without reactivation is the most important prognostic factor for survival and treatment-related mortality in stem cell transplantation from unrelated donors using pretransplant in vivo T-cell depletion with anti-thymocyte globulin. Br J Haematol 2001;113:1060–1071

88. Eapen M, Horowitz MM, Klein JP et al. Higher mortality after allogeneic peripheral-blood transplantation compared with bone marrow in children and adolescents: the Histocompatibility and Alternate Stem Cell Source Working Committee of the International Bone Marrow Transplant Registry. J Clin Oncol 2004;22:4872–4880

89. Miflin G, Russell NH, Hutchinson RM et al. Allogeneic peripheral blood stem cell transplantation for haematological malignancies – an analysis of kinetics of engraftment and GVHD risk. Bone Marrow Transplant 1997;19:9–13

90. Ringden O, Remberger M, Runde V et al. Peripheral blood stem cell transplantation from unrelated donors: a comparison with marrow transplantation. Blood 1999;94:455–464

91. Remberger M, Ringden O, Blau IW et al. No difference in graft-versus-host disease, relapse, and survival comparing peripheral stem cells to bone marrow using unrelated donors. Blood 2001;98:1739–1745

92. Storek J, Gooley T, Siadak M et al. Allogeneic peripheral blood stem cell transplantation may be associated with a high risk of chronic graft-versus-host disease. Blood 1997;90:4705–4709

93. Scott MA, Gandhi MK, Jestice HK et al. A trend towards an increased incidence of chronic graft-versus-host disease following allogeneic peripheral blood progenitor cell transplantation: a case controlled study. Bone Marrow Transplant 1998;22:273–276

Collection and processing of marrow and blood hematopoietic stem cells

Michele Cottler-Fox, Matthew Montgomery and John Theus

CHAPTER 24

Introduction

The technique described for marrow collection by Thomas & Storb in 1970[1] has undergone few major changes. Historically, transplant physicians have aimed to acquire $2-4 \times 10^8$ nucleated cells/kg recipient body weight for an unmanipulated allogeneic marrow graft, and $1-3 \times 10^8$ nucleated cells/kg for an unmanipulated autologous graft.[2] In general, this number of cells may be acquired with a collection of 10–20 ml of marrow/kg recipient body weight, although donors under the age of 20 years may have significantly more cells per volume harvested, while those over the age of 60 years may have significantly fewer.[3] When deciding how much marrow to harvest, it is imperative to know whether a graft will undergo manipulation, and what the cell loss associated with processing is likely to be, in order to harvest sufficient cells to ensure an adequate graft.

Hematopoietic progenitor/stem cell (HPC) grafts are currently obtained from human marrow, peripheral blood or cord blood. Collection of marrow from cadaveric human donors is also feasible,[4,5] and cadaveric donor marrow has been documented to engraft in the related recipient.[6] It is also possible to derive a graft from fetal liver,[7] or through tissue culture expansion of a minimal cell dose obtained from one of the sources listed above.[8] While many centers are primarily using grafts obtained by leukapheresis of peripheral blood due to generally larger yields as well as for patient comfort and convenience, traditional marrow harvest still has several potential benefits over peripheral blood stem cell (PBSC) collection, including a decreased incidence of chronic graft-versus-host disease (GvHD), as well as potentially better long-term marrow function due to the presence of mesenchymal stromal cells that are exclusive to the bone marrow niche. Other cell populations of potential interest to blood and marrow transplant or regenerative medicine which are exclusive to or more prevalent in marrow include: macrophages, reticular endothelial cells, endothelial progenitor cells, fibroblasts, adipocytes, and osteogenic progenitor cells.[9,10]

Bone marrow collection

When to harvest

Marrow from a related donor is generally harvested at the recipient's transplant center on the day of transplant. Marrow from an unrelated volunteer donor may be harvested on the day of transplant if transport time to the recipient is no more than 24 hours. Alternatively, an unrelated volunteer donor may be harvested on the day before transplant in order to allow the product to arrive on the planned day of infusion. Autologous marrows are usually cryopreserved, so that timing of the harvest is rarely a problem. However, with short conditioning regimens for transplant such as high-dose melphalan, some centers store the autologous marrow at 4°C in the liquid state for up to 48 hours.[11] Storage at room temperature is not recommended (Read, personal communication).

Although frozen allogeneic grafts have been used less commonly due to fear of HPC loss, successful engraftment has been reported with such grafts.[6,12]

Risks of marrow harvest

General, spinal and epidural anesthesia have all been utilized successfully. The major risks of harvest are associated with the induction of anesthesia. These include non-fatal cardiac arrest, pulmonary embolus, aspiration pneumonia, ventricular tachycardia and cerebral infarction.[13] At least one fatality in an older donor as a result of cardiac arrest is known but has never been fully reported.[14] The Seattle transplant team has reported that 27% of allogeneic donors have a complicating event, of which 92% may be considered minor, i.e. bacteremia, local infection at harvest sites, postoperative fever, fractured iliac crest, broken aspiration needle requiring surgical removal, transient pressure neuropathies from hematomas at harvest sites and spinal headache.[15] Approximately half of the serious complications in this series were related to anesthesia.

Heldal et al assessed patient complaints, as well as procedure-related risks, following either marrow donation or blood HPC donation and found that patients felt that blood HPC donation was significantly less burdensome than marrow donation, and that most would choose blood HPC donation if asked to donate again.[16] They also summarized the most common problems associated with blood HPC donation (low back pain, myalgia, skeleton pain, and headache) and marrow harvest (low back pain, limpness, anorexia/nausea and dizziness).[16]

Small-volume harvests (≤200 ml) are being carried out for use in regenerative medicine (cardiac muscle repair, orthopedic trauma), where local anesthesia will suffice.

Harvest technique

In general, an adequate harvest may be obtained from the posterior superior iliac crests in adults. Alternative sites which may be utilized in addition include the anterior iliac crests, sternum and, in a donor less than 1 year old, the tibia. Thus, after anesthesia is induced, the donor is usually placed first in the prone position on pillows to support the hips and lower rib cage, allowing the diaphragm free movement, or on an adjustable spinal frame, as is used for laminectomy. Harvest in the lateral position has also been described.[17]

After a sterile field has been prepared, the marrow is aspirated into a syringe which has been rinsed with preservative-free heparin or which may contain a heparinized solution. It has been suggested that no more than 3–5 ml should be collected per aspirate, as more than this is simply blood and increases the number of T-cells in a harvest and leads to a larger volume harvest to acquire an adequate number of stem cells.[18] The skin over the iliac crests is quite flexible, so that an average harvest of 1–1.5 liters may only require three or four skin punctures per iliac crest. Many different styles of needle have been used for harvest with varying degrees of comfort and success,[19] including disposable needles. It has become common to use disposable plastic syringes rather than glass as originally described, to avoid leaving the harvest field covered in splinters if a syringe weakens with use and breaks, and to avoid potential transfer of infectious agents should there be a sterilization failure.

Aspirated marrow is expelled into a container holding heparinized fluid. Tissue culture medium was originally used, but more recently a buffered saline solution approved for human use, such as Plasmalyte-A® or Normosol®, has been used. How much heparin to use per harvest, and whether it should be preservative free or not, remain controversial since the range of products used successfully is wide. The container itself was originally a stainless steel or glass beaker, but a commercial collection bag with attached filters is available (Baxter Fenwal, Deerfield, IL). If the Fenwal kit is not used, then some other means must be found to filter out bone spicules and to break up cell clumps after the harvest. After the harvest is filtered, many centers add citrate in a volume equal to 10% of the collection for further anticoagulation.

After the harvest

At the end of the harvest, the aspiration sites are bandaged with a pressure dressing, and analgesia is supplied as needed. Ice applied in the immediate postoperative and recovery room period may be useful to reduce swelling and pain. In any event, it is rare for a donor to need more than minor analgesics such as acetaminophen (paracetamol) with codeine or oxycodone for more than a few days following harvest.

Marrow harvests were inpatient procedures for many years following the development of marrow transplantation. However, the desire to decrease hospital costs led to the study of marrow harvesting as an outpatient procedure.[20,21] Today, if the patient is prepared to be admitted to the hospital in the event of hypotension, excessive pain or unexpected complications of harvest, the majority of autologous and allogeneic donors may be discharged within 12 hours of harvest.

Alternative sources of marrow

Surgically resected ribs, cadaveric vertebral bodies and complete ilia are potential sources of marrow.[22] The principle in such a harvest is to open the bone, expose the marrow-rich cavity, and remove the marrow into a buffered salt solution containing DNase but no heparin.[23] Gentle agitation releases cells from the bone matrix, and the cell suspension is then washed, filtered and prepared for use or cryopreservation. Alternatively, marrow may be initially pressed out of the bone into a sterile fluid. Although only a single cadaveric marrow transplant has been reported,[6] it is possible that there would be less graft-versus-host disease with cadaveric marrow since it contains fewer T-cells than does marrow aspirated from a living donor.[24] This approach has been considered as a means of inducing immune tolerance for solid organ transplants.[25]

Marrow transport

Marrow arrives from the operating room to the processing laboratory in a standard blood transfer bag of 600–2000 ml volume, bearing a label identifying the donor and recipient (if it is a related donor), as well as the fluid and anticoagulant solution into which it has been collected. Unrelated donor marrow is labeled with an identifying number, rather than the donor name, and is hand carried by a courier from the operating room at the harvest center to the processing laboratory at the transplant center. Unrelated donor marrow may be transported on wet ice or without coolant in an insulated container, and should arrive at the recipient's transplant center within 24 hours of harvest. Since marrows are collected and transported worldwide, it is common for the marrow courier to arrive outside regular working hours. Thus, if processing is required, the receiving laboratory may need to have personnel on call 24 hours a day.

Collection of hematopoietic progenitor/stem cells from blood

Mobilization of HPC

HPC mobilization and collection have several advantages over traditional marrow harvesting but also involve several distinct risks. Whereas marrow harvesting primarily poses risks related to anesthesia and the invasive nature of the harvest, leukapheresis of mobilized HPC entails risks not only with the actual leukapheresis procedure, including those of establishing venous access, but also with the preparative regimens employed for mobilization. Until recently, most comparisons of HPC collection and marrow harvesting have looked at mobilized peripheral progenitors versus steady-state, i.e. unmobilized, marrow. To address this discrepancy, many groups have begun to compare stem cell collections by both techniques following mobilization for all patient groups. Their findings, paired with basic research into the nature and function of the bone marrow niche, suggest a definite role for traditional marrow harvest.

Initiating collection

Although it is possible to begin collecting on a fixed day after mobilizing chemotherapy or growth factors alone, optimal timing of the initiation of collection is best based on the number of circulating CD34+ HPC in the donor's peripheral blood. These levels can be monitored daily by flow cytometry using either a commercially available single-platform system such as ProCount (Becton-Dickson, Mt View, CA) or StemKit (Beckman-Coulter, Fullerton, CA) or by using the ISHAGE method and an automated cell counter, which is a dual-platform system. The single-platform method has the advantage of allowing direct comparisons between institutions, which is difficult with standard flow cytometry.[26]

Other methods currently being studied include using a standard Sysmex (Kobe, Japan) automated cell counter equipped with an Immature Information channel (IMI), which calculates HPC based on cell size, density and lysis resistance.[27] In addition, since not all HPC express surface CD34,[28] another method involves staining with the Aldecount® reagent to assess intracytosolic aldehyde dehydrogenase activity, present in both CD34+ and CD34– cells.[29]

Predictive formula

Typically, a value of 5–20 CD34+ cells/μl, using a single-platform system, is felt to be optimal for beginning collection. While many centers use this result alone, others employ a predictive formula using the test value to give an estimation of the collection yield:

$$\text{\#CD34+ cells desired} = \frac{\text{\# of l blood to process} \times \text{CD34+ cells/}\mu l \times \text{machine collection efficiency}}{\text{patient weight in kg}}$$

The usual goal of apheresis is to provide a graft for transplant with 2–4×10^6 CD34+ cells/kg in a single procedure[30,31] although some centers routinely aim to collect enough for a tandem transplant if the patient has a diagnosis of myeloma.

Variables affecting mobilization

Many factors have been shown to influence the ability of a patient to mobilize HPC prior to transplant. Poor mobilization is currently defined as a collection of $< 2.0 \times 10^6$ CD34+ cells/kg.[32,33] In the myeloma population, age greater than 70, over 12 months of chemotherapy, and platelet counts $>200 \times 10^9$/l have been associated with poor mobilization.[34,35] In the acute leukemia population, baseline blood CD34+ cell count, CD34+ cells in the peripheral blood on the day of apheresis, and lack of fever or infection have been shown to be the most significant variables.[36] Finally, the mobilization regimen, degree of marrow involvement, and history of radiation therapy have shown clinical significance.[37,38]

Mobilization regimens

Mobilization using chemotherapy and growth factors together has been shown to be significantly more effective than with either alone.[37] Although many chemotherapeutic agents have been used, cyclophosphamide is commonly used, followed shortly thereafter with one or more growth factor regimens[39,40] as described below.

G-CSF and GM-CSF

G-CSF (granulocyte colony-stimulating factor) and GM-CSF (granulocyte-macrophage colony-stimulating factor) are the agents currently used most frequently for mobilization. Both agents have been shown to increase release of proteolytic enzymes from mature neutrophils in the bone marrow that serve to disrupt the anchoring of the more immature HPC, thus allowing their egress into the periphery.[41] Cyclophosphamide exhibits a similar effect on the marrow microenvironment and is thus very effective when used in conjunction with these regimens. GM-CSF has been shown to have inferior ability to mobilize HPC compared to G-CSF as well as to have greater toxicity.[42] Both agents can cause bone pain, nausea, vomiting, diarrhea, insomnia, chills, fevers, and night sweats,[43] which account for the major risks associated with peripheral stem cell collection when compared to marrow harvest. GM-CSF has shown a greater incidence of fever as well as increased length of hospital stay.[40,44] However, in poorly mobilizing patients, GM-CSF together with G-CSF have been shown to increase CD34+ yields and therefore may be of some benefit in this population. The optimal collection times following the administration of G-CSF have been shown to be between 4 and 12 hours.[45,46]

Erythropoietin

Erythropoietin (EPO) has been postulated to augment mobilization of stem cells due to the presence of small numbers of EPO receptors on their surfaces, which are thought to positively affect survival due to increases in antiapoptotic proteins following activation.[47] When used in conjunction with G- or GM-CSF, the effects may be additive,[48] although not all studies have been able to show such an effect.[49,50]

Stem cell factor

Stem cell factor (SCF), when used in combination with G-CSF, has been shown by some researchers to increase mobilization as well as to speed recovery in transplant recipients.[51,52] Others, however, have not shown this effect.[53] SCF has significant drawbacks, including severe allergic reactions and need for patient monitoring after administration, which have hindered its use.[54]

AMD-3100

AMD-3100 (Mozobil, Genzyme, CA) is a newer agent originally designed for the treatment of HIV infection. It acts as a reversible inhibitor of the CD34+ cell chemokine receptor, CXCR4. The CXCR4 receptor associates with its ligand, stromal-derived factor 1 (SDF-1) to mediate stem cell homing, trafficking, and retention.[51,55] Once CXCR4 has been bound by AMD-3100, the ability of HPC to migrate toward and adhere to the bone marrow niche is impaired, resulting in increased numbers of these progenitors in the circulation. When used in conjunction with G-CSF, the results have been synergistic with no increase in toxicity.[56] To date, most studies of AMD-3100 have been performed on healthy volunteers[57] or patients diagnosed with non-Hodgkin's lymphoma or multiple myeloma.[56]

GROβ/CXCL2

The GROβ chemokines interact with the CXCR2 receptors of neutrophils, causing release of matrix metalloproteinase-9 (MMP-9), which is one of the three primary enzymes involved in the bone marrow matrix degradation necessary for HPC egress, the other two enzymes being neutrophil elastase (NE) and cathepsin G (CG). It has been established that G-CSF administration increases levels of these enzymes in the marrow environment.[41] These compounds all degrade SDF-1, thus disrupting the SDF-1/CXCR4 axis necessary for HPC retention in the marrow and therefore favoring HPC release.[51] While G-CSF leads to increases in the enzyme concentrations in the marrow compartment, the plasma compartment is not significantly affected.[58] In contrast, GROβ leads to significant increases in the concentrations of MMP-9, NE, and CG in the plasma, without significant effects on the marrow compartment.[58]

Pelus et al have shown through a series of intricate experiments,[58,59] studying different enzyme/receptor blockades and inhibitions in mice and non-human primates, that the important factor in GROβ-mediated mobilization is the increase in plasma MMP-9 levels due to release from mature, peripheral neutrophils. They have noted that the exact mechanism by which plasma MMP-9 leads to the significant augmentation of G-CSF mediated HPC release from the marrow is not completely understood. However, they hypothesize that peripheral MMP-9 levels may disrupt endothelial cell junctions, which, when coupled with the marrow effects of G-CSF, lead to enhanced egress of HPC. Of clinical interest is the observation that the effects of GROβ are noticeable within 15–30 minutes of administration and can increase yields of HPC well over 200-fold. In addition, the grafts obtained from combined G-CSF and GROβ mobilization show significant repopulation advantages compared with normal bone marrow cells or HPC mobilized by G-CSF alone. While this research thus far has only been undertaken in mice and non-human primates, positive results in humans are promising. Pelus et al[58] suggest that the addition of GROβ, particularly in poor mobilizers, could decrease potential toxicity from higher G-CSF doses and significantly augment collections.

Timing of HPC collection relative to growth factor administration

Many studies have shown that collection of ≥ 2–2.5×10^6 CD34+ cells/kg provides a reasonable graft for a successful transplant, defined as adequate neutrophil and platelet recovery within 14 days after transplant.[32,34,37,38] Using the predictive formula, this goal may be achieved efficiently by initiating collection when the prediction is $\geq 1 \times 10^6$ CD34+ cells/kg. The collection should capture as much of the mobilization peak as is possible following growth factor administration. For standard non-pegylated G-CSF, the peak of mobilization correlates with the drug half-life of approximately 3–4 hours.[60] Pegylated G-CSF, however, has a much longer half-life of approximately 33 hours[60] and may therefore allow a greater degree of flexibility in administration and collection. It should be noted, however, that the pegylated form, while potentially more convenient due to fewer administrations, also sacrifices some of the ability to control, or 'fine tune' the peak of mobilization possible with a shorter acting agent such as standard G-CSF (Cottler-Fox, personal observation). AMD-3100 has shown a peak of mobilization at approximately 6 hours following administration and therefore works very well in conjunction with G-CSF, which shows similar kinetics.[56,61]

Remobilization

Approximately 5–30% of patients fail the initial mobilization attempt,[62,63] i.e. collection of at least $2–2.5 \times 10^6$ CD34+ cells/kg in their first collection. Many options have been investigated to deal with mobilization and collection in this subset of difficult-to-mobilize patients, including the addition of bone marrow harvesting to PBSC mobilization,[63] or second (and sometimes even a third) attempts at mobilization with modifications of the preparative regimens.[62,64] Results from these investigations have shown that it is worthwhile to attempt further mobilizations in this group of patients and that toxicity is not significantly increased by increasing dosages of growth factors.[65,66] It has been observed, however, that dosages of G-CSF at or above 8 µg/kg twice daily lead to significantly higher degrees of bone pain, headache and fatigue in healthy donors.[67] As such, these patients may require much stricter monitoring for signs and symptoms of toxicity.

Remobilization of peripheral blood HPC versus marrow harvest

Data regarding patients failing initial mobilization attempts have varied. Some studies have shown that subsequent marrow harvest has little clinical benefit and increases patient morbidity compared to repeated attempts at peripheral collection.[63,68] Another study, however, found that engraftment and hospital stays were comparable with the two regimens.[69]

Marrow versus peripheral blood as a source of hematopoietic progenitor/stem cells

Most studies comparing bone marrow harvesting with PBSC collection have looked at steady-state, unstimulated marrow. The question therefore remained as to what effects, if any, might be seen when comparing standard mobilized PBSC collections with growth factor-stimulated marrow harvests. The former studies have shown clear benefits to peripheral stem cell collections, i.e. ease of collection, few adverse events, rapid engraftment, and shorter hospital stays.[70,71] The latter studies, however, have not demonstrated such clear advantages to PBSC collection. It has been shown that bone marrow grafts may possess unique cell populations that aid in engraftment and hematopoietic reconstitution superior to peripherally acquired grafts.

Graft contents

Grafts derived from stimulated bone marrow have been shown to possess a distinct population of progenitor cells, the mesenchymal stromal cells (MSC), which are not found in blood progenitor cell collections.[72] In one study, ex vivo expansion of this subset followed by infusion led to neutrophil and platelet recovery at days +8 and +9 respectively, with no increased toxicity.[73] In addition to MSC, bone marrow also contains macrophages, reticular endothelial cells, endothelial progenitor cells, fibroblasts, adipocytes and osteogenic progeni-

tor cells, which provide various integrins, matrix receptors, growth factors and cell-to-cell interactions essential for hematopoiesis and progenitor cell differentiation.[74,75]

Graft yields

Marrow stimulated with G-CSF has been shown to have significantly higher numbers of mononuclear cells and more rapid engraftment compared to unstimulated marrow, thus showing the beneficial effect of mobilization protocols for bone marrow harvests.[76] Elfenbein et al performed a meta-analysis which showed a median value of 2.6 (1.0–6.4) $\times 10^6$ CD34+ cells in peripheral blood collections versus 1.5 (0.6–2.3) $\times 10^6$ CD34+ cells in stimulated marrow harvests.[77]

Engraftment and outcomes

The meta-analysis of Elfenbein ultimately concluded that in randomized controlled trials, the potential for successful engraftment and disease-free survival was equivalent between G-CSF stimulated marrow and blood progenitor cells.[77] In addition, the same investigators found that in HLA-identical allograft recipients, marrow-derived HPC showed engraftment equivalent to blood-derived HPC with no more cost or complications when compared to performing two leukapheresis procedures.[78] Weisdorf et al studied engraftment in Hodgkin's and non-Hodgkin's lymphoma patients and found no significant differences in either engraftment or length of hospital stay when comparing blood or bone marrow stimulated with G- or GM-CSF.[79]

Processing of marrow and blood hematopoietic progenitor/stem cell collections

Volume reduction

In many centers, an ABO-matched allogeneic marrow was originally transported directly from the operating room after harvest to the bedside, where it was infused through a central line. In such cases, the only potential complications to the recipient are related to the volume infused, the dose of heparin it contains, and the possibility that, despite filtering, cell clumps may cause respiratory difficulty. Today, it is more common to take the product to the processing lab so that quality assurance samples may be taken for enumeration of nucleated cells, viability of HPC, enumeration of HPC, and microbiologic testing as well as ABO/Rh confirmation. In cases where the volume collected would be enough to cause problems with fluid overload, the volume may be reduced by centrifugation and removal of plasma. This will increase the hematocrit of the final product, but should not present a clinical problem as long as the marrow is infused over an appropriate time period (3–4 hours). In cases where the marrow donor plasma contains a clinically significant antibody against cellular elements of the recipient (i.e. alloagglutinins against ABO or other red blood cell antigens in red blood cell mismatched transplants), donor plasma may be removed.

Red blood cell depletion

In the case of an ABO major mismatched allogeneic marrow transplant (where the recipient has alloagglutinins against a donor red blood cell antigen), the simple removal of red blood cells will prevent acute hemolysis. In the past, it was feared that this marrow manipulation might interfere with engraftment, for which reason recipient alloagglutinins were removed by vigorous plasmapheresis of the recipient, by plasma exchange over an immunoadsorbent column, or by infusing a small amount of incompatible red blood cells to adsorb out the recipient alloagglutinins in vivo just prior to marrow infusion. However, as red blood cell removal has been shown to involve minimal white blood cell (i.e. HPC) loss, it is now more common to remove red blood cells using one of the following methods:[80]

- starch sedimentation
- repeated dilution with compatible red blood cells
- buffy coat preparation
- mononuclear cell separation.

Red blood cells removed from an allogeneic or autologous marrow may also be reinfused into the donor after the harvest.

Starch sedimentation

Marrow containing heparin is mixed with 6% hydroxyethyl starch at a ratio of 8:1, after which the red blood cells are allowed to sediment as a function of gravity with the blood transfer bag in the inverted position (entry port side down). After 30–180 minutes, the sedimented red blood cells are removed into a secondary bag. The original bag contains approximately 75% of the original nucleated marrow cells for transplantation, as well as 5–25 ml of the original red blood cells. This volume of incompatible red blood cells is still capable of causing a hemolytic transfusion reaction, for which reason other techniques are commonly preferred to sedimentation.

Repeated dilution with compatible red blood cells

After a white blood cell-rich cell concentrate has been prepared by sedimentation, the remaining incompatible red blood cells may be decreased by diluting the cells with a unit of recipient-compatible, irradiated, leukocyte-depleted red blood cells and 150 ml of recipient-compatible plasma, if possible from the marrow donor. The product is then allowed to re-sediment, reducing the total of incompatible red blood cells to < 10 ml while retaining 85% of nucleated white blood cells. This procedure is time-consuming, however, and most processing laboratories today would choose instead to go directly to a method for concentrating white blood cells.

Buffy coat preparation

Buffy coat preparation is often the first step towards additional processing for T-cell depletion, tumor cell purging or cryopreservation for both marrow and blood HPC collections. A white blood cell-rich concentrate, the buffy coat, is prepared by centrifuging the original product using a standard blood bank centrifuge, a blood cell washer, or any of the apheresis devices currently available. Approximately 80% of nucleated cells from the marrow are retained, while simultaneously reducing the volume and red blood cell concentration by 80%. Although this is an adequate method of volume reduction for cryopreservation of marrow and blood HPC, and a good preliminary step towards a mononuclear cell separation of marrow, it is not recommended where red blood cell contamination may interfere with chemical or immunologic purging methods.

Mononuclear cell separation

Mature myeloid elements may be removed from a buffy coat using manual or automated methods, with or without density-gradient materials[80] such as albumin, Ficoll and Percoll. Such agents remove essentially all red blood cell and myeloid elements, leaving only mononuclear (morphologic lymphocyte + monocyte populations) portions of the graft. While this is of great importance for the economic feasibility and success of purging protocols for autologous transplantation, and of T-cell depletion for allogeneic transplantation, it remains a problem that upwards of 30% of the original HPC of a graft may be lost. In order to offset this loss, and to maintain adequate numbers of such

cells after separation procedures, it is necessary to collect considerably more than are needed for the final graft.

Cryopreservation

Autologous marrow and blood HPC are usually cryopreserved for later use. Cells to be cryopreserved may be aliquoted into small vials, or they may be placed into freezing bags with a capacity of 30–200 ml. If the bag to be frozen requires heat sealing, it is imperative to remove all air prior to sealing, as air in the bag may cause it to explode on thawing, when the air expands rapidly but the bag has not yet become flexible.

Addition of cryoprotectant

Dimethylsulfoxide (DMSO) is the cryoprotective agent most widely used to cryopreserve hematopoietic stem cells at present. DMSO is a universal solvent capable of stabilizing cell membranes under rapidly changing conditions, preventing intracellular ice crystal formation during freezing and heat release during the period of phase transition. DMSO has been described as toxic to stem cells at room temperature, for which reason investigators have emphasized the need to add it at 4°C to cells prior to controlled-rate freezing and to begin cryopreservation quickly thereafter. A final concentration of 10% DMSO with albumin or human serum is commonly used, with some centers using hydroxyethyl starch to help stabilize cell membranes and reduce the amount of DMSO used to 5%.

A new cryopreservative, Cryostor™ (BioLife Solutions Inc., Corning, NY), is also available. This compound modulates cellular biochemistry during the freezing process and is free of serum, proteins, and DMSO.

Methods of cryopreservation

Freezing has traditionally been performed in a controlled-rate freezer, using liquid nitrogen to decrease the temperature at a rate of 1–2°C/min until a phase transition occurs, during which heat is given off by the solution, followed by an extra burst of liquid nitrogen to prevent an increase in temperature. After this, the temperature drop is adjusted to 5–10°C/min until the mixture has reached a temperature of approximately −120°C.

An alternative to controlled-rate freezing is so-called 'dump' freezing.[81] In this technique a freeze mix containing DMSO, albumin or human serum and hydroxyethyl starch is added to cells and the product is placed into a −80°C freezer.

Storage conditions

After cryopreservation, the products are removed from the freezing apparatus and stored either in the liquid (−196°C) or vapor (−156°C) phase of a liquid nitrogen freezer, or in a mechanical (−80°C) freezer. Marrow frozen with a controlled-rate freezer and infused after more than 11 years in liquid nitrogen storage has resulted in good hematopoietic reconstitution,[82] but the products which have been subjected to 'dump' freezing and stored at −80°C may deteriorate more rapidly.[81]

Recent investigations have shown that certain cells derived from the bone marrow can lose function due to cryopreservation. In a study by Shepherd et al the investigators took peripherally collected HPC capable of endothelial differentiation and subjected them to cryopreservation with DMSO followed by thawing and infusion into rats subjected to hindlimb ischemia, and then measured the cells for their angiogenic capabilities.[83] They found two distinct populations of endothelial progenitors: endothelial progenitor cells (EPCs) capable of vascular regeneration in culture, and circulating angiogenic cells (CACs), which precede EPCs and stimulate angiogenesis via secretion of vascular endothelial growth factor (VEGF). The investigators found that cryopreservation had no effects on the functional abilities of CACs but that EPCs were only rarely recovered after thawing. While this study used peripherally collected HPC, it is possible that the impact of freezing on bone marrow-derived HPC may show similar results. This question remains to be answered.

Thawing and infusion

A number of studies have shown that rapid thawing is desirable for the survival of HPC.[84] Thawing may be performed in a temperature-controlled water bath, or in a sterile basin using sterile saline heated to 37–40°C prior to use. Once thawed, the cells are commonly infused directly and rapidly, via a central venous access device. Each bag is infused over roughly 15 minutes to avoid the supposed DMSO toxicity to stem cells. Immediate side-effects associated with rapid infusion of stem cell products may include volume overload, bradycardia (the result of cold cardioplegia), nausea and vomiting (the result of the unpleasant taste of DMSO via direct nerve stimulation from the product in blood), fever, tachycardia, hypotension or hypertension (the result of lysed granulocytes if the product is not a clean mononuclear product), CNS toxicity including confusion and seizures, and allergic reactions ranging from urticaria to anaphylaxis (related to plasma proteins and/or DMSO). Most, if not all, of these problems may be avoided by volume-reducing the products after collection, and giving antiemetics, diphenhydramine and/or hydrocortisone prior to infusing stem cells. Renal dysfunction related to red cell hemolysis is a delayed problem which may be seen with infusion of stem cell products, for which reason some centers give prophylactic mannitol and furosemide along with HPC.[85] Recently, it has been suggested that much of the toxicity is actually related to white cell lysis, rather than to DMSO.

Alternatively, the thawed product may be processed to remove DMSO prior to infusion and to reduce the volume. This is not a widely accepted maneuver, however, due to concern for stem cell loss. It is also possible to thaw rapidly and then dilute the product with a sterile buffered saline solution prior to infusion, and then infuse the product slowly at room temperature (E. Areman, personal communication, 1996). While this allows the processing laboratory to deal with potential bag breakage in the most efficient manner, it increases the volume infused and may require the use of DNase to avoid cell clumping.

Product assessment/quality assurance

Since there is thought to be a threshold dose for stem cells above which rapid hematopoietic reconstitution can be expected, it is important to evaluate graft quality. Grafts were originally evaluated solely on the basis of total nucleated cells infused per kilogram recipient body weight, with fewer nucleated cells believed to be needed in autologous transplantation than allogeneic. However, the total nucleated cell count is only a surrogate for those cells which reconstitute hematopoiesis, and much effort has been expended to define a more appropriate threshold dose.

Until recently, the most commonly used assay for reconstituting ability of a graft was the growth of the day 14 granulocyte-macrophage colony-forming unit (GM-CFU) in semi-solid culture media. Threshold doses for CFU-GM differ widely, but have been said to be in the range of $0.1–1 \times 10^4$/kg for marrow. Unfortunately, culture conditions have varied among laboratories, making comparisons difficult. Further, since the cultures cannot be counted until 14 days after a harvest, real-time evaluation of a graft was impossible. For this reason, most centers now use flow cytometry-based enumeration of cells using the CD34 cell-surface marker found on HPC to determine the suitability of a graft for transplantation. Here, too, technical problems originally made comparisons between centers difficult, but a standard method is now available (ISHAGE) and at present a dose of at least 2.0×10^6 CD34+ cells/kg is considered clinically acceptable,

since engraftment reliably occurs within 14–21 days of infusion, without growth factor support.

While all processing laboratories enumerate grafts in one of the above-named fashions prior to cryopreservation, many also evaluate viability of cells after thawing (in the United States this is also mandated by the College of American Pathologists if the product is held for more than 4 hours before cryopreservation). This may be done by flow cytometry using propidium iodide or 7AAD to show non-viable cells among CD34+ cells, or using the ALDH assay (Aldacount®, Aldagen, Durham, NC). Trypan blue has also been used, but calculating viable infused stem cells in this way is indirect and imprecise.

Finally, microbiologic evaluation of a graft for contamination resulting from the collection or processing procedures may be performed. While some feel that all grafts should be subjected to bacterial and fungal cultures both initially and after processing, others have pointed out that:

- results are often not available until after the infusion
- cultures are expensive
- due to the small volumes which most processing laboratories are willing to sacrifice for cultures, results may be invalid
- infusion of contaminated grafts has not been reported to be associated with ill effects in the recipients.[87]

Nonetheless, the American FDA, under Title 21 requirements, states that all tissue-based products, such as marrow grafts, be screened in a way that prevents the transmission of communicable diseases.[87]

Conclusion

Basic research into the nature of bone development and innervation has shown a critical interplay between osteoblasts, vascular endothelium, extracellular matrix and sympathetic innervation.[88,89] Murine and human osteoblasts have been shown to produce G-CSF, GM-CSF, VEGF and SDF-1.[89,90] Katayama et al have shown that G-CSF acts directly on sympathetic neurones in the marrow, causing release of noradrenaline, which suppresses SDF-1 production by osteoblasts, thus favoring stem cell egress.[89]

The results of such experiments can be interpreted in several ways. These mechanisms might be the basis behind G-CSF driven mobilization of HPC into the blood. However, they also point out the key interplay between marrow microenvironment and progenitor cell homing and differentiation. Considering that stem cell transplantation usually follows some degree of marrow ablation, could peripheral blood HPC homing and reconstitution be improved by the addition of bone marrow? Studies such as that of Lazarus et al[73] seem to suggest that concurrent infusion of blood HPC and cells unique to the bone marrow may show benefits over either method alone. The risks of marrow harvest have to be balanced against patient variables and co-morbidities, but marrow harvest, though on the decline, is far from becoming an antiquated and obsolete procedure.

References

1. Thomas ED, Storb R. Technique for human marrow grafting. Blood 1970;36:507–511
2. Klingemann HG. Collection, processing and infusion of marrow. In: Deeg H, Klingemann H, Phillips G (eds) A guide to bone marrow transplantation. Springer-Verlag, New York, 1988
3. Deeg HJ. Bone marrow and hematopoietic stem cell transplantation: sorting the chaff from the grain. In: Areman E, Deeg H, Sacher R (eds) Bone marrow and stem cell processing: a manual of current techniques. Davis, Philadelphia, 1992
4. Ferrebee JW, Atkins L, Lochte HL et al. The collection, storage and preparation of viable cadaver marrow for intravenous use. Blood 1959;14:140–147
5. Mugashimi H, Terasaki P, Sueyoshi A. Bone marrow from cadaver donors for transplantation. Blood 1985;65:392–396
6. Blazar BR, Lasky LC, Perentesis JP et al. Successful donor cell engraftment in a recipient of bone marrow from a cadaveric donor. Blood 1986;6:1655–1660
7. Touraine JL. In utero transplantation of fetal liver stem cells in humans. Blood Cells 1991;17:379–387

8. Zimmerman TM, Williams SF, Bender JG et al. Clinical use of selected and expanded peripheral blood CD34+ cells: a preliminary report of feasibility and safety. J Haematother 1995;4:527–529

9. Devine SM, Hoffman R. Role of mesenchymal stem cells in hematopoietic stem cell transplantation. Curr Opin Hematol 2000;7:358–363

10. Pittenger MF, Mackay AM, Beck SC et al. Multilineage potential of adult human mesenchymal stem cells. Science 1999;284:143–146

11. Burnett A, Tansey P, Hills C et al. Haematological reconstitution following high dose and supralethal chemoradiotherapy using stored, non-cryopreserved autologous bone marrow. Br J Haematol 1983;54:309–316

12. Gluckman E, Broxmeyer HE, Auerbach AD et al. Hematopoietic reconstitution in a patient with Fanconi's anemia by means of umbilical cord blood from an HLA identical sibling. N Engl J Med 1989;321:1174–1178

13. Buckner CD, Clift RA, Sanders JE et al. Marrow harvesting from normal donors. Blood 1984;64:630–634

14. Bortin MM, Buckner CD. Major complications of marrow harvesting for transplantation. Exp Haematol 1983;11:916–921

15. Petersen FB, Buckner CD, Bolonesi B et al. Marrow harvesting from normal donors. Exp Haematol 1990;18:676

16. Heldal D, Brinch L, Tjonnfjord G et al. Donation of stem cells from blood or bone marrow: results of a randomized study on safety and complaints. Bone Marrow Transplant 2002;29:479–486

17. Wilson RE. Techniques of human bone marrow procurement by aspiration from living donors. N Engl J Med 1959;261:781–785

18. Batinic D, Marusic M, Pavletic Z et al. Relationship between differing volumes of bone marrow aspirates and their cellular composition. Bone Marrow Transplant 1990;6:103–107

19. Cottler-Fox M. Bone marrow collection techniques. In: Areman E, Deeg H, Sacher R (eds) Bone marrow and stem cell processing: a manual of current techniques. Davis, Philadelphia, 1992

20. Brandwein JM, Callum J, Rubinger M et al. An evaluation of outpatient bone marrow harvesting. J Clin Oncol 1989;7:648–650

21. Dicke KA, Hood DL, Hanks S et al. A marrow harvest procedure under local anesthesia. Exp Haematol 1995;23:1229–1232

22. Haurani Fl, Repplinger E, Tocantis LM. Attempts at transplantation of human bone marrow in patients with acute leukemia and other marrow depletion disorders. Am J Med 1960;28:794–806

23. Sharp TG, Sachs DH, Matthews JG et al. Harvest of human bone marrow directly from bone. J Immunol Methods 1984;69:187–195

24. Saunders EF, Kapelushnik J, Solh H et al. Graft vs host disease is reduced in allogeneic bone marrow transplantation using marrow obtained surgically. Blood 1990;76 (Suppl 1):563

25. Barber WH, Diethelm AG, Laskow DA et al. Use of cryopreserved donor bone marrow in cadaver kidney allograft recipients. Transplantation 1989;47:66–71

26. Rivadeneyra-Espinoza L, Perez-Romano B, Gonzalez-Flores A et al. Instrument- and protocol-dependent variation in the enumeration of CD34+ cells by flow cytometry. Transfusion 2006;46:530–536

27. Suh C, Kim S, Kim SH et al. Initiation of peripheral blood progenitor cell harvest based on peripheral blood hematopoietic progenitor cell counts enumerated by the Sysmex SE9000. Transfusion 2004;44:1762–1768

28. Dao MA, Arevelo J, Nolta JA. Reversibility of CD34 expression on human hematopoietic stem cells that retain the capacity for secondary reconstitution. Blood 2003;101:112–118

29. Hess DA, Wirthlin L, Craft TP et al. Selection based on CD133 and high aldehyde dehydrogenase activity isolates long-term reconstituting human hematopoietic stem cells. Blood 2006;107:2162–2169

30. Bender JG, To LB, Williams S, Schwartzberg LS. Defining a therapeutic dose of peripheral blood stem cells. J Hematother 1992;1:329–341

31. Weaver CH, Hazelton B, Birch R et al. An analysis of engraftment kinetics as a function of the CD34 content of peripheral blood progenitor cell collections in 692 patients after the administration of myeloablative chemotherapy. Blood 1995;86:3961–3969

32. Cottler-Fox M, Lapidot T. Mobilizing the older patient with myeloma. Blood Rev 2006;20:43–50

33. Koenigsmann M, Jentsch-Ullrich K, Mohren M et al. The role of diagnosis in patients failing peripheral blood progenitor cell mobilization. Transfusion 2004;44:777–784

34. Tricot G, Jagannath S, Vesole Det al. Peripheral blood stem cell transplants for multiple myeloma: identification of favorable variables for rapid engraftment in 225 patients. Blood 1995;85:588–596

35. Morris CL, Siegel E, Barlogie B et al. Mobilization of CD34+ cells in elderly patients (>/=70 years) with multiple myeloma: influence of age, prior therapy, platelet count and mobilization regimen. Br J Haematol 2003;120:413–423

36. Pastore D, Specchia G, Mestice A et al. Good and Poor CD34+ cell mobilization in acute leukemia: analysis of factors affecting the yield of progenitor cells. Bone Marrow Transplant 2004;33:1083–1087

37. Bensinger W, Appelbaum F, Rowley S et al. Factors that influence collection and engraftment of autologous peripheral-blood stem cells. J Clin Oncol 1995;13:2547–2555

38. Fu P, Bagai RK, Meyerson H et al. Pre-mobilization therapy blood CD34+ cell count predicts the likelihood of successful hematopoietic stem cell mobilization. Bone Marrow Transplant 2006;38:189–196

39. Olavarria E, Kanfer EJ. Selection and use of chemotherapy with hematopoietic growth factors for mobilization of peripheral blood progenitor cells. Curr Opin Hematol 2000;7:191–196

40. Ballestrero A, Ferrando F, Garuti A et al. Comparative effects of three cytokine regimens after high-dose cyclophosphamide: G-CSF, GM-CSF, and sequential interleukin-3 and GM-CSF. J Clin Oncol 1999;17:1296–1303

41. Copelan EA. Hematopoietic stem-cell transplantation. N Engl J Med 2006;354:1813–1826

42. Weaver CH, Schulman KA, Buckner CD. Mobilization of peripheral blood stem cells following myelosuppressive chemotherapy: a randomized comparison of filgrastim, sargramostim, or sequential sargramostim and filgrastim. Bone Marrow Transplant 2001;2(suppl): S23-S29

43. Anderlini P, Przepiorka D, Seong D et al. Clinical toxicity and laboratory effects of G-CSF mobilization and blood stem cell apheresis from normal donors, and analysis of charges for the procedures. Transfusion 1996;36:590–595

44. Peters WP, Rosner G, Ross M et al. Comparative effects of GM-CSF and G-CSF on priming peripheral blood progenitor cells for use with autologous bone marrow after high-dose chemotherapy. Blood 1993;81:1709–1719

45. Watts MJ, Addison I, Ings SJ et al. Optimal timing for collection of PBPC after glycoslyated G-CSF administration. Bone Marrow Transplant 1998;21:365–368

46. Stroncek DF, Matthews CL, Follmann D, Leitman SF. Kinetics of G-CSF-induced granulocyte mobilization in healthy subjects: effects of route of administration and addition of dexamethasone. Transfusion 2002;42:597–602

47. Testa U, Fossati C, Samoggia P et al. Expression of growth factor receptors in unilineage differentiation culture of purified hematopoietic progenitors. Blood 1996;88:3391–3406

48. Olivieri A, Offidani M, Cantori I et al. Addition of erythropoietin to granulocyte colony-stimulating factor after priming chemotherapy enhances hemopoietic progenitor mobilization. Bone Marrow Transplant 1995;16:765–770

49. Perillo A, Ferrandina G, Pierelli L et al. Cytokines alone for PBPC collection in patients with advanced gynaecological malignancies: G-CSF vs. G-CSF plus EPO. Bone Marrow Transplant 2004;34:743–744

50. Sautois B, Baudoux E, Salmon JP et al. Administration of erythropoietin and granulocyte colony-stimulating factor in donor/recipient pairs to collect peripheral blood progenitor cells (PBPC) and red blood cell units for use in the recipient after allogeneic PBPC transplantation. Haematologica 2001;86:1209–1218

51. Lapidot T, Petit I. Current understanding of stem cell mobilization: the roles of chemokines, proteolytic enzymes, adhesion molecules, cytokines, and stromal cells. Exp Haematol 2002;30:973–981

52. Dawson MA, Schwarer AP, Muirhead JL et al. Successful mobilization of peripheral blood stem cells using recombinant human stem cell factor in heavily pretreated patients who have failed a previous attempt with a granulocyte colony-stimulating factor-based regimen. Bone Marrow Transplant 2005;36:389–396

53. Da Silva MG, Pimentel P, Carvalhais A et al. Ancestim (recombinant human stem cell factor, SCF) in association with filgrastim does not enhance chemotherapy and/or growth factor-induced peripheral blood progenitor cell (PBPC) mobilization in patients with a prior insufficient PBPC collection. Bone Marrow Transplant 2004;34:683–691

54. Costa JJ, Demetri GD, Harrist TJ et al. Recombinant human stem cell factor (Kit Ligand) promotes human mast cell and melanocyte hyperplasia and functional activation in vitro. J Exp Med 1996;183:2681–2686

55. Fricker SP, Anastassov V, Cox J et al. Characterization of the molecular pharmacology of AMD3100: A specific antagonist of the G-protein coupled chemokine receptor, CXCR4. Biochem Pharmacol 2006;72:588–596

56. Flomenberg N, Devine SM, DiPersio JF et al. The use of AMD3100 plus G-CSF for autologous hematopoietic progenitor cell mobilization is superior to G-CSF alone. Blood 2005;106:1867–1874

57. Liles WC, Rodger E, Broxmeyer HE et al. Augmented mobilization and collection of CD34+ hematopoietic cells from normal human volunteers stimulated with granulocyte-colony-stimulating factor by single-dose administration of AMD3100, a CXCR4 antagonist. Transfusion 2005;45:295–300

58. Pelus LM, Bian H, King AG et al. Neutrophil-derived MMP-9 mediates synergistic mobilization of hematopoietic stem and progenitor cells by the combination of G-CSF and the chemokines GROβ/CXCL2 and GROβT/CXCL2₇₄. Blood 2004;103:110–119

59. Fukuda S, Bian H, King A, Pelus L. The chemokine GROb mobilizes early hematopoietic stem cells characterized by enhanced homing and engraftment. Blood 2007;110:860–869

60. Hosing C, Qazilbash MH, Kebriaei P et al. Fixed-dose single agent pegfilgrastim for peripheral blood progenitor cell mobilization in patients with multiple myeloma. Br J Haematol 2006;133:533–537

61. Broxmeyer HE, Orschell CM, Clapp DW et al. Rapid mobilization of murine and human hematopoietic stem and progenitor cells with AMD3100, a CXCR4 antagonist. J Exp Med 2005;201:1307–1318

62. Boeve S, Strupeck J, Creech S, Stiff PJ. Analysis of remobilization success in patients undergoing autologous stem cell transplants who fail an initial mobilization: risk factors, cytokine use and cost. Bone Marrow Transplant 2004;33:991–1003

63. Goterris R, Hernandez-Boluda JC, Teruel A et al. Impact of different strategies of second-line stem cell harvest on the outcome of autologous transplantation in poor peripheral blood stem cell mobilizers. Bone Marrow Transplant 2005;36:847–853

64. Lefrere F, Levy V, Makke J et al. Successful peripheral blood stem cell harvesting with granulocyte colony-stimulating factor alone after previous mobilization failure. Haematologica 2004;89:1532–1534

65. Winter JN, Lazarus HM, Rademaker A et al. Phase I/II study of combined granulocyte colony-stimulating factor administration for the mobilization of hematopoietic progenitor cells. J Clin Oncol 1996;14:277–286

66. Gazitt Y. Comparison between granulocyte colony-stimulating factor and granulocyte-macrophage colony-stimulating factor in the mobilization of peripheral blood stem cells. Curr Opin Hematol 2002;9:190–198

67. Kroger N, Renges H, Sonnenberg S et al. Stem cell mobilization with 16 μg/kg vs 10 μg/kg of G-CSF for allogeneic transplantation in healthy donors. Bone Marrow Transplant 2002;29:727–730

68. Stiff PJ. Management strategies for the hard-to-mobilize patient. Bone Marrow Transplant 1999;23(suppl. 2): S29–S33

69. Lemoli RM, DeVivo A, Damiani D et al. Autologous transplantation of G-CSF-primed bone marrow is effective in supporting myeloablative chemotherapy in patients with hema-

tologic malignancies and poor peripheral blood stem cell mobilization. Blood 2003;102:1595–1600

70. Beyer J, Schwella N, Zingsem J et al. Hematopoietic rescue after high-dose chemotherapy using autologous peripheral-blood progenitor cells or bone marrow: a randomized comparison. J Clin Oncol 1995;13:1328–1335

71. Schmitz N, Linch DC, Dreger P et al. Randomized trial of filgrastim-mobilized peripheral blood progenitor cell transplantation versus autologous bone-marrow transplantation in lymphoma patients. Lancet 1996;347:353–357

72. Lazarus HM, Haynesworth SE, Gerson SL, Caplan AI. Human bone marrow-derived mesenchymal (stromal) progenitor cells (MPCs) cannot be recovered from peripheral blood progenitor cell collections. J Hematother 1997;6:447–455

73. Lazarus HM, Haynesworth SE, Gerson SL et al. Ex vivo expansion and subsequent infusion of human bone marrow-derived stromal progenitor cells (mesenchymal progenitor cells): implications for therapeutic use. Bone Marrow Transplant 1995;16:557–564

74. Devine SM, Hoffman R. Role of mesenchymal stem cells in hematopoietic stem cell transplantation. Curr Opin Hematol 2000;7:358–363

75. Pittenger MF, Mackay AM, Beck SC et al. Multilineage potential of adult human mesenchymal stem cells. Science 1999;284:143–146

76. Damiani D, Fanin R, Silvestri F et al. Randomized trial of autologous filgrastim-primed bone marrow transplantation vs. filgrastim-mobilized peripheral blood stem cell transplantation in lymphoma patients. Blood 1997;90:36–42

77. Elfenbein GJ, Sackstein R. Primed marrow for autologous and allogeneic transplantation: A review comparing primed marrow to mobilized blood and steady-state marrow. Exp Haematol 2004;32:327–339

78. Elfenbein GJ, Sackstein R, Oblon DJ. Do G-CSF mobilized, peripheral blood-derived stem cells from healthy, HLA-identical donors really engraft more rapidly than do G-CSF primed, bone marrow-derived stem cells? No! Blood Cells Mol Dis 2004;32; 106–111

79. Weisdorf D, Miller J, Verfaillie C et al. Cytokine-primed bone marrow stem cells vs. peripheral blood stem cells for autologous transplantation: a randomized comparison of GM-CSF vs. G-CSF. Biol Blood Marrow Transplant 1997;3:217–223

80. Spitzer TR. Bone marrow component processing. In: Areman E, Deeg H, Sacher R (eds) Bone marrow and stem cell processing: a manual of current techniques. Davis, Philadelphia, 1992

81. Stiff PJ. Simplified bone marrow cryopreservation using dimethyl sulfoxide and hydroxyethyl starch as cryoprotectants. In: Gee AP (ed) Bone marrow processing and purging: a practical guide. CRC Press, Boca Raton, 1991

82. Aird WC, Labopin M, Gorin N, Antin JH. Long-term cryopreservation of human bone marrow. Blood 1990;76(suppl 1):525

83. Shepherd RM, Capoccia BJ, Devine SM et al. Angiogenic cells can be rapidly mobilized and efficiently harvested from the blood following treatment with AMD3100. Blood 2006;108:3662–3667

84. Gorin NC. Cryopreservation and storage of stem cells. In: Areman E, Deeg H, Sacher R (eds) Bone marrow and stem cell processing: a manual of current techniques. Davis, Philadelphia, 1992

85. Davis J, Rowley S, Santos GW. Toxicity of autologous bone marrow graft infusion. Prog Clin Biol Res 1990;330:531–540

86. Rowley SD, Davis J, Dick J et al. Bacterial contamination of bone marrow grafts intended for autologous and allogeneic bone marrow transplantation. Transfusion 1988;28:109–112

87. American Code of Federal Regulations. §1271 subpart D. 2006

88. Aguila HL. Regulation of hematopoietic niches by sympathetic innervation. BioEssays 2006;28:687–691

89. Katayama Y, Battista M, Wei-Ming K et al. Signals from the sympathetic nervous system regulate hematopoietic stem cell egress from bone marrow. Cell 2006;124:407–421

90. Taichman RS, Emerson SG. The role of osteoblasts in the hematopoietic microenvironment. Stem Cells 1998;16:7–15

Vascular access

John Oram and Andrew Bodenham

CHAPTER 25

Introduction

Vascular access for stem cell transplantation is required at different time points; firstly for harvesting, secondly for cytoreductive therapy, and thirdly for the ongoing support required by these high-risk patients. It is possible to provide almost all of this therapy through peripheral catheters. However, vein sites soon run out as each vein is sequentially used, and this patient population has often been the subject of previous intensive intravenous therapy. We will therefore concentrate on central venous catheters (CVCs), and in particular those capable of providing long-term venous access.

There are a multitude of devices available and choice depends on intended purpose, predicted duration of use and local expertise. This chapter aims to provide a summary of the devices available, their indications and contraindications, and a practical guide to their insertion and use.

Types of catheter

A number of options are available for venous access. The choice of device depends on the patient, the proposed use, and the length of time for which access will be needed. Apheresis requires two points of access. This can be achieved with two separate catheters or by using a device which incorporates two lumens. There are many devices which can achieve this for either short- or long-term use. After harvesting, patients will require access for ongoing support through transfusions, fluid, nutrition and antibiotics. A long-term catheter is usually the best solution to this. Knowledge of all the options, and the advantages and disadvantages of each, is necessary to ensure that the correct choice is made.

Physics of flow through catheters

A simple understanding of flow dynamics is required in order to appreciate the properties of the catheters as related to flow. The dimensions of the catheter are related to flow by the Hagen–Poiseuille equation:

$$\text{Flow} = \frac{Pr^4\pi}{8\eta L}$$

P = pressure
r = radius
η = viscosity
L = length

This equation basically shows that flow is proportional to the fourth power of the radius, and inversely proportional to length i.e. short,

wide-bore catheters allow higher flow rates. Similarly, as viscosity increases, flow will be reduced.

These factors must be taken into account when choosing devices for any specific purpose.

Short-term catheters

Simple peripheral catheters

Simple peripheral venous cannulae provide rapid access to the venous system. They are available in a range of sizes depending on the intended use. These devices are prone to infection and become easily dislodged. Extravasation is common, as is thrombosis, and hence their lifespan is often limited to little more than a few days. Short, large-bore catheters can provide high flow rates as explained above. These are suitable for outflow and reinfusion during apheresis. They will not be discussed further as they are common, and well understood by most practicing doctors.

'Short-term' CVCs

These are inserted into a large vein and then travel short distances through the vein to lie in the central circulation. A range of styles is available depending on the required purpose. The most common type is 15–20 cm long with 3–4 lumens contained in a smooth body of approximately 14 gauge. CVCs allow safe infusion of irritant drugs into large veins and can be used for blood sampling. Although the external diameter is quite large, each internal lumen is small and long and maximal flow rates may be low. Cases of these 'bursting' when high pressure is applied have been reported.

If high infusion and outflow rates are required, then devices designed for hemodialysis are suitable. These are dual-lumen, large-bore catheters which allow very high flow rates (~200–300 ml/min). They are best inserted by the right internal jugular or femoral routes as they do not traverse corners easily.

CVCs can be inserted relatively quickly and, with the advent of ultrasound, with minimal complications. If the vein has been entered easily and no resistance encountered, it is often assumed that the line tip will pass into the right atrium. However, inadequate positioning is relatively common and can cause the same problems as those encountered with peripherally inserted central catheters (PICC) (see later), although movement post insertion is less common.

Short-term CVCs can stay in place for a longer period of time than can peripheral lines, if they are well cared for, but they rarely last more than 2–3 weeks. If it is anticipated that treatment is likely to be needed for more than 3 weeks, then a tunneled or other long-term access device may be more appropriate.

Long-term catheters

Peripherally inserted central catheters (PICCs)

The term PICC encompasses all catheters inserted peripherally, which are then threaded through the lumen of the vein so that the tip lies in a central vein. They are generally inserted at the antecubital fossa or just above and pass through the arm to end in the right atrium or superior vena cava (SVC). As the tip of the line lies centrally, these lines are suitable for infusion of irritant drugs. They are not usually tunneled and do not generally have an anchoring cuff.

PICCs provide a solution to central access with limited complications related to insertion. Unfortunately, the premature failure rate for these lines is as high as 21%.[1] These devices are long, with a small internal diameter, and as such they cannot be used for rapid infusions of blood products. It can also be difficult to sample blood from them, and they are not suited to apheresis. Double-lumen lines are available, but these have even smaller diameters.

PICC are reasonably easy to insert. A range of kits is available, using similar insertion techniques. Usually, a large cannula or splitting sheath is inserted into an antecubital fossa vein and the catheter is then inserted through this cannula to a premeasured depth (estimated by measurements against the chest wall or with X-ray screening). The cannula is removed from the vein and either sits on the line or is removed via a detachable hub assembly. The main practical problems relate to obtaining adequate positioning of the line tip (see below), and passing the line through the clavipectoral fascia (often made easier by abducting the arm).

Problems obtaining adequate positioning of the line tip during insertion, and subsequent movement of the line tip as the patient moves their arm are common. Incorrect initial position occurs in up to 40% of cases and can only be avoided with fluoroscopic screening.[1-3] Movement of the tip post insertion can be by as much as 9 cm and can result in an increase in complications.[4,5] The incidence of thrombosis rises to 60% if the line tip lies in either the subclavian or brachiocephalic vein (compared to 21% if it lies in the SVC or right atrium).[6] Movement post insertion can cause arrhythmias if the line enters the heart, or damage to the vessel wall as the line tip moves against the endoluminal surface of the vein.

Tunneled central venous lines

These devices are the most common type of long-term venous access device in current use for stem cell transplantation cases. They consist of a soft, pliable catheter which is inserted into one of the central veins and then tunneled under the skin to an exit site distant to the venepuncture site. A Dacron cuff attached to the line lies in the tunnel and produces a local fibrotic reaction which anchors the cuff and catheter to the tissues. Since their introduction by Broviac in 1973,[7] a number of similar devices with a range of features has been used. Tunneled lines can stay in the circulation with minimal complications for many months or even years.

Hickman lines are essentially the same as Broviac lines, but with a larger internal lumen. They are the most common type of long-term device in use today. Derivatives of these are common, and double- and triple-lumen lines have increased their range of application.

Large-bore implantable devices are available such as **Tesio lines** which consist of two large-bore parallel tunneled catheters. They are usually used for renal replacement therapy, with one limb being used as the arterial side and one as the venous, but are equally suitable for apheresis.

Valved catheters have a valve at their distal tip (Groschong), or proximally which requires either a negative or positive pressure (up to 80 mmHg) to open and pressurized systems to infuse. They cannot be used to measure central venous pressure. This valve prevents backflow of blood into the line, and hence reduces the need for heparin locks. It can also prevent air embolism. Double-lumen versions are available.

Implantable ports consist of a tunneled venous line connected to an access device which is inserted subcutaneously, often on the chest wall. A special non-coring needle is required to access the thick port membrane. The catheter has a relatively low internal diameter which limits maximum flow rates. These devices are sometimes more acceptable to patients as they are completely subcutaneous when not being used and hence are more cosmetically pleasing. They also allow the patient to swim or bathe and have the lowest rates of infection for long-term access devices. These advantages progressively disappear as the need for access moves from intermittent injection to continuous infusions over days and weeks. The continued presence of the access needle breaches protective skin barriers and makes the device more like a Hickman-type catheter with the disadvantage of lower flow rates and the inconvenience of a stiff needle protruding from the device, with risks of dislodgment and extravasation. Table 25.1 summarizes the properties of the various lines available.

Sites of access

The choice of site depends on many factors. Different sites have different benefits and disadvantages, although there is little objective evidence on this issue. Choice may be limited by thrombotic complications of previous lines, anatomic variability and presence of localized pathology. Hence, the operator should have a detailed knowledge of the anatomy and risks relevant to each site. The following is a brief summary of the advantages and disadvantages of the commonly used sites.

Jugular

Internal or external jugular veins can be used on either side of the neck. The internal jugular vein has advantages in that it is relatively superficial and on the right side there is a straight insertion line from

Table 25.1 Line characteristics

Type of line	Duration of use	Pros	Cons
Peripheral	2–3 days	Cheap, easy to inset. Few major complications	Very short lifespan. Cannot be used for irritant drugs
PICC	Months	Easy to insert	Difficult to control tip position. Low infusion rates
Short-term central	Up to 3 weeks	Can be used for sampling and infusing	Limited lifespan due to infections
Tunneled central line	Months to years	Very long lifespan. Access for sampling and infusing to the central circulation	Expensive; high flows difficult to achieve
Tunneled port	Months to years	Completely internal system. Cosmetically pleasing	Access device needed with skin puncture each time. Expensive. Limited flows

the skin through to the long axis of the SVC, providing the most reliable catheter tip position in blind procedures. Lines inserted via the left-sided vessel have two 'corners' to negotiate and hence do not always achieve satisfactory central positions.

The position of the internal jugular is traditionally described as lying lateral to the carotid, and various landmark techniques have been used to guide insertion. Unfortunately, the position of the vessel in relation to the carotid is not reliable,[8] rendering landmark techniques potentially hazardous. Internal jugular lines can be uncomfortable for patients, and tunneled devices pass over the clavicle and can be unsightly. The internal jugular is thought to have the lowest risk of thrombosis.[9] Thrombosis is often occult, due to collateral flow through the contralateral side.

Subclavian/infraclavicular axillary

The subclavian vein has traditionally been accessed by passing a needle deep to the clavicle and puncturing the vein as it passes between the clavicle and first rib. It is possible to access the vein more laterally, before it passes under the clavicle. Landmark techniques have been advocated for this, but positioning is very variable and ultrasound guidance is usually required to facilitate a more lateral puncture to what is technically the axillary vein. The advantage of the more lateral position is that the artery and ribcage are further from the vein, and hence complications related to damage to these structures are less frequent, and it is possible to apply pressure directly to the vein (or artery) if hemorrhage does occur.[10]

These routes are comfortable for the patient, and provide direct access to the central circulation. Right-sided lines have a shorter, more direct route into the SVC than left-sided ones, and may have a lower risk of thrombosis than those inserted from the left, but this may reflect left-sided catheters being left too short.[11] Lines inserted into the subclavian may have a higher risk of thrombosis than internal jugular lines but this may reflect in part the easier clinical recognition of this problem due to a swollen arm.

Femoral

Femoral veins are relatively easy to access in slim patients and early complication rates are low. Again, the position of the vein is more variable than traditional anatomic teaching would suggest. Landmark techniques should be used with caution. Discomfort can be a problem as the line is inserted close to a skin crease. Infection rates can be high. Tunneled lines inserted via the femoral route are usually brought up to exit the skin on the abdominal wall (Fig. 25.1). We tend to limit the use of this site for long-term access to patients with SVC obstruction or thrombosis. Table 25.2 gives a summary of the different sites of access.

Right-sided versus left-sided lines

While it is important to appreciate the advantages of each site, it is also important to realize the difference between the different sides. This is less relevant in femoral access, but has a significant impact on lines inserted into the chest. Lines inserted into the right side of the chest generally have a shorter intravascular course and lie more parallel to the long axis of the vessel. There is some anecdotal evidence to suggest that this results in a lower risk of thrombosis. Left-sided lines have to traverse the innominate vein and hence have a longer intravascular portion. These lines will enter the SVC at an angle and may point against the lateral wall of the vessel, increasing the risk of perforation (see below for a discussion of line tip position).

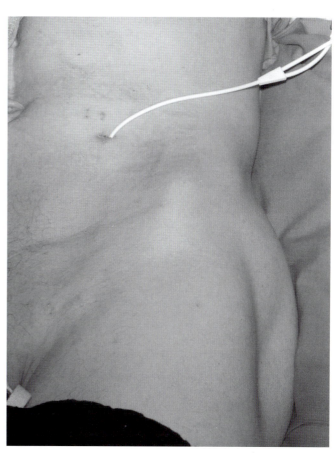

Figure 25.1
Femoral Hickman line. Line is inserted via the left femoral vein, tunneled onto the anterior abdominal wall. This approach can be used in cases of SVC obstruction.

Table 25.2 Sites of access

Site	Jugular	Subclavian/axillary	Femoral
Ease of insertion	Easily identifiable landmarks, but variable position	Can be difficult, ultrasound needed for axillary access	Variable position in relation to artery
Comfort	Movement associated with turning head means limited comfort	More comfortable	Close to skin crease, less comfortable
Proximity to arteries	Very close to carotid	Lies close to the artery medially, but further away in more lateral approaches	Very close to femoral artery, but easy to apply pressure
Proximity to nerves	Vagus at risk medially, brachial plexus laterally, sympathetics	Brachial plexus	Femoral nerve
Infection risk	Potentially higher than subclavian as difficult to clean in skin crease	Lower	High
Pneumothorax risk	Moderate	Significant	None

Other options for central access

When all the routine sites have been used and are no longer suitable for recannulation, it is possible to access deeper veins. The portal vein, internal mammary vein, cephalic vein, pudendal vein, gonadal vein, and azygos veins have all been successfully cannulated.[12–15] Techniques involving direct puncture of the inferior vena cava (IVC) have also been used.[16] These routes are clearly not for the inexperienced operator and may require surgical cut-down rather than a percutaneous approach. Equally, radiologic stenting of narrowed central veins may restore patency of previously damaged sites. Difficult cases should be discussed with experienced staff who have the knowledge and expertise to resolve such problems.

Construction of catheters

Catheters consist of a number of components bonded together to form a single unit capable of lying within tissue without producing an inflammatory reaction. They must be chemically and immunologically inert, non-thrombogenic and soft and flexible enough to reduce any mechanical damage that movement may incur. Most currently available catheters are made of silicon rubber impregnated with radio-opaque materials.

Addition of anticoagulant coatings in an attempt to reduce thrombotic complications has been largely unsuccessful. Antibiotic-bonded lines have been shown to reduce the incidence of catheter colonization,[17–19] but there is still debate about effects on bacteremia or mortality. There are now antimicrobial-coated catheters for both short- and long-term usage.

Use of ultrasound

Guidelines have been drawn up on this issue in the UK,[20] which suggest routine use of ultrasound for all internal jugular lines, although insufficient evidence has been found to recommend the technology for use at other sites. However, it has been shown that the course of vessels at all common sites for vascular access can vary. Landmark techniques will fail even the most experienced operator if the vessel differs greatly from its predicted position, and ultrasound can help to identify this. UIltrasound can be used at all sites of access and provides a quick, easy, non-invasive method of vein identification. It also allows the operator to confirm patency of the vessel and can be used to guide the needle into the vessel and, more importantly, away from other structures.[21]

While it is important to maintain knowledge of landmark techniques for emergencies, we feel that ultrasound should be used wherever possible.

Insertion technique

General measures

Insertions can be performed a number of ways. We will describe techniques for short-term or tunneled devices for insertion by the percutaneous route.

Formal written consent should be obtained for all elective procedures, and verbal explanation given as a minimum in more acute situations. The procedure should take place under strict asepsis, with facilities for resuscitation from complications, and enough space for the operator and an assistant. It is possible to insert lines on the ward but it is difficult to maintain asepsis and resuscitation equipment is often limited. Operating theaters or radiology suites are usually the better option, and the use of fluoroscopic guidance makes such a facility almost mandatory.

1. Sedation is administered as appropriate to the individual patient. Occasional patients may require a general anesthetic.
2. Identify the vein with ultrasound techniques. After an appropriate site for vascular access is chosen, the skin is prepared and draped as for a formal surgical procedure. Local anesthetic with adrenaline is administered by local infiltration, to provide complete anesthesia of the operative site.
3. The vein is punctured with direct ultrasound visualization and a flexible J-tip wire is passed into the vessel. The wire is fluoroscopically screened to ensure that it has passed centrally to the required depth, and its internal length is measured to guide catheter length.
4. A small incision is made at the proposed exit site, and at the point where the wire exits the skin.
5. The tunneler is then inserted at the exit site and gently advanced subcutaneously towards the vein entry site and the wire. The flushed catheter is attached to the tunneler and is pulled through, so that the line now lies in a subcutaneous tunnel. The line is positioned so that the cuff sits well inside the tunnel to reduce the risk of cuff extrusion through the exit site.
6. The line is cut to length according to previous measurements from a correctly sited guidewire using fluoroscopy. A stiff dilator with a peel-away sheath is passed over the wire and advanced into the vein. The dilator and wire are removed, and the line is advanced through the sheath into the vein. The sheath is then withdrawn and split away to leave the line lying in the vein.
7. Correct positioning of the line is adjusted and confirmed by fluoroscopy.
8. The skin incisions are sutured and anchoring devices are fixed in place.
9. A routine chest X-ray is performed to document the position of the line tip and any procedural complications.

Choice of exit site

Choice of exit site depends on cosmetic considerations and the presence of local disease. In women with large breasts and in obese patients, it is important to take into account traction on the exit site which will occur when the patient stands or sits up, which will tend to pull the line out, shortening the intravascular portion and changing the tip position.[22]

Choice of tip position

This is a matter of some debate. Traditionally, central catheters have been inserted into the SVC, but with the intention of keeping the tip above the pericardial reflection to reduce the risk of cardiac tamponade if it were to erode through the myocardial wall. The carina has been used as a radiologic landmark for the pericardial reflection.

Catheters inserted to this length can cause problems as they will have a relatively short course in the SVC. Lines inserted from either the subclavian or the left internal jugular vein will angulate on entering the SVC. If they do not have a long enough section in the SVC, they may move on coughing, abut against the vessel wall and increase the risk of pain, irritation, thromboses and vascular perforation. If a line is inserted further, it will tend to lie more in the long axis of the SVC, and its tip may lie within the right atrium, but overall this may present a lower risk[11,23,24] (Fig. 25.2).

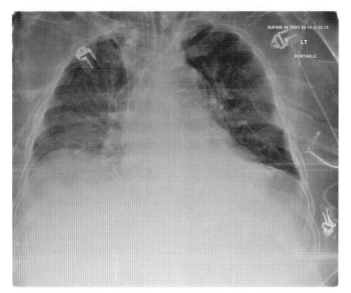

Figure 25.2
Long line and short line. Chest X-ray of a patient with two central lines. One lies high, above the pericardium but has the potential to perforate the SVC, whereas the longer line is below the pericardial reflection but lies in the long axis of the vessel and is less likely to cause perforation.

It is also worth noting that the pericardium can extend further up the SVC than previously thought, and hence higher positions do not necessarily reduce the risk of tamponade.[25–27]

Chest X-ray

Chest X-rays have been seen as a standard investigation after any central line has been inserted. The intention is to confirm correct positioning of the line and to detect any complications such as pneumothoraces. However, if a vessel has been entered under direct ultrasound guidance, and fluoroscopic screening has confirmed line position, the value of a routine CXR is debatable.[28,29]

Pneumothoraces from lines are often not visible on immediate postprocedure films, and may take some time to become apparent. In this situation a delayed film would be more useful, but even then it would not necessarily change care unless symptoms were present.

The anticoagulated patient

Anticoagulation can be either therapeutic or as a result of pathology. Patients with a coagulopathy should have appropriate corrective therapy prior to catheter insertion. The international normalized ratio (INR) should be less than 1.5, the platelet count should be in excess of 50×10^9/l, and the fibrinogen should be greater than 1 g/l.[30]

The approach to the anticoagulated patient depends upon the indication for anticoagulation and hence for how long it can be safely stopped. Ideally, anticoagulants should be stopped prior to the procedure and an appropriate interval left to allow all effects to wear off. This may not be possible in those cases where the risk of thrombotic problems is high, and periods without anticoagulation carry an increased risk. If anticoagulation has to be continued up to the time of catheter insertion, the patient should be converted to iv heparin and maintained at an appropriate activated partial thromboplastin time (APTT) ratio until the INR has normalized. Heparin can then be stopped prior to surgery and recommenced after hemostasis is achieved. If in doubt, the case should be discussed with the operator in advance of the procedure.

Complications

The complications associated with any specific catheter depend upon its type and insertion site. Complications can be divided into procedural (those occurring during or related to insertion), and late (those associated with the ongoing presence of the line).

Procedural complications

Hemorrhage

Bleeding can be related to puncture of the vein, inappropriate puncture of an artery, tear of an artery or vein, or leakage around a sited line. Bleeding from the subcutaneous tissues will usually settle with pressure and/or an additional suture. Bleeding from venous sites is usually easy to control if pressure can be applied to the vessel. As long as the hole is not too large, most bleeding will stop. Larger holes may require surgical repair and hence it is important to ensure that the guidewire has passed into the correct structure before it is dilated.

Hemorrhagic complications are more common in those patients with bleeding diatheses related to their primary diagnosis or to treatment. Significant local bleeding with hematoma formation, or bleeding into the chest or other sites requires urgent consultation with vascular or cardiothoracic surgeons and/or interventional radiologists, depending on the site.

Pneumothorax

Pneumothoraces are related to internal jugular and subclavian procedures. The apex of the lung can extend into the base of the neck for quite some distance. Care is needed to avoid the lung at these locations. The use of ultrasound, a high approach to internal jugular puncture and a more lateral approach to the subclavian area can ameliorate most of this risk.

Treatment of a pneumothorax depends on its size and symptoms and the clinical scenario. A large pneumothorax with symptoms needs draining, but smaller ones may not require any specific therapy. Guidelines do not exist for management of pneumothorax after line insertion. The operator should be contacted and referral made to the appropriate specialty (e.g. critical care, chest medicine or thoracic surgery).

Inadvertent arterial cannulation

Arterial puncture should be readily recognizable by the pulsatile blood flow from the needle; however, this has not always prevented the vessel from being cannulated. Catheters placed into the arterial tree can cause problems with bleeding at the site of insertion which may require vascular repair if large, and embolic problems distal to the insertion site. Emboli have particularly grave consequences if the line is placed into the carotid.

If arterial puncture occurs, the needle should be removed and pressure applied. If the line has been fully inserted into the artery then bleeding on removal is more problematic as the hole will be that much larger after dilatation. Advice should be sought from vascular surgeons or interventional radiologists before removing large cannulae from arteries. There may be problems in applying pressure to a carotid artery that has been punctured. The subclavian artery is not easily accessed for direct pressure. Surgical closure is rarely needed but becomes more necessary with the use of larger lines. Endovascular repair is often the technique of choice, if possible.

Dislodgment/cuff extrusion

Long-term catheters are held in place by a number of methods, but most have some form of cuff which elicits a fibrotic reaction and the line 'heals' into the tissue. This reaction can take 3–4 weeks to complete, particularly in the presence of chemotherapy and immunosuppression, and until this time the catheter is at great risk of falling out. A line that has moved significantly at its exit site will have moved at the tip, which may no longer be in a safe or suitable position. These lines may need reinserting. Lines that have moved so far that the cuff is extruding at the exit site may also need resiting.

Late complications

Infection

Infection of long-term catheters is common, with as many as 60% of patients having some form of infective complication during the lifespan of the device.[31-33] These infections range from trivial, superficial infections through to life-threatening bacteremia requiring intensive therapy. Infections can be subdivided, depending upon the infected area.

Exit site infection consists of a small area of cellulitis at this site. This is uncomfortable for the patient but rarely requires the line to be removed and is often easily treated with antibiotics.

Tunnel infection can be more serious and may require the line to be removed depending on the virulence of the organism. These infections can lead to abscess formation which will not settle while a foreign body (the catheter) is present. Following catheter removal, this infection will usually settle with antibiotics but severe cases may require surgical drainage of pus.

Catheter-related bacteremia is the most serious and potentially life-threatening infective complication, with mortality rates as high as 24%.[34] Diagnosis is difficult and the line may be prematurely removed when it is not the source of the bacteremia.

There is an association between the formation of intravascular thrombus and infection, and strategies aimed at reducing the thrombus rate have been associated with a reduction in catheter-related sepsis. Treatment of catheter-related sepsis is possible without removal of the catheter but relies on correct diagnosis of a fully sensitive pathogen. Removal of the line makes treatment easier, but may remove the only access site for administration of antibiotics. The decision to remove the line should be made on an individual basis. Differential cultures through the catheter and peripheral site may be helpful.

Catheter blockage

Catheter blockage can occur at any time after insertion and can be due to extraluminal compression or intraluminal blockage.

Pinch-off is the term applied to compression of subclavian lines as they get trapped between the clavicle and first rib (Fig. 25.3). This can cause decreased flow through the catheter, and over time can lead to fracture of the line. If the line fractures, the intravascular portion can embolize, with significant consequences. Early recognition of pinch-off is vital to prevent fracture. One of the early signs of impending

fracture is a change in catheter patency with alterations in arm position. Further indicators are listed below.

Other signs of pinch-off include:
- difficulty injecting or withdrawing
- pain in the shoulder during injection (due to extravasation of drugs)
- visible compression of the line on CXR (Figs 25.4, 25.5).

Intraluminal blockage is usually due to thrombosis, but can be due to incompatible drugs precipitating in the line. Prevention of blockage involves heparin flushes and locks, or the use of valved catheters which do not allow backflow of blood. Thrombolytic agents have been used with some success, the intention being to dissolve clot in the line without producing systemic thrombolysis. If the line is not completely blocked it is possible to infuse the thrombolytic agent very slowly. If the line is completely blocked it is more difficult to get the drug down the line to the clot. Two techniques are commonly used in this setting.
- Using a three-way tap, the syringe is sucked to collapse with one syringe. The tap is then turned to allow thrombolytic agent in a second syringe to be sucked back into the line as it re-expands.
- A syringe of thrombolytic agent can be attached to the blocked line and simply allowed to spread along it by diffusion.

The dose of urokinase used is 5000–10,000 units.[35] There are commercial preparations designed for this indication, although they are only obtainable on a named patient basis.[30]

Similar problems may occur due to organized clot forming a fibrin sleeve along the length of the catheter. Such blockage may be resolved

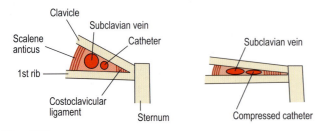

Figure 25.3
Mechanism of pinch-off. As the arm moves, the clavicle and first rib approximate. If the catheter lies between them it will be compressed. Over time this will damage the catheter, causing leaks and eventually fracture.

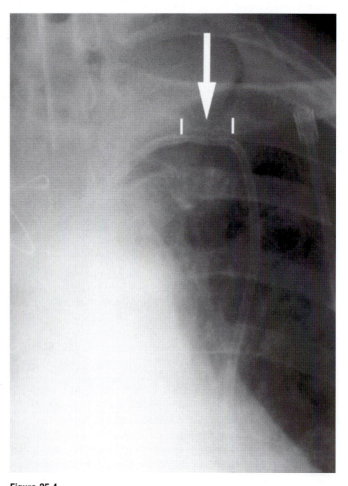

Figure 25.4
Scalloping (arrow). This image shows compression of a catheter between clavicle and first rib. This is typical of pinch-off. This appearance should prompt removal before complications occur.

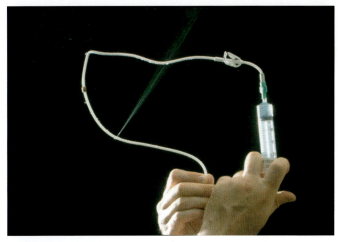

Figure 25.5
Perforated Hickman. The catheter from Fig. 25.4 after removal. Pinch-off has caused damage to the wall of the catheter, resulting in leakage of injectate.

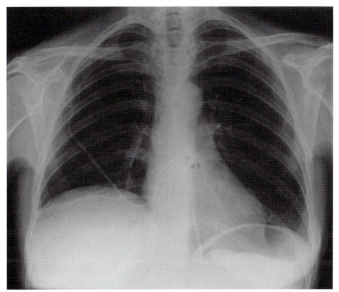

Figure 25.6
Migrating line. This Hickman line has migrated outwards after insertion. The tip now lies at the junction of the right subclavian and internal jugular veins. The catheter needs removing before it causes thrombosis.

with the use of fibrinolytic drugs as described above, or mechanical removal with a snare by radiologists.

Catheter damage

The external portion of long-term catheters can be repaired using kits from the manufacturer if the catheter is sterile and considered precious, i.e. other sites of access are unavailable or difficult. Advice should be sought.

Catheter tip migration

Catheter tip migration is relatively common post insertion and can result in increased risk of thrombosis and vascular perforation. Migration may be picked up incidentally on X-ray, or after the line has become difficult to aspirate or inject. Catheters whose tips have moved should be removed and resited to avoid ongoing complications. Figure 25.6 shows a tunneled line which has migrated out after insertion. It is not easy to move cuffed catheters back to their original positions with an aseptic technique. Intravascular loops of catheter can be manipulated by interventional radiology if they have migrated.

Intravascular thrombosis

Catheter-related thrombosis is common and is visible in up to 67% of cases in ultrasound studies, but it is often subclinical.[36] Sequelae are significant. Thrombus is thought to be a medium for infection and can also produce blockage of the major veins which can be life threatening.

Various strategies have been used to prevent the formation of thrombus. Warfarin, low molecular weight heparin and unfractionated heparin have all been shown to reduce the incidence of catheter-related thrombosis, but all produce a degree of anticoagulation which may be unacceptable. Low-dose warfarin regimens have been shown to be ineffective,[37,38] leaving clinicians to decide whether to offer no prophylaxis or therapeutic dose anticoagulation to patients considered at major risk. Heparin-bonded lines are available but have not been shown to be of benefit in long-term use.

Treatment of thrombosis does not necessarily involve removal of the line. Thrombolysis has been used successfully with the line left in situ. One consequence of thrombosis is long-term blockage of the vein. This is caused by organization of the clot, with limited recannulation. Blockage can result in distal edema due to locally high venous pressures, but obstructions in more central positions can result in SVC obstruction which can be life-threatening. In time, collaterals will open up, allowing normal flow, but sometimes the obstruction will need to be dilated with radiologically guided intravascular techniques.

Vessel perforation

This rare complication is most commonly the result of poorly placed central catheter tips. The most common situation is that of a catheter inserted on the left which enters the SVC at an angle and is left short, so that the tip presses into the lateral wall of the SVC. This can generally be avoided by ensuring that a long enough portion of the line lies in the long axis of the vessel.

The outcome of a catheter perforation depends upon:
- the size of the defect generated
- how quickly the event is discovered
- whether any substance was infused through the hole
- the nature of any substance infused through the hole.

Mediastinitis, hydrothorax and pericardial tamponade are recognized complications requiring specialist management.

Repeated procedures

Many patients will require more than one catheter during the course of their treatment. For these individuals, problems can become compounded, with procedures becoming progessively more difficult as sites become thrombosed and no longer useable. In infected cases, time should be allowed between removal and reinsertion procedures, if possible. Ultrasound permits identification of suitable sites in most cases, but more difficult cases may need venography, computed tomography (CT) or other imaging to ascertain patency of central veins. If no easily accessible central veins can be found then it may be possible to stent vessels under radiologic guidance, and specialist advice should be sought (Figs 25.7–25.9). In these cases, the peripheral vein can appear normal on ultrasound and may seem suitable for cannulation, but proximal blockage will result in inability to pass the guidewire or catheter centrally.

Line removal

Catheters should be removed either when they are no longer needed or when a complication which requires removal of the line occurs. In the latter situation, the decision is clinical and should take into account

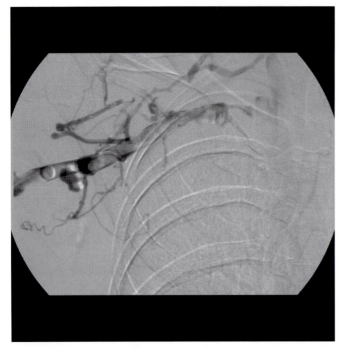

Figure 25.7
Subclavian blockage. Venogram of right-sided axillary/subclavian system. The axillary vein is obstructed and contrast can be seen flowing through collateral vessels.

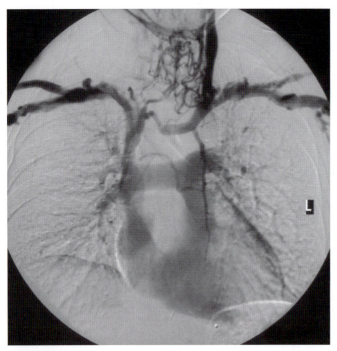

Figure 25.8
Contrast injected up both arms demonstrates blockage of the left innominate vein following long-term central venous catheterization. There is reflux of contrast up the left internal jugular vein and multiple venous collaterals.

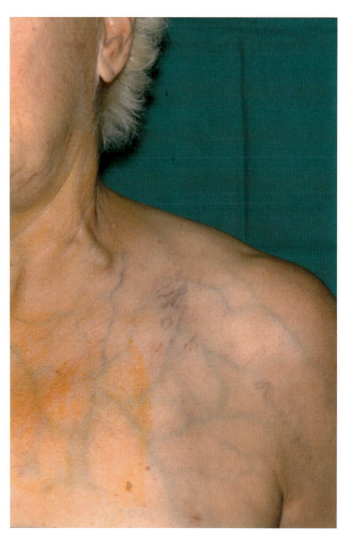

Figure 25.9
Surface appearance of a similar patient to Fig. 25.8. Distended collateral veins on the chest wall over the site of a previous central venous catheter should warn the operator of potential central vein obstruction. This patient had had a previous left subclavian catheter for long-term access which was removed due to blockage.

individual patient factors. A catheter is more likely to be removed if alternative sites for both long- and short-term access are available than if multiple previous lines have been sited and there are limited options for recannulation.

Catheters are removed with the patient supine to avoid air entry and subsequent embolization. Non-cuffed catheters are pulled out and pressure is then applied for 5–10 minutes and the exit site covered with an occlusive dressing. Catheter tips need only to be sent for culture if there is clinical suspicion of catheter-related sepsis.

Cuffed catheters that have only been in for a short time or those that are heavily infected may have a non-anchored cuff allowing removal by traction. Otherwise, after this time if excessive force is applied, pain and snapping of the catheter are likely.

Removal of established tunneled devices usually involves dissecting out the cuff from the tissue in which it has become embedded. This will require a local anesthetic. It is easy to cut the soft catheter during this process. Embolization of the intravascular portion of the line may then occur into the SVC, right atrium, right ventricle or pulmonary artery. Such fragments should be removed by radiologic snaring. It is vital to secure the venous section of the catheter before the cuff is dissected out (Fig. 25.10).

Following a small skin incision, blunt dissection is performed to expose the cuff and catheter. Removal of the venous section of the catheter first will secure it against embolization. The cuff can then be cut out from its adhesions and removed. Pressure should be applied over the venous puncture site in order to limit further bleeding.[39]

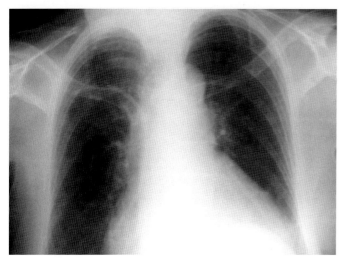

Figure 25.10
This chest X-ray shows a tunneled line where the external portion has been cut before the intravascular portion has been secured. The intravascular catheter section has migrated inwards and lies in the subclavian vein. It required radiology removal via the femoral vein.

Who should insert devices?

A large number of practitioners from a variety of different specialties insert catheters for both long- and short-term use. There is no evidence suggesting that any one group is better than another in terms of either a satisfactory result or complications. The current climate of competency-based training and revalidation suggests the need for a required standard to be reached, and then maintenance of adequate exposure to ensure good practice. As yet, there is no recognized training program or standard at which the trainee can be recognized as competent. Training is often supplied by local practitioners who have been deemed competent by years of practice. Core competencies should include the use of local anesthesia, intravenous sedation, the use of ultrasound and fluoroscopy, familiarity of access at all common insertion sites, and the recognition and management of common complications.

Insertion technique

Tunneled lines can be inserted percutaneously or via surgical cut-down. The percutaneous route is usually preferred for adult patients, performed under local anesthesia with supplemental intravenous sedation and analgesia. Cut-downs under general anesthesia are still routinely used for children in many centers. Studies have shown the percutaneous route to be superior for adult patients by a number of criteria, including:
- lower risk of infection
- fewer failed insertions
- reduction in theater time.

Surgical cut-downs can limit access to the vein for future cannulations.

Conclusion

Central venous access is a fundamental part of practice in the stem cell transplant population. An understanding of such devices, their complications and risk benefits is essential for safe practice in these vulnerable patients.

References

1. Merrill S, Peatross B, Grossman M et al. Peripherally inserted central venous catheters. Low-risk alternatives for ongoing venous access. Western J Med 1994;160:25–30
2. Duerksen D, Papineau N, Siemens J et al. Peripherally inserted central catheters for parenteral nutrition: a comparison with centrally inserted catheters. J Parenteral Enteral Nutr 1999;23:85–89
3. Ragasa J, Shah N, Watson R. Where antecubital catheters go: a study under fluoroscopic control. Anesthesiology 1989;71:378–380
4. Kalso E, Rosenberg P, Vuorialho M et al. How much do arm movements displace cubital central venous catheters? Acta Anaesthesiol Scand 1982;26:354–356
5. Nadroo A, Glass R, Lin J et al. Changes in upper extremity position cause migration of peripherally inserted central catheters in neonates. Pediatrics 2002;110:131–136
6. Kearns P, Coleman S, Wehner J. Complications of long arm catheters: a randomised trial of central versus peripheral tip location. J Parenteral Enteral Nutr 1996;20:20–24
7. Broviac J, Cole J, Scribner B. A silicone rubber right atrial catheter for prolonged parenteral alimentation. Surg Gynecol Obstet 1973;136:602–606
8. Caridi JG, Hawkins IF, Wiechman BN et al. Sonographic guidance when using the right internal jugular vein for central vein access. Am J Roentgenol 1998;171:1259–1263
9. Timsit JF, Farkas JC, Boyer JM et al. Central vein catheter-related thrombosis in intensive care patients: incidence, risks factors, and relationship with catheter-related sepsis. Chest 1998;114:207–213
10. Sharma A, Bodenham AR, Mallick A. Ultrasound-guided infraclavicular axillary vein cannulation for central venous access. Br J Anaesth 2004;93:188–192
11. Stonelake PA, Bodenham AR. The carina as a radiological landmark for central venous catheter tip position. Br J Anaesth 2006;96:335–340
12. Chuter T, Starker P. Placement of Hickman-Broviac catheters in the cephalic vein. Surg Gynecol Obstet 1988;166:163–164
13. Fukui S, Coggia M, Goeau-Brissonniere O et al. Introducing an implantable central venous catheter via the right pudendal vein. Presse Medicale 1995;24:1608–1609
14. Coit D, Turnbull A. Long term central vascular access through the gonadal vein. Surg Gynecol Obstet 1992;175:362–364
15. Patel N. Percutaneous translumbar placement of a Hickman catheter into the azygos vein. Am J Roetgenol 2000;175:1302–1304
16. Bennett J, Papadouris D, Rankin R, et al. Percutaneous inferior vena caval approach for long term central venous access. J Vasc Intervent Radiol 1997;8:851–855
17. Maki D, Stolz S, Wheeler S et al. Prevention of central venous catheter-related bloodstream infection by use of an antiseptic-impregnated catheter. Ann Intern Med 1997;127:257–266
18. Pai M, Pendland S, Danziger L. Antimicrobial-coated/bonded and -impregnated intravascular catheters. Ann Pharmacother 2001;35:1255–1263
19. Veenstra D, Saint S, Saha S et al. Efficacy of antiseptic-impregnated central venous catheters in preventing catheter-related bloodstream infection. A meta-analysis. JAMA 1999;281:261–267
20. National Institute for Clinical Excellence (NICE). Guidance on the use of ultrasound locating devices for central venous catheters. NICE Technology Appraisal. National Institute for Clinical Excellence, London, 2002:49
21. Chapman GA, Johnson D, Bodenham AR. Visualisation of needle position using ultrasonography. Anaesthesia 2006;61:148–158
22. Nazarian GK, Bjarnason H, Dietz CA Jr et al. Changes in catheter tip position when a patient is upright. J Vasc Intervent Radiol 1997;8:437–441
23. Gravenstein N, Blackshear RH. In vitro evaluation of relative perforating potential of central venous catheters: comparison of materials, selected models, number of lumens and angles of incidence to simulated membrane. J Clin Monitor 1991;7:1–6
24. McGee WT, Ackermann BL, Rouben LR et al. Accurate placement of central venous catheters: a prospective, randomized, multicenter trial. Crit Care Med 1993;21:1118–1123
25. Dailey R. Late vascular perforations by CVP catheters. J Emerg Med 1998;146:487–490
26. Puel V, Cudrey M, Le Metayer P et al. Superior vena cava thrombosis related to catheter malposition in cancer chemotherapy given through implanted ports. Cancer 1993;72:2248–2252
27. Schuster M, Nave H, Piepenbrock S et al. The carina as a landmark in central venous catheter placement. Br J Anaesth 2000;85:191–193
28. Lucey B, Varghese J, Haslam P et al. Routine chest radiographs after central line insertion: mandatory postprocedural evaluation or unnecessary waste of resources? Cardiovasc Intervent Radiol 1999;22:381–384
29. Gladwin M, Slonim A, Landucci D et al. Cannulation of the internal jugular vein: is postprocedural chest radiography always necessary? Crit Care Med 1999;27:1819–1823
30. Bishop L, Dougherty L, Bodenham A et al. Guidelines on the insertion and management of central venous access devices. Int J Lab Hematol 2007;29(4):261–278
31. Hartman G, Shochat S. Management of septic complications associated with Silastic catheters in childhood malignancy. Pediatr Infect Dis J 1987;6:1042–1047
32. Shaw J, Douglas R, Wilson T. Clinical performance of Hickman and Portacath atrial catheters. Aust NZ J Surg 1988;58:657–659
33. Greene F, Moore W, Strickland G et al. Comparison of a totally implantable access device for chemotherapy (Port-ACath) and long-term percutaneous catheterization (Broviac). Southern Med J 1988;81:580–603
34. Pittet D, Tarara D, Wenzel R. Nosocomial bloodstream infection in critically ill patients. Excess length of stay, extra costs and attributable mortality. JAMA 1994;271:1598–1601
35. Haire W, Lieberman R. Thrombosed central venous catheters: restoring function with 6-hour urokinase infusion after failure of bolus urokinase. J Parenteral Enteral Nutr 1992;16:129–132

36. Randolph A, Cook D, Gonzales C et al. Benefit of heparin in central venous and pulmonary artery catheters. A meta-analysis of randomized controlled trials. Chest 1998;113: 165–171

37. Couban S, Goodyear M, Burnell M et al. Randomized placebo-controlled study of low-dose warfarin for the prevention of central venous catheter-associated thrombosis in patients with cancer J Clin Oncol 2005;20:4063–4069

38. Young AM, Begum G, Billingham LJ et al, WARP Collaborative Group. WARP – a multi-centre prospective randomised controlled trial (RCT) of thrombosis prophylaxis with warfarin in cancer patients with central venous catheters (CVCs). Proceedings of the ASCO Annual Meeting 2005, 23 (16S): LBA8004. ASCO, Alexandria, Virginia

39. Galloway S, Bodenham AR. Safe removal of long-term cuffed Hickman-type catheters. Hosp Med 2003;64:120–123

High-dose regimens for autologous stem cell transplantation

Suzanne Fanning and John W Sweetenham

CHAPTER 26

Introduction

The use of high-dose therapy and autologous stem cell transplantation (ASCT) continues to evolve. In the last decade, improvements in supportive care for patients receiving ASCT have expanded the number of patients being offered this therapy. Randomized clinical trials have better defined the role of ASCT for certain hematologic malignancies such as leukemia and lymphoma. Large-scale randomized studies in solid tumors, especially breast cancer, have resulted in the almost total abandonment of this treatment strategy for some indications. The development of effective new therapies such as rituximab for B-cell lymphoma, imatinib for chronic myeloid leukemia and thalidomide and bortezomib for multiple myeloma have raised new questions concerning the use of ASCT in these diseases, and have also raised questions regarding the potential role of these agents as components of the preparative regimens prior to ASCT.

The use of ASCT for non-malignant conditions, including autoimmune disorders and amyloidosis, is now under investigation and has resulted in a new paradigm for preparative regimens, directed at providing immunosuppression rather than simply applying a dose escalation strategy to overcome relative drug resistance. Despite major advances in the understanding of the role of ASCT in various diseases, optimization of high-dose therapy in pre-autograft conditioning has been underinvestigated. Very few prospective randomized studies have compared various high-dose regimens for ASCT, and the rationale for the use of a particular regimen in a particular disease has been poorly developed. The use of identical regimens for ASCT in all subtypes of non-Hodgkin's and Hodgkin's lymphomas represents a good example of this phenomenon. Although optimal initial chemotherapy regimens for these diseases vary markedly, it is generally accepted that the same regimen can be used at the time of transplant, although there are virtually no data to support this approach. Development of conditioning regimens has therefore been largely empiric and partly derived from experience in allogeneic stem cell transplantation, especially for diseases such as acute myeloid leukemia.

Most high-dose regimens commonly used in ASCT have been based on classic concepts of dose response. Although some high-dose regimens are based on single agents such as melphalan, most combine several drugs with non-overlapping dose-limiting toxicities other than hematologic toxicity. Improvements in supportive care, in particular the use of peripheral blood progenitor cells and hematopoietic growth factors, have enabled the use of tandem transplant strategies, including high-dose sequential therapies. These approaches most commonly use consecutive autologous stem cell support, typically including a different, non-cross resistant high-dose regimen for each transplant to maximize the antitumor effect.

Recently, the use of non-myeloablative transplantation following an initial ASCT has also been investigated in some diseases including lymphoma. In this case, the initial high-dose regimen and subsequent ASCT are used as a 'cytoreductive' strategy to establish a state of minimal residual disease, after which a non-myeloablative allogeneic transplant is used. The second transplant exploits the graft-versus-tumor effect in an attempt to eradicate minimal residual disease. Again, in this situation, the high-dose regimen for ASCT will be chosen for its cytoreductive activity, but also to be non-cross resistant with the subsequent non-myeloablative conditioning regimen.

High-dose regimens for ASCT have been largely developed on an individual disease basis as follows.

Acute and chronic leukemias

The indications for ASCT in acute myelogenous leukemia (AML) have changed over the last decade. The current standard of care includes ASCT for patients in first complete response (CR1) with intermediate- to high-risk cytogenetics and relapsed patients following CR1 without a human leukocyte antigen (HLA)-matched related or unrelated donor.[1] As nearly one-third of patients do not have an HLA-matched donor, numerous patients undergo ASCT for AML. In a recent retrospective, observational database study, the results of 668 autotransplants were compared to 476 allotransplants in patients with AML in CR1 or CR2. ASCT had a significantly reduced transplant-related mortality (TRM), but at the expense of a much higher rate of relapse.[2] The conditioning regimens used in ASCT have, in many cases, been derived from those used in allogeneic hematopoietic stem cell transplant (HSCT), many of which have been based on the use of total-body irradiation (TBI).

Total-body irradiation (TBI)

TBI was initially used as conditioning for allogeneic transplantation in view of its ability to induce profound immunosuppression. Although this effect has no direct relevance to ASCT, preclinical models also demonstrated the activity of TBI as a cytoreductive regimen for myeloid leukemia. Early studies in animal models, subsequently repeated in clinical studies, showed that the use of fractionated TBI was associated with less potential for toxicity than single fraction treatment.[3–8] The widely used standard regimen developed as a result of these studies uses fractions of 2 Gy given twice per day for 3 days to a total of 12 Gy. Other hyperfractionated regimens have also been developed, in which 1.25 Gy are given three times per day for 3 days to a total of 15 Gy. These regimens allow repair of sublethal damage and thereby reduce the toxicity of TBI to normal tissues.

It is still not clear whether fractionation or hyperfractionation of TBI results in superior antileukemia activity. No studies addressing this issue have been performed in the setting of ASCT. The Seattle group has previously compared fractionated TBI to a total of 12 Gy with hyperfractionated TBI to 15.75 Gy in patients with acute and chronic myeloid leukemias undergoing allogeneic SCT.[9] The relapse rate was markedly lower in the hyperfractionated group (0 versus 37%), but this improvement in relapse rate was offset by much higher TRM. Interstitial pneumonitis is a major toxicity of TBI. The incidence of this complication can be reduced by adjusting dose rates of TBI, and by the use of lung shielding.

In the autologous setting, the use of TBI has raised concerns that sublethal damage to hematopoietic stem cells may result in genetic changes which predispose to subsequent myelodysplastic syndrome (MDS) and secondary leukemia. Although cytogenetic abnormalities have been reported in the marrow of patients undergoing ASCT with TBI-based regimens,[10] there are few data demonstrating an increased long-term risk of secondary AML/MDS specifically associated with TBI.

Chemotherapy/TBI combinations

TBI is no longer used as a single treatment modality prior to ASCT. Several regimens have been developed which combine TBI with various chemotherapy drugs, based on preclinical models which demonstrate higher leukemia cell kill when both modalities are used.

The standard combination of cyclophosphamide 60 mg/kg/day for 2 days followed by fractionated TBI after a brief rest period was developed on the basis of these experiments.[3,4,11] The use of a rest period was thought to be important to allow repair of sublethal damage to normal tissues prior to the use of TBI, although subsequent studies have failed to confirm this, and the two modalities are now typically given on consecutive days. Subsequent regimens have incorporated

additional or alternative drugs to cyclophosphamide, based on antileukemia activity and ability to cross the blood–brain barrier. Additional drugs include etoposide, cytarabine and melphalan. Results from studies using some of these regimens are summarized in Table 26.1.

Chemotherapy-only regimens

Multiple chemotherapy-only regimens have been developed for patients undergoing transplantation for leukemia. Again, most of these were initially developed for use in allogeneic transplantation and have subsequently been used in the autologous setting. Studies of chemotherapy-only regimens used for ASCT in leukemia are summarized in Table 26.1.

Chemotherapy-only regimens have potential advantages over TBI-based regimens, partly due to the lower potential for toxicity but also for practical, logistic reasons. TBI is not available in all centers, and chemotherapy-only regimens can therefore be used more widely. Additionally, chemotherapy-only regimens circumvent the necessity for scheduling for fractionated TBI and the requirement for patients to leave the transplant unit and therefore be exposed to a higher risk of infection.

The combination of busulfan with cyclophosphamide (Bu/Cy) was originally reported in the early 1980s and remains a standard conditioning regimen for ASCT in leukemias.[23] In a prospective, randomized trial comparing busulfan/cyclophosphamide to cyclophosphamide/TBI, efficacy and toxicity of these regimens were found to be similar, with a trend toward improved disease-free survival noted in those receiving cyclophosphamide/TBI for CR ≥ 2.[13] A retrospective analysis of 824 patients conditioned with these same regimens (Bu/CY vs CY/TBI) also reported similar results with regard to disease-free survival, TRM, and relapse incidence.[24]

Various Bu/Cy regimens have been reported in which doses of both drugs have been modified, although there are no comparative studies

Table 26.1 ASCT conditioning regimens for acute leukemia

Regimen	n	F/U	Results	Comment	Reference
Etoposide 60 mg/kg, Melphalan 140 mg/m², TBI 500–2400 cGy	145	96 mo.	OS : CR1 62%, CR2 36%	81% in CR1, no long-term survivors >CR2	12
CY/TBI Cyclophosphamide 120 mg/kg TBI 950–1440 Gy	18 43 190	24 mo. 39 mo. 84 mo.	DFS 50%, RR 43%, DFS for CR1 67%, ≥CR2 42% DFS approx 50% at 4-yr DFS 53%	AML in CR ≥ 1, CY/TBI with better 2-yr DFS for those >CR1 AML in CR1 AML in CR1	13 14 15
BuCy4 Busulfan 16 mg/kg, Cyclophosphamide 200 mg/kg	17 63 52 86	24 mo. 48 mo. 39 mo. 48 mo.	DFS 24%, RR 70%, DFS for CR1 50%, ≥CR2 9% DFS 35% DFS approx 50% at 4-yr DFS 44%	AML in ≥CR1 AML in CR1, not superior to standard chemotherapy AML in CR1 AML in CR1, no difference compared with standard chemotherapy	13 16 14 17
BuCy2 Busulfan 16 mg/mg, Cyclophosphamide 120 mg/kg	432	59 mo.	TRM 4%, OS 50%, LFS 46%, RI 44%	Retrospective comparison to BAVC, AML in CR1	18
BAVC BCNU 800 mg/m² Amsacrine 450 mg/m² Etoposide 450 mg/m² Cytarabine 900 mg/m²	94 60	89 mo. 60 mo.	TRM 11%, OS 47%, LFS 37%, RI 58% DFS 42% (projected at 10-yr)	Retrospective comparison to Bu/Cy2, AML in CR1 AML in CR2	18 19
BUMEL Busulfan (16 mg/kg) /Melphalan(180 mg/m²)	17	84 mo.	DFS 28%	AML CR1 68% TRM 11.7%	20 21
Idarubicin (20 mg/m² ci × 3 d) /Busulfan (16 mg/kg)	40		32 mo., 75% alive, 65% continuous CR	82% gr3/4 mucositis, TRM 0%	22
BU/VP16 Busulfan (16 mg/kg)/VP-16 (60 mg/kg)	22	84 mo.	DFS 46%	AML CR1 33% TRM 13.6%	21
BEM BCNU (300 mg/m²)/VP-16(2 g/m²)/Melphalan(160 mg/m²)	3	84 mo.		AML CR1 50%	21

RD, refractory disease.

of these regimens for patients receiving autologous transplants. Many other drugs have also been incorporated into preparative regimens for ASCT. Results of the use of some of these regimens are shown in Table 26.1. Few comparative studies of these regimens have been undertaken.

A restrospective analysis comparing the BAVC (BCNU (carmustine), amsacrine, etoposide and cytosine arabinoside) and Bu/Cy regimens revealed no difference in overall survival, but lower TRM with the BAVC regimen.[18] In patients over 60 years of age, ASCT using standard regimens including Bu/Cy2, BAVC, and 1-Bu was shown to be feasible, producing toxicity comparable to that seen in younger patients.[25]

The use of radiolabeled anti-CD33, anti-CD45 and anti-CD66 monoclonal antibodies has been studied in patients with acute myeloid leukemia undergoing allogeneic stem cell transplantation.[26–28] Their role in the preparative regimens of ASCT for AML has not yet been evaluated.

Myelodysplastic syndromes

Allogeneic stem cell transplantation, either myeloablative or non-myeloablative, is the more common form of transplantation in this patient population. While ASCT has been shown to be feasible, use in this disease has been limited by a high risk of relapse. In patients who lack an HLA-matched donor for allogeneic transplant, ASCT remains a viable alternative, with prolonged disease-free survival (DFS) observed in some cases. Table 26.2 lists the preparative regimens that have been investigated in MDS. The regimens used have been similar to those used in acute leukemias, and in general based on TBI or Bu/Cy. No comparative studies have been performed to identify an optimum regimen in this context.

Hodgkin's and non-Hodgkin's lymphomas

The use of high-dose therapy and ASCT is now well established for the management of patients with relapsed and refractory Hodgkin's (HL) and non-Hodgkin's lymphomas (NHL). The use of high-dose therapy in these diseases is discussed in Chapter 9. As with the acute leukemias, multiple combinations of drugs have been assessed as high-dose regimens for these diseases. Representative results from their use are summarized in Tables 26.3 and 26.4. Tandem transplantation has also been extensively investigated in this context and again, representative results are included in the tables.

Most centers have used the same regimen as high-dose therapy for both groups of diseases, and few studies have explored the potential role of different conditioning regimens in different histologic subtypes of lymphoma. Heterogeneity of patient populations with respect to histologic subtype and disease status at transplant is such that it is impossible to reach conclusions regarding the superiority of one high-dose regimen over another based on cross-trial comparisons.

The most widely used high-dose regimens for HL include cyclophosphamide and TBI, BEAM (carmustine, etoposide, cytarabine, melphalan), CBV (cyclophosphamide, carmustine, etoposide) and BEAC (carmustine, etoposide, cytarabine, cyclophosphamide). Doses of individual drugs in these regimens have evolved and several variants of each regimen are in regular use in different centers. In the absence of direct comparative trials, no optimum regimen has been defined for any specific subtype of HL and NHL, and decisions regarding choice of regimen have been based largely on the standard protocols active at particular centers.

Tandem transplant regimens have typically chosen different, non-cross resistant high-dose chemotherapy for each of the two cycles. As shown in Tables 26.3 and 26.4, Phase II studies with these regimens have typically shown superior results to those with single transplants, although this probably reflects selection bias for these more intensive regimens rather than true increased activity for tandem approaches.

Some retrospective studies have compared preparative regimens, with no difference in efficacy or toxicity noted between busulfan, melphalan, and thiotepa and radiation-based regimens,[33] and favorable outcomes predicted with BEAM.[36] Tandem transplantation for those with poor-risk disease (induction failure, refractory relapse, or relapse within 12 months of induction therapy) demonstrated a CR rate of 51%, with 74% 2-yr overall survival (OS)[40] in one series. Another study demonstrated feasibility of tandem transplant leading, in some patients, to prolonged remission.[41]

Monoclonal antibodies

The introduction of the chimeric anti-CD20 monoclonal antibody rituximab for the treatment of B-cell NHL has resulted in improved disease-free and overall survival rates for many subtypes of B-cell NHL. Numerous studies have now demonstrated that the addition of rituximab to chemotherapy improves outcomes in multiple clinical situations, including both aggressive and indolent subtypes of NHL, and in first-line treatment as well as salvage therapy.

More recently, rituximab has been combined with pretransplant, cytoreductive regimens such as ICE (ifosfamide, carboplatin, etoposide). Data from Phase II studies suggest that this approach may improve response rates prior to transplant, increase the number of patients who are rendered eligible for ASCT and improve the long-term outcome after transplant.[57]

Based on the increased efficacy of rituximab-based regimens, and the observed in vivo 'purging' effect of rituximab, which may reduce the risk of post-transplant relapse, this agent is now frequently incorporated into mobilization regimens and also into high-dose regimens. At present, few results are available from studies which have included rituximab in the peritransplant period.

Table 26.2 ASCT regimens for MDS

Regimen	n	F/U	Results	Comments	Reference
Cyclophosphamide 200 mg/m² /Busulfan 16 mg/kg	24	19 mo.	DFS 29 mo. OS 33 mo.	MDS in CR1, 55% high risk, 58% normal karyotype, TRM 12.5% (3/16 ABMT, 0/8 ASCT)	29
TBI/cyclophosphamide Cyclophosphamide/busulfan Non-TBI based regimens No regimen description	18 10 7 26	Median actuarial f/u: 3.6 years	4-year DFS 27.3%, 4-yr OS from CR 32.7%	35/61 in CR1, TRM of 35 pts in CR = 11%	30
TBI-based Non-TBI based Unknown	10 52 3		3-yr OS: 35%, 3-yr DFS: 32%, 5-yr RI: 58%	CR1 = 46, CR2 = 46, R/R = 6, TRM = 12%, significantly increased for age >40.	31

Table 26.3 ASCT regimens for Hodgkin's lymphoma

Regimen	n	F/U	Results	Comments	Reference
Bu/Cy/VP16 Busulfan 16 mg/kg Cyclophosphamide 120 mg/kg Etoposide 30–45 mg/kg	10	21 mo.	Phase II, 3-yr OS 43%, EFS 31%.	High-risk patients	32
TBI 12 Gy, Cyclophosphamide 60– 100 mg/kg, Etoposide 30–60 mg/kg	42 28	60 mo. 60 mo.	52% alive, 45% in remission, 38% relapsed OS 61%, PFS 43%	Relapsed, refractory HD Relapsed, refractory HD	33 34
Busulfan 12 mg/kg Melphalan 100 mg/m^2 Thiotepa 500 mg/m^2	50	41 mo.	52% alive, 46% in remission, 34% relapsed	Relapsed, refractory HD	33
BCNU 15 mg/kg Etoposide 60 mg/kg Cyclophosphamide 100 mg/kg	48	60 mo.	OS 50%, PFS 43%	Relapsed, refractory HD	34
TMJ Thiotepa 750 mg/m^2 Mitoxantrone 40 mg/m^{22} Carboplatin 1000 mg/m^2	37	91 mo.	Median survival 87 mo.	All patients with chemosensitive relapse	35
BEAM Carmustine 300 mg/m^2 Cytarabine 800–1600 mg/m^2 Etoposide 800–1200 mg/m^2 Melphalan 140 mg/m^2	42 21	60 mo. 37 mo.	OS 71% OS 81%	Advanced HD, BEAM associated with favorable outcome when compared to CBV and TBI-containing preparative regimens Primary refractory HD, ASCT superior to conventional chemotherapy	36 37
CBV Cyclophosphamide 1.8 g/m^2 Carmustine 600 mg/m^2 Etoposide 2.4 g/m^2	29	136 mo.	RR 43% TRM 26%	Primary refractory or relapsed HD	38
CBVP Cyclophosphamide 1.8 g/m^2 Carmustine 500 mg/m^2 Etoposide 2.4 g/m^2 Cisplatin 150 mg/m^2	71	136 mo.	RR 36% TRM 23%	Primary refractory or relapsed HD, less mucosal and hepatic toxicity than CBV	38
Tandem regimens					
Course 1: TMJ Thiotepa 750 mg/m^2 Mitoxantrone 40 mg/m^2 Carboplatin 1000 mg/m^2 Course 2: ICE Ifosfamide 16 g/m^2 Carboplatin 1800 mg/m^2 Etoposide 1800 mg/m^2	76	83 mo.	HD 32.14% long-term survival, DFS 7 mo., TRM 15.8%	NHL and HD patients with resistant lymphoma, 49 patients received both ASCT	39
Course 1: CBV + mito Mitoxantrone 30 mg/m^2 Course 2: Cytarabine 6 g/m^2 Melphalan 140 mg/m^2 TBI 12 Gy or busulfan 12–16 mg/kg	43	24 mo.	OS 65% for one ASCT, 74% after 2nd ASCT	ASCT following induction failure or very unfavorable relapse, 32 patients received 2nd ASCT	40
Course 1: BCNU 300 mg/m^2 Cyclophosphamide 4.5 g/m^2 Etoposide 1 g/m^2 Mitoxantrone 30–45 mg/m^2 Course 2: Busulfan 12 mg/kg Carboplatin 1.2 g/m^2 Melphalan 140 mg/m^2	9	18 mo.	RR 67%, CR maintained in 58%	Relapse <1 yr following initial treatment, toxicity associated with VOD and mucositis	41
Course 1: TMC Thiotepa 750 mg/m^2 Mitoxantrone 40 mg/m^2 Carboplatin 990 mg/m^2 Course 2: BEAM	10	10 mo.	Response rate 70% (CR 2, PR 5), TRM 20%	Primary progressive or relapsed/refractory HD	42
Course 1: Melphalan 140 mg/m^2 Course 2: BEAC Carmustine 300 mg/m^2 Etoposide 800 mg/m^2 Cytarabine 800 mg/m^2 Cyclophosphamide 6 g/m^2	8	60 mo.	OS 86%	Advanced HD	36

Table 26.4 ASCT regimens for NHL

Regimen	n	F/U	Results	Comments	Reference
BEAM Carmustine 300 mg/m² Etoposide 900–1200 mg/m² Cytarabine 1200–1600 mg/m² Melphalan 140 mg/m²	31 49 57	34 mo. 25 mo.	CR 100%, RR 39% and RFS 34 mo. (for patients in PR prior to ASCT) OS 45%, PFS 26% OS 47%, FF2F 25%	Relasped or refractory B-NHL Relapsed, low-intermediate grade B-NHL Relapsed or refractory B-NHL	43 36 44
BEAC Carmustine 300 mg/m² Etoposide 600 mg/m² Cytarabine 600 mg/m² Cyclophosphamide 105 mg/kg	44	63 mo.	RR 84%, OS 53%, EFS 46%	B-NHL with chemosensitive relapse, superior to standard chemotherapy	45
BCV BCNU 600 mg/m² Cyclophosphamide 2 g/m² x 3 d Etoposide 800 mg/m² d x 3 d	9		CR 100%, RFS: 6 mo.	Refractory B-NHL, CR after ASCT does not result in long-term control.	43
TBI (12 Gy) + Cyclophosphamide 120 mg/kg	11 4 21 62	4.2 yrs 15 mo. 25 mo.	5-yr PFS 64.7%(p,.0001) ORR = 100% (20CR, 1PR) Longer PFS(p = .0108), 3-yr OS 83%	Advanced follicular NHL, 1st remission PTCL, 1st remission (phase II) Mantle cell NHL, ASCT as 1st consolidation.	46 47 48
Bu/Cy/VP16 Busulfan 16 mg/kg Cyclophosphamide 120 mg/kg Etoposide 30–45 mg/kg	43	21 mo.	Phase II, OS 43%, EFS 31%.	High-risk patients	32
CBV Cyclophosphamide 4.8–7.2 g/m² Etoposide 1200–2400 mg/m² BCNU 300 mg/m²	16	34 mo.	Relapsed low-intermediate B-NHL	OS 45%, PFS 26%	36
TMJ Thiotepa Mitoxantrone Carboplatin	63	91 mo.	Median survival 107 mo.	50 patients with chemosensitive relapse, 13 patients in CR1	35

Radio-immunotherapy (RIT)

Regimen	n	F/U	Results	Comments	Reference
¹³¹I-tositumomab (0.75 Gy TDB)/BEAM	23	38 mo.	CR 57%, ORR 65%, OS 55%, EFS 39%	Chemoresistant relapse or refractory B-cell NHL, Phase I	49
⁹⁰Y-ibritumomab tiuxetan/BEAM	22 12	36 mo. 9 mo.	OS 60%, PFS 47% Relapse rate 17%	Phase I, heavily-pretreated Phase II	50 51
⁹⁰Y-ibritumomab tiuxetan (target 1000 cGy)/ Etoposide (40–60 mg/kg)/Cyclophosphamide (100 mg/kg)	31	22 mo.	OS 93%, DFS 80%	Phase I/II, TRM 6%, B-cell NHL	52
¹³¹I-labeled anti-CD22	21		Phase I/II, RR 33% (5CR, 2PR)	Relapsed B-cell NHL	53
¹³¹I-tositumomab	29 27	42 mo. Estimated 5-yr	RR 86%, CR 79%, OS 68 mo, PFS 42 mo. OS 67%, PFS 48%, TRM 3.7%	High relapse rate, but durable remissions seen. Comparison to conventional HDCT with improved results	54 55
¹³¹I-tositumomab/Etoposide (60 mg/kg)/ Cyclophosphamide (100 mg/kg)	52 16	Estimated 3-yr	Median f/u 2 yrs: 85% alive, 73% prog-free CR 91%, RR 100%, OS 93%, PFS 61%	Mantle cell Relapsed B-NHL	55

Tandem regimens

Regimen	n	F/U	Results	Comments	Reference
TMJ (course 1) Thiotepa Mitoxantrone Carboplatin ICE (course 2) Ifosfamide Carboplatin Etoposide	76	83 mo.	NHL 12.76% long-term survival, DFS 2 mo., TRM 15.8%	NHL and HD patients with resistant lymphoma, 49 patients received both ASCT	39
Course 1:Mitoxantrone 60–90 mg/m² Melphalan 140–180 mg/m² Course 2: Etoposide 1.5 g/m² Carboplatin 1.5 g/m²	25	24 mo.	CR > 90%, OS 79%, DFS 85% (for those in CR)	Initial treatment of aggressive B-NHL	56
Course 1: BCNU 300 mg/m² Cyclophosphamide 4.5 g/m² Etoposide 1 g/m² Mitoxantrone 30–45 mg/m² Course 2: Busulfan 12 mg/kg Carboplatin 1.2 g/m² Melphalan 140 mg/m²	15	18 mo.	Response rate 67%, CR maintained in 58%	Agressive B-NHL with poor prognostic factors, toxicity associated with VOD and mucositis	41
Course 1: TMC Thiotepa 750 mg/m², Mitoxantrone 40 mg/m² Carboplatin 990 mg/m² Course 2: BEAM	15	10 mo.	Response rate 46% (CR 5, PR 2), TRM 20%	Relapsed, aggressive B-NHL	42

RR, refractory relapse; TBD, total body dose; ORR, overall response rate; OS,overall survival; EFS, event-free survival; PFS, progression-free survival; PTCL, peripheral T-cell NHL.

Another antibody-based approach has been the use of radio-immunotherapy. This treatment combines anti-CD20 monoclonal antibodies with a radio-isotope, combining the therapeutic effect of monoclonal antibodies with targeted radiation, which has the advantage of maximizing the dose of radiation to the tumor and minimizing the dose to normal tissues. Two such radio-immunoconjugates have been assessed in NHL: ^{131}I-tositumomab (Bexxar) and ^{90}Y-ibritumomab tiuxetan (Zevalin). Both of these have also been investigated as components of high-dose regimens for ASCT, as single agents, and in combination with high-dose chemotherapy. Results of these studies are summarized in Table 26.4. Phase I and II studies have confirmed the feasibility of combining these agents with more standard high-dose regimens, without significant additional toxicity. Typically, the radio-immunoconjugate is given first, followed by a rest period, after which the patient is admitted for high-dose chemotherapy. Toxicities of combining these agents have generally been comparable with chemotherapy-only regimens and there have been no apparent differences in engraftment kinetics in patients receiving radio-immunoconjugates. Whether the inclusion of these agents will produce improvements in long-term disease-free and overall survival requires prospective randomized trials. One such study, comparing BEAM/^{131}I-tositumomab with BEAM/rituximab, is currently in progress.

Multiple myeloma and amyloidosis

The optimum conditioning regimen for multiple myeloma is considered by many to be melphalan 200 mg/m^2 (MEL200). High-dose melphalan, with or without TBI, remains the most commonly used regimen. In a study by Moreau et al, melphalan 200 mg/m^2 was shown to be superior to melphalan 140 mg/m^2 with 8 Gy TBI.[58] Several series have demonstrated that MEL200 is associated with less toxicity and that TBI does not provide additional long-term disease control.[59,60] With these regimens, overall response rates of up to 69% have been seen.[61] However, the success of these regimens is limited by side-effects including renal failure, hepatic veno-occlusive disease (VOD), sepsis, and pneumonitis. Regimens incorporating combination high-dose alkylating agents rely on dose–response characteristics and non-overlapping toxicities,[63,67] with the hope that maximizing cytoreduction will improve patient outcome.

Many regimens have been studied in the treatment of multiple myeloma and are listed in Table 26.5. Tandem ASCT, when administered in a timely fashion, has been shown in some series to be superior to single ASCT, with statistically significant improvements in both event-free survival (EFS) and OS.[74] In review of the long-term results of the University of Arkansas tandem ASCT experience, 21% of patients remained in CR or stable partial response (PR) at 9 years, while 65% had received treatment for relapsed disease. The median time from ASCT to relapse was 2.9 years, with a median survival from relapse of 2.4 years. Dose escalation of melphalan to 220 mg/m^2 in ASCT has shown increased response rates, although randomized comparisons to melphalan 200 mg/m^2 have not been completed.[58,72]

More recently, standard chemotherapy, without ASCT, has seen a resurgence with the incorporation of novel agents including thalidomide, lenolinamide, and botezomib. Results of these data are competitive with those of high-dose therapy followed by ASCT in multiple myeloma. Future prospective, randomized trials comparing these treatments are needed.

The use of ASCT in primary amyloidosis has been studied with similar conditioning regimens to multiple myeloma. Table 26.6 includes previous studies of preparative regimens for ASCT in primary amyloidosis. An increased TRM has been seen with ASCT compared to standard chemotherapy,[76] but retrospective data have suggested a survival benefit for ASCT.[77] Patients with amyloidosis are often cate-

gorized as good, intermediate, or poor risk. Previous studies have reported that patients with symptomatic cardiac involvement, two or more involved organs, and poor performance status are considered poor candidates for ASCT.[75,76,79] Comenzo & Gertz have recommended a risk-adapted approach to the treatment of patients with amyloid based on dose-related and age-related differences observed in retrospective data from the Mayo Clinic. This approach advises a conditioning regimen of melphalan 200 mg/m^2 for patients ≤60, melphalan 140 mg/m^2 for patients 61–70, and melphalan 100 mg/m^2 for patients >71 years.[80]

Solid tumors

The role of high-dose therapy and ASCT in various solid tumors remains uncertain and controversial. This subject is covered elsewhere in this text. At present, the use of ASCT in relapsed/refractory germ cell tumors is widespread, based largely on results of Phase II studies. In general, Phase III studies have not confirmed the superiority of this approach over conventional dose approaches (see Chapter 14). High-dose strategies have been assessed in Phase II studies for many other solid tumors. The use of ASCT for breast cancer, which was very widespread in the 1990s, has now been largely abandoned following publication of several studies showing no survival benefit to this approach compared with conventional-dose therapy (see Chapter 12). For reference, a list of high-dose regimens commonly used for solid tumors, and results from these regimens, are summarized in Table 26.7.

Autoimmune disorders

The use of stem cell transplantation in severe autoimmune diseases, while increasing in frequency, remains investigational and should be conducted in the setting of a clinical trial. Whether ASCT will prove to be beneficial in this patient population remains to be proven. In contrast to ASCT for hematologic malignancies, the goal of ASCT in this setting is not myeloablation but rather elimination of immune reactions through intense immunosuppression with subsequent regeneration of naïve T-lymphocytes derived from reinfused hematopoetic stem cells.[94] It is imperative to note the considerable heterogeneity among the various autoimmune disorders with regard to disease morbidity and associated end-organ disease. Some patients can be relatively asymptomatic, while the disease course in others is characterized by frequent relapse. Disease-modifying antirheumatic drugs (DMARDs) have improved the time to end-organ damage, but do not offer hope for cure.

The role of ASCT in autoimmune disorders has risen out of results from animal models with autoimmune diseases, as well as clinical observations of autoimmune disease response in patients treated for concomitant cancer. An inherent flaw in the study of ASCT for autoimmune diseases has been the heterogeneous and retrospective nature of trials published thus far. Review of the literature with regard to ASCT in this population reveals that each autoimmune disorder has its own measure of disease response to treatment. In multiple sclerosis, for example, one measure of treatment response is the extended disability status score (EDSS).[95] Table 26.8 reviews preparative regimens that have been used to treat various autoimmune disorders and their respective measurement of response scales. In Table 26.9, the preparative regimens are categorized as high, intermediate, and low intensity, based on degree of myeloablation.

Due to the potential for longer overall survival based on the underlying disease process, patients undergoing ASCT for autoimmune disorders should not be exposed to unacceptable TRM. To limit such

Table 26.5 ASCT preparative regimens for multiple myeloma

HDT	n	F/U	Results	Comment	Reference
Melphalan 200 mg/m²	57	17 mo.	Projected 12 mo.	Previously treated, RR 68%	63
	89		EFS 85%, OS 85%	Initial treatment, PFS 20 mo.	61
			CR 27%, PR 42%		
Melphalan 140 mg/m² + TBI 8–12 Gy	37		RFS 16 mo.	ASCT not recommended for resistant relapse.	63
	71	12 mo	OS 47 mo.	Longer median survival for patients with CR.	64
	74	41 mo.	27% CR	Previously untreated patients.	65
	213	76 mo.	46% PR	Not different from SDT, TRM 8/213	66
			38% CR or very good PR, median		
			EFS 27 mo.		
			7-yr		
			PFS 17%, OS 37%		
Thiotepa 450 mg/m² Busulfan 16 mg/kg Cyclophosphamide 120 mg/kg	97	45 mo.	CR 16%, PR 50%	PFS 21 mo.	61
Busulfan 12 mg/kg Etoposide 30 mg/kg Cyclophosphamide 120 mg/kg	26	30 mo.	CR 38%, PR/SD 58%, EFS 24 mo. OS 43 mo.	73% transplanted after primary therapy, 62% IIIA, 0% TRM	62
Melphalan 140 mg/m²	25			Longer median survival for patients with CR	64
Busulfan 16 mg/kg	15		CR 4, PR 2	Heavily pre-treated, TRM: 20%, Can be used in patients with renal disease	66
Busulfan 14 mg/kg Cyclophosphamide 120 mg/m² Bu 14–16 mg/kg Cy 120–174 mg/kg	104	26 mo.	OS 57 mo.	71% in first CR	69
	18			High incidence grade 3/4 toxicities with increased doses	70
Busulfan 12 mg/kg Melphalan 100 mg/m² Thiotepa 500 mg/m²	9				70
Thiotepa 750 mg/m²/ TBI 850 cGy	18		RFS 7 mo. OS 15 mo.		63
Busulfan 16 mg/m² Cyclophosphamide 120 mg/kg, TBI 6–10.5 Gy	36			No increased mortality with added TBI	70
Cyclophosphamide 6 g/m² Carboplatin 800 mg/m² Etoposide 1800 mg/m²	18		RR 22%	Heavily pretreated, relapsed disease, TRM 22%	71
Tandem regimens					
Melphalan 200 mg/m² Melphalan 200 mg/m² or 140 mg/m² + TBI 10 Gy	123	31 mo.	CR 40%, EFS 49 mo. OS 62+ mo.	TRM 4%, CR within 6 mo. of induction favorable prognostic feature	68
Melphalan 200 mg/m² Melphalan 220 mg/m²	85	54 mo.	EFS 35 mo.	High-risk de novo, RR 30.6%	72
Melphalan 100 mg/m² Melphalan 100 mg/m²	71	30 mo.	CR 19,34,47%, PR 77,86,88% after 1st, 2nd, and 3rd MEL100	0% TRM	73

Table 26.6 ASCT in primary amyloidosis

Regimen	N	F/U	Results	Comments	Reference
Mel 200 mg/m² Mel 140 + TBI, Mel 140 Mel 100	171		Responders with significantly longer median survival (12.6 mo. in non-responders, not yet reached in responders)	Retrospective, TRM 12%, Mel 200 and Mel 140 + TBI with significantly higher RR	75
Mel 200 Mel 140 + TBI Mel 140 Mel 100	63	44 mo.	2-yr OS 71%	4-yr 71% vs 41% (p < 0.001)	76
Mel 200 Mel 140 Mel 100	312		Improved 5-yr survival (median survival 54 mo.)	TRM 13%, highest among patients with CM	77
Melphalan 140–200 mg/m²	100	45 mo.	2-yr OS 54–60% (depending on oral course prior to ASCT)	Newly diagnosed patients, no benefit to 2 cycles of oral MP prior to ASCT	78

MP, melphalan/prednisone; CM, cardiomyopathy.

Table 26.7 ASCT preparative regimens for solid tumors

Solid tumor	Regimen	n	F/U	Results	Comment	Reference
Germ cell tumors-chemosensitive relapse	CEC: Cyclophosphamide Etoposide Carboplatin CarboPEC: Carboplatin AUC, d-7 Etoposide 450 mg/m² /d x 5 d Cyclophosphamide 1600 mg/m²/d x 5 d Mesna 3600 mg/m²/d x 5 d TVCa: Thiotepa 500 mg/m² Etoposide1000 mg/m² Carboplatin 1500 mg/m² (adjusted for renal function)	108 135 24	45 mo.	No difference in 1-yr CR rate compared with conventional chemo 3-yr EFS: 42% OS: 46% TRM 7%	1st line, inter/poor risk, phase III, May be role in patients without tumor marker decline on conventional chemo. Chemosensitive relapse. No benefit to ASCT over conventional treatment Phase I/II tandem ASCT trial with dose-adjusted carboplatin, 38% CR rate with durable response at 71 mo. f/u, 7% TRM.	81 82 83
Adult soft-tissue sarcomas	VIC: Ifosfamide 12 g/m² Etoposide 800 mg/m² Cisplatin 200 mg/m² Doxorubicin 75 mg/m² Ifosfamide 5 g/m² rhGM-CSF 250 μg/m² x 13 d Tandem ICE: Ifosfamide 3 g/m² x 5 d Carboplatin 400 mg/m² x 3 d Etoposide 500 mg/m² x 3 d	30 145 2	94 mo.	5-yr OS: 23% PFS: 21% No increase in OS Increased PFS following ASCT (p = 0.03) Some tumor regression, possible delay of progression	ASCT following CR vs. non-CR: OS 75% vs. 5% (p.001) Phase III, randomized. Case reports	84 85 86
Ovarian cancer	Cyclophosphamide/ carboplatin/mitoxantrone Cyclophosphamide/ carboplatin/thiotepa Ifosfamide/carbopatin Ifosfamide/carboplatin Other Melphalan 140 mg/m² Cyclophosphamide 120 mg/kg Melphalan 140 mg/m² Carboplatin 300 mg/m² x 4 d, Etoposide 250 mg/m² x 4 d, Melphalan 140 mg/m² Platinum-based Melphalan-based Platinum/melphalan Other Radiation Unknown Three consecutive ASCT: 1: Carboplatin AUC 20 Taxol 250 mg/m² 2: Topotecan 5 mg/m² Etoposide 600 mg/m² 3: Thiotepa 500 mg/m²	99 57 35 23 207 8 9 16 117 62 68 23 2 16 14	29 mo. 60 mo. 76 mo. 11.7 mo	2-yr PFS: 12% OS 35% 5-yr PFS: 29% OS: 45%, Results superior for patients with CPR at SLO CR+VGPR vs not: DFS 18 vs 9 mo.(p = 0.005), No difference in OS ORR: 50% (5CR, 2PR, SD 2), PFS: 7 mo. OS: 18 mo. TRM 0%	89% with stage III/IV at diagnosis, 49% in CR at transplant Chemosensitive EOC, FIGO stage III/IV, all pre-treated with carboplatin-based regimens Survival improved for patients in CR or VGPR (p = 0.0001) Phase I/II, pre-treated, advanced OC, 88% with persistant/recurrent disease	87 88 89 90
Brain tumors	Thiotepa 900 mg/m² BCNU 800 mg/m² Thiotepa 600 mg/m² Busulfan 12 mg/m² Cyclophosphamide 4 g/m²	39 114 7	80.5 mo. 89 mo.	PFS 78 mo. OS not reached OS: GBM 12 mo., OD 37 mo., AA 81 mo. CR: 6/7 after ASCT. 5 patients alive, relapse free at 5,8,24,36, and 42 mo. from diagnosis.	Phase II, anaplastic oligodenroglioma, consolidation following PCV. Radiotherapy followed ASCT, TRM 5/114 (4 with KPS 60%). Primary CNS lymphoma. 5/7 treated with HD-MTX prior to ASCT, 2/7 treated with ASCT for recurrent disease. No WBRT.	91 92 93

EOC, epithelial ovarian carcimona; CPR, complete pathologic response; SLO, second look operation; CR, complete remission; VGPR, very good partial response; GBM, glioblastoma multiforme; AA, anaplastic astrocytoma; TRM, treatment-related mortality; KPS, Karnofsky performance scale.

Table 26.8 ASCT preparative regimens for autoimmune disorders

Disease Preparative regimen	n	F/U	TRM	Markers of response	Comment	Reference
Multiple sclerosis						
BEAM*	85	16 mo.	8.2%	EDSS, MRI	PFS 74% at 3 yrs for primary	96
BEAM/ATG*	14	36 mo.	0%	EDSS, MRI, CSF, SNRS.	progressive, 66% for secondary	95
Cyclophosphamide/ATG*					progressive	
Cyclophosphamide/TBI/ATG*					9/14 with worse, 2/14 with improved,	
Busulfan ± cyclophosphamide ± ATG*					and 3/14 with stable EDSS	
Fludarabine/ATG*						
Cyclophosphamide 120 mg/kg						
TBI 10 Gy						
ATG 45 mg/kg						
Systemic sclerosis						
Cyclophosphamide 150–200 mg/kg	57	22.9 mo.	8.7%	Rodnan skin score	5-yr progression 48%, OS 72%	97
Cyclophosphamide 150–200 mg/kg/TBI*	19	14.7 mo.	15.7%	Rodnan skin score, mHAQ-DI	2-yr OS 79%, ORR 100%, decreased	98
Cyclophosphamide 150–200 mg/kg/TLI*					M/M with lung shielding	
Cyclophosphamide 150–200 mg/kg/ATG*						
Fludarabine alone*						
BCNU alone*						
Cyclophosphamide 120 mg/kg						
TBI 800 cGy						
ATG 45 mg/kg						
Rheumatoid arthritis						
Cyclophosphamide 200 mg/kg	62	16 mo.	0%	ACR criteria – 67% with 50% ACR	EBMT/ABMTR	99
Cyclophosphamide/ATG*	7			response; HAQ – significant reduction in		–
Cyclophosphamide/busulfan*	2			level of disability; Most restarted DMARD in		
Cyclophosphamide/ATG/TBI*	1			<6 mo. For persistant or recurrent disease		
Fludarabine/ATG*	1			with response.		
				DAS		
				HAQ		
Idiopathic thrombocytopenic purpura						
Cyclophosphamide 200 mg/kg	14	42 mo.	0%	Durable CR 2, PR 2	EBMT	100
Cyclophosphamide*	12		11.7%	Continuous remission 4		101

ACR, American College of Rheumatology; HAQ, Health Assessment Questionnaire; DAS, Disease Activity Score; MS, Multiple sclerosis; BEAM, BCNU, etoposide, cytosine arabinoside, melphalan; mHAQ-DI, modified Health Assessment Questionnaire Disability Index; ORR, overall response rate; SNRS, Scripps Neurological Rating Score; TLI, total lymph node irradiation.
* Dosing details not provided.

Table 26.9 Intensity of preparative regimens used in ASCT for autoimmune disease

Low-intensity
Cyclophosphamide alone
Melphalan alone
Fludarabine-based
Intermediate-intensity
BEAM
BEAM ± ATG
High-intensity
TBI-based
Busulfan + cyclophosphamide ± ATG

effects, preparative regimens used to treat these disorders must take into account toxicities of commonly used chemotherapeutic agents and radiation. These include pulmonary damage from carmustine, bleomycin, and TBI.[102] In a retrospective analysis of 234 patients in the Basel database, ASCT preparative regimens investigated for autoimmune disorders were grouped according to immunoablative intensities. Patients received different preparative regimens: high-intensity regimens (22%), intermediate-intensity regimens (32%), and low-

intensity regimens (46%). In this analysis, the 1-year TRM was significantly increased with use of a high-intensity regimen (22%), compared to 5% and 7% for intermediate- and low-intensity regimens, respectively (p = 0.008). There was no significant difference in progression or progression-free survival between groups. This stratification of low-, intermediate-, and high-intensity preparative regimens was also evaluated in a retrospective analysis by the EBMT. In this analysis of 473 patients with severe autoimmune diseases who underwent ASCT, 17% had high-intensity preparative regimens, 52% intermediate-intensity, and 31% low-intensity. TRM at 3 years was 7 ± 3%. Disease progression was increased with low- and intermediate-intensity regimens, but TRM was increased with high-intensity regimens.[103] Additionally, variability was noted with regard to disease progression among the autoimmune diseases treated with ASCT in this study.

Some preparative regimens should be avoided in certain autoimmune disorders. In systemic sclerosis, for example, radiation-based preparative regimens may result in increased pulmonary end-organ damage. Similarly, the BCNU component of the BEAM regimen may also result in pulmonary toxicity. Cyclophosphamide should be avoided in patients with cardiac dysfunction related to systemic disease due to risk of increased cardiac toxicity. While there are currently no comparative data from which to choose the best preparative regimen for ASCT in autoimmune disorders, high-dose cyclophosphamide (200 mg/kg) has been shown to be well tolerated and is thus far the most commonly used regimen in this patient population.

References

1. Nathan PC, Sung L, Crump M et al. Consolidation therapy with autologous bone marrow transplantation in adults with acute myeloid leukemia: a meta-analysis. J Natl Cancer Inst 2004;96:38–45
2. Lazarus HM, Perez WS, Klein JP et al. Autotransplantation versus HLA-matched unrelated donor transplantation for acute myeloid leukaemia: a retrospective analysis from the Center for International Blood and Marrow Transplant Research. Br J Haematol 2006; 132:755–769
3. Thomas ED, Buchner T, Clift RA et al. Marrow transplantation for acute non-lymphoblastic leukemia in first remission. N Engl J Med 1979;301:597–599
4. Thomas ED, Buchner CD, Banaji M et al. One hundred patients with acute leukemia with chemotherapy, total body irradiation and allogeneic marrow transplantation. Blood 1977;49:511–533
5. Clift RA, Buchner D, Appelbaum FR et al. Allogeneic marrow transplantation in patients with acute myeloid leukemia in first remission: a randomized trial of 2 irradiation regimens. Blood 1990;76:1867–1871
6. Socié G, Devergies A, Gerinsky T et al. Influence of fractionation of total body irradiation on complications and relapse rate for chronic myelogenous leukemia. Int J Radiat Biol Phys 1991;20:397–404
7. Oszahin M, Pene F, Touboul E et al. Total body irradiation before bone marrow transplantation. Results of two randomized instantaneous dose rates in 157 patients. Cancer 1992;69:2853–2865
8. Oszahin M, Belkacemi Y, Pene F et al. Interstitial pneumonitis following autologous bone marrow transplantation conditioned with cyclophosphamide and total body irradiation. Int J Radiat Biol Phys 1996;34:71–77
9. Deeg HJ, Flournoy N, Sullivan K et al. Cataracts after total body irradiation and marrow transplantation. Effect of dose fractionation. Int J Radiat Biol Phys 1984;10:957–964
10. Perot C, van den Akker J, Laporte J et al. Multiple chromosome abnormalities in patients with acute leukemia after autologous bone marrow transplantation using total body irradiation and marrow purged with mafosfamide. Leukemia 1993;7:509–515
11. Thomas ED. Total body irradiation regimens for marrow grafting. Int J Radiat Biol Phys 1990;19:1285–1288
12. Mollee P, Gupta V, Song K et al. Long-term outcome after intensive therapy with etoposide, melphalan, total body irradiation and autotransplant for acute myeloid leukemia. Bone Marrow Transplant 2004;12:1201–1208
13. Dusenbery KE, Daniels KA, McClure JS et al. Randomized comparison of cyclophosphamide-total body irradiation versus busulfan-cyclophosphamide conditioning in autologous bone marrow transplantation for acute myeloid leukemia. Int J Radiat Oncol Biol Phys 1995;31:119–128
14. Zittoun RA, Mandelli F, Willemze R et al. Autologous or allogeneic bone marrow transplantation compared with intensive chemotherapy in acute myelogenous leukemia. European Organization for Research and Treatment of Cancer (EORTC) and the Gruppo Italiano Malattie Ematologiche Maligne dell'Adulto (GIMEMA) Leukemia Cooperative Groups. N Engl J Med 1995;332:217–223
15. Burnett AK, Goldstone AH, Stevens RM et al. Randomised comparison of addition of autologous bone-marrow transplantation to intensive chemotherapy for acute myeloid leukaemia in first remission: results of MRC AML 10 trial. UK Medical Research Council Adult and Children's Leukaemia Working Parties. Lancet 1998;351:700–708
16. Cassileth PA, Harrington DP, Appelbaum FR et al. Chemotherapy compared with autologous or allogeneic bone marrow transplantation in the management of acute myeloid leukemia in first remission. N Engl J Med 1998;339:1649–1656
17. Harrousseau JL, Cahn JY, Pignon B et al. Comparison of autologous bone marrow transplantation and intensive chemotherapy as postremission therapy in adult acute myeloid leukemia. The Groupe Ouest-Est des Leucemies Aigues Myeloblastiques (GOELAM). Blood 1997;90:2978–2986
18. Fouillard L, Labopin M, Meloni G et al. Comparison of BAVC to BuCy regimens in autologous stem cell transplantation for adult patients with acute myeloid leukemia. Haematologica 2004;89:107–108
19. Meloni G, Vignetti M, Avvisati G et al. BAVC regimen and autograft for acute myelogenous leukemia in second complete remission. Bone Marrow Transplant 1996;18:693–698
20. Reiffers J, Stoppa AM, Attal M et al. Allogeneic vs autologous stem cell transplantation vs chemotherapy in patients with acute myeloid leukemia in first remission: the BGMT 87 study. Leukemia 1996;10:1874–1882
21. Martins C, Lacerda JF, Lourenco F et al. Autologous stem cell transplantation in acute myeloid leukemia. Factors influencing outcome. A 13 year single institution experience. Acta Med Port 2005;18:329–337
22. Ferrera F, Palmieri S, de Simone M et al. High-dose idarubicin and busulphan as conditioning to autologous stem cell transplantation in adult patients with acute myeloid leukaemia. Br J Haematol 2005;128:234–241
23. Santos GW, Tutschka PJ, Brokmeyer R et al. Marrow transplantation for acute non-lymphocytic leukemia after treatment with busulphan and cyclophosphamide. N Engl J Med 1983;309:1347–1353
24. Ringden O, Labopin M, Tura S et al. A comparison of busulphan versus total body irradiation combined with cyclophosphamide as conditioning for autograft or allograft bone marrow transplantation in patients with acute leukaemia. Acute Leukaemia Working Party of the European Group for Blood and Marrow Transplantation (EBMT). Br J Haematol 1996;93:637–645
25. Villela L, Sureda A, Canals C et al. Low transplant related mortality in older patients with hematologic malignancies undergoing autologous stem cell transplantation. Haematologica 2003;88:300–305
26. Matthews DC, Appelbaum FR, Eary JF et al. Phase I study of ^{131}I-anti-CD45 antibody plus cyclophosphamide and total body irradiation for advanced acute leukemia and myelodysplastic syndrome. Blood 1999;94:1237–1247
27. Burke JM, Caron PC, Papadopoulos EB et al. Cytoreduction with iodine-131-anti-CD33 antibodies before bone marrow transplantation for advanced myeloid leukemias. Bone Marrow Transplant 2003;32:549–556
28. Bunjes D. 188Re-labeled anti-CD66 monoclonal antibody in stem cell transplantation for patients with high-risk acute myeloid leukemia. Leuk Lymphoma 2002;43:2125–2131
29. Wattel E, Solary E, Leleu X et al. A prospective study of autologous bone marrow or peripheral blood stem cell transplantation after intensive chemotherapy in myelodysplastic syndromes. Groupe Francais des Myelodysplasies. Group Ouest-Est d'etude des Leucemies Aigues Myeloides. Leukemia 1999;13:524–529
30. de Witte T, Suciu S, Verhoef G et al. Intensive chemotherapy followed by allogeneic or autologous stem cell transplantation for patients with myelodysplastic syndromes (MDSs) and acute myeloid leukemia following MDS. Blood 2001;98:2326–2331
31. Kroger N, Brand R, van Beizen A et al. Autologous stem cell transplantation for therapy-related acute myeloid leukemia and myelodysplastic syndrome. Bone Marrow Transplant 2006;37:183–189
32. Hanel M, Kroger N, Sonnenberg S et al. Busulfan, cyclophosphamide, and etoposide as high-dose conditioning regimen in patients with malignant lymphoma. Ann Hematol 2002;81:96–102
33. Gutierrez-Delgado F, Holmberg L, Hooper H et al. Autologous stem cell transplantation for Hodgkin's disease: busulfan, melphalan and thiotepa compared to a radiation-based regimen. Bone Marrow Transplant 2003;32:279–285
34. Stiff P, Unger JM, Foreman SJ et al. The value of augmented preparative regimens combined with an autologous bone marrow transplant for the management of relapsed or refractory Hodgkin disease: a Southwest Oncology Group phase II trial. Biol Blood Marrow Transplant 2003;9:529–539
35. Waheed F, Kancherla R, Seiter K et al. High dose chemotherapy with thiotepa, mitoxantrone and carboplatin (TMJ) followed by autologous stem cell support in 100 consecutive lymphoma patients in a single centre: analysis of efficacy, toxicity and prognostic factors. Leuk Lymphoma 2004;45:2253–2259
36. Nachbaur D, Greinix HT, Koller E et al. Long-term results of autologous stem cell transplantation for Hodgkin's disease (HD) and low-/intermediate-grade B non-Hodgkin's lymphoma (NHL): a report from the Austrian Stem Cell Transplantation Registry (ASCTR). Ann Hematol 2005;84:462–473
37. Morabito F, Stelitano C, Luminaro S et al. The role of high-dose therapy and autologous stem cell transplantation in patients with primary refractory Hodgkin's lymphoma: a report from the Gruppo Italiano per lo Studio dei Linfomi (GISL). Bone Marrow Transplant 2006;37:283–288
38. Lavoie JC, Connors JM, Phillips GL et al. High-dose chemotherapy and autologous stem cell transplantation for primary refractory or relapsed Hodgkin lymphoma: long-term outcome in the first 100 patients treated in Vancouver. Blood 2005;106:1473–1478
39. Ahmed T, Rashid K, Waheed F et al. Long-term survival of patients with resistant lymphoma treated with tandem stem cell transplant. Leuk Lymphoma 2005;46:405–414
40. Brice P, Divine M, Simon D et al. Feasibility of tandem autologous stem-cell transplantation (ASCT) in induction failure or very unfavorable (UF) relapse from Hodgkin's disease (HD). SFGM/GELA Study Group. Ann Oncol 1999;10:1485–1488
41. Fitoussi O, Simon D, Brice P et al. Tandem transplant of peripheral blood stem cells for patients with poor-prognosis Hodgkins's disease or non-Hodgkin's lymphoma. Bone Marrow Transplant 1999;24:747–755
42. Glossman JP, Staak JO, Nogova JL et al. Autologous tandem transplantation in patients with primary progressive or relapsed/refractory lymphoma. Ann Hematol 2005;84: 517–525
43. Ferrara F, Viola A, Copia C et al. Therapeutic results in patients with relapsed diffuse large B cell Non-Hodgkin's lymphoma achieving complete response only after autologous stem cell transplantation. Hematol Oncol 2006;24:73–77
44. Josting A, Sieniawski M, Glossmann JP et al. High-dose sequential chemotherapy followed by autologous stem cell transplantation in relapsed and refractory aggressive non-Hodgkin's lymphoma: results of a multicenter phase II study. Ann Oncol 2005;16:1359–1365
45. Philip T, Guglielmi C, Hagenbeek A et al. Autologous bone marrow transplantation as compared with salvage chemotherapy in relapses of chemotherapy-sensitive non-Hodgkin's lymphoma. N Engl J Med 1995;333:1540–1545
46. Lenz G, Dreyling M, Schneignitz E et al. Myeloablative radiochemotherapy followed by autologous stem cell transplantation in first remission prolongs progression-free survival in follicular lymphoma: results of a prospective, randomized trial of the German Low-Grade Lymphoma Study Group. Blood 2004;104:2667–2674
47. Reimer P, Schertlin T, Rudiger T et al. Myeloablative radiochemotherapy followed by autologous peripheral blood stem cell transplantation as first-line therapy in peripheral T-cell lymphomas: first results of a prospective multicenter study. Hematol J 2004;5:304–311
48. Dreyling M, Lenz G, Hoster E et al. Early consolidation by myeloablative radiochemotherapy followed by autologous stem cell transplantation in first remission significantly prolongs progression-free survival in mantle-cell lymphoma: results of a prospective randomized trial of the European MCL Network. Blood 2005;105:2677–2684
49. Vose JM, Bierman PJ, Enke C et al. Phase I trial of iodine-131 tositumomab with high-dose chemotherapy and autologous stem-cell transplantation for relapsed non-Hodgkin's lymphoma. J Clin Oncol. 2005;23:461–467
50. Cilley J, Winter JN. Radioimmunotherapy and autologous stem cell transplantation for the treatment of B-cell lymphomas. Haematologica 2006;91:114–120
51. Fung HC, Forman SJ, Nademanee A et al. A new preparative regimen for older patients with aggressive CD-20 positive B-cell lymphoma utilizing standard dose Yttrium 90 ibritumomab tiuxetan radioimmunotherapy combined with high dose BEAM followed by autologous hematopoietic cell transplantation. Blood 2003;102:248a
52. Nademanee A, Forman SJ, Molina A et al. A phase 1/2 trial of high-dose yttrium-90-ibritumomab tiuxetan in combination with high-dose etoposide and cyclophosphamide followed by autologous stem cell transplantation in patients with poor-risk or relapsed non-Hodgkin lymphoma. Blood 2005;106:2896–2902

53. Vose JM, Colcher D, Gobar L et al. Phase I/II trial of multiple dose 131Iodine-MAb LL2 (CD22) in patients with recurrent non-Hodgkin's lymphoma. Leuk Lymphoma 2000;38:91–101

54. Liu SY, Eary JF, Petersdorf SH et al. Follow-up of relapsed B-cell lymphoma patients treated with iodine-131-labeled anti-CD20 antibody and autologous stem-cell rescue. J Clin Oncol 1998;16:3270–3278

55. Gopal AK, Gooley TA, Maloney DG et al. High-dose radioimmunotherapy versus conventional high-dose therapy and autologous hematopoietic stem cell transplantation for relapsed follicular non-Hodgkin lymphoma: a multivariable cohort analysis. Blood 2003;102:2351–2357

56. Ballestrero A, Calvio M, Ferrando F et al. High-dose chemotherapy with tandem autologous transplantation as part of the initial therapy for aggressive non-Hodgkin's lymphoma. Int J Oncol 2000;17:1007–1013

57. Kewalramani T, Zelenetz AD, Nimer SD et al. Rituximab and ICE as second line therapy before autologous stem cell transplantation for relapsed or primary refractory diffuse large B0-cell lymphoma. Blood 2004;103:3684–3688

58. Moreau P, Facon T, Attal M et al. Comparison of 200 mg/m^2 melphalan and 8 Gy total body irradiation plus 140 mg/m^2 melphalan as conditioning regimens for peripheral blood stem cell transplantation in patients with newly diagnosed multiple myeloma: final analysis of the Intergroupe Francophone du Myelome 9502 randomized trial. Blood 2002;99:731–735

59. Majolino I, Vignetti M, Meloni G et al. Autologous transplantation in multiple myeloma: a GITMO retrospective analysis on 290 patients. Gruppo Italiano Trapianti di Midollo Osseo. Haematologica 1999;84:844–852

60. Lahuerta JJ, Martinez-Lopez J, Grande C et al. Conditioning regimens in autologous stem cell transplantation for multiple myeloma: a comparative study of efficacy and toxicity from the Spanish Registry for Transplantation in Multiple Myeloma. Br J Haematol 2000;109:138–147

61. Anagnostopoulos A, Aleman A, Ayers G et al. Comparison of high-dose melphalan with a more intensive regimen of thiotepa, busulfan, and cyclophosphamide for patients with multiple myeloma. Cancer 2004;100:2607–2612

62. Cogle CR, Moreb JS, Leather HL et al. Busulfan, cyclophosphamide, and etoposide as conditioning for autologous stem cell transplantation in multiple myeloma. Am J Hematol 2003;73:169–175

63. Jagannath S, Vesole DH, Glenn L et al. Low-risk intensive therapy for multiple myeloma with combined autologous bone marrow and blood stem cell support. Blood 1992;80:1666–1672

64. Harousseau JL, Attal M, Divine M et al. Autologous stem cell transplantation after first remission induction treatment in multiple myeloma: a report of the French Registry on autologous transplantation in multiple myeloma. Blood 1995;85:3077–3085

65. Barlogie B, Jagganath S, Naucke S et al. Long-term follow-up after high-dose therapy for high-risk multiple myeloma. Bone Marrow Transplant 1998;21:1101–1107

66. Attal M, Harrousseau JL, Stoppa AM et al. A prospective, randomized trial of autologous bone marrow transplantation and chemotherapy in multiple myeloma. Intergroupe Francais du Myelome. N Engl J Med 1996;335:91–97

67. Mansi J, daCosta F, Viner C et al. High-dose busulfan in patients with myeloma. J Clin Oncol 1992;10:1569–1573

68. Barlogie B, Jagganath S, Naucke S et al. Long-term follow-up after high-dose therapy for high-risk multiple myeloma. Bone Marrow Transplant 1998;21:1101–1107

69. Toor AA, Ayers J, Strupeck J et al. Favourable results with a single autologous stem cell transplant following conditioning with busulphan and cyclophosphamide in patients with multiple myeloma. Br J Haematol 2004;124:769–776

70. Bensinger WI, Rowley SD, Demirere T et al. High-dose therapy followed by autologous hematopoietic stem-cell infusion for patients with multiple myeloma. J Clin Oncol 1996;14:1447–1456

71. Mehta J, Tricot G, Jagganath S et al. High-dose chemotherapy with carboplatin, cyclophosphamide and etoposide and autologous transplantation for multiple myeloma relapsing after a previous transplant. Bone Marrow Transplant 1997;20:113–116

72. Moreau P, Hullin C, Garban F et al. Tandem autologous stem cell transplantation in high-risk de novo multiple myeloma: final results of the prospective and randomized IFM 99–04 protocol. Blood 2006;107:397–403

73. Palumbo A, Triolo S, Argentino C et al. Dose-intensive melphalan with stem cell support (MEL100) is superior to standard treatment in elderly myeloma patients. Blood 1999;94:1248–1253

74. AttalM, Harrousseau JL, Facon T et al. Single versus double autologous stem-cell transplantation for multiple myeloma. N Engl J Med 2003;349:2495–2502

75. Gertz MA, Lacy MO, Dispenzieri A et al. Risk-adjusted manipulation of melphalan dose before stem cell transplantation in patients with amyloidosis is associated with a lower response rate. Bone Marrow Transplant 2004;34:1025–1031

76. Skinner M, Sanchorawala V, Seldin DC et al. High-dose melphalan and autologous stem-cell transplantation in patients with AL amyloidosis: an 8-year study. Ann Intern Med 2004;140:85–93

77. Dispenzieri A, Kyle R, Lacy MO et al. Superior survival in primary systemic amyloidosis patients undergoing peripheral blood stem cell transplantation: a case-control study. Blood 2004;103:3960–3963

78. Sanchorawala V, Wright DG, Seldin DC et al. High-dose intravenous melphalan and autologous stem cell transplantation as initial therapy or following two cycles of oral chemotherapy for the treatment of AL amyloidosis: results of a prospective randomized trial. Bone Marrow Transplant 2004;33:381–388

79. Comenzo RL, Vosburgh E, Falk RH et al. Dose-intensive melphalan with blood stem-cell support for AL (amyloid light-chain) amyloidosis: survival and responses in 25 patients. Blood 1998;91:3662–3670

80. Comenzo RL, Gertz MA. Autologous stem cell transplantation for primary systemic amyloidosis. Blood 2002;99:4276–4282

81. Barjorin DF, Nichols CR, Margolin KA et al. Phase III trial of conventional-dose chemotherapy alonme or with high-dose chemotherapy for metastatic germ cell tumors (GCT): a cooperative group trial by Memorial Sloan Kettering Cancer Center, ECOG, SWOG and CALGB. J Clin Oncol 2006;24:219s

82. Pico JL, Rosti G, Kramar A et al. A randomised trial of high-dose chemotherapy in the salvage treatment of patients failing first-line platinum chemotherapy for advanced germ cell tumours. Ann Oncol 2005;16:1152–1159

83. Chaudhary UB, Damon LE, Rugo HS et al. High-dose etoposide, thiotepa, and dose-adjusted carboplatin (TVCa) with autologous hematopoietic stem cell rescue as treatment of relapsed or refractory germ cell cancer. Am J Clin Oncol 2005;28:130–137

84. Blay JY, Bouhour D, Ray-Coquard I et al. High-dose chemotherapy with autologous hematopoietic stem-cell transplantation for advanced soft tissue sarcoma in adults. J Clin Oncol 2000;18:3643–3650

85. LeCesne A, Judson I, Crowther D et al. Randomized phase III study comparing conventional-dose doxorubicin versus high-dose doxorubicin plus ifosfamide plus recombinant human granulocyte-macrophage colony-stimulating factor in advanced soft tissue sarcomas: a trial of the European Organization for Research and Treatment of Cancer/Soft Tissue and Bone Sarcoma Group. J Clin Oncol 2000;18:2676–2684

86. Kozuka T, Kiura K, Katayama H et al. Tandem high-dose chemotherapy supported by autologous peripheral blood stem cell transplantation for recurrent soft tissue sarcoma. Anticancer Res 2002;22:2939–2944

87. Stiff PJ, Veum-Stone J Lazarus HM et al. High-dose chemotherapy and autologous stem-cell transplantation for ovarian cancer: an autologous blood and marrow transplant registry report. Ann Intern Med 2000;133:504–515

88. Bertucci F, Viens P, Delpero JR et al. High-dose melphalan-based chemotherapy and autologous stem cell transplantation after second look laparotomy in patients with chemosensitive advanced ovarian carcinoma: long-term results. Bone Marrow Transplant 2000;26:61–67

89. Ledermann JA, Herd R, Maraninchi D et al. High-dose chemotherapy for ovarian carcinoma: long-term results from the Solid Tumour Registry of the European Group for Blood and Marrow Transplantation (EBMT). Ann Oncol 2001;12:693–699

90. Tiersten A, Selleck M, Smith DH et al. Phase I/II study of tandem cycles of high-dose chemotherapy followed by autologous hematopoietic stem cell support in women with advanced ovarian cancer. Int J Gynecol Cancer 2006;16:57–64

91. Abrey LE, Childs BH, Paleologos N et al. High-dose chemotherapy with stem cell rescue as initial therapy for anaplastic oligodendroglioma: long-term follow-up. Neuro-oncology 2006;8:183–188

92. Durando X, Lemaire JJ, Tortochaux V et al. High-dose BCNU followed by autologous hematopoietic stem cell transplantation in supratentorial high-grade malignant gliomas: a retrospective analysis of 114 patients. Bone Marrow Transplant 2003;31:559–564

93. Cheng T, Forsyth P, Chauhdry T et al. High-dose thiotepa, busulfan, cyclophosphamide and ASCT without whole-brain radiotherapy for poor prognosis primary CNS lymphoma. Bone Marrow Transplant 2003;31:679–685

94. Snowden JA, Brooks PM, Biggs JC. Haemopoietic stem cell transplantation for autoimmune diseases. Br J Haematol 1997;99:9–22

95. Samijn JP, teBoekhorst PA, Mondria T et al. Intense T cell depletion followed by autologous bone marrow transplantation for severe multiple sclerosis. J Neurol Neurosurg Psychiatry 2006;77:46–50

96. Fassas A, Passweg JR, Anagnostopoulos A et al. Hematopoietic stem cell transplantation for multiple sclerosis. A retrospective multicenter study. J Neurol 2002;249:1088–1097

97. Farge D, Passweg J, van Laar JM et al. Autologous stem cell transplantation in the treatment of systemic sclerosis: report from the EBMT/EULAR Registry. Ann Rheum Dis 2004;63:974–981

98. McSweeney PA, Nash RA, Sullivan KM et al. High-dose immunosuppressive therapy for severe systemic sclerosis: initial outcomes. Blood 2002;100:1602–1610

99. Snowden JA, Passweg J, Moore JJ et al. Autologous hemopoietic stem cell transplantation in severe rheumatoid arthritis: a report from the EBMT and ABMTR. J Rheumatol 2004;31:482–488

100. Huhn RD, Fogarty PF, Nakamura R et al. High-dose cyclophosphamide with autologous lymphocyte-depleted peripheral blood stem cell (PBSC) support for treatment of refractory chronic autoimmune thrombocytopenia. Blood 2003;101:71–77

101. Passweg JR, Rabusin M, Musso M et al. Haematopoetic stem cell transplantation for refractory autoimmune cytopenia. Br J Haematol 2004;125:749–755

102. Burt RK, Patel D, Thomas J et al. The rationale behind autologous autoimmune hematopoietic stem cell transplant conditioning regimens: concerns over the use of total-body irradiation in systemic sclerosis. Bone Marrow Transplant 2004;34:745–751

103. Gratwohl A, Passweg J, Botelli-Tyndall C et al. Autologous hematopoietic stem cell transplantation for autoimmune diseases. Bone Marrow Transplant 2005;35:869–879

Myeloablative conditioning regimens for allogeneic stem cell transplantation

CHAPTER 27

James A Russell

Introduction

Selection of the conditioning or preparative treatment given before allogeneic stem cell transplantation depends on a number of factors including the disease being treated, the donor and the stem cell product to be given. Historically, it was believed that the regimen needed to be sufficiently immunosuppressive to prevent graft rejection and that it needed, in some circumstances, to provide 'space' in the recipient bone marrow. Finally, in the case of malignant disease, it should exert a profound cytotoxic effect on the cancer cells. In a condition such as severe aplastic anemia (SAA) immunosuppression is paramount. In other non-malignant diseases this would need to be accompanied by the ability to provide space in bone marrows with normal or increased cellularity. A transplant for malignancy could be seen essentially as a 'rescue' procedure allowing dose escalation of cytotoxic agents whose primary dose-limiting toxicity is on the bone marrow. In general, agents given in such doses would also achieve the immunosuppression required for engraftment, particularly in patients who had previously been exposed to cytotoxic therapy.

We now know that agents selected primarily for their immunosuppressive qualities, particularly if given with the high doses of progenitor cells which can be collected from peripheral blood, are capable of producing durable engraftment without myeloablation. For practical purposes, a myeloablative regimen could be seen as one which, when used for malignant disease, is given with the intent of achieving maximal tumor cell kill by the cytotoxic agents. For non-malignant disease, where regimens with myeloablative potential have traditionally been used, our understanding of the relative contributions of immunosuppression and creation of space in the recipient marrow is evolving and it could be that newer agents such as fludarabine may contribute to durable engraftment without myeloablation. However, non-malignant diseases for which regimens thought to be myeloablative have traditionally been used will be considered briefly in this chapter.

When given with stem cell rescue, the ability to escalate doses of agents used in myeloablative regimens is limited by their toxicity to organs and tissues other than the bone marrow. With unmanipulated (not T-depleted or CD34+ cell selected) transplants a major, if not the predominant, contribution to morbidity and mortality is that from graft-versus-host disease (GvHD). There is increasing evidence that dose escalation of cytotoxic agents may, in fact, increase mortality by a synergistic effect with acute GvHD, in particular perhaps by increasing cytokine release from tissue damage.[1] Improved GvHD prophylaxis may therefore be necessary for the high transplant-related mortality (TRM) historically associated with myeloablative regimens to be significantly reduced. The aim of the myeloablative regimen in

malignancy is to achieve the maximum possible antitumor effect while limiting toxicity (either 'regimen related' or from GvHD). In practice, the relative contributions of graft-versus-malignancy (GvM) and dose escalation may be difficult to determine in view of the complex interaction described above between GvHD, regimen-related toxicity, GvM, the direct tumor kill of cytotoxic agents and the diseases being treated.

Particularly in view of the increase in popularity of non-myeloablative regimens, it is important to emphasize that there is substantial evidence for the value of dose intensity at least in some malignancies. The first, of course, is the success of autologous transplants which depend solely on the principle of dose escalation. Secondly, there is evidence that relapse after allotransplant may be reduced by higher doses of cytotoxic agents such as total-body irradiation (TBI) for some diseases.[2] In this case, however, it is difficult to be absolutely sure how much this effect is due to a direct cytotoxic effect and how much to an impact on GvHD as described above.

Agents used in myeloablative combinations

Most of the more widely employed agents have in common the feature that hematologic toxicity is dose limiting when they are given without stem cell support. In addition, cytotoxic activity is dose dependent, thus achieving more tumor cell killing with increasing doses. The most commonly used have hitherto been TBI, cyclophosphamide, busulfan, and VP16 (etoposide). These agents share acute toxicities, in part related to their inherent cytotoxic activity. Short-term complications include nausea and vomiting, mucositis (particularly stomatitis and enteritis), hair loss and the sequelae of bone marrow suppression. Other side-effects are more agent specific (Table 27.1).

Total-body irradiation (TBI)

Total-body irradiation is a powerful immunosuppressant and cytotoxic agent and has been a component of some of the most widely used regimens since the early days of transplantation. The potential to penetrate sanctuary sites such as the central nervous system (CNS) may give TBI an advantage over some drugs. Radiation is delivered from a linear accelerator or a cobalt source used for routine cancer treatments. These machines need to be adapted to deliver TBI; such adaptation requires the patient to be sufficiently far from the source to allow the whole body to be included in a single field.

The effect of TBI depends largely on the dose rate, the total dose delivered and the number of fractions into which the total dose is divided.[2–6] Some earlier protocols involved delivering about 1000 cGy in a single fraction at a low dose rate. This required several hours to

Table 27.1 Cytotoxic agents in myeloablative conditioning protocols

Agent	Approximate upper limit of total dose#	Common scheduling	Organ-specific toxicity*		References to toxicity
			Short term (<3 mo)	Long term (>3 mo)	
Total-body irradiation	1400–1500 cGy	6–12 fractions over 3–4 days	Parotitis Skin erythema Xerostomia Interstitial pneumonitis	Cataracts Xerostomia Hypothyroidism Growth arrest Gonadal failure Delayed puberty Dental decay Second malignancies	5 92 93 93 94,96 95 90 8,97
Cyclophosphamide	200 mg/kg	Over 2–4 days	Cardiac failure Hemorrhagic cystitis	Cardiac failure	98,99
Busulfan po	16 mg/kg	4 days	Veno-occlusive disease Hemorrhagic cystitis Convulsions Skin erythema and pigmentation	Alopecia	30,100
Busulfan iv	12.8 mg/kg or 520 mg/m^2	Once to 4 times daily over 4 days			26
VP-16	60 mg/kg	Single dose	Hypotension Hepatotoxicity Hand-foot syndrome		101
Fludarabine	240–250 mg/m^2	iv over 4–6 days	Neurotoxicity		102
Melphalan	200–220 mg/m^2	Single dose			103
Ara-C	36 g/m^2	Up to q12h over 6 days	Cerebellar toxicity	Cerebellar toxicity	102
Thiotepa	600 mg/m^2	Single dose	Skin rash Renal Hepatic		104
Treosulfan	47 mg/m^2	Single dose			105

Upper limit will vary according to other components of regimen.
* Some effects are common to more than one agent.

administer and was inconvenient because of the time involved and the fact that patients would often vomit and be otherwise uncomfortable during the procedure. Subsequent refinements resulted in TBI being given at a somewhat higher dose rate, in multiple fractions, which appears to improve tolerability while maintaining the antitumor effect. Thus, some long-term effects such as cataracts and thyroid dysfunction seem to be less after fractionated schedules.[7,8] Dose escalation above about 1500 cGy has increased TRM with or without a compensatory effect on relapse.[9,10] Single doses as low as 500 cGy delivered at a high dose rate have been remarkably effective but no direct comparisons with fractionated schedules have been performed.[11] While dose and dose rate are closely monitored, the details of delivery vary in different institutions. Moreover, there may be changes over time in TBI dose rates when delivered from a cobalt source.

Cyclophosphamide

Cyclophosphamide is an alkylating agent which was originally used alone as conditioning for SAA in view of its powerful immunosuppressant effects. Cyclophosphamide is not strictly speaking a myeloablative agent, as primitive stem cells appear to lack the enzyme pathway necessary for activation. Cardiotoxicity is the main adverse effect limiting dose escalation. Cyclophosphamide metabolism is very variable, and high concentrations of metabolites are related to liver injury including veno-occlusive disease (VOD) or sinusoidal obstruction syndrome.[12] High doses should be administered with hydration and/or Mesna in order to minimize hemorrhagic cystitis.

Busulfan

Busulfan is an alkylating agent originally given qid by mouth, generally with cyclophosphamide in the so-called BuCy regimens.[13–15] Pharmacokinetic studies revealed very wide variations in exposure because

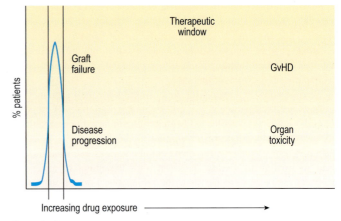

Figure 27.1
Relationship of exposure to clinical effects for a chemotherapeutic agent such as busulfan.

many patients vomited the drug, replacement was haphazard and intestinal absorption was very variable. In some diseases low drug exposures predisposed to failed engraftment and relapse whereas toxic effects, including VOD, were more common at high levels (Fig. 27.1).[16–20] Optimal therapeutic ranges have been established for oral busulfan.[20,21] Exposures within the desired range appeared to produce better outcomes in myeloid malignancy, leading to a recommendation of therapeutic drug monitoring (TDM) for oral busulfan. An iv form is now available which, when given qid, gives more patients exposures in ranges considered optimal for oral busulfan and better outcomes within these ranges.[22,23]

Intravenous busulfan given 12 hourly or once daily in myeloablative doses appears effective and well tolerated although no direct comparisons have been done.[24–26] Daily total exposures are similar to those achieved with qid dosing and the tolerable limit of daily exposure may also be much the same as for qid po busulfan even when combined with fludarabine instead of cyclophosphamide.[27] Because 10–15% of patients given iv busulfan based on weight may experience unacceptably high exposures, TDM is probably justifiable. The availability of an assay may mean that the delivery can be more rationally based than with other agents used in myeloablative regimens.

Although oral busulfan with TDM and dose adjustment could be as effective as the intravenous drug it may be more cumbersome, requiring more dose adjustments which are not always achieving the target and possibly expose more patients to the hazards of VOD. It is therefore becoming more difficult to justify the use of oral busulfan.

VP16 (etoposide)

VP16 (etoposide) is widely used in autotransplant regimens and may be more effective therapy for some leukemias than cyclophosphamide. Formerly given as a prolonged infusion at low concentration, it is now usually given in concentrated form as a short iv infusion.

Fludarabine

This purine analog is increasingly used because it is a powerful immunosuppressant, is effective in leukemias and is less toxic than cyclophosphamide. Total doses in current regimens have not exceeded 240–250 mg/m^2 because of concern regarding neurotoxicity at higher exposures.

Common myeloablative conditioning regimens

The above agents have been combined in a variety of myeloablative regimens. In some cases dose-finding studies have determined the upper limit of one or more or of the constituents. As with combination chemotherapy in general, the intent is to maximize the dose of the individual constituents while trying to avoid overlapping non-hematologic toxicity.

The cyclophosphamide and TBI (CyTBI) combination has the longest track record of any regimen for hematologic malignancy and perhaps remains the 'gold standard' against which others must be judged.

Busulfan was substituted for TBI in myeloablative regimens in order to avoid some of the toxicities of TBI and to develop drug-based protocols which could be used by centers without TBI facilities. Busulfan was originally given po at 1 mg/kg qid for 4 days, with cyclophosphamide at 200 mg/kg over 4 days (BuCy4). While effective, this regimen was quite toxic and reducing the cyclophosphamide dose to 120 mg/kg over 2 days (BuCy2) improved the tolerability of the combination.[14,15]

The major concern was a relatively high incidence of VOD which reached 50% in some centers.[28,29] Larger multicenter studies indicate a figure more in the order of 10%.[30] However, VOD is often fatal and attempts to prevent it have not been uniformly successful. The clearance of cyclophosphamide is decreased if given shortly after the last dose of busulfan so attention should be paid to the details of scheduling.[31]

In the BuCy2 combination iv busulfan is associated with less toxicity and early TRM than the oral form.[22, 32,33]

The combination of VP16 and TBI (VPTBI) has been explored particularly by the Stanford group and showed activity in leukemia at least comparable to other regimens.[34–37]

Recent studies have demonstrated that myeloablative doses of iv busulfan in conjunction with relatively high doses of fludarabine

provide a regimen with relatively low TRM.[24,26] The combination appears to be effective at least in AML and myelodysplasia (MDS).[24] Concerns that combining two potentially neurotoxic agents at high doses could result in unacceptable neurologic sequelae have not been substantiated.

Combinations of three or more of the above agents have been devised in order to provide more broadly based regimens combining cytotoxicity with the sparing of overlapping non-hematologic toxicity.[18,38,39] Additional drugs have been combined with each other and/or one or more of the above in myeloablative regimens. These include thiotepa,[40–43] treosulfan,[44] melphalan,[45–49] BCNU[50] and Ara-C.[51–53] However, in general the superiority of other combinations has been difficult to demonstrate; indeed, some studies have indicated worse results largely due to increased toxicity.[53–55]

Comparison of commonly used myeloablative regimens

The use of a particular myeloablative regimen in a transplant center depends on a number of factors including, for example, a particular research interest, involvement in multicenter studies requiring 'standard' regimens and other constraints such as the availability of TBI. The evolution of commonly used protocols has been somewhat haphazard and direct comparisons are relatively few. Comparative data are derived from a few randomized studies and information from large registries such as the CIBMTR and EBMT. Although there are limitations of registry-based comparisons, they may reflect outcomes in the 'real world' in comparison with those derived from randomized studies, where patient selection is quite rigorous, or from single center experiences. Registry data have been compared with results obtained in one or a few centers, but once again these need to be interpreted with some caution.

If an optimal myeloablative regimen were to be developed, it would somehow have to balance the beneficial effects of antitumor activity with the higher toxicity to be expected from dose escalation. While a GvM effect may be important in some diseases, this may often be at the expense of GvHD, still a major cause of morbidity and mortality. Moreover, survival as an endpoint needs to be viewed in the light of quality of life, often impaired by delayed effects of conditioning therapy and chronic GvHD. The ideal regimen might also involve the ability to monitor the delivery of agents to account for differences in pharmacokinetics.

Regimens for hematologic malignancies

Credible information comparing myeloablative regimens for hematologic malignancy is really limited to the leukemias. Unfortunately, some of these studies do not report outcomes for the different leukemias separately.

Randomized studies comparing CyTBI with BuCy2 for leukemia in general have indicated remarkable effectiveness of oral busulfan despite its very erratic pharmacokinetics. In general, BuCy2 has resulted in more VOD.[56] While registry data have indicated that CyTBI causes more interstitial pneumonitis,[57] a meta-analysis of randomized trials did not find this significant.[56] Perhaps variability in TBI techniques may account for these differences. The latter analysis also indicated that while CyTBI is not demonstrably superior overall, it is unlikely to be inferior to BuCy2. A randomized study of VP16TBI against BuCy2 indicated very similar outcomes in patients beyond first chronic phase of CML or first complete response (CR1) of acute leukemia.[58]

Chronic myelogenous leukemia (CML)

Randomized trials showed BuCy2 to be as well or better tolerated than CyTBI with equivalent final outcomes.[10, 59–61] Retrospective studies have also indicated that BuCy2 may be comparable to CyTBI.[62] Some reports observed a trend to less relapse after BuCy2.[60,62] Our increased understanding of the importance of graft-versus-leukemia effects (GvL) in CML has led to speculation that the dose intensity of the regimen may be of secondary importance. However, some studies with BuCy2 where the busulfan is given orally or iv have indicated that busulfan exposure seems to be important.[23] The fact that BuCy2 is convenient and at least as effective as TBI-based regimens in CML has led it to be standard regimen for this disease in many centers.

The use of imatinib as first-line therapy for most patients in chronic phase has altered the population of CML patients coming to allotransplant. Conceivably, these patients may need more intense cytoreduction but it will be some time before this can be established. Conversely, given the response of persistent or relapsed CML after transplant to donor lymphocytes or tyrosine kinase inhibitors, it will be critically important to minimize TRM.

Acute myelogenous leukemia (AML)

The results of randomized comparisons of BuCy2 and CyTBI have not been entirely consistent. A combined analysis of trials[8,63,64] devoted to or including AML patients demonstrated a non-significant trend to better projected survival and leukemia-free survival at 10 years with CyTBI.[61] Registry data indicate again that ultimate outcomes are very similar.[7,8,57,65] More relapse after BuCy2 compared with BuCy4 and CyTBI was seen in a pediatric series.[7] A similar effect, compensated for by a slight reduction in TRM, was observed in a CIBMTR report.[65] The VP16TBI combination seems active in AML and a randomized comparison with BuCy2 in advanced disease showed equivalent outcomes.[36,58] Recent reports of fludarabine and daily iv busulfan combinations with or without TBI have indicated good survival with low TRM for AML and MDS.[24,66] However, these regimens have not been directly compared to the alternatives and CyTBI should perhaps continue to be the reference for comparison. Another promising avenue is the addition of radiolabeled antibodies to provide enhanced radiation doses targeted to the bone marrow while sparing other tissues.[67]

Acute lymphoblastic leukemia (ALL)

There is a preference for TBI-containing regimens before transplants for ALL.[68,69] Most children with leukemia will therefore be exposed to TBI with the consequent late effects of growth retardation in particular. Survival is better after CyTBI than after BuCy2.[70–72] A recent analysis comparing outcomes in adults with ALL given VP16TBI with those for patients in the CIBMTR database treated with CyTBI acknowledges the problem of comparing individual center results with registry data.[35] Outcomes were similar in CR1 but for patients in CR2 it may be better to increase the dose of TBI from 1200 to 1320 cGy with Cy or to substitute VP16 for Cy. The VP16TBI combination is now being used as standard conditioning in multigroup studies of ALL.

Other hematologic malignancies

Allogeneic transplantation is increasingly being applied to other hematologic malignancies including chronic lymphocytic leukemia, lymphomas and multiple myeloma. The advantages of using myeloablative regimens over less intense protocols are not well established. Many patients are relatively old and/or have been heavily pretreated with chemotherapy, irradiation and often autologous transplants. Historically, TRM has tended to be high with myeloablative regimens but possibly this may improve with better patient selection and GvHD prophylaxis. However, it is difficult to make a solid recommendation for one regimen over another.

Non-malignant disease

Non-malignant diseases provide particular challenges for selection of conditioning regimens. Hematologic disorders such as SAA and thalassemia occur in the context of largely intact cell-mediated immunity and resistance to engraftment may be enhanced by previous transfusion. Myeloablative conditioning is aimed simply at providing sufficient immunosuppression for engraftment while attempting to avoid long-term complications of agents such as TBI. Additionally, there is no benefit from GvHD.

Severe aplastic anemia (SAA)

Aplastic anemia was the first disease to be successfully transplanted in significant numbers. Initially, high doses of cyclophosphamide were used alone for conditioning. It became clear that presensitization by multiple transfusions, particularly from family members, increased the risk of rejection.[73] This is now less of an issue with sibling transplants which can be done soon after diagnosis but may influence outcomes of alternative donor transplants. Immunosuppressants such as antithymocyte globulins (ATG) may facilitate engraftment in addition to reducing GvHD.[74] Further addition of a single fraction of 200 cGy TBI has proved sufficient to allow engraftment of stem cells from most unrelated donors.[75] An alternative approach is to avoid irradiation and substitute some of the cyclophosphamide with fludarabine.[76,77]

β-Thalassemia

The transplant program in Pesaro has pioneered the development of effective drug-based regimens for thalassemia.[78] Graft failure has been somewhat more common than in hematologic malignancy, perhaps related in part to multiple transfusions.[79] A regimen of 14 mg/kg busulfan with 200 mg/kg cyclophosphamide has been suitable for the majority of patients in Class 1 and 2. Cyclophosphamide doses may need to be reduced for Class 3 disease although rejection may be more frequent. Even with intensive regimens there is a significant incidence of autologous reconstitution. Complete engraftment may depend as much on immunosuppression and the immunologic effect of the graft as on the ability of conditioning to eradicate recipient hemopoiesis. Whether agents such as fludarabine can replace some of the other drugs to improve tolerability and maintain engraftment remains to be seen but early case reports are encouraging.[80–82]

Metabolic disorders

Once again, these conditions have proven somewhat more refractory to engraftment than the hematologic malignancies. There is a preference for chemotherapy regimens because of the significant long-term effects of TBI in children. There may be promise in non-myeloablative transplants particularly as full donor engraftment may not be necessary for amelioration of some of these disorders.[83]

Modification of conditioning according to stem cell product and donor

In both malignant and non-malignant disorders, engraftment may be influenced by the degree of matching and relatedness of the donor and also by the product infused, particularly the progenitor cell dose. Recovery may be compromised by in vitro T-cell depletion which involves some loss not only of stem cells but also of lymphocytes which may facilitate engraftment.[84–86] Immunosuppression can be enhanced by increasing TBI dose or by adding total lymphoid irradiation[87–89] or other agents. Engraftment from cord blood is significantly influenced by the progenitor cell doses infused and tends to result in slower recovery than other sources, particularly in adults. Most regimens are TBI or busulfan based and many include ATG.[90]

As matching techniques have become more sophisticated there is currently little evidence that cytotoxic conditioning appropriate for a matched sibling transplant should be modified for a limited degree of mismatching and/or for an unrelated donor. It may be rational, however, to add immune suppression such as ATG in order to modify GvHD as well as facilitating engraftment. Most haploidentical transplants from family members have been heavily T-cell depleted, both in vivo and in vitro. The resistance to engraftment is offset somewhat by high doses of infused donor cells and many regimens have used quite intense conditioning in addition to ATG in this setting.[40] On the other hand, unmanipulated haploidentical transplants appear to engraft well with conventional conditioning and ATG.[91]

References

1. Antin JH, Ferrara JL. Cytokine dysregulation and acute graft-versus-host disease. Blood 1992;80(12):2964–2968
2. Clift RA, Buckner CD, Appelbaum FR et al. Allogeneic marrow transplantation in patients with acute myeloid leukemia in first remission: a randomized trial of two irradiation regimens. Blood 1990;76(9):1867–1871
3. Brochstein JA, Kernan NA, Groshen S et al. Allogeneic bone marrow transplantation after hyperfractionated total-body irradiation and cyclophosphamide in children with acute leukemia. N Engl J Med 1987;317(26):1618–1624
4. Deeg HJ, Sullivan KM, Buckner CD et al. Marrow transplantation for acute nonlymphoblastic leukemia in first remission: toxicity and long-term follow-up of patients conditioned with single dose or fractionated total body irradiation. Bone Marrow Transplant 1986;1(2):151–157
5. Demirer T, Petersen FB, Appelbaum FR et al. Allogeneic marrow transplantation following cyclophosphamide and escalating doses of hyperfractionated total body irradiation in patients with advanced lymphoid malignancies: a Phase I/II trial. Int J Radiat Oncol Biol Phys 1995;4:1103–1109
6. Thomas ED, Clift RA, Hersman J et al. Marrow transplantation for acute nonlymphoblastic leukemia in first remission using fractionated or single-dose irradiation. Int J Radiat Oncol Biol Phys 1982;8(5):817–821
7. Michel G, Gluckman E, Esperou-Bourdeau H et al. Allogeneic bone marrow transplantation for children with acute myeloblastic leukemia in first complete remission: impact of conditioning regimen without total-body irradiation – a report from the Societe Francaise de Greffe de Moelle. J Clin Oncol 1994;12(6):1217–1222
8. Ringden O, Remberger M, Ruutu T et al. Increased risk of chronic graft-versus-host disease, obstructive bronchiolitis, and alopecia with busulfan versus total body irradiation: long-term results of a randomized trial in allogeneic marrow recipients with leukemia. Nordic Bone Marrow Transplantation Group. Blood 1999;93(7):2196–2201
9. Alyea E, Neuberg D, Mauch P et al. Effect of total body irradiation dose escalation on outcome following T-cell-depleted allogeneic bone marrow transplantation. Biol Blood Marrow Transplant 2002;8(3):139–144
10. Clift RA, Radich J, Appelbaum FR et al. Long-term follow-up of a randomized study comparing cyclophosphamide and total body irradiation with busulfan and cyclophosphamide for patients receiving allogeneic marrow transplants during chronic phase of chronic myeloid leukemia. Blood 1999;94(11):3960–3962
11. Fyles GM, Messner HA, Lockwood G et al. Long-term results of bone marrow transplantation for patients with AML, ALL and CML prepared with single dose total body irradiation of 500 cGy delivered with a high dose rate. Bone Marrow Transplant 1991;8(6):453–463
12. DeLeve LD, Shulman HM, McDonald GB. Toxic injury to hepatic sinusoids: sinusoidal obstruction syndrome (veno-occlusive disease). Semin Liver Dis 2002;22(1):27–42
13. Copelan EA, Deeg HJ. Conditioning for allogeneic marrow transplantation in patients with lymphohematopoietic malignancies without the use of total body irradiation. Blood 1992;80(7):1648–1658
14. Santos GW. Busulfan and cyclophosphamide versus cyclophosphamide and total body irradiation for marrow transplantation in chronic myelogenous leukemia – a review. Leuk Lymphoma 1993;11(suppl 1):201–204
15. Tutschka PJ, Copelan EA, Klein JP. Bone marrow transplantation for leukemia following a new busulfan and cyclophosphamide regimen. Blood 1987;70(5):1382–1388
16. Copelan EA, Bechtel TP, Avalos BR et al. Busulfan levels are influenced by prior treatment and are associated with hepatic veno-occlusive disease and early mortality but not with delayed complications following marrow transplantation. Bone Marrow Transplant 2001;27(11):1121–1124
17. Grochow LB, Jones RJ, Brundrett R et al. Pharmacokinetics of busulfan: correlation with veno-occlusive disease in patients undergoing bone marrow transplantation. Cancer Chemother Pharmacol 1989;25(1):55–61
18. Kroger N, Zabelina T, Sonnenberg S et al. Dose-dependent effect of etoposide in combination with busulfan plus cyclophosphamide as conditioning for stem cell transplantation in patients with acute myeloid leukemia. Bone Marrow Transplant 2000;26(7):711–716
19. Ljungman P, Hassan M, Bekassy AN et al. High busulfan concentrations are associated with increased transplant-related mortality in allogeneic bone marrow transplant patients. Bone Marrow Transplant 1997;20(11):909–913
20. Slattery JT, Clift RA, Buckner CD et al. Marrow transplantation for chronic myeloid leukemia: the influence of plasma busulfan levels on the outcome of transplantation. Blood 1997;89(8):3055–3060
21. Deeg HJ, Storer B, Slattery JT et al. Conditioning with targeted busulfan and cyclophosphamide for hemopoietic stem cell transplantation from related and unrelated donors in patients with myelodysplastic syndrome. Blood 2002;100(4):1201–1207
22. Andersson BS, Gajewski J, Donato M et al. Allogeneic stem cell transplantation (BMT) for AML and MDS following i.v. busulfan and cyclophosphamide (i.v. BuCy). Bone Marrow Transplant 2000;25(suppl 2):S35–38
23. Andersson BS, Thall PF, Madden T et al. Busulfan systemic exposure relative to regimen-related toxicity and acute graft-versus-host disease: defining a therapeutic window for i.v. BuCy2 in chronic myelogenous leukemia. Biol Blood Marrow Transplant 2002;8(9):477–485
24. de Lima M, Couriel D, Thall PF et al. Once-daily intravenous busulfan and fludarabine: clinical and pharmacokinetic results of a myeloablative, reduced-toxicity conditioning regimen for allogeneic stem cell transplantation in AML and MDS. Blood 2004;104(3):857–864
25. Fernandez HF, Tran HT, Albrecht F et al. Evaluation of safety and pharmacokinetics of administering intravenous busulfan in a twice-daily or daily schedule to patients with advanced hematologic malignant disease undergoing stem cell transplantation. Biol Blood Marrow Transplant 2002;8(9):486–492
26. Russell JA, Tran HT, Quinlan D et al. Once-daily intravenous busulfan given with fludarabine as conditioning for allogeneic stem cell transplantation: study of pharmacokinetics and early clinical outcomes. Biol Blood Marrow Transplant 2002;8(9):468–476
27. Geddes M, Kangarloo SB, Naveed F et al. High busulfan exposure is associated with worse outcomes in a daily i.v. busulfan and fludarabine allogeneic transplant regimen. Biol Blood Marrow Transplant 2008;14(2):220–228
28. Jones RJ, Lee KS, Beschorner WE et al. Venoocclusive disease of the liver following bone marrow transplantation. Transplantation 1987;44(6):778–783
29. McDonald GB, Hinds MS, Fisher LD et al. Veno-occlusive disease of the liver and multi-organ failure after bone marrow transplantation: a cohort study of 355 patients. Ann Intern Med 1993;118(4):255–267
30. Carreras E, Bertz H, Arcese W et al. Incidence and outcome of hepatic veno-occlusive disease after blood or marrow transplantation: a prospective cohort study of the European Group for Blood and Marrow Transplantation. European Group for Blood and Marrow Transplantation Chronic Leukemia Working Party. Blood 1998;92(10):3599–3604
31. Slattery JT, Kalhorn TF, McDonald GB et al. Conditioning regimen-dependent disposition of cyclophosphamide and hydroxycyclophosphamide in human marrow transplantation patients. J Clin Oncol 1996;14(5):1484–1494
32. Kashyap A, Wingard J, Cagnoni P et al. Intravenous versus oral busulfan as part of a busulfan/cyclophosphamide preparative regimen for allogeneic hematopoietic stem cell transplantation: decreased incidence of hepatic venoocclusive disease (HVOD), HVOD-related mortality, and overall 100-day mortality. Biol Blood Marrow Transplant 2002;8(9):493–500
33. Thall PF, Champlin RE, Andersson BS. Comparison of 100-day mortality rates associated with i.v. busulfan and cyclophosphamide vs other preparative regimens in allogeneic bone marrow transplantation for chronic myelogenous leukemia: Bayesian sensitivity analyses of confounded treatment and center effects. Bone Marrow Transplant 2004;33(12):1191–1199
34. Jamieson CH, Amylon MD, Wong RM et al. Allogeneic hematopoietic cell transplantation for patients with high-risk acute lymphoblastic leukemia in first or second complete remission using fractionated total-body irradiation and high-dose etoposide: a 15-year experience. Exp Hematol 2003;31(10):981–986
35. Marks DI, Forman SJ, Blume KG et al. A comparison of cyclophosphamide and total body irradiation with etoposide and total body irradiation as conditioning regimens for patients undergoing sibling allografting for acute lymphoblastic leukemia in first or second complete remission. Biol Blood Marrow Transplant 2006;12(4):438–453
36. Snyder DS, Chao NJ, Amylon MD et al. Fractionated total body irradiation and high-dose etoposide as a preparatory regimen for bone marrow transplantation for 99 patients with acute leukemia in first complete remission. Blood 1993;82(9):2920–2928
37. Snyder DS, Negrin RS, O'Donnell MR et al. Fractionated total-body irradiation and high-dose etoposide as a preparatory regimen for bone marrow transplantation for 94 patients with chronic myelogenous leukemia in chronic phase. Blood 1994;84(5):1672–1679
38. Kroger N, Kruger W, Wacker-Backhaus G et al. Intensified conditioning regimen in bone marrow transplantation for Philadelphia chromosome-positive acute lymphoblastic leukemia. Bone Marrow Transplant 1998;22(11):1029–1033
39. Zander AR, Berger C, Kroger N et al. High dose chemotherapy with busulfan, cyclophosphamide, and etoposide as conditioning regimen for allogeneic bone marrow transplantation for patients with acute myeloid leukemia in first complete remission. Clin Cancer Res 1997;3(12 Pt 2):2671–2675
40. Aversa F, Tabilio A, Velardi A et al. Treatment of high-risk acute leukemia with T-cell-depleted stem cells from related donors with one fully mismatched HLA haplotype. N Engl J Med 1998;339(17):1186–1193
41. Bibawi S, Abi-Said D, Fayad L et al. Thiotepa, busulfan, and cyclophosphamide as a preparative regimen for allogeneic transplantation for advanced myelodysplastic syndrome and acute myelogenous leukemia. Am J Hematol 2001;67(4):227–233
42. Cahn JY, Bordigoni P, Souillet G et al. The TAM regimen prior to allogeneic and autologous bone marrow transplantation for high-risk acute lymphoblastic leukemias: a cooperative study of 62 patients. Bone Marrow Transplant 1991;7(1):1–4
43. Zecca M, Pession A, Messina C et al. Total body irradiation, thiotepa, and cyclophosphamide as a conditioning regimen for children with acute lymphoblastic leukemia in first or

second remission undergoing bone marrow transplantation with HLA-identical siblings. J Clin Oncol 1999;17(6):1838–1846

44. Hilger RA, Baumgart J, Scheulen ME et al. Pharmacokinetics of treosulfan in a myeloablative combination with cyclophosphamide prior to allogeneic hematopoietic stem cell transplantation. Int J Clin Pharmacol Ther Toxicol 2004;42(11):654–655

45. Bordigoni P, Esperou H, Souillet G et al. Total body irradiation-high-dose cytosine arabinoside and melphalan followed by allogeneic bone marrow transplantation from HLA-identical siblings in the treatment of children with acute lymphoblastic leukaemia after relapse while receiving chemotherapy: a Societe Francaise de Greffe de Moelle study. Br J Haematol 1998;102(3):656–665

46. Deconinck E, Cahn JY, Milpied N et al. Allogeneic bone marrow transplantation for high-risk acute lymphoblastic leukemia in first remission: long-term results for 42 patients conditioned with an intensified regimen (TBI, high-dose Ara-C and melphalan). Bone Marrow Transplant 1997;20(9):731–735

47. Helenglass G, Powles RL, McElwain TJ et al. Melphalan and total body irradiation (TBI) versus cyclophosphamide and TBI as conditioning for allogeneic matched sibling bone marrow transplants for acute myeloblastic leukemia in first remission. Bone Marrow Transplant 1988;3(1):21–29

48. Locatelli F, Pession A, Bonetti F et al.Busulfan, cyclophosphamide and melphalan as conditioning regimen for bone marrow transplantation in children with myelodysplastic syndromes. Leukemia 1994;8(5):844–849

49. Przepiorka D, Khouri I, Thall P et al. Thiotepa, busulfan and cyclophosphamide as a preparative regimen for allogeneic transplantation for advanced chronic myelogenous leukemia. Bone Marrow Transplant 1999;23(10):977–981

50. Zander AR, Culbert S, Jagannath S et al. High dose cyclophosphamide, BCNU, and VP-16 (CBV) as a conditioning regimen for allogeneic bone marrow transplantation for patients with acute leukemia. Cancer 1987;59(6):1083–1086

51. Coccia PF, Strandjord SE, Warkentin PI et al. High-dose cytosine arabinoside and fractionated total-body irradiation: an improved preparative regimen for bone marrow transplantation of children with acute lymphoblastic leukemia in remission. Blood 1988;71(4):888–893

52. Petersen FB, Appelbaum FR, Buckner CD et al. Simultaneous infusion of high-dose cytosine arabinoside with cyclophosphamide followed by total body irradiation and marrow infusion for the treatment of patients with advanced hematological malignancy. Bone Marrow Transplant 1988;3(6):619–624

53. Woods WG, Ramsay NK, Weisdorf DJ et al. Bone marrow transplantation for acute lymphocytic leukemia utilizing total body irradiation followed by high doses of cytosine arabinoside: lack of superiority over cyclophosphamide-containing conditioning regimens. Bone Marrow Transplant 1990;6(1):9–16

54. Kanda Y, Sakamaki H, Sao H et al. Effect of conditioning regimen on the outcome of bone marrow transplantation from an unrelated donor. Biol Blood Marrow Transplant 2005;11(11):881–889

55. Mengarelli A, Lori A, Guglielmi C et al. Standard versus alternative myeloablative conditioning regimens in allogeneic hematopoietic stem cell transplantation for high-risk acute leukemia. Haematologica 2002;87(1):52–58

56. Hartman AR, Williams SF, Dillon JJ. Survival, disease-free survival and adverse effects of conditioning for allogeneic bone marrow transplantation with busulfan/cyclophosphamide vs total body irradiation: a meta-analysis. Bone Marrow Transplant 1998;22(5):439–443

57. Ringden O, Labopin M, Tura S et al. A comparison of busulphan versus total body irradiation combined with cyclophosphamide as conditioning for autograft or allograft bone marrow transplantation in patients with acute leukemia. Acute Leukemia Working Party of the European Group for Blood and Marrow Transplantation (EBMT). Br J Haematol 1996;93(3):637–645

58. Blume KG, Kopecky KJ, Henslee-Downey JP et al. A prospective randomized comparison of total body irradiation-etoposide versus busulfan-cyclophosphamide as preparatory regimens for bone marrow transplantation in patients with leukemia who were not in first remission: a Southwest Oncology Group study. Blood 1993;81(8):2187–2193

59. Clift RA, Buckner CD, Thomas ED et al. Marrow transplantation for chronic myeloid leukemia: a randomized study comparing cyclophosphamide and total body irradiation with busulfan and cyclophosphamide. Blood 1994;84(6):2036–2043

60. Devergie A, Blaise D, Attal M et al. Allogeneic bone marrow transplantation for chronic myeloid leukemia in first chronic phase: a randomized trial of busulfan-cytoxan versus cytoxan-total body irradiation as preparative regimen: a report from the French Society of Bone Marrow Graft (SFGM). Blood 1995;85(8):2263–2268

61. Socie G, Clift R, Blaise D et al. Busulfan plus cyclophosphamide compared with total-body irradiation plus cyclophosphamide before marrow transplantation for myeloid leukemia: long-term follow-up of 4 randomized studies. Blood 2001;98(13):3569–3574

62. Kim I, Park S, Kim B K et al. Allogeneic bone marrow transplantation for chronic myeloid leukemia: a retrospective study of busulfan-cytoxan versus total body irradiation-cytoxan as preparative regimen in Koreans. Clin Transplant 2001;15(3):167–172

63. Blaise D, Maraninchi D, Archimbaud E et al. Allogeneic bone marrow transplantation for acute myeloid leukemia in first remission: a randomized trial of a busulfan-Cytoxan versus Cytoxan-total body irradiation as preparative regimen: a report from the Group d'Etudes de la Greffe de Moelle Osseuse. Blood 1992;79(10):2578–2582

64. Blaise D, Maraninchi D, Michallet M et al. Long-term follow-up of a randomized trial comparing the combination of cyclophosphamide with total body irradiation or busulfan as conditioning regimen for patients receiving HLA-identical marrow grafts for acute myeloblastic leukemia in first complete remission. Blood 2001;97(11):3669–3671

65. Litzow MR, Perez WS, Klein JP et al. Comparison of outcome following allogeneic bone marrow transplantation with cyclophosphamide-total body irradiation versus busulphan-cyclophosphamide conditioning regimens for acute myelogenous leukemia in first remission. Br J Haematol 2002;119(4):1115–1124

66. Savoie ML, Balogh A, Chaudhry MA et al. The influence of adding low-dose (400 cGy) total body irradiation (TBI) on outcomes of allogeneic stem cell transplantation for acute myelogenous leukemia (AML) with myeloablative conditioning incorporating daily intravenous busulfan, fludarabine and low-dose antithymocyte globulin. Blood 2005;106: abstract 2733

67. Pagel JM, Appelbaum FR, Eary JF et al. 131I-anti-CD45 antibody plus busulfan and cyclophosphamide before allogeneic hematopoietic cell transplantation for treatment of acute myeloid leukemia in first remission. Blood 2006;107(5):2184–2191

68. Heinzelmann F, Ottinger H, Muller C H et al. Total-body irradiation – role and indications: results from the German Registry for Stem Cell Transplantation (DRST). Strahlentherapie und Onkologie 2006;182(4):222–230

69. Yanada M, Naoe T, Iida H et al. Myeloablative allogeneic hematopoietic stem cell transplantation for Philadelphia chromosome-positive acute lymphoblastic leukemia in adults: significant roles of total body irradiation and chronic graft-versus-host disease. Bone Marrow Transplant 2005;36(10):867–872

70. Bunin N, Aplenc R, Kamani N et al. Randomized trial of busulfan vs total body irradiation containing conditioning regimens for children with acute lymphoblastic leukemia: a Pediatric Blood and Marrow Transplant Consortium study. Bone Marrow Transplant 2003;32(6):543–548

71. Davies SM, Ramsay NK, Klein JP et al. Comparison of preparative regimens in transplants for children with acute lymphoblastic leukemia. J Clin Oncol 2000;18(2): 340–347

72. Granados E, de la Camara R, Madero L et al. Hematopoietic cell transplantation in acute lymphoblastic leukemia: better long term event-free survival with conditioning regimens containing total body irradiation. Haematologica 2000;85(10):1060–1067

73. Storb R, Champlin RE. Bone marrow transplantation for severe aplastic anemia. Bone Marrow Transplant 1991;8(2):69–72

74. Kahl C, Leisenring W, Deeg HJ et al. Cyclophosphamide and antithymocyte globulin as a conditioning regimen for allogeneic marrow transplantation in patients with aplastic anemia: a long-term follow-up. Br J Haematol 2005;130(5):747–751

75. Deeg HJ, O'Donnell M, Tolar J et al. Optimization of conditioning for marrow transplantation from unrelated donors for patients with aplastic anemia after failure of immunosuppressive therapy. Blood 2006;108:1485–1491

76. Bacigalupo A, Locatelli F, Lanino E et al. Fludarabine, cyclophosphamide and anti-thymocyte globulin for alternative donor transplants in acquired severe aplastic anemia: a report from the EBMT-SAA Working Party. Bone Marrow Transplant 2005;36(11):947–950

77. Srinivasan R, Takahashi Y, McCoy JP et al. Overcoming graft rejection in heavily transfused and allo-immunised patients with bone marrow failure syndromes using fludarabine-based haematopoietic cell transplantation. Br J Haematol 2006;133(3):305–314

78. Lucarelli G, Andreani M, Angelucci E. The cure of thalassemia by bone marrow transplantation. Blood Rev 2002;16(2):81–85

79. Lucarelli G, Clift RA, Galimberti M et al. Marrow transplantation for patients with thalassemia: results in class 3 patients. Blood 1996;87(5):2082–2088

80. Hongeng S, Pakakasama S, Chuansumrit A et al. Outcomes of transplantation with related- and unrelated-donor stem cells in children with severe thalassemia. Biol Blood Marrow Transplant 2006;12(6):683–687

81. Shenoy S, Grossman W J, DiPersio J et al. A novel reduced-intensity stem cell transplant regimen for nonmalignant disorders. Bone Marrow Transplant 2005;35(4):345–352

82. Zhu K E, Gu J, Zhang T. Allogeneic stem cell transplantation from unrelated donor for class 3 beta-thalassemia major using reduced-intensity conditioning regimen. Bone Marrow Transplant 2006;37(1):111–112

83. Horn B, Baxter-Lowe L-A, Englert L et al Reduced intensity conditioning using intravenous busulfan, fludarabine and rabbit ATG for children with nonmalignant disorders and CML. Bone Marrow Transplant 2006;37(3):263–269

84. Marmont AM, Horowitz MM, Gale RP et al. T-cell depletion of HLA-identical transplants in leukemia. Blood 1991;78(8):2120–2130

85. Martin PJ, Hansen JA, Torok-Storb B et al. Graft failure in patients receiving T cell-depleted HLA-identical allogeneic marrow transplants. Bone Marrow Transplant 1988;3(5):445–456

86. Patterson J, Prentice HG, Brenner MK et al. Graft rejection following HLA matched T-lymphocyte depleted bone marrow transplantation. Br J Haematol 1986;63(2):221–230

87. Down J D, Tarbell N J, Thames H D et al. Syngeneic and allogeneic bone marrow engraftment after total body irradiation: dependence on dose, dose rate, and fractionation. Blood 1991;77(3):661–669

88. Ferrara JL, Michaelson J, Burakoff SJ et al. Engraftment following T cell-depleted bone marrow transplantation. III. Differential effects of increased total-body irradiation on semi-allogeneic and allogeneic recipients. Transplantation 1988;45(5):948–952

89. Soiffer RJ, Mauch P, Tarbell NJ et al. Total lymphoid irradiation to prevent graft rejection in recipients of HLA non-identical T cell-depleted allogeneic marrow. Bone Marrow Transplant 1991;7(1):23–33

90. Rocha V, Labopin M, Sanz G et al. Transplants of umbilical-cord blood or bone marrow from unrelated donors in adults with acute leukemia. N Engl J Med 2004; 351(22):2276–8225

91. Lu D P, Dong L, Wu T et al. Conditioning including antithymocyte globulin followed by unmanipulated HLA-mismatched/haploidentical blood and marrow transplantation can achieve comparable outcomes with HLA-identical sibling transplantation. Blood 2006;107(8):3065–3073

92. Buchali A, Feyer P, Groll J et al. Immediate toxicity during fractionated total body irradiation as conditioning for bone marrow transplantation. Radiother Oncol 2000;54(2):157–162

93. Kolb HJ, Bender-Gotze C 1990 Late complications after allogeneic bone marrow transplantation for leukemia. Bone Marrow Transplant 1990;6(2): 61–72

94. Weiner RS, Horowitz MM, Gale RP et al. Risk factors for interstitial pneumonia following bone marrow transplantation for severe aplastic anemia. Br J Haematol 1989;71(4):535–543

95. Sanders JE, Pritchard S, Mahoney P et al. Growth and development following marrow transplantation for leukemia. Blood 1986;68(5):1129–1135

96. Sanders JE, Hawley J, Levy W et al. Pregnancies following high-dose cyclophosphamide with or without high-dose busulfan or total-body irradiation and bone marrow transplantation. Blood 1996;87(7):3045–3052

97. Giorgiani G, Bozzola M, Locatelli F et al. Role of busulfan and total body irradiation on growth of prepubertal children receiving bone marrow transplantation and results of treatment with recombinant human growth hormone. Blood 1995;86(2): 825–831

98. Gardner SF, Lazarus HM, Bednarczyk EM et al. High-dose cyclophosphamide-induced myocardial damage during BMT: assessment by positron emission tomography. Bone Marrow Transplant 1993;12(2):139–144

99. Kupari M, Volin L, Suokas A et al. Cardiac involvement in bone marrow transplantation: electrocardiographic changes, arrhythmias, heart failure and autopsy findings. Bone Marrow Transplant 1990;5(2): 91–98

100. Vassal G, Deroussent A, Hartmann O et al. Dose-dependent neurotoxicity of high-dose busulfan in children: a clinical and pharmacological study. Cancer Res 1990; 50(19):6203–6207

101. Blume KG, Forman SJ, O'Donnell MR et al. Total body irradiation and high-dose etoposide: a new preparatory regimen for bone marrow transplantation in patients with advanced hematologic malignancies. Blood 1987;69(4):1015–1020

102. Cheson BD, Vena DA, Foss FM et al. Neurotoxicity of purine analogs: a review. J Clin Oncol 1994;12(10):2216–2228

103. Samuels BL, Bitran JD. High-dose intravenous melphalan: a review. J Clin Oncol 1995;13(7): 1786–1799

104. Devetten MP, Qazilbash MH, Beall CL et al. Thiotepa and fractionated TBI conditioning prior to allogeneic stem cell transplantation for advanced hematologic malignancies: a phase II single institution trial. Bone Marrow Transplant 2004;34(7):577–580

105. Scheulen ME, Hilger RA, Oberhoff C et al. Clinical phase I dose escalation and pharmacokinetic study of high-dose chemotherapy with treosulfan and autologous peripheral blood stem cell transplantation in patients with advanced malignancies. Clin Cancer Res 2000;6(11):4209–4216

Reduced-intensity conditioning for allogeneic stem cell transplantation

Hanna Jean Khoury and Douglas R Adkins

Introduction

With the introduction of chemotherapy in the 1950s, treatments for patients with hematologic malignances began to aim for curative intents. Encouraging in vitro concentration-dependent drug-specific patterns of cytotoxicity[1,2] and dose escalation-induced reversal of drug resistance in human tumor model systems led to the development and subsequent successful implementation of dose-intense therapy supported by hematopoietic stem cells. This approach allowed escalation of radiation and/or chemotherapy doses beyond the limiting marrow toxicity, and to the limit of acceptable organ toxicity. It led to long-term remissions and even cures in patients with chemosensitive and chemorefractory relapsed hematologic malignancies.[3,4]

However, in contrast to the autologous transplant setting, dose escalation of the conditioning followed by allogeneic stem cell transplantation is associated with improvements in disease-free survival (DFS) but does not always translate into better survivals due to inevitable transplant-related morbidity and mortality (TRM).[5,6] Very early on, TRM was recognized as a major limiting factor for the success of allogeneic transplantation,[7] and several multivariable predictive models were developed to estimate the risk of post-transplant death.[8–11] Older age and the co-morbidities which are often associated with it[12–16] remain the major limiting factors for the application of transplantation to a large number of patients who might otherwise benefit from this treatment modality. Indeed, SEER data for 2000–2003 showed that median age at diagnosis for acute leukemia is 67 years, with approximately 15% diagnosed between ages 55 and 64, 21% between 65 and 74, 24% between 75 and 84, and 10% in patients older than 85.[17]

In the late 1980s and early 1990s, better understanding of the immunomodulatory effects of the allogeneic T-cells refined the role of the allograft, initially perceived merely as an antidote to high-dose therapy. Key observations from allografts carried out in patients with chronic myeloid leukemia (CML)[18–23] showed high relapse rates in syngeneic and T-cell depleted transplants as compared to T-cell replete sibling transplants, low relapse rates in patients who develop chronic graft-versus-host disease (GvHD), and durable remissions effectively achieved after donor lymphocyte infusion (DLI) for post-transplant relapses. These observations, and others, dramatically impacted upon the perceived 'raison d'être' of the conditioning regimen and opened the door for reduced-intensity conditioning (RIC) regimens.

What is a reduced-intensity conditioning regimen?

First attempts to reduce the intensity of the allograft conditioning regimen were pioneered, in the late 1970s, by the Hôpital Saint Louis

transplant team (Paris) in patients with Fanconi anemia (FA). Allografts in FA patients were complicated by severe cyclophosphamide toxicity and early lethal acute GvHD,[24] which led to reductions in both the doses of cyclophosphamide (20 mg/kg) and irradiation (500 cGy), as well as radiation field (thoracoabdominal). This modified preparative regimen was associated with successful donor cell engraftment and a marked reduction in TRM and GvHD.[25] Similarly, in other diseases where cytoreduction was not necessary, such as severe aplastic anemia, the immunosuppressive properties of the conditioning regimen (cyclophosphamide, antithymocyte globulin) were explored, with successful engraftment of allogeneic stem cells and low TRM.[26,27]

Reduction of conditioning intensity can be achieved by dose de-escalation or changes in drug delivery of existing agents such as total body irradiation (TBI)[28–31] or busulfan[32] or by incorporating newer agents that selectively target the lymphohematopoietic system (fludarabine, alentuzamab[33,34] or antithymocyte globulin[35]). The goal of these modified conditionings is not only to reduce non-hematologic toxicities but to rely on the immunomodulatory effects of the donor T-lymphocytes to eradicate residual malignant cells (graft-versus-tumor). It is through immunosuppression rather than complete eradication of the recipient's hematopoiesis that these conditionings allow the co-existence of donor and recipient cells (chimerism, also called 'mixed chimerism') and reversible myelosuppression in case of graft failure ('non-myeloablative'). This chimeric status can subsequently be converted to full donor cell engraftment with DLI.[36]

No consensus defining qualifying doses for reduced-intensity regimens exists. The following criteria, adopted by the National Marrow Donor Program, are generally accepted and include a total dose of TBI of <500 cGy (single dose) or 800 cGy (fractionated), <9 mg/kg total busulfan dose, <140 mg/m^2 total melphalan dose, <10 mg/kg total thiotepa dose, and BEAM conditioning (BCNU, cytosine arabinoside, etoposide and melphalan). In the absence of clear-cut defined doses separating myeloablative conditioning (MAC) from RIC, those preparative regimens are perhaps better viewed as part of a spectrum (Fig. 28.1).

Outcomes after reduced-intensity conditioning regimens

There are no prospective randomized trials comparing RIC to MAC to date. Therefore, limitations and biases must be considered with the interpretations of prospective single-institution Phase II trials and retrospective analyses comparing outcomes of RIC to MAC transplants. These variables include, among others, patient selection, response to induction or salvage therapy (or timing of loss of response), disease status at the time of transplantation, scheduled administration of DLIs,

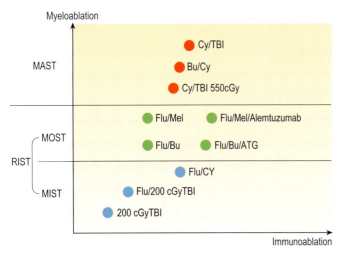

Figure 28.1
Diagram showing intensity of each regimen. The x-axis indicates the degree of immunoablation and the y-axis degree of myeloablation. RIST, reduced-intensity stem cell transplantation; MIST, minimal-intensity stem cell transplantation; MOST, moderate-intensity stem cell transplantation; MAST, myeloablative stem cell transplantation.

changes over time in immunosuppressive drugs, source of stem cells, age of donor and recipient, short follow-up, and variability of immunosuppressive or cytotoxic agents used in the conditioning regimen.

Toxicities

RIC focuses mainly on the reduction of TRM and indeed, a favorable *early* toxicity profile is observed with RIC,[37] including reduced early infectious,[38] fungal,[39] viral,[40] pulmonary,[41] gastrointestinal and hepatic[42] complications. Additionally, and due to lower hematologic toxicity, the duration of neutropenia and the number of units of blood product transfused are reduced[43] which translates into decreased duration or even complete abrogation of initial hospitalization, and reduction in early costs.[44]

Graft-versus-host disease

The pathophysiology of GvHD is complex. This disorder is in part mediated by interactions of T-cells with the microenvironment, which is significantly influenced by the intensity of the conditioning regimen. Therefore, in theory, conditioning regimens which minimally alter the microenvironment should prompt a milder 'cytokine storm' and therefore reduced incidences of GvHD. Given the non-selective alloreactivity of donor T-cells, separating graft-versus-tumor from graft-versus-host disease remains a formidable challenge. Additionally, various conditioning regimens have incorporated scheduled DLI, which adds yet another layer of complexity in the interpretation of the incidence of GvHD.

When compared with MAC, the overall incidence of acute GvHD (grades II–IV) is somewhat lower after RIC[37,45] but severe (grades III–IV) acute GvHD, especially after sibling transplants, and chronic GvHD remain unchanged. Acute GvHD post-RIC is associated with increases in TRM while chronic GvHD appears to offer protection against relapses, both accounting for recurrent hospitalizations and increased late costs.[44]

Survival

Many reviews have summarized survival outcomes (disease-free and overall survival) after RIC for various hematologic disorders.[46–50] Generally, no particular RIC regimen appears to be superior, median

follow-up is 1 year in most studies, up to 3 years in a few, and better outcomes are reported in patients transplanted in remission and in patients with indolent disorders. The following section provides a non-exhaustive but practical summary derived from published studies of RIC followed by related or unrelated peripheral blood or bone marrow stem cell transplantation.

RIC for *acute myeloid leukemia (AML) and myelodysplastic syndromes (MDS)* is associated with reduction in early non-relapse mortality (5–10% by day 100). However, the advantages of reduced TRM with RIC are balanced, in patients transplanted with residual disease, by an increased risk of death from relapse. Disease-free and overall survivals averaging 30–45%, and as high as 70% for AML patients transplanted in first complete remission, have been reported. Conditionings have incorporated fludarabine with cyclophosphamide, melphalan, busulfan, cytosine arabinoside or TBI and combined with either antithymocyte globulin or alemtuzamab.

Recent studies from the European Group for Blood and Marrow Transplantation (EBMT) compared outcomes of RIC and MAC in patients older than 50 years of age with AML[37] (315 RIC vs 407 MAC) or MDS[51] (215 RIC vs 621 MAC) receiving HLA-identical hematopoietic stem cell transplantation (HSCT). Fludarabine/busulfan and a low-dose TBI-based regimen were the predominant conditioning regimens for both AML and MDS. Median follow-up for the RIC group was 13 and 38 months for AML and MDS, respectively. Both groups (RIC and MAC) in both studies had comparable risks for relapse (cytogenetic risk group and disease status at transplant); however, RIC patients were older, transplanted more recently, and more frequently with peripheral blood stem cells rather than marrow. On multivariate analysis, both acute GvHD (II–IV) (22% vs 31% for AML and 43% vs 58% for MDS) and 2-year TRM (18% vs 32% for AML, 22% vs 32% for MDS) were lower with RIC transplants. However, high rates of relapses (41% vs 24%, p = 0.003) were associated with RIC transplantation, and leukemia-free and overall survivals were comparable in the two groups (40–47% for AML and 33–39% for MDS). These two studies, despite limitations associated with their retrospective nature, are mature, include a large number of patients, and clearly highlight pitfalls of RIC, i.e. reduced non-relapse mortality and increased relapse rates.

With the introduction of very effective targeted therapy using imatinib mesylate[52] in early 2000, the number of transplants performed in patients with *chronic myeloid leukemia* decreased significantly.[53] Initial single-institution Phase II trials of RIC for CML reported very encouraging outcomes;[54,55] however, both large single-center[56,57] and registry data reported a rather disappointingly low disease-free survival (33% in the EBMT study), especially in patients transplanted in first chronic phase (50–60%). Although graft-versus-leukemia (GvL) is very potent in CML, and molecular remissions can be successfully induced with RIC transplants,[58] it is unclear why those patients do not benefit from RIC conditioning similarly to those receiving MAC. It is important to note that initial experience with RIC transplants in CML was complicated by high rejection rates;[57] additionally, imatinib-resistant CML cells may be less sensitive to the GvL effects.[59]

Allogeneic HSCT for *lymphoid malignancies* has traditionally been offered early to patients with predictable poor prognosis and those who fail to mobilize adequate numbers of stem cells for autografting or later for refractory or relapsed disease post-autologous HSCT. In small series, *large cell non-Hodgkin's lymphoma* patients with chemosensitive non-bulky disease after a failed autologous HSCT, who underwent RIC allograft, had durable remissions (40–50% short-term disease-free survivals),[60–63] especially if full donor engraftment was established early.[64] Better outcomes are observed in more indolent lymphoid malignancies (50–70% short-term disease-free survivals) such as low-grade non-Hodgkin's lymphoma,[65] mantle cell lymphoma[66,67] and chronic lymphocytic leukemia.[68,69]

Despite major advances in the treatment of *multiple myeloma*, this plasma cell disorder remains incurable, and transplants using MAC are complicated by high TRM. RIC allografts for relapsed myeloma are associated with low TRM and modest progression-free survivals (20–30%),[70,71] while better outcomes (DFS of approximately 50%) appear to be achievable when RIC is performed earlier in the course of the disease and after a debulking autograft.[72] Enthusiasm for RIC in *acute lymphoblastic leukemia* was tempered by the limited efficacy of the GvL effect in this disease[73] and by data from the Center of International Blood and Marrow Transplant Research (CIBMTR) showing superiority of conventional TBI/cyclophosphamide to non-TBI or TBI regimens containing lower than 1200 cGy doses,[74] suggesting that dose intensity may play a role in the success of transplantation in this disease. Nevertheless, reports of RIC in acute lymphoblastic leukemia show that this approach is feasible, associated with donor cell engraftment and reduced early TRM and toxicities.[75]

Special interests in harnessing the graft-versus-tumor effects arose in cancers that are both resistant to standard therapies and have strong immunogenic properties, such as *renal cell cancer*. Initial experience with RIC allografts in patients with advanced renal cell carcinoma showed that this approach was feasible, and associated with stabilization and in some cases regression of tumors.[76] However, enthusiasm for this treatment modality waned quickly as responses were not sustained and GvHD was a major cause of morbidity and mortality.[77]

Allogeneic HSCT is a curative therapy for patients with *hemoglobinopathies*,[78–81] and given the high morbidity and mortality associated with MAC, great hopes were raised with the development of RIC and the availability of cord blood as a source of stem cells for transplantation.[82] Published reports are limited and sustained donor cell engraftment remains a significant challenge.[83]

To whom should we offer a reduced-intensity conditioning allograft?

These newer transplant preparative regimens suggest that if a graft can be 'less dramatically' established (by avoiding the cytokine storm commonly associated with MAC[84]), the positive effects of the allogeneic cells could be preserved and TRM associated with MAC regimens avoided. This treatment modality would therefore be more broadly applied, especially for patients not eligible for MAC. This hope is reflected by the trend in the number of RIC transplants reported to the CIBMTR (Fig. 28.2). Based on current data, it is conceivable that only patients in remission and patients with indolent disorders benefit the most from RIC. GvHD nevertheless remains a significant problem and is perhaps the major limiting factor in older transplant recipients. For patients in remission at the time of transplant, the choice between MAC and RIC is a dilemma, especially in younger patients not enrolled on a clinical trial. In these particular conditions, early advantages of RIC need to be balanced against its undetermined long-term benefits, and the long track record of experience with MAC.

Where are we heading with reduced-intensity conditioning?

Given the limitations associated with RIC, new approaches are currently being investigated to tackle post-transplant relapses. These include post-transplant consolidation or maintenance using targeted therapy with kinase inhibitors for bcr-abl, flt-3 ITD or c-kit positive malignancies or monoclonal antibodies for CD20+ or CD33+ malignancies; enhancing donor cell immunomodulation in the recipient (post-transplant cytokines and/or vaccinations), in the donor (using tumor-specific anti-idiotype vaccine) prior to stem cell collection, or in vitro by novel graft engineering techniques to expand specific cell subpopulations (e.g. mesenchymal stem cells). Finally, antitumor immunotherapy can only be safely and more broadly implemented once the Achilles heel of allogeneic transplantation, i.e. GvHD, is effectively separated from the graft-versus-tumor effects.

References

1. Saijo N. Chemotherapy: the more the better? Overview. Cancer Chemother Pharmaco 1997;40(Suppl):S100–S106
2. Frei EI, Canellos GP. Dose: a critical factor in cancer chemotherapy. Am J Med 1980;69:585–595
3. Sweetenham JW, Carella AM, Taghipour G et al. High-dose therapy and autologous stem-cell transplantation for adult patients with Hodgkin's disease who do not enter remission after induction chemotherapy: results in 175 patients reported to the European Group for Blood and Marrow Transplantation. J Clin Oncol 1999;17:3101–3109
4. Lazarus HM, Rowlings PA, Zhang MJ et al. Autotransplants for Hodgkin's disease in patients never achieving remission: a report from the Autologous Blood and Marrow Transplant Registry. J Clin Oncol 1999;17:534–545
5. Clift RA, Buckner CD, Appelbaum FR et al. Allogeneic marrow transplantation in patients with acute myeloid leukemia in first remission: a randomized trial of two irradiation regimens. Blood 1990;76:1867–1871
6. Clift RA, Buckner CD, Thomas ED et al. Marrow transplantation for chronic myeloid leukemia: a randomized study comparing cyclophosphamide and total body irradiation with busulfan and cyclophosphamide. Blood 1994;84:2036–2043
7. Thomas ED, Storb R, Clift RA et al. Bone marrow transplantation. N Engl J Med 1975;292:832–843, 895–902
8. Charlson ME, Pompei P, Ales KL, MacKenzie CR. A new method of classifying prognostic comorbidity in longitudinal studies: development and validation. J Chron Dis 1987;40:373–383
9. Sorror ML, Maris MB, Storer B et al. Comparing morbidity and mortality of HLA-matched unrelated donor hematopoietic cell transplantation after nonmyeloablative and myeloablative conditioning: influence of pretransplant comorbidities. Blood 2004;104:961–968
10. Sorror ML, Maris MB, Storer B et al. Hematopoietic cell transplantation (HCT)-specific comorbidity index: a new tool for risk assessment before allogeneic HCT. Blood 2005;106:2912–2919
11. Parimon T, Au DH, Martin PJ et al. A risk score for mortality after allogeneic hematopoietic cell transplantation. Ann Intern Med 2006;144:407–414
12. Feinstein AR. The pre-therapeutic classification of co-morbidity in chronic disease. J Chron Dis 1970;23:455–468
13. Extermann M. Measurement and impact of comorbidity in older cancer patients. Crit Rev Oncol Hematol 2000;35:181–200
14. Extermann M. Measuring comorbidity in older cancer patients (review). Eur J Cancer 2000;36:453–471
15. Yancik R, Wesley MN, Ries LAG et al. Comorbidity and age as predictors of risk for early mortality of male and female colon carcinoma patients. Cancer 1998;82:2123–2134
16. Extermann M, Overcash J, Lyman GH et al. Comorbidity and functional status are independent in older cancer patients. J Clin Oncol 1998;16:1582–1587
17. http://SEER.cancer.gov
18. Gratwohl A, Brand R, Apperley J et al. Graft-versus-host disease and outcome in HLA-identical sibling transplantations for chronic myeloid leukemia. Blood 2002;100:3877–3886
19. Barrett AJ, Ringden O, Zhang MJ et al. Effect of nucleated marrow cell dose on relapse and survival in identical twin bone marrow transplants for leukemia. Blood 2000;95:3323–3327
20. Ringden O, Hermans J, Labopin M et al. The highest leukaemia-free survival after allogeneic bone marrow transplantation is seen in patients with grade I acute graft-versus-host

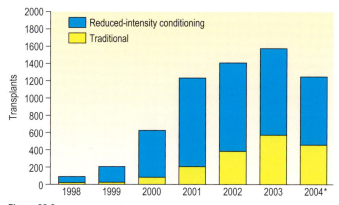

Figure 28.2
Reduced-intensity conditioning allogeneic transplants, registered with the CIBMTR, 1998–2004. *Data incomplete.

disease. Acute and Chronic Leukaemia Working Parties of the European Group for Blood and Marrow Transplantation (EBMT). Leuk Lymphoma 1996;24:71–79

21. Goldman JM, Gale RP, Horowitz MM et al. Bone marrow transplantation for chronic myelogenous leukemia in chronic phase. Increased risk for relapse associated with T-cell depletion. Ann Intern Med 1988;108:806–814
22. Kolb HJ, Mittermuller J, Clemm C et al. Donor leukocyte transfusions for treatment of recurrent chronic myelogenous leukemia in marrow transplant patients. Blood 1990;76: 2462–2465
23. Collins RH Jr, Shpilberg O, Drobyski WR et al. Donor leukocyte infusions in 140 patients with relapsed malignancy after allogeneic bone marrow transplantation. J Clin Oncol 1997;15:433–444
24. Gluckman E, Devergie A, Schaison G et al. Bone marrow transplantation in Fanconi anaemia. Br J Haematol 1980;45:557–564
25. Gluckman E, Devergie A, Dutreix J. Radiosensitivity in Fanconi anaemia: application to the conditioning regimen for bone marrow transplantation. Br J Haematol 1983;54: 431–440
26. Gluckman E, Devergie A, Benbunan A et al. Bone marrow transplantation in severe aplastic anemia using cyclophosphamide and thoracoabdominal irradiation. Progr Clin Biol Res 1984;148:325–333
27. Stucki A, Leisenring W, Sandmaier BM et al. Decreased rejection and improved survival of first and second marrow transplants for severe aplastic anemia (a 26-year retrospective analysis). Blood 1998;92(8):2742–2749
28. McSweeney PA, Niederwieser D, Shizuru JA et al. Hematopoietic cell transplantation in older patients with hematologic malignancies: replacing high-dose cytotoxic therapy with graft-versus-tumor effects. Blood 2001;97:3390–3400
29. Maris MB, Niederwieser D, Sandmaier BM et al. HLA matched unrelated donor hematopoietic cell transplantation after nonmyeloablative conditioning for patients with hematologic malignancies. Blood 2003;102:2021–2030
30. Lowsky R, Takahashi T, Liu YP et al. Protective conditioning for acute graft-versus-host disease. N Engl J Med 2005;353:1321–1331
31. Hallemeier C, Girgis M, Blum W et al. Outcomes of adults with acute myelogenous leukemia in remission given 550 cGy of single-exposure total body irradiation, cyclophosphamide, and unrelated donor bone marrow transplants. Biol Blood Marrow Transplant 2004;10:310–319
32. Kashyap A, Wingard J, Cagnoni P et al. Intravenous versus oral busulfan as part of a busulfan/cyclophosphamide preparative regimen for allogeneic hematopoietic stem cell transplantation: decreased incidence of hepatic venoocclusive disease (HVOD), HVOD-related mortality, and overall 100-day mortality. Biol Blood Marrow Transplant 2002;8: 493–500
33. Ho AY, Pagliuca A, Kenyon M et al. Reduced-intensity allogeneic hematopoietic stem cell transplantation for myelodysplastic syndrome and acute myeloid leukemia with multilineage dysplasia using fludarabine, busulphan and alemtuzumab (FBC) conditioning. Blood 2004;104:1616–1623
34. van Besien K, Artz A, Smith S et al. Fludarabine, melphalan, and alemtuzumab conditioning in adults with standard-risk advanced acute myeloid leukemia and myelodysplastic syndrome. J Clin Oncol 2005;23:5728–5738
35. Mohty M, Bay JO, Faucher C et al. Graft-versus-host disease following allogeneic transplantation from HLA identical sibling with antithymocyte globulin-based reduced intensity preparative regimen. Blood 2003;102:470–476
36. Marks DI, Lush R, Cavenagh J et al. The toxicity and efficacy of donor lymphocyte infusions given with reduced-intensity conditioning allogeneic stem cell transplantation. Blood 2002;100:3108–3114
37. Aoudjhane M, Labopin M, Gorin NC et al. Comparative outcome of reduced intensity and myeloablative conditioning regimen in HLA identical sibling allogeneic haematopoietic stem cell transplantation for patients older than 50 years of age with acute myeloblastic leukaemia: a retrospective survey from the Acute Leukaemia Working Party (ALWP) of the European group for Blood and Marrow Transplantation (EBMT). Leukemia 2005;19: 2304–2312
38. Junghanss C, Marr KA, Carter RA et al. Incidence and outcome of bacterial and fungal infections following nonmyeloablative compared with myeloablative allogeneic hematopoietic stem cell transplantation: a matched control study. Biol Blood Marrow Transplant 2002;8:512–520
39. Fukuda T, Boeckh M, Carter RA et al. Risks and outcomes of invasive fungal infections in recipients of allogeneic hematopoietic stem cell transplants after nonmyeloablative conditioning. Blood 2003;102:827–833
40. Junghanss C, Boeckh M, Carter RA et al. Incidence and outcome of cytomegalovirus infections following nonmyeloablative compared with myeloablative allogeneic stem cell transplantation, a matched control study. Blood 2002;99:1978–1985
41. Fukuda T, Hackman RC, Guthrie KA et al. Risks and outcomes of idiopathic pneumonia syndrome after nonmyeloablative and conventional conditioning regimens for allogeneic hematopoietic stem cell transplantation. Blood 2003;102:2777–2785
42. Hogan Maris M, Storer B et al. Hepatic injury after nonmyeloablative conditioning followed by allogeneic hematopoietic stem cell transplantation: a study of 193 patients. Blood 2004;103:78–84
43. Weissinger F, Sandmaier BM, Maloney DG et al. Decreased transfusion requirements for patients receiving nonmyeloablative compared with conventional peripheral blood stem cell transplants from HLA-identical siblings. Blood 2001;98:3584–3588
44. Cordonnier C, Maury S, Esperou H et al. Do minitransplants have minicosts? A cost comparison between myeloablative and nonmyeloablative allogeneic stem cell transplant in patients with acute myeloid leukemia. Bone Marrow Transplant 2005;36:649–654
45. Mielcarek M , Martin PJ, Leisenring W et al. Graft-versus-host disease after nonmyeloablative versus conventional hematopoietic stem cell transplantation. Blood 2003;102: 756–762
46. Antin JH. Stem cell transplantation – harnessing of graft-versus-malignancy. Curr Opin Hematol 2003;10:440–444
47. Kassim AA, Chinratanalab W, Ferrara JL, Mineishi S. Reduced-intensity allogeneic hematopoietic stem cell transplantation for acute leukemias: 'what is the best recipe?' Bone Marrow Transplant 2005;36:565–574
48. Burroughs L, Storb R. Low-intensity allogeneic hematopoietic stem cell transplantation for myeloid malignancies: separating graft-versus-leukemia effects from graft-versus-host disease. Curr Opin Hematol 2005;12:45–54
49. Scott BL, Sandmaier BM. Outcomes with myeloid malignancies. Hematology Am Soc Hematol Educ Program 2006;381–389
50. Khouri IF. Reduced-intensity regimens in allogeneic stem-cell transplantation for non-Hodgkin lymphoma and chronic lymphocytic leukemia. Hematology Am Soc Hematol Educ Program 2006;390–397
51. Martino R, Lacobelli S, Brand R al. Retrospective comparison of reduced intensity conditioning and conventional high dose conditioning for allogeneic hematopoietic stem cell transplantation using HLA identical sibling donors in myelodysplastic syndromes. Blood 2006;108:836–846
52. Druker BJ, Guilhot F, O'Brien SG et al. Five-year follow-up of patients receiving imatinib for chronic myeloid leukemia. N Engl J Med 2006;355:2408–2417
53. Gratwohl A, Baldomero H, Frauendorfer K, Urbano-Ispizua A, for the Joint Accreditation Committee of the International Society for Cellular Therapy ISCT and the European Group for Blood and Marrow Transplantation EBMT (JACIE). EBMT activity survey 2004 and changes in disease indication over the past 15 years. Bone Marrow Transplant 2006;37;1069–1085
54. Or R, Shapira MY, Resnick Y et al. Nonmyeloablative allogeneic stem cell transplantation for the treatment of chronic myeloid leukemia in first chronic phase. Blood 2003;101: 441–445
55. Khoury H, Adkins D, Brown R et al. Low transplant-related complications in patients with chronic myeloid leukemia undergoing allogeneic stem cell transplantation with a low dose (550 cGy) total body irradiation conditioning. Biol Blood Marrow Transplant 2001;7:352–358
56. Kerbauy FR, Storb R, Hegenbart U et al. Hematopoietic cell transplantation from HLA-identical sibling donors after low-dose radiation-based conditioning for treatment of CML. Leukemia 2005;19:990–997
57. Baron F, Maris MB, Storer BE et al. HLA-matched unrelated donor hematopoietic cell transplantation after nonmyeloablative conditioning for patients with chronic myeloid leukemia. Biol Blood Marrow Transplant 2005;11:272–279
58. Uzunel M, Mattson J, Brune M et al. Kinetics of minimal residual disease and chimerism in patients with chronic myeloid leukemia after nonmyeloablative conditioning and allogeneic stem cell transplantation. Blood 2003;101:469–472
59. Weisser M. Schmid C, Schoch C et al. Resistance to pretransplant imatinib therapy may adversely affect the outcome of allogeneic stem cell transplantation in CML. Bone Marrow Transplant 2005;36:1017–1018
60. Escalon MP, Champlin RE, Saliba RM et al. Nonmyeloablative allogeneic hematopoietic transplantation: a promising salvage therapy for patients with non-Hodgkin's lymphoma whose disease has failed a prior autologous transplantation. J Clin Oncol 2004;22: 2419–2423
61. Branson K, Chopra R, Kottaridis PD et al. Role of nonmyeloablative allogeneic stem cell transplantation after failure of autologous transplantation in patients with lymphoproliferative malignancies. J Clin Oncol 2002;20:4022–4031
62. Faulkner RD, Craddock C, Byrne JL et al. BEAM alemtuzumab reduced-intensity allogeneic stem cell transplantation for lymphoproliferative diseases: GVHD, toxicity, and survival in 65 patients. Blood 2004;103:428–434
63. Tanimoto TE, Kusumi E, Hamaki T et al. High complete response rate after allogeneic hematopoietic stem cell transplantation with reduced-intensity conditioning regimens in advanced malignant lymphoma. Bone Marrow Trnsplant 2003;32:131–137
64. Bishop MR, Whit-Shan Hou J, Wilson WH. Establishment of early donor engraftment after reduced-intensity allogeneic hematopoietic stem cell transplantation to potentiate the graft-versus-lymphoma effect against refractory lymphomas. Biol Blood Marrow Transplant 2003;9:162–169
65. Morris E, Thomson K, Craddock C et al. Outcomes after alemtuzumab-containing reduced-intensity allogeneic transplantation regimen for relapsed and refractory non-Hodgkin lymphoma. Blood 2004;104:3865–3871
66. Khouri I, Lee MS, Saliba RM et al. Nonablative allogeneic stem-cell transplantation for advanced/recurrent mantle-cell lymphoma. J Clin Oncol 2003;21:4407–4412
67. Maris MB, Sandmaier BM, Storer BE et al. Allogeneic hematopoietic cell transplantation after fludarabine and 2 Gy total body irradiation for relapsed and refractory mantle cell lymphoma. Blood 2004;104:3535–3542
68. Pavletic SZ, Khouri IF, Haagenson M et al. Unrelated donor marrow transplantation for B-cell chronic lymphocytic leukemia after using myeloablative conditioning: results from the Center for International Blood and Marrow Transplant Research. J Clin Oncol 2005;23:5788–5794
69. Sorror ML, Maris MB, Sandmaier GM et al. Hematopoietic cell transplantation after nonmyeloablative conditioning for advanced chronic lymphocytic leukemia. J Clin Oncol 2005;23:3819–3829
70. Gerull S, Goerner M, Benner A et al. Long-term outcome of nonmyeloablative allogeneic transplantation in patients with high-risk multiple myeloma. Bone Marrow Transplant 2005;36:963–969
71. Crawley C, Lalancette M, Szydlo R et al. Outcomes for reduced-intensity allogeneic transplantation for multiple myeloma: an analysis of prognostic factors from the Chronic Leukaemia Working Party of the EBMT. Blood 2005;105:4532–4539
72. Maloney DG, Molina AJ, Sahebi F et al. Allografting with nonmyeloablative conditioning following cytoreductive autografts for the treatment of patients with multiple myeloma. Blood 2003;102:3447–3454
73. Collins RH Jr, Shpilberg O, Drobyski WR et al. Donor leukocyte infusions in 140 patients with relapsed malignancy after allogeneic bone marrow transplantation. J Clin Oncol 1997;15:433–444
74. Davies SM, Ramsay NKC, Klein JP et al. Comparison of preparative regimens in transplants for children with acute lymphoblastic leukemia. J Clin Oncol 2000;18:340–347

75. Hamaki T, Kami M, Kanda Y et al. Reduced-intensity stem-cell transplantation for adult acute lymphoblastic leukemia: a retrospective study of 33 patients. Bone Marrow Transplant 2005;6:549–556

76. Childs R, Chernoff A, Contentin N et al. Regression of metastatic renal cell carcinoma after nonmyeloablative allogeneic peripheral blood stem cell transplantation. N Engl J Med 2000;343:750–758

77. Rini BI, Zimmerman T, Stadler WM et al. allogeneic stem cell transplantation of renal cell cancer after nonmyeloablative chemotherapy: feasibility, engraftment and clinical results. J Clin Oncol 2002;20:2017–2024

78. Thomas ED, Buckner CD, Sanders JE et al. Marrow transplantation for thalassaemia. Lancet 1982;2:227–229

79. Lucarelli G, Galimberti M, Polchi P et al. Bone marrow transplantation in patients with thalassemia. N Engl J Med 1990;322:417–421

80. Walters MC, Patience M, Leisenring W et al. Bone marrow transplantation for sickle cell disease. N Engl J Med 1996;335:369–376

81. Vermylen C, Cornu G, Ferster A et al. Haematopoietic stem cell transplantation for sickle cell anaemia: the first 50 patients transplanted in Belgium. Bone Marrow Transplant 1998;22:1–6

82. Locatelli F, Rocha V, Reed W et al, for the Eurocord Transplant Group. Related umbilical cord blood transplantation in patients with thalassemia and sickle cell disease. Blood 2003;101:2137–2143

83. Fleischauer K, Locatelli F, Zecca M et al. Graft rejection after unrelated donor hematopoietic stem cell transplantation for thalassemia is associated with non-permissive HLADPB1 disparity in host-versus-graft direction. Blood 2006;107:2984–2992

84. Ferrara JL. Cytokine dysregulation as a mechanism of graft versus host disease. Curr Opin Immunol 1993;5:794–799

Transplants from unrelated or mismatched family donors

Rupert Handgretinger

CHAPTER 29

Introduction

Allogeneic transplantation is increasingly used for the treatment of various malignant and non-malignant diseases. Currently, the donor of choice is a healthy human leukocyte antigen (HLA)-identical matched sibling. HLA antigens are inherited en bloc and each individual has two HLA haplotypes. According to the Mendelian laws governing dominant genetic inheritance, each offspring has a 25% chance of inheriting the same haplotypes as another offspring. With the tendency to smaller families in Northern America and Europe, the likelihood of identifying a matched sibling donor (MSD) is approximately 25%. Therefore, enormous efforts have been made to increase the pool of HLA-identical unrelated volunteer donors by establishing national and international registries of volunteer donors. For patients for whom no HLA-matched unrelated volunteer donor can be identified in the registries, transplantation with a haploidentical donor has become a realistic option. With the improvements in HLA typing methods and the identification of highly matched donors (9/10 or 10/10 HLA allele-matched donors), the outcome of matched unrelated transplants has improved significantly, and survival rates are virtually the same as for matched sibling transplants.

Transplants from unrelated donors

While MSD are still the preferred choice, matched unrelated donors (MUD) are increasingly identified for those patients who do not have a MSD. With better HLA typing techniques, there is no major difference in the clinical outcome after MSD and MUD transplants in children[1-3] or adults.[4,5] This chapter will discuss practical clinical issues, such as selection of an appropriate conditioning regimen (myeloablative versus non-myeloablative), selection of bone marrow or peripheral blood stem cells (PBSC) as stem cell source, graft-versus-host disease (GvHD) prophylaxis schemes and transplant indications for malignant and non-malignant diseases in children and adults.

Conditioning regimens: myeloablative versus non-myeloablative

The preparative regimen should have a cytotoxic, antileukemia effect, but should also provide adequate immunosuppression in order to ensure engraftment. The most commonly used preparative regimes prior to allogeneic transplantation for leukemia include various doses (12 Gy to 15.75 Gy) of fractionated total-body irradiation (TBI) and cyclophosphamide, with or without the addition of etoposide, cytarabine, thiotepa or fludarabine. Non-TBI based chemotherapy-only regimens with busulfan/cyclophosphamide/cytarabine have been suc-cessfully employed in adults with high-risk acute myelogenous leukemia.[6] Other non-TBI based less intensive regimens have been reported to facilitate safe engraftment with acceptable toxicity.[7,8] Less aggressive, non-myeloablative stem cell transplantation regimens have been designed especially for patients who could not otherwise tolerate a conventional myeloablative regimen. Such regimens range from minimal, to facilitate engraftment (fludarabine plus low-dose TBI),[9-11] to more intensive but still non-myeloablative (reduced-intensity conditioning, or RIC), such as reduced doses of fludarabine plus busulfan,[11] treosulfan and fludarabine[8] or others.[12,13]

The rationale behind non-myeloablative stem cell transplantation is to reduce transplant-related toxicity and mortality while inducing an optimum graft-versus-leukemia (GvL) effect by donor alloreactive effector cells.[14] This form of transplantation is mostly used in adult and elderly patients who are at higher risk for anticipated post-transplant toxicity. The data for children with leukemia remain insufficient to conclude that the reduced cytotoxic antileukemia effect of the preparative regimen is counterbalanced by an increased antileukemia effect of the allograft, and should therefore only be used in the context of controlled clinical trials.

Bone marrow versus PBSC as the stem cell source

The decision concerning whether to donate bone marrow or PBSC is primarily that of the donor. Prior to the availability of granulocyte colony-stimulating growth factor (G-CSF), bone marrow harvested under general anesthesia was exclusively used as a stem cell source. The discovery and clinical use of G-CSF and granulocyte-macrophage colony-stimulating growth factor (GM-CSF) led to the observation that CD34+ bone marrow (BM) stem cells can be mobilized in large numbers into the peripheral bloodstream[15,16] and that mobilized PBSCs can completely reconstitute hematopoiesis.[17] PBSCs are collected with a single or repeated leukaphereses on an outpatient basis and are therefore becoming more and more the donor's preferred mode of donation.

PBSCs are preferred by physicians particularly in the context of RIC regimens in order to facilitate engraftment via the larger number of T-lymphocytes contained in the graft, and to exert a maximum antileukemic effect.[18] The higher number of T-cells in PBSC is most likely to be responsible for the higher incidence of extensive chronic GvHD in recipients of unrelated PBSC transplants.[19] A more pronounced GvL effect might be counterbalanced by the increased transplant-related complications and lower survivals seen in adult acute lymphoblastic leukemia (ALL) patients allografted with matched unrelated PBSC compared to bone marrow recipients.[20] More promising data have been reported in pediatric patients with ALL who received mobilized peripheral blood positively selected CD34+ cells from matched unrelated donors.[21] A similar approach was used in pediatric patients with severe aplastic anemia, with long-term survivals of 88%.[22]

Prophylaxis of GvHD

GvHD is still a major cause of mortality after matched unrelated transplantation. The most commonly used pharmacologic prophylaxis of GvHD consists of ciclosporin and post-transplant methotrexate. Additional prophylactic use of antithymocyte globulin[23] or alemtuzumab[24] will reduce the incidence of acute and chronic GvHD. In addition, partial ex vivo removal of T-lymphocytes from the bone marrow graft is an effective method of decreasing the incidence of GvHD.[25–27] Many techniques for T-cell depletion are available, based on either physical methods or more or less specific antibody-based anti-T-cell directed methods.[28] A method described more recently is indirect T-cell depletion by positive selection of CD34+ or CD133+ stem cells from PBSC with or without T-cell add-back.[21,22,29,30] The employed method might be of importance, since it has been shown that depletion methods based on narrow rather than broad anti-T-cell specificities might have an advantage in patients with leukemia.[28]

Indications

Due to the comparable outcomes after MSD and MUD transplants, the indications for transplantation from a MUD donor are similar to those for a transplant from a MSD. The most common indications are acute myeloid leukemia, acute lymphoblastic leukemia, the myelodysplastic syndromes, chronic myeloid leukemia and severe aplastic anemia. In pediatric patients particularly, there are a number of nonmalignant and inherited disorders which can be potentially cured by allogeneic transplantation. These disorders include hemoglobinopathies, immunodeficiencies, inherited disorders of metabolism and aplastic marrow disorders.

When considering a MUD transplant for a patient, a number of factors have to be taken into account in order to determine the risk–benefit ratio of the transplant procedure. These factors include patient age, the underlying disease, disease status and intensity of previous chemotherapy treatments. Only with all this information can a recommendation for or against MUD transplantation be given to the patient.

Acute lymphoblastic leukemia

Children

International studies of childhood ALL carried out between 1986 and 1998 in developed countries have achieved 5-year event-free survival rates ranging from 63% to 83%[31] or even higher.[32] Allogeneic transplantation is therefore only applicable to smaller subpopulations of children with ALL and should be considered in patients in first complete response (CR1) with high-risk features such as certain translocations (MLL-AF4, hypodiploidy (<45 chromosomes), induction failure (5% or more leukemic cells) and minimal residual disease (MRD) of more than 1% after 4–6 weeks of first-line therapy).[33–35] Early clearance of leukemia cells, as measured by morphologic criteria[36] or flow cytometry,[35] seems to be an important prognostic factor.

A recent study reviewing cases of a Philadelphia chromosome (Ph)-positive ALL from 10 study groups between 1986 and 1996 showed that transplantation of marrow from an HLA-matched related donor yields a significantly better outcome in these patients than does chemotherapy alone.[37] The majority of transplants are performed in relapsed patients in CR2 or beyond, given the fact that the probability of leukemia-free survival with chemotherapy alone is only in the range of 10–40%.[38] Older age at relapse (>10–15 years of age) and a short

CR1 result in lower rates of leukemia-free survival (LFS).[39] Patients with bone marrow relapse while receiving therapy or early after treatment have a poor outcome with chemotherapy alone[40,41] and should proceed to transplant. Patients with early or late relapse of T-ALL have a poor prognosis and transplantation for this subgroup is recommended.[41,42] About two-thirds of patients with late extramedullary relapse, and about one-third of those with early extramedullary relapse or late non-T-marrow relapse or early combined non-T relapses, can be rescued by chemotherapy. However, the persistence of high-level MRD after appropriate relapse therapy in these patients has been reported to identify patients at risk of subsequent relapse.[43] The importance of MRD determination is further documented by the observation that patients with detectable MRD before transplant have a poorer outcome than do those with no detectable MRD.[44]

The role of transplantation in infant ALL is controversial. Most of these patients have rearrangements of the MLL gene in chromosome 11q23 and an associated poor outcome,[45] and allogeneic transplantation does not seem to improve the prognosis for this subgroup.[46] Since no difference has been observed in the outcome after matched related or matched unrelated transplantation,[2] MUD transplants are a valuable option for all children with ALL in whom it is indicated and for whom no HLA-matched sibling can be identified.

Adults

The role of MUD transplants in adult patients with ALL has to be seen in the context of various factors, such as patient age, leukemia subtype and status of disease. Although advances in the chemotherapeutic treatment of adult ALL have improved the outcome over the last decade,[47] the LFS survival rates are in the range of 30–40% and are lower compared to childhood ALL.[48,49] Favorable results of allogeneic transplantation for standard-risk ALL patients in CR1 have been reported.[50] For patients with high-risk ALL, such as those presenting with high-risk cytogenetics (t(9;22) and t(4;11)), MUD transplants will increase disease-free survival (DFS).[51] Comparable results have been obtained in patients in CR1 receiving either a matched related or matched unrelated transplant.[4] Patients with relapsed disease in CR2 will benefit from an allogeneic transplant, and comparable results have also been obtained in patients in CR2 or more using either an HLA-matched related or unrelated donor.[5] The outcome of transplantation is less favorable in patients with refractory disease.[52] The role of the stem cell source is not clear and inferior survivals have been reported in ALL patients who received PBSC grafts compared to bone marrow.[20] Non-myeloablative conditioning regimens might enable this treatment modality to be offered to patients with a high risk of TRM but there are no successful alternatives to myeloablative conditioning in younger ALL patients.[53]

Acute myeloid leukemia (AML)

Children

With conventional chemotherapy alone, up to 45% of children and adolescents with AML survive for 5 years or longer without relapse.[54,55] Certain cytogenetic abnormalities have prognostic value, and patients with complex karyotypes, such as −5, del(5q), −7, or 3q abnormalities, might benefit from transplantation.[56] In the largest randomized trial to date comparing allogeneic bone marrow transplant (BMT), autologous BMT and aggressive postremission chemotherapy for AML, investigators indicated that in adolescents and children, allogeneic BMT in first remission is the treatment of choice when a matched related donor is available,[57] although similar, good survival rates have been reported by the UK MRC group (56% at 7 years) with chemotherapy alone,[58] and allogeneic transplantion in CR1 could be restricted to patients with higher risk features.

Allogeneic HSCT is the therapy of choice for most patients with relapses of AML.[59] Advanced disease phase and cytogenetic abnormalities at time of transplantation have been associated with decreased survival and increased risk of relapse.[60] Since outcomes of matched related and matched unrelated transplants are comparable,[61] MUD transplants for children and adolescents with high-risk AML in CR1 should be considered, and most patients with relapsed AML should proceed to an allogeneic transplant in CR2.

Adults

The role of MUD BMT for adult patients with AML in CR1 is controversial. For patients with adverse cytogenetics, an improved outcome has been demonstrated in patients in CR1 after allo-BMT,[62] while other studies have failed to show a benefit.[63] In a larger study, cytogenetics had no influence on the outcome for 161 primary AML patients undergoing MUD BMT.[64] A chemotherapy-only preparative regimen for high-risk AML patients followed by MUD transplant was associated with a lower TRM and demonstrated promising outcomes,[65] indicating an advantage for proceeding early to unrelated transplantation for patients with poor-prognosis features of AML in CR1. Allogeneic transplants should also be considered for younger patients with postremission positive MRD levels.[66] Improvements in supportive care and the use of RIC conditioning regimens have allowed older patients to receive an allogeneic BMT.[67,68] In another retrospective study comparing autologous and allogeneic BMT in patients with AML in CR1 or CR2, a lower risk of relapse after MUD BMT was counterbalanced by a higher TRM rate, and autotransplants offered a higher 3-year survival for patients in CR1 and CR2.[69] The outcome of patients in more than CR2 or with refractory disease is dismal, and MUD BMT might offer the only chance of cure.[70–72]

Chronic myeloid leukemia (CML)

Children

Allogeneic transplantation from a MSD or MUD donor offers long-term disease-free survival and it is still the treatment of choice for this patient population in chronic phase.[73] A shorter time between diagnosis and transplantation results in a better outcome.[74] One study comparing the use of PBSC with BM found the former method to have a significant survival advantage (1000-day overall survival (OS) of 94% vs 66%).[75] A 3-year OS of 65% after MUD transplants with a myeloablative conditioning regimen has been described.[76] In this study, however, 55% of the MUD transplants were performed more than 1 year after diagnosis and were associated with a higher TRM (31% in chronic phase 1 (CP1) and 46% in advanced phase). Relapse rates were higher in advanced-phase patients, especially after MSD transplants. The outcomes for patients in advanced phase were a 3-year OS of 46% for MSD, and 39% for MUD transplants. In an early pediatric study, the 12-year OS for patients transplanted within 3 years of diagnosis with MSD and MUD donors was 62%.[77] RIC conditioning regimens and the known sensitivity of CML to immunologic approaches such as donor lymphocyte infusions (DLI) might decrease TRM and increase long-term survival.[78,79] However, the efficacy of RIC needs to be confirmed in larger studies in pediatric studies comparing RIC and myeloablative approaches.

Given the observations that the outcome of MUD transplants might be poorer when performed >1 year after diagnosis, pediatric patients with a MSD or well-matched MUD donor should proceed to an allogeneic transplantation within 1 year from diagnosis.[80]

Adults

As in pediatric patients, allogeneic transplantation remains the only known curative treatment for CML in adult patients. Donor availability, toxicity of the procedure and the age of the patients limit this approach. However, better HLA typing strategies of MUD donors and the increasing use of RIC regimens are improving the outcome of transplantation. Factors predicting survival at diagnosis such as molecular and biologic features[81] or risk assessment score for the outcome of transplantation involving age at transplantation, disease stage, donor type, donor–recipient gender combination and interval from diagnosis to transplantation may help to identify the best treatment strategies.[82] In addition to the disease stage, age has been shown to influence outcome of unrelated transplants.[73] For patients >40–50 years of age in chronic-phase CML, survival is similar after MSD or MUD transplantation,[73,83,84] and a DFS of >70% was reported for patients less than 50 years of age who were transplanted within 1 year of diagnosis.[73] The optimum stem cell source (PBSC versus BM) is still controversial. While two studies have found an advantage of PBSC over BM,[75,85] another retrospective study of MUD transplants in all phases of CML found no differences in rates of GvHD, relapse and survival.[86]

Since the long-term outcome of imatinib needs to be established, allogeneic transplantation with standard or RIC conditioning with a well-matched MUD donor is a reasonable approach, especially for younger, newly diagnosed patients.[87]

Myelodysplastic syndromes

Children

The prognosis of most children with myelodysplastic syndrome (MDS) is poor, and hematopoietic stem cell transplantation (HSCT) is currently the therapy of choice.[88,89] Patients who are most likely to do better without transplantation are also those who respond best to allogeneic transplantation.[90] This group includes patients with refractory anemia (RA), refractory anemia with ringed sideroblasts (RARS) and those with normal cytogenetics. The children most likely to benefit from transplantation are those with refractory anemia with excess blasts (RAEB), refractory anemia with excess blasts in transformation (RAEB-t), an age younger than 2 years, and a hemoglobin F level of 10% or higher.[91] The rarity of this disease requires international studies by co-operative groups, such as the European Working Group of MDS in Childhood (EWOG-MDS), in order to find the best treatment options. The timing of transplantation and whether or not induction chemotherapy should precede transplantation are controversial. Patients with RAEB-t have a high relapse rate if transplanted without preceding chemotherapy, whereas those with less than 5% blasts do better with HSCT performed in the absence of induction chemotherapy.[88,92] A large, prospective study of children with MDS found that patients with RAEB-t often do as well as those with AML when treated with AML therapy at diagnosis, including transplant when an HLA-matched sibling is available.[93] On the other hand, children with RA or RAEB do very poorly with standard AML therapy and should be considered for allogeneic transplantation.[94,95]

The optimal treatment for juvenile myelomonocytic leukemia (JMML) is not clearly established. Conventional chemotherapy is unlikely to eradicate the stem cell abnormality, but it may ameliorate the disease, and a transplant offers the greatest likelihood for cure.[96] The success is limited primarily by the tendency of this disease to relapse.[97]

Adults

Allogeneic transplantation is also the only curative option for adult patients with myelodysplastic syndrome. Since MDS is more frequent in older patients, conventional transplantation approaches are limited by the age of the patients. Due to the progress in molecular HLA typing, outcomes after transplants from unrelated donors matched by high-resolution HLA typing are comparable to those with genotypically identical siblings.[98–100] Conditioning regimens not incorporating high-dose TBI are reducing the TRM and various RIC regimens have been described with different results.[101–104] Various factors, such as age, co-morbid conditions, stage of disease, type of donors and others should be taken into account when the decision to proceed to allogeneic transplantation is made. For patients with therapy-related myelodysplastic syndrome, allogeneic transplantation is the only chance of long-term cure for this disease. However, the results in children and adults are less encouraging due to the high TRM and relapse rate.[105,106]

Aplastic anemia

Graft failure, toxicity and GvHD are the main problems of unrelated transplants for aplastic anemia. In a larger series of Japanese patients, all of whom received a MUD transplant, the probability of overall survival at 5 years was 56%. Unfavorable factors were transplantation more than 3 years after diagnosis, patient more than 20 years of age, absence of antithymocyte globulin in the conditioning regimen and HLA-A or B mismatch, as determined by molecular HLA typing.[107] Novel conditioning regimens might have a favorable impact.[108] Partial T-cell depletion was associated with a lower incidence of GvHD in children.[109] Comparable outcomes of matched related and alternative donor stem cell transplantation in children have been observed[110] and allogeneic transplantation should be encouraged early after failure of front-line immunosuppressive therapy.[111] Use of large numbers of purified stem cells obtained from mobilized peripheral blood from MUD donors might allow avoidance of serious complications, and promising results have been reported in pediatric patients.[22]

Non-malignant diseases

This patient group is mainly composed of pediatric patients with inherited disorders, such as hemoglobinopathies, immunodeficiencies and inborn errors of metabolism. Promising results have been obtained in patients grafted from MUD donors with various non-malignant disorders, and the results are comparable to those obtained after MSD transplants.[3,112,113] The good results of MUD BMT, especially in children, support the use of alternative donors for those patients who lack an HLA-identical sibling.

Transplantation using haploidentical donors

Rationale for haploidentical transplantation

The main reason for haploidentical transplantation is lack of a matched sibling or matched unrelated volunteer donor. Compared to matched unrelated donor transplantation, a haploidentical donor can be identified in the shortest time, without delaying treatment of the patient. In malignant diseases particularly, some patients experience disease progression during the time taken for the unrelated donor search and will ultimately not proceed to a potentially life-saving transplant. The exact number of patients lost during the time taken to identify a suitably HLA-matched unrelated donor is unknown, since no prospective studies addressing this question have been performed to date. Clearly, the inclusion of mismatched family members into the donor pool would allow almost all patients to proceed to a transplant in the necessary time frame.

Haploidentical transplantation can not only be performed in a timely manner, but crossing the HLA barrier might also induce a stronger graft-versus-leukemia effect. While this has been shown in animal models,[114] data in the human setting are less clear. At the beginning of haploidentical transplantation, a putative stronger GvL effect might have been masked by the intensive prophylaxis or treatment of GvHD.[115] With increasingly effective T-cell depletion by either CD34+ selection[116] or CD3+ depletion,[117] haploidentical transplants can be performed with complete absence of, or with only moderate pharmacologic GvHD prophylaxis.[118] It has already been convincingly demonstrated that alloreactive natural killer (NK) cells can exert an impressive antileukemia effect in adults with AML[119] or in pediatric patients with ALL.[120] Other effector cells with potential antileukemia activity and without GvHD-inducing alloreactivity might also play a role. Examples of such cell populations are natural killer cells[121] or gamma/delta T-lymphocytes.[122] It can be anticipated that ongoing research in this area will further harness the antileukemia efficacy of haploidentical effector cells without increasing the risk of GvHD.

Another advantage of haploidentical transplantation is the continuous availability of the same motivated donor after transplantation. With the development of sophisticated, large-scale clinical cellular therapy methods, post-transplant strategies using donor-derived cells have become a reality and will play an even more important role in the future. Such strategies include the post-transplant infusion of NK cells[123,124] or virus-specific T-lymphocytes.[125] Other future strategies might include CD4+/CD25+ T-regulatory cells to induce tolerance[126] or T-cells depleted of alloreactive cells to improve immune reconstitution or antileukemia effects.[127] Finally, the generation of leukemia-specific donor-derived T-lymphocytes can be envisaged.[128]

The concept of alloreactive natural killer (NK) cells

While much effort has been expended to identify the perfect HLA-matched donor, the concept of alloreactive NK cells in transplantation proposes a NK-mediated antileukemia effect particularly in the HLA-mismatched setting (the perfect mismatch) in the absence of GvHD.[129] In addition, it has been shown in animal models that alloreactive NK cells not only exert an antileukemia effect, but that they are also able to facilitate engraftment across the HLA barrier and can even reduce the risk of GvHD by eliminating residual host-derived antigen-presenting dendritic cells.[130]

The concept of alloreactive NK cells in allogeneic transplantation is based on the 'missing self' hypothesis, which has been proposed by Karre et al.[131] This hypothesis proposes that NK cells are, in contrast to T-lymphocytes, activated by the absence of self HLA class I molecules on the surface of target cells. The discovery of the killer cell immunoglobulin-like receptors (KIR) and the generation of monoclonal antibodies for their identification[132] allowed a detailed analysis of the system of inhibitory and activating receptors on NK cells. KIRs are expressed on subsets of NK cells and are receptors for certain HLA class I alleles. The binding of the HLA allele to its receptor induces an inhibitory signal, and the NK cells cannot exert their effector function. However, in the absence of the corresponding HLA alleles, NK cells are not inhibited and become cytotoxic. The 'missing self' hypothesis predicted that in any individual, the NK cells must have at least one inhibitory receptor for a self HLA class I allele.[133] It is therefore conceivable that in an HLA-mismatched transplant situation, the likelihood is very high that the KIRs expressed on the donor-derived NK cells have no corresponding inhibitory HLA class I allele and will become cytotoxic towards the host-derived target cells. While donor-derived allogeneic T-cells would attack the GvHD target organs such as skin, gut or liver, alloreactive NK cells exert their effector function only against host-derived hematopoietic cells and therefore do not induce GvHD.[130] A well-characterized interaction between KIR and HLA antigens is the inhibition of NK cells via CD158a (receptor for

HLA alleles Cw 2,4,5,6 and others, group 2) and CD158b (receptor for HLA alleles Cw 1,3,7,8 and others, group 1).[121,129]

Based on the concept that NK cells must have at least one inhibitory HLA class I allele, selection of NK-alloreactive donors based on the HLA class I mismatch between donor and recipient has been proposed.[134] However, this concept has been challenged recently and it was shown that KIR-expressing NK cell subsets exist in healthy individuals which do not have the corresponding inhibitory HLA class I ligand.[135] Therefore, the prediction of NK alloreactivity using HLA class I typing alone would lead to incorrect results in a number of donors, and it was suggested that the donor's KIR repertoire on the NK cells be directly determined using either flow cytometry or PCR-based methods.[136]

The overall significance of the KIR system in allogeneic, and particularly haploidentical, transplantation is not yet completely clear. Besides the KIR system there are other systems which are either inhibitory or activating, and the final status of the NK effector cells is composed of the sum of many known and unknown inhibiting or activating signals. In addition, it has been shown that antibody-mediated cellular cytotoxicity can override the KIR-mediated inhibition of NK cells.[137] The role of alloreactive NK cells in transplantation should therefore be further investigated in controlled clinical trials.

Graft manipulation strategies in haploidentical transplantation

Over time, a variety of methods have been described for the depletion of T-lymphocytes in haploidentical transplantation. Early on, the methods available, such as anti-T-cell antibodies plus complement, were mostly used with bone marrow, and they rarely exceeded a 2–3 log T-cell depletion.[115] With the concept of the 'megadose' approach,[138] bone marrow was replaced more and more by G-CSF mobilized peripheral stem cells as a stem cell source.[139] With G-CSF induced mobilization, the number of PBSC harvested CD34+ stem cells is much higher than that obtained from bone marrow, and 'megadoses' of 10×10^6 CD34+ cells/kg can be obtained. However, antibody/complement-based T-cell depletion methods were not effective with PBSC, since the number of mononuclear cells to be processed is much higher with this product compared to bone marrow. Therefore, new processing technologies had to be developed which allow large numbers of cells to be processed.[116]

Currently, large numbers of T-cell depleted mobilized peripheral stem cells are used as a stem cell source in most haploidentical transplants. For T-cell depletion, CD34+ selection was introduced, and T-cell depletion of more than 5 logs can be accomplished with this method, thus allowing haploidentical transplantation with no pharmacologic GvHD prophylaxis.[118] From the experience to date, infusion of less than 25,000 T-cells/kg recipient body weight is safe, and no additional GvHD prophylaxis is necessary. If the T-cell number is between 25,000 and 50,000/kg, the risk of GvHD may be higher. Patients receiving more than 50,000 T-cells/kg should receive moderate pharmacologic GvHD prophylaxis.

A method described more recently is the negative depletion of CD3+ T-lymphocyte (CD3 depletion), or CD3+ T- and CD19+ B-lymphocyte (CD3/19 depletion).[117] In contrast to CD34+ selection, the negative depletion approach retains, besides the stem cells, all other cells which are not CD3+ and CD19+, such as NK cells, dendritic cells, monocytes and myeloid cells. With such grafts, large numbers of CD56+ NK cells are transplanted with the stem cells to induce an alloreactive NK-mediated GvL effect. Compared to the CD34+ selection method, T-cell depletion is slightly less effective, with a log depletion of 3.5–4. Short courses of post-transplant pharmacologic GvHD prophylaxis may therefore be necessary, depending on the

number of residual T-lymphocytes. In this context, it is important to mention that determination of the absolute number of T-lymphocytes remaining in the graft requires experience with detecting rare populations by flow cytometry.[140] Another interesting approach to non-T-cell depleted haploidentical transplantation is the use of a combination of G-CSF primed bone marrow together with PBSC.[141]

Donor selection

In most haploidentical transplants, the donor will share one haplotype with the patient. With most pediatric transplants, one of the parents is used as the donor, whereas in the majority of adult recipients the donor is the patient's sibling. While most mismatched family donors share a full haplotype, there are family donors who are only mismatched at two or one antigens. The degree of HLA mismatch between recipient and donor does not seem to play a clinical role in the context of extensive T-cell depletion by CD34+ selection.[118]

Donor selection according to NK alloreactivity is being actively researched in the context of haploidentical transplantation. The ligand–ligand method uses HLA typing of the donor to predict the KIR receptor repertoire on the donor's NK cells,[134] whereas the receptor–ligand method determines the donor's KIR repertoire directly by PCR-based genotyping by flow cytometry.[136] It has recently been shown that predicted NK alloreactivity based on the receptor–ligand model is a more accurate method of predicting antileukemic effect compared to basing it on the ligand–ligand model.[120,136] In addition, other more classic donor selection criteria such as CMV status of donor and recipient or crossmatch results are also considered. There are insufficient data to address the role of age, sex or multiparous female donors fully in the context of the available T-cell depletion methods.

In the context of non-T-cell depleted mismatched related transplantation, it has been shown that recipients of non-inherited maternal antigen mismatched (NIMA) sibling donor stem cells had less acute GvHD.[142] However, transplant-related mortality was higher in recipients of maternal or paternal donor grafts. In other non-T-cell depleted SCTs, the incidence of grade II–IV GvHD was higher in patients with NIMA mismatched donors, whereas a lower rate of GvHD was seen in recipients of grafts from NIMA mismatched donors in the GvHD direction.[143,144]

Immune reconstitution, infections and infection prophylaxis

After haploidentical transplantation, patients experience varying periods of immunoincompetence which can cause significant morbidity and mortality.[145] Immune reconstitution can be further hampered by acute and chronic GvHD or by their treatment. Although rapid expansion of donor-derived NK cells is usually seen within weeks following transplantation,[146,147] it is the impaired and delayed T-cell mediated immunity, mainly characterized by a low CD4+ helper T-cell count, which is responsible for the high susceptibility to infections.[148] In a recent retrospective comparative analysis of a pediatric patient population, T-cell phenotypes, T-cell repertoire and the number of T-cell receptor excision circles (TREC) were analyzed in recipients of CD3-depleted haploidentical PBSC after TBI-based myeloablative or non-TBI based RIC conditioning.[149] Significantly faster immune reconstitution was seen in the early post-transplant period in those patients who received the RIC conditioning, and no fatal infectious complications were observed, whereas in the TBI-conditioned patients T-cell recovery was delayed. Faster immune reconstitution has also been reported in a smaller group of adults after RIC conditioning and transplantation of CD3-depleted haploidentical PBSC.[147] Non-TBI based RIC regimens may therefore encourage rapid immune reconstitution after haploidentical transplantation. Since RIC regimens may be associated with less mortality but higher relapse rates, controlled clinical studies should be performed to evaluate the influence of the conditioning regimens on overall survival.

Prevention and management of opportunistic viral, bacterial and fungal infections remain major challenges in haploidentical transplantation. Major causes of therapy failure are, in particular, viral infections with cytomegaloviruses (CMV), adenoviruses (ADV) and Epstein–Barr viruses (EBV). Other viruses such as herpes viruses, HHV-6, and BK viruses should also be considered when the situation is clinically unclear. Recipient and donor CMV status should be considered in the prevention of CMV infection, and patients at risk for CMV infection can receive either prophylactic or pre-emptive treatment.[150] Reactivation of adenoviruses also occurs frequently in recipients of CD34+ positively selected or CD3 T-cell depleted PBSC.[151] Quantitative real-time PCR methods measuring adenovirus copy numbers in blood are available[152] and allow successful pre-emptive treatment with cidofovir.[153]

EBV-associated lymphoproliferative disease (EBV-LPD) is another serious complication after allogeneic transplantation.[154] Since EBV-LPD is mostly of donor B-cell origin, the most effective method of prevention is to remove all mature B-lymphocytes from the graft. The methods used currently for T-cell depletion in haploidentical transplantation, either CD34+ selection or CD3/19 depletion, result in effective B-cell depletion, and donor-derived EBV-LPS has rarely been described. If ex vivo B-cell depletion cannot be performed, in vivo depletion by anti-CD20 antibodies at the time of stem cell infusion might be an option. In a series of 25 patients who received CD3-depleted PBSC and a single dose of anti-CD20 antibody at day 0 prior to the graft infusion, no EBV-LPS was observed.[155] As in other viral infections, early, quantitative detection of EBV-DNA in plasma using real-time PCR analysis and pre-emptive therapy with anti-CD20 antibodies might decrease the high mortality rate otherwise associated with this complication.[156,157] Despite all these measures, a significant proportion of patients will not respond sufficiently to antiviral therapy. Therefore, adoptive immunotherapy strategies have been developed, with donor-derived ex vivo expanded virus-specific T-cells, and ex vivo generated adenovirus-specific T-cells have been used successfully after haploidentical transplantation for the prevention and treatment of ADV-associated diseases.[125]

Haploidentical transplantation for malignant diseases

Haploidentical transplantation is still considered an experimental treatment for patients who lack an HLA-identical donor and such transplants should therefore be carried out in the context of controlled clinical studies. Most haploidentical transplants have been performed in patients with advanced stages of refractory hematologic malignancies after myeloablative conditioning, and promising results have been obtained using CD34+ positively selected grafts in adult patients with AML,[119] in pediatric patients with ALL[158] and in children with acute leukemia.[159,160] In another study using unmanipulated haploidentical blood and marrow stem cells, the results were comparable to HLA-identical sibling transplantation.[161] In addition to myeloablative conditioning regimens, non-myeloablative approaches using unmanipulated HLA 2–3 antigen-mismatched haploidentical stem cells have been conducted, with promising results.[162] Fast engraftment and low toxicity have been observed in adults with high-risk or refractory disease with CD3/CD19-depleted PBSC using a non-TBI based less intensive conditioning regimen.[147] Less intensive conditioning regimens and CD3/CD19-depleted PBSC were associated with low toxicity and a low incidence of infections.[155,163]

Due to the susceptibility of solid tumor target cells to alloreactive NK-mediated cytotoxicity,[164] pilot studies in patients with pediatric solid tumors have been initiated.[165] Another interesting approach is the infusion of haploidentical NK cells after low-intensity chemotherapy in a non-transplant setting.[166] The use of less intensive conditioning regimens and newer anti-infection strategies should improve outcome of haploidentical transplantation, and further clinical research is necessary to determine the optimum times and patients for such a procedure.[167]

Haploidentical transplantation for non-malignant diseases

While haploidentical transplants have mostly been carried out on adult and pediatric patients with advanced or refractory hematologic malignancies, haploidentical transplants using T-cell depleted haploidentical bone marrow have been used in children with immunodeficiencies.[168] With the development of newer and more effective T-cell depletion methods, haploidentical transplantation has become a realistic option, especially for pediatric patients with non-malignant hematologic or genetic diseases. The positive selection of CD34+ stem cells has been used in limited numbers of patients with severe aplastic anemia,[169] hemoglobinopathies,[170] osteopetrosis[171] and other disorders.[118,172] Further attempts to reduce toxicity and mortality by RIC regimens and to improve immune reconstitution will make haploidentical transplantation a realistic option in the absence of a suitable HLA-matched donor for patients who can potentially be cured of their underlying non-malignant disease.

Future directions for haploidentical transplantation

Overcoming the HLA barrier by using donor-derived cell components such as alloreactive NK cells and T-regulatory cells, and inducing tolerance while fully harnessing the antimalignancy effect are major challenges for the future. Better understanding of the biology of the mechanisms responsible for delayed immune reconstitution will hopefully lead to therapeutic approaches, including soluble factors, or the adoptive transfer of antigen-specific T-cells, to rapidly restore the T-cell repertoire. Since most of these strategies require donor-derived cells, the continued availability and motivation of haploidentical donors will be crucial if the full potential of haploidentical transplantation is to be successfully exploited.

References

1. Eapen M, Rubinstein P, Zhang MJ et al. Comparable long-term survival after unrelated and HLA-matched sibling donor hematopoietic stem cell transplantations for acute leukemia in children younger than 18 months. J Clin Oncol 2006;24:145–151
2. Al-Kasim FA, Thornley I, Rolland M et al. Single-centre experience with allogeneic bone marrow transplantation for acute lymphoblastic leukaemia in childhood: similar survival after matched-related and matched-unrelated donor transplants. Br J Haematol 2002;116: 483–490
3. Gustafsson A, Remberger M, Winiarski J, Ringden O. Unrelated bone marrow transplantation in children: outcome and a comparison with sibling donor grafting. Bone Marrow Transplant 2000;25:1059–1065
4. Kiehl MG, Kraut L, Schwerdtfeger R et al. Outcome of allogeneic hematopoietic stem-cell transplantation in adult patients with acute lymphoblastic leukemia: no difference in related compared with unrelated transplant in first complete remission. J Clin Oncol 2004;22: 2816–2825
5. Dahlke J, Kroger N, Zabelina T et al. Comparable results in patients with acute lymphoblastic leukemia after related and unrelated stem cell transplantation. Bone Marrow Transplant 2006;37:155–163
7. Kroger N, Bornhauser M, Ehninger G et al. Allogeneic stem cell transplantation after a fludarabine/busulfan-based reduced-intensity conditioning in patients with myelodysplastic syndrome or secondary acute myeloid leukemia. Ann Hematol 2003;82:336–342
8. Kroger N, Shimoni A, Zabelina T et al. Reduced-toxicity conditioning with treosulfan, fludarabine and ATG as preparative regimen for allogeneic stem cell transplantation (alloSCT) in elderly patients with secondary acute myeloid leukemia (sAML) or myelodysplastic syndrome (MDS). Bone Marrow Transplant 2006;37:339–344
9. Niederwieser D, Maris M, Shizuru JA et al. Low-dose total body irradiation (TBI) and fludarabine followed by hematopoietic cell transplantation (HCT) from HLA-matched or mismatched unrelated donors and postgrafting immunosuppression with cyclosporine and

mycophenolate mofetil (MMF) can induce durable complete chimerism and sustained remissions in patients with hematological diseases. Blood 2003;101:1620–1629

10. Hegenbart U, Niederwieser D, Sandmaier BM et al. Treatment for acute myelogenous leukemia by low-dose, total-body, irradiation-based conditioning and hematopoietic cell transplantation from related and unrelated donors. J Clin Oncol 2006;24:444–453

11. Or R, Shapira MY, Resnick I et al. Nonmyeloablative allogeneic stem cell transplantation for the treatment of chronic myeloid leukemia in first chronic phase. Blood 2003;101:441–445

12. Kusumi E, Kami M, Yuji K et al. Feasibility of reduced intensity hematopoietic stem cell transplantation from an HLA-matched unrelated donor. Bone Marrow Transplant 2004;33:697–702

13. Uzunel M, Remberger M, Sairafi D et al. Unrelated versus related allogeneic stem cell transplantation after reduced intensity conditioning. Transplantation 2006;82:913–919

14. Giralt S, Estey E, Albitar M et al. Engraftment of allogeneic hematopoietic progenitor cells with purine analog-containing chemotherapy: harnessing graft-versus-leukemia without myeloablative therapy. Blood 1997;89:4531–4536

15. Socinski MA, Cannistra SA, Elias A et al. Granulocyte-macrophage colony stimulating factor expands the circulating haemopoietic progenitor cell compartment in man. Lancet 1988;1:1194–1198

16. Siena S, Bregni M, Brando B et al. Circulation of CD34+ hematopoietic stem cells in the peripheral blood of high-dose cyclophosphamide-treated patients: enhancement by intravenous recombinant human granulocyte-macrophage colony-stimulating factor. Blood 1989;74:1905–1914

17. Schmitz N, Dreger P, Suttorp M et al. Primary transplantation of allogeneic peripheral blood progenitor cells mobilized by filgrastim (granulocyte colony-stimulating factor). Blood 1995;85:1666–1672

18. Maris MB, Niederwieser D, Sandmaier BM et al. HLA-matched unrelated donor hematopoietic cell transplantation after nonmyeloablative conditioning for patients with hematologic malignancies. Blood 2003;102:2021–2030

19. Remberger M, Beelen DW, Fauser A et al. Increased risk of extensive chronic graft-versus-host disease after allogeneic peripheral blood stem cell transplantation using unrelated donors. Blood 2005;105:548–551

20. Garderet L, Labopin M, Gorin NC et al. Patients with acute lymphoblastic leukaemia allografted with a matched unrelated donor may have a lower survival with a peripheral blood stem cell graft compared to bone marrow. Bone Marrow Transplant 2003;31:23–29

21. Lang P, Handgretinger R, Niethammer D et al. Transplantation of highly purified CD34+ progenitor cells from unrelated donors in pediatric leukemia. Blood 2003;101:1630–1636

22. Benesch M, Urban C, Sykora KW et al. Transplantation of highly purified CD34+ progenitor cells from alternative donors in children with refractory severe aplastic anaemia. Br J Haematol 2004;125:58–63

23. Meijer E, Bloem AC, Dekker AW et al. Effect of antithymocyte globulin on quantitative immune recovery and graft-versus-host disease after partially T-cell-depleted bone marrow transplantation: a comparison between recipients of matched related and matched unrelated donor grafts. Transplantation 2003;75:1910–1913

24. von dem Borne PA, Beaumont F, Starrenburg CW et al. Outcomes after myeloablative unrelated donor stem cell transplantation using both in vitro and in vivo T-cell depletion with alemtuzumab. Haematologica 2006;91:1559–1562

25. Meijer E, Cornelissen JJ, Lowenberg B, Verdonck LF. Antithymocyteglobulin as prophylaxis of graft failure and graft-versus-host disease in recipients of partially T-cell-depleted grafts from matched unrelated donors: a dose-finding study. Exp Hematol 2003;31:1026–1030

26. Bunin N, Aplenc R, Leahey A et al. Outcomes of transplantation with partial T-cell depletion of matched or mismatched unrelated or partially matched related donor bone marrow in children and adolescents with leukemias. Bone Marrow Transplant 2005;35:151–158

27. Pavletic SZ, Carter SL, Kernan NA et al. Influence of T-cell depletion on chronic graft-versus-host disease: results of a multicenter randomized trial in unrelated marrow donor transplantation. Blood 2005;106:3308–3313

28. Champlin RE, Passweg JR, Zhang MJ et al. T-cell depletion of bone marrow transplants for leukemia from donors other than HLA-identical siblings: advantage of T-cell antibodies with narrow specificities. Blood 2000;95:3996–4003

29. Kobbe G, Fenk R, Neumann F et al. Transplantation of allogeneic CD34+-selected cells followed by early T-cell add-backs: favorable results in acute and chronic myeloid leukemia. Cytotherapy 2004;6:533–542

30. Lang P, Bader P, Schumm M et al. Transplantation of a combination of CD133+ and CD34+ selected progenitor cells from alternative donors. Br J Haematol 2004;124:72–79

31. Pui CH, Campana D, Evans WE. Childhood acute lymphoblastic leukaemia–current status and future perspectives. Lancet Oncol 2001;2:597–607

32. Pui CH, Evans WE. Treatment of acute lymphoblastic leukemia. N Engl J Med 2006;354:166–178

33. Heerema NA, Nachman JB, Sather HN et al. Hypodiploidy with less than 45 chromosomes confers adverse risk in childhood acute lymphoblastic leukemia: a report from the children's cancer group. Blood 1999;94:4036–4045

34. Johansson B, Moorman AV, Haas OA et al. Hematologic malignancies with t(4;11)(q21;q23)–a cytogenetic, morphologic, immunophenotypic and clinical study of 183 cases. European 11q23 Workshop participants. Leukemia 1998;12:779–787

35. Coustan-Smith E, Sancho J, Behm FG et al. Prognostic importance of measuring early clearance of leukemic cells by flow cytometry in childhood acute lymphoblastic leukemia. Blood 2002;100:52–58

36. Sandlund JT, Harrison PL, Rivera G et al. Persistence of lymphoblasts in bone marrow on day 15 and days 22 to 25 of remission induction predicts a dismal treatment outcome in children with acute lymphoblastic leukemia. Blood 2002;100:43–47

37. Arico M, Valsecchi MG, Camitta B et al. Outcome of treatment in children with Philadelphia chromosome-positive acute lymphoblastic leukemia. N Engl J Med 2000;342:998–1006

38. Henze G, Fengler R, Hartmann R et al. Six-year experience with a comprehensive approach to the treatment of recurrent childhood acute lymphoblastic leukemia (ALL-REZ BFM 85). A relapse study of the BFM group. Blood 1991;78:1166–1172

39. Woolfrey AE, Anasetti C, Storer B et al. Factors associated with outcome after unrelated marrow transplantation for treatment of acute lymphoblastic leukemia in children. Blood 2002;99:2002–2008

40. Bleakley M, Shaw PJ, Nielsen JM. Allogeneic bone marrow transplantation for childhood relapsed acute lymphoblastic leukemia: comparison of outcome in patients with and without a matched family donor. Bone Marrow Transplant 2002;30:1–7

41. Borgmann A, von Stackelberg A, Hartmann R et al. Unrelated donor stem cell transplantation compared with chemotherapy for children with acute lymphoblastic leukemia in a second remission: a matched-pair analysis. Blood 2003;101:3835–3839

42. Uderzo C, Dini G, Locatelli F et al. Treatment of childhood acute lymphoblastic leukemia after the first relapse: curative strategies. Haematologica 2000;85:47–53

43. Eckert C, Biondi A, Seeger K et al. Prognostic value of minimal residual disease in relapsed childhood acute lymphoblastic leukaemia. Lancet 2001;358:1239–1241

44. Bader P, Hancock J, Kreyenberg H et al. Minimal residual disease (MRD) status prior to allogeneic stem cell transplantation is a powerful predictor for post-transplant outcome in children with ALL. Leukemia 2002;16:1668–1672.

45. Pui CH, Behm FG, Downing JR et al. 11q23/MLL rearrangement confers a poor prognosis in infants with acute lymphoblastic leukemia. J Clin Oncol 1994;12:909–915

46. Pui CH, Gaynon P, Boyett JM et al. Outcome of treatment in childhood acute lymphoblastic leukaemia with rearrangements of the 11q23 chromosomal region. Lancet 2002;359:1909–1915

47. Xie Y, Davies SM, Xiang Y et al. Trends in leukemia incidence and survival in the United States (1973–1998). Cancer 2003;97:2229–2235

48. Hoelzer D, Gokbuget N. Recent approaches in acute lymphoblastic leukemia in adults. Crit Rev Oncol Hematol 2000;36:49–58

49. Hoelzer D, Gokbuget N. New approaches to acute lymphoblastic leukemia in adults: where do we go? Semin Oncol 2000;27:540–559

50. Rowe JM, Buck G, Fielding A et al. In adults with standard-risk acute lymphoblastic leukemia (ALL) the greatest benefit is achieved from an allogeneic transplant in first complete remission (CR) and an autologous transplant is less effective than conventional consolidation/maintenance chemotherapy: final results of the International ALL Trial (MRC UKALL XII/ECOG E2993). ASH Annual Meeting Abstracts. Blood 2006;108:2

51. Thiebaut A, Vernant JP, Degos L et al. Adult acute lymphocytic leukemia study testing chemotherapy and autologous and allogeneic transplantation. A follow-up report of the French protocol LALA 87. Hematol Oncol Clin North Am 2000;14:1353–1366

52. Johny A, Song KW, Nantel SH et al. Early stem cell transplantation for refractory acute leukemia after salvage therapy with high-dose etoposide and cyclophosphamide. Biol Blood Marrow Transplant 2006;12:480–489

53. Martino R, Giralt S, Caballero MD et al. Allogeneic hematopoietic stem cell transplantation with reduced-intensity conditioning in acute lymphoblastic leukemia: a feasibility study. Haematologica 2003;88:555–560

54. Hurwitz CA, Mounce KG, Grier HE. Treatment of patients with acute myelogenous leukemia: review of clinical trials of the past decade. J Pediatr Hematol Oncol 1995;17:185–197

55. Woods WG, Kobrinsky N, Buckley JD et al. Timed-sequential induction therapy improves postremission outcome in acute myeloid leukemia: a report from the Children's Cancer Group. Blood 1996;87:4979–4989

56. Wells RJ, Arthur DC, Srivastava A et al. Prognostic variables in newly diagnosed children and adolescents with acute myeloid leukemia: Children's Cancer Group Study 213. Leukemia 2002;16:601–607

57. Woods WG, Neudorf S, Gold S et al. A comparison of allogeneic bone marrow transplantation, autologous bone marrow transplantation, and aggressive chemotherapy in children with acute myeloid leukemia in remission. Blood 2001;97:56–62

58. Stevens RF, Hann IM, Wheatley K, Gray RG. Marked improvements in outcome with chemotherapy alone in paediatric acute myeloid leukaemia: results of the United Kingdom Medical Research Council's 10th AML trial. MRC Childhood Leukaemia Working Party. Br J Haematol 1998;101:130–140

59. Aladjidi N, Auvrignon A, Leblanc T et al. Outcome in children with relapsed acute myeloid leukemia after initial treatment with the French Leucemie Aique Myeloide Enfant (LAME) 89/91 protocol of the French Society of Pediatric Hematology and Immunology. J Clin Oncol 2003;21:4377–4385

60. Nemecek ER, Gooley TA, Woolfrey AE et al. Outcome of allogeneic bone marrow transplantation for children with advanced acute myeloid leukemia. Bone Marrow Transplant 2004;34:799–806

61. Hongeng S, Krance RA, Bowman LC et al. Outcomes of transplantation with matched-sibling and unrelated-donor bone marrow in children with leukaemia. Lancet 1997;350:767–771

62. Chalandon Y, Barnett MJ, Horsman DE et al. Influence of cytogenetic abnormalities on outcome after allogeneic bone marrow transplantation for acute myeloid leukemia in first complete remission. Biol Blood Marrow Transplant 2002;8:435–443

63. Ferrant A, Labopin M, Frassoni F et al. Karyotype in acute myeloblastic leukemia: prognostic significance for bone marrow transplantation in first remission: a European Group for Blood and Marrow Transplantation study. Acute Leukemia Working Party of the European Group for Blood and Marrow Transplantation (EBMT). Blood 1997;90:2931–2938

64. Sierra J, Storer B, Hansen JA et al. Unrelated donor marrow transplantation for acute myeloid leukemia: an update of the Seattle experience. Bone Marrow Transplant 2000;26:397–404

65. Ayash LJ, Ratanatharathorn V, Braun T et al. Unrelated donor bone marrow transplantation using a chemotherapy-only preparative regimen for adults with high-risk acute myelogenous leukemia. Am J Hematol 2007;82:6–14

66. Laane E, Derolf AR, Bjorklund E et al. The effect of allogeneic stem cell transplantation on outcome in younger acute myeloid leukemia patients with minimal residual disease detected by flow cytometry at the end of post-remission chemotherapy. Haematologica 2006;91:833–836

67. de Lima M, Giralt S. Allogeneic transplantation for the elderly patient with acute myelogenous leukemia or myelodysplastic syndrome. Semin Hematol 2006;43:107–117
68. Niederwieser D, Lange T, Cross M et al. Reduced intensity conditioning (RIC) haematopoietic cell transplants in elderly patients with AML. Best Pract Res Clin Haematol 2006;19:825–838
69. Lazarus HM, Perez WS, Klein JP et al. Autotransplantation versus HLA-matched unrelated donor transplantation for acute myeloid leukaemia: a retrospective analysis from the Center for International Blood and Marrow Transplant Research. Br J Haematol 2006;132:755–769
70. Schmid C, Schleuning M, Schwerdtfeger R et al. Long-term survival in refractory acute myeloid leukemia after sequential treatment with chemotherapy and reduced-intensity conditioning for allogeneic stem cell transplantation. Blood 2006;108:1092–1099
71. Blum W, Bolwell BJ, Phillips G et al. High disease burden is associated with poor outcomes for patients with acute myeloid leukemia not in remission who undergo unrelated donor cell transplantation. Biol. Blood Marrow Transplant 2006;12:61–67
72. Litzow MR. Progress and strategies for patients with relapsed and refractory acute myeloid leukemia. Curr Opin Hematol 2007;14:130–137
73. Hansen JA, Gooley TA, Martin PJ et al. Bone marrow transplants from unrelated donors for patients with chronic myeloid leukemia. N Engl J Med 1998;338:962–968
74. van Rhee RF, Szydlo RM, Hermans J et al. Long-term results after allogeneic bone marrow transplantation for chronic myelogenous leukemia in chronic phase: a report from the Chronic Leukemia Working Party of the European Group for Blood and Marrow Transplantation. Bone Marrow Transplant 1997;20:553–560
75. Elmaagacli AH, Basoglu S, Peceny R et al. Improved disease-free-survival after transplantation of peripheral blood stem cells as compared with bone marrow from HLA-identical unrelated donors in patients with first chronic phase chronic myeloid leukemia. Blood 2002;99:1130–1135
76. Cwynarski K, Roberts IA, Iacobelli S et al. Stem cell transplantation for chronic myeloid leukemia in children. Blood 2003;102:1224–1231
77. Creutzig U, Ritter J, Zimmermann M, Klingebiel T. [Prognosis of children with chronic myeloid leukemia: a retrospective analysis of 75 patients]. Klin Padiatr 1996;208:236–241
78. Chakraverty R, Peggs K, Chopra R et al. Limiting transplantation-related mortality following unrelated donor stem cell transplantation by using a nonmyeloablative conditioning regimen. Blood 2002;99:1071–1078
79. Kolb HJ, Mittermuller J, Clemm C et al. Donor leukocyte transfusions for treatment of recurrent chronic myelogenous leukemia in marrow transplant patients. Blood 1990;76:2462–2465
80. Pulsipher MA. Treatment of CML in pediatric patients: should imatinib mesylate (STI-571, Gleevec) or allogeneic hematopoietic cell transplant be front-line therapy? Pediatr Blood Cancer 2004;43:523–533
81. Huntly BJ, Reid AG, Bench AJ et al. Deletions of the derivative chromosome 9 occur at the time of the Philadelphia translocation and provide a powerful and independent prognostic indicator in chronic myeloid leukemia. Blood 2001;98:1732–1738
82. Gratwohl A, Hermans J, Goldman JM et al. Risk assessment for patients with chronic myeloid leukaemia before allogeneic blood or marrow transplantation. Chronic Leukemia Working Party of the European Group for Blood and Marrow Transplantation. Lancet 1998;352:1087–1092
83. Davies SM, DeFor TE, McGlave PB et al. Equivalent outcomes in patients with chronic myelogenous leukemia after early transplantation of phenotypically matched bone marrow from related or unrelated donors. Am J Med 2001;110:339–346
84. Weisdorf DJ, Anasetti C, Antin JH et al. Allogeneic bone marrow transplantation for chronic myelogenous leukemia: comparative analysis of unrelated versus matched sibling donor transplantation. Blood 2002;99:1971–1977
85. Elmaagacli AH, Beelen DW, Opalka B et al. The risk of residual molecular and cytogenetic disease in patients with Philadelphia-chromosome positive first chronic phase chronic myelogenous leukemia is reduced after transplantation of allogeneic peripheral blood stem cells compared with bone marrow. Blood 1999;94:384–389
86. Remberger M, Ringden O, Blau IW et al. No difference in graft-versus-host disease, relapse, and survival comparing peripheral stem cells to bone marrow using unrelated donors. Blood 2001;98:1739–1745
87. Radich JP, Olavarria E, Apperley JF. Allogeneic hematopoietic stem cell transplantation for chronic myeloid leukemia. Hematol Oncol Clin North Am 2004;18:685–702
88. Anderson J.E, Appelbaum FR, Storb R. An update on allogeneic marrow transplantation for myelodysplastic syndrome. Leuk Lymphoma 1995;17:95–99
89. Cheson BD, Bennett JM, Kantarjian H et al. Report of an international working group to standardize response criteria for myelodysplastic syndromes. Blood 2000;96:3671–3674
90. Luger S, Sacks N. Bone marrow transplantation for myelodysplastic syndrome – who? when? and which? Bone Marrow Transplant 2002;30:199–206
91. Passmore SJ, Hann IM, Stiller CA et al. Pediatric myelodysplasia: a study of 68 children and a new prognostic scoring system. Blood 1995;85:1742–1750
92. Sutton L, Chastang C, Ribaud P et al. Factors influencing outcome in de novo myelodysplastic syndromes treated by allogeneic bone marrow transplantation: a long-term study of 71 patients. Societe Francaise de Greffe de Moelle. Blood 1996;88:358–365
93. Woods WG, Barnard DR, Alonzo TA et al. Prospective study of 90 children requiring treatment for juvenile myelomonocytic leukemia or myelodysplastic syndrome: a report from the Children's Cancer Group. J Clin Oncol 2002;20:434–440
94. Davies SM, Wagner JE, DeFor T et al. Unrelated donor bone marrow transplantation for children and adolescents with aplastic anaemia or myelodysplasia. Br J Haematol 1997;96:749–756
95. Anderson JE, Anasetti C, Appelbaum FR et al. Unrelated donor marrow transplantation for myelodysplasia (MDS) and MDS-related acute myeloid leukaemia. Br J Haematol 1996;93:59–67
96. Niemeyer CM, Arico M., Basso G et al. Chronic myelomonocytic leukemia in childhood: a retrospective analysis of 110 cases. European Working Group on Myelodysplastic Syndromes in Childhood (EWOG-MDS). Blood 1997;89:3534–3543
97. MacMillan ML, Davies SM, Orchard PJ et al. Haemopoietic cell transplantation in children with juvenile myelomonocytic leukaemia. Br J Haematol 1998;103:552–558
98. Deeg HJ, Storer B, Slattery JT et al. Conditioning with targeted busulfan and cyclophosphamide for hemopoietic stem cell transplantation from related and unrelated donors in patients with myelodysplastic syndrome. Blood 2002;100:1201–1207
99. Flomenberg N, Baxter-Lowe LA, Confer D et al. Impact of HLA class I and class II high-resolution matching on outcomes of unrelated donor bone marrow transplantation: HLA-C mismatching is associated with a strong adverse effect on transplantation outcome. Blood 2004;104:1923–1930
100. Petersdorf EW, Malkki M. Human leukocyte antigen matching in unrelated donor hematopoietic cell transplantation. Semin Hematol 2005;42:76–84
101. Russell JA, Tran HT, Quinlan D et al. Once-daily intravenous busulfan given with fludarabine as conditioning for allogeneic stem cell transplantation: study of pharmacokinetics and early clinical outcomes. Biol Blood Marrow Transplant 2002;8:468–476
102. de Lima M, Anagnostopoulos A, Munsell M et al. Nonablative versus reduced-intensity conditioning regimens in the treatment of acute myeloid leukemia and high-risk myelodysplastic syndrome: dose is relevant for long-term disease control after allogeneic hematopoietic stem cell transplantation. Blood 2004;104:865–872
103. de Lima M, Couriel D, Thall PF et al. Once-daily intravenous busulfan and fludarabine: clinical and pharmacokinetic results of a myeloablative, reduced-toxicity conditioning regimen for allogeneic stem cell transplantation in AML and MDS. Blood 2004;104:857–864
104. Ho AY, Pagliuca A, Kenyon M et al. Reduced-intensity allogeneic hematopoietic stem cell transplantation for myelodysplastic syndrome and acute myeloid leukemia with multilineage dysplasia using fludarabine, busulphan, and alemtuzumab (FBC) conditioning. Blood 2004;104:1616–1623
105. Yakoub-Agha I, de La SP, Ribaud P et al. Allogeneic bone marrow transplantation for therapy-related myelodysplastic syndrome and acute myeloid leukemia: a long-term study of 70 patients-report of the French society of bone marrow transplantation. J Clin Oncol 2000;18:963–971
106. Woodard P, Barfield R, Hale G et al. Outcome of hematopoietic stem cell transplantation for pediatric patients with therapy-related acute myeloid leukemia or myelodysplastic syndrome. Pediatr Blood Cancer 2006;47:931–935
107. Kojima S, Matsuyama T, Kato S et al. Outcome of 154 patients with severe aplastic anemia who received transplants from unrelated donors: the Japan Marrow Donor Program. Blood 2002;100:799–803
108. Gupta V, Ball SE, Sage D et al. Marrow transplants from matched unrelated donors for aplastic anaemia using alemtuzumab, fludarabine and cyclophosphamide based conditioning. Bone Marrow Transplant 2005;35:467–471
109. Bunin N, Aplenc R, Iannone R et al. Unrelated donor bone marrow transplantation for children with severe aplastic anemia: minimal GVHD and durable engraftment with partial T cell depletion. Bone Marrow Transplant 2005;35:369–373
110. Kennedy-Nasser AA, Leung KS, Mahajan A et al. Comparable outcomes of matched-related and alternative donor stem cell transplantation for pediatric severe aplastic anemia. Biol Blood Marrow Transplant 2006;12:1277–1284
111. Passweg JR, Perez WS, Eapen M et al. Bone marrow transplants from mismatched related and unrelated donors for severe aplastic anemia. Bone Marrow Transplant 2006;37:641–649
112. Svenberg P, Remberger M, Svennilson J et al. Allogeneic stem cell transplantation for nonmalignant disorders using matched unrelated donors. Biol Blood Marrow Transplant 2004;10:877–882
113. Willasch A, Hoelle W, Kreyenberg H et al. Outcome of allogeneic stem cell transplantation in children with non-malignant diseases. Haematologica 2006;91:788–794
114. Truitt RL, Rimm AA, Saltzstein EC et al. Graft-versus-leukemia for AKR spontaneous leukemia-lymphoma. Transplant Proc 1976;8:569–574
115. Henslee-Downey PJ, Abhyankar SH, Parrish RS et al. Use of partially mismatched related donors extends access to allogeneic marrow transplant. Blood 1997;89:3864–3872
116. Schumm M, Lang P, Taylor G et al. Isolation of highly purified autologous and allogeneic peripheral CD34+ cells using the CliniMACS device. J Hematother 1999;8:209–218
117. Barfield RC, Otto M, Houston J et al. A one-step large-scale method for T- and B-cell depletion of mobilized PBSC for allogeneic transplantation. Cytotherapy 2004;6:1–6
118. Handgretinger R, Klingebiel T, Lang P et al. Megadose transplantation of purified peripheral blood CD34+ progenitor cells from HLA-mismatched parental donors in children. Bone Marrow Transplant 2001;27:777–783
119. Aversa F, Terenzi A, Tabilio A et al. Full haplotype-mismatched hematopoietic stem-cell transplantation: a phase II study in patients with acute leukemia at high risk of relapse. J Clin Oncol 2005;20:3447–3454
120. Leung W, Iyengar R, Turner V et al. Determinants of antileukemia effects of allogeneic NK cells. J Immunol 2004;172:644–650
121. Farag SS, Fehniger TA, Ruggeri L et al. Natural killer cell receptors: new biology and insights into the graft-versus-leukemia effect. Blood 2002;100:1935–1947
122. Lamb LS Jr, Henslee-Downey PJ, Parrish RS et al. Increased frequency of TCR gamma delta + T cells in disease-free survivors following T cell-depleted, partially mismatched, related donor bone marrow transplantation for leukemia. J Hematother 1996;5:503–509
123. Passweg JR, Koehl U, Uharek L et al. Natural-killer-cell-based treatment in haematopoietic stem-cell transplantation. Best Pract Res Clin Haematol 2006;19:811–824
124. Triplett B, Handgretinger R, Pui CH, Leung W. KIR-incompatible hematopoietic-cell transplantation for poor prognosis infant acute lymphoblastic leukemia. Blood 2006;107:1238–1239
125. Feuchtinger T, Matthes-Martin S, Richard C et al. Safe adoptive transfer of virus-specific T-cell immunity for the treatment of systemic adenovirus infection after allogeneic stem cell transplantation. Br J Haematol 2006;134:64–76
126. Wichlan DG, Roddam PL, Eldridge P et al. Efficient and reproducible large-scale isolation of human CD4+ CD25+ regulatory T cells with potent suppressor activity. J Immunol Methods 2006;315:27–36

127. Wehler TC, Nonn M, Brandt B et al. Targeting the activation-induced antigen CD137 can selectively deplete alloreactive T cells from antileukemic and antitumor donor T-cell lines. Blood 2007;109:365–373

128. Houtenbos I, Westers TM, Dijkhuis A et al. Leukemia-specific T-cell reactivity induced by leukemic dendritic cells is augmented by 4-1BB targeting. Clin Cancer Res 2007;13:307–315

129. Ruggeri L, Capanni M, Casucci M et al. Role of natural killer cell alloreactivity in HLA-mismatched hematopoietic stem cell transplantation. Blood 1999;94:333–339

130. Ruggeri L, Capanni M, Urbani E et al. Effectiveness of donor natural killer cell alloreactivity in mismatched hematopoietic transplants. Science 2002;295:2097–2100

131. Karre K, Ljunggren HG, Piontek G, Kiessling R. Selective rejection of H-2-deficient lymphoma variants suggests alternative immune defence strategy. Nature 1986;319:675–678

132. Moretta L, Moretta A. Killer immunoglobulin-like receptors. Curr Opin Immunol 2004;16:626–633

133. Ruggeri L, Aversa F, Martelli MF, Velardi A. Allogeneic hematopoietic transplantation and natural killer cell recognition of missing self. Immunol Rev 2006;214:202–218

134. Ruggeri L, Mancusi A, Burchielli E et al. Natural killer cell recognition of missing self and haploidentical hematopoietic transplantation. Semin Cancer Biol 2006;16:404–411

135. Grau R, Lang KS, Wernet D et al. Cytotoxic activity of natural killer cells lacking killer-inhibitory receptors for self-HLA class I molecules against autologous hematopoietic stem cells in healthy individuals. Exp Mol Pathol 2004;76:90–98

136. Leung W, Iyengar R, Triplett B et al. Comparison of killer Ig-like receptor genotyping and phenotyping for selection of allogeneic blood stem cell donors. J Immunol 2005;174:6540–6545

137. Lang P, Barbin K, Feuchtinger T et al. Chimeric CD19 antibody mediates cytotoxic activity against leukemic blasts with effector cells from pediatric patients who received T-cell-depleted allografts. Blood 2004;103:3982–3985

138. Reisner Y, Martelli MF. Tolerance induction by 'megadose' transplants of CD34+ stem cells: a new option for leukemia patients without an HLA-matched donor. Curr Opin Immunol 2000;12:536–541

139. Aversa F, Tabilio A, Velardi A et al. Treatment of high-risk acute leukemia with T-cell-depleted stem cells from related donors with one fully mismatched HLA haplotype. N Engl J Med 1998;339:1186–1193

140. Schumm M, Handgretinger R, Pfeiffer M et al. Determination of residual T- and B-cell content after immunomagnetic depletion: proposal for flow cytometric analysis and results from 103 separations. Cytotherapy 2006;8:465–472

141. Huang X, Liu DH, Liu KY et al. Haploidentical hematopoietic stem cell transplantation without in vitro T-cell depletion for the treatment of hematological malignancies. Bone Marrow Transplant 2006;38:291–297

142. van Rood JJ, Loberiza FR Jr, Zhang MJ et al. Effect of tolerance to noninherited maternal antigens on the occurrence of graft-versus-host disease after bone marrow transplantation from a parent or an HLA-haploidentical sibling. Blood 2002;99:1572–1577

143. Ichinohe T, Uchiyama T, Shimazaki C et al. Feasibility of HLA-haploidentical hematopoietic stem cell transplantation between noninherited maternal antigen (NIMA)-mismatched family members linked with long-term fetomaternal microchimerism. Blood 2004;104:3821–3828

144. Obama K, Utsunomiya A, Takatsuka Y, Takemoto Y. Reduced-intensity non-T-cell depleted HLA-haploidentical stem cell transplantation for older patients based on the concept of feto-maternal tolerance. Bone Marrow Transplant 2004;34:897–899

145. Parkman R, Weinberg KI. Immunological reconstitution following bone marrow transplantation. Immunol Rev 1997;157:73–78

146. Handgretinger R, Lang P, Schumm M et al. Immunological aspects of haploidentical stem cell transplantation in children. Ann NY Acad Sci 2001;938:340–357

147. Bethge WA, Haegele M, Faul C et al. Haploidentical allogeneic hematopoietic cell transplantation in adults with reduced-intensity conditioning and CD3/CD19 depletion: fast engraftment and low toxicity. Exp Hematol 2006;34:1746–1752

148. Storek J, Gooley T, Witherspoon RP et al. Infectious morbidity in long-term survivors of allogeneic marrow transplantation is associated with low CD4 T cell counts. Am J Hematol 1997;54:131–138

149. Chen X, Hale GA, Barfield R et al. Rapid immune reconstitution after a reduced-intensity conditioning regimen and a CD3-depleted haploidentical stem cell graft for paediatric refractory haematological malignancies. Br J Haematol 2006;135:524–532

150. Hebart H, Brugger W, Grigoleit U et al. Risk for cytomegalovirus disease in patients receiving polymerase chain reaction-based preemptive antiviral therapy after allogeneic stem cell transplantation depends on transplantation modality. Blood 2001;97:2183–2185

151. Feuchtinger T, Richard C, Pfeiffer M et al. Adenoviral infections after transplantation of positive selected stem cells from haploidentical donors in children: an update. Klin Pediatr 2005;217:339–344

152. Gu Z, Belzer SW, Gibson CS et al. Multiplexed, real-time PCR for quantitative detection of human adenovirus. J Clin Microbiol 2003;41:4636–4641

153. Yusuf U, Hale GA, Carr J et al. Cidofovir for the treatment of adenoviral infection in pediatric hematopoietic stem cell transplant patients. Transplantation 2006;81:1398–1404

154. Gottschalk S, Rooney CM, Heslop HE. Post-transplant lymphoproliferative disorders. Annu Rev Med 2005;56:29–44

155. Hale GA, Kasow KA, Madden R et al. Mismatched family member donor transplantation for patients with refractory hematologic malignancies: long-term followup of a prospective clinical trial. ASH Annual Meeting Abstracts. Blood 2006;108:3137

156. van Esser JW, van der Holt B, Meijer E et al. Epstein–Barr virus (EBV) reactivation is a frequent event after allogeneic stem cell transplantation (SCT) and quantitatively predicts EBV-lymphoproliferative disease following T-cell-depleted SCT. Blood 2001;98:972–978

157. Wagner HJ, Cheng YC, Huls MH et al. Prompt versus preemptive intervention for EBV lymphoproliferative disease. Blood 2004;103:3979–3981

158. Klingebiel T, Handgretinger R, Lang P et al. Haploidentical transplantation for acute lymphoblastic leukemia in childhood. Blood Rev 2004;18:181–192

159. Hale GA, Kasow KA, Gan K et al. Haploidentical stem cell transplantation with CD3 depleted mobilized peripheral blood stem cell grafts for children with hematologic malignancies. ASH Annual Meeting Abstracts. Blood 2005;106:2910

160. Marks DI, Khattry N, Cummins M et al. Haploidentical stem cell transplantation for children with acute leukaemia. Br J Haematol 2006;134:196–201

161. Lu DP, Dong L, Wu T et al. Conditioning including antithymocyte globulin followed by unmanipulated HLA-mismatched/haploidentical blood and marrow transplantation can achieve comparable outcomes with HLA-identical sibling transplantation. Blood 2006;107:3065–3073

162. Ogawa H, Ikegame K, Yoshihara S et al. Unmanipulated HLA 2–3 antigen-mismatched (haploidentical) stem cell transplantation using nonmyeloablative conditioning. Biol Blood Marrow Transplant 2006;12:1073–1084

163. Lang P, Schumm M, Greil J et al. A comparison between three graft manipulation methods for haploidentical stem cell transplantation in pediatric patients: preliminary results of a pilot study. Klin Paediatr 2005;217:334–338

164. Re F, Staudacher C, Zamai L et al. Killer cell Ig-like receptors ligand-mismatched, alloreactive natural killer cells lyse primary solid tumors. Cancer 2006;107:640–648

165. Lang P, Pfeiffer M, Muller I et al. Haploidentical stem cell transplantation in patients with pediatric solid tumors: preliminary results of a pilot study and analysis of graft versus tumor effects. Klin Paediatr 2006;218:321–326

166. Miller JS, Soignier Y, Panoskaltsis-Mortari A et al. Successful adoptive transfer and in vivo expansion of human haploidentical NK cells in patients with cancer. Blood 2005;105:3051–3057

167. Zuckerman T, Rowe JM. Alternative donor transplantation in acute myeloid leukemia: which source and when? Curr Opin Hematol 2007;14:152–161

168. Friedrich W, Muller SM. Allogeneic stem cell transplantation for treatment of immunodeficiency. Springer Semin Immunopathol 2004;26:109–118

169. Woodard P, Cunningham JM, Benaim E et al. Effective donor lymphohematopoietic reconstitution after haploidentical CD34+-selected hematopoietic stem cell transplantation in children with refractory severe aplastic anemia. Bone Marrow Transplant 2004;33:411–418

170. Woodard P, Jeng M, Handgretinger R et al. Summary of symposium: the future of stem cell transplantation for sickle cell disease. J Pediatr Hematol Oncol 2002;24:512–514

171. Schulz AS, Classen CF, Mihatsch WA et al. HLA-haploidentical blood progenitor cell transplantation in osteopetrosis. Blood 2002;99:3458–3460

172. Caillat-Zucman S, Le DF, Haddad E et al. Impact of HLA matching on outcome of hematopoietic stem cell transplantation in children with inherited diseases: a single-center comparative analysis of genoidentical, haploidentical or unrelated donors. Bone Marrow Transplant 2004;33:1089–1095

Management of the older patient

CHAPTER 30

Andrew S Artz and William B Ershler

Introduction

Allogeneic hematopoietic stem cell transplantation (HSCT) has the potential to eradicate otherwise incurable hematologic malignancies. Historically, the toxicities of standard myeloablative conditioning regimens restricted application to patients less than 50 years of age.[1] Such age barriers limit the benefit of HSCT to a relatively small number of patients since the median age of most hematologic malignancies is in the late seventh decade of life and older adults have more aggressive disease for which standard chemotherapy has limited efficacy. Major advances in the last decade in conditioning regimens and supportive care have facilitated extension of HSCT to adults 50 years old and over. Determining whether or not to pursue HSCT in older adults remains difficult. Emerging tools that enable a better prediction of HSCT tolerance may become useful in deciding which older patients will benefit from this approach, but, to date, this remains an unresolved research question.

In this chapter, we will briefly discuss some features of the biology of aging relevant to transplantation and review prior and current research on this issue.

The biology of aging

It is a central theme in gerontology that aging is not a disease. Nonetheless, functional declines accompany normal aging but these are usually insufficient to account for symptoms and should be considered separate from disease. For example, kidney function decline with age is well recognized[2] yet clinical consequences in the absence of a disease or exposure to a nephrotoxic agent are uncommon. Similarly, there are age-associated qualitative and quantitative changes within the bone marrow. Marrow stem cells are fewer and proliferative potential of progenitor cells is less.[3–5] However, anemia is uncommon in the absence of disease, as are neutropenia and thrombocytopenia. In fact, in rodents, serial transplantation of marrow has indicated that there is enough regenerative capacity to sustain life for several generations.[4] There have also been distinct changes in measurable immune functions described with age[6] but the clinical consequences of these are minimal or even non-existent in the absence of disease. Marrow functional reserves in the context of aging and transplantation will be discussed below.

Although aging is not a disease, physiological alterations accompanying aging may make an individual susceptible to disease. For example, those described for the immune system, although not primarily a problem, may render an individual susceptible to reactivation of tuberculosis[7,8] or herpes zoster[9] and less capable of responding to influenza vaccine with protective titers of antibody.[10,11] The immune decline, however, is not of sufficient magnitude or duration to account for the increased incidence of cancer in old people.[12,13] In fact, we[14] and others[15–17] have shown in experimental models that immune senescence, paradoxically, is associated with reduced tumor growth and spread (see below). Nevertheless, the immune deficiency that occurs in patients as a result of disease (or the treatment thereof) is likely to be more profound and result in consequences such as opportunistic infection.

Lifespan

Over the past century there has been dramatic improvement in median survival, most of which can be attributed to modern sanitation, refrigeration and other public health measures including vaccination and antibiotics.[18] Early deaths have been diminished and more individuals are reaching old age. In the United States today, life expectancy now approaches 80 years.[19]

Gerontologists draw a major distinction between median and maximum survival, the latter of which is more likely to reflect interventions that influence biological aging rather than disease. The oldest human being alive today is approximately 120 years old, a record that has remained stable for the past century during which adequate records have been maintained. In the laboratory, similar limits have been established for a variety of species. Drosophila, free of predators, can live 30 days, whereas C57BL/6 mice in a laboratory environment and allowed to eat a healthy diet *ad libitum* may survive 40 months. Interestingly, unlike the public health initiatives in humans, experimental interventions in lower species have been associated with a prolongation of maximum survival. In drosophila, for example, transgenic offspring producing extra copies of the free radical scavenging enzymes superoxide dismutase and catalase survived about 33% longer than controls.[20] In mammalian species, the only experimental intervention that characteristically prolongs maximum survival is the restriction of caloric intake. In fact, dietary restriction (DR) has become a common experimental paradigm exploited in the investigation of primary processes of aging, reviewed in ref 21.

Briefly, DR typically involves a reduction of 30–40% in caloric intake, with careful attention to the provision of adequate amounts of essential nutrients. It is associated with both a delay in the acquisition of age-related diseases and a reduction in the rate of achieving certain established biomarkers of aging (i.e. retardation in primary aging). Furthermore, DR significantly reduces the incidence of cancer in cancer-prone animals whether the carcinogen is viral or chemical. The critical questions remain: what is the mechanism of the DR effect, and will it be applicable to higher species? With regard to the latter, there are now at least four comprehensive and interactive studies within the United States in which DR is being examined in non-human primates, and most recently in humans.[22] Although it appears that the calorie-restricted monkeys are assuming a more youthful phenotype in a variety of physiological measures,[23,24] it is too early to predict whether maximum survival will be affected.

Immunity and aging

There is a well-characterized deficit in immune function with advancing age (for review, see ref 6), but as mentioned above, the consequences are not fully established. It is apparent that otherwise healthy older individuals are more susceptible to reactivation of tuberculosis[7,8] or herpes zoster,[9] and responses to vaccines, such as the commercially available and widely used influenza hemagglutinin, are lower.[25,26] However, it has been postulated that other age-associated diseases, such as cancer,[27] atherosclerosis,[28] diabetes[29] and even Alzheimer's disease[30,31] have been related to the immune decline with age.

What can be said with confidence is that there are changes in T-cell function with age that result in decreased proliferation when measured in vitro.[32] When studied as a population, there appears to be an accumulation of T-cells with the surface characteristics of memory cells and a correspondingly diminished absolute number of naïve T-cells.[6] Qualitative defects in T-cell function are commonly reported[33–35] but B-cell function, including the capacity to make antibody, remains intact, although certain intrinsic alterations have been noted.[36] Immunoregulatory functions are affected by the aging process and paraproteinemia, and autoantibodies are increasingly observed with each advancing decade. The paraproteinemia may be an indicator of dysregulated immunity, but it is considered not to be an antecedent of multiple myeloma.[37,38] However, myeloma does increase in incidence in geriatric populations and it must be distinguished from the benign paraproteinemia of aging. Typically, this is accomplished by examination of bone marrow, skeletal X-rays, renal function and serial determinations of paraprotein level.[37]

Another indication of dysregulated immune function is the alterations in certain key cytokines, measured in plasma, culture supernatants or in the appropriate tissue microenvironment. Notably and consistently, interleukin-2 (IL-2) levels and function decrease with age,[39] and IL-6 levels increase.[40] The decline in IL-2 may account for a significant component of the measured decline in T-cell function, and the increased IL-6 has been implicated in the pathogenesis of certain age-associated diseases including osteoporosis, Alzheimer's disease and cancer.[41]

Immune senescence and tumor growth

There is a curious association of immune competence and experimental tumor growth that has been of some interest to both gerontologists and oncologists. It has been long recognized that certain tumors, particularly breast and prostate (but also, to a lesser extent, lung and colon), appear clinically less aggressive in older people.[42] This has proven to be difficult to establish using tumor registry data, perhaps reflecting the more likely existence of co-morbidities and less aggressive screening, diagnostic and therapeutic efforts afforded to elderly patients. Nonetheless, it is clear in certain experimental animal models that slower tumor growth, fewer metastases and longer survival are observed in old hosts.[16,43] Several explanations have been postulated, including less vigorous angiogenic response or other microenvironmental or extracellular matrix 'soil' factors, but experimental evidence has supported the paradoxical role of immune senescence. Thus, old animals reconstituted with the syngeneic immune system of young donors, either by thymus and spleen[44] or bone marrow[45] transplantation, develop more rapid and aggressive tumor growth, whereas young animals irradiated and reconstituted with old immune cells have tumor growth characteristics that resemble old control animals. These

observations have led to the re-evaluation of the immune enhancement hypothesis, as originally proposed by Prehn and colleagues.[46,47]

Bone marrow function and aging

In a classic series of experiments performed in mice three decades ago, Harrison demonstrated that hematopoietic stem cells transplanted into myeloablated recipients would continue to produce large numbers of differentiated blood cells for a period well in excess of the lifespan of the donor.[4,48] That there is a limit to this replicative capacity was demonstrated by serial transplantation experiments in which the original bone marrow graft was passaged through a series of recipients, but not indefinitely. Depending on the mouse strain, the number of sequential transfers was approximately five, but the number was less if the original donor was an old animal.[49–51] The question of whether these findings are relevant to normal aging remains to be determined, but certainly marrow reserve should not be considered indefinite and conceivably, aging coupled with life-long environmental exposures could contribute to late-life cytopenias that are occasionally observed (particularly anemia) and for which other explanations are not readily apparent.[52,53]

Hematologic diseases and aging

Epidemiology

Hematologic malignancies are generally diseases of the elderly, as the median age for most of these diseases hovers around 65–70 years of age. Acute myeloid leukemia (AML), the most common indication for allogeneic transplant, is an important example. Compared to adults 20–24 years of age, the incidence of AML is almost threefold higher for adults 50–54 years and 13-fold higher for those 70–74 years (http://seer.cancer.gov/csr/1975_2000/sections.html).

Increased life expectancy in developed countries has led to a 'graying' of society such that the proportion of older adults has risen. Around 16% of people were 60 or older in 1995, while approximately 27% will be 60 years or older in 2050. Consequently, we can expect not only more cases of hematologic malignancy in the elderly, but the median age for patients with hematologic malignancies will rise.

Disease biology and outcomes

Pursuing hematopoietic stem cell transplantation for hematologic diseases rests on the premise that standard non-transplant therapy has a low likelihood of long-term disease control. Older age is strongly associated with adverse biologic disease characteristics. For example, AML in older adults more typically has unfavorable cytogenetics, increased expression of the multidrug resistance protein, and antecedent myelodysplasia.[54,55] Consequently, complete remission rates for AML in the elderly are only 30–50% and median survival is generally less than 1 year, as recorded by co-operative group trials of selected older patients undergoing intensive therapy.[54,56,57] One recent co-operative group analysis of AML in adults 60 years and older placed 5-year survival at only 6.6%.[56] United States Medicare data reveal an abysmal median survival of only 2 months for older AML patients.[58] Aucte lymphoblastic leukemia (ALL) in older adults leads to similar poor outcomes. Among 759 patients enrolled in Cancer and Leukemia Group B (CALGB) studies between 1988 and 2002, striking age-related differences exist. Overall survival at 3 years was 58% for those <30 years, 38% for 30–59 years, and 12% for patients 60 years and older.[59] Furthermore, data derived from co-operative group trials likely underestimate the poor outcomes in older adults since only the most fit elderly are enrolled.[60] The aggressive nature and high prevalence of hematologic malignancies coupled with often inadequate therapy account for the observation that 77% of all leukemia deaths in the United States in 2003 occurred in patients 60 years and over.[61]

Evaluation of older adults for allogeneic hematopoietic stem cell transplant

HSCT indications

Hematologic malignancies unlikely to be eradicated by conventional chemotherapy continue to be the primary indication for HSCT in older adults, with aplastic anemia representing the most common non-malignant condition. In general, the most common disease indications are: AML, ALL, chronic myeloid leukemia (CML), lymphoma and myelodysplasia. Specifically, leukemia accounts for 78% of HSCT based upon recent EBMT registry data.[62] In light of the aggressive and incurable nature of most leukemias in older adults, HSCT must be considered a treatment option. Yet, no randomized or prospective trials exist in older adults comparing HSCT to standard therapy to guide clinicians on the precise benefits of HSCT. Thus, clinicians must infer from data gathered from younger patients with similar disease features (e.g. AML in first complete remission with adverse cytogenetics) and make decisions regarding appropriate therapy. Without sufficient clinical trial evidence, and with only rudimentary understanding of the physiology of aging, many clinicians have been reluctant to offer HSCT for fear of doing more harm than good. Whereas in young adults, disease prognosis (assuming donor availability) primarily dictates the HSCT decision, in older adults there is an added need to estimate transplant tolerance. To date, there has been no validated clinical instrument to effectively accomplish this task.

Tolerability

Standard myeloablative conditioning regimens for HSCT result in serious extramedullary toxicities to liver, intestine, and lung, and thus the procedure was initially restricted to fit patients, typically less than 50 years of age. In addition to the adverse consequences of high-dose chemotherapy or radiation, other required medications, such as those to minimize graft-versus-host disease (GvHD) or prevent infection, may also add considerable toxicity. Thus, as recently as the 1980s, HSCT studies rarely enrolled adults 50 years or older.[1,63]

HSCT numbers in older adults

Rapid advances in the field of HSCT enhancing transplant tolerability and reducing acute transplant-related mortality (TRM, i.e. non-relapse mortality) have altered the transplant landscape. Initially, a few series indicated feasibility in selected older adults.[64] The Center for International Blood and Marrow Transplantation (CIBMTR) now reports that approximately 13% of allogeneic transplants performed are for patients older than 50 years of age (www.cibmtr.org/ABOUT/NEWS/2006May.pdf). While the proportion of older adults who receive an HSCT remains very low relative to younger subjects, the rate of rise has been most marked in older adults. The future growth of HSCT is likely to occur in older adults.

Factors promoting HSCT in older adults

Although reduced-intensity conditioning (RIC) has been central to promoting HSCT for older adults, other factors, often less appreciated, have enhanced HSCT utilization (Table 30.1).

Table 30.1 Factors contributing to the increasing use of transplantation for older adults

Factor	Example or explanation
Reduced-intensity conditioning	Non-ablative preparative regimens
Supportive care	CMV monitoring and prophylaxis
Peripheral blood stem cells	Hastens hematologic recovery
GvHD prophylaxis	Mini-methotrexate, T-cell depletion
Donor pool	Donor registries facilitate availability of unrelated donors
Risk stratification tools	Co-morbidity scores for predicting tolerance rather than age alone
Patient health	Older adults healthier and have longer life expectancy than prior generation
Societal attitudes	Patient and physician attitudes on the desire to receive treatment when older

Reduced-intensity conditioning

RIC regimens have been widely credited for the increased tolerance of HSCT and expansion to older cohorts. The European Bone Marrow Transplantation Registry (EBMTR) reports 31% of allogeneic transplants now incorporate RIC, whereas RIC before 1999 was rare.[62] RIC permits engraftment while retaining graft-versus-leukemia effects and reducing acute transplant-related toxicities.[65–67] Regimen intensity and toxicities vary widely, but in general, acute toxicity has been appreciably reduced. Considering differences in regimen intensity, supportive care, and patient heterogeneity, it is not surprising that when using RIC, TRM varies widely, even among older adults, ranging from 3% to 55%.[68–79] While reducing regimen intensity and/or increasing immunosuppression to enhance tolerability, such manipulations reduce long-term disease control.[80] Higher dose intensity decreases relapse rates[68,81,82] which must be counterbalanced with increased complications.

Donors

The likelihood of finding a matched unrelated donor has risen dramatically over the past decade. Donors in the National Marrow Donors Program (NMDP) have rapidly risen to approximately 5.5 million, which, when coupled with advances in HLA typing, has made unrelated donor transplantation more feasible and successful.[83,84]

Other factors promoting HSCT in older adults

There have been additional measures enhancing outcomes in general, including more tolerable immune suppression, infusion of peripheral blood progenitor cells (to hasten hematologic recovery), and improved supportive care. In composite, these have been instrumental in expanding HSCT to older adults[85] (see Table 30.1). For example, improved detection and treatment of the most problematic infections such as cytomegalovirus (CMV) and aspergillosis have been of critical importance.[86–89]

Another factor relates to societal attitudes. Expectations for a 70-year-old today include a decade and a half more of expected survival. Although the incidence of co-morbidity rises with age, older persons today are healthier than prior generations,[90] thus making a greater proportion of patients at a given age eligible for intensive therapy. The rise in autografts (which primarily employ myeloablative conditioning) for adults 50 years and over indicates the influence of factors other than RIC in promoting transplantation in older adults. Although not separable, these factors have arguably been more influential than just RIC preparative regimens. For example, 20% of autograft patients are now over 60 years of age. Between 1998 and 2003, CIBMTR data show that only 26% of recipients between 50 and 59 years received non-ablative grafts and slightly over half of recipients 60–69 years of age (Table 30.2). While the definitions of non-ablative grafts may be debated, clearly many HSCTs in older adults in the modern era employ myeloablative preparative regimens.

Donor selection for older adults

Advancing age of the donor has negative effects on transplant outcome. In a large registry study of 6978 unrelated bone marrow transplants, Kollman and colleagues showed that when the donor was 45 years or older, recipients were more likely to experience acute GvHD, chronic GvHD, and inferior overall survival.[91] Even with RIC, advancing age of the sibling donor may lead to a worse outcome.[92]

Increasing donor age has been associated with decreased allograft stem cell yields.[93] Similarly, autografts in older adults have reduced stem cell collection numbers.[94] Not surprisingly, older donor age is also associated with graft failure.[95] Yet, there remain incomplete quantitative data on stem cells and age, and thus no specific recommendations regarding donor age have been established. Also, of note, CMV seropositivity prevalence is higher among older adults[96] and this may also account for some of the less favorable outcomes with advanced-age donors.

These data raise the challenging question of whether one should consider selecting a young unrelated donor over an older matched sibling donor. Transplant timing and insurance often dictate the use of an immediately available HLA-identical related donor over the delays in procuring an unrelated donor. Cord blood cells offer the opportunity for quick procurement of a donor although data are sparse among older adults. The longer duration of neutropenia associated with cord blood cell grafts remains a worrisome complication, especially for older patients where infection risk may be higher, and some have previously experienced long durations of neutropenia from prior therapy.

In our experience, procuring sibling donors for older adults poses unique challenges. Siblings will generally be older and may have concurrent health problems complicating or excluding donation. Not infrequently, the donor examination in older adults uncovers a new medical problem requiring further evaluation for donor safety. As a consequence, unanticipated delays may occur.

Table 30.2 HCST for older adults: published experience

| Author/Year | Age | | Donor | n | Regimen | Disease | TRM |
	Median	Range					Day (D)/year
Ditschkowski 2006[100]		50–67	Sib and MUD	214	Flu/cy/TBI Bu/cy Flu/cy/treo	Heme malig.	100 D, 13–30% 1 yr, 21–46%
Kroger 2006[103]	60	44–70	Sib and MUD	26	Flu/treo/ ATG	MDS, AML	100 D, 28%
Wallen 2005*[104]	63	60–68	Sib	52	Ablative regimens	Heme malig. MDS 67%	100 D, 27% 3 yr, 43%
Gupta 2005[102]	64	61–70	Sib	24	Flu/TBI	MDS, AML	100 D, 8% 2 yr, 25%
Corradini 2005[98]	59	55–69	Sib	160	Flu/thio/cy	Heme malig.	5 yr, 19%
Shimoni 2005[78]	58	56–66	MUD	36	Flu/bu/treo or Mel/ATG or Camp	Heme malig.	1 yr, 39%
Alyea 2005[68]	58	51–70	Sib and MUD	71	Flu/bu	Heme malig.	100 D, 6%
Weisser 2004[105]	51	45–62	Sib MUD	35	Flu/cy/TBI/ ATG	CML	100 D, 11% 1 yr, 29%
Alyea 2005[68]	54	51–66	Sib MUD	81	TBI/cy Bu/cy	Heme malig.	100 D, 30%
Shapira 2004[151]	63	60–67	Sib MUD	17	Flu/bu Flu/TBI, Bu alone	Heme malig.	100 D, 33%
Bertz 2003[67]	64	60–70	Sib MUD	19	Flu/mel/ carmustine +/– ATG	Myeloid	1 yr, 22%
Wong 2003[152]	59	55–69	Sib MUD	29	Flu/mel, Flu/bu +/– ATG for MUD	Myeloid	1 yr, 55%
de la Camara 2002[99]	53	50–59	Sib	32	Bu/cy TBI/cy	Myeloid	100 D, 9%
Deeg 2000*[72]	59	55–66	Sib	50	Bu/cy TBI/cy Bu/TBI	MDS	2 yr, 39%
Du 1998[101]		51–59	Sib	59	Bu/cy TBI/cy	Heme. malig	100 D, 24% 1 yr, 36%
REGISTRY STUDY							
Yanada 2004[106]	52	50–67		398			100 D, 17% 1 yr, 35%

* may report on similar patients.
TRM, transplant-related mortality; Sib, sibling donor; MUD, matched unrelated donor; Treo, treosulfan; Flu, fludarabine; Bu, busulfan; cy, cyclophosphamide; TBI, total body irradiation; ATG, antithymocyte globulin; Camp, alemtuzumab (CAMPATH); MDS, myelodysplastic syndromes; AML, acute myeloid leukemia; Heme malig., hematologic malignancies.

Outcomes

Early registry data indicated unfavorable outcomes for older transplant recipients,[97] yet only 80 of the over 2000 registered transplant patients were 50 years or older. Since that report, over a dozen sites have examined their HSCT experience in the context of advancing patient age.[67,68,72,78,79,98–106] Yet, the median age for all studies was below 65 years and patients were only rarely transplanted beyond 69 years of age. AML and myelodysplastic syndromes (MDS) represented the commonest indications, and regimen intensity varied from non-ablative to fully myeloablative. Many, but not all preparative regimens incorporated fludarabine. Limited insight into survival and disease control can be surmised due to variation in regimens, secular trends, and disease features. However, the toxicity as measured by TRM is instructive. TRM at day 100 in older adults ranged from 6% to 33% and was up to 55% at 1 year. Several authors highlighted the impact of GvHD on outcome.[99,100,106] GvHD occurs more commonly in older adults.[107] Ditschkowski and colleagues[100] showed by multivariable analysis that acute GvHD grades II–IV correlated with increased TRM and inferior survival (p < 0.0001). These data raise the concern that GvHD might not only be more frequent in older adults, but that it has a more detrimental impact as well. Although it is commonly postulated that modern transplantation procedures can be applied safely to patients over 50 years old,[72,79,99] a recent Japanese registry study found an association of age over 50 years with transplant-related and overall mortality.[106]

Clinical results

While most authors conclude that HSCT is feasible in older adults, supporting data are very limited and/or inconclusive. For instance, the definition of 'older' is often quite varied and has included in some series patients primarily between the ages of 40 and 60 years. In this transitional age group, an assessment of physical function and co-morbidities might distinguish those who require special attention on the basis of age.[73,108,109] Thus, as has been the case for cancer clinical investigation in general, the failure to enroll older subjects disallows confident extrapolation of trial results to the management of older patients.[110,111] In the field of transplantation, where a small number of transplants are performed among the large number of older patients diagnosed with hematologic malignancies, such selection bias is likely to be amplified. Patients must be sufficiently well to visit an HSCT center, meet criteria for HSCT, and remain alive long enough for insurance approval and donor identification. We have previously shown that unrecognized patient selection has a powerful and independent impact on HSCT outcome.[112]

Although disease factors are commonly reported and adjustments in planned treatment made, a more comprehensive assessment of health status may prove useful in clinical decision making. Unfortunately, almost no study offers details on health status, such as co-morbidities or performance status. Several recent studies highlighting the role of co-morbidities and functional status now offer a more precise method of estimating tolerance than age alone.[113,114]

Estimation of transplant tolerance

With the limited available evidence from clinical trials, potential benefits for a specific disease indication in older adults are estimated from results from younger subjects with similar disease features (e.g. disease type, remission status, disease features) and transplant characteristics (e.g. donor relation, degree of HLA matching, graft characteristics, CMV serologic status, GvHD prophylaxis, infectious disease supportive care). However, tolerance or risk of toxicity among older HSCT recipients remains largely unknown. Thus, a challenging paradox arises in that older age reduces transplant tolerance but chronologic age is likely to be an insufficient criterion for exclusion from HSCT. A certain percentage of older patients will tolerate transplant well, but we have yet to develop an index sufficiently sensitive to identify that subset. In this regard, measures of health status have considerable value in gauging toxicity and may be of prognostic value. Transplant-related mortality represents the most objective and least biased outcome in quantifying tolerance. Organ toxicity, quality of life, and GvHD are potentially quantifiable results, but the data remain limited in the context of age. Therefore, we focus primarily on TRM as a surrogate indicator of tolerance.

Age

On average, TRM rises (with advancing age) from both regimen toxicities and GvHD,[115–117] although many studies in selected populations show no difference in older adults. We recently evaluated the role of age and health status among 105 consecutively enrolled subjects with hematologic malignancies given a uniform reduced-intensity regimen with fludarabine, melphalan, and in vivo alemtuzumab T-cell depletion.[118] Sixty percent were at least 50 years of age. Older patients fared worse, with increased TRM on univariate analysis (p = 0.05). After adjusting for health and disease status, age differences were even more pronounced (hazard ratio (HR) = 3.2, p = 0.01), hinting that age may have an independent impact on outcome. Thus, while no age limits can be strictly applied, HSCT is infrequently undertaken in patients 60 years or older and rarely in those 70 years or greater.

Novel methods of estimating HSCT tolerance

Numerous measures have been tested in non-transplant settings to capture health status and predict outcome, including co-morbidity, functional measures, nutritional status, emotional state, socio-economic considerations, and genetic predisposition. In non-transplant oncology cohorts, simple methods of clinical assessment of health status have demonstrated remarkable ability to predict regimen toxicity and overall survival. Transplant physicians have begun to draw upon such measures, focusing primarily on co-morbid conditions and performance status (as a measure of functional status).

Co-morbidity

Co-morbid conditions are those co-existing medical diagnoses such as atherosclerosis, diabetes or cirrhosis, which in composite may significantly influence engraftment, toxicity and survival. In our parochial way, we naturally assign the malignancy as the primary and other diseases as co-morbidities. However, under certain circumstances, the co-existing illnesses may be of greater importance, rendering aggressive cancer treatment (HSCT in this case) of no value.

Routine clinical testing

Prior to transplantation, patients commonly undergo tests of pulmonary, liver, kidney, and cardiac functions, but experience has shown that these have limited value in predicting transplant outcome.[119] Such baseline testing, on the other hand, may offer greater predictive value for the older or less healthy prospective transplant recipient. Furthermore, organ-directed testing may facilitate the selection of a conditioning regimen or supportive care that minimizes toxicity while maintaining therapeutic efficacy (e.g. minimizing busulfan exposure with abnormal liver transaminases).

Co-morbidity Indices

Instruments have been developed and validated which predict various medical outcomes based upon an organized list of co-morbid conditions.[120–124] Typically, the number of medical conditions is tabulated and a summary score created. Although originally developed for epidemiologic studies, these assessments have become a central component of geriatric patient assessment and are also being tested in various clinical settings, including HSCT.

The Charlson Co-morbidity Index (CCI) is one of the most widely employed and simplest instruments.[125,126] Other indices validated in oncology include the Kaplan-Feinstein (KF),[127] Index of Co-existent Disease (ICED),[128] Cumulative Illness Rating Scale (CIRS),[129] reviewed in reference 110. Less sensitive scales (CCI and KF) are simpler and easier to apply, particularly for chart review, whereas more comprehensive measures (ICED, CIRS) may require more time and effort and/or prospective identification of conditions (CIRS).

Charlson Co-morbidity Index

Investigators from Seattle published the first evaluation of a validated co-morbidity medical index (CCI) on outcome after allogeneic transplant. In two simultaneous publications they reported that the CCI had moderate predictive value in recipients of related donor or unrelated donor allografts following non-ablative regimens.[108,109] Elevated CCI scores were found in over 50% of the recipients of non-ablative grafts but were infrequent in recipients of ablative conditioning. The high prevalence of high CCI scores was not surprising, since recipients of non-ablative conditioning regimens are older and less fit. CCI scores of 3 or greater, the typical threshold used in other studies showing adverse outcomes, were present in only 8–18% for non-ablative allografts and predicted for both grade IV toxicity and worse TRM. In contrast, a subsequent series by Sorror and colleagues retrospectively reviewing a large cohort of HSCT recipients at the Fred Hutchinson Cancer Center showed a much lower prevalence and predictive value of the CCI.[130] Eighty-seven percent of recipients had a normal pretransplant CCI (i.e. CCI = 0), and only 3% a CCI of 3 or greater. They found CCI scores were not statistically associated with increased non-relapse mortality although scores of 3 or above were associated with inferior survival.

Investigators at MD Anderson presented an abstract mirroring these results,[131] demonstrating that high CCI scores predicted for TRM among patients with MDS/AML receiving an allograft. We also reported similar findings among recipients of a fludarabine, melphalan, alemtuzumab regimen.[132] The CCI was >0 in only 27% of the 105 patients and an elevated score did not predict for TRM. Thus, in the context of HSCT, the CCI suffers from ceiling effects (most patients have normal scores) and appears to lack discriminative capacity.[73,85,108,109,113,131–133] Nevertheless, the CCI signifies an advance over single-organ objective testing in the ability to predict outcome and define high-risk patients.

Kaplan-Feinstein

We also analyzed the added benefit of the Kaplan-Feinstein Scale (KF) since it may be more sensitive but still amenable to chart review. KF identified one or more co-morbid conditions in 47% (49/105) (p < 0.0001 for the difference).[114] Scores of 2 or greater were present in 11% (12/105) by CCI compared to 24% (25/105) by KF (p = 0.004). Age was associated with increased co-morbidity as measured by CCI or KF. Among patients 50 years and over, a co-morbid condition was found in 37% by CCI and 57% by KF, compared to 12% by CCI and 31% by KF for younger subjects (p = 0.005 for CCI and p = 0.008 for KF between younger and older subjects). Thus, KF was more sensitive, and co-morbidity occurred more frequently in older subjects, even among the select subset who received HSCT.

Hematopoietic Cell Transplantation-Specific Co-morbidity Index

The Seattle Group extended their findings on the CCI to develop a more sensitive and validated index specific to allogeneic transplant.

This hematopoietic cell transplantation-specific co-morbidity index (HCT-CI) added individual co-morbid conditions and abnormal laboratory parameters (e.g. serum creatinine, abnormal pulmonary function testing) that predicted worse outcome on univariate analysis, to the standard CCI score.[113] Discriminative capacity was enhanced as the range of scores was 0–11 for the HCT-CI compared to 0–4 for the CCI. The HCT-CI scored diagnoses in 62% of patients compared to only 12% using the CCI. Only scores of 3 or greater on the HCT-CI (present in 28% of this high-risk cohort) predicted a worse outcome. At 2 years, TRM was increased (HR = 3.5, 95% confidence interval (CI) 2.0–6.3) and overall survival was less (HR = 2.7, 95% CI 1.8–4.1).

Functional assessment

In addition to an assessment of co-morbidity, geriatricians have demonstrated the value of functional assessment gauging health status and predicting clinical outcomes.[134] The concept is not new, in fact oncologists rely on assessments of performance status (PS), such as the Karnofsky score or the Eastern Co-operative Oncology Group Performances Scale (ECOG PS), both of which might be considered a short form of functional assessment. In fact, Karnofsky and ECOG PS have excellent interobserver and intraobserver reliability.[135] For the purposes of patient assessment prior to HSCT, developing and validating an expanded functional assessment instrument are currently under way. Such an expanded assessment would be likely to include measures of daily activity (e.g. can the person cook for themselves?) and performance-based measures, such as a timed walk. In other clinical settings, combining multiple functional measures permits prognostic assessment even in high-functioning adults.[136,137] Among older adults, measurable functional impairments are frequent[123] and highly predictive of outcome, independent of co-morbid conditions.[134,138] Similarly, functional status and co-morbidity independently predict toxicity and survival in older cancer patients.[120,121,139]

For such an expanded assessment to become standard of care for HSCT, it would be essential that it show added value over the standard Karnofsky or ECOG PS. These measures have not been frequently reported in HSCT studies, but when they have, PS remains a powerful, and probably underappreciated, predictor of HSCT survival.[73,132,140–142] ECOG PS ≥ 2 appears a critical threshold, where adverse outcomes are strongly increased. However, even among older or less fit HSCT recipients, PS ≥ 2 is found in less than 10% of subjects.[74,114] In one study of non-HSCT subjects, Repetto and colleagues found 37% of subjects with PS < 2 had limitations in normal daily activities (i.e. abnormal instrumental activities of daily living),[121] affirming the concept that additional measures of functional impairment may supplement overall assessment and thereby improve prognostic evaluation. No studies of functional measures, other than PS, have yet to be reported in the HSCT setting.

Combining PS and co-morbidity

To increase sensitivity in recognizing patients at high risk of reduced transplant tolerance, we capitalized on the independent impact of co-morbidity and PS.[114] We evaluated 105 recipients of a reduced-intensity preparative regimen of fludarabine, melphalan, and alemtuzumab. Established high-risk features of KF co-morbidity score of >3 or an ECOG PS = 2 (eligibility for the protocol was limited to a PS of ≤2) were allocated to the high-risk group. However, many subjects fell into an intermediate category of PS = 1 and KF = 1–2, traditionally considered lower risk. By placing transplant recipients with both KF and PS scores above 0 in the high-risk group, we found the combined measure useful for predicting TRM (HR = 4.6, 95% CI 2.1–10.2) and overall survival (OS) (HR = 3.2, 95% CI 1.8–6.2) (Table 30.3). The 6-month cumulative incidence of TRM was 50% for high-risk

Table 30.3 Multivariate analysis of pretransplant factors on outcome

Characteristic*	Transplant-related mortality		Overall survival	
	HR	p-value	HR	p-value
Age ≥50 years	3.2	0.01	2.2	0.016
Disease status (active)	2.5	0.04	3.3	0.0009
Donor, unrelated	1.1	0.76	1.8	0.05
Donor, mismatch	3.5	0.03	2.7	0.04
Prior transplant	4.1	0.007	2.8	0.002
DLCO <78	1.4	0.35	1.9	0.03
Ejection fraction <55%	0.92	0.84	1.4	0.31
Charlson Co-morbidity Index ≥1	0.94	0.88	1.5	0.2
Kaplan-Feinstein ≥1	2.0	0.08	2.5	0.004
Performance status ≥1	2.3	0.03	2.3	0.006
Risk group, high†	4.6	0.0002	3.4	0.0001

* Adjusted for age, disease risk, HLA mismatch, and prior transplant, when applicable.
† Risk group combines the Kaplan-Feinstein Scale and performance status.

compared to 15% for low-risk patients (p = 0.001). After adjustment for disease status, the differences in the overall cumulative incidence of TRM (p = 0.0002) and OS (p = 0.0001) persisted (see Table 30.3). Finally, this high-risk group was predictive when restricting the analysis to older adults, although the sample size was small.

Interestingly, results were fairly similar to the Seattle HCT-CI, and both identified about 25% of patients who would be considered at high risk for TRM. Further, both scales predicted for worse overall survival, even after adjusting for disease status. Such studies have laid the groundwork for future investigation aimed at predicting transplant tolerance.

Other domains

Additional considerations in health status determination of older individuals include mental status, emotional status, social support, geriatric syndromes, and nutrition. More recently, proinflammatory cytokines, such as C-reactive protein (CRP) or interleukin 6, have become an important tool in risk stratifying older adults for important outcomes such as functional decline, increased cardiac events, and increased mortality.[143–145] While not studied as a pretransplant predictor for HSCT, changes in CRP from baseline to after conditioning have been shown to strongly predict HSCT outcome.[146,147]

The impact of these domains on HSCT outcome remains unknown in older adults. Comprehensive geriatric assessments incorporating domains in addition to co-morbid conditions and functional status outside the HSCT setting can identify additional problems and possibly improve outcome.[148,149] Future studies are warranted with complete geriatric assessment for older and/or at-risk individuals of poor HSCT tolerance. The considerable acute and chronic toxicities from HSCT place a tremendous physiologic stress on patients which may unmask subtle abnormalities, leading to potentially devastating complications. For example, dementia is strongly associated with advancing age and highly predicts for hospital delirium. Delirium is a common complication after HSCT, occurring in up to 50% of HCT recipients.[150] Cognitive evaluation of older adults may thus indicate delirium risk and allow preventive strategies.

Additional value of health status measures

The prediction of TRM and survival in HSCT recipients by health status measures has an obvious role for individual decision making.

Patients can be more accurately counseled regarding the precise risks of transplant, and potentially the risk/benefit ratio. The health measures also hold promise for generalizability of study results. Knowing the health status of individuals should enhance comparisons across studies and identify precisely which older adults should be considered for HSCT.

Determining health status measures, such as by a modification of the comprehensive geriatric assessment to estimate transplant tolerance, has become an active research issue. There remain many unanswered questions requiring prospective investigation. Can monitoring or treatment of pretransplant limitations improve outcome? Will alterations in the treatment regimen (RIC and/or T-cell depletion) mitigate complications in high-risk patients? Most importantly, will the decision to pursue HSCT be influenced by the additional information afforded by such an assessment?

Conclusion

Allografts are increasingly being used to treat hematologic malignancies in older adults. Although age alone should not be a contraindication to HSCT, the precise risk/benefit ratio for older adults in general remains undefined. Certain older adults can undergo allogeneic transplant with reasonable tolerance and reasonably good success. We have learned that chronological age and assessment of performance status (i.e. ECOG or Karnofsky) provide some predictive value but a more refined assessment that includes measures of co-morbidity and physical function is likely to enhance estimates of transplant risk and inform decision making. The question is more than academic; the number of patients for whom HSCT offers the greatest likelihood of treatment success will be growing exponentially over the next several decades and there remains a lack of evidence on how best to proceed with transplantation recommendations.

References

1. Storb R, Thomas ED. Allogeneic bone-marrow transplantation. Immunol Rev 1983;71:77–102
2. Lindeman RD. Overview: renal physiology and pathophysiology of aging. Am J Kidney Dis 1990;16(4):275–282
3. Geiger H, van Zant G. The aging of lympho-hematopoietic stem cells. Nat Immunol 2002;3(4):329–333
4. Harrison DE. Proliferative capacity of erythropoietic stem cell lines and aging: an overview. Mechanisms of ageing and development 1979;9(5–6):409–426
5. Harrison DE, Astle CM, Stone M. Numbers and functions of transplantable primitive immunohematopoietic stem cells. Effects of age. J Immunol 1989;142(11):3833–3840
6. Miller RA. The aging immune system: primer and prospectus. Science 1996;273(5271):70–74
7. Dubrow EL. Reactivation of tuberculosis: a problem of aging. J Am Geriatr Soc 1976;24(11):481–487
8. Nagami PH, Yoshikawa TT. Tuberculosis in the geriatric patient. J Am Geriatr Soc 1983;31(6):356–363
9. Schmader K. Herpes zoster in the elderly: issues related to geriatrics. Clin Infect Dis 1999;24(3):736–739.
10. Goodwin K, Viboud C, Simonsen L. Antibody response to influenza vaccination in the elderly: a quantitative review. Vaccine 2006;24(8):1159–1169
11. Potter JM, O'Donnel B, Carman WF et al. Serological response to influenza vaccination and nutritional and functional status of patients in geriatric medical long-term care. Age Ageing 1999;28(2):141–145
12. Balducci L, Aapro M. Epidemiology of cancer and aging. Cancer Treat Res 2005;124:1–15
13. Kaesberg PR, Ershler WB. The importance of immunesenescence in the incidence and malignant properties of cancer in hosts of advanced age. J Gerontol 1989;44(6):63–66
14. Ershler WB, Gamelli RL, Moore AL et al. Experimental tumors and aging: local factors that may account for the observed age advantage in the B16 murine melanoma model. Exp Gerontol 1984;19(6):367–376
15. Rockwell S. Effect of host age on the transplantation, growth, and radiation response of EMT6 tumors. Cancer Res 1981;41(2):527–531
16. Stjernsward J. Age-dependent tumor-host barrier and effect of carcinogen-induced immunodepression on rejection of isografted methylcholanthrene-induced sarcoma cells. J Natl Cancer Inst 1966;37(4):505–512
17. Yuhas JM, Pazmino NH, Proctor JO, Toya RE. A direct relationship between immune competence and the subcutaneous growth rate of a malignant murine lung tumor. Cancer Res 1974;34(4):722–728

18. Christensen K, Vaupel JW. Determinants of longevity: genetic, environmental and medical factors. Journal of internal medicine 1996;240(6):333–341

19. Oeppen J, Vaupel JW. Demography. Broken limits to life expectancy. Science 2002;296(5570):1029–1031

20. Orr WC, Sohal RS. Extension of life-span by overexpression of superoxide dismutase and catalase in Drosophila melanogaster. Science 1994;263(5150):1128–1130

21. Masoro EJ. Overview of caloric restriction and ageing. Mechanisms of ageing and development 2005;126(9):913–922

22. Heilbronn LK, de Jonge L, Frisard MI et al. Effect of 6-month calorie restriction on biomarkers of longevity, metabolic adaptation, and oxidative stress in overweight individuals: a randomized controlled trial. JAMA 2006;295(13):1539–1548

23. Blanc S, Schoeller D, Kemnitz J et al. Energy expenditure of rhesus monkeys subjected to 11 years of dietary restriction. J Clin Endocrinol Metab 2003;88(1):16–23

24. Mattison JA, Roth GS, Lane MA, Ingram DK. Dietary restriction in aging nonhuman primates. Interdisciplin Topics Gerontol 2007;35:137–158

25. Powers DC, Sears SD, Murphy BR et al. Systemic and local antibody responses in elderly subjects given live or inactivated influenza A virus vaccines. J Clin Microbiol 1989;27(12):2666–2671

26. Smith NM, Shay DK. Influenza vaccination for elderly people and their care workers. Lancet 2006;368(9549):1752–1753

27. Gatti RA, Good RA. Aging, immunity, and malignancy. Geriatrics 1970;25(9):158–168

28. Bulychev VV. [Longevity, atherosclerosis and cellular immunity.] Klin Med (Mosk) 1993;71(5):51–54

29. Lehuen A, Bendelac A, Bach JF, Carnaud C. The nonobese diabetic mouse model. Independent expression of humoral and cell-mediated autoimmune features. J Immunol 1990;144(6):2147–2151

30. Hull M, Fiebich BL, Lieb K et al. Interleukin-6-associated inflammatory processes in Alzheimer's disease: new therapeutic options. Neurobiol Aging 1996;17(5):795–800

31. Hull M, Strauss S, Berger M et al. The participation of interleukin-6, a stress-inducible cytokine, in the pathogenesis of Alzheimer's disease. Behav Brain Res 1996;78(1):37–41

32. Gillis S, Kozak R, Durante M, Weksler ME. Immunological studies of aging. Decreased production of and response to T cell growth factor by lymphocytes from aged humans. J Clin Invest 1981;67(4):937–942

33. Effros RB, Cai Z, Linton PJ. CD8 T cells and aging. Crit Rev Immunol 2003;23(1–2):45–64

34. Globerson A, Effros RB. Ageing of lymphocytes and lymphocytes in the aged. Immunol Today 2000;21(10):515–521

35. Grubeck-Loebenstein B, Wick G. The aging of the immune system. Adv Immunol 2002;80:243–284

36. Stephan RP, Sanders VM, Witte PL. Stage-specific alterations in murine B lymphopoiesis with age. Int Immunol 1996;8(4):509–518

37. Blade J, Rosinol L. Smoldering multiple myeloma and monoclonal gammopathy of undetermined significance. Curr Treatment Options Oncol 2006;7(3):237–245

38. Kyle RA, Rajkumar SV. Monoclonal gammopathy of undetermined significance. Br J Haematol 2006;134(6):573–589

39. Thoman ML, Weigle WO. Lymphokines and aging: interleukin-2 production and activity in aged animals. J Immunol 1981;127(5):2102–2106

40. Ershler WB, Sun WH, Binkley N et al. Interleukin-6 and aging: blood levels and mononuclear cell production increase with advancing age and in vitro production is modifiable by dietary restriction. Lymphokine Cytokine Res 1993;12(4):225–230

41. Ershler WB, Keller ET. Age-associated increased interleukin-6 gene expression, late-life diseases, and frailty. Annu Rev Med 2000;51:245–270

42. Holmes FF. Clinical evidence for a change in tumor aggressiveness with age. Semin Oncol 1989;16(1):34–40

43. Ershler WB, Stewart JA, Hacker MP et al. B16 murine melanoma and aging: slower growth and longer survival in old mice. J Natl Cancer Inst 1984;72(1):161–164

44. Tsuda T, Kim YT, Siskind GW et al. Role of the thymus and T-cells in slow growth of B16 melanoma in old mice. Cancer Res 1987;47(12):3097–3100

45. Ershler WB, Moore AL, Shore H, Gamelli RL. Transfer of age-associated restrained tumor growth in mice by old-to-young bone marrow transplantation. Cancer Res 1984;44(12 Pt 1):5677–5680

46. Prehn RT. The immune reaction as a stimulator of tumor growth. Science 1972;176(31):170–171

47. Prehn RT, Lappe MA. An immunostimulation theory of tumor development. Transplant Rev 1971;7:26–54

48. Harrison DE. Normal function of transplanted mouse erythrocyte precursors for 21 months beyond donor life spans. Nature: New Biol 1972;237(76):220–222

49. Siminovitch L, Till JE, McCulloch EA. Decline in colony-forming ability of marrow cells subjected to serial transplantation into irradiated mice. J Cell Physiol 1964;64:23–31

50. Ogden DA, Mickliem HS. The fate of serially transplanted bone marrow cell populations from young and old donors. Transplantation 1976;22(3):287–293

51. Janzen V, Forkert R, Fleming HE et al. Stem-cell ageing modified by the cyclin-dependent kinase inhibitor p16INK4a. Nature 2006;443(7110):421–426

52. Artz AS, Fergusson D, Drinka PJ et al. Mechanisms of unexplained anemia in the nursing home. J Am Geriatr Soc 2004;52(3):423–427

53. Guralnik JM, Eisenstaedt RS, Ferrucci L et al. Prevalence of anemia in persons 65 years and older in the United States: evidence for a high rate of unexplained anemia. Blood 2004;104(8):2263–2268

54. Appelbaum FR, Gundacker H, Head DR et al. Age and acute myeloid leukemia. Blood 2006;107(9):3481–3485

55. Leith CP, Kopecky KJ, Godwin J et al. Acute myeloid leukemia in the elderly: assessment of multidrug resistance (MDR1) and cytogenetics distinguishes biologic subgroups with remarkably distinct responses to standard chemotherapy. A Southwest Oncology Group study. Blood 1997;89(9):3323–3329

56. Farag SS, Archer KJ, Mrozek K et al. Pretreatment cytogenetics add to other prognostic factors predicting complete remission and long-term outcome in patients 60 years of age or older with acute myeloid leukemia: results from Cancer and Leukemia Group B 8461. Blood 2006;108(1):63–73

57. Rowe JM, Andersen JW, Mazza JJ et al. A randomized placebo-controlled phase III study of granulocyte-macrophage colony-stimulating factor in adult patients (>55 to 70 years of age) with acute myelogenous leukemia: a study of the Eastern Cooperative Oncology Group (E1490). Blood 1995;86(2):457–462

58. Menzin J, Lang K, Earle CC et al. The outcomes and costs of acute myeloid leukemia among the elderly. Arch Intern Med 2002;162(14):1597–1603

59. Larson RA. Management of acute lymphoblastic leukemia in older patients. Semin Hematol 2006;43(2):126–133

60. Ershler WB, Longo DL. A report card for geriatric oncology: borderline pass, improvement needed. J Gerontol 2006;61(7):688

61. Jemal A, Siegel R, Ward E et al. Cancer statistics, 2006. CA Cancer J Clin 2006;56(2):106–130

62. Gratwohl A, Baldomero H, Frauendorfer K, Urbano-Ispizua A. EBMT activity survey 2004 and changes in disease indication over the past 15 years. Bone Marrow Transplant 2006;37(12):1069–1085

63. Clift RA, Buckner CD, Appelbaum FR et al. Allogeneic marrow transplantation in patients with acute myeloid leukemia in first remission: a randomized trial of two irradiation regimens. Blood 1990;76(10):1867–1871

64. Clift RA, Appelbaum FR, Thomas ED. Treatment of chronic myeloid leukemia by marrow transplantation. Blood 1993;82(7):1954–1956

65. Giralt S, Estey E, Albitar M et al. Engraftment of allogeneic hematopoietic progenitor cells with purine analog-containing chemotherapy: harnessing graft-versus-leukemia without myeloablative therapy. Blood 1997;89(12):4531–4536

66. Slavin S, Nagler A, Naparstek E et al. Nonmyeloablative stem cell transplantation and cell therapy as an alternative to conventional bone marrow transplantation with lethal cytoreduction for the treatment of malignant and nonmalignant hematologic diseases. Blood 1998;91(3):756–763

67. Bertz H, Potthoff K, Finke J. Allogeneic stem-cell transplantation from related and unrelated donors in older patients with myeloid leukemia. J Clin Oncol 2003;21(8):1480–1484

68. Alyea EP, Kim HT, Ho V et al. Comparative outcome of nonmyeloablative and myeloablative allogeneic hematopoietic cell transplantation for patients older than 50 years of age. Blood 2005;105(4):1810–1814

69. Canals C, Martino R, Sureda A et al. Strategies to reduce transplant-related mortality after allogeneic stem cell transplantation in elderly patients: Comparison of reduced-intensity conditioning and unmanipulated peripheral blood stem cells vs a myeloablative regimen and CD34+ cell selection. Exp Hematol 2003;31(11):1039–1043

70. Couriel DR, Saliba RM, Giralt S et al. Acute and chronic graft-versus-host disease after ablative and nonmyeloablative conditioning for allogeneic hematopoietic transplantation. Biol Blood Marrow Transplant 2004;10(3):178–185

71. de Lima M, Couriel D, Thall PF et al. Once-daily intravenous busulfan and fludarabine: clinical and pharmacokinetic results of a myeloablative, reduced-toxicity conditioning regimen for allogeneic stem cell transplantation in AML and MDS. Blood 2004;104(3):857–864

72. Deeg HJ, Shulman HM, Anderson JE et al. Allogeneic and syngeneic marrow transplantation for myelodysplastic syndrome in patients 55 to 66 years of age. Blood 2000;95(4):1188–1194

73. Giralt S, Thall PF, Khouri I et al. Melphalan and purine analog-containing preparative regimens: reduced-intensity conditioning for patients with hematologic malignancies undergoing allogeneic progenitor cell transplantation. Blood 2001;97(3):631–637

74. Gomez-Nunez M, Martino R, Caballero MD et al. Elderly age and prior autologous transplantation have a deleterious effect on survival following allogeneic peripheral blood stem cell transplantation with reduced-intensity conditioning: results from the Spanish multicenter prospective trial. Bone Marrow Transplant 2004;33(5):477–482

75. Hamaki T, Kami M, Kim SW et al. Reduced-intensity stem cell transplantation from an HLA-identical sibling donor in patients with myeloid malignancies. Bone Marrow Transplant 2004;33(9):891–900

76. Martino R, Caballero MD, Simon JA et al. Evidence for a graft-versus-leukemia effect after allogeneic peripheral blood stem cell transplantation with reduced-intensity conditioning in acute myelogenous leukemia and myelodysplastic syndromes. Blood 2002;100(6):2243–2245

77. Picardi A, Fabritiis Pd P, Cudillo L et al. Possibility of long-term remission in patients with advanced hematologic malignancies after reduced intensity conditioning regimen (RIC) and allogeneic stem cell transplantation. Hematol J 2004;5(1):24–31

78. Shimoni A, Kroger N, Zabelina T et al. Hematopoietic stem-cell transplantation from unrelated donors in elderly patients (age >55 years) with hematologic malignancies: older age is no longer a contraindication when using reduced intensity conditioning. Leukemia 2005;19(1):7–12

79. Wong R, Giralt SA, Martin T et al. Reduced-intensity conditioning for unrelated donor hematopoietic stem cell transplantation as treatment for myeloid malignancies in patients older than 55 years. Blood 2003;102(8):3052–3059

80. Martino R, Iacobelli S, Brand R et al. Retrospective comparison of reduced intensity conditioning and conventional high dose conditioning for allogeneic hematopoietic stem cell transplantation using HLA identical sibling donors in myelodysplastic syndromes. Blood 2006;108(3):836–846

81. de Lima M, Anagnostopoulos A, Munsell M et al. Nonablative versus reduced-intensity conditioning regimens in the treatment of acute myeloid leukemia and high-risk myelodysplastic syndrome: dose is relevant for long-term disease control after allogeneic hematopoietic stem cell transplantation. Blood 2004;104(3):865–872

82. Slattery JT, Clift RA, Buckner CD et al. Marrow transplantation for chronic myeloid leukemia: the influence of plasma busulfan levels on the outcome of transplantation. Blood 1997;89(8):3055–3060

83. Kiehl MG, Kraut L, Schwerdtfeger R et al. Outcome of allogeneic hematopoietic stem-cell transplantation in adult patients with acute lymphoblastic leukemia: no difference in related compared with unrelated transplant in first complete remission. J Clin Oncol 2004;22(14):2816–2825
84. Weisdorf DJ, Anasetti C, Antin JH et al. Allogeneic bone marrow transplantation for chronic myelogenous leukemia: comparative analysis of unrelated versus matched sibling donor transplantation. Blood 2002;99(6):1971–1977
85. van Besien K, Artz A, Stock W. Unrelated donor transplantation over the age of 55. Are we merely getting (b)older? Leukemia 2005;19(1):31–33
86. Herbrecht R, Denning DW, Patterson TF et al. Voriconazole versus amphotericin B for primary therapy of invasive aspergillosis. N Engl J Med 2002;347(6):408–415
87. Kline J, Pollyea DA, Stock W et al. Pre-transplant ganciclovir and post transplant high-dose valacyclovir reduce CMV infections after alemtuzumab-based conditioning. Bone Marrow Transplant 2006;37(3):307–310
88. Ljungman P, de la Camara R, Milpied N et al. Randomized study of valacyclovir as prophylaxis against cytomegalovirus reactivation in recipients of allogeneic bone marrow transplants. Blood 2002;99(8):3050–3056
89. Nichols WG, Corey L, Gooley T et al. Rising pp65 antigenemia during preemptive anti-cytomegalovirus therapy after allogeneic hematopoietic stem cell transplantation: risk factors, correlation with DNA load, and outcomes. Blood 2001;97(4):867–874
90. Manton KG, Corder L, Stallard E. Chronic disability trends in elderly United States populations: 1982–1994. Proc Natl Acad Sci USA 1997;94(6):2593–2598
91. Kollman C, Howe CW, Anasetti C et al. Donor characteristics as risk factors in recipients after transplantation of bone marrow from unrelated donors: the effect of donor age. Blood 2001;98(7):2043–2051
92. Mehta J, Gordon LI, Tallman MS et al. Does younger donor age affect the outcome of reduced-intensity allogeneic hematopoietic stem cell transplantation for hematologic malignancies beneficially? Bone Marrow Transplant 2006;38(2):95–100
93. Engelhardt M, Bertz H, Wasch R, Finke J. Analysis of stem cell apheresis products using intermediate-dose filgrastim plus large volume apheresis for allogeneic transplantation. Ann Hematol 2001;80(4):201–208
94. Morris CL, Siegel E, Barlogie B et al. Mobilization of CD34+ cells in elderly patients (>/=70 years) with multiple myeloma: influence of age, prior therapy, platelet count and mobilization regimen. Br J Haematol 2003;120(3):413–423
95. Davies SM, Kollman C, Anasetti C et al. Engraftment and survival after unrelated-donor bone marrow transplantation: a report from the national marrow donor program. Blood 2000;96(13):4096–4102
96. Broers AE, van der Holt R, van Esser JW et al. Increased transplant-related morbidity and mortality in CMV-seropositive patients despite highly effective prevention of CMV disease after allogeneic T-cell-depleted stem cell transplantation. Blood 2000;95(7):2240–2245
97. Ringden O, Horowitz MM, Gale RP et al. Outcome after allogeneic bone marrow transplant for leukemia in older adults. JAMA 1993;270(1):57–60
98. Corradini P, Zallio F, Mariotti J et al. Effect of age and previous autologous transplantation on nonrelapse mortality and survival in patients treated with reduced-intensity conditioning and allografting for advanced hematologic malignancies. J Clin Oncol 2005;23(27):6690–6698.
99. de la Camara R, Alonso A, Steegmann JL et al. Allogeneic hematopoietic stem cell transplantation in patients 50 years of age and older. Haematologica 2002;87(9):965–972
100. Ditschkowski M, Elmaagacli AH, Trenschel R et al. Myeloablative allogeneic hematopoietic stem cell transplantation in elderly patients. Clin Transplant 2006;20(1):127–131
101. Du W, Dansey R, Abella EM et al. Successful allogeneic bone marrow transplantation in selected patients over 50 years of age – a single institution's experience. Bone Marrow Transplant 1998;21(10):1043–1047
102. Gupta V, Daly A, Lipton JH et al. Nonmyeloablative stem cell transplantation for myelodysplastic syndrome or acute myeloid leukemia in patients 60 years or older. Biol Blood Marrow Transplant 2005;11(10):764–772
103. Kroger N, Shimoni A, Zabelina T et al. Reduced-toxicity conditioning with treosulfan, fludarabine and ATG as preparative regimen for allogeneic stem cell transplantation (alloSCT) in elderly patients with secondary acute myeloid leukemia (sAML) or myelodysplastic syndrome (MDS). Bone Marrow Transplant 2006;37(4):339–344
104. Wallen H, Gooley TA, Deeg HJ et al. Ablative allogeneic hematopoietic cell transplantation in adults 60 years of age and older. J Clin Oncol 2005;23(15):3439–3446
105. Weisser M, Schleuning M, Ledderose G et al. Reduced-intensity conditioning using TBI (8 Gy), fludarabine, cyclophosphamide and ATG in elderly CML patients provides excellent results especially when performed in the early course of the disease. Bone Marrow Transplant 2004;34(12):1083–1088
106. Yanada M, Emi N, Naoe T et al. Allogeneic myeloablative transplantation for patients aged 50 years and over. Bone Marrow Transplant 2004;34(1):29–35
107. Carlens S, Ringden O, Remberger M et al. Risk factors for chronic graft-versus-host disease after bone marrow transplantation: a retrospective single centre analysis. Bone Marrow Transplant 1998;22(8):755–761
108. Diaconescu R, Flowers CR, Storer B et al. Morbidity and mortality with nonmyeloablative compared with myeloablative conditioning before hematopoietic cell transplantation from HLA-matched related donors. Blood 2004;104(5):1550–1558
109. Sorror ML, Maris MB, Storer B et al. Comparing morbidity and mortality of HLA-matched unrelated donor hematopoietic cell transplantation after nonmyeloablative and myeloablative conditioning: influence of pretransplantation comorbidities. Blood 2004;104(4):961–968
110. Extermann M. Measurement and impact of comorbidity in older cancer patients. Crit Rev Oncol Hematol 2000;35(3):181–200
111. Talarico L, Chen G, Pazdur R. Enrollment of elderly patients in clinical trials for cancer drug registration: a 7-year experience by the US Food and Drug Administration. J Clin Oncol 2004;22(22):4626–4631
112. Artz AS, van Besien K, Zimmerman T et al. Long-term follow-up of nonmyeloablative allogeneic stem cell transplantation for renal cell carcinoma: The University of Chicago Experience. Bone Marrow Transplant 2005;35(3):253–260
113. Sorror ML, Maris MB, Storb R et al. Hematopoietic cell transplantation-specific comorbidity index: a new tool for risk assessment before allogeneic HCT. Blood 2005;106(8):2912–2919
114. Artz AS, Pollyea DA, Kocherginsky M et al. Performance status and comorbidity predict transplant-related mortality after allogeneic hematopoietic cell transplantation. Biol Blood Marrow Transplant 2006;12(9):954–964
115. Cahn JY, Labopin M, Schattenberg A et al. Allogeneic bone marrow transplantation for acute leukemia in patients over the age of 40 years. Acute Leukemia Working Party of the European Group for Bone Marrow Transplantation (EBMT). Leukemia 1997;11(3):416–419
116. Klingemann HG, Storb R, Fefer A et al. Bone marrow transplantation in patients aged 45 years and older. Blood 1986;67(3):770–776
117. Przepiorka D, Smith TL, Folloder J et al. Risk factors for acute graft-versus-host disease after allogeneic blood stem cell transplantation. Blood 1999;94(4):1465–1470
118. Artz AS. Comorbidity and beyond: pre-transplant clinical assessment. Bone Marrow Transplant 2005;36(6):473–474
119. Alamo J, Shahjahan M, Lazarus HM et al. Comorbidity indices in hematopoietic stem cell transplantation: a new report card. Bone Marrow Transplant 2005;36(6):475–479
120. Firat S, Bousamra M, Gore E, Byhardt RW. Comorbidity and KPS are independent prognostic factors in stage I non-small-cell lung cancer. Int J Radiat Oncol Biol Phys 2002;52(4):1047–1057
121. Repetto L, Fratino L, Audisio RA et al. Comprehensive geriatric assessment adds information to Eastern Cooperative Oncology Group performance status in elderly cancer patients: an Italian Group for Geriatric Oncology Study. J Clin Oncol 2002;20(2):494–502
122. Yancik R, Ganz PA, Varricchio CG, Conley B. Perspectives on comorbidity and cancer in older patients: approaches to expand the knowledge base. J Clin Oncol 2001;19(4):1147–1151
123. Yancik R, Havlik RJ, Wesley MN et al. Cancer and comorbidity in older patients: a descriptive profile. Ann Epidemiol 1996;6(5):399–412
124. Yancik R, Wesley MN, Ries LA et al. Effect of age and comorbidity in postmenopausal breast cancer patients aged 55 years and older. JAMA 2001;285(7):885–892
125. Charlson M, Szatrowski TP, Peterson J, Gold J. Validation of a combined comorbidity index. J Clin Epidemiol 1994;47(11):1245–1251
126. Charlson ME, Pompei P, Ales KL, MacKenzie CR. A new method of classifying prognostic comorbidity in longitudinal studies: development and validation. J Chronic Dis 1987;40(5):373–383
127. Kaplan MH, Feinstein AR. The importance of classifying initial co-morbidity in evaluating the outcome of diabetes mellitus. J Chronic Dis 1974;27(7–8):387–404
128. Imamura K, McKinnon M, Middleton R, Black N. Reliability of a comorbidity measure: the Index of Co-Existent Disease (ICED). J Clin Epidemiol 1997;50(9):1011–1016
129. Linn BS, Linn MW, Gurel L. Cumulative Illness Rating Scale. J Am Geriatr Soc 1968;16(5):622–626
130. Sorror M, Maris M, Diaconescu R, Storb R. Lessened severe graft-versus-host after 'minitransplantations'. Blood 2005;105(6):2614
131. Shahjahan M, Alamo J, de Lima M, Khouri I. Effect of comorbidities on allogeneic hematopoietic stem cell transplant outcomes in AML/MDS patients in first complete remission. Biol Blood Marrow Transplant 2004;10(suppl):1
132. van Besien K, Artz A, Smith S et al. Fludarabine, melphalan, and alemtuzumab conditioning in adults with standard-risk advanced acute myeloid leukemia and myelodysplastic syndrome. J Clin Oncol 2005;23(24):5728–5738
133. Pollyea DA, Artz AS, Stock W et al. Clinical predictors of transplant related mortality after reduced intensity conditioning allogeneic stem cell transplantation (RIST). Blood 2004;104(11):Abstract 1145
134. Inouye SK, Peduzzi PN, Robison JT et al. Importance of functional measures in predicting mortality among older hospitalized patients. JAMA 1998;279(15):1187–1193
135. Roila F, Lupattelli M, Sassi M et al. Intra and interobserver variability in cancer patients' performance status assessed according to Karnofsky and ECOG scales. Ann Oncol 1991;2(6):437–439
136. Guralnik JM, Ferrucci L, Simonsick EM et al. Lower-extremity function in persons over the age of 70 years as a predictor of subsequent disability. N Engl J Med 1995;332(9):556–561
137. Reuben DB, Seeman TE, Keeler E et al. Refining the categorization of physical functional status: the added value of combining self-reported and performance-based measures. J Gerontol 2004;59(10):M1056–M1061
138. Lee SJ, Lindquist K, Segal MR, Covinsky KE. Development and validation of a prognostic index for 4-year mortality in older adults. JAMA 2006;295(7):801–808
139. Extermann M, Overcash J, Lyman GH et al. Comorbidity and functional status are independent in older cancer patients. J Clin Oncol 1998;16(4):1582–1587
140. Sayer HG, Kroger M, Beyer J et al. Reduced intensity conditioning for allogeneic hematopoietic stem cell transplantation in patients with acute myeloid leukemia: disease status by marrow blasts is the strongest prognostic factor. Bone Marrow Transplant 2003;31(12):1089–1095
141. van Besien K, Sobocinski KA, Rowlings PA et al. Allogeneic bone marrow transplantation for low-grade lymphoma. Blood 1998;92(5):1832–1836
142. Wong R, Shahjahan M, Wang X et al. Prognostic factors for outcomes of patients with refractory or relapsed acute myelogenous leukemia or myelodysplastic syndromes undergoing allogeneic progenitor cell transplantation. Biol Blood Marrow Transplant 2005;11(2):108–114
143. Harris TB, Ferrucci L, Tracy RP et al. Associations of elevated interleukin-6 and C-reactive protein levels with mortality in the elderly. Am J Med 1999;106(5):506–512
144. Masotti L, Ceccarelli E, Forconi S, Cappelli R. Prognostic role of C-reactive protein in very old patients with acute ischaemic stroke. J Intern med 2005;258(2):145–152
145. Penninx BW, Kritchevsky SB, Newman AB et al. Inflammatory markers and incident mobility limitation in the elderly. J Am Geriatr Soc 2004;52(7):1105–1113
146. Min CK, Kim SY, Eom KS et al. Patterns of C-reactive protein release following allogeneic stem cell transplantation are correlated with leukemic relapse. Bone Marrow Transplant 2006;37(5):493–498

147. Schots R, Kaufman L, van Riet I et al. Proinflammatory cytokines and their role in the development of major transplant-related complications in the early phase after allogeneic bone marrow transplantation. Leukemia 2003;17(6):1150–1156

148. Extermann M, Meyer J, McGinnis M et al. A comprehensive geriatric intervention detects multiple problems in older breast cancer patients. Crit Rev Oncol Hematol 2004;49(1):69–75

149. Silverman M, Musa D, Martin DC et al. Evaluation of outpatient geriatric assessment: a randomized multi-site trial. J Am Geriatr Soc 1995;43(7):733–740

150. Fann JR, Alfano CM, Burington BE et al. Clinical presentation of delirium in patients undergoing hematopoietic stem cell transplantation. Cancer 2005;103(4):810–820

151. Shapira MY, Resnick IB, Bitan M et al. Low transplant-related mortality with allogeneic stem cell transplantation in elderly patients. Bone Marrow Transplant 2004;34(2):155–159

152. Wong JM, Collins K. Telomere maintenance and disease. Lancet 2003;362(9388):983–988

PART 4

POST-TRANSPLANT CARE

Transfusion medicine support for stem cell transplantation

Sumithira Vasu and Charles Bolan

Introduction

Transfusion medicine plays a vital role in the supportive care of patients undergoing hematopoietic stem cell transplantation (HSCT), with a spectrum of applications including donor peripheral blood stem cell (PBSC) collection, cellular processing, granulocyte transfusions, donor lymphocyte infusions, and the evaluation of immunohematologic issues in ABO-mismatched and other transplant situations. In turn, HSCT poses unique challenges for transfusion medicine, since transplant recipients may require substantial transfusion support due to cytopenias associated with toxic medications, decreased marrow reserve, infection, and malignancy, and may also exhibit competing donor and recipient immune and hematopoietic systems which carry their own distinct set of red cell, leukocyte and platelet antigens.

This chapter describes the services provided by transfusion medicine to ensure safe and effective blood component therapy, and the role of transfusion medicine in the evaluation and management of transfusion complications. The application of blood bank procedures and tests, and approaches to the management of unique challenges in HSCT such as those posed by blood group incompatibility between donor and recipient are also discussed.[1]

Blood component transfusion:

Overview

A basic understanding of the normal body distribution of blood constituents is an important aid towards understanding transfusion requirements and responses in transplant recipients. The standard blood volume for a normal adult may be estimated at 70 ml/kg, or approximately 5 liters in a 70-kg individual. In terms of body cellular reserve, most of the red cell mass and 75–80% of platelets are in the intravascular space, with the remainder residing in the spleen and marrow. In contrast, the majority of lymphocytes and granulocytes are extravascular in distribution. Thus, a 500 ml whole-blood donation by a healthy donor provides approximately 200 ml of packed red cells, 250–300 ml of plasma and 5.5×10^{10} platelets, with the exact contribution depending on the specific composition within an individual at the time of donation. In turn, for a recipient with a 5-liter blood volume, a 2–3% increase in the hematocrit (HCT) is expected from transfusion of a unit of packed red blood cells (RBC) obtained from a single donor. However, a clinically significant response in the degree of thrombocytopenia or granulocytopenia that is associated with HSCT patients requires transfusion of much more than the amount of platelets and granulocytes derived from a single 500 ml unit. Hence, granulocytes for transfusion are collected by apheresis procedures which provide

cells by processing larger blood volumes from single donors, while platelet components are collected either by apheresis from a single donor or by pooling the platelet content of multiple whole-blood units into a single product.

An overview of blood component therapy is provided in Table 31.1. In practice, the logistic management of red blood cell, fresh frozen plasma (FFP) and cryoprecipitate transfusion is simplified by the relatively long shelf-life of these products, even in settings where recipient red blood cell compatibility is complicated by antibody formation, requiring selective recruitment of compatible donors. However, the short shelf-life of platelets (5–7 days) and granulocytes (<24 hours) can significantly complicate transfusion support, which may become practically impossible in patients with multiple antibodies to common human leukocyte antigen (HLA) or neutrophil antigens. In these instances, and in those involving rare red blood cell types, close communication between the transfusion medicine service and the primary clinical team is critical to ensure the best possible therapy with granulocytes and HLA-matched platelets.

Red blood cells

Red blood cells, commonly referred to as 'packed RBCs' (PRBC), are the cells remaining after plasma and buffy coat are removed by centrifugation of one unit of whole blood. Depending on the anticoagulant preservative solution and the bag used to collect the unit, each unit of PRBC has an approximate volume of 350 ml and HCT of approximately 60–65%, and is expected to raise the HCT by 3%, or Hgb by 1 g/dl, in an adult without active bleeding or hemolysis. Liquid red cells are stored at 1–6°C for 35–42 days, depending on the anticoagulant solution. As storage time increases, the free hemoglobin and the potassium content increase in the supernatant, and the product may become less effective. As with platelets and granulocytes, the freshest infusion may be most desirable but least practical due to demands for infectious disease and compatibility testing, labeling and clerical checking, and other practical blood banking requirements.

Red cell transfusions are indicated for severe anemia due to active bleeding, red cell destruction, marrow hypoplasia or replacement of chronic losses. Patients receiving HSCT have heterogeneous causes of anemia and associated co-morbid conditions and hence no single standard indication for red cell transfusion applies to transplant recipients. In general, patients with a hemoglobin level greater than 9 g/dl do not require transfusion, while those with hemoglobin <7 g/dl benefit from transfusion. Patients with coronary heart disease have been shown to have reduced mortality when the hemoglobin is maintained at greater than 9–10 gm/dl.[2] Transplant recipients with a minor ABO-incompatible donor are at increased risk for immune hemolysis and may benefit from maintaining a hemoglobin level greater than

Table 31.1 Blood components: usual dose and volume

Product	Volume of one unit	Factors to replace	Dose
FFP	200–225 ml	II, V, VII, VIII, IX, X, XI	10–20 ml/kg
Cryoprecipitate	5–15 ml	Fibrinogen, factor VIII, vWF, factor XIII	1 unit/10 kg body weight
Platelets i. Single-donor apheresis platelets	180–400 ml	$3–9 \times 10^{11}$ platelets	Adults: administered as 6–8 equivalent units*
ii. Random donor platelets	35–60 ml	5.5×10^{10} platelets/unit	
RBCs	250–350 ml	RBCs	Varies

* One unit of random donor platelets contains at least 5.5×10^{10} platelets. The usual adult dose is at least 3×10^{11} platelets, which is equivalent to 6 random donor platelet units. Hematologic/oncologic patients almost always receive apheresis platelets. Each apheresis pack contains anywhere from 3 to 9×10^{11} platelets. The apheresis pack may be split so as to provide at least 3×10^{11} platelets for each patient (which is equivalent to 6 random donor platelet units).

9 g/dl.[3] Therefore, the decision to transfuse an individual patient should be based not just on the hemoglobin level, but on age, co-morbid factors, presence of active bleeding and underlying disease.

Red blood cells may be frozen in the presence of a cryoprotective agent such as glycerol. This method is used to store stockpiles of red cells with rare phenotypes. Once thawed, the unit must be washed to remove the glycerol and must then be used within 24 hours; licensed rejuvenation solutions may prolong the post-thaw shelf-life to 14 days at 4°C. Frozen red cells have decreased concentrations of plasma, potassium and other solutes which may reduce the incidence of adverse reactions associated with liquid RBC transfusion.

Fresh frozen plasma (FFP)

One unit of FFP contains all the coagulation factors present in fresh blood at the time of donation, in a volume of approximately 200–250 ml volume. FFP may be derived by apheresis or by separation of plasma from one unit of whole blood, and must be stored at −18°C within 6–8 hours of collection. FFP must be ABO compatible with the patient's RBCs but can be administered without regard to Rh type. Since FFP does not contain red cells, Rh immune globulin is not indicated when plasma from an Rh-positive donor is transfused to an Rh-negative patient. FFP is indicated in coagulation factor deficiencies, reversal of warfarin therapy and during massive transfusion in selected patients.[4,5] In patients who receive PRBC massive transfusion (greater than one blood volume transfused in 24 hours), coagulation factor deficiency may occur due to dilution and coagulation parameters must be carefully followed. FFP is also used as the replacement solution for plasma exchange in thrombotic thrombocytopenic purpura.

The time required to thaw FFP is about 30–40 minutes, and this fact, along with the volume of FFP required to treat factor deficiencies associated with liver disease and warfarin toxicity may limit applicability of FFP in certain settings. Concomitant use of hemostatic agents such as Novo-seven may be considered. In clinical practice, FFP is frequently overutilized, without appreciation of potential toxicities including transfusion-related acute lung injury (TRALI) and allergic reactions.

Cryoprecipitate

Cryoprecipitate is the insoluble portion produced when FFP has been thawed at 1–6°C. Each unit of cryoprecipitate has a volume of 10–15 ml, and contains approximately 80 units of factor VIII/vWF, 200–300 mg of fibrinogen and factor XIII at a concentration that is increased from 1.5–4 times that in plasma. Similar to FFP, cryoprecipitate must be ABO compatible with the patient's RBC but can be administered without regard to Rh type. Cryoprecipitate is mainly used in situations with documented hypofibrinogenemia, as may occur in disseminated intravascular coagulation (DIC) and massive transfusion.[6] Ten to 20 units are normally pooled and infused, with repeat doses based on measurements of fibrinogen concentration. Its use as a hemostatic agent for uremia has been largely supplanted by DDAVP (desmopressin), estrogens, and red cell transfusions or erythropoietin therapy to maintain the hemoglobin greater than 10 g/dl.[7]

Platelets

The two principal methods by which platelets are collected differ in terms of donor exposure, a fact that might be expected to lead to differences in patient outcomes[8] but which has been surprisingly difficult to associate with significant differences in randomized studies.[9]

Random donor platelets are separated by centrifugation from individual whole blood, and contain approximately 5.5×10^{10} platelets in a volume of 50 ml. The actual number of platelets varies from unit to unit, and the relatively small number of platelets in each unit requires pooling (usually of at least six units) to generate a dose sufficient to treat an adult recipient.

Single-donor apheresis platelets are collected by processing approximately 1–1.5 donor blood volumes (4–7 liters depending on weight) on a cell separator machine, and are essentially a suspension of platelets in plasma. Theoretically, this method might decrease the incidence of infection and alloimmunization by decreasing donor exposures, although studies have not shown a difference between random donor platelets and single-donor platelets.[9] However, a recent retrospective analysis of 716 oncology and transplant patients showed that prestorage leukoreduction of red cells and platelet components decreased the incidence of HLA alloimmunization and platelet refractoriness.[10] Single-donor apheresis platelets are increasingly used in the United States, especially in large academic medical centers which may support hematopoietic transplant programs.[8] Each apheresis component contains at least 3×10^{11} platelets suspended in a volume of approximately 300 ml. Due to advances in technique, nearly all platelet-pheresis devices produce components that are leukocyte depleted (contain less than 1×10^6 white blood cells). Thus, plateletpheresis components do not require the use of a white cell reduction filter to ensure a leukocyte-depleted component. Plateletpheresis is the preferred method of collection of platelet components from HLA-selected community donors or HLA-matched family donors due to the provision of a larger platelet dose with each donation, as well as the potential for repeat collections at more frequent intervals for the support of the severely thrombocytopenic, alloimmunized transplant recipient.

Platelets are stored at 20–24°C for 5–7 days, depending on the collection method, and undergo testing for bacterial contamination in addition to other more routine pathogen detection tests prior to release. The practical implications of bacterial testing (see below) are that release of platelet components to inventory may be delayed for at least 24 hours after collection. Occasionally, in case of emergency need for HLA-matched components, the patient's physician and the transfusion medicine physician may agree to emergency release of components prior to completion of testing. The plasma content associated with platelet transfusions may have significant clinical impact, as a source of allergic reactions or as a cause of immune hemolysis in cases of minor ABO incompatibility (see below).

Platelet membranes possess antigens of the ABO and HLA systems, as well as distinct platelet membrane antigens such as HPA1 through HPA5. ABO compatibility between donor and recipient is preferred, but not required. Antibodies against ABO antigens (i.e. recipient iso-hemagglutinins in major ABO-mismatched platelet transfusions) can result in modest to moderate reductions in transfusion increments, while antibodies against HLA (in HLA-alloimmunized recipients) or against HPA1 through HPA5 (in cases of post-transfusion purpura – see below) result in severe reductions in post-transfusion platelet count increments.

Platelet products may be washed to remove plasma as a prophylactic measure to reduce symptoms in cases of recurrent allergic transfusion reactions. However, the loss of platelets associated with washing may range from 15% to 55%. Platelet products may also undergo volume reduction for use in children; this is done by centrifugation and removal of platelet-poor plasma. All platelet products contain viable lymphocytes, and components intended for use in HSCT recipients must be irradiated to prevent transfusion-associated graft-versus-host disease (GvHD) (see below).

Because apheresis-derived as well as random donor 'pooled' platelets contain small quantities of red blood cells (up to 1–2 ml), donor and recipient Rh incompatibility may be clinically important when the donor is Rh (D) positive and the recipient is Rh (D) negative. Since stem cell transplant recipients may require multiple transfusions, it may not be feasible to maintain support for an individual patient exclusively with Rh-matched platelets; by necessity, it is common practice to provide Rh-positive platelets to Rh-negative patients. In this instance, Rh immunoglobulin can be given to prevent Rh alloimmunization (see under Rh immune globulin).

Most platelet transfusions are used prophylactically for prevention of bleeding rather than for treatment of active bleeding, and this decision to transfuse platelets depends on the clinical condition of the patient, the underlying disease, the functional ability of native platelets and the platelet count. In the absence of specific guidelines for HSCT recipients, published guidelines for platelet transfusions in oncology patients are generally followed. These suggest that a threshold of 10,000/µl for prophylactic platelet transfusion in stable adult patients receiving therapy for acute leukemia is safe and appropriate in the absence of bleeding, fever, or requirements for anticoagulation or invasive procedures.[11] For those patients with signs of hemorrhage, fever and sepsis, the transfusion trigger is a platelet count of 20,000/µl, while a platelet count of 40,000–50,000/µl is recommended prior to surgery. Bone marrow biopsies can be safely performed at counts of less than 20,000/µl.

Platelet transfusions should always be followed by a 1-hour post-transfusion assessment of the recipient's platelet count to document response or diagnose refractoriness, and as a critical guide for future transfusion and platelet selection. The platelet count should increase by 30,000–60,000/µl after transfusion of 4×10^{11} platelets (6–8 units) in an average-sized adult recipient. Platelet transfusions (and granulocyte transfusions) should not be administered within 2–4 hours of amphotericin-based preparations due to the risk of severe lung injury.[12]

For a more precise determination of response to platelet transfusion, the corrected count increment (CCI) should be used (Fig. 31.1), in which case the platelet refractory state may be defined as a CCI of 5000 or less after two consecutive ABO-compatible platelet transfusions. Common causes of platelet refractoriness are shown in Figure 31.2, broadly classified as being due to either immune-mediated or non-immune mediated etiologies. Immunologic causes include HLA alloimmunization, idiopathic thrombocytopenic purpura (ITP), major ABO incompatibility, and post-transfusion purpura (PTP). Patients with ITP[13] and those who have received ABO-incompatible platelets may show reduced but detectable increments to transfusions, while those with HLA alloimmunization and post-transfusion purpura may demonstrate no increment, or at times a decrease in the post-transfusion count compared with the pretransfusion count. Non-immunologic causes such as fever and 'older' platelets generally produce more modest decrements in platelet transfusion responses, while sepsis and

$$CCI = \frac{\text{Body surface area (m}^2) \text{ x Platelet count increment}}{\text{No. of platelets transfused}}$$

E.g. If 6 units of platelets are transfused, the dose is $6 \times 5.5 \times 10^{10} = 3.3 \times 10^{11}$ platelets (Each unit contains 5.5×10^{10} platelets).
If BSA is 1.4 m^2, the pre-transfusion count is 2000/mcl and the 1 hr post-transfusion count is 27,000/mcl, then the CCI would be:

$$CCI = \frac{1.4 \times (27,000 - 2000) \times 10^{11}}{6 \times 5.5 \times 10^{10}}$$

CCI = 10,606 platelets/m^2

The refractory state is defined as a CCI of < 5000 platelets/m^2 after two consecutive ABO-compatible platelet transfusions.

Figure 31.1
Calculation of corrected count increment (CCI).

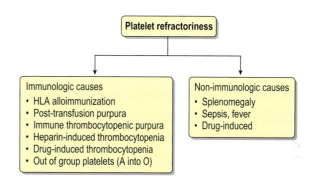

Figure 31.2
Outline of causes of platelet refractoriness. In general, immune conditions cause more severe refractoriness than non-immune causes. CCI is determined as shown in Fig. 31.1.

splenomegaly may result in more significant decreases,[14] especially in severe cases.

Considerations in the management of the refractory patient include:
- addressing correctable, clinical factors associated with refractoriness
- assessing response after at least one transfusion of fresh, ABO compatible products
- evaluation for medications that may produce thrombocytopenia such as vancomycin, sulfonamides (including bactrim), amphotericin, cephalosporins, penicillins. Consider evaluation for drug-dependent antibodies with an experienced reference laboratory when clinically indicated
- performing an HLA antibody screen; if positive, support with HLA selected platelets or with appropriate related donors. Consider empiric HLA selection strategies if the clinical history is consistent with HLA alloimmunization in the absence of testing
- in cases with continued refractoriness, considering platelet cross-matching or evaluation for platelet specific antibodies[15]
- careful review of transfusion history including ABO type, platelet dose, platelet age, and donor HLA types if available, with transfusion medicine staff.

Several laboratory techniques are available for the detection of patient antibodies to HLA antigens or platelet-specific antigens. Some assays may allow for the quantitation of antibodies to HLA antigens given as a percentage of panel reactivity (%PRA). Further analysis may permit identification of antibodies to specific antigens. However, such results are dependent on the individual assay and may vary between laboratories. The method of evaluation of HLA and other platelet-associated antibodies should be based upon patient needs and should be agreed upon by the clinical, laboratory, and transfusion services. Providing HLA-matched products is a resource-intensive venture for the transfusion service due to requirements for donor HLA typing, and establishment of selection algorithms for donor recruitment or use of appropriate platelet products in inventory. As noted above, after an HLA-selected volunteer completes the donation, up to 48 hours may be routinely required prior to release of the product into the inventory in order to complete viral and bacterial testing.

Historical practice has focused on selection of HLA-compatible platelets by matching within cross-reactive epitope groups (CREG) if an exact HLA match is not available. However, more recently, 'triplet matches' or 'epitope matches' have come into practical use,[16] based on experience with solid organ transplantation and computerized algorithms (HLA Matchmaker, University of Pittsburgh). Such approaches calculate the number of mismatches either in triplet or epitope format between donor and recipient, with less than 12 triplet mismatches considered as a potential HLA-matched donor, which may expand the pool of donors likely to provide an appropriate platelet increment. Hence, early involvement with the transfusion medicine service and HLA laboratory is crucial.

In situations where an HLA-selected donor is difficult to obtain or when antibody testing results are pending, the identification of HLA types associated with prior platelet transfusions that have produced adequate CCI may assist with selection of other HLA-matched products while testing is pending. The persistence of HLA alloimmunization following transplantation or chemotherapy tends to decay over time, in contrast to the situation in patients with aplastic anemia. Thus, follow-up testing and re-evaluation may identify transplant recipients for whom the degree of alloimmunization has lessened, and point toward a broader number of donors with potentially HLA-compatible platelets.

The prognosis of HLA alloimmunization depends on the underlying disease; in chemotherapy-induced myelosupression, it tends to decrease with time. In aplastic anemia, it tends to persist. The absence of a strict dose–response relationship has been demonstrated with HLA alloimmunization;[17] some patients tend to form antibodies while others do not,[17,18] despite multiple transfusions.

ABO-incompatible platelets

For transfusion of red cells, ABO compatibility is critical since a mismatch is potentially fatal. However, ABO matching of platelet transfusions is less critical, although platelets carry A and B substance and plasma contains anti-A or anti-B isohemagglutinins. The amount of incompatible plasma usually results in a positive direct antibody test (DAT), but rarely causes hemolysis. Restricting transfusions to blood group-specific platelets puts pressure on an already stressed inventory system due to the 5-day shelf-life of platelets. Each transfusion service has its own policy based on the demands of its hospital and the logistics of the transfusion service.

Major ABO incompatibility

When group A or B platelets are transfused into O patients, some groups have noted shortened survival of platelets.[19]

Minor ABO incompatibility

In these cases, donor plasma is incompatible with the recipient red cells. Plasma from some group O donors with high-titer anti-A and anti-B isohemagglutinins can cause hemolytic transfusion reactions when transfused into group A or B patients.[19] Some centers in Europe screen their platelet donors for the presence of high-titer isohemagglutinins and exclude them from donating platelets if titers exceed a certain level. Sadani et al reported a fatal hemolytic reaction after transfusion of repeat ABO-incompatible platelets.[20] Currently, the risk of severe hemolysis is estimated at 1 per 9000 minor ABO-mismatched platelet transfusions,[21] although there is widespread acceptance that this complication is underappreciated.[22] Pediatric recipients are at higher risk of this complication, and transfusion services generally provide ABO-compatible platelets to this higher risk group. Two ways of reducing this complication are to screen and defer donors with high isohemagglutinin titers or to wash all platelets from group O donors intended for transfusion into non-group O recipients.[23]

Granulocytes

Effective transfusion therapy using granulocyte components requires considerable planning and co-ordination between clinical teams and transfusion medicine services due to requirements for precollection medical stimulation of the donor, the relatively limited pool of available donors, need for specialized apheresis technology to perform the collection, and short shelf-life of the collected component. Granulocyte components are not approved by the Food and Drug Administration as a licensed blood component, and only specialized blood centers generally collect these components, often as part of research protocols.

In the 1970s, granulocyte transfusions were used mainly to treat fulminant bacterial and fungal infections in children.[24,25] With improvements in antibacterial and antifungal agents, interest in granulocyte transfusion waned for many years. More recently, the ability to boost granulocyte yields by steroid and granulocyte colony-stimulating factor (G-CSF) administration of the donor has renewed interest in the use of granulocyte transfusions in adult patients,[26] generally those with profound neutropenia and life-threatening bacterial or fungal infections. Following G-CSF and dexamethasone stimulation of the donor, apheresis yields of $4–8 \times 10^{10}$ granulocytes are routinely obtained, a fivefold increase over that achieved with steroid administration alone. Since G-CSF and dexamethasone must be taken by the donor on the evening prior to the apheresis collection,[27] scheduling of the donor may require several days of advance notice. Concerns about the long-term safety of repeat G-CSF and steroid administration to volunteer community donors continue to limit the widespread availability of this specialized component. Lastly, although transfusion of G-CSF and steroid-mobilized granulocyte concentrates typically raises the recipient neutrophil count by 1000–2000 cells/μl within 1 hour after transfusion, controlled trials of the impact of this modality on resolution of infection have not been completed.

Granulocyte concentrates are rich in donor plasma, platelets, red cells, and lymphocytes and other mononuclear cells, in addition to neutrophils, and have a volume of approximately 250–500 ml of plasma. Hence, granulocyte components may be associated with the types of transfusion reaction seen with any of these blood constituents. Febrile reactions are common, as are adverse pulmonary events. Pulmonary toxicity may be acute or chronically progressive, and the pulmonary status of the recipient should be closely monitored during granulocyte therapy (see below). Due to the red cell content, granulocyte products must be ABO and cross-match compatible with the recipient. Due to the mononuclear cell content, granulocyte products must be irradiated if administered to recipients at risk for transfusion-associated GvHD (TA-GvHD). Although there is not complete consensus on whether there is an increased risk of severe pulmonary reactions associated with concurrent administration of granulocytes and amphotericin,[12,28,29–31] it seems most prudent based on current evidence not to administer granulocyte components within 4 hours of amphotericin or amphotericin-based preparations. Granulocyte components should never be passed through leukocyte depletion filters. If the intended recipient is CMV seronegative and immunosuppressed, CMV-seronegative donors are preferred, if available.[32,33]

Granulocyte transfusions are most likely to produce benefit in severely neutropenic patients with life-threatening fungal or antimicrobial-resistant infections,[34,35] where eventual marrow recovery is expected. A complete blood count (CBC) with white blood cell differential should be obtained in the recipient before and after each transfusion, and the increment in both absolute neutrophil count (ANC) and platelet count assessed, as development of HLA alloimmunization may be indicated by blunted responses in either neutrophil or platelet cell lines. Thus, a baseline HLA antibody screen should be obtained prior to initiation of therapy, and repeated if increments in ANC or platelet count are not observed. If the patient is HLA alloimmunized, selection of HLA-compatible donors may be possible if the spectrum of antibody formation is not extensive. The risk of severe pulmonary reactions increases in recipients with antibodies to HLA or neutrophil antigens.

The use of prophylactic granulocyte transfusions obtained from family member PBSC donors has been used in some centers to reduce the period of neutropenia following stem cell infusion for HSCT, resulting in fewer numbers of febrile days and fewer days requiring antibiotics. However, this approach has not been shown to produce a survival benefit.[36] As noted above, rapid recruitment of community donors may be difficult in emergency situations or when the recipient has significant alloimmunization, in which case the PBSC or marrow donor, if medically stable, may be an optimal donor (see below).

Due to the narrow focus of potential efficacy and the myriad logistical, technical, and clinical considerations involved in granulocyte transfusion support, physicians considering this modality should contact their transfusion service promptly to begin collaborative planning. Factors to consider may include any of the following.

- Underlying disease, expected period of neutropenia
- Source of suspected infection, likelihood of response to antimicrobial agents
- Recipient weight, ABO blood type, red cell alloantibodies
- Evidence of HLA alloimmunization
- Pulmonary reserve
- Timely availability of either community or related donors
- Transfusion service granulocyte collection capability: G-CSF/ steroid versus steroid donor administration; donor availability, start time for granulocyte support

Complications of transfusion therapy

Complications associated with transfusion of blood components range from those which are frequent and mild, such as most allergic reactions, to those that are less common but potentially fatal, such as transfusion-related acute lung injury (TRALI) or hemolytic transfusion reactions. Although immunologic complications rather than infection are the most common cause of minor as well as severe reactions at the present time, many clinicians focus on risks of infection when considering the risk versus benefit of transfusion support. The clinical features, mechanism, and management of common transfusion reactions are shown in Table 31.2.

It is essential that in all cases of suspected transfusion reactions, the transfusion be stopped and patient evaluated to determine the cause of reaction. With the exception of mild allergic transfusion reactions, such as itching, transfusion of the implicated component should not be restarted. In all cases, the transfusion service must be promptly notified. Classification of transfusion complications is shown in Figure 31.3, and described in the following sections according to those which are immune mediated or caused by other means.

Immune-mediated complications

Hemolytic transfusion reactions

These reactions can be immediate or delayed in onset. *Immediate hemolysis* occurs when preformed recipient antibodies destroy donor

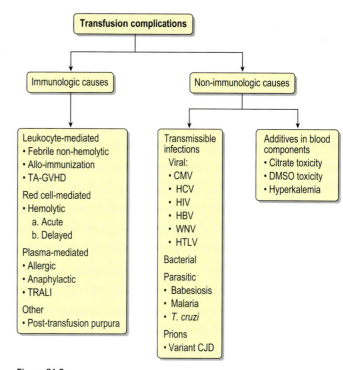

Figure 31.3

Types of transfusion reactions. Most transfusion reactions are acute in onset, with the exception of delayed hemolytic transfusion reaction and post-transfusion purpura, which usually happen 5–10 days after transfusion.

erythrocytes, as happens when an ABO-mismatched unit is accidentally transfused. Patients may complain of fevers or back pain, and hypotension and hematuria are commonly but not uniformly observed. Immediate hemolytic reactions are mediated by naturally occurring anti-A or anti-B isohemagglutinins which fix complement onto ABO-incompatible red cells, with the potential to cause rapid intravascular hemolysis, activation of complement and cytokine cascades, DIC, shock and renal failure in the most severe cases. Since fever is the most common presenting symptom, transfusions should be stopped in all febrile reactions and the possibility of hemolysis evaluated. In particular, the occurrence of hemolysis in transplant recipients with donor ABO incompatibility warrants careful consideration and evaluation for hemolysis throughout the immediate and subacute period of recovery from the conditioning regimen (see below).

Delayed hemolytic transfusion reaction

Delayed hemolytic transfusion reactions (DHTR) are caused by an anamnestic antibody response in the recipient precipitated by re-exposure to a non-ABO red cell antigen previously introduced by transfusion, transplantation or pregnancy. The antibody, often of the Kidd or Rh system, may be undetectable on pretransfusion testing but often increases rapidly in titer following the transfusion. DHTR due to a variety of red cell antigens have been extensively reported, and may be as high as 3.7% in patients undergoing HSCT.[37] In one center's experience, red cell alloantibody formation to non-ABO antigens was more frequently seen in ABO-mismatched transplants; the preparative regimen/GvHD prophylaxis did not influence the development of these alloantibodies.[37] Hemolytic reactions associated with infusion of donor immune cells are discussed under blood group incompatibility.[38–40]

Febrile, non-hemolytic transfusion reactions (FNHTR)

These occur in 0.5–1% of all transfusions, and are associated with leukocyte antibodies in the patient which react with transfused

Table 31.2 Transfusion reactions

Reaction type	Clinical features	Etiology	Most common blood component	Treatment	Prevention/work-up
Febrile, non-hemolytic	Temperature rise >1° C, chills	Cytokines in plasma or in supernatant of stored products	Non-leukodepleted RBCs, platelets	Stop the transfusion; acetaminophen. Premedicate with acetaminophen for future transfusions or use leukoreduced products	Notify blood bank; product will be sent for bacterial culture
Allergic	Erythema, urticaria, pruritus, laryngeal edema in severe cases	Allergen in donor plasma	Any plasma containing product – FFP, platelets, RBCs	Stop the transfusion; administer iv antihistamines. Only reaction where transfusion can be restarted if symptoms resolve in 30 minutes	Premedicate with iv H1 and H2 blockers; if two successive reactions occur despite optimal dose of antihistamines, consider washed products
Anaphylactic/ anaphylactoid	Hypotension, wheezing, respiratory distress, stridor, tachypnea, tachycardia, abdominal pain, diarrhea	Recipient antibodies to allergen in donor plasma; recipient is IgA deficient or has anti-IgA	Any plasma-containing product	Epinephrine, steroids	Premedicate with antihistamines, glucocorticoids. Use washed products. In IgA-deficient patients, use plasma from IgA-deficient donors
TRALI (transfusion-related acute lung injury)	Respiratory distress, hypoxemia, hypotension within 6 hours after transfusion (Popovsky); bio-active lipid particles in stored products (Silliman), usually resolves with supportive care in 24 hours	Donor HLA antibodies and neutrophil antibodies	RBC, plasma and platelets	Supportive care, mechanical ventilation if severe	Blood bank may test for HLA/neutrophil antibodies in the implicated donors
Hemolytic	Fever, hypotension, back pain, DIC, hemoglobinuria, renal failure, elevated LFTs	ABO or phenotypically mismatched blood	RBC, occasionally platelets	Supportive care	Provide phenotypically matched blood
Citrate toxicity	Perioral numbness, tingling, nausea, vomiting, tetany; in severe cases cardiac arrest	Citrate-induced hypocalcemia; Citrate is infused either as anticoagulant during apheresis or in the FFP administered as a replacement fluid	FFP	Slow the infusion of citrate/FFP; check ionized calcium; give IV calcium chloride/gluconate	Identify patients at increased risk and institute empiric calcium administration (e.g. women with low BMI and mechanically ventilated patients)
DMSO toxicity	Nausea, vomiting, cough, hypotension, arrhythmia, fever, chills, hemoglobinuria	DMSO is used as cryopreservative in bone marrow	PBSC, DLI, any frozen cellular product (not FFP)	Slow or stop the infusion; supportive care; restart infusion if symptoms resolve	Antihistamines, washed cellular infusions

In all suspected transfusion reactions, stop the transfusion while maintaining the intravenous access and notify the blood bank.

leukocytes. The symptoms of fever, chills, malaise, headache, nausea or vomiting may be initially indistinguishable from more severe hemolytic reactions, and hence the transfusion must be stopped and the transfusion service notified to initiate work-up of a hemolytic reaction. The incidence of FNHTR has decreased with increasing use of leukodepleted blood components.[41]

Allergic reactions

Mild allergic reactions occur in to 1–3% of transfusions, and are mediated by plasma proteins or cytokines. Symptoms such as hives, wheezing and pruritus are generally mild, occur during or shortly after transfusion, and can usually be managed with antihistamine agents (H1 blockers such as diphenhydramine or H2 blockers such as cimetidine).[42] In particularly nettlesome cases, symptoms may be reduced or prevented by washing cellular blood products, a modality that may reduce the plasma content by 98% but which may also be associated with a concomitant 20–40% loss in the platelet content of platelet

components (see below). In contrast to febrile non-hemolytic transfusion reactions, leukoreduction does not reduce the incidence of allergic reactions.[41]

Anaphylactic reactions are more severe but much less common reactions that occur in 1 in 20,000–47,000 units transfused. Symptoms include sudden onset of flushing, chills, vomiting, diarrhea, hypotension, generalized edema, coughing, stridor, and laryngeal edema. Of note, patients with congenital IgA deficiency may develop anaphylactic reactions when transfused with plasma from healthy, non-IgA deficient donors. The majority of IgA-deficient subjects, however, do not experience serious reactions following transfusion, and blood support in these patients should be individualized on a case-by-case basis.[43] IgA deficiency should be diagnosed by measuring IgA levels on a pretransfusion sample; recent transfusions may result in passive transfer of IgA, giving a false-negative result. Transfusions to IgA-deficient patients experiencing reactions may require products from IgA-deficient donors. If IgA-deficient blood products are not available, washed or frozen-deglycerolized products can be used.[44]

TRALI (transfusion-related acute lung injury)

TRALI refers to non-cardiogenic pulmonary edema occurring within 1–6 hours after transfusion of plasma-containing blood products. The incidence of TRALI is estimated at 1 in every 4500 transfusions, and has a fatality rate of 5–8%. TRALI is currently considered the leading cause of transfusion-related death.[45] Symptoms include tachypnea, dyspnea, hypotension and fever; hypoxia may be profound and the chest radiograph demonstrates diffuse pulmonary infiltrates. Patients usually recover within 24 hours with supportive care.

There are two hypotheses for the etiology of TRALI.[46] One proposed mechanism implicates donor antileukocyte antibodies directed against either HLA or neutrophil antigens as the cause of TRALI, since these may be found in 50–90% of implicated units. The higher frequency of HLA antibodies in multiparous women has led to the practice in some countries of utilizing plasma derived only from male donors. The second hypothesis implicates biologically active lipids and neutrophil priming as the cause of TRALI. In this model, two insults result in TRALI: one from sepsis, trauma or other injury results in the priming of neutrophils and their adherence to pulmonary endothelium; the other insult arises from biologically active lipids formed in stored blood products which activate the neutrophils in the lung, leading to sequestration and pulmonary endothelial damage. In this model, patients at highest risk are those with other co-morbid medical conditions who receive blood products close to shelf outdate. Thus, mild cases of TRALI are often not recognized. In all suspected cases of TRALI, the transfusion service should be notified to allow for testing of the product/donor and possible deferral of the donor from future donations.

Post-transfusion purpura

Post-transfusion purpura (PTP) is a rare complication of blood transfusion characterized by the precipitous onset of severe thrombocytopenia and absolute refractoriness to platelet transfusions. PTP occurs 3–12 days after blood transfusion, often in a multiparous female or previously transfused recipient.[47] The exact mechanism is uncertain, but involves anamnestic formation of an alloantibody against transfused platelets which then destroys both transfused and recipient platelets, resulting in both severe thrombocytopenia and transfusion refractoriness. PTP generally resolves spontaneously in 2 weeks. However, more rapid responses occur following high-dose intravenous immunoglobulin (IVIG) or plasmapheresis therapy, either of which is indicated urgently to reduce the risk of significant bleeding. The diagnosis is suggested by the occurrence of profound thrombocytopenia and refractoriness to platelet transfusions in the appropriate clinical setting. Recipients are also refractory to antigen-negative platelet transfusions. The diagnosis is supported by platelet antigen genotyping and platelet antibody identification, performed in an experienced reference laboratory.[15] The diagnosis may be confounded by other conditions causing thrombocytopenia in the post-transplant patient. However, cases responsive to appropriate intervention have been described.[48] In contrast to HLA alloimmunization and sepsis, the degree of thrombocytopenia is more severe. Several polymorphisms of platelet antigens associated with post-transfusion purpura have been reported in different ethnic populations.[49]

Transfusion-associated graft-versus-host disease

TA-GvHD is a rare, but life-threatening adverse effect of transfusion, which is entirely preventable if appropriate policies for irradiation of transfused blood products are effectively implemented.[50] TA-GvHD is mediated by engraftment and proliferation of immunocompetent donor lymphocytes, resulting in fever, rash, diarrhea, liver function abnormalities and severe pancytopenia, within 3–30 days after transfusion. Patients at risk include immunocompromised populations, such as patients with primary immunodeficiencies, with hematologic malignancies, receiving chemotherapy, and following HSCT. Immunocompetent patients receiving blood components from first-degree family relatives are also at risk. TA-GvHD is prevented by prophylactic irradiation of cellular products with 2500 cGy.[51] Leukoreduction does not prevent TA-GvHD. There is no treatment for TA-GvHD once it occurs. Diagnosis is confirmed when HLA testing reveals additional lymphocyte HLA types consistent with those from donors who provided transfused blood components.[52] The clinical features of TA-GvHD are compared to transplantation-related GvHD in Table 31.3.

Infectious complications of transfusion

Since the recognition of human immunodeficiency virus (HIV) as a transfusion-transmissible agent, tremendous advances have been made in the screening and testing of volunteer donors to enhance the bacteriologic and virologic safety of blood products. However, concerns about infectious complications of transfusion continue to influence the effective use of blood components. Current issues involve estimation of the extremely low risk of transmission of known agents such as hepatitis B and C viruses and HIV, for which sensitive laboratory tests are available, as well as the assessment and prevention of other, new or emerging agents which might be transmissible through blood transfusion. At present, blood component testing in the United States includes use of seven serologic and three DNA-based tests to detect HIV-1/2, hepatitis B and C viruses, HTLV-I/II, West Nile virus, *Treponema pallidum* (syphilis), and *Trypansoma cruzi* (Chagas' disease) (Table 31.4). Current risks of transmission of most of these agents are too low to accurately measure and are estimated based on mathematical modeling (Table 31.5).[53,54] However, emerging, existing and

Table 31.3 Characteristics of post-transplant acute GvHD and transfusion-associated GvHD

Features	HSCT–Acute GVHD	TA-GVHD
Time of onset	Within first 100 days of transplant	2–30 days post transfusion
Symptoms	Rash, diarrhea	Rash, diarrhea
Lab abnormalities	Elevated LFTs, minimal pancytopenia	Elevated LFTs, marked pancytopenia
Mortality	10–15%	80–100%

Table 31.4 Tests used to detect transfusion-transmitted infections

Transfusion-transmitted infection	Serologic test	Detection of viral DNA
HIV-1/2	Anti-HIV-1/2 ELISA	Nucleic acid test
HBV	HBsAg and anti-HBc Elisa	
HCV	Anti-HCV ELISA	Nucleic acid test
West Nile virus	–	Nucleic acid test
HTLV-I/II	Anti-HTLV-1/2 ELISA	–
Treponema pallidum (syphilis)	RPR flocculation test or anti-*T. pallidum* agglutination test	–
Trypansoma cruzi (Chagas')	Anti-*T. cruzi* ELISA	

The testing for most transfusion-transmitted viruses involves detection of both antibody (past infection) and viral DNA. Detection of viral DNA helps detect infections during window-period. ELISA, enzyme linked immunosorbent assay; HBsAg, hepatitis B surface antigen; anti-HBc, antibodies to hepatitis B core antigen.

Table 31.5 Estimated risk of transfusion-transmitted viral disease[1]

Virus	Risk per transfusion
HIV 1 and 2	1: 2,000,000–3,000,000
Hepatitis C	1: 1,000,000–2,000,000
Hepatitis B	1: 58,000–200,000
HTLV 1 and II	1 : 641,000
West Nile virus	Ranges between 1.46 : 10,000 and 12.33 : 10,000

[1]The risks shown here are those calculated after implementation of nucleic acid testing.

re-emerging infections such as parvovirus B19, dengue virus, human herpes virus (HHV)-8 may also be poised to threaten blood safety.[55] In addition, there is currently no licensed assay available for detection of prion disorders.[56] Until reliable and safe methods for pathogen inactivation of blood products are available, potential transfusion-transmitted infection will continue to be a threat to a zero-risk blood supply.[57]

Strategies to improve blood safety may also impact upon blood availability, since they may involve more stringent donor screening, selection and deferral procedures, testing for infectious agents with additional serologic, nucleic-acid and other methods, efforts to enforce more judicious transfusion practices, and pathogen reduction technologies Approaches to pathogen reduction include technologies designed to be effective against viruses, bacterial, and protozoan agents. Consideration of these modalities should include the degree of pathogen reduction, the potential impact of product pooling, and potential for immunologic and other side-effects.[58,59]

Solvent detergent-treated FFP (SD-FFP) and methylene-blue light treated plasma (MBLT) are offered in Europe. SD-FFP is prepared by pooling about 2000–2500 units of ABO-identical FFP; the process results in a reduction of factor V, VIII, vWF multimers and plasmin inhibitors but does not significantly reduce the infectivity of non-lipid encapsulated viruses such as parvovirus. In turn, reductions in fibrinogen, factors V, VIII, IX and XI occur with MBLT plasma. Approaches to pathogen reduction of platelet components include photochemical inactivation using amtosalen HCI and UVA light,[60] which inactivates bacteria and several transfusion-transmitted viruses. Data from available randomized clinical trials indicate that amtosalen/UVA treatment of platelets results in a preparation that has normal hemostatic function, but reduced platelet recovery and survival. This method is licensed in Europe.[61]

Cytomegalovirus (CMV)

Transfusion-transmitted CMV is a significant concern in HSCT recipients. The risk of transfusion-transmitted CMV infection can be decreased either by the use of seronegative blood products or by using leukodepleted products. Since a substantial portion of blood donors are CMV positive, it is sometimes difficult to provide only CMV-seronegative products. Alternatively, since leukocytes are considered as the reservoir of CMV, leukodepleted products have been utilized as an alternative to CMV-seronegative products.

Because transfusion-transmitted CMV may occur despite the use of seronegative components due to donation during the 'serosilent' window period, CMV NAT testing using PCR methods has been studied. However, a large cross-sectional study of 1000 US donors utilizing two well-validated PCR assays demonstrated that CMV DNA is only rarely detectable in seropositive donors.[62] Hence, the use of CMV PCR assays with optimal performance characteristics may not increase blood safety from CMV transmission beyond a level provided by serologic screening tests.

The efficacy of the reduction in CMV transmission by use of CMV serologically negative versus leukodepleted blood products is a matter

of debate. Bowden et al[63] found no statistically significant difference in CMV infection in a study of 502 bone marrow transplant (BMT) recipients between those prospectively randomized to receive leukodepleted or CMV-seronegative products. The probability of developing CMV disease by day 100 after transplantation was 0% among recipients of seronegative components, compared to 1.2% among recipients of leukodepleted products (p = 0.25); survival also was not different. More recently, Nichols et al[64] followed a cohort of 807 seronegative recipients of autologous and allogeneic BMTs over two time periods, finding that transfusion-transmitted CMV was significantly higher when CMV-untested/leukoreduced products were used compared to CMV-seronegative products. However, the higher risk of transmission did not result in a higher risk of actual CMV disease since prospective monitoring for CMV antigenemia and pre-emptive ganciclovir therapy resulted in a very low risk of morbidity or mortality from CMV disease. These findings are consistent with results of a recent meta-analysis by Vamvakas[65] which showed:

- a small but real risk of acquiring CMV infection whether CMV-seronegative or CMV-untested, WBC leukoreduced products are used
- the risk of CMV transmission may be increased with the administration of CMV-untested, leukocyte-reduced products
- any increased risk of transfusion-transmitted CMV infection may not necessarily translate into an appreciable increase in CMV-related mortality and morbidity.

Bacterial contamination

In contrast to transfusion-transmitted viral agents, bacterial contamination of cellular products is a more common and more serious cause of transfusion complications, accounting for up to 10% of transfusion-related deaths.[66] Bacterial contamination is particularly troublesome for platelets, which are stored at room temperature and more susceptible to rapid bacterial growth following collection. The current risk to a recipient receiving contaminated platelets may be 10–1000 times higher than the combined risk of transfusion-transmitted viruses.[67] In previous studies, approximately 1 in 3000 units of platelet concentrates was shown to be contaminated, with a risk of a severe septic transfusion reaction of approximately 1 in 50,000 platelets, and 1 in 500,000 red blood cells transfused. A more recent study showed a contamination rate of 1 in 5157 apheresis platelet products.[68] Symptoms include high-grade fevers and chills during or right after the transfusion.

Bacterial testing of platelets is currently performed to reduce these risks,[69] with several automated, continuous incubation and detection systems in use which rely on the detection of CO_2 production or O_2 consumption by actively metabolizing bacteria in the initial 24-hour period after collection.[70] Implementation of bacterial testing for platelet components has been reported to decrease septic transfusion reactions in centers adopting this technology when compared to historical rates,[71] but results in an additional delay before products are released into the transfusion services inventory for administration to patients.

Transfusion-transmitted prion disease

In response to the variant CJD (vCJD) epidemic (mad cow disease) in the UK, a surveillance system was set up between the UK national vCJD surveillance unit and UK national blood service. Of the 23 known individuals who received a blood transfusion from a person who subsequently developed vCJD, three cases of vCJD have been reported, confirming the transmissibility by transfusion.[72–74] Donors with a travel history indicating potential exposure to bovine spongiform encephalopathy (BSE) may be debarred from blood donation when returning to countries without BSE infection; however, there is currently no assay available for prion detection in asymptomatic donors. Epidemiologic evidence does not suggest that sporadic CJD is transmitted by transfusion.

Other agents

Parvovirus B-19 can cause potentially severe bone marrow suppressive effects in immunocompromised patients;[75] it is not inactivated by the solvent detergent method that renders pooled plasma free of the major lipid-enveloped agents.[76] Testing of parvoviral titers is currently done in some countries. However, no method reliably prevents transmission of this agent and the diagnosis in a recipient is based on clinical presentation.

A number of protozoal species may be transmitted by transfusion, including malaria, which may be the most frequently transfusion-transmitted agent worldwide. In non-endemic areas, infections with babesia species and trypanosomes may occur in accordance with shifting population demographics and disease activity. Babesia species, transmitted via tick bites, may cause severe infection and intravascular hemolysis similar to malaria, for which immunocompromised, aged and asplenic patients are particularly at risk.[77] Chagas' disease, caused by the protozoal parasite *Trypanosoma cruzi*, is transmitted by the reduviid bug, with an estimated 19 million infected individuals living in South and Central America and parts of Mexico. Transfusion-transmitted Chagas' disease may therefore occur in parts of North America due to population migration.[55] In the United States, an enzyme immunoassay test for blood screening has now been instituted.

Toxicity from additive solutions and storage

Transfusion complications may also occur due to additive solutions and other factors related to storage. *DMSO* (dimethyl sulfoxide), is a solvent used as a cryoprotectant for hematopoietic stem cells, which is quickly distributed to all the tissues after administration and produces a characteristic garlic odor when metabolized.[78] Anaphylactoid symptoms after DMSO administration are common, due to the release of histamine. Other side-effects include nausea, vomiting, fever, chills, cough, diarrhea, flushing, headache and hemolysis, and cardiovascular toxicity includes bradycardia or tachycardia, heart block, and hemodynamic instability (hypotension or hypertension). Antihistamine prophylaxis is routinely recommended prior to the administration of DMSO. Slowing the infusion or increasing the time between infusions of different aliquots may also minimize toxicity.[79]

Citrate toxicity can be observed in patients undergoing plasma exchange, large-volume leukapheresis for collection of autologous or allogeneic mononuclear cells, or massive transfusion, due to citrate contained in the anticoagulant storage or apheresis solutions. Initial symptoms include perioral tingling, numbness and tingling in the extremities, which can progress rapidly to include tetany and cardiovascular arrest. Ionized calcium levels should be closely monitored, and intravenous calcium replaced accordingly.[79,80]

Hyperkalemia may occur with rapid transfusion of older blood products to very small bodyweight patients, due to the exponential increase in potassium concentration in the supernatant of stored blood products over time.[81,82] These reactions can be prevented by using fresh products or washed products, and are assessed by measurement of serum potassium levels. Treatment with calcium can provide a cardioprotective effect.

Blood bank practices

Leukocyte depletion

Donor leukocyte-mediated febrile non-hemolytic transfusion reactions, alloimmunization and CMV infection associated with infusion of contaminated red blood cell and platelet products may be significantly reduced through leukodepletion, either at the time of component preparation ('prestorage leukodepletion') or at the time of transfusion by the use 'bedside' filters.[83] Leukodepleted products are indicated for hematopoietic stem cell recipients, hematologic malignancies, congenital immunodeficiency syndromes, and hemoglobinopathies. Due to logistic difficulties in providing leukodepleted products to selected patient populations and to reactions associated with the use of filtration at the time of administration, many blood centers and hospitals are moving towards use of 'universal prestorage leukoreduction'.[10] By the standards of the American Association of Blood Banks, a leukodepleted product has to contain less than 5×10^6 WBCs in platelet pheresis units and red blood cells, while European standards require less than 1×10^6 WBCs. Compared with non-leukocyte depleted blood components, those that are leukocyte-depleted significantly reduce the incidence of FNHTR and CMV transmission, and may also reduce, but not eliminate, the risk of PTP.[84]

Washed red cells and platelet products

Washing is a process in which cells are suspended in an electrolyte solution and processed to remove up to 99% of plasma. Washed blood products should be reserved for management of otherwise unmanageable allergic plasma reactions, due to a 20–40% reduction in the platelet content of platelet products and complications associated with additional cell manipulation. The shelf-life of red cells after washing decreases to 24 hours, while that of washed platelets decreases to 4 hours.

Irradiation

Irradiation of red cells and platelets prevents TA-GvHD (as described above). Due to the numbers of immunosuppressed patients at risk in tertiary cancer centers, universal irradiation is used in all major centers, and has been recommended for more widespread application in other settings. The dose for irradiation should be at least 2500 cGy. Although platelet survival is not affected,[85] red cells may have shortened survival times in circulation if not transfused shortly after irradiation.

Use of Rh immune globulin

Rh immune globulin (RhIg) is indicated to prevent alloimmunization of Rh-negative recipients exposed to Rh-positive blood, and is available in intramuscular or intravenous preparations. RhIg is a plasma-derived product and is not risk free.[86] It is traditionally administered by transfusion services to prevent sensitization and formation of an anti-D alloantibody for Rh (D)-negative women who have an Rh (D)-positive fetus. Consideration for the use of RhIg usually occurs in two settings:

- to prevent formation of anti-D in Rh (D)-negative patients following exposure to Rh (D)-positive platelets and granulocytes.[87] The usual dose contains 300 ug of anti-D which covers an exposure of 15 ml of Rh-positive RBC
- to treat post-HSCT immune thrombocytopenic purpura in Rh (D)-positive patients.

The use of RhIg following Rh-incompatible platelet transfusion deserves special attention. The incidence of anti-D alloimmunization after the transfusion of platelets from Rh (D)-positive donors to Rh (D)-negative recipients has been reported to be between 0% and 19%.[19,88] Cid reported that hematology patients, because of intense immunosuppression from chemotherapy, will not form anti-D and that support with Rh-incompatible platelet products would be considered safe.[89] This author reported no anti-D formation in 22 Rh (D)-positive patients with hematologic diseases after a median follow-up of 8 weeks.[90] These patients received platelet concentrates prepared from whole blood. In contrast, platelet pheresis-derived platelets have been reported to contain a mean of 3 ml of RBC, although recent reports suggest that a much smaller RBC content is present.[91] At present, there are no consensus recommendations regarding RhIg immune prophylaxis for HSCT patients.

Serologic studies

Along with their associated historical significance and essential nature in everyday blood banking procedures, traditional serologic assays such as those used to determine ABO blood type may be useful in the management of HSCT recipients.

Assessment of the forward type detects the presence of A or B antigens on the patient's RBCs using commercial antisera (i.e. anti-B, anti-A) as outlined in Table 31.6. With this approach, 4+ indicates strong agglutination and 0 indicates no agglutination; intermediate degrees of clumping are assigned numbers 3, 2 and 1. This technique allows for detection of as little as 5% antigen-positive red cells in peripheral blood; smaller populations may be observed by light microscopy. The presence of different ABO red cell phenotypes (mixed field) may be possible for detection of red blood cell chimerism with sensitivity similar to molecular techniques for lymphocytes and white blood cells.

Assessment of the reverse type detects the presence of antibodies in the patient plasma with commercial reagent red cells. Assay results are scored as outlined in Table 31.7. The antibodies to ABO antigens, termed isohemagglutinins, become detectable within months after birth and may result in severe hemolysis in ABO-mismatched hemolytic transfusion reactions as well as in HSCT with donor–recipient ABO incompatibility.

Isohemagglutinin titers

The strength of the isohemagglutinin measured with the reverse type can be further assessed as a titer using serial dilutions of the sample plasma.

Table 31.6 Forward typing to detect blood group

Patient RBCs + anti-A	Patient RBCs + anti-B	Patient ABO type
4+	0	A
0	4+	B
4+	4+	AB
0	0	O

Patient's RBCs are allowed to react with reagent antisera. Agglutination is recorded in ascending order of reactivity from 0 to 4+. For example, a patient whose type is AB has both A and B antigens and hence will react with reagent anti-A and anti-B. The final determination of ABO type is done with the concurrent interpretation of forward and reverse types.

Table 31.7 Reverse typing to detect blood group

Patient plasma + group A RBCs	Patient plasma + group B RBCs	Patient ABO type
4+	0	B
0	4+	A
4+	4+	O
0	0	AB

Patient's plasma is allowed to react with reagent red blood cells. The plasma usually has naturally occurring antibodies (IgM) which agglutinate reagent red cells; reactivity is recorded in ascending order of strength from 0 to 4+. For example, a patient with blood group AB will not have any naturally occurring antibodies and hence will not react with reagent A and B red cells.

Direct antibody test (DAT)

The DAT detects in vivo coating of patient RBCs with either IgG or complement with the use of polyvalent antihuman globulin obtained from rabbits sensitized to human IgG and complement. The patient RBC can be further tested with specific antisera to determine whether coating is due to IgG or complement, and the eluate of the red cell may be analyzed to determine the specificity of the antibody (anti-A, anti-B or against other blood group antigens). When excessive amounts of antibody are present in serum, available antigenic sites on RBCs become saturated and antibody may be detected in serum using the indirect antibody test.

A positive DAT does not by itself indicate active, ongoing hemolysis in the absence of clinical signs or other laboratory findings, for which the following clinical correlations may be helpful.

- Does the patient have clinical or laboratory evidence of hemolysis?
- Did the patient receive a hematopoietic stem cell transplant from a donor with ABO or other blood group incompatibility? (consider passenger lymphocyte syndrome or other hemolytic interaction)
- Has the patient been recently transfused with packed RBCs? (if yes, consider delayed hemolytic reaction)
- Has the patient received platelets or granulocytes from ABO-incompatible donors?
- Is the indirect antibody screen also positive?
- Is the patient receiving penicillin, cephalosporin, or other medications associated with autoimmune hemolytic anemia?
- Has the patient recently received anthymocyte globulin (ATG), IVIG or Rh immune globulin or other preparations which may contain antibodies to red cell antigens?
- Is there a discrepancy in forward/reverse type of the patient?

Additional considerations

Management of donor–recipient blood group incompatibility

ABO incompatibility

Donor–recipient ABO incompatibility in HSCT requires careful evaluation and follow-up due to its association with significant post-transplant immunohematologic events, which include prolonged reticulocytopenia and immune-mediated hemolysis that may be of sufficient severity to result in death.[92] Because the genes coding for the ABO blood groups and HLA system are on different chromosomes, ABO incompatibility may occur between HLA-matched related family members as well as with unrelated HSCT donors.[92]

The immunobiology of the ABO blood group system differs from other blood groups in several key respects. Unlike other blood group antigens, humans form antibodies to ABO antigens lacking on their own cells within the first year of life; these antibodies are termed isohemagglutinins. Isohemagglutinins include IgM antibodies and other immunoglobulins, which may be of high titer and have the potential to fix complement and cause cell lysis when combined with red cell surface antigens.[93] ABO antigens are also expressed on the cell surface of primitive erythroid cells, and on cells of other tissues throughout the body,[94] a fact which accounts for the very high impact of major ABO incompatibility in solid organ transplantation due to the risk of graft rejection.[93]

It is essential that the presence of an ABO-incompatible HSCT donor be identified early to allow the cell processing laboratory to apply graft processing procedures for removal of RBC from major ABO-incompatible donors and to reduce the plasma content of minor

ABO-incompatible donors. Similarly, the transfusion service must be aware of ABO incompatibility to allow appropriate interpretation of post-transplant serologic testing, and must consider ABO incompatibility throughout the peritransplant period for appropriate selection of blood products (Table 31.8).

In HSCT patients, ABO incompatibility is defined as 'major' when the immune system of the recipient produces/can produce antibodies against the donor cells, and as 'minor' when the immune system of the donor produces/can produce antibodies against the recipient. In bidirectional mismatch, both the donor and recipient can produce antibodies against each other. Following graft infusion, the impact of ABO incompatibility depends on a variety of factors including time after transplant, conditioning regimen,[95] graft source,[3] GvHD prophylaxis,[80,96] and whether major, minor or bidirectional incompatibility is present.[92] Although ABO incompatibility has been proposed to have an adverse effect on HSCT outcomes in certain settings,[97] other studies have not observed a clinically significant adverse effect due to this condition.[98,99]

Minor ABO-incompatible transplants

The most profound risk of post-transplant immune hemolysis is associated with donor–recipient minor ABO incompatibility due to rapid production of anti-recipient isohemagglutinins by donor-derived immune cells,[96] an event referred to as the passenger lymphocyte syndrome.[92] Hemolysis in this setting generally occurs from day 4 to day 14 of transplant and may result in death.[3,100] As described in solid organ transplantation,[101] the severity of passenger lymphocyte-mediated hemolysis is related to the lymphocyte content of the graft (PBSC > marrow >> cord blood in HSCT) and use of ciclosporin alone as GvHD prophylaxis; the risk is increased with the use of unre-

lated donors in HSCT[102] and may be further aggravated in this setting by donor cytokine administration prior to PBSC collection (Fig. 31.4).

Some centers have advocated the use of a pretransplant red cell exchange in minor ABO-incompatible HSCT to lower the amount of donor-incompatible red cells prior to transplant.[103] However, red cell exchange therapy in this setting can cause significant adverse events, such as TRALI and allergic reactions.[103] In addition, a substantial fraction (25–40%) of residual recipient cells remains in the recipient circulation following red cell exchange procedures using 6–8 units of packed red cells in adults.[3] Thus, prophylactic red cell exchange therapy does not eliminate hemolytic complications such as renal failure, which may occur due to the passenger lymphocyte syndrome in HSCT.[102] In all cases, aggressive peritransplantation monitoring with daily CBC testing and therapy with donor-compatible red cells to maintain a hemoglobin level greater than 9.5 g/dl should be practiced in all patients at risk.[3] Serial monitoring with post-transplant DAT testing has poor positive and negative predictive value for identifying hemolysis,[92] and does not obviate the need for aggressive transfusion support.

Major ABO incompatibility

Recipients having major ABO incompatibility with the HSCT donor may develop pure red cell aplasia (PRCA) following HSCT. Post-HSCT PRCA in this setting occurs due to:

* conversion to donor hematopoiesis (loss of recipient hematopoiesis)[94]
* inhibition of donor hematopoiesis due to persistent circulation of recipient-type anti-donor isohemagglutinins and the presence of incompatible ABO antigens on donor erythroid-forming cells.[104]

Patients who receive reduced-intensity conditioning regimens may not exhibit decreased overall erythropoietic function despite persistent circulation of recipient isohemagglutinins and inhibition of donor erythropoiesis due to autologous hematopoiesis. In the setting of major ABO mismatch between donor and recipient, overall post-HSCT erythropoietic function depends on the relationship between the rate of disappearance of anti-donor isohemagglutinins (which depends on the

Table 31.8 Choice of blood components in ABO-incompatible transplants

Major ABO mismatch

The recipient has preformed antibodies against the donor's RBC. Recipients are at risk of immediate hemolysis, pure red cell aplasia and delayed hemolytic reactions

Recipient	Donor	Preferred choice of RBC	Platelets/plasma
O	A	O	A
O	B	O	B
O	AB	O	AB
A	AB	O	AB
B	AB	O	AB

Minor ABO mismatch

The donor can generate antibodies against the recipient's RBC. Recipients are at risk of delayed hemolytic transfusion reactions from 'passenger lymphocytes' in the graft.

Recipient	Donor	Preferred choice of RBC	Platelets/plasma
A	O	O	A
B	O	O	B
AB	O	O	AB
AB	A	O, A	AB
AB	B	O, B	AB

Bidirectional mismatch

Recipients are at risk of immediate and delayed hemolysis.

Recipient	Donor	Preferred choice of RBC	Platelets/plasma
A	B	O	AB
B	A	O	AB

O type RBCs are usually provided either from the start of conditioning or from the transplant date, depending on individual transfusion service policies.

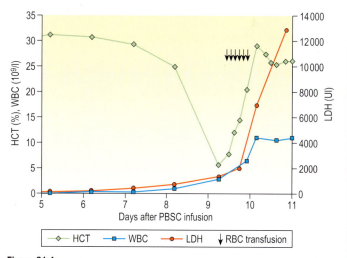

Figure 31.4
Hemolysis secondary to passenger lymphocyte syndrome in a 58-year-old group A positive male with CLL, who received a PBSC graft from his HLA-matched, group O daughter. On day 8 and 9 post-transplant, a precipitous drop in HCT occurred along with a rise in LDH, fever, hemodynamic instability and renal insufficiency. Although the hematocrit responded to group O red cells, cardiopulmonary arrest occurred; neurological function did not recover and the patient died on day 16. Serologic testing revealed that donor-type anti-A isohemagglutinins were the cause of massive immune hemolysis. Potential risk factors for hemolysis in this case included use of ciclosporin alone as anti-GvHD prophylaxis, use of PBSC instead of marrow as the HSCT graft source, and use of a non-HLA matched sibling donor. Reproduced with permission from Bolan et al.[3]

pretransplant titer and the intensity of transplant conditioning regimen), the effectiveness of pretransplant recipient erythropoiesis, and the timing of the conversion to donor erythropoiesis (Fig. 31.5). Patients receiving reduced-intensity conditioning may be at higher risk of PRCA due to prolonged persistence of recipient isohemagglutinin-pro-

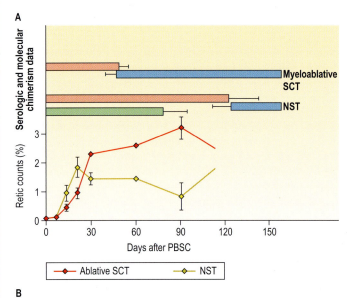

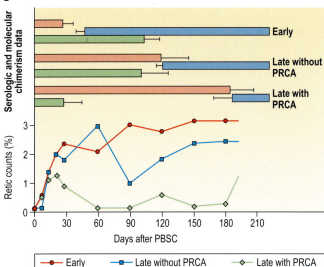

Figure 31.5

Recovery of reticulocyte counts as evidence of overall erythropoietic function following major ABO-incompatible SCT following myeloablative and non-myeloablative (NST) conditioning. The appearance of donor red cell chimerism was assessed by forward typing for major ABO-incompatible donor RBC in recipient blood, while the persistence of recipient-type anti-donor isohemagglutinins was measured by reverse typing as described in the text. Symbols are (pink bars) host anti-donor isohemagglutinin above 1+; (blue bars) detectable donor RBC chimerism; (green bars) detectable host myeloid chimerism. Laboratory analysis for the degree of host myeloid chimerism after myeloablative SCT was not performed. Top portion (a) shows that reticulocyte counts initially recover more slowly after myeloablative SCT than after NST, but reticulocyte counts after NST decreased significantly at the time of conversion to full donor myeloid chimerism, reflecting loss of autologous erythropoiesis at a time when persistent host anti-donor isohemagglutinin activity inhibited the onset of donor RBC chimerism. Error bars (±SEM) are shown at points with significant differences between NST and myeloablative SCT (p < 0.05). Bottom portion (b) illustrates the impact of the timing of these relationships in NST patients. In those with persistent recipient type anti-donor isohemagglutinins and delayed donor RBC chimerism, full donor myeloid chimerism occurred significantly sooner in those with PRCA compared with those without PRCA. The time intervals between conversion to full donor myeloid chimerism and a decrease in host anti-donor isohemagglutinins to 1+ or lower were significantly different among these three groups. Reproduced with permission from Bolan et al.[3]

ducing plasma cells, and disparities in the timing and degree of graft-mediated effects against different recipient cell populations.[105] Although PRCA may respond to manipulation of GvHD prophylaxis or donor lymphocyte infusions, these measures may also induce GvHD; transfusion support with recipient-compatible PRBC alone may be indicated since PRCA eventually resolves. Patients with major ABO incompatibility may also develop post-transplant hemolysis due to isohemagglutinin effects against circulating donor RBC. However, this event is generally milder in comparison to minor ABO-mediated hemolysis.[92]

Persistent recipient-derived isohemagglutinins disappear more rapidly after unrelated donor transplantation, consistent with a greater graft-versus-host effect.[106,107] Following major ABO-incompatible transplants, the blood type, DAT and anti-donor antibody titers should be monitored closely. Until the DAT becomes negative, the recipient is supported with group O red cells.

Rh

As with the ABO blood groups, the inheritance of Rh antigens is also independent of the HLA antigen complex, and hence D mismatch can occur in HLA-matched allogeneic HSCT. Unlike ABO isohemagglutinin antibodies, Rh alloantibody formation usually does not occur without prior exposure through pregnancy, transfusion or transplantation. The terms *alloimmune* and *autoimmune* should be used carefully with regard to antibodies that develop after transplantation.[92] An antibody produced by the recipient's immune system in response to donor RBC antigen is termed alloantibody; also an antibody produced by engrafted donor cells against recipient RBC antigens is an alloantibody. Donor-mediated anti-donor antibodies and recipient-mediated anti-recipient antibodies can be appropriately referred to as autoantibodies.

Different possibilities can occur in Rh (D)-mismatched HSCT. While Rh-mismatched transplants can cause immune hemolysis, PRCA and other cytopenias do not occur and Rh incompatibility is not usually a clinically significant consideration for successful HSCT.[92]

Minor Rh (D) mismatch

An Rh (D)-positive recipient of an Rh (D)-negative HSCT donor may develop a de novo anti-D *alloantibody* (donor mediated) since residual Rh-positive RBC may circulate for months after conditioning and stimulate antibody production by donor immune cells. In this setting, transfusion support consists of donor type RBCs or Rh (D)-negative RBCs. If the HSCT donor has preformed anti-D at the time of transplant, immediate hemolysis after graft infusion can be prevented by removing plasma from the PBSC product; mild hemolysis similar in timing to minor ABO-incompatible passenger lymphocyte-mediated hemolysis may also occur.[96] Generally, however, the appearance of anti-D in the recipient circulation occurs much more slowly. Esteve et al reported appearance of anti-D in the recipient 7 months after HSCT.[108] In a case reported by Franchini et al, anti-D was detected in the recipient on day +35;[109] increased transfusion requirements and evidence of hemolysis were noted.

Major Rh (D) mismatch

In this setting, an Rh (D)-negative recipient undergoes HSCT from an Rh-positive donor. Rh antigens are not expressed on primitive erythroid-forming cells,[94] and PRCA has not been reported to occur in this setting.[110] Berkman et al reported successful engraftment of Rh-positive marrow in an Rh-negative recipient with anti-D.[111]

Other blood group antigen mismatches

Delayed, but not fatal hemolysis may also occur due to donor–recipient mismatch in other blood group systems. Lopez et al reported DHTR on days 21, 35 and 160 after PBSCT due to multiple recipient-derived red cell alloantibodies (anti-Jkb, anti-K).[39] Zupanska et al reported formation of anti-Di(b) after ABO-matched PBSCT.[40]

Serologic monitoring was not predictive of hemolysis. PRCA has not been described due to donor–recipient blood group incompatability except following major ABO-incompatible HSCT.

Pediatric patients

Because of their small blood volume, pediatric transfusion dose is based on the child's weight instead of a whole number of units. Appropriate transfusion support for pediatric patients extends far beyond simple consideration of children as 'small adults', due to the specific immunology and diseases of children, in addition to logistical considerations associated with body size. Irradiation and leukoreduction should be carefully considered in the pediatric patient, and ABO- and Rh (D)-compatible platelets are transfused when possible. Additional guidelines are available from recent reviews.[112,113]

Use of hemostatic drugs

A variety of pharmacologic agents are available to augment hemostasis in patients who are refractory to transfusion, for whom compatible blood products cannot be obtained, or who have bleeding despite transfusion.[114] For example, measures including red cell transfusions, use of estrogens or DDAVP may be useful in patients with uremia, while antifibrinolytic agents such as amicar are indicated for cases involving excess local or systemic fibrinolysis. More recently, use of recombinant factor VII, initially developed to treat hemophilia patients with inhibitors, has been increasingly applied in major surgery, trauma and transplant patients with global coagulation defects due to its potent hemostatic effects including increased platelet function, thrombin generation, and antifibrinolysis.[115–117] A randomized trial comparing different doses of recombinant factor VII and placebo did not find clinically significant improvements in control of bleeding following HSCT.[118] However, a large body of anecdotal studies and evidence from randomized trials is consistent with substantial benefits in certain settings.[119] Combination therapy of recombinant factor VII with concomitant platelet transfusions has been described to be efficacious in alloimmunized, thrombocytopenic patients with severe hemorrhage.[120] Recombinant factor VIIa and other hemostatic agents may exhibit significant toxicity, especially when used in repeated doses or in settings with active thrombosis, and their use should be carefully considered in all patients.[119]

HSCT patients who refuse blood transfusion

HSCT in this group of patients is a challenging procedure since they do not accept transfusion of blood products, but may accept bone marrow or peripheral blood stem cell support. The degree and nature of transfusion support that is acceptable may vary from patient to patient, and the transplant physicians should initiate a careful discussion with the patient, family, religious advisors, blood bank, and hospital ethics and legal personnel prior to undertaking HSCT. Mazza et al reported that myeloablative stem cell transplants have been successfully performed without transfusion support in a variety of hematologic malignancies.[121] Zenz et al reported a successful reduced-intensity conditioning transplant in a patient with CML.[122] Ciurea noted that employing blood conservation methods and erythropoietin prior to conditioning chemotherapy can be used to limit life-threatening anemia.[123] Conservation practices suggested by these authors include:

- using pediatric tubes for blood sampling
- decreasing frequency of blood sampling to every other day
- using a closed system return of the waste blood after drawing blood
- providing daily folic acid, iron supplementation and weekly vitamin K

- giving aminocaproic acid when the platelet count is below 30,000/µl and using gastrointestinal prophylaxis with a proton-pump inhibitor.

Use of family donors for post-HSCT granulocyte/platelet support

Post-transplant management of cytopenias and HLA alloimmunization may be improved with use of HLA-matched family members for platelet pheresis or as granulocyte donors. Additional factors must be considered when the family member has previously served as the marrow or PBSC donor, such as anemia following marrow donation and a 50–75% decrease in blood platelet counts following PBSC donation. Platelet counts also decrease significantly following platelet pheresis. Substantial recovery of counts may occur within 48–72 hours in some individuals; however, the response varies and the donor CBC should be followed carefully in this situation. In some cases, products may have to be released without viral testing, while in all cases, communication with the transfusion service is essential to ensure safe, effective donations, and to maintain adherence to applicable regulations when utilizing family donors for post-HSCT transfusion support. American Association of Blood Bank standards allow 24 granulocyte or platelet pheresis donations per year, with at least 72 hours between successive donations. Appropriate irradiation practices must be followed to prevent TA-GvHD.

Treatment of iron overload

Therapeutic phlebotomy is a safe and effective method to treat transfusion-related iron overload in long-term survivors following successful treatment of marrow failure states[124,125] and malignant disease.[126] Transfusional siderosis can cause significant organ damage in the liver and heart, and may be an important cause of other post-transplant complications such as infection.[127] In patients with post-transplant hemoglobin levels in the lower range, erythropoietin can be given to continue phlebotomy. When low hemoglobin levels prevent initiation of phlebotomy, iron chelation therapy is an effective alternative.[128] Subcutaneous or intravenous administration of deferoxamine is widely used. Because of its relatively short half-life, continuous infusions are necessary using one of the above-mentioned routes. Of note, patients receiving deferoxamine may be at increased risk of infection with mucormycosis and yersinia.[129,130] More recently, orally effective iron chelators have become available which have been shown to be well tolerated and to possess similar efficacy to intravenous chelation in initial randomized studies in patients with non-transplantation related transfusion overload.[131,132]

Conclusion

Transfusion medicine support is essential for proper care of the HSCT patient. A variety of therapeutic blood components and other treatment modalities is available. Although not as prominent as HSCT donor–recipient immunologic interactions, similar but more distant relationships between the HSCT patient and blood donor(s) may have very high impact on overall outcomes. Early and continued communication between clinical teams and transfusion medicine services can help avert transfusion complications and streamline the institution of appropriate transfusion therapy.

Acknowledgment

The authors acknowledge Susan F Leitman MD, Deputy Chief, Department of Transfusion Medicine, Clinical Center, National Institutes of Health, Bethesda MD, 20892, for her review of this chapter and many helpful suggestions during the preparation of this work.

References

1. Popovsky MA, Triulzi D. The role of the transfusion medicine consultant. Am J Clin Pathol 1996;105:798–801
2. Wu WC, Rathore SS, Wang Y et al. Blood transfusion in elderly patients with acute myocardial infarction. N Engl J Med 2001;345:1230–1236
3. Bolan CD, Childs RW, Procter JL et al. Massive immune haemolysis after allogeneic peripheral blood stem cell transplantation with minor ABO incompatibility. Br J Haematol 2001;112:787–795
4. Consensus conference. Fresh-frozen plasma. Indications and risks. JAMA 1985;253: 551–553
5. O'Shaughnessy DF, Atterbury C, Bolton MP et al. Guidelines for the use of fresh-frozen plasma, cryoprecipitate and cryosupernatant. Br J Haematol 20041;126:11–28
6. Ness PM, Perkins HA. Cryoprecipitate as a reliable source of fibrinogen replacement. JAMA 1979;241:1690–1691
7. Mannucci PM. Hemostatic drugs. N Engl J Med 1998;339:245–253
8. Ness PM, Campbell-Lee SA. Single donor versus pooled random donor platelet concentrates. Curr Opin Hematol 2001;8:392–392
9. Leukocyte reduction and ultraviolet B irradiation of platelets to prevent alloimmunization and refractoriness to platelet transfusions. The Trial to Reduce Alloimmunization to Platelets Study Group. N Engl J Med 1997;337:1861–1869
10. Seftel MD, Growe GH, Petraszko T et al. Universal prestorage leukoreduction in Canada decreases platelet alloimmunization and refractoriness. Blood 2004;103:333–339
11. Schiffer CA, Anderson KC, Bennett CL et al. Platelet transfusion for patients with cancer: clinical practice guidelines of the American Society of Clinical Oncology. J Clin Oncol 2001;19:1519–1538
12. Wright DG, Robichaud KJ, Pizzo PA, Deisseroth AB. Lethal pulmonary reactions associated with the combined use of amphotericin B and leukocyte transfusions. N Engl J Med 1981;304:1185–1189
13. Carr JM, Kruskall MS, Kaye JA, Robinson SH. Efficacy of platelet transfusions in immune thrombocytopenia. Am J Med 1986;80:1051–1054
14. Slichter SJ, Davis K, Enright H et al. Factors affecting posttransfusion platelet increments, platelet refractoriness, and platelet transfusion intervals in thrombocytopenic patients. Blood 2005;105:4106–4114
15. McFarland JG. Detection and identification of platelet antibodies in clinical disorders. Transfus Apher Sci 2003;28:297–305
16. Nambiar A, Duquesnoy RJ, Adams S et al. HLA Matchmaker-driven analysis of responses to HLA-typed platelet transfusions in alloimmunized thrombocytopenic patients. Blood 2006;107:1680–1687
17. Dutcher JP, Schiffer CA, Aisner J, Wiernik PH. Alloimmunization following platelet transfusion: the absence of a dose-response relationship. Blood 1981;57:395–398
18. Dutcher JP, Schiffer CA, Aisner J, Wiernik PH. Long-term follow-up patients with leukemia receiving platelet transfusions: identification of a large group of patients who do not become alloimmunized. Blood 1981;58:1007–1011
19. Lozano M, Cid J. The clinical implications of platelet transfusions associated with ABO or Rh(D) incompatibility. Transfus Med Rev 2003;17:57–68
20. Sadani DT, Urbaniak SJ, Bruce M, Tighe JE. Repeat ABO-incompatible platelet transfusions leading to haemolytic transfusion reaction. Transfus Med 2006;16:375–379
21. Mair B, Benson K. Evaluation of changes in hemoglobin levels associated with ABO-incompatible plasma in apheresis platelets. Transfusion 1998;38:51–55
22. Murphy MF, Hook S, Waters AH et al. Acute haemolysis after ABO-incompatible platelet transfusions. Lancet 1990;335:974–975
23. Pierce RN, Reich LM, Mayer K. Hemolysis following platelet transfusions from ABO-incompatible donors. Transfusion 1985;25:60–62
24. Winston DJ, Ho WG, Gale RP. Therapeutic granulocyte transfusions for documented infections. A controlled trial in ninety-five infectious granulocytopenic episodes. Ann Intern Med 1982;97:509–515
25. Herzig RH, Herzig GP, Graw RG Jr et al. Successful granulocyte transfusion therapy for gram-negative septicemia. A prospectively randomized controlled study. N Engl J Med 1977;296:701–705
26. Liles WC, Huang JE, Llewellyn C et al. A comparative trial of granulocyte-colony -stimulating factor and dexamethasone, separately and in combination, for the mobilization of neutrophils in the peripheral blood of normal volunteers. Transfusion 1997;37: 182–187
27. Liles WC, Rodger E, Dale DC. Combined administration of G-CSF and dexamethasone for the mobilization of granulocytes in normal donors: optimization of dosing. Transfusion 2000;40:642–644
28. Boxer LA, Ingraham LM, Allen J et al. Amphotericin-B promotes leukocyte aggregation of nylon-wool-fiber-treated polymorphonuclear leukocytes. Blood 1981;58:518–523
29. Karp DD, Ervin TJ, Tuttle S et al. Pulmonary complications during granulocyte transfusions: incidence and clinical features. Vox Sang 1982;42:57–61
30. Dana BW, Durie BG, White RF, Huestis DW. Concomitant administration of granulocyte transfusions and amphotericin B in neutropenic patients: absence of significant pulmonary toxicity. Blood 1981;57:90–94
31. Bow EJ, Schroeder ML, Louie TJ. Pulmonary complications in patients receiving granulocyte transfusions and amphotericin B. Can Med Assoc J 1984;130:593–597
32. Nichols WG, Price T, Boeckh M. Donor serostatus and CMV infection and disease among recipients of prophylactic granulocyte transfusions. Blood 2003;101:5091–5092
33. Vij R, Dipersio JF, Venkatraman P et al. Donor CMV serostatus has no impact on CMV viremia or disease when prophylactic granulocyte transfusions are given following allogeneic peripheral blood stem cell transplantation. Blood 2003;101:2067–2069
34. Hubel K, Dale DC, Engert A, Liles WC. Current status of granulocyte (neutrophil) transfusion therapy for infectious diseases. J Infect Dis 2001;183:321–328
35. Strauss RG. Therapeutic granulocyte transfusions in 1993. Blood 1993;81:1675–1678
36. Oza A, Hallemeier C, Goodnough L et al. Granulocyte-colony-stimulating factor-mobilized prophylactic granulocyte transfusions given after allogeneic peripheral blood progenitor cell transplantation result in a modest reduction of febrile days and intravenous antibiotic usage. Transfusion 2006;46:14–23
37. de la Rubia J, Arriaga F, Andreu R et al. Development of non-ABO RBC alloantibodies in patients undergoing allogeneic HPC transplantation. Is ABO incompatibility a predisposing factor? Transfusion 2001;41:106–110
38. Nussbaumer W, Schwaighofer H, Gratwohl A et al. Transfusion of donor-type red cells as a single preparative treatment for bone marrow transplants with major ABO incompatibility. Transfusion 1995;35:592–595
39. Lopez A, de la Rubia J, Arriaga F et al. Severe hemolytic anemia due to multiple red cell alloantibodies after an ABO-incompatible allogeneic bone marrow transplant. Transfusion 1998;38:247–251
40. Zupanska B, Zaucha JM, Michalewska B et al. Multiple red cell alloantibodies, including anti-Dib, after allogeneic ABO-matched peripheral blood progenitor cell transplantation. Transfusion 2005;45:16–20
41. Paglino JC, Pomper GJ, Fisch GS et al. Reduction of febrile but not allergic reactions to RBCs and platelets after conversion to universal prestorage leukoreduction. Transfusion 2004;44:16–24
42. Geiger TL, Howard SC. Acetaminophen and diphenhydramine premedication for allergic and febrile nonhemolytic transfusion reactions: good prophylaxis or bad practice? Transfus Med Rev 2007;21:1–12
43. Sandler SG. How I manage patients suspected of having had an IgA anaphylactic transfusion reaction. Transfusion 2006;46:10–13
44. Sandler SG, Zantek ND. Review: IgA anaphylactic transfusion reactions. Part II. Clinical diagnosis and bedside management. Immunohematology 2004;20:234–238
45. Bueter M, Thalheimer A, Schuster F et al. Transfusion-related acute lung injury (TRALI) – an important, severe transfusion-related complication. Langenbecks Arch Surg 2006;391:489–494
46. Swanson K, Dwyre DM, Krochmal J, Raife TJ. Transfusion-related acute lung injury (TRALI): current clinical and pathophysiologic considerations. Lung 2006;184:177–185
47. Shulman NR, Aster RH, Leitner A, Hillier MC. Immunoreactions involving platelets v post-transfusion purpura due to a complement-fixing antibody against a genetically controlled platelet antigen. A proposed mechanism for thrombocytopenia and its relevance in 'autoimmunity'. J Clin Invest 1961;40:1597–1620
48. Evenson DA, Stroncek DF, Pulkrabek S et al. Posttransfusion purpura following bone marrow transplantation. Transfusion 1995;35:688–693
49. Rozman P. Platelet antigens. The role of human platelet alloantigens (HPA) in blood transfusion and transplantation. Transpl Immunol 2002;10:165–181
50. Leitman SF, Holland PV. Irradiation of blood products. Indications and guidelines. Transfusion 1985;25:293–303
51. Klein HG. Transfusion-associated graft-versus-host disease: less fresh blood and more gray (Gy) for an aging population. Transfusion 2006;46:878–880
52. Warren LJ, Simmer K, Roxby D et al. DNA polymorphism analysis in transfusion-associated graft-versus-host disease. J Paediatr Child Health 1999;35:98–101
53. Stramer SL, Glynn SA, Kleinman SH et al. Detection of HIV-1 and HCV infections among antibody-negative blood donors by nucleic acid-amplification testing. N Engl J Med 2004;351:760–768
54. Busch MP, Glynn SA, Stramer SL et al. A new strategy for estimating risks of transfusion-transmitted viral infections based on rates of detection of recently infected donors. Transfusion 2005;45:254–264
55. Kotton CN. Zoonoses in solid-organ and hematopoietic stem cell transplant recipients. Clin Infect Dis 2007;44:857–866
56. Ironside JW. Variant Creutzfeldt-Jakob disease: risk of transmission by blood transfusion and blood therapies. Haemophilia 2006;1(suppl):8–15
57. Alter HJ, Stramer SL, Dodd RY. Emerging infectious diseases that threaten the blood supply. Semin Hematol 2007;44:32–41
58. Seghatchian J, de Sousa G. Pathogen-reduction systems for blood components: the current position and future trends. Transfus Apher Sci 2006;35:189–196
59. Solheim BG, Seghatchian J. Update on pathogen reduction technology for therapeutic plasma: an overview. Transfus Apher Sci 2006;35:83–90
60. Roback JD, Conlan M, Drew WL et al. The role of photochemical treatment with amotosalen and UV-A light in the prevention of transfusion-transmitted cytomegalovirus infections. Transfus Med Rev 2006;20:45–56
61. Ciaravi V, McCullough T, Dayan AD. Pharmacokinetic and toxicology assessment of INTERCEPT (S-59 and UVA treated) platelets. Hum Exp Toxicol 2001;20:533–550
62. Roback JD, Drew WL, Laycock ME et al. CMV DNA is rarely detected in healthy blood donors using validated PCR assays. Transfusion 2003;43:314–321
63. Bowden RA, Slichter SJ, Sayers M et al. A comparison of filtered leukocyte-reduced and cytomegalovirus (CMV) seronegative blood products for the prevention of transfusion-associated CMV infection after marrow transplant. Blood 1995;86:3598–3603
64. Nichols WG, Price TH, Gooley T, Corey L, Boeckh M. Transfusion-transmitted cytomegalovirus infection after receipt of leukoreduced blood products. Blood 2003;101:4195–4200
65. Vamvakas EC. Is white blood cell reduction equivalent to antibody screening in preventing transmission of cytomegalovirus by transfusion? A review of the literature and meta-analysis. Transfus Med Rev 2005;19:181–199
66. Brecher ME, Hay SN. Bacterial contamination of blood components. Clin Microbiol Rev 2005;18:195–204
67. Blajchman MA, Goldman M, Baeza F. Improving the bacteriological safety of platelet transfusions. Transfus Med Rev 2004;18:11–24
68. Fang CT, Chambers LA, Kennedy J et al. Detection of bacterial contamination in apheresis platelet products: American Red Cross experience, 2004. Transfusion 2005;45:1845–1852
69. Cid J, Lozano M. Improving the bacteriological safety of platelet transfusions. Transfus Med Rev 2004;18:235–236
70. Dunne WM Jr, Case LK, Isgriggs L, Lublin DM. In-house validation of the BACTEC 9240 blood culture system for detection of bacterial contamination in platelet concentrates. Transfusion 2005;45:1138–1142

71. Ramirez-Arcos S, Jenkins C, Dion J et al. Canadian experience with detection of bacterial contamination in apheresis platelets. Transfusion 2007;47:421–429

72. Hewitt PE, Llewelyn CA, Mackenzie J, Will RG. Creutzfeldt-Jakob disease and blood transfusion: results of the UK Transfusion Medicine Epidemiological Review study. Vox Sang 2006;91:221–230

73. Llewelyn CA, Hewitt PE, Knight RS et al. Possible transmission of variant Creutzfeldt-Jakob disease by blood transfusion. Lancet 2004;363:417–421

74. Wroe SJ, Pal S, Siddique D et al. Clinical presentation and pre-mortem diagnosis of variant Creutzfeldt-Jakob disease associated with blood transfusion: a case report. Lancet 2006;368:2061–2067

75. Azzi A, Morfini M, Mannucci PM. The transfusion-associated transmission of parvovirus B19. Transfus Med Rev 1999;13:194–204

76. Azzi A, Ciappi S, Zakvrzewska K et al. Human parvovirus B19 infection in hemophiliacs first infused with two high-purity, virally attenuated factor VIII concentrates. Am J Hematol 1992;39:228–230

77. Alter HJ, Stramer SL, Dodd RY. Emerging infectious diseases that threaten the blood supply. Semin Hematol 2007;44:32–41

78. Rowley SD, Anderson GL. Effect of DMSO exposure without cryopreservation on hematopoietic progenitor cells. Bone Marrow Transplant 1993;11:389–393

79. Dzik WH, Kirkley SA. Citrate toxicity during massive blood transfusion. Transfus Med Rev 1988;2:76–94

80. Bolan CD, Cecco SA, Wesley RA et al. Controlled study of citrate effects and response to i.v. calcium administration during allogeneic peripheral blood progenitor cell donation. Transfusion 2002;42:935–946

81. Bansal I, Calhoun BW, Joseph C et al. A comparative study of reducing the extracellular potassium concentration in red blood cells by washing and by reduction of additive solution. Transfusion 2007;47:248–250

82. Weiskopf RB, Schnapp S, Rouine-Rapp K et al. Extracellular potassium concentrations in red blood cell suspensions after irradiation and washing. Transfusion 2005;45:1295–1301

83. Trial to Reduce Alloimmunization to Platelets Study group. Leukocyte reduction and ultraviolet B irradiation of platelets to prevent alloimmunization and refractoriness to platelet transfusions. N Eng J Med 1997;337:1861–1868

84. Williamson LM, Stainsby D, Jones H et al. The impact of universal leukodepletion of the blood supply on hemovigilance reports of posttransfusion purpura and transfusion-associated graft-versus-host disease. Transfusion 2007;47:1455–1467

85. Read EJ, Kodis C, Carter CS, Leitman SF. Viability of platelets following storage in the irradiated state. A pair-controlled study. Transfusion 1988;28:446–450

86. Hong F, Ruiz R, Price H et al. Safety profile of WinRho anti-D. Semin Hematol 1998;35(suppl 1):9–13

87. Stroncek DF, Procter JL, Moses L et al. Intravenous Rh immune globulin prevents alloimmunization in D− granulocyte recipients but obscures the detection of an allo-anti-K. Immunohematology 2001;17:37–41

88. McLeod BC, Piehl MR, Sassetti RJ. Alloimmunization to RhD by platelet transfusions in autologous bone marrow transplant recipients. Vox Sang 1990;59:185–189

89. Cid J. Platelet transfusions from D+ blood donors to D-patients with hematologic diseases: an update. Transfusion 2003;43:1759–1760

90. Cid J, Lozano M. Risk of Rh(D) alloimmunization after transfusion of platelets from D+ donors to D− recipients. Transfusion 2005;45:453–454

91. Atoyebi W, Mundy N, Croxton T et al. Is it necessary to administer anti-D to prevent RhD immunization after the transfusion of RhD-positive platelet concentrates? Br J Haematol 2000;111:980–983

92. Petz LD. Immune hemolysis associated with transplantation. Semin Hematol 2005;42:145–155

93. Eastlund T. The histo-blood group ABO system and tissue transplantation. Transfusion 1998;38:975–988

94. Wada H, Suda T, Miura Y et al. Expression of major blood group antigens on human erythroid cells in a two phase liquid culture system. Blood 1990;75:505–511

95. Bolan CD, Leitman SF, Griffith LM et al. Delayed donor red cell chimerism and pure red cell aplasia following major ABO-incompatible nonmyeloablative hematopoietic stem cell transplantation. Blood 2001;98:1687–1694

96. Hows J, Beddow K, Gordon-Smith E et al. Donor-derived red blood cell antibodies and immune hemolysis after allogeneic bone marrow transplantation. Blood 1986;67:177–181

97. Worel N, Kalhs P, Keil F et al. ABO mismatch increases transplant-related morbidity and mortality in patients given nonmyeloablative allogeneic HPC transplantation. Transfusion 2003;43:1153–1161

98. Rowley SD, Liang PS, Ulz L. Transplantation of ABO-incompatible bone marrow and peripheral blood stem cell components. Bone Marrow Transplant 2000;26:749–757

99. Klumpp TR, Herman JH, Ulicny J et al. Lack of effect of donor-recipient ABO mismatching on outcome following allogeneic hematopoietic stem cell transplantation. Bone Marrow Transplant 2006;38:615–620

100. Worel N, Greinix HT, Keil F et al. Severe immune hemolysis after minor ABO-mismatched allogeneic peripheral blood progenitor cell transplantation occurs more frequently after nonmyeloablative than myeloablative conditioning. Transfusion 2002;42:1293–1301

101. Ramsey G. Red cell antibodies arising from solid organ transplants. Transfusion 1991;31:76–86

102. Gajewski JL, Petz LD, Calhoun L et al. Hemolysis of transfused group O red blood cells in minor ABO-incompatible unrelated-donor bone marrow transplants in patients receiving cyclosporine without posttransplant methotrexate. Blood 1992;79:3076–3085

103. Worel N, Greinix HT, Supper V et al. Prophylactic red blood cell exchange for prevention of severe immune hemolysis in minor ABO-mismatched allogeneic peripheral blood progenitor cell transplantation after reduced-intensity conditioning. Transfusion 2007;47:1494–1502

104. Barge AJ, Johnson G, Witherspoon R, Torok-Storb B. Antibody-mediated marrow failure after allogeneic bone marrow transplantation. Blood 1989;74:1477–1480

105. Griffith LM, McCoy JP Jr, Bolan CD et al. Persistence of recipient plasma cells and anti-donor isohaemagglutinins in patients with delayed donor erythropoiesis after major ABO incompatible non-myeloablative haematopoietic cell transplantation. Br J Haematol 2005;128:668–675

106. Mielcarek M, Leisenring W, Torok-Storb B, Storb R. Graft-versus-host disease and donor-directed hemagglutinin titers after ABO-mismatched related and unrelated marrow allografts: evidence for a graft-versus-plasma cell effect. Blood 2000;96:1150–1156

107. Lee JH, Lee JH, Choi SJ et al. Changes of isoagglutinin titres after ABO-incompatible allogeneic stem cell transplantation. Br J Haematol 2003;120:702–710

108. Esteve J, Alcorta I, Pereira A et al. Anti-D antibody of exclusive IgM class after minor Rh(D)-mismatched BMT. Bone Marrow Transplant 1995;16:632–633

109. Franchini M, de Gironcoli M, Gandini G et al. Transmission of an anti-RhD alloantibody from donor to recipient after ABO-incompatible BMT. Bone Marrow Transplant 1998;21:1071–1073

110. Cid J, Lozano M, Fernandez-Aviles F et al. Anti-D alloimmunization after D-mismatched allogeneic hematopoietic stem cell transplantation in patients with hematologic diseases. Transfusion 2006;46:169–173

111. Berkman EM, Caplan SN. Engraftment of RH-positive marrow in a recipient with RH antibody. Transplant Proc 1977;9(suppl 1):215–218

112. Gibson BE, Todd A, Roberts I et al. Transfusion guidelines for neonates and older children. Br J Haematol 2004;124:433–453

113. Roseff SD, Luban NL, Manno CS. Guidelines for assessing appropriateness of pediatric transfusion. Transfusion 2002;42:1398–1413

114. Bolan CD, Klein HG. Blood component and pharmacologic therapy of hemostatic disorders. In: Kitchens C, Kessler C, Alving B (eds) Consultative hemostasis and thrombosis (2nd edn). Harcourt Health Sciences, New York, 2007:461–490

115. Goodnough LT, Lublin DM, Zhang L et al. Transfusion medicine service policies for recombinant factor VIIa administration. Transfusion 2004;44:1325–1331

116. Mathew P, Simon TL, Hunt KE, Crookston KP. How we manage requests for recombinant factor VIIa (NovoSeven). Transfusion 2007;47:8–14

117. Grounds RM, Bolan C. Clinical experiences and current evidence for therapeutic recombinant factor VIIa treatment in nontrauma settings. Crit Care 2005;9:S29-S36

118. Pihusch M, Bacigalupo A, Szer J et al. Recombinant activated factor VII in treatment of bleeding complications following hematopoietic stem cell transplantation. J Thromb Haemost 2005;3:1935–1944

119. Roberts HR, Monroe DM, White GC. The use of recombinant factor VIIa in the treatment of bleeding disorders. Blood 2004;104:3858–3864

120. Savani BN, Dunbar CE, Rick ME. Combination therapy with rFVIIa and platelets for hemorrhage in patients with severe thrombocytopenia and alloimmunization. Am J Hematol 2006;81:218–219

121. Mazza P, Prudenzano A, Amurri B et al. Myeloablative therapy and bone marrow transplantation in Jehovah's Witnesses with malignancies: single center experience. Bone Marrow Transplant 2003;32:433–436

122. Zenz T, Dohner H, Bunjes D. Transfusion-free reduced-intensity conditioned allogeneic stem cell transplantation in a Jehovah's witness. Bone Marrow Transplant 2003;32:437–438

123. Ciurea S, Beri R, Dobogai L et al. The use of blood conservation methods in addition to erythropoietin allows myeloablative allogeneic stem cell transplantation without the use of blood products. Bone Marrow Transplant 2006;37:325–327

124. Angelucci E, Brittenham GM, McLaren CE et al. Hepatic iron concentration and total body iron stores in thalassemia major. N Engl J Med 2000;343:327–331

125. Angelucci E, Muretto P, Lucarelli G et al. Phlebotomy to reduce iron overload in patients cured of thalassemia by bone marrow transplantation. Italian Cooperative Group for Phlebotomy Treatment of Transplanted Thalassemia Patients. Blood 1997;90:994–998

126. Franchini M, Gandini G, Veneri D et al. Efficacy and safety of phlebotomy to reduce transfusional iron overload in adult, long-term survivors of acute leukemia. Transfusion 2004;44:833–837

127. Jastaniah W, Harmatz P, Pakbaz Z et al. Transfusional iron burden and liver toxicity after bone marrow transplantation for acute myelogenous leukemia and hemoglobinopathies. Pediatr Blood Cancer 2008;50(2):319–324

128. Cohen AR. New advances in iron chelation therapy. Hematology Am Soc Hematol Educ Program 2006;42–47

129. Boelaert JR, de Lochy M, Van CJ et al. Mucormycosis during deferoxamine therapy is a siderophore-mediated infection. In vitro and in vivo animal studies. J Clin Invest 1993;91:1979–1986

130. Green NS. Yersinia infections in patients with homozygous beta-thalassemia associated with iron overload and its treatment. Pediatr Hematol Oncol 1992;9:247–254

131. Piga A, Galanello R, Forni GL et al. Randomized phase II trial of deferasirox (Exjade, ICL670), a once-daily, orally-administered iron chelator, in comparison to deferoxamine in thalassemia patients with transfusional iron overload. Haematologica 2006;91:873–880

132. Vichinsky E, Onyekwere O, Porter J et al. A randomised comparison of deferasirox versus deferoxamine for the treatment of transfusional iron overload in sickle cell disease. Br J Haematol 2007;136:501–508

The transplant pharmacopeia

Stephen O Evans

CHAPTER 32

Introduction

This chapter provides an overview of the main classes of medicines used in the treatment of patients undergoing stem cell transplantation. It is not intended to be exhaustive, and further referenced sources should be used if clarification is required.

Antibacterials

This group of drugs comprises a large portion of this chapter, reflecting their importance in both the prevention and treatment of life-threatening infections in the immunocompromised host.

Aminoglycosides

These are a group of naturally occurring or semi-synthetic polycationic compounds with poor oral bio-availability of less than 1%. Distribution after parenteral administration is in the extracellular fluid. They are broadly bactericidal agents and interact synergistically with the pencillins against certain organisms. Aminoglycosides can cause concentration-related nephrotoxicity and ototoxicity, and hence, appropriate plasma level monitoring and dose–dose interval titration are required when they are administered systemically (Table 32.1).

Neuromuscular blockade is another adverse effect of this class of antibacterials, but it is usually only a problem in patients who are receiving muscle relaxants or anesthetics or in those who have myasthenia gravis.

They are used in combination with a β-lactam for empirical treatment of febrile neutropenia, although reviews of the literature suggest equivalent efficacy of monotherapy (with a β-lactam) with less toxicity.[2] They are also used for treatment of severe sepsis from gram-negative pathogens and for specific infections including bacterial endocarditis and tuberculosis (streptomycin; see below).

Aminoglycosides in common clinical use include the following.

Gentamicin

This is widely used, often dosed daily at 5–7 mg/kg.[3] (Higher doses should be based on lean body weight.) As for all systemic aminoglycosides, dose reductions are required in elderly patients and in those with renal impairment. With confirmed *Pseudomonas aeruginosa* infections, gentamicin must be combined with an anti-pseudomonal penicillin or cephalosporin.

Amikacin

This is useful for treating infections due to gentamicin-resistant organisms, and is dosed at 15 mg/kg/day, maximum daily dose 1.5 g, and a maximum cumulative dose per course of 15 g.[4]

Neomycin

This is too toxic for parenteral use. It can be used topically, usually in combination with other antibacterials, or it can be given orally as part of a selective gut decontamination regimen.[5]

Tobramycin

This has greater activity against *P. aeruginosa* than does gentamicin, and can be used systemically for severe infections caused by susceptible organisms. It is particularly useful in treating pulmonary colonization with *P. aeruginosa* and is given by inhalation[6] at the licensed dose of 300 mg bd.[4]

Streptomycin

This was the first aminoglycoside identified. It is highly toxic to the vestibular system and is reserved for drug-resistant tuberculosis in combination with other agents. It is administered by intramuscular injection only and its use would therefore be problematic in hematology patients who are likely to have disordered hemostasis.

Antipseudomonal penicillins

These penicillins are derived from either benzylpenicillin or ampicillin and possess activity against *P. aeruginosa*. Two of the commercially available agents have been combined with β-lactamase inhibitors (piperacillin + tazobactam, and ticarcillin + clavulanic acid).

They are used in serious infections caused by susceptible organisms, and in the empiric treatment of febrile neutropenia or severe infections in patients with impaired or suppressed host defenses.

Piperacillin + tazobactam (Tazocin®)

Licensed in the UK for the treatment of febrile neutropenia in combination with an aminoglycoside, at a dose of 4.5 g iv 6 hourly.[4] More studies are suggesting that monotherapy is sufficient in the empiric setting.[7] Tazocin also has broad-spectrum activity against many aerobic and anaerobic organisms. The most common adverse effects reported are nausea, diarrhea, vomiting and rash.

Ticarcillin + clavulanic acid (Timentin®)

Licensed in the UK for the treatment of severe infections in hospitalized patients. The recommended doses are 3.2 g 6–8 hourly, with a maximum frequency of 4 hourly. Timentin has been studied in neutropenic patients with leukemia in combination with an aminoglycoside and has been shown to have similar efficacy to ceftazidime + aminoglycoside in the empiric setting.[8] It is worth noting that prolonged treatment with clavulanic acid is associated with a greater risk of cholestatic jaundice, particular in the elderly.[9]

Table 32.1 Relative toxicity index* of aminoglycosides (based on Price et al[1])

	Vestibular	Auditory	Renal
Streptomycin	4	1	<1
Neomycin	1	4	4
Gentamicin	3	2	2
Tobramycin	2	2	2

* 1–4; least to most toxic.

Antistaphylococcal penicillins

This group of penicillins is stable to staphylococcal β-lactamases and therefore has activity against penicillinase-producing *Staph. aureus*. A number of drugs in this class are used clinically in different parts of the world. Nafcillin and oxacillin are used in North America, and flucloxacillin and cloxacillin in Europe.

They are used in the treatment of proven or suspected staphylococcal infections where the causative organism is susceptible to the agent. Severe infections, such as those affecting bone, joints and heart valves, are treated with intravenous therapy, often in combination with other agents.

Flucloxacillin

This is widely used in the UK and is well absorbed orally. Dosing is dependent on the site and severity of infection and ranges from 250 mg po 6 hourly to intravenous doses of 12 g per day in divided doses.[9] Flucloxacillin has been associated with hepatic disorders, and when treatment lasts more than 14 days, patients should be closely monitored.

Antituberculous drugs

Drugs that have activity against tuberculosis include the following: capreomycin, cycloserine, ethambutol, isoniazid, pyrizinamide, rifabutin, rifampicin and streptomycin. Other agents are effective against mycobacterium that belong to different classes of antibacterials and will be discussed elsewhere. Tuberculosis and non-tuberculous mycobacterial infections have been reported with a 0.8% incidence in allogeneic stem cell transplant recipients in one survey.[10]

Capreomycin

Reserved for multidrug-resistant tuberculosis and used in combination with other agents. Ototoxicity is reported, along with pain at injection sites. It is given as a deep intramuscular injection daily for the first 2–4 months and then 2–3 times per week.

Cycloserine

Used as part of a combination approach in multidrug-resistant tuberculosis. Central nervous system toxicity has been observed in the early phase of treatment and is associated with high peak plasma concentrations as a result of renal impairment.

Ethambutol

Has activity against several species of mycobacteria and forms part of quadruple therapy for tuberculosis where resistance to isoniazid is suspected. Optic neuritis is the most important adverse effect and treatment should be discontinued if signs of ocular toxicity develop. Ethambutol is dosed at 15 mg/kg per day.

Isoniazid

Used in both the treatment and prophylaxis of tuberculosis; neurologic side-effects can occur, but these can be prevented with pyridoxine. Patients should be monitored for liver toxicity. Treatment and prophylaxis doses are 300 mg a day.

Pyrazinamide

Used in the early phase of tuberculosis treatment, and its activity is limited to *M. tuberculosis*. Severe liver toxicity is uncommon but more likely in patients with pre-existing liver disease. Monitoring is required., and doses of 2 g per day for 2 months are standard in adults weighing over 50 kg.

Rifabutin

A rifamycin with activity similar to rifampicin, with the exception of being more active against the *Mycobacterium avium* complex, and used to prevent such infection in patients with low CD4 counts. Rifabutin is also used to treat non-tuberculosis mycobacterial disease in combination with other agents. Doses range from 300 mg daily in the prophylactic setting, up to 600 mg a day for treatment. Uveitis is rare, but is more common if patients are taking concomitant fluconazole or macrolide antibiotics and, as with all rifamycins, body secretions will be colored orange-red.

Rifampicin

Its clinical applications other than against tuberculosis encompass treatment of staphylococcal infections including MRSA and chemoprophylaxis of meningococcal meningitis. Rifampicin is used in combination with unrelated antibiotics because of the risk of the emergence of resistant mutants. A potent inducer of hepatic cytochrome P_{450} microsomal enzymes, rifampicin interacts with numerous drugs (Table 32.2).

Skin reactions are common, along with gastrointestinal disturbances, liver function test derangement and pink staining of body fluids. Patients taking rifampicin on an intermittent schedule may rarely experience a 'flu' like syndrome developing after 3–6 months of treatment. Adult doses vary depending on the indication, and range from 450 mg to 1.2 g daily, with larger doses being divided.

Carbapenems (ertapenem, imipenem and meropenem)

This group of antibacterials is characterized by its potent activity against a wide range of gram-positive and -negative organisms and in its resistance to hydrolysis by β-lactamases. Meropenem and imipenem + cilastin are extensively used and studied in neutropenic patients.

Ertapenem

A highly active agent against most gram-negative pathogens, with the notable exception of *P. aeruginosa*. Empiric monotherapy in the neutropenic patient is therefore not recommended with this agent. Nausea and vomiting are the most common side-effects and the drug is dosed intravenously at 1 g daily (24-hour dosing interval).

Imipenem + cilastin

Imipenem is rapidly metabolized by dehydropetidase I; cilastin inhibits this enzyme and is also a renal protectant. It does not exhibit any antibacterial activity. It is used to treat a broad range of serious infections, although it is not recommended in patients with central nervous system involvement. The main toxicities are confusion and seizures and the incidence is greater with high doses or renal impairment. Recommended dosing is 1–2 g/day in 3–4 divided doses (maximum dose 4 g a day).

Table 32.2 Antibacterial drug interactions (not exhaustive)

Antibiotic class	Interacting drug	Mechanism of interaction	Effect	Clinical recommendation
Aminoglycosides	Calcineurin inhibitors – ciclosporin and tacrolimus	Additive toxicities	Increased nephrotoxicity	Monitor very closely. Avoid combinations where possible
	Cytotoxics – platinum	Additive toxicities	Increased nephrotoxicity	Ensure patient has appropriate pre and post hydration. With mannitol diuresis, careful monitoring required
	Diuretics (loop)	Additive toxicities	Nephrotoxicity and ototoxicity potentiated	Some reports in literature with furosemide – monitor closely
	Neuromuscular blockers	Additive effect	Increase in neuromuscular blockade	Very close monitoring – potentially fatal interaction
Penicillins	Methotrexate	Competition for tubular excretion (postulated but not demonstrated in studies)	Reduced methotrexate excretion	Avoid concomitant use where possible. Monitor for methotrexate toxicity
Antituberculous drugs Rifamycins (rifampicin and rifabutin)	Antiarrhythmics – disopyramide, quinidine and propafenone	Liver enzyme induction	Accelerated metabolism Reduced plasma levels of antiarrhythmics	Dose of antiarrhythmics will need to be increased
	Anticoagulants – coumarins	Liver enzyme induction	Accelerated metabolism Reduced anticoagulant effect	Close monitoring and dose titration required
	Antiepileptics	Liver enzyme induction	Accelerated metabolism and reduced plasma levels of antiepileptics	Phenytoin – monitor levels and titrate to patient Carbamazepine – monitor levels and titrate to patient
	Antifungals (triazoles – itraconazole, fluconazole, voriconazole and posaconazole) Caspofungin	Liver enzyme induction (rifamycins) and inhibition (azoles)	Accelerated metabolism Reduced plasma levels of azoles, increased plasma levels of rifamycins	Itraconazole – avoid if possible (significant reduction in azole levels with both rifampicin and rifabutin) Fluconazole – increase dose with rifampcin, decrease dose of rifabutin (increases risk of uveitis) Voriconazole – avoid with rifampicin. Increase dose with rifabutin and monitor for toxicity Posaconazole – avoid with both rifamycins if possible Caspofungin – consider increasing dose with rifampicin
	Diuretics – eplerenone	Liver enzyme induction	Accelerated metabolism Reduced plasma levels	Avoid combination
	Estrogens and progestogens	Liver enzyme induction	Accelerated metabolism Reduced plasma levels	Avoid combination
	Sirolimus	Liver enzyme induction	Accelerated metabolism Reduced plasma levels	Avoid combination
Isoniazid	Carbamazepine	Liver enzyme inhibition and additive toxicities	Decreased clearance, increased plasma levels (increased risk of hepatotoxicity)	Close monitoring, plasma levels and liver function tests
	Phenytoin	Liver enzyme inhibition	Decreased clearance, increased plasma levels	Close monitoring of plasma levels and phenytoin toxicity
Carbapenems Imipenem with cilastin	Ganciclovir	Additive toxicities	Increased risk of convulsions	Avoid combination
Glycopeptides Vancomycin	Ciclosporin	Additive toxicities	Increase in nephrotoxicity	Monitor levels of both agents and monitor renal function closely
Macrolides* (Erythromycin and clarithromycin)	Pentamidine (parenteral erythromycin)	Additive toxicities	Increased risk of ventricular arrhythmias	Avoid combination
	Quinolones (moxifloxacin) (parenteral erythromycin)	Additive toxicities	Increased risk of ventricular arrhythmias	Avoid combination
	Sirolimus	Liver enzyme inhibition	Decreased clearance, increase in sirolimus levels	Avoid combination
	Statins (simvastatin and atorvastatin)	Liver enzyme inhibition	Decreased clearance, increase in statin plasma levels. Increased risk of myopathies	Avoid combination
	Theophylline	Liver enzyme inhibition	Decreased clearance, increase in theophylline levels	Requires close monitoring of plasma levels and theophylline toxicities

Meropenem

Stable to dehydropeptidases. It has been studied in the transplant population as first-line empiric therapy.[11] The incidence of central nervous system toxicity is lower than with imipenem, and high doses can be used to treat meningitis; adult dose range 1–2 g 8 hourly.

Cephalosporins

This comprises a vast group of agents containing over 100 semi-synthetic compounds which are not all currently marketed. They are β-lactam antibiotics with varying spectrums of cover. Overuse has been associated with a higher risk of *Clostridium difficile*-associated diarrhea as compared to that seen with other classes of antibiotics.[12] Here, the agents likely to be used in the hemato-oncology setting will be addressed.

Cefotaxime

Has historically been studied and used as an empiric agent in the neutropenic setting.[13] Good CNS penetration lends itself to the treatment of bacterial meningitis. Dose range 2–12 g/day depending on the severity of the infection.

Ceftriaxone

This is a broad-spectrum agent with a long plasma half-life compared to other agents. It is given as a single daily dose and is licensed in the UK for treatment of infections in neutropenic patients. Adverse effects are similar to those seen with other broad-spectrum cephalosporins and include nausea, vomiting, diarrhea (pseudomembranous colitis) and rashes. Dosing is 2–4 g/day for severe infections.

Ceftazidime

Highly active against *P. aeruginosa* and other gram-negative pathogens, and less active against *Staph. aureus* compared to other cephalosporins. Some studies show equivalence to tazocin as empiric monotherapy in hematology patients.[14] It is dosed at 2 g 8 hourly in the immunocompromised or meningitis settings.

Glycopeptides and other agents active against gram-positive organisms

A chemically complex group of compounds with activity restricted to gram-positive pathogens due to lack of penetration of the cell wall of gram-negative microbes. Glycopeptides have activity against methicillin-resistant strains of *Staph. aureus*. Most bacterial resistance to glycopeptides has been seen with enterococci.

New agents with activity against resistant gram-positive pathogens are in clinical use, with more in development. Linezolid, an oxazolidinone, and daptomycin, a lipopeptide, are giving clinicians more choice in the fight against MRSA.

Teicoplanin

A complex of several glycopeptide molecules, but due to size it does not cross the blood–brain barrier. Unlike with vancomycin, drug-level monitoring is not mandatory; the manufacturer does recommend this for optimizing therapy, but it is rarely done. Dose adjustment is required in patients with renal impairment and there are reports of drug-induced thrombocytopenia. Dosing in severe infections is 400 mg every 12 hours for three doses (iv/im) followed by 400 mg daily.

Vancomycin

This was first discovered in the 1950s and is still the only glycopeptide approved for human use in the USA. Rapid intravenous infusion is associated with a histamine-related reaction called 'red man' syndrome, resulting in severe pain and necrosis. Slow, intermittent infusion or continuous infusion is therefore recommended in some settings.[15] Therapeutic monitoring is required. Nephrotoxicity may occur with treatment in excess of 3 weeks and ototoxicity where plasma levels have been above 50 mg/l. Vancomycin is available as an oral preparation for treatment of antibiotic-induced colitis, dosed at 125 mg 6 hourly for 2–7 days. Systemic dosing is usually around 2 g daily in 2–4 divided doses.

Daptomycin

A lipopeptide, recently licensed in the UK for the treatment of complicated skin and soft tissue infections. Recent studies have shown promising results in staphylococcal bacteremias and endocarditis.[16] The main toxicities observed to date are muscle related, with the manufacturers recommending creatinine phosphokinase (CPK) measurements at baseline and throughout treatment. Daptomycin is dosed at 4 mg/kg iv once a day for treatment of skin and soft tissue infections.

Linezolid

An oxazolidinone, licensed in the UK for treatment of both hospital- and community-acquired pneumonia where a gram-positive organism is the likely pathogen, and for skin and soft tissue infections. Despite some initial evidence of bone marrow suppression, experience is building in neutropenic patients.[17] The most commonly reported toxicities include nausea, vomiting, diarrhea and taste disturbance. Peripheral and optic neuropathy have been reported where courses in excess of 28 days have been given. Linezolid causes mild, reversible inhibition of monoamine oxidase, and certain drugs should therefore be avoided or, if used, closely monitored (see Table 32.2).

Macrolides

These have broad-spectrum antimicrobial activity particularly against intracellular pathogens such as *Legionella, Chlamydia* and *Rickettsia* spp.

Toxicity varies between drugs. The most common side-effects are gastrointestinal, and liver function can be adversely affected.

Azithromycin

Has a long plasma half-life, enabling once-daily dosing, and is well tolerated compared to other macrolides. Clinical indications include upper and lower respiratory infections, skin and soft tissue infections, and treatment of parasitic infections such as toxoplasmosis. Dosing is indication based at 250–500 mg daily for 3 days.

Clarithromycin

This is more potent than erythromycin against common pathogens and available as both intravenous and oral preparations. Used to treat atypical respiratory tract infections including community-acquired pneumonias. Dosing is 250–500 mg 12 hourly orally, and 500 mg 12 hourly by iv infusion.

Erythromycin

Has variable absorption and nausea and vomiting can limit its oral use. The intravenous preparation must be well diluted and given slowly to avoid irritation. Indications for use are similar to the other macrolides and include campylobacter. Oral doses in adults range from 250 mg to 1 g 6 hourly and as an iv infusion, 50 mg/kg/day in four divided doses.

Metronidazole

A nitroimidazole with activity against a range of bacteria, protozoa and some helminths that depend on anaerobic metabolism. It is dosed at 400–800 mg tds orally, or 500 mg tds iv.

Aztreonam

The only monobactam licensed for use in humans in Europe. It is active against gram-negative organisms and has been used in combination in the empiric treatment of febrile neutropenia. Intravenous doses range from 1 g to 8 g daily in equally divided doses.

Penicillins

Amoxicillin

A generally well-tolerated antibiotic commonly used in wide of variety of clinical settings. It is unstable to most β-lactamases and its spectrum is extended with the addition of clavulanic acid (co-amoxiclav). It is dosed orally from 250 to 500 mg 8 hourly, with larger doses for specific indications. Intravenous dosing is from 500 mg 8 hourly to 1 g every 6 hours.

Ampicillin

Has a similar spectrum of activity to amoxicillin but causes more gastrointestinal upset with oral use. *Listeria monocytogenes* is susceptible and is usually treated in combination with an aminoglycoside. Oral dosing is 250 mg to1 g 6 hourly, and intravenous administration ranges from 500 mg 6 hourly to 2 g 4 hourly for meningitis.

Benzylpenicillin

A group 1 penicillin available as a parenteral preparation. It has a low toxicity profile although central nervous system toxicity is associated with high-dose treatment where cerebrospinal fluid concentrations are >10 mg/l. It is used in the treatment of streptococcal infections and meningococcal meningitis and dosed at 1.2–14.4 g in 2–4 divided doses.

Phenoxymethylpenicillin (penicillin V)

This is an oral agent with a limited spectrum of activity similar to that of benzylpenicillin. Clinical use is in infections that have responded to benzylpenicillin, or in the treatment of non-serious streptococcal infections. Dosing is 250 mg to 1 g 6 hourly.

Polymixins

Colistimethate sodium

This is the only polymixin available for systemic use. It is inactive against gram-positive organisms although most enterobacteria are susceptible. Nephrotoxicity is the most serious adverse effect and neurotoxicity has been observed in patients with renal impairment. It is dosed at 1–2 million units 8 hourly either nebulized or by intravenous injection.

Colistin sulfate

Used as part of selective gut decontamination. Doses vary from 1.5 to 3 million units three times daily.

Quinolones

Ciprofloxacin

A fluoroquinolone with the greatest potency against enterobacteria. Bacterial resistance has been demonstrated where the drug is used extensively.[18] It is used as an alternative to an aminoglycoside as part of a less nephrotoxic combination. It is dosed orally at 250–750 mg 12 hourly or 200–400 mg 12 hourly by the iv route.

Moxifloxacin

Possesses greater activity against gram-positive organisms than does ciprofloxacin. It is also active against a range of atypical pathogens but has no *Pseudomonas* cover. It is only available as an oral agent in the UK, and is dosed at 400 mg daily.

Sulfonamides/combinations

Co-trimoxazole (trimethoprim and sulfamethoxazole)

Indicated for the treatment and prophylaxis of *Pneumocystis jiroveci* pneumonia (PJP) (formerly *Pneumocystis carinii*). Guidelines recommend at least 6 months of prophylaxis post allogeneic and autologous SCT.[19] Co-trimoxazole is used to treat rare infections such as nocardiasis and toxoplasmosis, and infections due to resistant organisms such as *Stenotrophomonas maltophilia*. Standard prophylaxis orally is 480 mg bd thrice weekly. The treatment dose for PJP by mouth or intravenous infusion is 120 mg/kg in 2–4 divided doses. For treatment of other infections, the dose is 960–1440 mg 12 hourly.

Sulfadiazine

Used in combination with pyrimethamine in the treatment of proven or suspected toxoplasmosis. It is dosed intravenously at 1–1.5 g q4–6 hours.

Tetracyclines

Doxycycline

This has useful activity against a range of organisms including nocardia and mycoplasma spp. It is only available orally. Doses range from100 mg daily to 200 mg bd, depending on indication.

Tigecycline

A new, broad-spectrum agent which includes MRSA and extended spectrum β-lactamase (ESBL)-producing organisms. It is licensed for the treatment of complicated skin and soft tissue infections and is dosed iv at 100 mg load and then 50 mg 12 hourly.

Antifungals

This class of anti-infectives is commonly used in both the prophylaxis and treatment of fungal infections in the transplant setting. Invasive infections are associated with significant morbidity and mortality in this high-risk population.

Azoles

Fluconazole

Active against a range of fungi. Its clinical use is limited more to the prophylaxis and treatment of *Candida* infections, particularly where *Candida albicans* is implicated. Fluconazole also has activity against most strains of *Cryptococcus neoformans* but has no action against *Aspergillus*. Doses range from 50 mg daily orally up to 800 mg a day iv for the treatment of candidemia in the neutropenic patient. 400 mg a day is the licensed oral dose for prophylaxis of fungal infections in immunocompromised patients although many transplant centers would now use an azole with activity against molds.

Itraconazole

Possesses activity against both molds and yeasts and is licensed for both the treatment and prevention of invasive fungal infections. The Committee for the Safety of Medicines recommends caution when itraconazole is prescribed to patients at high risk of heart failure as it has negative inotropic properties. Itraconazole has also been associated with hepatotoxicity and a host of drug–drug interactions (Table 32.3).

Itraconazole solution (capsule formulation poorly absorbed) is licensed for the prevention of deep fungal infections in patients with a hematologic malignancy undergoing bone marrow transplantation, at a dose of 2.5 mg/kg twice a day. The intravenous formulation is licensed for the second-line treatment of aspergillosis and cryptococcosis at a dose of 200 mg twice a day for 2 days followed by once-daily dosing.

Posaconazole

The most recent azole on the market. It is licensed for salvage treatment of invasive fungal infections, including aspergillosis and rarer molds, and for the prophylaxis of invasive fungal infections in patients receiving remission-induction chemotherapy for acute myelogenous leukemia or myelodysplastic syndromes likely to cause prolonged neutropenia, resulting in a high risk of invasive fungal infections. It is also used for HSCT recipients who are receiving high-dose immunosuppressive therapy for GvHD and who are at high risk of developing invasive fungal infections.[4] Posaconazole is only available as an oral solution. The treatment dose is 400 mg twice a day and prophylaxis 200 mg three times a day.

Voriconazole

The only azole currently licensed for primary treatment of invasive aspergillosis and available in both oral and intravenous formulations. The oral dose is 400 mg twice daily for two doses followed by 200 mg twice daily. Intravenous dosing is 6 mg/kg twice daily for two doses, followed by 4 mg/kg twice daily.

Polyenes

Amphotericin B

The only polyene licensed for the treatment of invasive fungal infections. It is associated with toxic effects including infusion-related reactions and nephrotoxicity. Lipid preparations have been developed to enable higher doses to be delivered, with significantly less toxicity. Ambisome® is the only liposomal preparation, and is the market leader in the UK and Europe. It is licensed at a treatment dose of 3 mg/kg once a day by intravenous infusion (increasing gradually from 1 mg/kg per day after an initial test dose of 1 mg). Ambisome is also licensed for the empiric treatment of febrile neutropenia unresponsive to broad-spectrum antibiotics, although this strategy is being replaced by a pre-emptive approach, with certain antifungals initiated upon more specific clinical/diagnostic parameters, including

Table 32.3 Main interactions of azole antifungals

Antifungal	Interacting drug	Mechanism of interaction	Effect	Clinical recommendation
Fluconazole	Analgesics – celecoxib	Liver enzyme inhibition	Increase in celecoxib plasma levels	Halve celecoxib dose
	Anticoagulants –coumarins	Liver enzyme inhibition	Decreased clearance, increased anticoagulant effect	Close monitoring; may result in a dose reduction
	Antiepileptics – carbamazepine	Liver enzyme inhibition	Increase in carbamazepine levels	Monitor carbamazepine levels
	Antiepileptics – phenytoin	Liver enzyme inhibition	Increase in phenytoin levels	Monitor phenytoin levels
	Ciclosporin	Liver enzyme inhibition	Increase in ciclosporin levels	Monitor ciclosporin levels, consider dose reduction
	Diuretics – eplerenone	Liver enzyme inhibition	Increase in eplerenone levels	Reduce dose of eplerenone
	Theophylline	Liver enzyme inhibition	Increase in theophylline levels	Requires close monitoring of plasma levels and theophylline toxicities
Itraconazole	Antiarrhythmics – quinidine	Liver enzyme inhibition	Increase risk of ventricular arrhythmias	Avoid combination
	Anticoagulants – coumarins as per fluconazole			
	Antiepileptics – carbamazepine	Liver enzyme induction	Accelerated metabolism Reduced plasma levels of itraconazole	Monitor itraconazole levels
	Antiepileptics – phenytoin	Liver enzyme induction	Accelerated metabolism Reduced plasma levels of itraconazole	Avoid combination
	Anxiolytics – midazolam	Liver enzyme inhibition	Increase in midazolam levels	Monitor for excessive sedation
	Barbiturates – phenobarbitone	Liver enzyme induction	Accelerated metabolism Reduced plasma levels of itraconazole	Avoid combination
Voriconazole	Calcium channel blockers	Additive toxicities/ activity	Increase in negative inotropic effect	Avoid combination
	Cardiac glycosides – digoxin	Liver enzyme inhibition	Increase in digoxin levels	Monitor digoxin levels- and toxicity
	Ciclosporin – as per fluconazole			
	Cytotoxics – busulfan, cyclophosphamide	Inhibition of metabolism	Increase in toxicity	Avoid concomitant use
	Cytotoxics – vinca alkaloids	Inhibition of metabolism	Increase in toxicity	Avoid concomitant use
	Sirolimus	Liver enzyme inhibition	Increase in sirolimus levels	Avoid combination
	Statins – atorvastatin and simvastatin	Liver enzyme inhibition	Increase in statin levels with increased risk of myopathy	Avoid combination
	Tacrolimus	Liver enzyme inhibition	Increase in tacrolimus levels	Monitor levels closely

high-resolution computed tomography and serial fungal antigen testing.[20]

Echinocandins

Caspofungin

An echinocandin with activity against most *Candida* species and *Aspergillus*. It is licensed for the empiric treatment of presumed fungal infections in patients with febrile neutropenia and in the salvage setting in proven/probable invasive aspergillosis. Caspofungin is dosed at a 70 mg load, followed by 50 mg a day (70 mg if >80 kg body weight) by intravenous infusion.

Others

Flucytosine

Active against yeasts and has been used in combination with amphotericin B in the treatment of cryptococcal meningitis, at a dose of 200 mg/kg daily in four divided dose by intravenous infusion. Plasma monitoring is mandatory in patients with renal impairment.

Antiprotozoals

A summary of some of the agents used in the stem cell transplant population is given below. A number of the antibacterials discussed previously have activity against a range of protozoa, but the following have yet to be mentioned.

Quinine

Used in the treatment of falciparum malaria, particularly in cerebral malaria where chloroquine resistance is suspected. The oral dose is 600 mg every 8 hours for 7 days. It can be given intravenously if the patient is seriously ill, with a 20 mg/kg loading dose over 4 hours, followed by a maintenance dose 8 hours later of 10 mg/kg over 4 hours, every 8 hours (all doses are capped at a weight of 70 kg).

Choloroquine

Reserved for the chemoprophylaxis of malaria in areas where chloroquine-resistant falciparum malaria is uncommon. It is used in combination with proguanil at a weekly dose of 300 mg. Proguanil is dosed at 200 mg a day.

Pyrimethamine

Used in combination with sulfadiazine to treat toxoplasmosis infections. It is dosed at a 20 mg load, followed by 50–100 mg once daily orally and given with folinic acid to reduce the risk of bone marrow suppression.

Pentamidine

Used to treat a range of protozoa infections including visceral leishmaniasis and trypanosomiasis, and the fungal infection *Pneumocystis jiroveci*. The treatment dose for pneumocystis is by the iv route at a daily dose of 4 mg/kg, or via inhalation using suitable equipment at a dose of 600 mg a day. In the treatment of PJP, use is limited to severe disease in patients who have failed or cannot tolerate co-trimoxazole due to systemic side-effects.

Mefloquine

Active against chloroquine-resistant falciparum malaria and recommended as chemoprophylaxis for travelers on route to areas where resistance is endemic. Adverse affects have been reported and include neuropsychiatric reactions. Adult prophylaxis is 250 mg once weekly.

Antivirals

This section will exclude the antiretrovirals and focus on the remaining drugs that are commonly used in the stem cell transplant setting.

Aciclovir

Used for the prophylaxis and treatment of herpes simplex and varicella zoster infections.It has poor activity against cytomegalovirus. Oral absorption is around 20%.
- Herpes simplex prophylaxis in the immunocompromised patient: 200–400 mg four times daily orally (local practice 400 mg three times a day). 5 mg/kg every 8 hours by intravenous infusion. Treatment dose: 400 mg five times a day for 5 days.
- Varicella and herpes zoster, treatment: 800 mg five times a day for 7 days, 10 mg/kg every 8 hours by intravenous infusion.
- Simplex encephalitis: 10 mg/kg every 8 hours by intravenous infusion.

Valaciclovir

A prodrug of aciclovir indicated for the prophylaxis and treatment of herpes simplex and herpes zoster infections.[4] Dosing is as follows. Treatment of herpes zoster: 1000 mg three times daily for 7 days; 1 g has been shown to be equivalent to 5 mg/kg of intravenous aciclovir.[21] Treatment of herpes simplex: 500 mg twice daily for 5 days. For initial episodes, which can be more severe, treatment may have to be extended to 10 days. Suppression (prevention) of herpes simplex infection: for immunocompromised patients the dose is 500 mg twice daily.

Ganciclovir

Possesses a broader activity against herpes-type viruses as compared to aciclovir, as it is a potent anti-cytomegalovirus agent. It is dosed by intravenous infusion at 5 mg/kg 12 hourly in patients with good renal function who have CMV viremia and/or when CMV infection is clinically manifested or suspected. Ganciclovir is, however, myelosuppressive.

Valganciclovir

An oral prodrug of ganciclovir and 900 mg bd is equivalent to an iv treatment dose. It is not yet licensed for the pre-emptive treatment of CMV infection post allogeneic stem cell transplant but experience is growing.[22]

Foscarnet

Used as an alternative to ganciclovir in patients with low leukocyte counts or in suspected viral resistance, for both CMV and mucocutaneous herpes simplex virus (HSV) infections, unresponsive to aciclovir in immunocompromised patients.

Dosing for the treatment of CMV is dependent on renal function; the full dose is 60 mg/kg every 8 hours. Monitoring of electrolytes is mandatory, and supplementary hydration is recommended.

Cidofovir

Usually reserved for third-line treatment of CMV infection and highly nephrotoxic, Pre- and post-hydration are required, along with probenecid to ensure adequate renal clearance to prevent kidney damage. Cidofovir is initially dosed at 5 mg/kg weekly for the first 2 weeks, then weekly thereafter. Cidofovir is also reported to have activity against adenovirus.[23]

Ribavirin

Has antiviral activity against the respiratory viruses parainfluenza and respiratory syncytial virus (RSV), and also against hepatitis C. Ribavirin is licensed for use by the aerosol route in the treatment of RSV infection; 6 g is administered via a small particle aerosol generator over at least 6 hours, in three divided doses.

Cytotoxic agents

The focus will be on cytotoxics used in transplant conditioning, GvHD prophylaxis and/or treatment of steroid-refractory GvHD.

Alkylators

Busulfan

Often the alkylator of choice in conditioning protocols for myeloid malignancies. The intravenous preparation has largely superseded the oral preparation, offering predictable dosing and therefore conferring less risk of hepatic veno-occlusive disease. It is dosed at 0.8 mg/kg every 6 hours for 16 doses, followed by cyclophosphamide in the full-intensity setting. Data recently published suggest a single daily dose of 3.2 mg/kg is both safe and effective.[24] Patients receiving busulfan should be commenced on an anticonvulsant such as phenytoin or clonazepam 12 hours before the first dose and continued until 24 hours after the last dose, to prevent seizures as busulfan has demonstrated proconvulsant properties. Busulfan has been combined with other agents in conditioning regimens, such as fludarabine in the reduced-intensity setting.[25]

Carmustine (BCNU)

Used as part of the B*E*AM conditioning protocol for autografting lymphoma patients. BEAM plus alemtuzumab has been reported in the reduced-intensity allogeneic setting.[26] High doses of carmustine have been linked to pulmonary fibrosis. Lung function tests may be useful in screening and for follow-up in patients who have respiratory deficit or prior mediastinal radiation prior to BEAM.

Cyclophosphamide

Forms the basis of many full-intensity transplant conditioning protocols. When administered with total-body irradiation (TBI), it is usually dosed at 60 mg/kg on two consecutive days. High-dose cyclophosphamide requires concomitant hydration and the use of mesna to reduce the effects of the urotoxic metabolite, acrolein. Patients should also be monitored for macro- and microscopic hematuria.

Melphalan

The agent of choice for autografting in the myeloma setting. Doses above 140 mg/m^2 are thought to be myeloblative.[4] Aggressive hydration is given to ensure maximal renal clearance (although spontaneous degradation probably accounts for a significant proportion of high-dose clearance).[26] Gastrointestinal side-effects are very common with high-dose therapy and include nausea, mucositis manifested as stomatitis and diarrhea.

Antimetabolites

Cytarabine (Ara-C)

Forms part of the BE*A*M protocol.[27] Its main side-effects include sore eyes and central nervous system problems such as cerebellar ataxia.

Fludarabine

Used as a key component of many reduced-intensity transplant regimens with agents such as melphalan and alemtuzumab.[28] Doses vary but are usually 25–30 mg/m^2 for 5 days. The lymphotoxic activity of fludarabine is immunosuppressive rather than myeloablative.

Methotrexate

Used along with ciclosporin for the prevention of GvHD following sibling allogeneic SCT, according to the Seattle protocol,[29] and is dosed at 15/10/10/10 mg/m^2 on days +1, 3, 6 and 11, followed by folinic acid rescue. Weekly dosing has also been used in steroid-refractory GvHD.[30] Its immunosuppressive properties are thought to be mediated through activity on adenosine.

Pentostatin

A purine analog with antilymphoproliferative properties. It has been used in the treatment of GvHD,[31] with some success.

Etoposide

Forms part of the B*E*AM protocol and is also used as a single agent with TBI as conditioning for allogeneic transplantation[32] at a dose of 60 mg/kg. Side-effects include severe gastrointestinal toxicity, and metabolic acidosis has been reported.

Immunosuppressants

This ever-growing group of drugs plays a critical role in allogeneic stem cell transplantation. However, the powerful effects of these drugs do place recipients at risk of serious complications.

Calcineurin inhibitors

Ciclosporin

Initially used in solid organ transplantation in the 1970s. It is the key immunosuppressant in many transplant centers. The licensed dose is 3–5 mg/kg/day by intravenous infusion, from day −1 until oral maintenance begins. Ciclosporin is often combined with short-course methotrexate (see above) in the sibling allogeneic setting. Ciclosporin is a drug with a narrow therapeutic window, and maintaining serum levels within a predetermined range is important to ensure appropriate immune suppression without toxicity. A number of side-effects are associated with its use, the more common ones including tremor, headache, nausea, hypertension, hypomagnesemia and disturbances of both renal and liver function. Other serious but rarer side-effects include hemolytic uremic syndrome. Ciclosporin is mainly metabolized in the liver, and drug interactions commonly affect its handling (Table 32.4).

Tacrolimus

An alternative to ciclopsorin. It is unlicensed in the bone marrow transplant (BMT) setting but is extensively used for the prophylaxis and treatment of GvHD. It is available as intravenous and oral formulations and as a topical preparation for skin GvHD.[33]

Intravenous administration is 0.03–0.04 mg/kg/day as a 24-hour continuous infusion; doses as high as 0.15 mg/kg/day iv have been used as starting doses in some trials.[34]

Oral administration is 0.06 mg/kg bd starting dose, or 4–5 times the daily iv dose divided into two oral doses if converting from iv. Tacrolimus, like ciclosporin, is nephrotoxic and in solid organ transplantation secondary diabetes mellitus has been observed. Trough whole-blood levels are monitored and its interaction profile is similar to ciclosporin.

Table 32.4 Immunosuppressant drug interactions (not exhaustive)*

Immunosuppressant	Interacting drug	Mechanism of interaction	Effect	Clinical recommendation
Ciclosporin	ACE inhibitors and angiotensin II antagonists	Additive toxicities	Increased risk of hyperkalemia	Monitor potassium levels
	Analgesics – NSAIDs	Additive toxicities Interference with diclofenac handling	Increased risk of nephrotoxicity Increase in diclofenac levels	Monitor closely Halve dose of diclofenac
	Antidepressants – St John's wort	Liver enzyme induction	Decrease in ciclosporin levels	Avoid combination
	Antiepileptics- carbamazepine	Liver enzyme induction	Decrease in ciclosporin levels	Monitor ciclosporin levels closely
	Antiepileptics – phenytoin	Liver enzyme induction	Decrease in ciclosporin levels	Monitor ciclosporin levels closely
	Barbiturates	Liver enzyme induction	Decrease in ciclosporin levels	Monitor ciclosporin levels closely
	Bile acids – ursodeoxycholic acid	Interference with absorption of ciclosporin	Increased ciclosporin levels	Monitor ciclosporin levels closely
	Calcium channel blockers – diltiazem and verapamil	Interference with metabolism of ciclosporin	Increased ciclosporin levels	Monitor ciclosporin levels closely
	Cardiac glycosides – digoxin	Interference with digoxin handling	Increased digoxin levels	Monitor digoxin levels and toxicity
	Corticosteroids – high-dose methylprednisolone	Interference with metabolism of ciclosporin	Increased ciclosporin levels (risk of convulsions)	Monitor ciclosporin levels closely
	Cytoxics – doxorubicin	Additive toxicities	Increased risk of neurotoxicity	Monitor closely, avoid if possible
	Cytoxics – melphalan	Additive toxicities	Increased risk of nephrotoxicity	Monitor closely
	Diuretics – potassium-sparing and aldosterone antagonists	Additive toxicities	Increased risk of hyperkalemia	Monitor potassium levels
	Grapefruit juice	Interference with absorption and metabolism of ciclosporin	Increased ciclosporin levels	Avoid combination
	Hormone antagonists – danazol	Interference with metabolism of ciclosporin	Increased ciclosporin levels	Monitor ciclosporin levels closely
	Hormone antagonists – octreotide	Interference with metabolism of ciclosporin	Decrease in ciclosporin levels	Monitor ciclosporin levels closely
	Metoclopramide	Interference with metabolism of ciclosporin	Increased ciclosporin levels	Monitor ciclosporin levels closely
	Progestogens	Interference with metabolism of ciclosporin	Increased ciclosporin levels	Monitor ciclosporin levels closely
	Statins	Additive toxicities	Increased risk of myopathy	Monitor closely
	Tacrolimus	Additive toxicities	Increase in toxicities related to calcineurin inhibitors	Avoid combination
Sirolimus	Calcium channel blockers – diltiazem and verapamil as per ciclosporin			
	Grapefruit juice – as per ciclosporin			
Tacrolimus	Analgesics – NSAIDs as per ciclosporin			
	Antidepressants – St John's wort as per ciclosporin			
	Calcium channel blockers – diltiazem and nifedipine	Interference with metabolism of tacrolimus	Increase in tacrolimus levels	Monitor tacrolimus levels closely
	Ciclosporin	Additive toxicities	Increase in ciclosporin levels and toxicities	Avoid combination
	Diuretics – as per ciclosporin			
	Grapefruit juice – as per ciclosporin			

*Excludes antibacterial and antifungal interactions, as these are detailed in Tables 32.2 and 32.3.

Others

Corticosteroids

Utilized in the treatment of acute GvHD, initially in high doses, with rapid tapering as soon as there is a response. The intravenous route is used in patients with significant gastrointestinal involvement, with methylprednisolone being given at 1–2 mg/kg until response.

Mycophenolate mofetil (MMF)

A prodrug metabolized in the liver into the active moiety mycophenolic acid (MPA). MPA inhibits a key enzyme involved in the de novo synthesis of purines used in the proliferation of B- and T-lymphocytes. MMF has been used as both an alternative and an adjunct to calcineurin inhibitors in the prophylaxis and treatment of GvHD.[35] Dosing ranges from 1 to 1.5 g twice a day and oral bio-availabilty is good in approximately 94% of cases.[4] Intravenous and oral doses are usually interchangeable. Side-effects include GI toxicity and myelosuppression.

Sirolimus

This is not a calcineurin inhibitor, despite its name; its activity is mediated by inhibition of the mammalian target of the rapamycin (mTOR) pathway. Unlike calcineurin inhibitors, it is not nephrotoxic and is administered as a daily dose. No parenteral formulation is available. Sirolimus, like mycophenolate, has been used in combination with calcineurin inhibitors or as single agent in both the treatment[36] and prophylaxis of GvHD.[37]

Monoclonal antibodies

An ever-increasing number of antibodies is being used in oncology, and a number are used in stem cell transplantation.

Alemtuzumab

Also known as CAMPATH, this is an anti-CD52 monoclonal antibody used in conditioning regimens for sibling allografts, matched and mismatched unrelated donor transplants. Dosing varies but is usually in the order of 50–100 mg, split over 5 days.[25,38]

Basiliximab

A chimeric anti-CD25 monoclonal antibody (it binds to the α-subunit of the activated IL-2 receptor) which has been studied in the treatment of steroid-refractory GvHD.[39] The dose used was 40 mg a week for 2–3 doses along with steroids and ciclosporin.

Daclizumab

A humanized anti-CD25 monoclonal antibody which has also been studied in steroid-refractory GvHD as monotherapy,[40] and in combination with infliximab.[41] Daclizumab has been dosed at 1 mg/kg on day 1, 4, 8, 15 and 22.

Infliximab

A chimeric monoclonal antibody that binds to soluble and transmembrane forms of tumor necrosis factor alpha (TNF-α). It has been studied in the treatment of steroid-refractory GvHD in combination with daclizumab.[41] Infliximab was administered as a weekly infusion at a dose of 10 mg/kg, for four doses. Due to the profound nature of the resulting immunosuppression, treatment doses of antifungals were given as prophylaxis.

Inolimomab

A murine anti-CD25 monoclonal antibody that has been studied in the treatment of steroid-refractory GvHD.[42]

Rituximab

An anti-CD20 monoclonal antibody which has been used both in conditioning for acute lymphoblastic leukemia[43] and for the treatment of chronic GvHD.[44]

Polyclonal antibodies

Antilymphocyte globulin (ALG) and *antithymocyte globulin* (ATG) are purified antibodies produced in response to human T-cells and have been used in transplant conditioning and treatment for refractory GvHD; to date, the antibodies have been derived from rabbit or horse material. The nomenclature of these compounds is product specific, and dosing schedules vary for prophylaxis of GvHD.[45] These

antibodies have also been used in treatment of refractory GvHD.[46] They may now be superseded in some centers by monoclonal alternatives which are associated with fewer adverse effects.

Supportive care

This section includes a brief overview of the drugs that ameliorate the side-effects from treatment with intensive chemotherapy/radiotherapy.

Anticonvulsants

Phenytoin is used to prevent seizures in patients receiving busulfan.[4]

Antiemetics

Antihistamines

Cyclizine can be given orally or intravenously, dosed at 50 mg every 8 hours. It can also be given as a continuous subcutaneous infusion (unlicensed in the UK).

Benzodiazepines

Lorazepam is useful in anticipatory sickness due to its amnesic, sedative and anxiolytic effects. It is usually dosed at 0.5–1 mg prior to chemotherapy.

Corticosteroids

Dexamethasone is useful in preventing delayed sickness after highly emetogenic chemotherapy. Its use is limited in transplantation due to the side-effect profile and link to invasive fungal infections.[47]

Dopamine antagonists

Domperidone is an alternative to metoclopramide with a reduced incidence of extrapyramidal side-effects. It acts locally on gut and is dosed orally, 10–20 mg 3–4 times daily.

Levomepromazine is a class 1 antipsychotic and has useful activity in refractory nausea and vomiting at low doses. Doses range from 3.125 mg up to 25 mg daily and can be given orally or via the subcutaneous route.

Metoclopramide acts centrally and locally, and risk of extrapyramidal side-effects increases in the young and the elderly. Doses of up to 20 mg 6 hourly can be used for severe nausea.

5HT$_3$ antagonists

Granisetron and *ondansetron* have been shown to be effective in preventing nausea and vomiting following TBI.[48] Granisetron is usually dosed at 1–2 mg up to twice a day (although a maximum of 9 mg/24 hours is licensed). It is available as oral and intravenous preparations. Ondansetron is dosed at 8 mg twice daily orally. More frequent dosing may be necessary, and continuous intravenous infusions as well as bolus infections can be administered.

Growth factors

Recombinant technology has enabled the development of exogenous growth factors which have assisted stem cell transplantation.

Granulocyte colony-stimulating factors are used to mobilize donor peripheral stem cells for allogeneic transplantation, and the patient's own stem cells for rescue after high-dose chemotherapy. They are also used post transplant to aid the engraftment process, especially in patients with concomitant infections. The ASCO guidelines 2006 recommend that growth factors be used following autologous transplantation and not routinely in the allogeneic setting.[49]

Filgrastim (recombinant G-CSF) is licensed to mobilize healthy donors at a dose of 10 μg/kg daily for 4–5 days by sc injection, and to mobilize patients undergoing autologous transplantation 10 μg/kg are given for 5–7 days, or if following chemotherapy, 5 μg/kg until collection.[4] Post transplant, filgrastim is usually dosed at 5 μg/kg daily until engraftment.

Lenograstim is the glycosylated form of recombinant G-CSF. It is licensed for PBSC mobilization at a dose of 10 μg/kg daily for 6–7 days alone, or 5 μg/kg daily (150 iu/m^2) after chemotherapy and after transplant.

Pegfilgrastim is pegylated filgrastim which has a significantly extended plasma half-life. It is not licensed in the mobilization/transplant setting to date, although a number of studies have been carried out.[50,51]

Molgramostim, or granulocyte macrophage colony-stimulating factor (GM-CSF), has been used post chemotherapy for PBSC mobilization.[52] A licensed preparation is not available in the UK.

Palifermin is a recombinant keratinocyte growth factor (KGF) used to decrease the incidence, duration and severity of oral mucositis following myeloablative chemotherapy requiring autologous stem cell support.[4] It is dosed at 60 mg/kg for three doses before and after myeloablative chemotherapy and given by intravenous injection.

Erythropoietins

Recombinant erythropoietin has been used in the post-transplant setting to reduce transfusion requirements although this is by no means standard practice.[53]

Miscellaneous

Defibrotide is a single-stranded polydeoxyribonucleotide that has anti-thrombin and fibrinolytic properties on small vessels, without significant effects on systemic coagulation. It is used on a named patient basis in the UK for the prevention and treatment of veno-occlusive disease (sinusoidal obstructive syndrome, SOS).[54,55] Dosing ranges from 5 to 60 mg/kg in divided doses. Defibrotide has also been used for the treatment of thrombotic thrombocytopenic purpura (TTP).[56]

References

1. Price KE, Godfrey JC. Effect of structural modifications on the biological properties of aminoglycoside antibiotics containing 2-deoxystreptamine. Adv Appl Microbiol 1974;18:191–307

2. Paul M, Soares-Weiser K, Leibovici L. Beta lactam monotherapy versus beta lactam-aminoglycoside combination therapy for fever with neutropenia: systematic review and meta-analysis. BMJ 2003;326:1111

3. Freeman CD, Nicolau DP, Belliveau PP et al. Once-daily dosing of aminoglycosides: review and recommendations for clinical practice. J Antimicrob Chemother 1997;39:677–686

4. Electronic Medicines Compendium: http://emc.medicines.org.uk

5. Bosi A, Fanci R, Pecile P et al. Aztreonam versus colistin-neomycin for selective decontamination of the digestive tract in patients undergoing bone marrow transplantation: a randomized study. J Chemother 1992;4:30–34

6. Denton M, Wilcox MH. Antimicrobial treatment of pulmonary colonization and infection by *Pseudomonas aeruginosa* in cystic fibrosis patients. J Antimicrob Chemother 1992;40:468–474

7. Bow EJ, Rotstein C, Noskin GA et al. A randomized, open label, multicenter comparative study of the efficacy and safety of piperacillin-tazobactam and cefepime for the empirical treatment of febrile neutropenic episodes in patients with hematologic malignancies. Clin Infect Dis 2006;43:447–459

8. Fanci R, Paci C, Leoni F et al. Ticarcillin-clavulanic acid plus amikacin versus ceftazidime plus amikacin in the empirical treatment of fever in acute leukemia: a prospective randomized trial. J Chemother 2003;15:253–259

9. British National Formulary, 52nd edn. 2006, BMA and RPS Publishing

10. Cordonnier C, Martino R, Trabasso P et al. Mycobacterial infection: a difficult and late diagnosis in stem cell transplant recipients. Clin Infect Dis 2004;38:1229–1236

11. Reich G, Cornely OA, Sandherr M et al. Empirical antimicrobial monotherapy in patients after high-dose chemotherapy and autologous stem cell transplantation: a randomised, multicentre trial. Br J Haematol 2005;130:265–270

12. Gifford AH, Kirkland KB. Risk factors for Clostridium difficile-associated diarrhea on an adult hematology-oncology ward. Eur J Clin Microbiol Infect Dis 2006;25:751–755

13. Hoffken G, Pasold R, Pfluger KH et al. An open, randomized, multicentre study comparing the use of low-dose ceftazidime or cefotaxime, both in combination with netilmicin, in febrile neutropenic patients. German Multicentre Study Group. J Antimicrob Chemother 2000;44:367–376

14. Harter C, Schulze B, Goldschmidt H et al. Piperacillin/tazobactam vs ceftazidime in the treatment of neutropenic fever in patients with acute leukemia or following autologous peripheral blood stem cell transplantation: a prospective randomized trial. Bone Marrow Transplant 2006;37:373–379

15. Wysocki M, Delatour F, Faurisson F et al. Continuous versus intermittent infusion of vancomycin in severe Staphylococcal infections: prospective multicenter randomized study. Antimicrob Agents Chemother 2001;45:2460–2467

16. Fowler VG Jr, Boucher HW, Corey GR et al. Daptomycin versus standard therapy for bacteremia and endocarditis caused by Staphylococcus aureus. N Engl J Med 2006;355:653–665

17. Jaksic B, Martinelli G, Perez-Oteyza J et al. Efficacy and safety of linezolid compared with vancomycin in a randomized, double-blind study of febrile neutropenic patients with cancer. Clin Infect Dis 2006;42:597–607

18. Frere P, Hermanne JP, Debouge MH et al. Changing pattern of bacterial susceptibility to antibiotics in hematopoietic stem cell transplant recipients. Bone Marrow Transplant 2002;29:589–594

19. Rizzo JD, Wingard JR, Tichelli A et al. Recommended screening and preventive practices for long-term survivors after hematopoietic cell transplantation: joint recommendations of the European Group for Blood and Marrow Transplantation, the Center for International Blood and Marrow Transplant Research, and the American Society of Blood and Marrow Transplantation. Biol Blood Marrow Transplant 2006;12:138–151

20. Morrisey CO, Slavin MA. Antifungal strategies for managing invasive aspergillosis: The prospects for a pre-emptive treatment strategy. Med Mycol 2006;44(suppl):333–348

21. Hoglund M, Ljungman P, Weller S. Comparable aciclovir exposures produced by oral valaciclovir and intravenous aciclovir in immunocompromised cancer patients. J Antimicrob Chemother 2001;47:855–861

22. Ayala E, Greene J, Sandin R et al. Valganciclovir is safe and effective as pre-emptive therapy for CMV infection in allogeneic hematopoietic stem cell transplantation. Bone Marrow Transplant 2006;37:851–856

23. Neofytos D, Ojha A, Mookerjee B et al. Treatment of adenovirus disease in stem cell transplant recipients with cidofovir. Biol Blood Marrow Transplant 2007;13:74–81

24. Madden T, de Lima M, Thapar N et al. Pharmacokinetics of once-daily IV busulfan as part of pretransplantation preparative regimens: a comparison with an every 6-hour dosing schedule. Biol Blood Marrow Transplant 2007;13:56–64

25. Ho AY, Pagliuca A, Kenyon M et al. Reduced-intensity allogeneic hematopoietic stem cell transplantation for myelodysplastic syndrome and acute myeloid leukemia with multilineage dysplasia using fludarabine, busulphan, and alemtuzumab (FBC) conditioning. Blood 2004;104:1616–1623

26. Nieto Y, Vaughan WP. Pharmacokinetics of high-dose chemotherapy. Bone Marrow Transplant 2004;33:259–269

27. Mills W, Chopra R, McMillan A et al. BEAM chemotherapy and autologous bone marrow transplantation for patients with relapsed or refractory non-Hodgkin's lymphoma. J Clin Oncol 1995;13:588–595

28. Delgado J, Thomson K, Russell N et al. Results of alemtuzumab-based reduced-intensity allogeneic transplantation for chronic lymphocytic leukemia: a British Society of Blood and Marrow Transplantation Study. Blood 2006;107:1724–1730

29. Storb R, Deeg HJ, Pepe M et al. Methotrexate and cyclosporine versus cyclosporine alone for prophylaxis of graft-versus-host disease in patients given HLA-identical marrow grafts for leukemia: long-term follow-up of a controlled trial. Blood 1989;73:1729–1734

30. de Lavallade H, Mohty M, Faucher C et al. Low-dose methotrexate as salvage therapy for refractory graft-versus-host disease after reduced-intensity conditioning allogeneic stem cell transplantation. Haematologica 2006;91:1438–1440

31. Bolanos-Meade J, Jacobsohn DA, Margolis J et al. Pentostatin in steroid-refractory acute graft-versus-host disease. J Clin Oncol 2005;23:2661–2668

32. Schmitz N, Gassmann W, Rister M et al. Fractionated total body irradiation and high-dose VP 16–213 followed by allogeneic bone marrow transplantation in advanced leukemias. Blood 1988;72:1567–1573

33. Eckardt A, Starke O, Stadler M et al. Severe oral chronic graft-versus-host disease following allogeneic bone marrow transplantation: highly effective treatment with topical tacrolimus. Oral Oncol 2004;40:811–814

34. Nash RA, Antin JH, Karanes C et al. Phase 3 study comparing methotrexate and tacrolimus with methotrexate and cyclosporine for prophylaxis of acute graft-versus-host disease after marrow transplantation from unrelated donors. Blood 2000;96:2062–2068

35. Krejci M, Doubek M, Buchler T et al. Mycophenolate mofetil for the treatment of acute and chronic steroid-refractory graft-versus-host disease. Ann Hematol 2005;84:681–685

36. Johnston LJ, Brown J, Shizuru JA et al. Rapamycin (sirolimus) for treatment of chronic graft-versus-host disease. Biol Blood Marrow Transplant 2005;11:647–649

37. Cutler C, Antin JH. Sirolimus for GVHD prophylaxis in allogeneic stem cell transplantation Biol Blood Marrow Transplant 2005;11:47–55

38. Faulkner RD, Craddock C, Byrne JL et al. BEAM-alemtuzumab reduced-intensity allogeneic stem cell transplantation for lymphoproliferative diseases: GVHD, toxicity, and survival in 65 patients. Blood 2004;103:428–434

39. Funke VA, de Medeiros CR, Setubal DC et al. Therapy for severe refractory acute graft-versus-host disease with basiliximab, a selective interleukin-2 receptor antagonist. Bone Marrow Transplant 2006;37:961–965

40. Bordigoni P, Dimicoli S, Clement L et al. Daclizumab, an efficient treatment for steroid-refractory acute graft-versus-host disease. Br J Haematol 2006;135:382–385

41. Srinivasan R, Chakrabarti S, Walsh T et al. Improved survival in steroid-refractory acute graft versus host disease after non-myeloablative allogeneic transplantation using a daclizumab-based strategy with comprehensive infection prophylaxis. Br J Haematol 2004;124:777–786

42. Pinana JL, Valcarcel D, Martino R et al. Encouraging results with inolimomab (anti-IL-2 receptor) as treatment for refractory acute graft-versus-host disease. Biol Blood Marrow Transplant 2006;12:1135–1141

43. Kebriaei P, Saliba RM, Ma C et al. Allogeneic hematopoietic stem cell transplantation after rituximab-containing myeloablative preparative regimen for acute lymphoblastic leukemia. Bone Marrow Transplant 2006;38:203–209

44. Cutler C, Miklos D, Kim HT et al. Rituximab for steroid-refractory chronic graft-versus-host disease. Blood. 2006;108:756–762

45. Bacigalupo A. Antilymphocyte/thymocyte globulin for graft versus host disease prophylaxis: efficacy and side effects. Bone Marrow Transplant 2005;35:225–231

46. MacMillan ML, Weisdorf DJ, Davies SM et al. Early antithymocyte globulin therapy improves survival in patients with steroid-resistant acute graft-versus-host disease. Biol Blood Marrow Transplant 2002;8:40–46

47. Raman T, Marik PE. Fungal infections in bone marrow transplant recipients. Exp Opin Pharmacother 2006;7:307–315

48. Spitzer TR, Friedman CJ, Bushnell W et al. Double-blind, randomized, parallel-group study on the efficacy and safety of oral granisetron and oral ondansetron in the prophylaxis of nausea and vomiting in patients receiving hyperfractionated total body irradiation. Bone Marrow Transplant 2000;26:203–210

49. Smith TJ, Khatcheressian J, Lyman GH et al. Recommendations for the use of white blood cell growth factors: an evidence-based clinical practice guideline. J Clin Oncol 2006;24:3187–3205

50. Hosing C, Qazilbash MH, Kebriaei P et al. Fixed-dose single agent pegfilgrastim for peripheral blood progenitor cell mobilisation in patients with multiple myeloma. Br J Haematol 2006;133:533–537

51. Martino M, Pratico G, Messina G et al. Pegfilgrastim compared with filgrastim after high-dose melphalan and autologous hematopoietic peripheral blood stem cell transplantation in multiple myeloma patients. Eur J Hematol 2006;77:410–415

52. Kopf B, de Giorgi U, Vertogen B. A randomized study comparing filgrastim versus lenograstim versus molgramostim plus chemotherapy for peripheral blood progenitor cell mobilization. Bone Marrow Transplant 2006;38:407–412

53. Ivanov V, Faucher C, Mohty M et al. Early administration of recombinant erythropoietin improves hemoglobin recovery after reduced intensity conditioned allogeneic stem cell transplantation. Bone Marrow Transplant 2005;36:901–906

54. Dignan F, Gujral D, Ethell M et al. Prophylactic defibrotide in allogeneic stem cell transplantation: minimal morbidity and zero mortality from veno-occlusive disease. Bone Marrow Transplant 2007;40(1):79–82

55. Richardson PG, Murakami C, Jin Z et al. Multi-institutional use of defibrotide in 88 patients after stem cell transplantation with severe veno-occlusive disease and multisystem organ failure: response without significant toxicity in a high-risk population and factors predictive of outcome. Blood 2002;100:4337–4343

56. Corti P, Uderzo C, Tagliabue A et al. Defibrotide as a promising treatment for thrombotic thrombocytopenic purpura in patients undergoing bone marrow transplantation. Bone Marrow Transplant 2002;29:542–543

Nutrition support

CHAPTER 33

Louise Henry and Gayle Loader

Introduction

Maintaining good nutritional status is an important clinical aim following hemopoietic stem cell transplantation (HSCT). Underweight patients experience increased mortality and length of hospital stay following transplantation.[1-4] Recent clinical guidelines highlight the importance of good nutritional management of transplant patients and advocate a multidisciplinary approach involving medical teams, nursing staff, dietitians and catering staff.[5]

Many factors may impair a patient's ability to meet their nutritional requirements and maintain a good nutritional status.[6] Effective nutritional screening prior and during admissions is beneficial in identifying those patients requiring intensive nutrition support.[5] Active nutrition support is necessary in preventing and reversing weight loss and in aiding full recovery of the hematopoietic and immune systems prior to transplant, during hospitalization and, in some cases, for several months after discharge home.[7] Artificial nutrition support such as enteral and parenteral nutrition plays an important role if patients are unable to ingest sufficient fluid and nutrients.

Nutritional assessment

Patients should be assessed prior to hospital admission, throughout hospitalization and on subsequent outpatient appointments.[6] This ensures early identification of nutritional problems and hopefully allows instigation of measures to prevent deterioration in nutritional status.

Pretransplant assessment

The purpose of a pretransplant nutritional assessment is to ascertain overall nutritional status and to identify potential risk factors such as food allergies or intolerances, and the initiation of therapeutic or alternative diets.[8] It is an opportunity to obtain baseline anthropometric measurements and a dietary history.[9] Patients should be alerted to the possibility of eating difficulties during the post-HSCT period, and alternative methods of nutrition support and any food restrictions in operation on the ward should be explained. Patients who have lost 10–20% of their body weight should endeavor to regain this before transplant. Nutritional intervention at this point is aimed at increasing protein and calorie intake by administering commercial enteral supplements or initiating artificial nutrition support prior to transplantation. Since anorexia and other eating difficulties can persist for months post transplant,[10,11] patients should be advised to try to gain extra weight in the 2–4 weeks prior to HSCT.

Post-transplant assessment

Assessment of nutritional status can be particularly problematic in the early post-transplant period.[6] Several methods of assessment are described in research literature concerning nutrition in relation to hemopoietic transplant. However, many of these are unreliable and inaccurate and therefore of questionable validity (Table 33.1).

Development of a prognostic nutritional index for HSCT patients would greatly assist in identifying patients at risk of malnutrition and in monitoring the efficacy of nutrition support. Locally agreed, validated screening tools are the most practical way of assessing and monitoring patients during their inpatient admission and afterwards.

Food record charts can further assist in the monitoring of oral intake and can be an invaluable tool in quantifying changes in intake during an inpatient stay, giving early notice if oral intake begins to tail off.

Nutritional requirements

These are detailed in Table 33.2.

Factors affecting nutritional status

There are many factors influencing the nutritional status of patients undergoing transplant.

Underlying disease

The underlying disease state that has led to the patient undergoing transplantation may influence nutritional requirements. For example, patients with advanced chronic myeloid leukemia (CML) can present with anorexia and weight loss.[12,13] This is in contrast to patients suffering from other hematologic malignancies who rarely present with cachexia. In patients with myeloma, there is a risk of renal failure, which can have significant detrimental effects on nutritional intake and status.[14]

The nutritional impact of lymphoma at diagnosis depends largely on the anatomic site affected and the disease subtype. Celiac disease has been linked to the development of enteropathy-associated T-cell lymphoma, and risk of weight loss is increased if a gluten-free diet is not strictly adopted.[15] The presence of B symptoms (fever, weight loss and sweating) has significant implications for nutritional status. Gastrointestinal symptoms including early satiety, nausea and vomiting are associated with gastrointestinal lymphomas. Patients with lymphomas of the oropharyngeal area can present with significant weight loss and dysphagia and may need early referral for nutrition support.

Table 33.1 Methods of nutritional assessment

Measure	Limitations
Weight	Reflects fluid and electrolyte changes during the immediate post-transplant period. Weight may increase or remain stable despite loss of lean body mass Sequential measures after discharge home are useful as an indicator of nutritional status[6]
Anthropometric measurements	Skinfold measurements can be problematic (and therefore inaccurate) due to fluid and electrolyte imbalance Not sensitive to change Open to intraobserver error May result in severe bruising in patients with low platelet levels[19]
Biochemical measures	Measures such as serum albumin and transferrin are not reliable indicators of nutritional status as they are influenced by factors such as the use of blood products, sepsis and GvHD[100–102] Hematologic and immunologic measures do not reflect nutritional status in such patients
Nitrogen balance	Not practical to measure losses especially in the presence of diarrhea or urinary incontinence Insensitive measure as influenced by renal or hepatic impairment, inactivity Impossible to achieve positive nitrogen balance in critically ill patients

Table 33.2 Nutritional requirements

Nutrient	Estimated requirement
Energy	Currently unclear whether requirements are affected following HSCT Quantifying requirements is difficult as several small studies contradict each other with requirements being recorded as ranging from 30–50 kcal per kg. A starting point of 30–35 kcal per kg is suggested[85,102–104] Increases in theoretical energy requirements are often counterbalanced by a reduction in activity levels Energy requirements are also influenced by age, gender, type of transplant, i.e. allogeneic or autogenic, and the presence of sepsis or GvHD due to increased cell turnover Estimates of energy requirements may have to be adjusted according to changes in activity following discharge from hospital
Nitrogen	Following HSCT, patients experience marked protein catabolism due to increased protein turnover and leucine oxidation[105] Individual protein requirements are related to age and body size Protein requirements are also influenced by the use of medication such as corticosteroids, and the presence of sepsis and GvHD Requirements are thought to be approximately twice the recommended daily allowance for protein and nitrogen although adults may require 0.17–0.25 nitrogen per kg body weight, particularly during septic episodes[9,19,106] Excessively high nitrogen intakes are not advisable as it is unlikely that the nitrogen will be assimilated, particularly during sepsis and critical illness Sufficient energy is required for nitrogen to be utilized properly Cunningham et al[107] suggest that maintaining some level of activity is essential in the preservation of lean body mass
Vitamins and minerals	There is little information concerning the micronutrient requirements for this patient group Requirements for vitamins A, D, E, K, folic acid, ascorbic acid, B complex and biotin may be increased following HSCT[108] Antila et al[109] have suggested that zinc requirements may also be slightly increased Medication such as ciclosporin increases requirements for some minerals such as magnesium[21] Oral supplementation can be difficult as appropriate micronutrient supplements are poorly tolerated due to the low palatability of the preparations and tablets and frequent gastrointestinal discomfort or poor absorption Significant micronutrient deficiencies can rarely be successfully altered by dietary manipulation alone, particularly in the acute setting due to differences in bio-availability and absorption

Central nervous system lymphomas may be associated with confusion which can decrease the desire to eat and drink.

Cytoreductive treatment and type of transplant

The type of chemotherapy regimen and the use of total-body irradiation will influence the nature and severity of post-transplant complications and hence may induce adverse effects on nutritional status. Generally, patients receiving total-body irradiation (TBI) experience worse mucositis and more diarrhea and are at greater risk of developing thickened secretions, all of which can greatly compromise nutritional status.[10,16–17] Papadopoulou et al[18] found that children who received TBI required parenteral nutrition for longer periods and experienced more significant weight loss than did those children receiving chemotherapy only. Patients undergoing allogeneic transplant are also at risk of developing graft-versus-host disease (GvHD), which can have adverse effects on nutritional status.[19–22]

Side-effects of treatment likely to affect nutritional status

Anorexia/loss of appetite

Etiology
- Can be as a consequence of depression and anxiety or social factors such as isolation, limited income and lack of access to cooking facilities, unfamiliar hospital food[23]
- Fatigue
- Pain
- As a side-effect of medication, e.g. analgesia, some antibiotics
- As a consequence of other treatment side-effects such as nausea and vomiting, dry mouth, food aversions, diarrhea, constipation

Management
The underlying cause should be established and intervention planned on this basis.
- Pharmacologic interventions
  - Megestrol acetate[24]
  - Corticosteroids[25]
- Non-pharmacologic interventions
- Dietary advice for patients
  - Eat small, frequent meals
  - Eat foods high in energy and protein
  - Fortify foods by adding foods such as skimmed milk powder, oil, butter, sugar, and honey. Glucose polymer powders and protein supplements are available on prescription
  - Avoid 'filling up' with low-energy and protein-density foods (e.g. jelly, tea, coffee)
  - Separate drinks from meals to avoid early satiety
  - Time meals for when appetite best; generally this is breakfast time with a progressive decrease in appetite as the day progresses
  - Take nutritional supplements when appetite is poor, e.g. in the evening
  - Alcohol can stimulate the appetite[26]
  - Exercise may stimulate the appetite

– Eat in a pleasant environment, e.g. away from unpleasant odors and sounds. Eating in a day room rather than at the bedside may help.

If anorexia is persistent and accompanied by weight loss of 10%, consider enteral tube feeding.

- Social factors
  – Refer to social services for assessment of benefit entitlement, housing issues
  – Refer to occupational therapist for advice regarding adaptation of cooking equipment, management of fatigue
  – Refer to psychologic support services if patient is depressed/overly anxious

Nausea and vomiting

Etiology

Multifactorial etiology and often related to chemotherapy agents, antibiotics, opiates, ciclosporin and other medication, e.g. oral potassium preparations. Can be associated with thickened secretions, diarrhea or constipation and GvHD.[27] Severe, intractable vomiting may also indicate bowel obstruction. Intractable vomiting will lead to a reduction in nutrient intake and jeopardize nutritional status.

Management

The underlying cause should be established and intervention planned on this basis.

- Pharmacologic management
  – Routine use of antiemetics. Often a combination is required. Antiemetics should be given at appropriate time intervals to ensure maximum efficacy. Specific modes of action of antiemetics should be matched to symptoms to allow maximum action
- Dietary advice and non-pharmacologic management
  – Relax before eating and encourage rest after eating
  – Avoid food odors. Advise patient to move away from the kitchen, and from areas where food is prepared
  – Cold or room-temperature foods have fewer odors
  – Eat small frequent snacks/meals
  – Try sucking boiled sweets or chewing gum
  – Suck peppermints or try peppermint cordial
  – Reduce greasy, fatty foods as they delay gastric emptying
  – Try fizzy drinks (they can induce belching, which can help relieve symptoms of nausea)
  – Try drinks or foods containing ginger (ginger is traditionally thought to have antiemetic properties)
  – Fresh air from an open window or a walk outside may be beneficial

Consider parenteral feeding if vomiting is persistent and intractable. It may be advisable to minimize oral intake if vomiting is severe, to prevent aspiration.

Stomatitis/mucositis/esophagitis

Oral mucositis usually occurs 4–10 days after conditioning therapy and may persist for 34 weeks.[6,16,22] Improvement coincides with engraftment, and complete recovery commonly occurs within 20 days.[28] Limits the physical ability to eat by affecting ability to chew and swallow. Often affects taste perceptions.

Etiology

- Chemotherapy particularly if accompanied by TBI
- *Candida* and other oral infections
- GvHD.

Management

- Pharmacologic management
  – Regular mouth care is vital to attenuate mucositis[20]

– Topical anesthesia
– Opiates (oral and/or intravenous)
– New generation of medication is being developed to protect patients from mucositis, e.g. recombinant human keratinacyte growth factor (palifermin) and amifostine.[29–31] Once efficacy and safety have been clearly established, they are likely to be used extensively

- Dietary advice and non-pharmacologic management
  – Use soft toothbrush
  – Avoid spicy and rough-textured foods
  – Choose bland, cool, soft foods
  – Use gravies and sauces to moisten foods
  – Try ice lollies/flavored ice cubes
  – Avoid alcohol as can act as an irritant
  – Use nutritional supplement drinks (most can be frozen if desired)
  – Early placement of enteral feeding tube will increase tolerance
  – Consider the use of artificial nutrition support if patient is likely to have severe mucositis for more than 5 days

Xerostomia

Xerostomia can greatly affect nutritional intake. Xerostomia alters the patient's perception of their ability to swallow and therefore affects the comfort of eating and food choices.[32] Mastication and oral manipulation of food become difficult.[33]

Xerostomia can also lead to increased dental plaque and caries caused by a lack of buffering capacity, lowered salivary pH and decreased physical flushing of the oral cavity.[34]

Saliva plays an important role in taste sensation and therefore patients with xerostomia often complain of disturbed taste and associated lack of desire to eat. This is further exacerbated by an increased risk of oral fungal infections.[35]

Etiology

- As a result of TBI. May be long term or permanent. The majority of patients do recover saliva production within 2–3 months
- May be associated with use of opiates and some antiemetics
- Dehydration
- Chronic oral GvHD

Management

- Pharmacologic interventions
  – Frequent mouthwashes. Mouthwashes containing alcohol should be avoided
  – Saliva stimulants, e.g. pilocarpine[36]
  – Saliva substitutes, e.g. Biotene Oralbalance, BioXtra[37]
  – Long-term xerostomia requires regular dental treatment and topical fluoride to prevent or reduce dental decay
- Dietary advice and non-pharmacologic interventions
  – Try increasing liquids with foods, e.g. sauces and gravies, sips of drinks between mouthfuls of food
  – Suck on ice cubes or ice lollies. Try flavoring with citrus fruits or juices
  – Suck slices of citrus fruits
  – Suck boiled sweets
  – Avoid dry foods, i.e. bread and cakes
  – Chew sugar-free gum[38]
  – For persistently thickened secretions it may be necessary to consider nasogastric or gastrostomy tube feeding

Dysgeusia

A loss or alteration in the sense of taste can severely reduce the desire for food.[39]

Etiology

- Chemotherapy agents may change taste perception
- Xerostomia and mucositis exacerbate symptoms
- TBI
- Opiates and certain antibiotics

Management

- Pharmacologic management
  - Regular mouth care
- Dietary advice and non-pharmacologic management
  - Concentrate on foods that are pleasant tasting
  - Encourage patient to experiment with foods not usually liked
  - Use condiments and sauces
  - Marinate meats. If this fails then substitute with protein from dairy foods or beans and pulses
  - Suggest alternatives to foods often affected, e.g. try hot squash or milky drinks in place of tea and coffee
  - Eat cold foods

Diarrhea/malabsorption

The incidence and severity of diarrhea are variable. Patients suffering from diarrhea will experience a significant decrease in nutritional status and well-being.[18] They can also become deficient in specific nutrients.

Etiology

- Chemotherapy. Exacerbated if in conjunction with TBI
- 'Gut sterilization'
- Infection
- GvHD

Management

- Pharmacologic interventions
  - In absence of infection, antidiarrheal agents should be administered
  - Fluid losses should be replaced with iv fluids
- Dietary advice and non-pharmacologic interventions
  - Small frequent meals
  - Avoid large, fatty heavy meals
  - Some patients may benefit from a decrease in insoluble fiber intake (e.g. high bran-containing cereals, dried fruit)
  - Patients with persistent, high-volume diarrhea may require parenteral nutrition and 'bowel rest'

Constipation

Can cause early satiety and nausea/vomiting.

Etiology

- Analgesia
- Immobility
- Decreased oral intake
- Dehydration

Management

- Pharmacologic interventions
  - Establish likely cause and rule out bowel obstruction
  - Laxatives
- Dietary advice and non-pharmacologic interventions
  - Increase fluid intake
  - Increase dietary fiber intake (it is not recommended that pure bran is added to foods). However, generally this is not adequate to resolve constipation in the sick patient
  - Encourage gentle exercise

GvHD

Little research exists concerning the effects of acute or chronic GvHD on nutritional status or appropriate dietary management. Patients suffering from chronic GvHD often have a low body mass index (BMI).[40] Corticosteroid therapy often leads to an increase in appetite, which may reduce the impact on nutritional status, although it can also mask weight loss and muscle wastage by causing fluid gain and edema. High-dose steroids may also lead to hyperglycemia, which may further compromise nutritional status.

GvHD affecting the skin

Where food intake is poor or weight loss continues, patients should be encouraged to use nutritional supplements and may benefit from overnight supplementary nasogastric feeding.

GvHD affecting the gut

This may cause profuse diarrhea and malabsorption leading to deterioration in nutritional status. Enteral tube feeding can be tried, and an elemental or semi-elemental peptide feed may be best tolerated. If the feed is not absorbed parenteral nutrition (PN) should be given. Specialist anti-GvHD dietary strategies have been suggested.[41] However, their efficacy has not been well researched. It has been suggested that such patients may benefit from a low allergen diet, but these diets can be difficult to follow and due to their limited nature it might be difficult to meet nutritional requirements. Recent research suggests that enteral tube feeding can be safely used,[42] although a peptide feed may be indicated to facilitate absorption.

GvHD affecting the liver

When GvHD affects the liver, it can be difficult to maintain nutritional status. Patients often experience anorexia, frequently accompanied by early satiety. PN is likely to adversely affect liver function.[43] It is therefore advisable to encourage nutritional supplements and consider nasogastric feeding. There is no research to support the use of a low-fat diet.

Patients with veno-occlusive disease often experience similar side-effects and may also benefit from nasogastric feeding. PN is not indicated because of difficulties with fluid balance and the likelihood of it causing further liver function abnormalities.

Dietary restrictions for the immunocompromised patient

Historically, patients undergoing a bone marrow transplant were required to follow very restrictive sterile or 'low microbial' diets.[44,45] Sterile diets are now rarely used in the UK as there is limited evidence to suggest any benefit from this level of restriction, and the preparation techniques used make the diet impractical, unpalatable, limiting and expensive to prepare.[46]

Little empirical research exists concerning the efficacy and optimum composition of the 'neutropenic' diet. In recent years, a number of audits have been conducted to determine current practice in UK transplant centers.[47–49] These have shown disparity between the practices of different centers. Rees has suggested a consensus guideline to help rationalize restrictions and limit the variations in practice in different centers, thus reducing confusion for patients and staff who often move between hospitals.[49] However, there remains a lack of good-quality research in this area and debate continues concerning the level of restriction required since these audits highlight common practice rather than evidence-based practice.

Currently, all patients receiving high-dose chemotherapy or a stem cell transplant are encouraged to follow basic food hygiene guidelines for at least the first 3–6 months or until they stop taking immunosuppressants. These guidelines are based on the reduction of risk for

Table 33.3 Sources of food-borne micro-organisms in the UK food chain

Micro-organism	Food sources
Salmonella (*S.enteritidis*, *S.typhimurium*)	Eggs, poultry, meat products, soft and mold ripened cheeses
Campylobacter (*C. jejuni*)	Milk (particularly unpasteurized or doorstep milk pecked by birds), chicken, salads
Escherichia coli	Meat products (cross-contamination between raw and cooked meats is a significant risk), unpasteurized milk
Staphylococcus aureus	Cross-contamination of cooked meats, hard cheese. Foods kept warm and not eaten immediately
Listeria monocytogenes	Unpasteurized milk, soft cheeses, paté, salads, ice cream
Cryptosporidium	Raw fruit and vegetables, ice from ice machines
Pseudomonas aeruginosa	Bottled non-carbonated water
Small round structured viruses (SRSV)	Shellfish, pre-prepared salads, raw fruit and vegetables
Enteroviruses (hepatitis A)	Food contaminated by personal hygiene practices, e.g. shellfish, fruit, salads, ice

immunocompromised patients and are formulated from information regarding food-borne infections in the general population[50] (see Table 33.3 for most common sources of food poisoning). General food hygiene guidance should be given to patients and their families, and food-handling practices in the hospital setting should aim to minimize the risk of acquiring food-borne infection. It is important that patients and staff are given sufficient education and support to enable them to follow the required guidelines (Fig. 33.1).[45]

Many centers also recommend additional food restrictions for patients with neutropenia. These so-called 'neutropenic' diets may operate at different levels depending upon the neutrophil count and are designed to eliminate any potential sources of bacteria, virus or fungi from the food (Tables 33.4a, 33.4b). These restrictions are based upon studies investigating microbiology of common foods, i.e. fresh, uncooked fruit and vegetables,[51–53] products containing raw or lightly cooked eggs,[54] shellfish and smoked fish,[55] and bottled water.[56]

Methods of providing nutrition support

Historically, parenteral nutrition (PN) has been the method of choice for patients undergoing bone marrow transplantation.[45,57,58] Research in the 1980s and 1990s mainly concerned the use of PN, with many proponents advocating routine, prophylactic use.[7] There is need for further nutrition research in light of the effects of the reduced-intensity conditioning regimens and improvement in symptom management.[31,59,60] The routine, automatic use of parenteral nutrition is not clinically indicated unless the patient is unable to meet nutritional requirements via the oral or enteral routes.[61–65] Enteral tube feeding has become more commonplace in the UK centers although little empirical research exists to support the use of tube feeding, particularly in preference to PN.[57,66] Where research has been undertaken, the studies have been small with poor study design and mainly in the pediatric setting.[67–69] At best, it is possible to conclude from this research that nasogastric feeding in this patient group is feasible and probably safe.[42,68,70–73] Many questions remain to be answered regarding its use.

The aim of nutrition support

The aim of nutrition support is normally maintenance rather than repletion of body cell mass, as for the majority of patients nutritional status is good at the onset of treatment. When intake is likely to be

Shopping
- Avoid damaged packaging
- Avoid shops where raw and cooked foods are stored together
- Where possible buy pre-packaged deli items
- Avoid food from large containers
- Buy chilled and frozen foods last and get them home as soon as possible

Storage
- Fridges should be between 0 and 5°C
- Freezers should be kept below −18°C
- Overloading fridges and freezers will raise the temperature and should be avoided
- Cooked food should be stored at the top of the freezer
- Raw or defrosting meat and fish should be stored at the bottom of the fridge
- Eggs should be stored in the fridge
- Always use food within best before or use by dates
- Never refreeze thawed food

Food Preparation
- Wash hands with warm water and soap prior to handling food
- Wash hands again after using the toilet, sneezing, touching pets, dirty washing, rubbish, hair or face, ready-made or raw food
- Use separate towels for drying hands and dishes
- Cover any cuts or grazes with waterproof plasters
- Keep pets away from work surfaces, dishes and food
- Ensure cloths are regularly bleached, disinfected or changed
- Avoid cross-contamination by using different chopping boards and utensils for raw and cooked foods
- Disinfect work surfaces regularly
- Wash raw food before eating
- Wash can tops before opening

Cooking
- Cook all food thoroughly until the center meets 70°C for at least 2 minutes and it is piping hot
- Meat should be cooked until the juices run clear
- Pre-heat the oven to ensure food is cooked at the required temperature
- Follow manufacturer's instructions and do not reduce cooking times
- Thaw meat and fish in the fridge as bacteria quickly replicate at room temperature
- Do not reheat cooked food
- Microwaves can lead to uneven temperature and should only be used for defrosting
- Do not put hot food in the fridge as this increases the temperature of all the food stored in the fridge

Figure 33.1
Food hygiene advice.

inadequate for more than 7 days, intensive nutrition support should be instigated.[5,74]

Oral nutrition

As symptom management continues to improve, it is likely that there will be an increasing emphasis on the use of oral nutrition in maintaining the nutritional status of this patient group. Generally, patients require foods with high energy and protein density with snacks between meals if they are to meet their nutritional requirements. The 'Healthy Eating' guidelines for the general public are not applicable to this patient population. Patients may become afraid to eat, anticipating nausea, vomiting or pain.[75] Others may refuse to eat, since eating is the one function over which they still have control.

Oral nutritional support is easier if the food service is flexible enough to provide food and drink when patients want it. An audit of

Table 33.4a Foods restricted for patients following high-dose chemotherapy or stem cell transplantation with neutrophil counts below $0.5 \times 10^9/l$ at the Royal Marsden

Uncooked fruit, salads and vegetables
Uncooked herbs, spices and pepper
Uncooked cheese
Unpasteurized honey
Bottled water/non-drinking water
Paté
Unpasteurized dairy products
Live or bio yoghurts
Raw or undercooked eggs
Raw or undercooked meat, fish and poultry (including shellfish)

Table 33.4b Foods restricted for patients following high-dose chemotherapy or stem cell transplantation with neutrophil counts above $0.5 \times 10^9/l$ at the Royal Marsden

Soft ripened cheese, e.g. Brie, Camembert, goat's cheese
Blue-veined cheese, e.g. Danish blue, Stilton
Raw or lightly cooked shellfish
Raw or undercooked meats, poultry or fish, e.g. smoked salmon, Parma ham, sushi or rare meat
Raw or undercooked eggs, e.g. home-made mayonnaise, mousse, egg nog, meringue or hollandaise sauce
Paté and fish pastes (fresh or deli varieties only)
Probiotics, live or bio yoghurts
All unpasteurized dairy products

food request patterns demonstrated that patients requested 40% of their food between 5 pm and midnight, a time when food availability is often reduced.[75]

The use of oral nutritional intake confers considerable cost benefit compared to more intensive methods of nutrition support[76] although it does require a high level of input from the dietetic, nursing and catering staff. Patients generally do far better and are more compliant with dietary advice when they have increased contact from supportive staff.[10]

To aid in the provision of a nutritionally adequate diet, most patients will need to take sip feeds and nutritional supplements. Wide ranges of supplements are available in a variety of styles (milk-type, juice, soup and pudding). Many are nutritionally complete and can be used to replace or supplement meals. Supplements can be served cold or warm and may be modified to improve taste and texture. There is also a variety of modular supplements including glucose polymers and protein powders that can be used to fortify foods. The use of supplements should be carefully monitored.

Despite a wide range of flavors there remain several hurdles to supplement consumption, including taste fatigue, poor palatability, early satiety and problems with texture. Few studies have considered the role and effectiveness of dietary advice and/or nutritional supplement sip feeds in cancer patients.[77]

Whilst many patients will be able to maintain good levels of oral intake throughout the transplant period, when food intake meets less than 50% of their estimated energy and protein requirements, and is likely to remain so for more than 7 days, or a patient continues to lose weight, more intensive nutrition support is indicated.

Enteral tube feeding (ETF)

Enteral tube feeding involves the insertion of a feeding tube and the infusion of commercially produced, nutritionally complete feeds into the gastrointestinal tract. It is indicated in patients who are unable to take adequate oral diet due to anorexia, dysphagia or mucositis.

The role of enteral tube feeding in HSCT remains unclear. Historically, several objections to nasogastric feeding have been cited, including poor gut function and inadequate absorption, severe esophagitis, mucosal and gastric erosion by nasogastric tubes, risk of bleeding and detrimental effect on body image.[78] The use of fine-bore polyurethane feeding tubes, platelet cover if the patient is thrombocytopenic, and early insertion of the tube (i.e. prior to mucositis) may facilitate safe, effective feeding. To overcome issues of acceptance, compliance and effect on body image, patients should be prepared from the outset that tube placement is a standard part of their treatment. For patients with diarrhea or malabsorption there is a wide range of specialist feeds that can be used for various nutritional needs, for example, peptide feeds for those with malabsorption.

Quantifying the benefits of enteral tube feeding over parenteral feeding is difficult. No firm recommendations can be made due to the paucity of evidence.[57] However, extrapolating from the field of critical care medicine, it is suggested that early instigation of enteral feeding and prolonged enteral feeding during illness help to maintain gut function and reduce the risk of passage of bacteria across the intestinal mucosa. In considering nutrition support in oncology overall, several studies have indicated that enteral tube feeding causes fewer infectious complications when compared to parenteral nutrition.[61,79,80] The limited research available certainly demonstrates that enteral tube feeding is feasible and considerably cheaper than PN. It is also relatively easy to provide at home after discharge and could therefore theoretically facilitate earlier discharge from the ward. On a practical level, patients can have a large number of their oral medications administered via the tube, thus removing some of the daily burden of taking medication.

Practical aspects of enteral tube feeding

- *Type of feeding tube.* A variety of tubes are available. The choice of tube will depend on the anticipated length of time of feeding, gut function, etc. (Table 33.5). Nasogastric tubes should be made from polyurethane as these tubes can remain in situ for longer than PVC tubes without causing gastric erosion.
- *Timing of tube insertion.* In some institutions, nasogastric feeding tubes are prophylactically placed prior to transplant. An ideal time is in the days leading up to the transplant when the patient is already on the ward but not suffering from mucositis.
- *Type of* feed. A wide variety of commercially produced, sterile, low-lactose, gluten-free tube feeds are available. Most are nutritionally complete in 1500 ml.
  - Standard polymeric feeds. These contain whole protein as the nitrogen source, carbohydrate and hydrolyzed fat as the energy source. The standard feeds generally provide 1 kcal per ml and have a nitrogen content of 5–7 g per liter.
  - High energy/nitrogen feeds. These provide 1.5–2 kcal per ml and have increased nitrogen content. They tend to be hypertonic and can therefore cause diarrhea. These feeds are useful when feeding patients on fluid restriction, or as overnight supplementary feeding.
  - Fiber feeds. Fiber-containing feeds may be useful if the patient is suffering from diarrhea as they encourage the production of short-chain fatty acids.
  - Elemental/peptide feeds. These feeds may be better absorbed by patients suffering from severe mucositis or GvHD affecting the

Table 33.5 Enteral tube feeding

Type of tube	Method of insertion	Indication	Contraindication
Nasogastric tube	Bedside insertion	Patient is unable to achieve an adequate oral intake, e.g. due to mucositis, nausea, xerostomia Patient requires short-term feeding	Non-functioning GI tract Severe, intractable vomiting Severe mucositis Profuse diarrhea
Nasojejunal tube	Insertion under X-ray guidance or endoscopically. Usually given in conjunction with prokinetic agents	Patient is unable to achieve an adequate oral intake, e.g. due to mucositis, nausea, xerostomia Patient requires short-term feeding Patient has delayed gastric emptying	Non-functioning GI tract Severe, intractable vomiting Severe mucositis Profuse diarrhea
Gastrostomy tube	Endoscopically, radiologically or surgically	Patients requiring long-term tube feeding (i.e. >6 weeks)	Non-functioning GI tract GvHD affecting GI tract[60] Severe, intractable vomiting Severe mucositis Profuse diarrhea
Jejunostomy	Surgical	Patients with poor gastric emptying requiring long-term feeding	Non-functioning GI tract GvHD affecting the GI tract Not able to tolerate general anesthetic* Profuse diarrhea

* If the patient requires a jejunostomy tube but is not able to undergo a general anesthetic and alternative would be insertion of a PEJ tube (a percutaneous endoscopically placed jejunostomy).

gut. Protein is in the form or amino acids or peptides. However, these feeds are hypertonic and may exacerbate diarrhea.

- *Method of feed administration.* The appropriate feed can be delivered using 'bolus' feeding, 'gravity drip' feeding or administered using a dedicated feeding pump. The choice of delivery system will be dependent on gut function and whether feeding is a sole source of nutrition or an adjunct to normal food intake. For the majority of HSCT patients a relatively low rate of feed delivered over a long period is usually indicated with a transfer to overnight feeding when food intake begins to improve.
- *Monitoring feeding.* Monitoring needs multidisciplinary involvement if it is to be complete and effective. Several areas should be monitored including weight, fluid balance, biochemistry (an initial phosphate level is useful to highlight patients at risk of re-feeding syndrome) and bowel function.
- *Discontinuing tube feeds.* The tube feed should be phased out gradually as oral intake and nutritional status improve. It is useful to set realistic targets with patients and to encourage progress. Ideally the patient should be taking 50% of their estimated energy and protein requirements orally before feeds are stopped. Patients that have finished tube feeding will require follow-up and support from the dietitian. Weight should be routinely monitored.
- *Home enteral* feeding. This is widely used in the UK and relatively easy to organize. Many patients benefit from a short period of home enteral feeding following discharge from the ward.

Possible complications of enteral tube feeding

These are detailed in Table 33.6.

Parenteral nutrition (PN)

This is the intravenous administration of sterile, nutritionally complete solutions containing nitrogen, carbohydrate, lipid, vitamins, and minerals. It can be very effective in delivering precise quantities of nutrients and has no impact on GI symptoms. Enteral feeding should always be viewed as preferable to the parenteral route, and every effort should be made to use the gastrointestinal tract. Failure to stimulate the gastrointestinal tract may lead to marked atrophic changes in the bowel and pancreas, and can contribute to the occurrence of cholestasis and GvHD.[81–83] Enteral nutrition (EN) and 'standard care' (i.e. hydration/no nutrition support) are associated with a lower risk of infection than PN.[79,80] However, mortality and the risk of infection tend to be increased with 'standard care' compared with PN in a mal-

nourished patient population.[79] What is not clear at present is whether it is a case of EN having fewer complications than PN or whether EN is inherently better than PN.[79,84] It is a safe assumption that PN is not necessarily superior to enteral tube feeding and that it should be reserved for patients in whom enteral feeding has failed.[80,85]

Practical aspects of PN

Indications for PN

- GI tract not functioning, e.g. in complete bowel obstruction, severe diarrhea, intractable vomiting
- All methods of enteral nutrition have been considered and are not possible, e.g. jejunostomy feeding is not possible
- Complete bowel rest is required, e.g. acute grade IV GvHD affecting the gut
- Total nutrient requirements cannot be met using the enteral route only, due to limited absorption/tolerance of enteral feed, e.g. severe diarrhea, severe nausea and vomiting

Contraindications for PN

- Well-nourished patient who is likely to resume oral intake within 7 days
- GI tract is functioning (consider using all available routes of enteral feeding, e.g. nasogastric feeding, nasojejunal feeding)
- Lack of vascular access
- Severe hepatic abnormalities
- Patient has a very poor prognosis (research in the field of oncology suggests that the benefits of PN are often outweighed by undesirable side-effects and complications of PN in patients with advanced disease)[86–88]

PN is not of benefit if it is to be given for less than 7 days. In such circumstances it is likely that the risks and financial costs of PN outweigh any benefits that the patient might experience.

Access

PN can be administered via a central or peripheral line.

Administration

PN is generally administered using an iv infusion pump to maintain steady flow, which in turn may avoid occlusion of the line and help minimize complications such as fluid imbalance and hyperglycemia. Cyclic administration of PN is advisable (i.e. feeding over 18 hours or less) as it provides a period free from infusion to allow physiotherapy and time for a shower.[89]

Table 33.6 Complications of enteral feeding

Complication	Cause	Solution
Tube related		
Tube displacement	Patient accidentally/deliberately removes tube	Tape tube securely to patient's nose or cheek
Tube in incorrect position	Position not checked on insertion/monitored regularly	If it is a recurrent problem consider gastrostomy. Always check NG tube position by aspirating or X-ray. Monitor tube position
Tube blockage	Failure to flush feeding tube regularly or promptly. Inadequate flushing, i.e. using too small a volume. Administration of medication via the tube	To avoid this problem flush tube with 30–50 ml of water before and after feeding or medication. If medication is to be administered via the tube then ensure it is in liquid form or finely crushed. If the tube is blocked try soda water/Coke/sodium bicarbonate/spirits/pancreatic enzymes to try to unblock tubes
Mucosal erosion/sinusitis	Local damage to the nasal area or throat by the feeding tube. Common when Ryles tubes are used	Use polyurethane, fine-bore NG tubes. Consider changing to a gastrostomy tube
Leakage of gastric/jejunal fluid at tube site	Incorrect dressing or needless dressing of the wound. Erosion around the stoma site (especially if balloon catheters used)	Ensure that the site of insertion is allowed to heal or dressed in the appropriate dressing (refer to hospital wound care or stoma care nurse for advice). Avoid using catheters in place of specially designed tubes
Infection at insertion site	Incorrect dressing, no antibiotic cover given following insertion, poor technique when handling the tube	Ensure that the patient received 'antibiotic cover' after tube insertion. Ensure that appropriate dressings have been used and that the patient understands how to care for the site, e.g. wash hands before touching the site, etc. Swab site and treat infection. Avoid using tube until infection is clear
GI complications		
Aspiration	Regurgitation of feed due to poor gastric emptying. Incorrect placement of the tube	Give medication to improve gastric emptying, e.g. metoclopramide 1. Check tube placement 2. Try intermittent feeding 3. Try transpyloric feeding or jejunostomy feeding 4. Ensure patient has head at 45°
Nausea and vomiting	Generally related to disease/treatment, e.g. chemotherapy. Could be due to poor gastric emptying or rapid infusion of feed	Ensure appropriate antiemetics have been prescribed Reduce infusion rate Change from bolus feeding to intermittent feeding
Diarrhea	Could be due to antibiotic therapy, other medication such as chemotherapy, laxatives. Could be disease related, e.g. pancreatic insufficiency secondary to cystic fibrosis. Could be due to gut infection, microbial contamination of feed or equipment	Give antidiarrheal agent Discontinue antibiotics if possible Change to an iso-osmolar feed Reduce infusion rate Ensure that microbiologic contamination of feed or equipment is not likely Check to see if the patient is receiving laxatives Check stool appearance/content to see if malabsorption. Change to peptide feed in absence of GI infection (send stool sample) Try a fiber-containing feed
Constipation	Could be due to inadequate fluid intake, immobility, use of opiates and other medication causing gastric stasis, excessive use of antidiarrheal agents or bowel obstruction	Check fluid balance Suggest laxatives, bulking agents Encourage patient to be as mobile as possible Check if patient is in bowel obstruction – if yes then discontinue feed ?? Try fiber-containing feed
Abdominal distension	Poor gastric emptying, rapid infusion of feed, constipation or diarrhea	Reduce rate of infusion, prescribe gastric motility agents, encourage patient to be mobile. Check for constipation or diarrhea
Metabolic hyperglycemia	Underlying diabetes mellitus or insulin resistance as a result of 'stress response'	Regular monitoring of blood sugars and appropriate medication, e.g. sliding-scale insulin

Overfeeding

It is advisable to avoid overfeeding, particularly when commencing PN, as this can cause additional physical stress and may lead to fluid and electrolyte abnormalities as well as to changes in liver function. It is therefore advisable to start feeding at 30 kcal per kg and review this depending upon changes in clinical condition and nutritional status.

Composition

Most hospitals store a range of 'standard' PN bags, and if possible the patient should be given one of these. Where compounding units exist, the PN can be made to order. The dietitian should be involved in estimating requirements and should work closely with the medical team and pharmacist.

- The sources of energy used in PN are carbohydrate and lipid. Carbohydrate is a relatively cheap source of energy, well metabolized and has good nitrogen-sparing effect. However, excessive glucose administration can lead to lipogenesis, fatty liver, and problems controlling blood sugars (especially if the patient is physiologically stressed). Lipids are generally used in all PN solutions and should aim to provide 30–50% of total energy. Fat-free PN is not routinely recommended.

- Nitrogen is in the form of amino acids. There are still no clear guidelines as to what constitutes an optimum amino acid profile for PN. It is likely that some 'non-essential' amino acids are, in fact, essential during illness, and debate continues concerning the value of supplementing PN amino acid solutions with additional glutamine, carnitine, extra-branched chain amino acids, etc.

- Vitamins, minerals and trace elements are usually added in preformed compounds such as Cernavit, Vitlipid, Solvito and Additrace.

Monitoring

It is essential that the patient receiving PN is adequately monitored. Monitoring should place particular emphasis on fluid balance, biochemistry and hematology and changes in clinical condition. Due to the high volume of glucose in PN solutions, it is necessary to monitor blood sugars regularly.

Discontinuing PN

When possible many clinicians aim to run enteral feeds and PN concurrently. This in theory helps maintain gut function and facilitates the transition from PN to tube feeding. Decrease in PN should be matched by an increase in enteral intake (food or feed). PN should not stop until the patient is managing to have 50% of requirements via the enteral route.

Home parenteral feeding

This is complex and expensive to provide and needs the involvement of a specialist PN feeding team. It should only be used after careful consideration and the failure of other forms of nutrition support and is rarely indicated post HSCT.

Possible complications of PN

These are shown in Table 33.7.

PN-related infections can be reduced if a dedicated line is used. Breaking the line for drug administration or blood sampling may lead to contamination of nutrient solutions.

Displacement of a catheter may also be a problem.

Glutamine

Current research findings concerning the role of glutamine supplementation (both oral and parenteral) in patients undergoing HSCT are inconclusive.[57,65,66,90–93]

Diet and nutrition as a treatment for malignancy

At present, there is no evidence that a particular food or diet can cure cancer. A wide range of articles, books, internet sites and complemen-

Table 33.7 Possible metabolic complications of PN

Complication	Cause	Action required
Hyperglycemia[80]	Underlying diabetes mellitus Increased insulin resistance secondary to stress response Excessive glucose administration Excessively fast glucose infusion	Administer insulin Reduce glucose infusion rate Provide some kcal in the form of lipid Reduce total kcal given
Hypoglycemia	Excessive insulin infusion Rebound hypoglycemia if PN containing high levels of glucose is abruptly stopped	Reassess insulin requirements Reduce infusion rate of PN for the last 2 hours of feeding
Dehydration or overhydration	Miscalculation of fluid losses/intake	Adjust fluid volume provided from PN More concentrated dextrose and lipid solutions may be used, and sodium may be eliminated or reduced from PN[100]
Hypophosphatemia	Re-feeding syndrome (i.e. additional phosphate is required for malnourished patients) Excessive glucose infusion	Provide additional phosphate (10 mmol phosphate per 1000 kcal)[110] Increase % kcal from lipid
Hypokalemia	Increased potassium requirements secondary to stoma losses/diarrhea Given excess of glucose and insulin Re-feeding malnourished patients	Provide additional potassium Increase % of kcal from lipid
Hypernatremia	Multifactorial: water depletion, excessive sodium load with medication	Correct fluid imbalance and review drugs
Hyponatremia	Multifactorial: fluid overload, excessive GI or fistula losses	Check fluid balance and monitor fistula losses
Essential fatty acid deficiency	Lipid-free PN	Provide fat in PN. Administer walnut oil orally
Vitamin and trace elements deficiency (e.g. selenium, chromium)	Increased requirements	Monitor levels and provide supplements as necessary
Uremia	Renal failure, excess nitrogen load and high levels of catabolism	Check fluid balance Reduce nitrogen load
Hepatic dysfunction	May be seen after a few weeks' feeding. Cause unknown although could be: underlying liver disease or hepatotoxic drugs, cholestasis, excessive glucose infusion, essential fatty acid deficiency, continuous feeding, suppression of gut hormones	May resolve spontaneously or may continue and require cessation of feeding Investigate for other possible causes of liver dysfunction, e.g. disease, drug side-effects Decrease glucose infusion/increase lipid infusion Feed with an 8–14 hour break Administer a small amount of enteral feeding to stimulate gut function
Cholelithaisis	Prolonged PN Lack of enteral intake	Try to maintain small enteral intake, e.g. small amounts of food or NG feed at 10–20 ml/hour
Polymyopathy	Long-term PN ? Due to essential fatty acid or selenium deficiency	Provide lipid in PN Assess selenium levels and supplement
Metabolic bone disease	? Cause ? excess vitamin D ? excess aluminum ? inadequate calcium or phosphate	Provide additional calcium and phosphate

Table 33.8 Relative advantages and disadvantages of methods of nutrition support

Methods of feeding	Advantages	Disadvantages
Oral nutrition support	Helps maintain gut function Non-invasive Low risk of infection Low cost	Can be difficult to eat adequate quantities Requires access to a flexible catering service with supportive staff Can be difficult to provide the patient's preferred foods in a hospital setting Pressure on patient to eat perhaps when not feeling like eating Difficult to achieve adequate intake if patient is vomiting or has severe nausea
Enteral tube feeding	Helps maintain gut function Relatively low cost Wide range of feeds available to meet clinical needs Low risk of infection from administration of feed provided 'clean techniques' are used Patients can put medication down the tube	Requires placement of feeding tube Feeding tubes tend to be visible Painful to insert nasogastric tube if patient is suffering from mucositis Risk of infection from PEG/jejunostomy site Nasogastric tubes can be easily displaced particularly if the patient suffers from intractable vomiting If diarrhea is profuse may not absorb adequate volumes of feed
Parenteral nutrition	Guaranteed delivery of nutrients Does not stimulate/affect the GI tract Can be used if patient has non-functioning GI tract	Increased risk of infection Increased risk of metabolic abnormalities Does not protect GI tract mucosa Requires venous access Expensive Not easily done as an outpatient

tary or alternative therapists make unrealistic claims on the benefits of following particular diets or taking certain supplements. For the patient, the information can be misleading. Many confuse the findings of epidemiologic nutrition research into the etiology of cancer with the role of diet as a treatment for cancer. Patients are often advised that the body should be 'starved' to cure the cancer or that the cancer is a toxin that can be removed by dietary 'detoxification'.[94] There is often a great deal of emphasis placed upon patients taking responsibility for their own cure. Advice is often to follow a vegan diet with a high fruit, vegetable and grain content, to avoid caffeine, alcohol, and 'processed' foods. This is often also accompanied by the use of expensive vitamin, mineral and other supplements. If a patient has entered upon this type of nutrition regimen, all supplements should be checked for potential drug–nutrient interactions and potential toxicities.

The benefits in terms of returning control to the patient and promoting self-help must be balanced against the practical difficulties and financial cost of such diets, their low nutrient density, the potential for toxicities from the nutritional supplements prescribed, and the feelings of guilt experienced by patients if they fail to adhere to strict regimes.[94]

Discharge planning and follow-up

Patients often experience difficulties with food intake and deterioration of nutritional status following discharge home.[10,11] Compliance with dietary advice given on the ward declines, and many patients will have failed to regain their pretreatment weight a year after transplant[10] (Table 33.9).

On discharge patients should be advised on:
- basic food hygiene
- the avoidance of 'high-risk' foods
- the importance of maintaining nutritional status
- the principles of a high-energy/high-protein diet.

As long-term follow-up studies highlight the importance of ongoing nutrition support and monitoring patients, there should be systems in place that ensure that outpatients are weighed regularly. This information should be recorded sequentially and in a place where it is easily accessible to the multidisciplinary team. The use of oral nutritional support and enteral tube feeding is particularly effective in the outpatient setting and relatively easy to arrange. Home parenteral nutrition is rarely, if ever, indicated and due to the practical difficulties and costs involved, should only be used after careful consideration and the failure of other forms of nutrition support.

Table 33.9 Factors which may potentially affect nutritional status following discharge from hospital

Anorexia
Somnolence
Xerostomia/altered saliva
Taste changes
Depression/anxiety
GvHD

On discharge, patients who have undergone HSCT or high-dose chemotherapy may benefit from attending a multidimensional rehabilitation program. This provides an opportunity for patients to share experiences, and to access information and support from a range of healthcare professionals in an informal setting. Topics and activities usually covered include nutrition, exercise, relaxation sessions and fatigue management in addition to discussion on the psychosocial aspects of life post transplant. Such programs have been shown to be popular with patients, have a positive impact on quality of life and assist with fatigue management.[95–99]

References

1. Deeg HJ, Seidel K, Bruemmer B et al. Impact of patient weight on non-relapse mortality after marrow transplantation. Bone Marrow Transplant 1995;15:461–468
2. Horsley P, Bauer J, Gallagher B. Poor nutritional status prior to peripheral blood stem cell transplantation is associated with increased length of hospital stay. Bone Marrow Transplant 2005;35:1113–1116
3. Le Blanc K, Ringden O, Remberger M. A low body mass index is correlated with poor survival after allogeneic stem cell transplantation. Haematologica 2003;88:1044–1052
4. Raynard B, Nitenberg G, Gory-Delabaere et al. Summary of the standards, options and recommendations for nutritional support in patients undergoing bone marrow transplantation. Br J Cancer 2003;89:101–106
5. National Institute for Clinical Excellence. Guidelines 2003: Nutrition support in adults. National Institute for Clinical Excellence, London
6. Keenan AM. Nutritional support of the bone marrow transplant patient. Nurs Clin North Am 1989;24:383–392
7. Weisdorf S, Lysne J, Wind D et al. Positive effect of prophylactic total parenteral nutrition on long term outcome of bone marrow transplantation. Transplantation 1987;43:833–838
8. Buchsel PC, Whedon MB. Bone marrow transplantation. Administrative and clinical strategies. Jones and Bartlett, London, 1995
9. Dickson B, Barale KV. Section 2: nutritional assessment. In: Lenssen P, Aker SN (eds) Nutritional assessment and management during marrow transplantation. A resource manual. Murray, Seattle, 1985:45–63
10. Iestra JA, Fibbe WE, Zwinderman AH. Body weight recovery, eating difficulties and compliance with dietary advice in the first year after stem cell transplantation: a prospective study. Bone Marrow Transplant 2002;29:417–424

11. Lenssen P, Sherry ME, Cheney CL et al. Prevalence of nutrition-related problems among long-term survivors of allogeneic marrow transplantation. J Am Dietet Assoc 1990;90:835–842
12. Savage DG, Szydlo RM, Goldman JM. Clinical features in 430 patients with chronic myeloid leukaemia seen at a referral centre over a 16 year period. Br J Haematol 1997;96:111–116
13. Sessions J. Monitoring your patients with chronic myeloid leukemia. Am J Health-System Pharm 2006;63(23 suppl 8): S5–9
14. Bossola M, Tazza L, Giungi S, Luciani G. Anorexia in hemodialysis patients: an update. Kidney Int 2006;70:417–422
15. Catassi C, Bearzi I, Holmes G. Association of celiac disease and intestinal lymphomas and other cancers. Gastroenterology 2005;128: S79-S86
16. Sonis ST, Oster G, Fuchs H et al. Oral mucositis and the clinical and economic outcomes of hematopoietic stem-cell transplantation. J Clin Oncol 2001;19:2201–2205
17. Zerbe MB. Parkerson SG, Ortlieb ML. Relationship between oral mucositis and treatment variables in bone marrow transplant patients. Cancer Nurs 1992;15:196–205
18. Papadopoulou A, Nathavitharana KA, Williams MD. Diarrhea and weight loss after bone marrow transplantation in children. Pediatr Hematol Oncol 1994;11:601–611
19. Aker S N, Lenssen P, Darbinian J. Nutritional assessment in the marrow transplant patient. Nutrition Support Serv 1983;3:22–27
20. Moe G, Aker SN, Schubert MM. Section 4: enteral management. In: Lenssen P, Aker SN (eds) Nutritional assessment and management during marrow transplantation. A resource manual. Murray, Seattle, 1985:31–44
21. Stern JM, Lenssen P. Food and nutrition services for the BMT patient. In: Buchsel PC, Whedon MB (eds) Bone marrow transplantation. Administrative and clinical strategies. Jones and Bartlett, London, 1995
22. Vera-Llonch M, Oster G, Ford C M et al. Oral mucositis and outcomes of allogeneic hematopoietic stem-cell transplantation in patients with hematologic malignancies. Support Care Cancer 2007;15(5):491–496
23. Schmale AH. Psychological aspects of anorexia. Cancer 1979;43:2087–2092
24. Femia RA, Goyette RE. The science of megestrol acetate delivery: potential to improve outcomes in cachexia. Bio Drugs 2005;19:179–187
25. Yavuzsen T, Davies MP, Walsh D. Systematic review of the treatment of cancer-associated anorexia and weight loss. J Clin Oncol 2005;23:8500–8511
26. Yeomans MR, Hails NJ, Nesic JS. Alcohol and the appetizer effect. Behav Pharmacol 1999;10:151–161
27. Wu D, Hockenberry DM, Brentnall TA et al. Persistent nausea and anorexia after marrow transplantation: a prospective study of 78 patients. Transplantation 1998;66: 1319–1324
28. Ford R, Ballard B. Acute complications after bone marrow transplantation. Semin Oncol Nurs 1988;4:15–24
29. McDonnell AM, Lenz KL. Palifermin: role in the prevention of chemotherapy- and radiation-induced mucositis. Ann Pharmacother 2007;41:86–94
30. Spencer A, Horvath N, Gibson J. Prospective randomised trial of amifostine cytoprotection in myeloma patients undergoing high-dose melphalan conditioned autologous stem cell transplantation. Bone Marrow Transplant 2005;35:971–977
31. Stiff PJ, Emmanouilides C, Bensinger WI et al. Palifermin reduces patient-reported mouth and throat soreness and improves patient functioning in the hematopoietic stem-cell transplantation setting. J Clin Oncol 2006;24:5186–5193
32. Logemann JA, Smith CH, Pauloski BR et al. Effects of xerostomia on perception and performance of swallow function. Head Neck 2003;23:317–321
33. Hamlet S, Faull J, Klein B et al. Mastication and swallowing in patients with postirradiation xerostomia. Int J Palliat Nurs 1997;37:789–796
34. Chambers MS, Garden AS, Kies MS, Martin JW. Radiation-induced xerostomia in patients with head and neck cancer: pathogenesis, impact on quality of life, and management. Head Neck 2004;26:796–807
35. Dahlya MC, Redding SW, Dahlya RS. Oropharyngeal candiadiasis caused by non-albicans yeast in patients receiving external beam radiotherapy for head and neck cancer. Int J Radiat Oncol Biol Phys 2003;57:79–83
36. Singhal S, Powles R, Treleaven J et al. Pilocarpine hydrochloride for symptomatic relief of xerostomia due to chronic graft versus host disease or total body irradiation after bone marrow transplantation for hematologic malignancies. Leuk Lymphoma 1997;24:539–543
37. Shahdad SA, Taylor C, Barclay SC et al. A double blind, crossover study of Biotene Oralbalance and BioXtra systems as salivary substitutes in patients with post-radiotherapy xerostomia. Eur J Cancer Care 2005;14:319–326
38. Davies AN. A comparison of artificial saliva and chewing gum in the management of xerostomia in patients with advanced cancer. Palliat Med 2000;14:197–203
39. Boock CA, Reddick JE. Taste alterations in bone marrow transplant patients. J Am Dietet Assoc 1991;9:1121–1122
40. Jacobsohn DA, Margolis J, Doherty J et al. Weight loss and malnutrition in patients with chronic graft-versus-host disease. Bone Marrow Transplant 2002;29:231–236
41. Gauvreau JM, Lenssen P, Cheney CL et al. Nutritional management of patients with intestinal graft-versus-host disease. J Am Dietet Assoc 1981;79:673–675
42. Imataki O, Nakatani S, Hasegawa T et al. Nutritional support for patients suffering from intestinal graft-versus-host disease after allogeneic hematopoietic stem cell transplantation. Am J Hematol 2006;81:747–752
43. Payne-James J, Grimble G, Silk D (eds). Artificial nutrition support in clinical practice. Edward Arnold, London, 1995
44. Aker SN, Cheney CL. The use of sterile and low microbial diets in ultraisolation environments. J Parenteral Enteral Nutr 1983;7:390–397
45. Lipkin AC, Lenssen P, Dickons BJ. Nutrition issues in hematopoietic stem cell transplantation: state of the art. Nutr Clin Pract 2005;20:423–439
46. Pryke DC, Taylor RR. The use of irradiated food for immunosuppressed hospital patients in the United Kingdom. J Hum Nutr Dietet 1995;8:411–436
47. Bibbington A, Wilson P, Jones M. Audit of nutritional advice given to bone marrow transplant patients in the United Kingdom. Clin Nutr 1993;12:230–235
48. Pattison AJ. Review of current practice in 'clean' diets in the UK. J Hum Nutr Dietet 1993;6:3–11
49. Rees W. Low microbial diets in immunocompromised patients. Br J Cancer Manage 2005;2:21–23
50. Adak GK, Long SM, O'Brian SJ. Trends in indigenous foodborne disease and deaths, England and Wales:1992–2000. Gut 2002;51:832–841
51. Konowalchuk J, Speirs JL, Pontefract RD, Bergeron G. Concentration of enteric viruses from water with lettuce extract. Appl Microbiol 1974;28:717–719
52. Kominos SD, Copeland CE, Grosiak B, Postic B. Introduction of Pseudomonas aeruginosa into a hospital via vegetables. Appl Microbiol 1972;24:567–570
53. Sivapalasingam S, Friedman CR, Cohen L, Tauxe RV. Fresh produce: a growing cause of outbreaks of foodborne illness in the United States, 1973 through 1997. J Food Prot 2004;67:2342–2353
54. Mokhtari A, Moore CM, Yang H et al. Consumer-phase Salmonella enterica serovar enteritidis risk assessment for egg-containing food products. Risk Anal 2006;26:753–768
55. Gudmundsdottir S, Roche SM, Kristinsson KG, Kristjansson M. Virulence of Listeria monocytogenes isolates from humans and smoked salmon, peeled shrimp, and their processing environments. J Food Prot 2006;69:2157–2160
56. Bischofberger T, Cha SK, Schmitt R et al. The bacterial flora of non-carbonated, natural mineral water from the springs to reservoir and glass and plastic bottles. Int J Food Microbiol 1990;11:51–71
57. Murray SM, Pindoria S. Nutrition support for bone marrow transplant patients. Cochrane Database Systematic Review 2002;CD002920
58. Tartarone A, Wunder J, Romano G et al. Role of parenteral nutrition in cancer patients undergoing high-dose chemotherapy followed by autologous peripheral blood progenitor cell transplantation. Tumori 2005;91:237–240
59. Martino R, Caballero M, Simon J et al. Evidence for a graft-verse-leukemia effect after allogeneic peripheral blood stem cell transplantation with reduced-intensity conditioning in acute myelogenous leukaemia and myelodysplastic syndromes. Blood 2002;100: 2243–2245
60. McSweeney P, Niederwieser D, Shizuru J et al. Hematopoietic cell transplantation in older patients with hematological malignancies:replacing high-dose cytotoxic therapy with graft-versus-tumor effects. Blood 2001;97:3390–3400
61. Arfons LM, Lazarus HM. Total parenteral nutrition and hematopoietic stem cell transplantation: an expensive placebo? Bone Marrow Transplant 2005;36:281–288
62. Cetin T, Arpaci F, Dere Y et al. Total parenteral nutrition delays platelet engraftment in patients who undergo autologous hematopoietic stem cell transplantation. Nutrition 2002;18:599–603
63. Cutler C, Li S, Kim HT. Mucositis after allogeneic hematopoietic stem cell transplantation: a cohort study of methotrexate- and non-methotrexate-containing graft-versus-host disease prophylaxis regimens. Biol Blood Marrow Transplant 2005;11:383–388
64. Roberts SR, Miller JE. Success using PEG tubes in marrow transplant recipients. Nutr Clin Pract 1998;13:74–78
65. Sykorova A, Horacek J, Zak P. A randomized, double blind comparative study of prophylactic parenteral nutritional support with or without glutamine in autologous stem cell transplantation for hematological malignancies – three years' follow-up. Neoplasma 2005;52:476–482
66. Ardens J, Bodoky G, Bozzetti F et al. ESPEN guidelines on enteral nutrition: non surgical oncology. Clin Nutr 2006;25:245–259
67. Papadopoulou A, MacDonald A, Williams MD et al. Enteral nutrition after bone marrow transplantation. Arch Dis Child 1997;77:131–136
68. Ringwald-Smith K, Krance R, Strcklin L. Enteral nutrition support in a child after bone marrow transplant. Nutr Clin Pract 1995;10:140–143
69. Sefcick A, Anderton D, Byrne JL et al. Naso-jejunal feeding in allogeneic bone marrow transplant recipients: results of a pilot study. Bone Marrow Transplant 2001;28: 1135–1139
70. Seguy D, Berthon C, Micol JB et al. Enteral feeding and early outcomes of patients undergoing allogeneic stem cell transplantation following myeloablative conditioning. Transplantation 2006;82:835–839
71. Hopman GD, Pena EG, Le Cessie S et al. Tube feeding and bone marrow transplantation. Med Pediatr Oncol 2003;40:375–379
72. Langdana A, Tully N, Molloy E. Intensive enteral nutrition support in paediatric bone marrow transplantation. Bone Marrow Transplant 2001;27:741–746
73. Pietsch JB, Ford C, Whitlock JA. Nasogastric tube feedings in children with high-risk cancer: a pilot study. Pediatr Hematol Oncol 1999;21:111–114
74. Arends J. Cancer patients need safe and efficient nutrition. Krankenpfl J 2005;43:130
75. Gauvreau JM, Cheney CL, Aker SN et al. Food intake patterns and food service requirements on a marrow transplant unit. J Am Dietet Assoc 1989;89:367–372
76. Pritchard C, Duffy S, Edington J et al. Enteral nutrition and oral nutrition supplements: a review of the economics literature. J Parenteral Enteral Nutr 2006;30:52–59
77. Baldwin C, Parsons T, Logan S. Dietary advice for illness-related malnutrition in adults. Cochrane Database Systematic Reviews 2001; CD002008
78. Hermann VM, Petruska PJ. Nutrition support in bone marrow transplant recipients. Nutr Clin Pract 1993;8:19–27
79. Braunschweig CL, Levy P, Sheean PM et al. Enteral compared with parenteral nutrition, a meta-analysis. Am J Clin Nutr 2001;74:534–542
80. Sheean PM, Freels SA, Helton WS et al. Adverse clinical consequences of hyperglycemia from total parenteral nutrition exposure during hematopoietic stem cell transplantation. Biol Blood Marrow Transplant 2006;2 :656–664
81. Hughes CA, Dowling RH. Speed of onset of adaptive mucosal hypoplasia and hypofunction in the intestine of parenterally fed rats. Clin Sci 1980;59:317–327
82. Mattsson J, Westin S, Edlund S. Poor oral nutrition after allogeneic stem cell transplantation correlates significantly with severe graft-versus-host disease. Bone Marrow Transplant 2006;38:629–633
83. Strasser SI, Shulman HM, McDonald GB. Cholestasis after hematopoietic cell transplantation. Clin Liver Dis 1999;3:651–668

84. Klein S, Koretz RL. Nutrition support in patients with cancer: what do the data really show? Nutr Clin Pract 1994;9:91–100

85. Szeluga DJ, Stuart RK, Brookmeyer R et al. Nutritional support of bone marrow transplant recipients: a prospective, randomized clinical trial comparing total parenteral nutrition to an enteral feeding program. Cancer Res 1987;47:3309–3316

86. Bozzetti F, Cozzaglio L, Biganzoli E et al. Quality of life and length of survival in advanced cancer patients on home parenteral nutrition. Clin Nutr 2002;21:281–288

87. Gallagher-Allred CR. Nutritional care of the terminally ill. Aspen Publishers, Maryland, 1989

88. MacGeer AJ, Detsky AS, O'Rourke K. Parenteral nutrition in cancer patients undergoing chemotherapy: a meta analysis. Nutrition 1990;6:233–240

89. Reed MD, Lazarus HM, Herzig RH et al. Cyclic parenteral nutrition during bone marrow transplantation in children. Cancer 1983;51:1563–1570

90. Aquino VM, Harvey AR, Garvin JH et al. A double-blind randomized placebo-controlled study of oral glutamine in the prevention of mucositis in children undergoing hematopoietic stem cell transplantation: a pediatric blood and marrow transplant consortium study. Bone Marrow Transplant 2005;36:611–616

91. Blijlevens NM, Donnelly JP, Naber AH et al. A randomised, double-blinded, placebo-controlled, pilot study of parenteral glutamine for allogeneic stem cell transplant patients Support Care Cancer 2005;13:790–796

92. Scloerb PR, Amare M. Total parenteral nutrition with glutamine in bone marrow transplantation and other clinical applications (a randomised, double blind studyJ Parenteral Enteral Nutr 1993;17:407–413

93. Zeigler TR, Young LS, Benfell K et al. Clinical and metabolic efficacy of glutamine supplemented parenteral nutrition after bone marrow transplantation. Ann Intern Med 1992;116:821–828

94. Cunningham RS, Herbert V. Nutrition as a component of alternative therapy. Semin Oncol Nurs 2000;16:163–169

95. Carlston LE, Smith D, Russell J et al. Individualised exercise program for the treatment of severe fatigue in patients after allogeneic hematopoietic stem cell transplant: a pilot study. Bone Marrow Transplant 2006;37:945–954

96. Kim SD, Kim HS. Effects of a relaxation breathing exercise on fatigue in hemopoietic stem cell transplantation patients. J Clin Nurs 2005;14:51–55

97. Korstjens I, Mesters I, van der Peet E et al. Quality of life of cancer survivors after physical and psychological rehabilitation. Eur J Cancer Prev 2006;15:541–547

98. Losito J, Murphy S, Thomas M. The effects of group exercise on fatigue and quality of life during cancer treatment. Oncol Nurs Forum 2006;33:821–825

99. van Weert E, Hoekstra-Weebers J, Grol B et al. A multidimensional cancer rehabilitation program for cancer survivors: effectiveness on health-related quality of life. J Psychosom Res 2006;58:485–496

100. Barzaghi A, Rovelli A, Piroddi A et al. Six years experience of total parenteral nutrition in children with hematological malignancies at a single center: management: efficacy and complications. Pediatr Hematol Oncol 1996;13:349–358

101. Muscaritoli M, Conversano L, Cangiano C et al. Biochemical indices may not accurately reflect changes in nutritional status after allogeneic bone marrow transplantation. Nutrition 1995;11:433–436

102. Taveroff A, McArdle AH, Rybka WB. Reducing parenteral energy and protein intake improves metabolic homeostasis after bone marrow transplantation. Am J Clin Nutr 1991;6:1087–1092

103. Duggan C, Bechard L, Donovan K et al. Changes in resting energy expenditure among children undergoing allogeneic stem cell transplantation. Am J Clin Nutr 2003;78:104–109

104. Geibig CB, Owens JP, Mirtallo JM. Parenteral nutrition for marrow transplant recipients: evaluation of increased nitrogen dose. J Parenteral Enteral Nutr 1991;15:184–188

105. Keller U, Kraenzlin E, Gratwohl A et al. Protein metabolism assessed by 1–13C leucine infusions in patients undergoing bone marrow transplantation. J Parenteral Enteral Nutr 1990;14:480–484

106. Driedger L, Burstall CD. Bone marrow transplantation: dietitian's experience and perspective. J Am Dietet Assoc 1987;87:1387–1388

107. Cunningham BA, Morris G, Cheney CL et al. Effects of resistive exercise on skeletal muscle in marrow transplant recipients receiving total parenteral nutrition. J Parenteral Enteral Nutr 1986;10:558–563

108. Cunningham BA. Section 5: Parenteral management. In: Lenssen P, Aker SN (eds) Nutritional assessment and management during marrow transplantation. A resource manual. Murray, Seattle, 1985:45–63

109. Antila HM, Salo MS, Kirvela O et al. Serum trace element concentrations and iron metabolism in allogeneic bone marrow transplant recipients. Ann Med 1992;24:55–59

110. Thompson JS, Hodges RE. Preventing hypophosphataemia during total parenteral nutrition. J Parenteral Enteral Nutr 1984;8:137–139

Barrier precautions, prophylaxis and neutropenic fever

CHAPTER 34

Unell Riley

Introduction

Infections during stem cell transplantation arise in three ways.

- From endogenous flora already present in the patient. During neutropenia, this accounts for 80% of infections. A study has shown that half of these are acquired during hospital stay.[1]
- From exogenous infection that the patient has acquired from an outside source.
- With reactivation of infection from organisms dormant within the host which become active because of his/her immunocompromised state.

In the pre-engraftment phase of the transplant, prophylaxis involves attempting to reduce infections arising from the host's own flora, suppressing reactivation of infections and reducing acquisition of exogenous flora.

Suppression of endogenous flora

Prior to engraftment, the combination of neutropenia and damage to the normal anatomic barriers renders patients at particular risk from their own, endogenous flora. Attempts should therefore be made to reduce the microbial load. General measures include proper maintenance of the integument and suppression of skin and mucosal microbes. Typical regimens include daily chlorhexidine washes or showers to reduce the possible risk of skin colonization by potential pathogens such as *Staphylococcus aureus* and *Corynebacterium jeikeium*. Long-term central venous catheters result in prolonged disruption of the normal anatomic barrier and therefore need particular attention to their care. They should be inserted in an aseptic manner.[2–4] There is little evidence that the use of a glycopeptide such as vancomycin reduces the risk of infection.[5–7] A sterile, transparent, semi-permeable polyurethane dressing should be used to cover the catheter site. This should be changed every 7 days, or sooner if it is no longer intact or if moisture has collected under the dressing. The line should be cleaned at dressing change with an aqueous solution of chlorhexidine. Skin-tunneled intravascular catheters should be dressed until fully healed and the stitches have been removed. Manipulation of the line should be kept to a minimum, and any procedures involving the line should make use of an aseptic technique. Shaving prior to catheter insertion should be discouraged since it may cause abrasion to the skin and lead to colonization or infection.[4]

The oropharynx is a significant source of infection in a neutropenic patient, and oral hygiene is therefore very important. A dental examination should be carried out well before the bone marrow transplant and any dental work that is necessary should be performed approximately 1 month before the transplant to allow sufficient time for full healing. Brushing the teeth with a soft toothbrush is acceptable if it does not lead to gum damage. Suppression of oropharyngeal flora can be achieved by the use of regular chlorhexidine mouthwashes.

The main approach has been to attempt to develop effective antibacterial chemoprophylaxis regimens. Initially, intestinal decontamination was used. This approach could be subdivided into total or partial decontamination, depending upon whether anaerobic bacterial flora were preserved. Total intestinal decontamination aims to completely suppress all endogenous intestinal flora, which are considered to be the main source of infection in neutropenic patients.[8,9] Antibiotics commonly used for this purpose were various combinations of oral vancomycin, gentamicin, colistin and neomycin. However, compliance among patients was poor due to the unpalatable nature of these agents and the fact that they caused gastrointestinal problems such as nausea and vomiting. Poor compliance could lead to general recolonization or to colonization with opportunistic organisms from the hospital environment, and resulted in failure to prevent infection.[9]

Selected decontamination aims to suppress all aerobic gastrointestinal flora but to preserve the anaerobic intestinal flora which are thought to be essential in preventing gut recolonization with hospital-acquired organisms, a process known as colonization resistance.[10] The gut flora require regular monitoring to detect early signs of bacterial regrowth or appearance of resistance organisms. Trimethoprim-sulfamethoxazole combination (co-trimoxazole) was initially tried in combination, usually with oral antifungals such as oral amphotericin or oral nystatin. Co-trimoxazole has been shown to be more effective than non-absorbable antibiotics in comparative trials.[11–14] Co-trimoxazole also provided some degree of systemic prophylaxis; however, it is not effective against *Pseudomonas aeruginosa*. It also has the disadvantage of prolonging the period of neutropenia due to bone marrow suppression and has therefore lost favor for use during neutropenia.

This concept of selective decontamination/systemic prophylaxis became more popular when the fluoroquinolones were developed. These drugs had the advantage of sparing the anaerobic flora, being more palatable to the patient, having activity against *Pseudomonas aeruginosa* and having little effect on recovering bone marrow. Also, since they achieve high blood levels at the recommended dosage, they have significant systemic prophylactic activity. Use of various quinolones such as ciprofloxacin,[15] ofloxacin,[16–18] norfloxacin[19,20] and perfloxacin[21] has been shown to be superior in reducing the incidence of gram-negative sepsis by comparative studies.

The concern about these drugs is their poor activity against gram-positive organisms such as coagulase-negative staphylococci and viridans streptococci; these organisms are increasingly the cause of sepsis in the neutropenic patient. In one review, quinolone prophylaxis was associated with an increased risk of streptococcal bacteremia.[22] The mortality rate from streptococcal infection in this review was similar to that from gram-negative septicemia. Two meta-analyses[23,24] confirmed that fluoroquinolone prophylaxis did reduce the incidence of gram-negative infections but not the incidence of gram-positive infections, and that it was occasionally associated with increased resistance to ciprofloxacin in gram-positive organisms.[25–27] They also failed to confirm that prophylaxis altered the incidence of febrile episodes or infection-related mortality. The European Organization for Research and Treatment of Cancer (EORTC) found that with the use of prophylaxis there was a decrease in the incidence of microbiologically documented infection episodes but a rise in the incidence of fever of unknown origin, suggesting that prophylaxis would merely be inhibiting the isolation of gram-negative isolates but not reducing the total number of infections.

With the increased importance of streptococcal infections, many have studied the combination of an antistreptococcal agent with a quinolone for prophylaxis. The addition of roxithromycin to ciprofloxacin has been shown to reduce the incidence of streptococcal infection,[28] and the addition of benzylpenicillin has also been suggested.[29] Further advances in fluoroquinolone development have produced drugs which have more gram-positive activity, such as levofloxacin, and a recent trial has shown a significant reduction in febrile episodes in patients treated with levofloxacin prophylaxis who are receiving chemotherapy for solid tumors and lymphoma.[30] A very recent meta-analysis showed that prophylaxis, ideally with a quinolone, reduces mortality in neutropenic patients.[31] However, the major drawback associated with the use of fluoroquinolones is the emergence of resistance in gram-negative organisms.

This class of antibiotics is not only used for prophylaxis in cancer patients but is also widely used in the outpatient setting for treating certain conditions, since these are the only oral antibiotics that can be used against *Pseudomonas* infections. They are also widely used in the community, other hospital departments, and in general practice and therefore have a wide impact on the microbial flora found in hospitals and in the community. There has been an increase in the incidence of ciprofloxacin resistance worldwide, including in the UK, with a rise in ciprofloxacin-resistant isolates in blood cultures being reported for all patient groups by hospitals in the UK.[32] This is already beginning to impact on cancer and transplant centers and inspection of the IATG-EORC database shows that during the period of fluoroquinolone prophylaxis, all *Escherichia coli* strains were sensitive to quinolones from 1983 to 1990. However, from 1990 to 1993, when fluoroquinolone prophylaxis was established, resistance increased by 27% with a concomitant increase in fluoroquinolone prophylaxis of 1.4–45%.[33–37]

The widespread use of fluoroquinolones has resulted in the emergence of bacteria not only resistant to fluoroquinolones but resistant to aminoglycosides and possessing extended spectrum β-lactamases.[32] At present, the Infectious Diseases Society of America (IDSA) does not recommend routine prophylaxis in neutropenia.

Antibiotic prophylaxis for capsulated bacterial infections

After engraftment, allogeneic bone marrow stem cell recipients appear to be at increased risk from bacteremia with capsulated bacteria, particularly in the presence of chronic graft-versus-host disease.[38] This is illustrated by the relatively high incidence of pneumococcal bacteremia, beginning at about 100 days post transplant.[39] This is probably due to two factors.

- The relative deficiency of the IgG₂ subclass in patients who have had a transplant, which may last for up to 2 years. Antibodies to type-specific polysaccharide antigens seem to be restricted to the IgG₂ class.[40]
- The presence of chronic graft-versus-host disease which can cause functional and structural hyposplenism.[41]

With the considerable risk of overwhelming pneumococcal septicemia, patients should receive life-long penicillin prophylaxis starting after engraftment, and they should also receive pneumococcal, *Neisseria meningitidis* Group C and *Haemophilus influenzae type b* immunization 9–12 months after their bone marrow transplant.[41,42] Allogeneic transplant patients need reimmunization with the 23-valent polysaccharide pneumococcal vaccine every 5 years after the first dose due to their impaired ability to mount an adequate immune response.

Reducing acquisition of exogenous flora

The environment

Protective isolation

The aim of protective isolation is to reduce the means by which the patient can acquire organisms from external sources. It is at its most effective when combined with decontamination techniques,[43] and thus hand washing/hand decontamination and the use of personal protective equipment are particularly important.

In its most basic form, protective isolation would consist of a naturally ventilated room with bathroom facilities. All items brought into the room would be thoroughly cleaned or disinfected and the patient nursed with reverse barrier techniques to reduce all likely routes of a nosocomial infection. The use of barrier nursing and protective isolation has been controversial but it is now a Joint Accreditation Committee of the International Society of Cellular Therapy and European Group for Blood and Marrow Transplantation (JACIE) recommendation that all patients who have had, or who are undergoing, a transplant procedure should be nursed in a single room. Walls and floors are not usually thought to be significant sources of nosocomial infection and thus regular cleaning with hot water and detergent of floors and surfaces is all that is usually required. However, there are incidences where the patient may be colonized with a particularly virulent or resistant organism which may contaminate the local environment or cause cross-infection to other patients. Examples of this are patients who are colonized with vancomycin-resistant enterococci, or patients with *Clostridium difficile* diarrhea. In these situations, it may be of benefit to perform daily rigorous cleaning of surfaces using a hypochlorite disinfectant to areas where healthcare workers have prolonged contact such as door handles and stethoscopes, which are kept in the patient's room.[45] Rooms should always be cleaned after they are vacated and before a new patient enters. Taps and sinks can become heavily colonized with environmental pseudomonads and thus should be regularly cleaned. Potted or cut plants should be discouraged since they are a potential source of bacterial or fungal spores, and stagnant water can be a potential reservoir for *Pseudomonas* spp.

Low-microbial diet

Since water and food may readily harbor exogenous microbes, it is essential that a low-microbial diet is provided for patients who are receiving gut prophylaxis. Although it is possible to provide totally sterile food by irradiating it, this may render food unpalatable. However, by providing a well-cooked diet, this problem may be overcome.[45] Since good nutrition is of paramount importance for these patients in their recovery, the aim is to provide the patient with a diet which is as attractive and palatable as possible,[46] so as to avoid the significant risks associated with total parenteral nutrition.

As water is a recognized source of environmental pseudomonads and *Acinetobacter* spp, the quality of drinking water should be closely monitored, and filtered or boiled water used whenever possible. Fresh, well-cooked and good-quality food should be brought to the patient for consumption as soon as possible after preparation. Cook-chill[47] or microwave methods of cooking are probably not suitable for the neutropenic patient, and dry foods are particularly unsuitable for such preparation. Only pasteurized milk or fruit juices should be used for the neutropenic patient and these should be discarded within 24 hours of opening. Since peppers and spices can be a potential source of bacteria and bacterial and fungal spores,[48] these should also be irradiated or added to food during cooking. Nuts, raw vegetables and salads, and raw unpeeled fruit should not be provided. Bread should be as fresh as possible. In the postengraftment period, patients should continue to receive advice regarding suitable foods because their cell-mediated immunodeficiency will continue to make them susceptible to infections such as *Listeria monocytogenes*.

A wide range of organisms can be transmitted as airborne pathogens. These include fungi such as *Aspergillus* and *Mucor* species, bacteria such as *Legionella* species and the protozoan *Pneumocystis jiroveci*, as well as a number of viruses. Outbreaks have occurred in the wards of neutropenic patients nursed in naturally ventilated siderooms, and this has been particularly seen as outbreaks of *Aspergillus* infections, particularly when hospital renovation is being carried out or when the ward is near building construction.[49–51]

Air filtration systems are designed to overcome these problems. The most effective and popular system is high-efficiency particulate air (HEPA) filtration.[52] This is thought to remove at least 99.97% of all particles which are $\geq 0.3\ \mu m$ in diameter. Therefore, such a system should remove all bacteria and fungi (and their spores) from the air, but not viruses. They have been used in a number of forms including specially designed laminar air flow cubicles[53] or plastic tent isolators.[54] Although there is good evidence to suggest that air flow filtration combined with other methods for reducing exogenous and endogenous microbial exposure does reduce the incidence of infection in bone marrow transplant patients,[55] it does not, however, eliminate fever and its greatest impact seems to be in reducing the incidence of *Aspergillus* infections.[56] Such units are expensive to install and maintain, and their cost-effectiveness has been questioned, but they would probably be considered mandatory where hospital construction or renovation is an issue.

Suppression of latent infection

The aim here is to reduce reactivation of latent infections. Most commonly, these are viral infections such as herpes viruses (HSV1, HSV2, VZV, CMV, EBV). Herpes simplex (HSV) can reactivate in the pre-engraftment phase and contribute to mucositis, and aciclovir prophylaxis is therefore often given in this period. Varicella zoster virus (VZV) can reactivate as disseminated zoster or shingles in the postengraftment phase, particularly during treatment for GvHD, and prophylaxis should be given then. Cytomegalovirus (CMV) reactivation/infection is usually managed pre-emptively, with weekly testing for CMV viremia by methods such as polymerase chain reaction (PCR). Patients with a history of tuberculosis (TB) or significant risk factors for TB, such as close contact with a person with known open TB, or HIV positive, should be considered for isoniazid chemoprophylaxis with pyridoxine during the pre-engraftment phase and for 6–12 months post engraftment.[57,58]

Parasitic infections can be a problem in this setting. Toxoplasmosis is an infrequent cause of infection after transplantation, occurring in 2–7% of patients who are seropositive before transplant.[59] Although the parasite can be transmitted in marrow or blood products, almost all cases are reactivation infections. Again, GvHD and its treatment are significant risk factors, especially in those patients not receiving co-trimoxazole prophylaxis for *Pneumocystis*. They should receive this if they have a seropositive donor.[60] Toxoplasmosis infection can present as meningoencephalitis, myocarditis or pneumonitis.

Other parasitic infections seen during transplantation are usually reactivations. *Clornorchis*, Chagas' disease, malaria, giardiasis, pulmonary microspororidiosis and *Acanthamoeba* meningoencephalitis[61–67] have all been reported during stem cell transplantation. Routine screening by blood smears or stool samples cannot exclude infection with these parasites.

Prophylaxis against *Pneumocystis jiroveci*

Pneumocystis jiroveci (formerly known as *Pneumocystis carinii*) is a known and accepted risk for people undergoing stem cell transplantation.[68] It is not only patients with malignant hematologic diseases who are at risk of *P. jiroveci* (*carinii*) pneumonia (PCP); this can also occur in patients with solid tumors undergoing transplantation.[69–72] The major chemotherapeutic risk factor is thought to be the prolonged use of corticoseroids[69] in these patients, but other immunosuppressant drugs such as fludarabine[73] may influence cell-mediated immunity sufficiently to increase the risk of PCP. The drug of choice for prophylaxis is co-trimoxazole,[74,75] given three times a week. However, inhaled pentamadine is preferred in some units due to the potential for co-trimoxazole to cause bone marrow suppression. Other alternatives are dapsone, or dapsone with pyrimethamine.

Table 34.1 lists the prophylactic medications suggested for postallograft patients, and Table 34.2 lists those suggested for postautograft patients.

Immunotherapy

Passive immunotherapy

This has involved the use of intravenous immunoglobulin (IVIG) to prevent and treat infections in bone marrow transplant recipients. In theory, intravenous immunoglobulin corrects immunoglobulin deficiencies as well as increasing the potential for opsonization and anti-endotoxin and virus neutralization. It may also augment activation of the complement system and immunoregulatory functions. However, a multicenter, randomized, double-blind placebo-controlled study[76] showed that immunoglobulin had no benefit over placebo; 92% of patients in the immunoglobulin group and 90% of patients in the placebo group had one or more infections, and the cumulative incidences of interstitial pneumonia, GvHD, transplant-related mortality and overall survival were similar. Another, earlier study confirmed these findings, and found no influence of immunoglobulin on the incidence of bacteremia on survival, obliterative bronchiolitis or on the incidence or mortality from chronic GvHD. Additionally, after stopping the IVIG, there appeared to be impaired recovery of endogenous humoral immunity.[77]

Some small studies have, however, shown an influence of immunoglobulin on the number of septicemia episodes[78] and have also suggested a reduced incidence of gram-negative infections in patients receiving immunoglobulin,[79] although this did not influence overall survival. Since there is no clearly defined role for the use of immunoglobulin in bone marrow stem cell recipients, its routine use is not currently recommended.[76,77]

Active immunization

A number of antibacterial vaccines have been developed. However, the immunocompromised bone marrow transplant recipient may well not mount an adequate response to them, as was demonstrated by an early, unsuccessful vaccine for *Pseudomonas aeruginosa*.[80] Although there is a similar, poor response to the polysaccharide-based vaccines for *Pneumococcus*, limited protection may still be provided[81] and

Table 34.1 Prophylaxis after allogeneic stem cell transplantation

For bacterial prophylaxis: penicillin V

Dose:
Children: 1–5 years 125 mg in 5 ml bd
6–16 years 250 mg bd
Adults: 250–500 mg bd

In event of penicillin allergy:
Erythromycin 250 mg bd or clarithromycin 250 mg daily (dose adjusted appropriately for pediatric patients)
Note: This should be continued for *life*.

If patient requires readmission for infection and broad-spectrum antibiotics are used, penicillin may be stopped during the course of antibiotics but must be reintroduced on completion of the course.

For fungal prophylaxis: itraconazole

Dose:
Children: 2.5 mg/kg orally bd
Adults: 2.5 mg/kg orally bd
Note: Oral liquid is preferable to capsules as it results in superior drug blood levels. In pediatrics, double the dose if using capsules. Best to dose adults in terms of body weight as audit showed that patients above 80 kg body weight do not always achieve adequate levels with the 'flat' dosing of 200 mg bd.

In adults: voriconazole 200 mg bd or posaconazole 200 mg tds in the event of intolerance to itraconazole
In pediatrics: voriconazole dose
2–12 years 200 mg bd
12–18 years <40 kg 200 mg bd for 2 doses, then 100 mg bd (can be increased to 150 mg bd if needed)
12–18 years >40 kg 400 mg bd for 2 doses, then 200 mg bd (can be increased to 300 mg bd if needed)
Note: This should continue for 6–12 months after SCT, until immunosuppressive therapy has ceased and blood count, including lymphocytes, has fully recovered. Azoles inhibit liver enzymes and ciclosporin levels may rise.

For pneumocystis prophylaxis

Adults: Monthly pentamidine inhalations started just prior to the recipient receiving the donor cells and continued until immunosuppressive therapy has ceased. After recovery of the platelet count to >50 × 10^9/l, and neutrophils >1, pentamidine can be switched to co-trimoxazole 80/400, either one tablet every day or two tablets daily on alternate days.
Children: Give pentamidine on day +28 if count not recovered. Co-trimoxazole recommenced at prophylactic dose when neutrophils >1.0 × 10^9/l for at least 3 days and platelets >30 × 10^9/l unsupported.

Dosage based on surface area:

Surface area	Co-trimoxazole	Trimethoprim	Sulfamethoxazole
0.5–0.75 m²	240 mg bd	40 mg bd	200 mg bd
0.76–1.0 m²	360 mg bd	60 mg bd	300 mg bd
Over 1.0 m²	480 mg bd	80 mg bd	400 mg bd

Note: The rationale for the earlier pentamidine is that co-trimoxazole can cause marrow depression and may inhibit engraftment.

Dapsone 100 mg daily may be used as an alternative to co-trimoxazole if patients are intolerant of this. In pediatric patients, dapsone 2 mg/kg (maximum dose 100 mg) once daily or 4 mg/kg weekly (maximum dose 200 mg) orally is recommended. Side-effects include fever, rash and hemolytic anemia. G6PD qualitative assay should be performed before starting dapsone therapy.

Prophylaxis should be continued for 6–12 months after SCT, until immunosuppressive therapy has ceased and blood count, including lymphocytes, has fully recovered. In the presence of c-GvHD it may be expedient to continue it for longer.

For viral prophylaxis

a) Herpes simplex (HSV) and varicella zoster
No prophylaxis if donor and recipient seronegative. If either is positive, aciclovir 400 mg tds in adults.

Aciclovir in pediatric patients
When changing to oral from iv route of administration:
    Patients <2 years old: 200 mg qds
    Patients >2 years old: 800 mg qds
Note: This should be continued for 6–12 months after SCT, until immunosuppressive therapy has ceased and blood count, including lymphocytes, has fully recovered.

b) Cytomegalovirus
No prophylaxis and no monitoring are necessary if donor and recipient are seronegative. If either is seropositive, weekly CMV PCRs to be carried out, which should be continued for 100 days, or for longer (>1 year) in patients with chronic GvHD and in those on continuing immunosuppression. If CMV PCR copies >3000, or are rising weekly from a lower level, commence ganciclovir 5 mg/kg bid or foscarnet 60 mg/kg tds.

c) Influenza
Preseasonal vaccination with attenuated viruses on a yearly basis, commencing 6–12 months after SCT (to include family members living with patient).

d) Hepatitis B
For all Hbs-Ag positive patients and those who are PCR (anti-core) positive, lamivudine 100 mg/od.

Note: This should be continued for 6–12 months after SCT, until immunosuppressive therapy has ceased and blood count, including lymphocytes, has fully recovered.

e) EBV
Levels should be monitored by PCR on a weekly basis in patients at risk and in those with unexplained fever. Treatment with rituximab should be commenced if levels rise above 40,000 copies/ml.

Table 34.2 Prophylaxis after autologous stem cell transplantation

Note: The risk of opportunistic infection correlates with immune reconstitution. Where T-cells are depleted by CD34 selection or when TBI has been used in conditioning, the highest risk of infectious complications is encountered. This should be taken into consideration when deciding whether prophylaxis should or should not be given.

Bacterial prophylaxis

Not routinely recommended once counts have recovered fully BUT penicillin V should be given for life if TBI was used in conditioning.

Dose:
Children: 1–5 years 125 mg in 5 ml bd
6–16 years 250 mg bd
Adults: 250–500 mg bd

In event of penicillin allergy:
Erythromycin 250 mg bid or clarithromycin 250 mg daily (check doses for pediatric patients).

Fungal prophylaxis

Itraconazole
Dose:
Children: 2.5 mg/kg orally bd
Adults: 2.5 mg/kg bd
Note: Use in patients at risk of invasive aspergillus (in particular, those with leukemia and lymphoma and those who have received TBI). Itraconazole oral liquid is preferable to capsules as it results in superior drug blood levels. In pediatrics, double the dose if using capsules.

Fluconazole
Adults: 100 mg daily in adults *not* at risk of invasive aspergillus (myeloma patients who have received high-dose melphalan conditioning).
Children: 3 mg/kg rounded up/down to nearest 50 mg if using capsules.
NB: Avoid azoles if using busulfan in conditioning regimes.

Note: This should continue for 3–6 months, until the blood count has fully recovered.

In pediatric patients with evidence of liver complications or recovering VOD, Ambisome 1 mg/kg iv three times a week may be continued on an outpatient basis.

Pneumocystis prophylaxis

Not routinely recommended after full recovery of counts. Should be considered for up to 6 months:

1. After fludarabine, 2-CDA or steroids
2. After graft manipulation
3. In patients with underlying leukemia or lymphoma
4. If TBI was used in conditioning.

Viral prophylaxis

a) Herpes simplex (HSV) and varicella zoster
Not routinely recommended once counts have fully recovered. Should be considered:

1. After fludarabine, 2-CDA or steroids
2. After graft manipulation
3. In patients with underlying leukemia or lymphoma
4. If TBI was used in conditioning,
5. In patients with a history of recurrent herpes infections.

When indicated:
Adults: aciclovir 400 mg tds
Children:
Patients <2 years old: 200 mg qds
Patients >2 years old: 800 mg qds

b) CMV
Routine monitoring not recommended. Prophylaxis not recommended.

c) Influenza
Preseasonal vaccination with attenuated viruses on a yearly basis, commencing 6–12 months after SCT.

d) Hepatitis B
For all Hbs-Ag positive patients lamivudine 100 mg/od, continued for not more than 3 months because of development of resistant strains.

immunization is recommended. Patients undergoing transplantation will also lose immunity to childhood infections and should be immunized 1–2 years after transplantation.

Recommended post-transplant immunization schedules are given in Chapter 35.

Immunomodulating agents

Stimulation of regenerating host defense mechanisms is a reasonable approach in neutropenic patients. Bone marrow colony-simulating factors such as G-CSF and GM-CSF have been used both to prevent febrile neutropenia and also to treat it.[82–86] Two meta-analyses recently performed[87,88] concluded that G-CSF and GM-CSF, when given prophylactically to cancer patients undergoing chemotherapy, reduced the risk of neutropenia, febrile neutropenia and infection. The Lyman study showed that infection-related mortality was also reduced.[87] The Cochrane analysis, looking at very pragmatic endpoints, found no significant advantage in outcome of the underlying disease.[88] G-CSF has been associated with a shortening of antibiotic days and duration of neutropenia in the treatment of established neutropenia.[89,90] A meta-analysis performed more recently, however, showed that there was no advantage in the widespread use of colony-stimulating factors to attempt to reduce the mortality due to febrile neutropenia.[91]

The American Society of Clinical Oncology has published guidelines[92] for the use of these agents, and recommends that they are only used prophylactically where the risk of a febrile neutropenia episode is greater than 40%, as would be the situation after stem cell transplantation. The use of these agents as adjuvant treatment in cases of febrile neutropenia should be limited to those patients who have severe neutropenia, in particular aplastic patients with uncontrolled underlying disease complicated by life-threatening bacterial or fungal infection.

References

1. Schimpff SC, Young VM, Greene WH et al. Origin of infection in acute non-lymphocytic leukemia. Significance of hospital acquisition of potential pathogens. Ann Intern Med 1972;77:707–714
2. CDC Guidelines. Guidelines for the prevention of intravascular catheter-related infections. MMWR 2002;51:RR-10
3. McGeeDC, Gould MK. Preventing complications of central venous catheterization. N Engl J Med 2003;348:1123–1133
4. Pratt R, Pellowe C, Wilson JA et al. National evidence-based guidelines for preventing healthcare-associated infections in NHS hospitals in England. J Hosp Infect 2007;65(suppl 1):S1–S64
5. McKee R, Dunsmuir R, Whitby M, Garden OJ. Does antibiotic prophylaxis at the time of catheter insertion reduce the incidence of catheter-related sepsis in intravenous nutrition? J Hosp Infect 1985;6:419–425
6. Ranson MR, Oppenheim BA, Jackson A et al. Double-blind placebo controlled study of vancomycin prophylaxis for central venous catheter insertion in cancer patients. J Hosp Infect 1990;15:95–102
7. Ljungman P, Hagglund H, Bjorkstrand B et al. Peroperative teicoplanin for prevention of gram-positive infections in neutropenic patients with indwelling central venous catheters: a randomized, controlled study. Support Care Cancer 1997;5:485–488
8. Donnely JP. Chemoprophylaxis for the prevention of bacterial and fungal infections. Cancer Treat Res 1995;79:45–82
9. Hathorn JW. Critical appraisal of antimicrobials for prevention of infections in immunocompromised hosts. Hematol Oncol Clin North Am 1993;7:1051–1099
10. Guiot HFL, van den Broak J, van der Meer JWM et al. Selective antimicrobial modulation of the intestinal flora of patients with acute nonlymphocytic leukemia. A double blind, placebo-controlled study. J Infect Dis 1983;147:615–623
11. Gualtieri RJ, Donowitz GR, Kaiser DL et al. Double-blind randomized study of prophylactic trimethoprim/sulfamethoxazole in granlocytopenic patients with hematologic malignancies. Am J Med 1983;74:934–940
12. Kramer BS, Carr DJ, Rand KH et al. Prophylaxis of fever and infection in adult cancer patients: a placebo-controlled trial of oral trimethoprim-sulfamethoxazole plus erythromycin. Cancer 1984;53:329–335
13. EORTC International Antimicrobial Therapy Project Group. Trimethoprim-sulphamethoxazole in the prevention of infection in neutropenic patients. J Infect Dis 1984;150:372–379
14. Watson JG, Jamieson B, Powles RC et al. Co-trimoxazole versus non-absorbable antibiotics in acute leukaemia. Lancet 1982;1:6–9
15. Arning M, Wolf HH, Aul C et al. Infection prophylaxis in neutropenic patients with acute leukaemia: a randomised, comparative study with ofloxacin, ciprofloxacin and co-trimoxazole/colistin. J Antimicrob Chemother 1990;26: S137-S142
16. Winston DJ, Ho WG, Bruckner DA et al. Ofloxacin versus vancomycin/polymyxin for prevention of infections in granulocytopenic patients. Am J Med 1990;88:36–42
17. Liang RHS, Ying RWH, Chum T-K et al. Ofloxacin versus co-trimoxazole for prevention of infection in neutropenic patients following cytotoxic chemotherapy. Antimicrob Agents Chemother 1990;34:215–218
18. Kern W, Kubble E. Ofloxacin versus trimethoprim-sulphamethoxazole for prevention of infection in patients with acute leukaemia and granulocytopenia. Infection 1991;19:73–80
19. Bow EJ, Rayner E, Louie TH. Comparison of norfloxacin with co-trimoxazole for infection prophylaxis in acute leukemia. Am J Med 1989;84:847–854
20. The GIMEMA Infection Programme. Prevention of bacterial infection in neutropenic patients with hematological malignancies. A randomised, multi-centre trial comparing norfloxacin with ciprofloxacin. Ann Intern Med 1991;115:7–12
21. Aravantinos G, Samonis G, Panidis D et al. Multicentric randomized comparative study of ceftazidime plus amikacin vs ceftazidime plus perfloxacin in the treatment of febrile neutropenia. Eur J Cancer 2001;37(suppl 6):353
22. Kern W, Kurrle E, Scheiser T. Streptococcal bacteraemia in adult patients with leukaemia undergoing aggressive chemotherapy: a review of 55 cases. Infection 1990;18:138–145
23. Engels EA, Lau J, Barza M. Efficacy of quinolone prophylaxis in neutropenic cancer patients: a meta-analysis. J Clin Oncol 1998;16:1179–1187
24. Cruciani M, Rampazzo R, Malena M et al. Prophylaxis with fluoroquinolones for bacterial infections in neutropenic patients: a meta-analysis. Clin Infect Dis 1996;23:795–805
25. Kotilainen P, Nikoskelainen J, Huovien P. Emergence of ciprofloxacin-resistant co-agulase negative staphylococcal skin flora in immunocompromised patients receiving ciprofloxacin. J Infect Dis 1990;161:41–44
26. Cornelissen JJ, de Graeff A, Verdonck LF et al. Imipenem versus gentamicin combined with either cefuroxime or cephalothin as initial therapy for febrile neutropenic patients. Antimicrob Agents Chemother 1992;36:801–807
27. Trucksis M, Hooper DC, Wolfson JS. Emerging resistance to fluoroquinolones in staphylococci: an alert. Ann Intern Med 1991;114:424–426
28. Rosenberg-Arska M, Dekker A, Verndonck L, Verhoef J. Prevention of bacteraemia caused by alpha-haemolytic streptococci by roxithromycin (RU-28965) in granulocytopenic patients receiving ciprofloxacin. Infection 1989;17:240–244
29. Guiot HFL, Peters WG, van der Broek PJ et al. Respiratory failure elicited by streptococcal septicaemia in patients with cytosine arabinoside, and its prevention by penicillin. Infection 1990;18:131–137
30. Cullen M, Steven N, Billingham L et al. Antibacterial prophylaxis after chemotherapy for solid tumors and lymphomas. N Engl J Med 2005;353:988–998
31. Gafter-Gvili A, Fraser A, Paul M, Leibovici L. Meta-analysis: antibiotic prophylaxis reduces mortality in neutropenic patients. Ann Intern Med 2005;142:979–995
32. Livermore DM. Minimising antibiotic resistance. Lancet Infect Dis 2005;5:450–459
33. Cometta A, Calandra T, Bille J et al. Escherichia coli resistant to fluoroquinolone prophylaxis in patients with cancer and neutropenia. N Engl J Med 1994;330:1240–1241
34. Kern WV, Andriof E, Oethinger M et al. Emergence of fluoroquinolone-resistant flora of cancer patients receiving norfloxacin prophylaxis. Antimicrob Agents Chemother 1996;40:503–505
35. Caratalla J, Fernandez-Sevilla A, Dominquez MA et al. Emergence of fluoroquinolone-resistant Escherichia coli at a cancer center. Antimicrob Agents Chemother 1994;38:681–687
36. Richard P, Delangle MH, Merrien D et al. Fluoroquinolone use and fluoroquinolone resistance: is there an association? Clin Infect Dis 1994;19:54–59
37. Gomez L, Garau J, Estrada C et al. Ciprofloxacin prophylaxis in patients with acute leukemia and granulocytopenia in an area with a high prevalence of ciprofloxacin resistant Escherichia coli. Cancer 2003;97:419–424
38. Aucouturier P, Barra A, Intrator L et al. Long lasting IgG subclass and antibacterial polysaccharide antibody deficiency after allogeneic bone marrow transplantation. Blood 1987;70:779–795
39. Winston DJ, Schiffman G, Wang DC et al. Pneumococcal infections after human bone marrow transplantation. Ann Intern Med 1979;91:835–841
40. Barrett DJ, Ayoub EM. IgG$_2$ subclass restriction of antibody to pneumococcal polysaccharides. Clin Exp Immunol 1986;63:127–134
41. Working Party of the British Committee for Standard in Haematology Clinical Haematology Task Force. Guidelines for the prevention and treatment of infection in patients with an absent or dysfunctional spleen. BMJ 1996;312:430–434
42. Davies JM, Barnes R, Milligan D. Update of guidelines for the prevention and treatment of infection in patients with an absent or dysfunctional spleen. Clin Med 2002;2:440–443
43. Nauseef WM, Maki DG. A study of the value of simple protective isolation in patients with granulocytopenia. N Engl J Med 1981;304:448–453
44. Wilcox MH, Fawley WN, Wigglesworth N et al. Comparison of the effect of detergent versus hypochlorite cleaning on environmental contamination and incidence of Clostridium difficile infection. J Hosp Infect 2003;54:109–114
45. Pryke DC, Taylor PR. The use of irradiated food for immunosuppressed hospital patients in the United Kingdom. J Human Nutr Diet 1995;8:411–416
46. Pattison AJ. Review of current practice in 'clean' diets in the UK. J Human Nutr Diet 1993;6:3–11
47. Chudasama Y, Hamilton-Miller JM, Maple PA. Bacteriological safety of cook-chill food at the Royal Free Hospital, with particular reference to Listeria. J Hosp Infect 1991;19:225–230
48. Bouakline A, Lacroix C, Roux N et al. Fungal contamination of food in hematology units. J Clin Microbiol 2000;38:4272–4273
49. Arnow PM, Anderson RL, Mainos PD, Smith EJ. Pulmonary aspergillosis during hospital renovation. Am Rev Resp Dis 1978;118:49–53
50. Opal SM, Asp AA, Cannady PB et al. Efficacy of infection control measures during a nosocomial outbreak of disseminated aspergillosis associated with hospital construction. J Infect Dis 1986;153:634–637
51. Rogers TR, Barnes RA. Prevention of airborne fungal infection in ummunocompromised patients. J Hosp Infect 1988;11(suppl A):515–520
52. Rhame FS, Streifel AJ, Kersey JH, McGlare PB. Intrinsic risk factors for pneumonia in the patient at risk of infection. Am J Med 1984;76:45–52
53. Buckner CD, Clift RA, Sanders JE et al. Protective environment for marrow transplant recipients. Ann Intern Med 1978;89:893–901
54. Watson JG, Rogers TR, Selwyn S, Smith RG. Evaluation of Vickers-Trexlar isolation in children undergoing bone marrow transplantation. Arch Dis Child 1977;52:563–568
55. Petersen FB, Buckner CD, Clift RA et al. Infectious complications in patients undergoing marrow transplantation: a prospective randomised study of the additional effect of decontamination and laminar air flow isolation among patients receiving prophylactic systemic antibiotics. Scand J Infect Dis 1987;19:559–567
56. Barnes RA, Rogers TR. Control of an outbreak of nosocomial aspergillosis by laminar airflow isolation. J Hosp Infect 1989;14:89–94
57. Roy V, Weisdorf D. Mycobacterial infections following bone marrow transplantation: a 20 year retrospective review. Bone Marrow Transplant 1997;19:467–470
58. Ip MSM, Yuen KY, Woo PCY et al. Risk factors for pulmonary tuberculosis in bone marrow transplant recipients. Am J Respir Crit Care Med 1998;158:1173–1177
59. Mele A, Paterson PJ, Prentice HG et al. Toxoplasmosis in bone marrow transplantation: A report of two cases and systematic review of the literature. Bone Marrow Transplant 2002;29:691–698
60. Advisory Committee on the Microbiological Safety of Blood and Tissues for Transplantation. MSBT guidance on the microbiological safety of human organs, tissues and cells used in transplantation. Department of Health, London, 2000
61. Lefrere F, Besson C, Daltry A et al. Transmission of Plasmodium falciparum by allogeneic bone marrow transplantation. Bone Marrow Transplant 1996;18:473–474
62. Dictar M, Sinagra A, Veron MT et al. Recipients and donors of bone marrow transplants suffering from Chagas' disease: Management and preemptive therapy of parasitemia. Bone Marrow Transplant 1998;21:391–393
63. Woo PC, Lie AK, Yuen K et al. Chonorchiasis in bone marrow transplant recipients. Clin Infect Dis 1998;27:382–384

64. Feingold JM, Abraham J, Bilgrami S et al. Acanthamoeba meningoencephalitis following autologous peripheral stem cell transplantation. Bone Marrow Transplant 1998;22:297–300

65. Anderlini P, Przepiorka D, Luna M et al. Acanthamoeba meningoencephalitis after bone marrow transplantation. Bone Marrow Transplant 1994;14:459–461

66. Okamoto S, Wakui M, Kobayashi H et al. Trichomonas foetus meningoencephalitis after allogeneic peripheral blood stem cell transplantation. Bone Marrow Transplant 1998;21:89–91

67. Kelkar R, Sastry PS, Kulkarni SS et al. Pulmonary microsporidial infection in a patient with CML undergoing allogeneic marrow transplant. Bone Marrow Transplant 1997;19: 179–182

68. Varthalitis I, Meunier F. Pneumocystis carinii pneumonia in cancer patients. Cancer Treat Rev 1993;19:387–413

69. Sepkowitz KA. Pneumocystis carinii pneumonia in patients without AIDS. Clin Infect Dis 1993;17:S416-S422

70. Sepkowitz KA, Brown AE, Telzak EE et al. Pneumocystis carinii pneumonia among patients without AIDS at a cancer hospital. JAMA 1992;267:832–837

71. Castagnola E, Dini G, Lanino E et al. Low CD4 lymphocyte count in a patient with P. carinii pneumonia after autologous bone marrow transplantation. Bone Marrow Transplant 1995;15:977–978

72. Kulke MH, Vanve EA. Pneumocystis carinii pneumonia in patients receiving chemotherapy for breast cancer. Clin Infect Dis 1996;25:215–218

73. Anaissie EJ, Kontoyiannis DP, O'Brien S et al. Infections in patients with chronic lymphocytic leukemia treated with fludarabine. Ann Intern Med 1998;129:559–566

74. Fishman JA. Treatment of infection due to Pneumocystis carnii. Antimicrob Agents Chemother 1998;42:1309–1314

75. Castagnola E, Zarri D, Caprion D et al. Cotrimoxazole prophylaxis of Pneumocystis carinii infection during the treatment of childhood acute lymphoblastic leukaemia – beware non compliance in older children and adolescents. Support Care Cancer 2001;9:552–553

76. Cordonnier C, Chevret S, Legrand M et al. Should immunoglobulin therapy be used in allogeneic stem cell transplantation? A randomised, double-blind, dose effect, placebo-controlled, multicenter trial. Ann Intern Med 2003;139:8–18

77. Sullivan KM, Storek J, Kopecky KJ et al. A controlled trial of long-term administration of intravenous immunoglobulin to prevent late infection and chronic graft-vs-host disease after marrow transplantation: clinical outcome and effect on subsequent immune recovery. Biol Blood Marrow Transplant 1996;2:44–53

78. Petersen FB, Bowden RA, Thornquist M et al. The effect of prophylactic intravenous immune globulin on the incidence of septicaemia in marrow transplant recipients. Bone Marrow Transplant 1987;2:141–148

79. Sullivan K, Kopecky K, Jocom J et al. Immunomodulatory and antimicrobial efficiency of intravenous immunoglobulin in bone marrow transplantation. N Engl J Med 1990;323:705–712

80. Young LS, Meyer RD, Armstrong D. Pseudomonas aeruginosa vaccine in cancer patients. Ann Intern Med 1973;79:518–527

81. Winston DJ, Ho WG, Schiffman G et al. Pneumococcal vaccination of recipients of bone marrow transplants. Arch Intern Med 1983;143:1735–1737

82. Dallorso S, Rondelli R, Messina C et al. Clinical benefits of granulocyte colony stimulating factor therapy after hematopoietic stem cell transplant in children: results of a prospective randomized trial. Haematologica 2002;87:1274–1280

83. Bishop MR, Tarantolo SR, Gella RB et al. A randomized, double-blind trial of filgrastim (granulocyte colony-stimulating factor) versus placebo following allogeneic blood stem cell transplantation. Blood 2000;96:80–85

84. Pui CH, Boyett JM, Hughes WT et al. Human granulocyte colony-stimulating factor after induction chemotherapy in children with acute lymphoblastic leukemia. N Engl J Med 1997;336:1781–1787

85. Hartmann LC, Tschetter LK, Habrmann TM et al. Granulocyte colony-stimulating factor in severe chemotherapy-induced febrile neutropenia. N Engl J Med 1997;336:1776–1780

86. Alonzo TA, Kobrinsky NL, Aledo A et al. Impact of granulocyte colony-stimulating factor use during induction for acute myelogenous leukaemia in children. A report from the Children's Cancer Group. J Pediatr Hematol Oncol 2002;24:627–635

87. Lyman GH, Kuderer NM, Djulbegovic B. Prophylactic granulocyte colony-stimulating factor in patients receiving dose-intensive cancer chemotherapy: a meta-analysis. Am J Med 2002;112:406–411

88. Bohlius J. Reiser M. Schwarzer G et al. Granulopoiesis-stimulating factors in the prevention of adverse effects in the therapeutic treatment of malignant lymphoma. Cochrane Database Syst Rev. 2002;4: CD003189

89. Mitchell PL, Morland B, Stevens MC. Granulocyte colony-stimulating factor in established febrile neutropenia: a randomized study of pediatric patients. J Clin Oncol 1997;15: 1163–1170

90. Garcia-Carbonero R, Mayordomo JI, Tornamira MV et al. Granulocyte colony-stimulating factor in the treatment of high-risk febrile neutropenia. A multicenter randomized trial. J Natl Cancer Inst 2001;93:31–38

91. Berghmans T, Paesmans M, Lafitte JJ et al. Therapeutic use of granulocyte and granulocyte-macrophage colony-stimulating factors in febrile neutropenic cancer patients: a systematic review of the literature with meta-analysis. Support Care Cancer 2002;10:181–188

92. Ozer H, Armitage JO, Bennett CL et al. 2000 update of recommendations for the use of hematopoietic colony-stimulating factors: evidence-based clinical practice guidelines. J Clin Oncol 2000;18:3558–3585

Reimmunization after stem cell transplantation

Kenneth Carson, Jayesh Mehta and Seema Singhal

CHAPTER 35

Introduction

Immunization represents one of the most cost-effective ways of preventing serious infectious diseases. While the terms 'vaccination' and 'immunization' are often used interchangeably, 'immunization' refers to the provision of immunity by any means, active or passive. Active immunization refers to stimulation of the host immune system through use of antigens in the form of a vaccine or toxoid preparation. Passive immunization refers to the use of exogenously derived antibody-containing preparations to provide temporary immune protection.[1]

While many different types of vaccines are available for use in practice, a number of them are specific to certain parts of the world, and only some vaccines are recommended for routine use. In the United States, for example, vaccines recommended for routine use in children include: diphtheria-tetanus-acellular pertussis (DTaP), influenzavirus, trivalent inactivated polio, measles-mumps-rubella (MMR), hepatitis A, hepatitis B, varicella, *Haemophilus influenzae* type b conjugate (Hib), and heptavalent pneumococcal conjugate.[2] Other vaccines recommended for selected populations include meningococcal and human papillomavirus.[3] Some vaccines are recommended before travel to endemic areas or are routinely used in other countries.[1]

Over time, most allograft and a large proportion of autograft recipients lose their immunity to poliovirus, tetanus, diphtheria, measles and other organisms.[4–6] Additionally, hematopoietic stem cell transplant (HSCT) recipients are at increased risk for developing infections with organisms such as *H. influenzae* and *S. pneumoniae*, for which vaccines are available.[7,8] For these reasons, it is essential to reimmunize HSCT recipients at appropriate intervals following transplant. This chapter will focus on the use of vaccinations to achieve active immunization post transplant. The use of immunoglobulin and prophylactic antibiotics or antiviral medications is beyond the scope of this chapter.

Systematic reimmunization after HSCT is an aspect of patient follow-up which is often neglected.[9] Surveys of reimmunization practices at transplant centers have found wide variations in utilization of post-transplant vaccination.[10,11] Of 45 centers surveyed in the United States by Henning et al, tetanus toxoid vaccination was the most common practice, with 88% of the surveyed centers routinely administering this to patients over the age of 7. Utilization of other vaccines such as hepatitis B was much less frequent.

Both the United States Centers for Disease Control (CDC) and the European Group for Blood and Marrow Transplantation (EBMT) have devised recommendations for vaccination after HSCT.[12,13] Since these guidelines were published, there have been numerous advances in vaccination technology, with the development of new and/or improved vaccines. These new vaccines will require careful study in patients after HSCT before evidence-based recommendations can be made regarding their routine use in this setting.

Principles of vaccinating blood and marrow transplant recipients

Immune reconstitution after HSCT follows a general pattern developing from immature to mature immune functions.[14–20] Immune reactivity during the first month post graft is extremely low. Cytotoxic and phagocytic functions recover by day 100, but the more specialized functions of the T- and B-lymphocytes may remain impaired for a year or even longer. After a period of time, the various components of the immune systems of most healthy marrow recipients begin to work synchronously, whereas the immune systems of patients with chronic graft-versus-host disease (GvHD) remain suppressed.

The use of blood-derived stem cells has largely supplanted traditional marrow transplantation due to faster immune reconstitution and greater ease of stem cell harvest.[21–23] As a result of the faster immune reconstitution and larger inoculum of cells infused during peripheral blood stem cell transplantation, it is possible that peripheral blood stem cell graft recipients may have an earlier and better response to vaccines. Unfortunately, many of the data available on post-transplant immunization have been gathered on recipients of marrow grafts. For the purposes of this chapter, it is assumed that recipients of peripheral blood stem cell grafts will respond in the same way as marrow graft recipients, with regard to post-transplant reimmunization.

The most important factor when considering vaccination after HSCT is the immune status of the patient. Inactive, subunit or recombinant vaccines may at worst be ineffective in HSCT patients, while live vaccines may be harmful or fatal in immunocompromised patients. Table 35.1 shows contraindications to live-attenuated vaccination after HSCT. Live vaccines that are contraindicated in immunocompromised patients are adenovirus, tuberculosis (Bacille Calmette–Guerin, BCG), oral polio, measles-mumps-rubella, typhoid (Ty21a), varicella, and yellow fever.

While inactive, subunit or recombinant vaccination is unlikely to harm patients, the timing of revaccination should be such that the patient can be expected to develop an immune response. This has resulted in specific guidelines for vaccination following transplant. Tables 35.2–35.4 contain a summary of vaccination recommendations from the CDC and EBMT. Available information on the use of individual vaccines post transplant is discussed below.

Inactivated, subunit and toxoid vaccines

Pertussis

The acellular pertussis vaccine has largely replaced the cellular pertussis vaccine due to an improved side-effect profile. While largely ignored until recently, pertussis is probably markedly underdiagnosed in the adult population. Ward et al[24] found the incidence of pertussis in unvaccinated control subjects in the United States over age the age of 15 to be 370 cases per 100,000 person-years, which extrapolates to over 1,000,000 cases in the United States annually.[24] The CDC has recently recommended a one-time dose of acellular pertussis, in the form of the DTaP vaccine, in all individuals aged 19–64, in place of the already recommended 10-year booster for tetanus-diphtheria.[3]

There are no data evaluating the efficacy and safety of the acellular pertussis vaccine in the HSCT setting, and no recommendation is made by either the CDC or EBMT at this time. Reports of pertussis infection following HSCT are also confined to a single case report, and that patient's clinical course was not severe.[25] Formal evaluation of the efficacy and safety of the acellular pertussis vaccine in HSCT recipients may support its use in the future. As an acellular vaccine, it is unlikely to cause significant side-effects or infectious complications in HSCT recipients.

Table 35.1 Contraindications to use of live-attenuated vaccines after HSCT

All allograft recipients for 2 years
All autograft recipients for 2 years
Patients on immunosuppressive therapy for any reason
Patients with chronic graft-versus-host-disease, whether requiring therapy or not
Patients suffering from recurrent malignancy after transplantation

Diphtheria

Diphtheria has emerged as a problem in a number of countries where immunization coverage has been high historically. These outbreaks have been characterized by high fatality rates, a high proportion of cases in adults, and an increased incidence of complications.[26] Most allograft recipients and a large proportion of autograft recipients will lose protective immunity to diphtheria.[27] Therefore, both the CDC and EBMT recommend repeating a series of three injections of the diphtheria toxoid vaccine. The two organizations have recommended slightly different dosing schedules.[12,13] All patients should then receive a diphtheria toxoid booster every 10 years thereafter. This vaccination schedule has been deliberately designed to coincide with the vaccination schedule for tetanus toxoid, as it is administered in a combined tetanus-diphtheria or DTaP vaccine.

Hepatitis A

Hepatitis A is a serious infection for which an inactivated vaccine exists. Vaccination is not recommended routinely in most developed countries due to the low annual incidence, but could be considered for patients living in or traveling to countries where this disease is endemic. Godoi et al showed that 23% of patients with antibodies to hepatitis A from presumed previous hepatitis A infection became seronegative 4 years after HSCT.[28] Therefore serum antibody titers could be used to guide reimmunization in patients living in endemic areas, with the inactivated hepatitis A vaccine being administered to patients

Table 35.2 Recommended schedule for inactivated, subunit or toxoid vaccine administration

Vaccine	CDC recommendation Doses and schedule (months after HSCT)	EBMT recommendation Doses and schedule (months after HSCT)	Antibody response	Comments
Diphtheria toxoid	3 doses at 12, 14, and 24 months	3 doses; the first at 6–12 months, and then two more 1–3 months apart	Good	Booster recommended at 10 years
Hepatitis B	3 doses at 12, 14, and 24 months	Start series at 6–12 months		
Hepatitis A	Not routinely indicated	2 doses; time unclear	Poor	
Influenzavirus	Annual; starting at 6 months	Annual, starting at 4–6 months	Good	Vaccinate household contacts for 1 year
Pertussis (acellular)	Consider with toxoid in children under age 7	Consider with toxoid in children under age 7	Unknown	Immunogenicity and efficacy post HSCT not studied
Polio (inactivated)	3 doses at 12, 14, and 24 months	3 doses; first at 6–12 months; then 1–3 months apart	Good	
Tetanus toxoid	Part of toxoid vaccine in above schedule	Part of toxoid vaccine in above schedule	Good	
Measles	1 dose at 24 months	1 dose at 24 months	Good	
Mumps	1 dose at 24 months	Not specified	Good	
Varicella zoster	Contraindicated	Consider at 2 years		

Table 35.3 Recommended schedule for bacterial vaccine administration

Vaccine	CDC recommendation Doses and schedule (months after HSCT)	EBMT recommendation Doses and schedule (months after HSCT)	Antibody response	Comments
Haemophilus influenzae (Hib)	3 doses at 12, 14, and 24 months	3 doses; the first at 6 months; and then two more 1–3 months apart	Good	
Pneumococcus polysaccharide	2 doses at 12 and 24 months	1 dose at 12 months	Poor	
Pneumococcus conjugate	Not specified	Consider in specific groups	Good	
Meningococcal polysaccharide	Consider in individuals at risk	Consider in individuals at risk	Good	
Meningococcal conjugate	Not specified	Not specified	Unknown	Immunogenicity and efficacy post HSCT not studied

Table 35.4 Recommended schedule for live-attenuated vaccine administration

Vaccine	CDC Recommendation Doses and schedule (months after HSCT)	EBMT Recommendation Doses and schedule (months after HSCT)	Antibody response
Measles	1 dose at 24 months	1 dose at 24 months	Good
Mumps	1 dose at 24 months	Not specified	Good
Rubella	1 dose at 24 months	Only in children and women of child-bearing potential	Good
Varicella zoster	Contraindicated	Consider at 2 years	

who become seronegative. Neither the CDC nor EBMT recommends routine vaccination for hepatitis A in HSCT recipients because of lack of clinical data.[12,13] The EBMT does suggest that the risk of side-effects due to the use of the vaccine is low, and therefore HSCT recipients could consider its use if they reside in or are traveling to endemic areas.[13]

Hepatitis B

While the risk of hepatitis B infection is low in many regions, the risks and morbidity of the infection in high-prevalence areas are considerable. Even in low-prevalence areas, there are a number of situations in which hepatitis B vaccination should be considered before HSCT, after transplant, or sometimes both. The simplest and most frequent situation occurs when hepatitis B vaccination is desired routinely according to government guidelines. For example, the CDC recommends hepatitis B vaccination for everyone under the age of 19 and adults with one or more risk factors.[2,3] This recommendation is then extended to the same population subgroups at an appropriate interval following transplantation, in accordance with the CDC guidelines.[12] The EBMT also recommends hepatitis B vaccination for HSCT recipients residing in countries where there is a policy recommending general hepatitis B vaccination.[13] Hepatitis B vaccination is not routinely recommended for all HSCT recipients.

Vaccination recommendations become more difficult – and somewhat empiric – when either the donor or the recipient of a HSCT is positive for the hepatitis B surface antigen (HBsAg). In the former instance, the EBMT recommends vaccination of the recipient prior to the transplant.[13] Unfortunately, completing the vaccination series is not always feasible before HSCT, due to the underlying disease process that is being treated with the transplant. Additionally, there is no evidence to suggest that this strategy helps avoid infection with the donor-transmitted hepatitis B virus. Hepatitis B surface antibody (anti-HBsAb) titers should be followed after transplantation, with the administration booster vaccine doses as necessary. When the recipient is HBsAg positive, the donor, if not already immune (either through a prior natural infection or after vaccination), should be immunized prior to stem cell collection because it is sometimes possible to resolve the hepatitis B carrier state in the patient through an allograft from an immune donor.[29] This also may not be feasible, especially in patients receiving stem cells from an unrelated donor.

The vaccination schedule outlined in Table 35.2 is intended for situations in which neither the donor nor the recipient is HBsAg positive. Clinicians should keep in mind that even under ideal circumstances, a proportion of patients do not respond to hepatitis B vaccination.[30]

Human papillomavirus

Human papillomavirus (HPV) is a common sexually transmitted disease. Persistent infection with certain types of HPV is associated with cervical cancer and genital warts. A vaccine developed recently covers HPV types 6, 11, 16, and 18, which are responsible for 70% of cervical cancer and 90% of genital warts.[31] This vaccine uses injec-

tion of empty viral capsids to establish immunity, and therefore should not be capable of causing infection in immunocompromised patients.[32] In June 2006 the CDC recommended vaccination with a series of three doses of HPV vaccine for all females aged 11–26. There are no available data evaluating efficacy or safety of this vaccine in the post-HSCT setting, but its use could be considered in the appropriate age group.

Influenzavirus

The influenzavirus continues to cause annual epidemics of respiratory disease throughout the world. Transplant recipients can acquire influenza infections during community epidemics, and secondary bacterial infections including pneumonia may have serious consequences.[33] Influenza vaccination within the first 6 months following HSCT has been found to be ineffective.[34] However, in patients receiving the vaccine 2 or more years after HSCT, the efficacy (over 60%) was similar to that described in non-immunocompromised hosts.[34] Given the low risk of side-effects, both the CDC and EBMT recommend use of the inactivated influenza vaccine annually in all HSCT recipients starting 6 months post transplant.[12,13] It is also worthwhile vaccinating household contacts of transplant recipients to prevent transmission of influenza through them to patients, especially for patients who are still in the early post-transplant phase.[13]

It is important to note that a live-attenuated influenza vaccine that is administered intranasally is available in some countries.[35] Like other live-attenuated vaccines, its use is contraindicated for at least 2 years after HSCT and potentially longer, depending on the immune status of the transplant recipient (see Table 35.1). Furthermore, use of the live-attenuated influenza vaccine should be discouraged in household contacts of transplant recipients due to transmission risk.

Poliovirus

Poliomyelitis remains endemic in four countries: Afghanistan, India, Nigeria, and Pakistan.[36] There are no active HSCT programs in Afghanistan or Nigeria, and those in Pakistan and India are small, with the annual number of transplantation procedures in the two countries well under 300. The number of individuals at risk in these countries is therefore small. However, cases that occur within endemic countries have the potential to spread to many other countries, due to the increased frequency of international travel. For this reason, reimmunization against polio is important elsewhere.

Ljungman et al found that although almost 70% of allograft recipients were seropositive to all poliovirus types a year after transplantation, roughly half the patients had experienced an at least fourfold decrease in antibody levels from their pretransplant levels.[37] Half of the patients receiving three doses of the inactivated polio vaccine responded, and the presence of chronic GvHD did not affect the response. Around 20% of autograft recipients were also found to have lost antibodies to at least one type of poliovirus a year after transplantation.[38] This time-dependent decrease in antibody levels continued in the second and third years in patients who were not revaccinated. A high proportion of seronegative patients reimmunized with three doses of the inactivated vaccine responded.[38] Based on these and other observations, the CDC and EBMT recommend revaccination with a series of three injections of the inactivated polio vaccine following HSCT.[12,13] The recommended timing of repeat vaccination differs slightly between them (see Table 35.2).

There are no published data on the use of the live-attenuated oral polio vaccine in HSCT recipients or their household contacts. Transmission of infection from an immunocompetent to an immunocompromised individual following administration of the live-attenuated polio vaccine has been reported,[39] and the oral polio vaccine should be avoided in both patients and their household contacts. In an effort to avoid vaccine-associated paralytic polio, the oral vaccine has not been used in the United States since 2000 and is no longer recommended for use in the general population by the CDC.[2,40]

Tetanus

Ljungman et al found that half of all patients who were immune to tetanus before allogeneic HSCT had lost their immunity by a year after transplantation, and all the patients who were not reimmunized with tetanus toxoid after HSCT were seronegative by 2 years.[41] A large proportion of autologous transplant recipients also lose protective immunity.[42] Response rates were relatively poor, and loss of immunity was common in patients immunized with one or two doses of tetanus toxoid after HSCT.[41] However, primary immunization with three doses of toxoid resulted in 100% response and sustained immunity.[41]

Both the CDC and EBMT recommend a series of three injections of the tetanus toxoid vaccine following transplantation.[12,13] The CDC recommends starting those vaccinations a year after HSCT, presumably because that was the timetable used in the first trials evaluating revaccination with tetanus toxoid after transplantation. Subsequent studies have shown that protective immunity can be established with vaccination as early as 6 months following HSCT.[43] This finding is reflected in the EBMT recommendations, which call for revaccination 6–12 months after HSCT. All patients should subsequently receive a tetanus toxoid booster 10 years after completion of the series of reimmunization vaccinations, in accordance with standard vaccination protocols.[2,3]

Bacterial vaccines

Haemophilus influenzae

Haemophilus influenzae accounts for a significant proportion of pulmonary infections in long-term survivors of HSCT.[44] However, unlike pneumococci, almost all severe disease is related to one capsular serotype (type b) and the conjugated Hib vaccine is very effective at preventing infections.[1]

The tetanus toxoid-conjugated Hib capsular polysaccharide vaccine is more immunogenic than the unconjugated, capsular polysaccharide vaccine and induces protective antibodies in 85% of allograft recipients, including IgG2-deficient patients.[45] Between 4 and 18 months after HSCT, response to the conjugate vaccine did not correlate with GvHD, immunosuppressive therapy, or the time of vaccination. Beyond 18 months from HSCT, response correlated with time (increasing efficacy with longer time interval).[45] Autograft as well as allograft recipients receiving a conjugate Hib vaccine at 12 and 24 months or only at 24 months developed protective antibodies 80% and 50% of the time, respectively.[46]

Donor and recipient immunization with the Hib-conjugate vaccine before HSCT resulted in higher antibody concentrations in patients as early as 3 months after HSCT compared with immunization of patients after HSCT.[47] Higher antibody levels in the early stages post transplant could potentially decrease the incidence of respiratory tract infections in patients with lung disease or chronic GvHD. No clear consensus has emerged on the optimal donor vaccination schedule.

Given the importance of this pathogen in the post-HSCT setting, both the CDC and EBMT recommend a series of three Hib vaccinations on slightly different schedules.[12,13]

Neisseria meningitides

While meningococcal infections can be severe in the post-HSCT setting, currently there are no recommendations for routine vaccination from the CDC or EBMT.[12,13] Vaccination could be considered, however, in patients who are otherwise at increased risk for meningococcal disease or in populations in which universal vaccination is recommended. For example, the CDC recommends meningococcal vaccination in children aged 11–12 years.[2] Evidence from a single study supports the immunogenicity of the tetravalent polysaccharide meningococcal vaccine in allogeneic HSCT recipients.[48] Since that study was published, a tetravalent conjugate vaccine has been licensed in the United States.[49] Like other conjugate vaccines, it is thought that this vaccine will provide more durable protection than the polysaccharide vaccine. However, it has yet to be tested in a systematic fashion in HSCT recipients.

Pneumococcus

Pneumococcal infections can cause significant morbidity following HSCT.[7,44,50] The incidence of invasive pneumococcal infections is markedly elevated after allogeneic transplant, especially when the post-transplant course is complicated by chronic GvHD.[7,50] While autologous transplant recipients have a lower risk of invasive pneumococcal infection than allogeneic, the risk is still increased over the normal population.[51]

Many studies have been done to evaluate the efficacy of numerous pneumococcal vaccine formulations following HSCT. Most of these studies were done on polysaccharide vaccines before the introduction of the heptavalent pneumococcal conjugate vaccine in 2000. Consequently, both the CDC and EBMT recommend use of the 23-valent polysaccharide vaccine after HSCT.

The 23-valent polysaccharide vaccine can induce antibody response 12 months or more after allogeneic HSCT.[52] Hammarstrom et al found that of patients who lost immunity to pneumococcus after transplant and were vaccinated with a polyvalent pneumococcal vaccine, 34% showed a rise in IgG2 antibodies, 28% an increase in IgG1, and 38% showed no response at all.[53] Furthermore, none of the patients with chronic GvHD showed an increase in IgG2 antibodies and 75% did not respond at all. While administration of more than one dose of the polysaccharide vaccine does not boost antibody levels,[46] the CDC does recommend two doses, at 12 and 24 months respectively, to 'provide a second chance for immunologic response among persons who failed to respond to the first dose'.[12] The EBMT guidelines still recommend a single dose of pneumococcal polysaccharide vaccine at 12 months.[13]

The heptavalent pneumococcal conjugate vaccine has not been extensively studied post HSCT. Molrine et al found that vaccination with the conjugate vaccine on a three-dose schedule (3, 6, and 12 months after transplantation) resulted in a significantly higher antibody response at 13 months compared to a single dose of the 23-valent polysaccharide vaccine at 12 months.[54] Protective immunity was achieved in 64–75% of patients receiving the conjugate vaccine.[54] Similar immunogenicity of the conjugated vaccine was observed in autologous transplant recipients.[55] Overall, these results are very encouraging and may ultimately result in uniform recommendations for the use of a conjugated pneumococcal vaccine. The CDC does not make a recommendation regarding use of conjugated pneumococcal vaccine,[12] and the EBMT suggests use could be considered in small children or patients with chronic GvHD.[13] The EBMT recommendation is coupled with a reminder that pneumococcal serotypes vary between countries, and the heptavalent vaccine serotypes were selected based on epidemiologic data from the United States.[13]

Live-attenuated vaccines

Measles

A substantial portion of allograft recipients and some autograft recipients, especially children, lose immunity to measles over time.[56] Measles remains an important pathogen in developing countries, and is responsible for sporadic outbreaks in developed countries as well.[57] While fatal cases of measles have been reported in HSCT recipients, they remain rare.[58] An outbreak in Brazil infected eight HSCT recipients, but all survived.[59]

As a live-attenuated vaccine, revaccination with the trivalent MMR vaccine can pose a risk to an immunocompromised recipient.[58] Current guidelines suggest vaccination after 2 years in patients who do not have any of the contraindications listed in Table 35.1. In the situation of a measles outbreak, the experience in Brazil suggests that vaccination can safely be performed as early as 1 year after HSCT in patients without other contraindications.[59] Both the EBMT and CDC guidelines recommend vaccination 24 months after transplant.[12,13]

Mumps

As with measles, a large number of allograft and autograft recipients lose immunity to mumps.[60] Mumps has not been described to be a serious problem specifically in HSCT patients, but vaccination should be considered in the absence of contraindications to live-attenuated vaccine. The CDC and EBMT differ in their recommendation for mumps vaccination, with the CDC suggesting vaccination 24 months after HSCT as part of the MMR vaccine and the EBMT stating that there is no indication for routine mumps vaccination after HSCT.[12,13]

Rubella

Like measles and mumps, many allograft and autograft recipients lose immunity to rubella.[60] Although rubella has not been reported to be a problem following HSCT, pregnancy is possible in a minority of transplant recipients.[61] The offspring of these women could be at risk for congenital rubella syndrome, and it would therefore be advisable to revaccinate women with child-bearing potential. The MMR vaccine has been administered to non-immunocompromised allograft recipients beyond 2 years from the transplant with development of immunity to rubella, and in autografted children.[60,62] The CDC recommends routine vaccination in appropriate patients 24 months after HSCT.[12] The EMBT recommends vaccination in women of child-bearing potential 24 months after HSCT to reduce the risk of congenital rubella syndrome.[23]

Varicella zoster virus (VZV)

As a live-attenuated vaccine, administration of varicella vaccine after HSCT runs the risk of serious infection. Recommendations from the CDC and EBMT diverge on this vaccine, with the CDC classifying it as contraindicated and the EBMT suggesting its use 2 years after HSCT in patients without contraindications to live-attenuated vaccination.[12,13] Studies evaluating use of the live-attenuated varicella vaccine after HSCT are confined to a single pilot study in which nine autolo-

gous transplant recipients were vaccinated 3–4 months after transplantation.[63] No systemic side-effects were observed, though one patient developed herpes zoster during follow-up. An experimental inactivated varicella vaccine has been evaluated specifically in HSCT recipients.[64] However, whether this vaccine is truly beneficial or not is unknown, particularly as aciclovir is very effective in preventing varicella zoster reactivation.[65]

Just as a primary varicella infection (chicken pox) results in VZV establishing latency in the dorsal root ganglia, the varicella vaccine virus (the Oka strain of VZV) can establish latency and reactivation may occur. With widespread varicella vaccination of children, some childhood immunization recipients will undergo transplantation – and may be at risk of herpes zoster through reactivation of the vaccine strain. This strain is sensitive to aciclovir and appropriate prophylactic use of aciclovir[65,66] should protect such individuals.

The Oka/Merck strain of live-attenuated VZV has been used to develop a zoster vaccine recently.[67] This vaccine is contraindicated in children and in immunocompromised adults.

Additional vaccines

A number of additional vaccines are used under specific circumstances in at-risk populations. The use of some of these vaccines remains controversial, even in healthy patients, and data examining their use after HSCT are very limited.

As a general rule, inactivated vaccines are safer than live-attenuated vaccines after HSCT. If a live-attenuated vaccine is the only available option, then its use should only be considered 2 years after HSCT in patients without any of the contraindications listed in Table 35.1. Patients who are ineligible for vaccination should be counseled on risk avoidance and/or restriction on travel to endemic areas. Until additional data are made available, there can be no evidence-based recommendations regarding the use of these other vaccines in the post-HSCT setting.

References

1. Keusch GT, Bart KJ, Miller M. Immunization principles and vaccine use. In: Kasper DL, Braunwald E, Fauci AS et al (eds) Harrison's principles of internal medicine, 16th edn. McGraw-Hill, New York, 2006
2. Centers for Disease Control and Prevention. Recommended childhood and adolescent immunization schedule – United States, 2006. MMWR 2005;54: Q1-Q4
3. Centers for Disease Control and Prevention. Recommended adult immunization schedule – United States, October 2006–September 2007. MMWR 2006;55: Q1-Q4
4. Ljungman P, Lewensohn-Fuchs I, Hammarstrom V et al. Long-term immunity to measles, mumps, and rubella after allogeneic bone marrow transplantation. Blood 1994;84: 657–663
5. Engelhard D, Handsher R, Naparstek E et al. Immune response to polio vaccination in bone marrow transplant recipients. Bone Marrow Transplant 1991;8:295–300
6. Li Volti S, Mauro L, di Gregorio F et al. Immune status and immune response to diphtheria-tetanus and polio vaccines in allogeneic bone marrow-transplanted thalassemic patients. Bone Marrow Transplant 1994;14:225–227
7. Kulkarni S, Powles R, Treleaven J et al. Chronic GVHD is associated with long term risk for pneumococcal infections in recipients of bone marrow transplants. Blood 2000;95:3683–3686
8. Aucouturier P, Barra A, Intrator L et al. Long lasting IgG subclass and antibacterial polysaccharide antibody deficiency after allogeneic bone marrow transplantation. Blood 1987;70: 779–785
9. Singhal S, Mehta J. Reimmunization after blood or marrow stem cell transplantation. Bone Marrow Transplant 1999;23:637–646
10. Henning KJ, White MH, Sepkowitz KA, Armstrong D. A national survey of immunization practices following allogeneic bone marrow transplantation. JAMA 1997;277:1148–1151
11. Brandt L, Broadbent V. A survey of recommendations given to patients going home after bone marrow transplant. Arch Dis Child 1994;71:529–531
12. Centers for Disease Control and Prevention. Guidelines for preventing opportunistic infections among hematopoietic stem cell transplant recipients. MMWR 2000;49(RR-10): 1–128
13. Ljungman P, Engelhard D, de la Camara R et al. Vaccination of stem cell transplant recipients: recommendations of the Infectious Diseases Working Party of the EBMT. Bone Marrow Transplant 2005;35:737–746
14. Lum LG. The kinetics of immune reconstitution after human marrow transplantation. Blood 1987;69:369–380

15. Symann M, Bosly A, Gisselbrecht C et al. Immune reconstitution after bone-marrow transplantation. Cancer Treat Rev 1989;16(suppl A): 15–19

16. Atkinson K. Reconstruction of the haemopoietic and immune systems after marrow transplantation. Bone Marrow Transplant 1990;5:209–226

17. Kelsey SM, Lowdell MW, Newland AC. IgG subclass levels and immune reconstitution after T cell-depleted allogeneic bone marrow transplantation. Clin Exp Immunol 1990;80:409–412

18. Storek J, Saxon A. Reconstitution of B cell immunity following bone marrow transplantation. Bone Marrow Transplant 1992;9:395–408

19. Storek J, Ferrara S, Ku N et al. B-cell reconstitution after human bone marrow transplantation: recapitulation of ontogeny? Bone Marrow Transplant 1993;12:387–398

20. Storek J, Witherspoon RP, Storb R. T cell reconstitution after bone marrow transplantation into adult patients does not resemble T cell development early in life. Bone Marrow Transplant 1995;16:413–425

21. Roberts MM, To LB, Gillis D et al. Immune reconstitution following peripheral blood stem cell transplantation, autologous bone marrow transplantation and allogeneic bone marrow transplantation. Bone Marrow Transplant 1993;12:469–475

22. Ottringer HD, Beelen DW, Scheulen B et al. Improved immune reconstitution after allo-transplantation of peripheral blood stem cells instead of bone marrow. Blood 1996;88:2775–2779

23. Powles R, Mehta J, Kulkarni S et al. Allogeneic blood and bone-marrow stem-cell transplantation in haematological malignant diseases: a randomised trial. Lancet 2000;355:1231–1237

24. Ward JI, Cherry JD, Change SJ et al. Efficacy of an acellular pertussis vaccine among adolescents and adults. N Engl J Med 2005;353:1555–1563

25. Kochethu G, Clark FJ, Craddock CF. Pertussis: should we vaccinate post transplant? Bone Marrow Transplant 2006;37:793–794

26. Galazka AM, Robertson SE, Oblapenko GP. Resurgence of diphtheria. Eur J Epidemiol 1995;11:95–105

27. Lum LG, Munn NA, Scanfield MS et al. The detection of specific antibody formation to recall antigens after human bone marrow transplantation. Blood 1986;67:582–587

28. Godoi ER, de Souza VA, Cakmak S et al. Loss of hepatitis A virus antibodies after bone marrow transplantation. Bone Marrow Transplant 2006;38:37–40

29. Ilan Y, Nagler A, Adler R et al. Ablation of persistent hepatitis B by bone marrow transplantation from a hepatitits B-immune donor. Gastroenterology 1993;104: 1818–1821

30. Struve J, Aronsson B, Frenning B et al. Intramuscular versus intradermal administration of a recombinant hepatitis B vaccine: a comparison of response rates and analysis of factors influencing the antibody response. Scand J Infect Dis 1992;24:423–429

31. www.cdc.gov/std/hpv/STDFact-HPV-vaccine.htm (accessed 1/15/2007)

32. Kousky LA, Ault KA, Wheeler CM et al. A controlled trial of a human papillomavirus type 16 vaccine. N Engl J Med 2002;347:1645–1651

33. Whimbey E, Elting LS, Couch RB et al. Influenza A virus infections among hospitalized adult bone marrow transplant recipients. Bone Marrow Transplant 1994;13: 437–440

34. Engelhard D, Nagler A, Hardan I et al. Antibody response to a two-dose regimen of influenza vaccine in allogeneic T-cell depleted and autologous BMT recipients. Bone Marrow Transplant 1993;11:1–5

35. Belshe RB, Mendelman PM, Treanor J et al. The efficacy of live attenuated, cold-adapted, trivalent, intranasal influenzavirus vaccine in children. N Engl J Med 1998;338:1405–1412

36. Pallansch MA, Sandhu HS. The eradication of polio – progress and challenges. N Engl J Med 2006;355:2508–2511

37. Ljungman P, Duraj V, Magnius L. Response to immunization against polio after allogeneic marrow transplantation. Bone Marrow Transplant 1991;7:89–93

38. Pauksen K, Hammarstrom V, Ljungman P et al. Immunity to poliovirus and immunization with inactivated poliovirus vaccine after autologous bone marrow transplantation. Clin Infect Dis 1994;18:547–552

39. Zuckerman M, Brink N, Kyi M, Tedder R. Exposure of immunocompromised individuals to health-care workers immunized with oral poliovaccine. Lancet 1994;343:985–986

40. www.cdc.gov/nip/diseases/polio/faqs.htm (accessed 1/27/2007)

41. Ljungman P, Wiklund-Hammarsten M, Duraj V et al. Response to tetanus toxoid immunization after allogeneic bone marrow transplantation. J Infect Dis 1990;162:496–500

42. Hammarstrom V, Pauksen K, Bjorkstrand B et al. Tetanus immunity in autologous bone marrow and blood stem cell transplant recipients. Bone Marrow Transplant 1998;22: 67–71

43. Parkkali T, Olander R-M, Ruutu T et al. A randomized comparison between early and late vaccination with tetanus toxoid vaccine after allogeneic BMT. Bone Marrow Transplant 1997;19:933–938

44. Lossos IS, Breuer R, Or R et al. Bacterial pneumonia in recipients of bone marrow transplantation. A five-year prospective study. Transplantation 1995;60:672–678

45. Barra A, Cordonier C, Preziosi MP et al. Immunogenicity of Haemophilus influenzae type b conjugate vaccine in allogeneic bone marrow recipients. J Infect Dis 1992;166:1021–1028

46. Guinan EC, Molrine DC, Antin JH et al. Polysaccharide conjugate vaccine responses in bone marrow transplant patients. Transplantation 1994;57:677–684

47. Molrine DC, Guinan EC, Antin JH et al. Donor immunization with Haemophilus influenzae type b (HIB)-conjugate vaccine in allogeneic bone marrow transplantation. Blood 1996;87:3012–3018

48. Parkkali T, Kayhty H, Lehtonen H et al. Tetravalent meningococcal polysaccharide vaccine is immunogenic in adult allogeneic BMT recipients. Bone Marrow Transplant 2001;27:79–84

49. Gardner P. Prevention of meningococcal disease. N Engl J Med 2006;355:1466–1473

50. Rege K, Mehta J, Treleaven J et al. Fatal pneumococcal infections following allogeneic bone marrow transplantation. Bone Marrow Transplant 1994;14:903–906

51. Engelhard D, Cordonnnier C, Shaw PJ et al. Early and late invasive pneumococcal infection following stem cell transplantation: a European Bone Marrow Transplantation survey. Br J Haematol 2002;117:444–450

52. Lortan JE, Vellodi A, Jurges ES et al. Class- and subclass-specific penumococcal antibody levels and response to immunization after bone marrow transplantation. Clin Exp Immunol 1992;88:512–519

53. Hammarstrom V, Pauksen K, Azinge J et al. Pneumococcal immunity and response to immunization with pneumococcal vaccine in bone marrow transplant patients: the influence of graft versus host reaction. Support Care Cancer 1993;1:195–199

54. Molrine DC, Antin JH, Guinan EC et al. Donor immunization with pneumococcal conjugate vaccine and early protective antibody responses following allogeneic hematopoietic stem cell transplantation. Blood 2003;101:831–836

55. Antin JH, Guinan EC, Avigan D et al. Protective antibody responses to pneumococcal conjugate vaccine after autologous hematopoietic stem cell transplantation. Biol Blood Marrow Transplant 2005;11:213–222

56. Ljungman P, Aschan J, Barkhot L et al. Measles immunity after allogeneic stem cell transplantation; influence of donor type, graft type, intensity of conditioning, and graft-versus host disease. Bone Marrow Transplant 2004;34:589–593

57. Parker AA, Staggs W, Dayan GH et al. Implications of a 2005 measles outbreak in Indiana for sustained elimination of measles in the United States. N Engl J Med 2006;355: 447–455

58. Kaplan L, Daum R, Smaron M et al. Severe measles in immunocompromised patients. JAMA 1992;267:1237–1241

59. Machado CM, Gancalves FB, Pannuti CS et al. Measles in bone marrow transplant recipients during an outbreak in Sao Paulo, Brazil. Blood 2002;99:83–87

60. Ljungman P, Fridell E, Lonnqvist B et al. Efficacy and safety of vaccination of marrow transplant recipients with a live attenuated measles, mumps, and rubella vaccine. J Infect Dis 1989;159:610–615

61. Singhal S, Powles R, Treleaven J et al. Melphalan alone prior to allogeneic bone marrow transplantation from HLA-identical sibling donors for hematologic malignancies: alloengraftment with potential preservation of fertility. Bone Marrow Transplant 1996;18:1049–1055

62. Pauksen K, Duraj V, Ljungman P et al. Immunity to and immunization against measles, rubella and mumps in patients after autologous bone marrow transplantation. Bone Marrow Transplant 1992;9:427–432

63. Ljungman P, Wang FZ, Nilsson C et al. Vaccination of autologous stem cell transplant recipients with live varicella vaccine: a pilot study. Support Care Cancer 2003;11: 739–741

64. Hata A, Hideomi A, Rinki M et al. Use of an inactivated varicella vaccine in recipients of hematopoietic-cell transplants. N Engl J Med 2002;347:26–34

65. Mehta J. Varicella vaccine in recipients of hematopoietic stem-cell transplants. N Engl J Med 2002;347:1624–1625

66. Trifilio S, Verma A, Mehta J. Antimicrobial prophylaxis in hematopoietic stem cell transplant recipients: heterogeneity of current clinical practice. Bone Marrow Transplant 2004;33:735–739

67. Oxman MN, Levin MJ, Johnson GR et al. A vaccine to prevent herpes zoster and postherpetic neuralgia in older adults. N Engl J Med 2005;352:2271–2284

Psychologic and supportive care issues in the transplant setting

Barry Quinn

Introduction

In the 1970s, stem cell transplantation was essentially seen as an experimental treatment for those who were terminally ill. Medical advances now enable people to be cured of their disease or to live longer in disease remission, with a reduction in treatment-related side-effects which were once much more common. These ongoing changes and advances in medical treatment must be matched by an expert team that is not only knowledgeable in transplant practice but is sensitive to the impact that the transplant procedure will have on the patient and his family. Although aware of the sometimes life-threatening nature of these procedures and the short- and long-term morbidity they may cause, the clinical team must also be mindful of the real hope that stem cell transplantation offers to many patients and their families.

This chapter aims to examine the impact on the patient and their family arising from transplant-related issues and complications. The demands of these procedures almost inevitably lead to profound physical, emotional, social and spiritual changes in the entire family unit, and practical approaches that the transplant team can use to support the patient and their family will be discussed in the context of the additional resources that can be utilized when such complications arise.

Despite careful preparation prior to undergoing a stem cell transplantation procedure, many patients, both adults and children, and their family members remain unprepared for the complications they may have to endure and the issues they may have to face during and after transplantation (Table 36.1). While addressing the benefits of the procedure, the transplant team should always forewarn the patient and their family about the possible side-effects and complications that may occur and the effects that these may have on their physical and psychologic well-being. This is always done in an atmosphere that offers reassurance and hope.

Ongoing medical developments have now made it possible for an increasing number of people to undergo transplantation. People with co-existing morbidities and of a relatively advanced age can now successfully undergo stem cell transplantation whereas previously this would not have been considered to be a viable treatment option. These advances, while bringing benefits to the patient, also make increasing demands of the transplant team. While continuing to be experts in their own field, the transplant team need to be aware of potential co-morbidity issues and must work closely with colleagues from other medical disciplines to ensure that these are adequately addressed. It should be recognized that, while many of the core skills of clinical transplantation will always be required, the care needs of a child with thalassemia major undergoing transplantation, for example, may differ in many ways from those of an adult undergoing transplantation for a malignant disease.

While many thousands of stem cell transplants are performed annually, each child or adult undergoing such a treatment is an individual who will respond to the demands of the procedure in their own way. It is important that the team appreciates what the illness means to the individual since, in this way, they may be in a better position to understand the individual's requests and wishes. Bury[1] describes illness as a 'biographical disruption' in which a person's life story is disturbed in the light of their illness, the treatment demands and the many changes that occur. Many of the assumptions which are taken for granted about a person's life may now be questioned as they face the uncertainty of transplantation. While disease is the medical diagnosis that is made by professionals (leukemia, breast cancer, arthritis and so on), illness is the personal experience of that disease and the impact it will have on that individual.[2]

From person to 'patient' – the transplant journey

A person undergoing transplantation and their family members will require support during each step of the treatment process, and each step will hold its own challenges and uncertainties.[3] Due to the acute nature of some diseases treated by stem cell transplantation, the patient and family may have had little time to come to terms with the implications of their disease and the changes it has brought, including the uncertain future. The patient and family are sometimes expected to adjust quite rapidly to what appears to them as the highly technical world of transplantation. They will be expected to adapt to rules and requirements which they may not always understand, as they begin to comprehend and gradually use the medical language employed by the medical team. They will learn to monitor blood results and other tests and begin to understand what these might mean in relation to their disease. It may seem to them that, since their initial diagnosis, they have had little opportunity to return to anything resembling normal life and now they are facing the next step of the treatment journey, the transplant procedure. So many changes appear to have been thrust upon them that there has been little time to reflect on the impact of these changes and demands.

Facing the decision to undergo transplantation in the light of the potential risks and benefits can be a difficult and uncertain time, which may include the problem of locating a suitable donor. The extensive preparation period as the person awaits transplantation may be filled with questions and concerns, and the support of the transplant team in recognizing and addressing these issues is essential. Each day of the transplant procedure can bring many changes as engraftment is awaited, and clear explanations from a knowledgeable and sensitive member of the team can do much to address a patient's concerns. It is also important that the team takes time to support and prepare the patient for discharge, since returning to life following transplantation can be a further time of uncertainty and concern as each person tries to deal with their situation without the 24-hour support of the clinical team upon which they have become dependent.

The support offered to both patient and family during the early period of transplantation will be required consistently in the subsequent stages of treatment and recovery. There may be inadequate support and preparation to enable the patient and family to return to a more normal way of life, or to allow the patient to adapt to being a person without a disease, following transplantation. One young woman being treated for leukemia described feeling a lack of support when the team had not always focused on her as a person. 'I think one of the things I would criticize about my treatment was that in the hematology ward, they treat your blood disease . . . and anything else that comes out, or is related, or you have . . . it is kind of matter of fact' (Rebecca).

Baker et al[4] demonstrated that a significant number of people who had undergone transplantation had difficulty in returning to their former roles and renegotiating social relationships. The period following discharge can be a time of great uncertainty as the individual tries to readjust to life following the demands of treatment. Studies have shown that patients and their families continue to deal with complications and concerns many years after the transplant period.[5,6]

The ability to adapt successfully to the challenges of transplantation is influenced by several factors. These include disease status, patient response to prior treatments, patient physical and psychologic characteristics and whether family and social support are present or absent. Team members will be required to use their skills to apply the medical benefits of care critically and wisely and in a supportive manner, aware of the changes the patient will face in each step of the treatment process.[7]

Symptom management

It is essential that an accurate diagnosis is made regarding any symptom, in order that appropriate treatment is commenced. This will include being able to identify the symptoms that are directly related to the transplant process and ones that may be caused by a co-morbidity. Many of the conditions that require symptom management are listed in Table 36.1, and a few will be discussed here.

Nausea and vomiting

While nausea and vomiting are common in the transplant setting, the distress that these symptoms can cause the patient may be overlooked. As with any symptom, the team should carefully assess the possible physical (infection, drug treatment/toxicity, graft-versus-host disease (GvHD)) and psychologic causes (increased anxiety, low mood).[3] Having identified the cause, nausea and vomiting may be managed by the use of both pharmacologic and non-pharmacologic interventions. The patient will often be able to report what antiemetics and non-pharmacologic approaches have been effective in the past. The pharmacologic approach should include use of a combination of antiemetics, which may include benzamides, benzodiazepines, phenothiazines, antihistamines, 5-HT3 receptor antagonists and butyrophenones.[8] Non-pharmacologic approaches may include relaxation, guided imagery, aromatherapy, distraction, and careful consideration of the timing and presentation of food. Practical measures will include having a vomit receiver and wipes close by, ensuring privacy, and monitoring effectiveness of antiemetic therapy while supporting and reassuring the patient that the sickness can be controlled. Upon dis-

Table 36.1 Complications and concerns

Early phase
Infections – bacterial, fungal, viral, protozoa
Gastrointestinal disturbance
Bone marrow depression
Acute graft-versus-host disease (GvHD)
Graft failure
Renal toxicity
Hemorrhagic cystitis
Interstitial pneumonitis
Sinusoidal obstruction syndrome
Cardiac failure
Neurologic toxicity
Psychologic and social issues, including separation from family roles and social events, uncertainty
Spiritual questioning – making sense
Late phase
Infections – cytomegalovirus, *Pneumocystis carinii (jirovecii)* pneumonia
Chronic GvHD
Chronic pulmonary complications
Endocrine – gonad failure, hypothyroidism
Cataracts
Sexual changes
Cardiac and renal complications
Secondary malignancies
Psychologic and social readjustment – returning to family and work life
Continuing making sense and spiritual concerns

Table 36.2 Mucosal damage secondary to cytotoxic treatment[11]

1. Initiation – mucosa appears normal but basal epithelium and submucosa are damaged
2. Primary damage response – reactive oxygen species (ROS) cause damage to DNA and promote further damage through inflammatory cytokines
3. Signal amplification – patient may have few symptoms, further damage caused by inflammatory cytokines
4. Ulceration – loss of mucosal integrity, painful lesions, bacteria may penetrate mucosa leading to systemic infection, further inflammatory cytokines produced in response to bacteria
5. Healing – may take weeks or months

charge, patients and their families should be encouraged to report any unresolved nausea and/or vomiting which, if prolonged, may lead to fluid and electrolyte imbalance and nutritional problems, possibly necessitating readmission.

Mucositis

Another common side-effect of transplantation, and one which is under-reported, is mucositis.[9] This distressing side-effect can affect any part of the gastrointestinal tract, leading to further complications, including inability to continue treatment, poor hydration, poor nutrition, pain and discomfort, diarrhea, infection and sepsis.[10] It is now understood that the pathobiology of mucositis involves five phases (Table 36.2), leading to a variety of visible and invisible mucosal changes. Visible signs range from mild erythema to severe ulceration, which may act as a portal for infection.[11] Severity will depend on a number of factors including previous oral health, age, type of conditioning regimen and other treatments.[11,12]

The management of mucositis depends on four key elements: reducing the damage, accurate assessment, good care of the mucosa, and appropriate treatment of symptoms, including adequate pain management. Each member of the team carrying out an assessment should use a recognized assessment tool and be trained in how to assess the mucosa.[9] Good oral care requires regular cleaning with a soft toothbrush to remove any debris, and the mucosa should be kept moist. If the patient is unable to use a toothbrush, regular oral rinses with water or normal saline will help.[13] There may be periods during treatment when the patient will need support to carry out their oral care. There are a variety of topical and systemic agents available that should be considered.[14] Any indication of infection arising from the mucosa or any other source should be treated according to the protocol agreed by the medical, pharmacy and microbiology teams. Good pain control through the use of topical or systemic analgesia, including patient-controlled analgesia, can relieve the distress of this symptom.

Bowel disturbance

Changes in bowel habit are frequently reported by patients and may include constipation, although it is much more common to see diarrhea in the transplant setting. As with other symptoms, it is important to accurately diagnose and treat the underlying cause, which may include infection, mucositis, GvHD, treatment-related causes or a combination of these. While treatment generally requires pharmacologic intervention and nutritional support, symptom management will also require team support. People who begin the transplant process as independent persons may find themselves very dependent on the nursing staff to help them meet the most basic needs of using the lavatory and personal hygiene requirements.

Infection

The individual is at risk of infection throughout the transplant process because of a compromised immune system. Careful monitoring for infection, and a quick and appropriate response are essential. The possibility of infection continues in the post-transplant period after engraftment, since T- and B-cells can take months or years to recover. Prolonged use of immunosuppressive drugs to prevent and treat GvHD in the allogeneic setting may also encourage infection. Patients may need to adjust family and social life to minimize the risk of infection, which may impact upon them and other members of the family and their circle of friends. Participation in certain activities may be restricted during recovery.

Patients must be carefully monitored for infections including cytomegalovirus, herpes zoster and respiratory viruses and are required to take prophylactic antiviral, antifungal and antibacterial treatment. The decision to continue such treatment should be guided by the type of transplant that the patient has undergone. The transplant team should work closely with the patient, their family and the local referring center and general practitioner to reduce the incidence of infection, monitor for occurrence, and to identify the source and instigate prompt treatment. Patients will also require advice on revaccination as immunity will be lost through the transplant process (see Chapter 35).

Graft-versus-host disease

In the allogeneic setting, patients are generally aware of the benefits that the graft-versus-tumor effect may bring, and while aware of the morbidity that GvHD can cause, they may underestimate the impact of this transplant side-effect. It can be very disheartening for a patient to face the rigors of the transplant process, only to be discharged home and find that they are facing daily life with the complications of GvHD, months and perhaps years post transplant. Although patients may be receiving medication to suppress the immune response and reduce the incidence and severity of GvHD, it may nevertheless still occur. In the acute stage the damage is generally limited to the skin, liver and gut but in the chronic stages of GvHD any organ can be affected.[15] Medical treatment normally involves combination therapy including steroids and T-cell suppressing drugs. The use of extracorporeal photopheresis may also be beneficial as a treatment measure for refractory sclerodermoid and lichenoid skin problems.[16]

Patients will need advice on monitoring for signs of GvHD and should be guided on how to deal with the side-effects this may cause. Simple advice on how to care for the organs that are affected is essential. Practical measures may include keeping the skin clean and moist, avoiding breaks to the skin, good wound care of broken skin and reducing exposure to the sun. Other practical measure may address camouflaging changes to the body, including the use of cosmetics to mask skin discoloration and the use of a wig or head covering. Advice on clothing to mask weight gain secondary to steroid therapy, or nutritional support to deal with weight loss and decrease in appetite is also often needed.

The team can sensitively give advice on how to deal with gastro-intestinal disturbance, including occasional or unexpected incontinence, such as having a change of clothing and by providing pads that are discreet and can be easily disposed of. Other simple measures may include advice such as sucking sweets and regular fluid intake to relieve a dry mouth, and the use of eye drops to alleviate dry eyes.

Patients have reported the difficulties and distress that GvHD has caused and how it has affected their personal, family and social life, many years following transplant.[6]

Fatigue

Studies have demonstrated that fatigue is common in the transplant setting, and causes significant distress to patients.[17,18] However, fatigue is sometimes inadequately addressed, and among all the other complications it may be seen as of low priority, or clinicians may be unaware of the problems that it can cause.

Fatigue has been defined as a subjective and unpleasant feeling that affects the whole person. It may range from mild tiredness to complete exhaustion, creating an unrelenting condition affecting the person's ability to function.[19] Fatigue can be caused by a number of factors arising from both the disease process and treatments. These include increased cytokine production, anemia, sleeplessness, depression, pain, nausea, vomiting, infection, malnutrition and breathlessness.[20] Fatigue may also be exacerbated by the many changes to the daily routine due to transplant demands. Fatigue in the transplant setting is different from the fatigue seen in everyday life, in that the former may seem relentless and is not relieved by sleep. Patients may also report problems with sleeping and inability to concentrate years following a transplant procedure.[21] It is important to identify the cause of fatigue in order to treat it appropriately or to address the underlying cause.

If fatigue is not addressed it can lead to a reduced quality of life for the patient, affecting every aspect of their life. One patient experienced overwhelming fatigue following transplantation when he returned home. Misunderstanding the symptom, he lived for weeks fearing his disease had relapsed. Simple measures, including an explanation of this complication, and regular assessment can greatly reassure the patient and their family. Practical solutions can be suggested, including gentle exercise, planning rest and sleep periods while conserving energy to do the most desired tasks, and finding methods to reduce stress and anxiety.[19,20] When fatigue is thought to be related to anemia, the decision to support the patient with blood products or erythropoietin should be made based not solely on hemoglobin level, but also on the impact that this is having on the individual patient.

Sexuality

There is always more that the clinical team can do to support patients and their partners with sexual and fertility concerns.[22] It may be difficult for a patient or their partner to raise their sexual concerns due to the sensitive and private nature of the subject in what can appear to be a busy medical environment. Sexuality is much more than just its physical expression. As Weiss said in 1992, 'Sexuality is about connecting our head with our gut through our heart. It is about genuinely caring for ourselves, finding ecstasy in simply being alive, and giving creative voice to our ideas and feelings. It is about bridging physical pleasures with spiritual awareness and serenity'.[23]

Any aspect of the human sexual response cycle including arousal, plateau, orgasm and resolution[24] can be affected by disease, transplant-related issues and the clinical environment. The transplant team need to sensitively approach the subject in order to prepare and support men and women regarding the physical and emotional changes they may experience during and after treatment. Changes may include low libido, erectile and ejaculation difficulties, vaginal dryness, vaginal stenosis, orgasm difficulties, changes in physique, low self-esteem and the effects that these changes will have on sexual expression. These are summarized in Table 36.3.

Specific suggestions to help address these changes may include advice on treating erectile dysfunction (pharmacologic interventions, appliances such as vacuum pumps), vaginal dryness and stenosis (lubrication, vaginal dilators). Hormone replacement therapy may help alleviate symptoms of early menopause. However, changes to sexuality are not only experienced on a physical level but may also affect the patient on an emotional and social level, causing doubts in self-worth and loss of self-confidence. The team needs to be mindful of these changes, which may not always be apparent. Other helpful suggestions may include planning times during the day when the person can have time to be alone or with their partner. Aware that the person may lack energy or have lost the desire for sex, it may be helpful to suggest that sexual intimacy such as cuddling, a hug, gentle sexual foreplay, going for a meal or to the theater may replace sexual intercourse for a time following transplantation.

Intensive therapy may be required for people who have continuing and severe difficulties, and in this case the person should be referred to a counselor specializing in sexual matters. The team needs to be sensitive to the needs of adolescents who may have only recently begun to discover and explore their own sexuality, now interrupted by the disease and treatment demands. It is important that an environment is created where this subject can be addressed (Table 36.4). Some patients will require detailed information while others want minimum information; the sensitive clinician is usually able to discern the level of information required.

Unfortunately, within the healthcare setting, the issue of sexual concerns continues to be either overlooked or inadequately addressed. This is due to a number of reasons, including the belief held by many healthcare professionals that they have to have all the answers.[25] While it is necessary that the team understand the possible effects of transplant-related treatments on sexuality and are aware of the resources available, often what is required is for patients to be allowed to simply express their concerns. The PLISSIT model (Table 36.5)[26] may be helpful in addressing sexual concerns.

Fertility

Previous treatment and the use of high doses of chemotherapy agents and total-body irradiation as part of the conditioning therapy in transplantation put the patient at high risk of gonadal failure, resulting in temporary or permanent loss of fertility. Prior to high-dose treatment, patients should be guided through the options for semen storage and embryo, egg, and ovarian/testicular tissue preservation (Table 36.6). In women, the risk of early ovarian failure is high, and while pregnancy post transplant may be achieved, there is an increased risk of spontaneous abortion. Schover speaks about 'empty arms', and the hidden pain of infertility, the loss that others may not see or witness.[25]

Although this will always be discussed prior to treatment, the impact of being infertile may only become apparent for the man or woman many months or years after the transplant.[27] While the focus was initially on successfully traversing the transplant process, following recovery this may now be directed towards attempting to return

Table 36.3 Sexual changes

- Changed physique
- Reduced self-esteem
- Increased fear/uncertainty
- Breathlessness
- Smells
- Fatigue
- Erectile problems, impotence
- Reduced sex drive
- Incontinence
- Infertility
- Premature menopause
- Vaginal dryness
- Infections
- Depression
- Loss of meaning
- Pain
- Dyspareunia
- *Relief*
- *Renewal*

Table 36.4 Addressing sexual concerns

Create an environment where sexuality is acknowledged and can be addressed
Plan time and ensure privacy
Introduce the topic sensitively as part of holistic care
Obtain permission from the patient to address this subject
Watch for cues
Learn how the disease and treatments can affect a person's sexuality and fertility
If appropriate, offer practical advice and alternatives to stereotypical sexual behavior
Be aware of fertility options available
Be sensitive to issues stemming from culture, religion, gender, sexual orientation, age
Make no assumptions
Have the courage to listen
Do not perpetuate stereotypical myths
Recognize your limitations
Examine personal attitudes and beliefs

Table 36.5 PLISSIT model[26]

P – permission (give patient permission to talk about sexual concerns)
LI – limited information (explain how the disease and treatments may affect sexuality)
SI – specific information (offer practical advice on how to deal with problems arising)
IT – intensive therapy (refer to specialist if problem is not resolving)

Table 36.6 Addressing infertility

Sperm banking
Egg storage
Embryo storage
Ovarian tissue preservation
Testicular tissue preservation
Egg donation
Sperm donation
Surrogacy
Adoption

Table 36.7 Complementary therapies

Massage
Reiki
Aromatherapy
Reflexology
Herbs
Homeopathy
Acupuncture
Autogenesis
Imagery
Touch and bodywork

to some kind of normality while conscious of the loss of fertility, a distressing time for many patients. The initial question of 'Why have I got this disease?' may turn to 'Why can I not have a child?'. Members of the transplant team can forewarn the patient that this may become a reality and encourage them to access counseling support and, if appropriate, expert fertility advice. It is important that patients and their partners have an opportunity to talk about any concerns surrounding fertility, and the transplant team should critically evaluate the advice they give. Special consideration needs to be given when considering the options available to enable the preservation of a child's fertility.

Complementary therapies

There has been increasing interest in the use of a variety of complementary therapies.[28,29] Some of these therapies have been used for centuries, and while there is a growing body of research demonstrating the benefits,[30–32] there is already extensive anecdotal evidence to indicate the physical, emotional and spiritual benefits they bring. In a European survey of people with cancer, many respondents reported the benefits they had received through these therapeutic approaches.[33] Today, an increasing number of people will have already used some of these therapies prior to becoming ill or undergoing any medical treatment.[34]

The therapies that bring benefit need to be clearly distinguished from those that may cause harm and give false hope to patients, leading to increased stress. The decision to access or continue with these therapies during the transplant and recovery phases may allow the patient to have some control over their care while addressing their physical, spiritual and psychologic needs. The team should be knowledgeable about the different complementary therapies available and how they work (Table 36.7) in order to support the patient in making

an informed decision based on the benefits or contraindications of a particular therapy in the clinical setting.

The use of aromatherapy oils, either as a burner left in the room or through massage, may help to alleviate both physical and psychologic symptoms, providing relief while at the same time complementing the medical interventions.[35] Twycross[36] highlights the benefit of simple touch, and distinguishes between the use of instrumental and expressive touch. The former is used to perform a clinical task (take a blood pressure reading), while the latter is used as an expression of care (touching someone's shoulder, holding someone's hand). A woman who had spent some time on a hematology ward undergoing treatment turned to the complementary therapist who was massaging her back and said, 'You know, you are the first person who has touched me since I came into hospital who has not taken something from me'. This woman's words may remind the clinical team of the demands of treatment and the need for caring touch.

The search to find meaning

Facing and undergoing a transplant procedure will bring changes on many levels to the person and their family. Any life-threatening illness or medical procedure may become a crisis time for the person, when questions about the meaning of life arise and the bonds of relationships are tested.[37] These changes can be disconcerting and sometimes uncomfortable as people learn to renegotiate family roles and daily activities. A transplant team can underestimate the impact that such changes can have on the individual and their family. Frankl claims that all human beings spend much of their lives trying to make sense of the world about them.[38] However, it may only be when something begins to go wrong, such as discovering one has a particular illness or one has to face life-threatening treatment, that a person becomes conscious of this search to find meaning in which everyone is involved. In the busy environment of transplantation, people are trying to make sense of day-to-day events and the effect these changes are having on their own life and the lives of those close to them.[39]

During this difficult and often traumatic time people describe re-examining their values and what is important to them.[40–42] People with a religious faith may find it helpful to talk with a priest, imam, rabbi or minister, while others may simply want quiet periods alone, to reflect or to do things that bring meaning to their lives. Due to the relationship that has developed over time, it is not unusual for the patient or family member to turn to a member of the clinical team for support during this period of questioning. The clinical team member will find it difficult to recognize or to support another in this search if that team member is unaware of their own search to find meaning and their own need for support.[39]

While not all human beings may choose to follow a religious tradition, all human beings are spiritual and have spiritual needs. Spirituality addresses the whole person and is everything that makes that person unique, including their successes and failures, their joys and sorrows, their strengths and weaknesses; it will include background, culture, work, school, home and social life. Frankl[38] describes the spiritual dimension as the deepest part of every human being, the search for meaning and value in any situation. While a patient may not have religious needs, the chaplaincy team is generally a good resource to help and support the other members of the transplant team in addressing spiritual concerns.

Addressing suffering and loss

Many patients who undergo medical treatments, including transplantation, talk about the loss of control they experience over a number of aspects of their lives. This loss of control may be expressed in the metaphors that patients use to describe their experiences of hospitalization and treatment. While some patients appreciate having the privacy of a room to themselves, the clinical rules of isolation have caused others to describe their experience as similar to being imprisoned. One young man who had been treated for leukemia came to see the intravenous drip stand as a constant reminder of his confinement and a symbol of his loss of freedom.

Suffering as part of the human condition is something that every person will experience at some point in their lives, and many people will come to experience suffering as they face the reality of illness.[35,43] Although medicine has a long history of being concerned with relieving suffering, the ability to address and deal with this has not always been achieved in the clinical setting. As stated by Barritt, 'One of the major shortcomings of technological medicine is that in the relentless search for cures for disease, the suffering of humans is relatively neglected'.[7]

With the rapid advances in medicine, there is a danger that the suffering of individuals may not be noticed or attended to; it is rare to see the word 'suffering' appear in the medical or nursing notes. Practitioners may feel uncomfortable simply being present with a person going through a difficult or painful time facing loss, if they are more used to diagnosing and treating (fixing) ailments.[36] Kearney[44] rightly states that sometimes the role of the doctor or nurse is to support the patient when there is nothing more to be done. Patients and their family know that members of the team cannot solve all problems but they do need reassurance that, at those difficult and uncertain moments, the team will be present to support them, and they will not be abandoned.[45] While there may come a time when certain medical treatments are no longer appropriate, there will never come a time when medical care and support should be withdrawn. The patient and family need to be reassured of that. While pain may be addressed by the clinical team, pain and suffering are different, although closely linked. 'People in pain frequently report suffering from pain when they feel out of control, when the pain is overwhelming, when the source of the pain is unknown, when the meaning of the pain is dire, or when the pain is apparently without end.'[43]

If the team only focuses on physical pain in the clinical setting, then it will fail to address the underlying emotional, social and spiritual pain that may be present.[44] If this underlying pain is ignored or not addressed, then it must find an expression in some form, and it may appear as physical pain. Good pain management cannot be adequately achieved unless we address all these aspects of pain.[46] While physical pain can be treated by medical intervention, the suffering of which Kearney speaks is not treatable in this way.

> *Not all human distress is responsive to the interventions of the medical model, as is the case with certain forms of psychological and existential suffering . . . It may be very challenging and difficult, but there will be times when team members will be required to support people who face difficult realities and indeed the suffering associated with the uncertainty of treatment.*[44]

The support required is not always about fixing the situation, but simply listening: 'If we want to support each other's inner lives, we must remember a simple truth: the human soul does not want to be fixed, it wants simply to be seen and heard'.[47]

Cassidy[45] describes this support in a different way when she talks of 'sharing the darkness' with another. These moments occur when a doctor or nurse is confronted with a painful situation and there appears to be nothing they can do to help. If the doctor or nurse can simply stay with that person during the uncomfortable and difficult time, then they will have shared a moment of that person's darkness, creating support.

Table 36.8 Addressing spiritual care

Being present versus carrying out a clinical task
Creating privacy and time
Truly hearing the person's story
Establishing a trusting relationship
Caring touch
Watching for cues
Being aware of the person's cultural and religious needs
Preparing for religious and cultural needs – rituals/diet/prayer times/clothing/washing/post-death care of the body
Support of chaplaincy team
Being aware of own spirituality
Caring for self and colleagues
Showing humility – 'I don't know'

Children diagnosed with cancer will have unique spiritual needs, which place them at risk of developing spiritual distress.[48] Children, like adults having to face the demands of treatment, may experience many losses, leading to depression and the feeling of being isolated from their normal life.[49] Children with spiritual concerns may not always express these problems in language used by adults. Nevertheless, these needs are there and must be addressed. Activities such as holding, comforting, playing with the child, providing relief from pain, and supporting parental involvement in the child's care can all help to address the child's spiritual needs. In her study, Callaghan[50] demonstrated that adolescents have their own spiritual needs as they try to make sense of their experiences. The young person's concerns may be addressed through creating an atmosphere of openness where the adolescent is free to express their philosophic and religious concerns. The adolescent may gain support through being in touch with their own peers who hold similar beliefs and values. The role of the team may be to simply listen and support the young person as they make sense of their changing world.

In the continuing debate about whether medicine and nursing should be practiced as a science or an art, Barritt[7] suggests that both aspects are required. Treating patients with dignity, respect and understanding can be demanding, but it is no more time-consuming, and it will be the quality of the caring team that the patient remembers. However, both the secular and increasingly technologic nature of healthcare may make it more difficult to recognize and attend to the spiritual needs of patients and their families.[35,51] Each member of the transplant team may be asked to perform the role of the 'skilled companion',[52] using their clinical and non-clinical skills to support the patient as they journey with them. No matter what clinical task is being performed, spiritual care and attending to someone's distress can be achieved when that person is given the carer's full attention.[36] Table 36.8 shows some helpful points that may guide the team in addressing spiritual care in the transplant setting. It should not be overlooked that spiritual care can often be expressed through the ordinary things – offering a cup of tea, offering to take the person to the prayer room, playing with a child, saying a simple greeting.

Donor support

National donor registries working with the World Marrow Donor Association have established very clear support mechanisms and guidelines to support and protect the unrelated donor. Unfortunately, there continues to be a lack of consistency in the support offered to donors who are related to the recipient. A family member may be asked to consider undergoing human leukocyte antigen (HLA) testing with a view to becoming a donor. In the majority of cases, a family member will be happy to undergo the matching process. However, the transplant team should be receptive to issues that may prevent a family member from wanting to undergo HLA typing that may lead to stem cell donation.[53] The donor should be given clear information about each aspect of the donating process so that they can make their own informed choice about whether to undergo testing, to proceed with donation and about whether they would prefer to undergo bone marrow or peripheral stem cell collection. No family member should feel coerced into donating by the transplant team.

This issue of coercion is made even more difficult in the pediatric setting when a young sibling is approached to consider being a donor for their sick brother or sister. Ideally, the donor should be supported by a clinical individual who is not a member of the transplant team. When this is not possible in smaller centers, someone from the team should be appointed to perform this supportive role. The team should have clear guidelines in place to enable them to support the donor and, if required, to ensure that the donor is referred to the relevant support agencies if they have been confronted with difficult news during HLA and viral testing.[54]

As long as the donating process is seen merely as a medical procedure, there is a danger that the team will neglect to address the emotional impact donation can have on both the recipient and the donor.[55] The team should be aware of the concerns and worries that may arise for the related donor following transplantation stemming from complications, including graft rejection, graft-versus-host disease, and recurring infections which may cause the recipient long-term morbidity and even death.[53] It is important that the transplant team is aware of these issues and is available to talk to the donor about their concerns. Each member of the transplant team should be sensitive to the issues that may arise, aware of the potential for coercion from family, and the other pressures that the related donor may face.

Survivorship

Following transplantation, there will be a period of readjustment for the patient and their family. A necessary part of the process for the patient post transplant is being able to reintegrate themselves into their family and social life, conscious of the events and treatments they have undergone.[4] Mullan[56] speaks of the 'seasons of survival', which gives some helpful insights into some of the issues a patient and their family may face during the treatment and post-treatment periods.

- Surviving the initial diagnosis and treatment.
- Extended survival: the period immediately after treatment ceases, a period when patients are most concerned about their disease returning or the treatment not working.
- Surviving with uncertainty: in this period the person begins to get on with life but is often reluctant to make long-term plans.
- Permanent survival: the period when it appears the disease has been permanently eradicated and the person recommences their life, conscious that things have changed.

Members of the transplant team can support the patient and their family during each of these stages. Some centers have developed a multiprofessional rehabilitation program to assist patients in the post-transplant period. This may be an opportunity to meet with other patients recovering and adjusting to life. In some cases, due to geographical distance, it may not be possible for patients to attend such programs. In such cases, a program could be developed which the patient can undertake in their own home environment. Such individual or group programs should address the physical, social and psychologic aspects of rehabilitation.

Many patients find it difficult to return to a 'normal life' following transplantation, particularly as they may need to make changes to their daily routine in order to facilitate the taking of daily medication, steps to avoid infections and making adjustments to address the side-effects of treatment.[57] While much of the focus may be on the patient, family members including parents, partners, siblings and children may need support. Just as the patient may develop a relationship of trust with team members, family members will often turn to the team for support. Family members may require support in adjusting to the patient's return to health or dealing with long-term complications. With support and guidance from the transplant team, family members can be a vital source of support for the person undergoing transplantation.

Due to the specialized nature of treatment, patients may have to travel long distances to undergo transplantation. While most patients are keen to be followed up by the transplant team, some of the follow-up care can be delivered at a more local hospital. The transplant team can support the local hospital and the local community team by passing on relevant information. Clearly established pathways and agreed care plans can facilitate the hospital and community teams in ensuring a smooth and safe transfer to home. Some aspects of transplantation are now being successfully delivered in an ambulatory setting. With adequate support and resources, patients and their families are required to spend less time in the hospital environment.

Relapse

Many patients going through the transplant procedure will at some stage of their treatment ask themselves 'Will it work for me?' and 'Will my disease return?'. While this question will often be uttered verbally, sometimes it may simply be seen on the concerned face of the patient as they await their daily blood results. Such questions will continue long after discharge from hospital.[4] Now out of the busy clinical environment and away from supportive staff, patients may ask themselves even more questions about their illness, and their concerns over relapse may be heightened. The need for close monitoring of the blood and marrow along with signs of organ toxicity is a reminder of this reality. Despite the advances in medicine, it is still very difficult to accurately predict the outcome of treatment and the possibility of the disease returning and the complications that may ensue.

Again, the transplant team should always be honest, while maintaining hope. In the case of relapse it is important that the team listens to the patient's needs and concerns. The patient should be supported to consider treatment options, including the choice of declining further medical treatment in favor of having a better quality of life for their remaining time, in their own home. Equally, there will be patients who want treatment no matter how poor the results are likely to be. A strong and caring team working together can address the difficult issue of relapse and offer realistic options, including non-medical approaches. It is essential that the transplant team works closely with the patient's local medical team, including the referring hospital, the community team and the palliative care services, throughout the treatment process and not only at the point when the disease advances.

There is an increased risk of a secondary malignancy due to the transplant treatment.[58] An increased incidence of post-transplant lymphoproliferative disorders, secondary myelodysplastic syndromes, and acute leukemia has been reported,[59] and there is also an increased risk of solid tumors, including melanoma, oral cavity cancers, liver, thyroid, bone and central nervous system.[17,60] With recipients living longer after transplantation, continued monitoring is required for secondary malignancies.[61] This reality should be addressed honestly without causing undue alarm.

Palliative care

Despite extensive developments in both palliative and transplant care, doctors, nurses and other members of the team in the transplant setting may still fail to see that palliative care, by its very definition, is not simply about care in the terminal stages of disease.[62] There is much that the palliative care approach can do to enhance patient and family care throughout the transplant journey.[63] In the UK, national guidelines require that a member of the palliative care team works closely with the hematology team when supporting a patient and their family with a malignant disease.[64] The concept and philosophy of palliative care can be introduced to the patient and family early on in the treatment pathway. In this way, should movement from curative options to terminal care be required, the transition may be less painful and difficult. While not every member of the transplant team is expected to be an expert in palliative care, they will be required to use palliative care skills, and should work closely with the palliative care specialists.[63]

Unfortunately, care of the dying patient in the transplant setting has often been overlooked, possibly because death may be due to treatment-related causes in patients who are usually young.[3] Table 36.9 shows the principles of palliative care which address the physical, psychologic, social and spiritual needs of patients and families.

Children

Particular attention needs to be given to children and teenagers undergoing transplantation, always mindful of the many life changes with which they may already be dealing. All children need security, and many of the changes brought on by diagnosis, hospital admission and treatment may cause some of that security to be obscured. It has been demonstrated that children enter into the transplant with a heightened level of distress which increases during the treatment period.[65] The same study showed that adolescents were at more risk of distress than younger children. It can be a particularly difficult time for a teenager who has begun to make the uncertain journey from childhood to adulthood to be dealing with the demands of treatment. The team should do everything it can to ensure that some of the child's routine is maintained. Children and teenagers may need support in renegotiating their re-entry into school and their circle of friends. The team, along with the young person and family members, should give consideration to the possibility of a small group of friends visiting in order to maintain some connection with ongoing life.

Some centers may discourage young children visiting the unit when a parent is undergoing transplantation, and such a decision needs to be taken in the light of the interruption that treatment has on family roles and connections. It may be worthwhile for each team member to reflect on how they would feel if they were separated from their children for a long period of time. The decision for children to visit

Table 36.9 Components of palliative care

Provides relief from pain and other distressing symptoms
Affirms life and regards dying as a normal process
Intends neither to hasten nor postpone death
Integrates the psychologic and spiritual aspects of patient care
Offers a support system to help patients to live as actively as possible until death
Offers a support system to help the family to cope during the patient's illness and in their own bereavement
Uses a team approach to address the needs of patients and their families, including bereavement counseling, if indicated
Will enhance quality of life, and may also positively influence the course of illness

should be made by the patient, who is sensitive to his or her own needs and the needs of their children, and in light of the unit's guidance on visiting. One young woman undergoing a transplant felt that she was able to maintain her role as a mother by undertaking the children's ironing during her treatment, while a young man maintained his father role by doing paintings for his children while in hospital.

Dying in the transplant setting

In his book *The loneliness of the dying*, Norbert Elias reminds us that today we live in societies that find death difficult to accept, and death is often presented as a failure.[66] Our way of dealing with death may be to push the dying to the edges of society. This approach to death and dying may also be seen in the transplant setting, where death following intensive treatment can seem like failure.

There may come a time when a difficult conversation about the continuation of treatment and the reality of dying needs to be addressed. The patient may or may not want to continue treatment. They may wish to decide whether they want to be ventilated or not in a critical care unit, knowing that the likelihood of coming off the ventilator is not realistic. In this case, a patient may choose to die being more aware of their surroundings. It is important that the team broaches the subject of dying. One of the skills demanding greatest sensitivity from an experienced doctor or nurse is knowing if, and when, it is appropriate to talk through the actual dying process with the patient and family members. Too many patients are not given the option of where they wish to die. The concerns over addressing the subject of death may be more to do with the team's own discomfort about dying than concern over upsetting the patient, who may already know that their own death is imminent. Once a patient has made known their wish of where they want to die, the team should do everything within its power to facilitate that request.

The team will need to decide which treatments may be required to maintain a life which is as comfortable as possible for the person and which should be stopped in order to facilitate the patient's request. Close working with the ward-based team, the community and hospice teams can make this transition from the transplant unit to home or hospice possible.

Caring for the team and clinical reflection

As stem cell transplantation advances, members of the team will continue to support patients and their families who are affected by treatment-related morbidities during the transplant process. Although many patients will be able to return to some normality following transplant, they will need support to adjust to the changes that have occurred. The team must face the reality that patients for whom they have cared over an extended period of time may die of their disease and/or transplant-related complications. Within the transplant setting, each practitioner needs to be sensitive to their own needs in order to continue responding to the needs of those for whom they care.[67] Formal and informal support can be found in many ways to meet the needs of individual team members. Each clinical practitioner needs to feel that their own role is valued and appreciated by the other members of the team. It is important that the voice of each team member is heard and respected at multiprofessional team meetings when discussing best treatments and care for patients.

With the increasing demands made on the team, it can be difficult to find time to reflect on clinical practice. While some transplant centers may have formal meetings to reflect on practice, others may carry this out in informal ways. These opportunities can be a time to address any concerns arising in the team while exploring ways to improve the care and treatment delivered. Johns[68] describes clinical reflection as an opportunity 'to rest in a quiet eddy amidst a fast flowing stream'. It is an opportunity for the team members to collectively or individually reflect on the work that they do, recognizing what they do well and identifying what they can do better, while supporting one another. Reflection continues to be an opportunity for practitioners to develop their clinical and caring skills, but it can also help the team to address the difficult and sometimes distressing aspects of the patient's experience. 'Being mindful is the exquisite ability to pay attention to self within the unfolding moment in such a way that one remains available to ease suffering and nurture growth.'[35]

It is through reflection on everyday clinical practice that the team can come to see that what they have perhaps perceived as routine practice is in reality sacred work.[35] To work as a member of the team in the field of stem cell transplantation as it continues to advance, and to support patients and their families is an exciting and challenging opportunity. Medical advances in every aspect of stem transplantation continue to extend hope to many more patients and their families. These exciting developments need to be matched by a transplant team that continues to support each other as they address the physical, psychologic, social and spiritual needs of those for whom they care.

References

1. Bury M. Chronic illness as a biographical disruption. Sociol Health Illness 1982;4:167–182
2. Radley A. Making sense of illness: the social psychology of health and disease. Sage Publications, London, 1994
3. Kiss A, Kainz M. Psychologic aspects. In: Apperley J, Carreras E, Gluckman E, Gratwohl A, Masszi T (eds) The EBMT handbook: haemopietic stem cell transplant. FSE, Genoa, 2004:353–363
4. Baker F, Zabora J, Polland A, Wingard J. Reintegration after bone marrow transplantation. Cancer Pract 1999;7:190–197
5. Molassiotis A, Morris P. Quality of life in patients with chronic myeloid leukaemia after unrelated donor bone marrow transplantation. Cancer Nurs 1989;22:340–349
6. Andryskowski MA, Bruehi S, Brady MJ, Henslee-Downey PJ. Physical and psychosocial status of adults one year after bone marrow transplantation: a prospective study. Bone Marrow Transplant 1995;15:837–844
7. Barritt P. Humanity in healthcare: the heart and soul of medicine. 2005; Radcliffe Publishing. Oxford
8. Dougherty L, Lister S. The Royal Marsden Hospital manual of clinical nursing procedures, 6th edn. Blackwell Publishing, Oxford, 2004
9. Quinn B, Stone R, Uhlenhopp M et al. Ensuring accurate oral mucositis assessment in the European Group for Blood and Marrow Transplantation prospective oral mucositis audit. Eur J Oncol Nurs 2007;11(suppl): 10–18
10. Stone R, Potting CM, Clare S et al. Management of oral mucositis at European transplantation centres. Eur J Oncol Nurs 2007;11(suppl): 3–10
11. Sonis ST. The pathobiology of mucositis. Nat Rev Cancer 2004;4:277–284
12. Blijlevens N, Donnelly J, de Pauw B. Mucosal barrier injury: biology, pathology, clinical counterparts and consequences of intensive treatment for haematologic malignancy: an overview. Bone Marrow Transplant 2000;25:1269–1278
13. Majorana A, Schubert MM, Porta F et al. Oral complications of paediatric haematopoietic cell transplantation: diagnosis and management. Support Care Cancer 2000;8:353–365
14. Rubenstein E, Douglas E, Schubert M et al. Clinical practice guidelines for the prevention and treatment of cancer therapy-induced oral and gastrointestinal mucositis. Cancer 2004;100(S9): 2026–2046
15. Vogelsang GB, Lee L, Bensen-Kennedy DB. Pathogenesis and treatment of graft versus host disease after bone marrow transplant. Ann Rev Med 2003;52:29–52
16. Seaton ED, Szydlo RM, Kanger E et al. Influence of extracorporeal photopheresis on clinical and laboratory parameters in chronic graft versus host disease and analysis of predictors of response. Blood 2003;102:1217–1223
17. Baker KS, DeFor TE, Burns LJ et al. New malignancies after blood and marrow stem cell transplantation in children and adults: incidence and risk factors. J Clin Oncol 2003;21:1352–1358
18. Kopp M, Schweigkofler H, Holzner B et al. Time after bone marrow transplantation as an important variable for quality of life: results of a cross-sectional investigation using two different instruments for quality of life assessments. Ann Hematol 1998;77:27–32
19. Ream E, Richardson A. Fatigue: a concept analysis. Int J Nurs Stud 1996;33:519–529
20. Mock V, Atkinson A, Barsevick A et al. NCCN practice guidelines for cancer-related fatigue. National Comprehensive Cancer Network. Oncology (Williston Park) 2000;14(11A): 151–161
21. Andryskowski MA, Carpenter JS, Greiner CB et al. Energy level and sleep quality following bone marrow transplantation. Bone Marrow Transplant 1997;20:669–679
22. Masters W, Johnson V. Human sexual response. Little, Brown, Boston, 1966
23. Weiss K. Women's experience of sex and sexuality. City Center, Hazeldon, MN, 1992
24. Quinn B. Sexual health in cancer care. Nurs Times 2003;99:32–34
25. Schover LR. Sexuality and fertility after cancer. John Wiley, New York, 1997
26. Annon J. The P-LI-SS-IT models. J Sex Educ Ther 1976;2:1–15
27. Socie G, Klingebiel T, Schwarze CP. Late complications of HSCT. In: Apperley J, Carreras E, Gluckman E, Gratwohl A, Masszi T (eds) The EBMT handbook: haemopietic stem cell transplant. FSE, Genoa, 2004:179–196
28. Royal College of Nursing. Complementary therapies in nursing midwifery and health visiting practice. RCN guidance on integrating complementary therapies into clinical care. Royal College of Nursing, London, 2003
29. House of Lords. Select Committee on Science and Technology. Complementary and alternative medicine. HL Paper 123. House of Lords London, 2000
30. Lively BT, Holiday-Goodman M, Black C, Arondekar B. Massage therapy for chemotherapy induced emesis. In: Rich GJ (ed) Massage therapy: the evidence for practice. Harcourt Brace, London, 2002
31. Wilkinson S. An evaluation of aromatherapy massage in palliative care. Palliati Med 1999;13:409–417
32. Wright S, Courtney C, Donnelly C et al. Clients' perceptions of the benefits of reflexology on their quality of life. Complement Ther Nurs Midwif 2002;8:69–76
33. Molassiotis A, Fernandez-Ortega P, Pud D et al. Use of complementary and alternative medicine in cancer patients: a European survey. Ann Oncol 2005;16:655–663
34. Corner J, Harewood J. Exploring the use of complementary and alternative medicine by people with cancer. Nurs Times 2004;9:101–109
35. Johns C. Becoming a transformational leader through reflection. Reflect Nurs Leadersh 2004;30:24–26
36. Twycross RG. Symptom management in advanced cancer. Int J Clin Oncol 2002;7:271–278
37. Bolen JS. Close to the bone: life-threatening illness and the search for meaning. Touchstone, New York, 1996
38. Frankl V. Man's search for meaning. Washington Square Press, New York, 1946
39. Quinn B. Cancer and the treatment: does it make sense to patients? Hematology 2005;10:325–328
40. Brennan J. Adjustment to cancer – coping or personal transition? Psycho-oncology 2001;10:1–18
41. Greenstein M, Breitbart W. Cancer and the experience of meaning: a group psychotherapy programme for people with cancer. Am J Psychother 2000;54:486–500
42. Steeves R. Patients who have undergone bone marrow transplantation: their quest for meaning. Oncol Nurs Forum 1992;19:899–905
43. Cassell EJ. The nature of suffering and the goals of medicine. Oxford University Press, New York, 1991
44. Kearney M. A place of healing: working with suffering in living and dying. Oxford University Press, Oxford, 2000
45. Cassidy S. Sharing the darkness. Darton, Longman and Todd, London, 1988
46. Barnard D. The promise of intimacy and fear of our own undoing. J Palliat Care 1995;11:22–26
47. Palmer P. The courage to teach. Jossey-Bass, San Francisco, 1998
48. Hart D, Schneider D. Spiritual care for children with cancer. Semin Oncol Nurs 1997;13:263–270
49. Fulton RA, Moore CM. Spiritual care of the school age child with a chronic condition. J Pediatr Nurs 1995;10:224–231
50. Callaghan DM. The influence of spiritual growth on adolescents' initiative and responsibility. Pediatr Nurs 2005;31:91–95
51. Le Shan L. Cancer as a turning point. Plume Books., New York, 1994
52. Campbell AV. Moderated love: a theology of professional care. SPCK, London, 1984
53. Christopher KA. The experience of donating bone marrow to a relative. Oncol Nurs Forum 2000;27:693–700
54. Clare S, Mank A, Stone B et al. A European survey of related donor care. Bone Marrow Transplant 2006;37: S274
55. Bywater L, Atkins S. A study of factors influencing patients' decisions to undergo bone marrow transplantation from a sibling or matched related donor. Eur J Oncol Nurs 2001;5:7–15
56. Mullan F. Seasons of survival: reflections of a physician with cancer. N Eng J Med 1985;313:270–273
57. Quinn B, Stephens M. Bone marrow transplantation. In: Kearney N, Richardson A (eds) Nursing patients with cancer: principles and practice. Elsevier, Edinburgh, 2006:329–352
58. Deeg HJ, Socie G. Malignancies after haematopoietic stem cell transplantation: many questions, some answers. Blood 1998;91:1833–1844
59. Socie G, Curtis RE, Deeg HJ et al. New malignant diseases after allogeneic marrow transplantation for childhood leukaemia. J Clin Oncol 2000;18:348–357
60. Curtis RE, Rowlings PA, Deeg J et al. Solid cancers after bone marrow transplantation. N Engl J Med 1997;336:897–904
61. Balsdon H, Craig JI. Bone marrow and peripheral stem cell transplantation. In: Booth S, Bruera E (eds) Palliative care consultations: haemato-oncology. Oxford University Press, Oxford, 2003:61–74
62. Jeffrey D, Owen R. Changing the emphasis from active curative care to active palliative care in haematology patients. In: Booth S, Bruera E (eds) Palliative care consultations: haemato-oncology. Oxford University Press, Oxford, 2003:153–176
63. National Institute for Clinical Excellence. Supportive and palliative care guidelines 2004. www.nice.org.uk
64. National Institute for Clinical Excellence. Improving outcomes in haemato-oncology cancer 2003. www.nice.org.uk
65. Phipps S, Dunavant M, Garvie PA et al. Acute health related quality of life in children undergoing stem cell transplantation. Descriptive outcomes. Bone Marrow Transplant 2002;29:425–434
66. Elias N. The loneliness of the dying. Continuum, London, 1985
67. Tschudin T. The emotional cost of caring. In: Brykczynska G (ed) Caring: the compassion and wisdom of nursing. Arnold, London, 1997:155–179
68. Johns C. Guided reflection: advancing practice: research in practice. Blackwell Publishing, Oxford, 2002

PART 5

MANAGEMENT OF POST-TRANSPLANT COMPLICATIONS

Graft failure

Michael Potter

Introduction

The traditional approach to transplantation involves myeloablative conditioning with chemotherapy and/or radiotherapy resulting in a subsequent period of obligate pancytopenia followed by recovery of hemopoiesis. In the setting of myeloablative or full-intensity conditioned (FIC) transplantation, myeloid engraftment is often defined as the first day that a neutrophil count of 0.5×10^9/l is achieved and sustained. Red cell and platelet engraftment implies independence from transfusion support. A platelet count of 20×10^9/l and/or 50×10^9/l sustained and transfusion independent are useful clinical definitions of megakaryocyte engraftment. Primary graft failure implies a failure to ever achieve these target values. Secondary graft failure implies an initial achievement of these parameters but subsequent cytopenias with a neutrophil count $<0.5 \times 10^9$/l and requirement for transfusions. The diagnosis of graft failure will also usually require bone marrow examination to demonstrate hypocellularity and lack of infiltration by the original malignant disease or another process.

These definitions of primary and secondary graft failure are applicable to both the allogeneic and autologous settings. In recent years, however, the introduction of non-myeloablative or reduced-intensity conditioning (RIC) allogeneic transplantation requires supplementary definitions of graft failure. Patients may no longer have an obligate period of pancytopenia following conditioning, and engraftment may be a seamless transition from recipient to donor hemopoiesis. In this case, graft failure may be better defined in terms of chimerism analysis with a failure to achieve or subsequent loss of donor chimerism.

The traditional definitions of graft failure may also not take into account deficiencies specific to individual lineages, e.g. red cell aplasia which is now well documented following allogeneic transplantation. There is also the concept of poor graft function, where the basic parameters of engraftment are fulfilled but blood counts may remain suboptimal for long periods of time, leading to potential complications. Both primary and secondary graft failure are usually evident within the first 6 months following transplantation, although late graft failure can occur and historically has been seen more commonly in patients with severe aplastic anemia and β-thalassemia major. In patients with malignant disease, late graft failure may herald subsequent relapse of the original clone.

Incidence of graft failure

Graft failure in the setting of autologous transplantation is a rare event in modern practice, with an incidence <1%.[1] The position with regard to allogeneic transplantation is more complex. In the standard setting of FIC HLA-identical sibling transplantation with no T-cell depletion, the rate of graft failure is of the order of 1–2%.[2] T-cell depletion increases the risk of graft failure.[3] Recipients of RIC transplants are also at higher risk of this complication.[4] Unrelated donor transplants and HLA-mismatched donor transplants (related/unrelated) may also be associated with a higher risk of graft failure.[2] For example, in the setting of a RIC transplant or a T-cell depleted FIC transplant with an HLA-mismatched donor transplant, graft failure rates of 5–30% may occur.[2-4]

The clinical impact of graft failure

The standard complications of graft failure include prolonged hospitalization, an increased risk of bacterial and fungal infection and risk of hemorrhage.[5,6] This may lead to an increased risk of transplant-related mortality. In addition, there is evidence that incomplete donor chimerism is associated with an increased relapse risk.[7]

Mechanisms of graft failure

In the allogeneic setting, the concept of an immunologic process causing graft rejection is well established. Historically, this is best described in the setting of allogeneic transplantation for patients with severe aplastic anemia[8] and may be in part attributed to alloimmunization from previous blood transfusions. An immunologic mechanism of graft failure or rejection is also associated more with recipients of HLA-mismatched and unrelated donor transplants than those with matched related donors. In the unrelated donor setting, it has been shown that HLA class II disparity between donor and recipient may not increase the rate of graft rejection but class I disparity, especially at the HLA C locus, is associated with this complication.[9,10] This is believed to be predominantly a T-cell mediated process involving donor cytotoxic T-cells, although there is also evidence for a natural killer (NK) cell-mediated graft rejection process.[11,12] Immunologic graft rejection is usually characterized by a transient process of donor engraftment followed by loss of donor cells and either a complete failure of hemopoiesis or a recovery of autologous reconstitution, the latter being more typical with RIC transplants.

Another mechanism of graft failure relates to the composition of the donor graft. Clearly, graft failure may be due to an inadequate number of transplanted hemopoietic stem cells in both the allogeneic and autologous setting. Many studies have been published indicating the requirement for engraftment in terms of mononuclear cell (MNC) numbers, and particularly CD34+ (stem cell) numbers, infused in both the allogeneic and autologous settings.[13–15] The commonly quoted threshold for prompt and reliable engraftment is the infusion of ≥2 ×

10^6 CD34 cells per kg of recipient body weight. This may represent a gross oversimplification, however, and it is difficult to define a lower limit for successful engraftment in clinical practice. The source of stem cells also needs to be taken into account. In the field of umbilical cord transplantation, satisfactory engraftment may be obtained with CD34 counts more than 1 log below the above figure.[16,17] CD34 numbers are clearly not the only determinant of engraftment in an infused stem cell product. The presence of other populations of cells, such as T-cells or even serum factors, may affect the engraftment process.[16] However, clinically the pace of engraftment is more rapid with peripheral blood stem cell transplantation than bone marrow transplantation, which, in turn, exceeds that seen in the setting of umbilical cord transplantation, and this is predominantly a CD34 numbers effect.

The quality of stem cell products in terms of engraftment potential may also be adversely affected by events occurring following collection of cells. Examples include prolonged storage prior to cryopreservation,[18] the cryopreservation process itself and subsequent thawing procedure,[19] in vitro manipulation of the graft (e.g. CD34 selection[3]), incubation with antibodies for T-cell depletion[20] or malignant cell purging.[21]

Host factors which may affect engraftment

Patients with certain diagnoses are at higher risk of graft rejection than others. This relates to the extent to which the patients have already received myelo- or immunosuppressive therapies, the number of transfusions of cellular products received and possible stromal defects in the marrow microenvironment associated with certain diagnoses. Patients with severe aplastic anemia and β-thalassemia major may have typically received tens or hundreds of units of cellular blood products prior to transplantation. This may have the effect of alloimmunization which increases the risk of graft failure.[8,22,23]

Patients with myeloproliferative disorders including chronic myeloid leukemia may have received little in the way of intensive chemotherapy prior to transplantation. The increased cellularity in the bone marrow of patients with myeloproliferative disorders coupled with the lack of intensive prior chemotherapy compared to patients with acute leukemia may increase the risk of graft failure in these diseases. Stromal abnormalities occur in myelofibrosis where the normal bone marrow stroma is replaced by a dense fibrotic reaction.[24] In severe aplastic anemia, it is possible that stromal defects contribute to the etiology of the disease in certain patients. If these are not corrected by transplantation, similar problems may ensue with the donor-derived hemopoiesis.[25] Finally, patients with moderate to massive splenomegaly at the time of transplantation may be at higher risk of graft failure.[24,26] This may be as a result of preferential donor engraftment in the spleen rather than the marrow and subsequent inefficient hemopoiesis coupled with the effects of hypersplenism.[26,27]

The intensity of the conditioning regimen may also affect the engraftment process. In the last 10 years there has been the successful introduction of RIC transplantation with non-myeloablative chemotherapy and/or low-dose total-body irradiation regimens. In simple terms, conditioning treatment needs to have two elements: myelosuppression and immune suppression. The myelosuppressive element creates space for the incoming donor hemopoiesis and the immunosuppressive element eradicates the potential for host-versus-graft immune reactions. The former element (myelosuppression) is substantially attenuated in RIC transplantation, with an associated increase in the potential for graft failure. Therefore, this is usually compensated for by increasing the immunosuppressive element of the conditioning regimen. In practice, this has usually been achieved by the use of fludarabine, a purine analog with very potent T-cell suppressive properties, in conjunction with non-myeloablative doses of chemotherapy – busulfan, melphalan or cyclophosphamide – or low-dose total-body irradiation.[28,29] In vivo administration of T-cell antibodies such as antithymocyte globulin (ATG) or alemtuzumab (CAMPATH-1H) prior to transplantation is an alternative approach with the potential additional benefit of reduction in graft-versus-host disease (GvHD) risk due to T-cell depletion of the incoming graft.[30,31]

Infections which occur in the early post-transplant phase may be a cause of non- or suboptimal engraftment. Certain viruses such as parvovirus may directly infect hemopoietic cell progenitors, leading to a failure of maturation. In particular, parvovirus targets erythroid progenitors and has been associated with pure red cell aplasia.[32] Many viruses, particularly those of the herpes group, have been shown to cause the potential for hemophagocytosis, which may be a cause of graft failure. Examples include the Epstein–Barr virus (EBV),[33] cytomegalovirus (CMV)[34] and human herpes virus 6 (HHV6).[35] Other viruses which may also stimulate hemophagocytosis include adenoviral[36] and influenza viral infections.[37]

Myelosuppressive drugs may also be a cause of graft failure or impairment. The choice of post-transplant immunosuppressive regimen may affect engraftment. Ciclosporin is generally considered to be 'protective' against graft failure by reducing the chance of a host-versus-graft immune-based rejection. Patients with aplastic anemia and β-thalassemia major generally receive prolonged treatment with ciclosporin A to at least 1 year post transplant to prevent late graft rejection in these high-risk disorders. Ciclosporin is often used with 3–4 injections of methotrexate. The latter increases the potency of post-transplant immune suppression and reduces the incidence of severe GvHD. However, methotrexate is also myelosuppressive and its use usually does lead to a delay in engraftment of neutrophils by around 7 days.[38] Other drugs may also have myelosuppressive effects. Co-trimoxazole, used for prophylaxis against Pneumocystis infections, may lead to macrocytosis and cytopenias.[39] Ganciclovir and its prodrug valganciclovir, used to prevent or treat CMV infection, are a commonly recognized cause of often severe myelosuppression.[40,41] Mycophenolate mofetil, which may be used for post-transplant immune suppression or in the treatment of GvHD, may also be myelosuppressive.[42] H2 antagonists have also been associated with graft failure.[43]

Rare causes of graft failure relate to nutritional factors such as folic acid deficiency, vitamin B12 deficiency and protein energy malnutrition. Delayed red cell engraftment, including rare cases of pure red cell aplasia, may also be seen in cases of ABO mismatched transplantation.[44]

Intensive T-cell depletion may delete subsets of donor T-cells which support engraftment. One such population of cells has been named 'veto cells'.[45,46] These have been described in animal models of transplantation and shown to counteract host-versus-graft immune-based rejection. This may account for the high rate of graft rejection seen in the T-cell depleted setting.

Donor factors which may affect engraftment

In the unrelated donor setting, male donors are usually preferred over female donors. There are several reasons for this. The collection of cells, particularly peripheral blood progenitor cells (PBPC) by pheresis, may be technically easier because of better venous access. A higher yield of stem cells may result because of this and increased donor weight. In female donors, alloimmunization from prior pregnancies may theoretically increase the potential for graft failure.[47] Donor age may also have an effect on cell yield and engraftment, and younger donors are generally preferred.

The cell source is also an important consideration. The yield of CD34+ cells is usually superior in peripheral blood rather than bone marrow collections. The composition of the graft may also be different, with a higher T-cell content and increased G-CSF driven myeloid progenitors. These differences may explain the significant improvements in the rate of neutrophil and platelet engraftment in recipients of PBPC transplantation compared to bone marrow transplantation (BMT).[48] In certain conditions, however, bone marrow may be a preferable source of hemopoietic progenitor cells to peripheral blood. An example of this is aplastic anemia where a superior outcome has been described with BMT. This is mainly related to a reduced incidence of chronic GvHD.[49]

The rate of graft failure is higher in the unrelated donor setting than the matched related donor setting.[2] Disparity at major and minor histocompatibility antigen loci is clearly a risk factor for an immune-based graft rejection.[2] However, as the Perugia group first demonstrated, it is possible to obtain full donor engraftment even in the haploidentical setting, provided a very immune suppressive conditioning protocol is used, together with a high CD34 content in the infused graft, together with intensive T-cell depletion to prevent the complications of acute and chronic GvHD.[50] In the unrelated umbilical cord setting, satisfactory donor engraftment is usually seen despite very low doses of CD34 cells infused and usually significant HLA mismatching. This may be a result of an enhanced in vivo proliferative capacity of umbilical cord-derived stem cells, or the presence of cellular or serum factors which enhance engraftment.

Approach to the patient with graft failure

Suspicions should be raised in the patient who has not engrafted neutrophils by day 21 or certainly day 28. The latter time-point may be more appropriate in recipients receiving post-transplant methotrexate, where engraftment is typically delayed. Initially, it is recommended that the details of the infused stem cells product are reviewed, including CD34 and MNC counts. The procedures undertaken in the cell processing laboratory should also be reviewed. It is good practice in the stem cell laboratory for a pilot vial of stem cells to be cryopreserved and stored with the bags for reinfusion. In the setting of graft failure, the pilot vial may be thawed and studies of cell viability and in vitro proliferative assays performed.

The patient should also undergo detailed clinical assessment. The drug chart should always be reviewed carefully. If possible, myelosuppressive drugs should be stopped. For example, in a patient requiring CMV therapy with ganciclovir or valganciclovir, foscarnet or cidofovir may be used as less myelosuppressive alternatives. Co-trimoxazole may be substituted with pentamidine for *Pneumocystis* prophylaxis. Relevant clinical signs include moderate or massive splenomegaly which has occasionally been described in association with graft failure, for example in myelofibrosis.

Appropriate tests for virology should be arranged including PCR assessment of EBV, CMV, parvovirus, adenovirus and HHV6 in particular. A bone marrow aspirate and trephine should be performed. This may show aplasia or hypoplasia, hemophagocytosis associated with viral infection, or infiltration by underlying disease in cases of hematologic malignancy. Virus-associated hemophagocytic syndrome may respond to treatment of the underlying virus and possibly to intravenous immunoglobulin infusion. Co-trimoxazole based immune suppression may be associated with megaloblastic changes in the marrow and treated with folinic acid.

Blood and/or marrow should also be sent for donor–recipient chimerism analysis. Historically, this has been assessed by ABO grouping in cases of ABO-mismatched transplants, or cytogenetic analysis including X-Y chromosome fluorescence in situ hybridization (FISH)

for sex-mismatched transplants. More recent tests include characterization of donor and recipient DNA by PCR of variable number of tandem repeats (VNTR) which allows assessment of chimerism even in sex-matched transplants.

In the allogeneic setting, graft failure is usually associated with loss of donor chimerism which may be complete or partial. Complete absence of donor chimerism usually implies an immune-based graft rejection process. The presence of graft failure in association with predominant donor chimerism may suggest an extrinsic source of marrow suppression, such as by a drug or virus.

Management of graft failure

Growth factor administration

Units differ as to their policies for the routine administration of growth factors such as granulocyte-colony stimulating factor (G-CSF) to transplant recipients. Large, retrospective registry studies have provided conflicting data as to whether this practice is beneficial or detrimental to patient survival.[51,52] A small advantage in terms of the pace of neutrophil engraftment may, however, be expected. In the author's unit, the routine use of G-CSF post transplant is reserved for patients receiving grafts with low CD34 content, such as in the setting of umbilical cord transplantation.

In patients with suspected primary or secondary graft failure, evidence supports a trial of G-CSF or granulocyte macrophage-colony stimulating factor (GM-CSF).[53] This is more likely to be successful where the cause of graft failure is related to an extrinsic factor (such as drug or viral toxicity) than to an intrinsic, immune-based rejection. Growth factors are often very useful in the management of patients with suboptimal myeloid engraftment caused by similar toxicities. Erythropoietin generally has a very limited role in the post-transplant setting.

Manipulation of immunosuppressive drugs

In the setting of allogeneic stem cell transplantation, the fact that immune suppression can be withdrawn with continued donor engraftment and absence of GvHD implies that bidirectional tolerance has been successfully achieved. Transplants have been performed without any post-transplant immune suppression, and successful donor engraftment can occur. In such cases, intensive T-cell depletion is required to prevent GvHD. In patients at high risk of immunologic graft rejection such as those with aplastic anemia or β-thalassemia major who have received intensive transfusion regimens prior to transplantation, prolonged administration of ciclosporin for at least 1 year is recommended. This implies that immunosuppressive therapy with ciclosporin is suppressing a host-versus-graft immune-based rejection.

In the case of a patient who is demonstrating signs of incipient or established graft failure, increasing immune suppression would therefore seem a logical therapeutic approach. This could be achieved by increasing the dose of drugs such as ciclosporin to the high end of the therapeutic range or by the addition of other drugs such as corticosteroids or mycophenolate mofetil. While this may be successful, particularly in cases of slow/progressive loss of donor chimerism, this maneuver is unlikely to correct established graft failure demonstrated by pancytopenia/marrow aplasia or by complete loss of donor chimerism. In the setting of a selective erythroid graft failure associated with ABO mismatch (this usually occurs in a blood group O recipient receiving transplantation from a blood group A or B donor with anti-A or anti-B antibodies lysing engrafting erythroid precursor cells in the marrow), increasing immune suppression may, however, be successful.[54]

Infusion of donor lymphocytes to correct graft failure

With the advent of RIC transplantation, and particularly if T-cell antibodies are used pretransplant as part of the conditioning regimen with a resulting in vivo T-cell depletion, there has been interest in monitoring lineage-specific chimerism. It has been demonstrated that progressive loss of T-cell donor chimerism can be associated with graft failure. In the RIC setting, this can be a progressive process, with or without restoration of autologous hemopoiesis. Progressive loss of donor T-cell chimerism may also be associated with the potential for increased relapse risk.[7] It has been demonstrated that this progressive loss of donor T-cell chimerism can be reversed by donor lymphocyte infusions (DLI).[55] DLI are often given in a graded, incremental and increasing dose schedule to minimize the risk of GvHD. In the context of complete graft failure with loss of donor myeloid cells, DLI is unlikely to restore full donor hemopoiesis.

Infusion of further donor stem cells without prior conditioning

Graft failure with loss of donor hemopoiesis may also be restored by a second infusion of donor stem cells.[56] In patients who have previously received bone marrow as a source of stem cells for transplantation, a second request is often made for G-CSF mobilized peripheral blood progenitor cells, as the expected dose of CD34+ cells and T-cells may be higher. A second transplant procedure with unmanipulated donor stem cells may be successful in reversing graft failure associated with a prior T-cell depleted transplant approach. Because of the high T-cell content of such infusions, however, there is a significant risk of GvHD, and consideration therefore needs to be given to appropriate post-transplant immune suppression. Alternatively, recipients may be given a T-cell antibody such as ATG or alemtuzumab (CAMPATH 1H) prior to infusion of donor stem cells. Another approach has been to CD34 select the second transplant or use other methods of in vitro T-cell depletion. In practice, the author has found that infusion of a second transplant without prior conditioning is most applicable to patients who have demonstrated graft failure with pancytopenia but still have evidence of donor hemopoiesis on chimerism analysis. In these cases, the graft failure may be a result of inadequate initial donor CD34 counts, or subsequent suppression of donor hemopoiesis by drugs or viral infections.

Administration of second donation of stem cells with prior conditioning

Clearly, this represents another approach in cases of established graft failure. A request may be made for a second donation of stem cells from the original donor, and a second transplant performed after further conditioning therapy.[57] In patients who have received an initial RIC approach, consideration may be given to increasing the intensity of immune or myelosuppression for the second transplant. For patients who have initially received a full-intensity approach, however, a second transplant procedure is usually performed with RIC, perhaps with emphasis on increased immune suppression, in order to minimize the toxicity of the second transplant procedure.[57]

In patients who have initially received a pan T-cell antibody in vivo prior to the first transplant or another method of T-cell depletion, second transplants for graft failure may be performed with no T-cell depletion as a means of promoting donor engraftment. Clearly, in this situation the risks of GvHD are considerably increased, and due consideration therefore needs to be given to adequate post-transplant immune suppression.

There is also the possibility of requesting a new donor for the second transplant.[58] In this setting, the patient will require further conditioning therapy along the lines discussed above, and this approach is occasionally successful.

A second donation of stem cells, usually from the original donor following conditioning therapy, is the author's preferred approach in cases of established graft failure with a total absence of donor chimerism (both T-cell and myeloid). A RIC approach is generally employed in this setting.

Finally, it is also possible to rescue patients with graft failure and complete loss of donor chimerism with reinfusion of prior stored autologous stem cells.[58] In this case, pretransplant conditioning is not required. Patients considered at high risk of graft failure may therefore be considered for pretransplant autologous back-up harvesting of marrow or peripheral blood stem cells. This includes recipients of mismatched related or unrelated donors and umbilical cord transplants. The main issue which needs to be considered here, however, is the prospect of an autologous graft contaminated by tumor cells, and this approach is therefore only recommended in patients who are known to be in complete remission in the setting of malignant disease.

Infusion of other cell products

Marrow-derived mesenchymal stem cells (MSC) have a range of biologic properties which may be of therapeutic value in the field of human transplantation. This includes the ability of MSCs to support human hemopoiesis.[59,60] Another interesting observation is the inhibitory effect of MSCs in in vitro models of mixed lymphocyte culture (MLC). This suggests an immunosuppressive effect of MSCs which may be exploited to clinical advantage. Early clinical studies of infusion of MSCs derived from donors or third parties (HLA matched or mismatched) have demonstrated a potential beneficial role in the treatment of acute GvHD and in treating or reducing the risk of graft failure in certain settings.[59,60] Randomized clinical trials are now under way.

References

1. Wannesson L, Panzarella T, Mikhael J, Keating A. Feasibility and safety of autotransplants with noncryopreserved marrow or peripheral blood stem cells: a systematic review. Ann Oncol 2007;18:623–632

2. Ottinger HD, Ferencik S, Beelen DW et al. Hematopoietic stem cell transplantation: contrasting the outcome of transplantations from HLA-identical siblings, partially HLA-mismatched related donors, and HLA-matched unrelated donors. Blood 2003;102: 1131–1137

3. Urbano-Ispizua A, Rozman C, Pimentel C et al. The number of donor CD3+ cells is the most important factor for graft failure after allogeneic transplantation of CD34+ selected cells from peripheral blood from HLA-identical siblings. Blood 2001;97: 383–387

4. Baron F, Baker JE, Storb R et al. Kinetics of engraftment in patients with hematologic malignancies given allogeneic hematopoietic cell transplantation after nonmyeloablative conditioning. Blood 2004;104:2254–2262

5. Offner F, Schoch G, Fisher LD et al. Mortality hazard functions as related to neutropenia at different times after marrow transplantation. Blood 1996;88:4058–4062

6. Morrison VA, Haake RJ, Weisdorf DJ. Non-candida fungal infections after bone marrow transplantation: risk factors and outcome. Am J Med 1994;96:497–503

7. Mattsson J, Uzunel M, Tammik L et al. Leukemia lineage-specific chimerism analysis is a sensitive predictor of relapse in patients with acute myeloid leukemia and myelodysplastic syndrome after allogeneic stem cell transplantation. Leukemia 2001;15: 1976–1985

8. Storb R, Thomas ED, Weiden PL et al. Aplastic anemia treated by allogeneic bone marrow transplantation: a report on 49 new cases from Seattle. Blood 1976;48:817–841

9. Petersdorf EW, Longton GM, Anasetti C et al. Association of HLA-C disparity with graft failure after marrow transplantation from unrelated donors. Blood 1997 1;89:1818–1823

10. Petersdorf EW, Kollman C, Hurley CK et al. Effect of HLA class II gene disparity on clinical outcome in unrelated donor hematopoietic cell transplantation for chronic myeloid leukemia: the US National Marrow Donor Program Experience. Blood 2001;98:2922–2929

11. Murphy WJ, Kumar V, Bennett M. Rejection of bone marrow allografts by mice with severe combined immune deficiency (SCID). Evidence that natural killer cells can mediate the specificity of marrow graft rejection. J Exp Med 1987;165:1212–1217

12. Jukes JP, Wood KJ, Jones ND. Natural killer T cells: a bridge to tolerance or a pathway to rejection? Transplantation 2007;84:679–681

13. Klaus J, Herrmann D, Breitkreutz I et al. Effect of CD34 cell dose on hematopoietic reconstitution and outcome in 508 patients with multiple myeloma undergoing autologous peripheral blood stem cell transplantation. Eur J Haematol 2007;78:11–28

14. Ringden O, Barrett AJ, Zhang MJ et al. Decreased treatment failure in recipients of HLA-identical bone marrow or peripheral blood stem cell transplants with high CD34 cell doses. Br J Haematol 2003;121:874–885

15. Weaver CH, Hazelton B, Birch R et al. An analysis of engraftment kinetics as a function of the CD34 content of peripheral blood progenitor cell collections in 692 patients after the administration of myeloablative chemotherapy. Blood 1995;86:3961–3969

16. Terakura S, Azuma E, Murata M et al. Hematopoietic engraftment in recipients of unrelated donor umbilical cord blood is affected by the CD34+ and CD8+ cell doses. Biol Blood Marrow Transplant 2007;13:822–830

17. Wagner JE, Barker JN, DeFor TE et al. Transplantation of unrelated donor umbilical cord blood in 102 patients with malignant and nonmalignant diseases: influence of CD34 cell dose and HLA disparity on treatment-related mortality and survival. Blood 2002;100:1611–1618

18. Antonenas V, Garvin F, Webb M et al. Fresh PBSC harvests, but not BM, show temperature-related loss of CD34 viability during storage and transport. Cytotherapy 2006;8:158–165

19. Fois E, Desmartin M, Benhamida S et al. Recovery, viability and clinical toxicity of thawed and washed haematopoietic progenitor cells: analysis of 952 autologous peripheral blood stem cell transplantations. Bone Marrow Transplant 2007;40:831–835

20. Hale G, Waldmann H. CAMPATH-1 monoclonal antibodies in bone marrow transplantation. J Hematother 1994;3:15–31

21. Alvarnas JC, Forman SJ. Graft purging in autologous bone marrow transplantation: a promise not quite fulfilled. Oncology (Williston Park) 2004;18:867–876

22. Lucarelli G, Galimberti M, Polchi P et al. Bone marrow transplantation in patients with thalassemia. N Engl J Med 1990;322:417–421

23. Novotny VM, van Doorn R, Witvliet MD et al. Occurrence of allogeneic HLA and non-HLA antibodies after transfusion of prestorage filtered platelets and red blood cells: a prospective study. Blood 1995;85:1736–1741

24. Guardiola P, Anderson JE, Bandini G et al. Allogeneic stem cell transplantation for agnogenic myeloid metaplasia: a European Group for Blood and Marrow Transplantation, Societe Francaise de Greffe de Moelle, Gruppo Italiano per il Trapianto del Midollo Osseo, and Fred Hutchinson Cancer Research Center Collaborative Study. Blood 1999;93: 2831–2838

25. Weber-Mzell D, Urban C, Benesch M et al. Durable remission following a third allogeneic stem cell transplantation in a patient with repeatedly relapsing SAA. The importance of stroma cells for sustained engraftment? Pediatr Transplant 2007;11:332–335

26. Helenglass G, Treleaven J, Parikh P et al. Delayed engraftment associated with splenomegaly in patients undergoing bone marrow transplantation for chronic myeloid leukaemia. Bone Marrow Transplant 1990;5:247–251

27. Pamphilon DH, Cornish JM, Goodman S et al. Successful second unrelated donor BMT in a child with juvenile chronic myeloid leukaemia: documentation of chimaerism using the polymerase chain reaction. Bone Marrow Transplant 1993;11:81–84

28. Slavin S, Nagler A, Naparstek E et al. Nonmyeloablative stem cell transplantation and cell therapy as an alternative to conventional bone marrow transplantation with lethal cytoreduction for the treatment of malignant and nonmalignant hematologic diseases. Blood 1998;91:356–363

29. Niederwieser D, Maris M, Shizuru JA et al. Low-dose total body irradiation (TBI) and fludarabine followed by hematopoietic cell transplantation (HCT) from HLA-matched or mismatched unrelated donors and postgrafting immunosuppression with cyclosporine and mycophenolate mofetil (MMF) can induce durable complete chimerism and sustained remissions in patients with hematological diseases. Blood 2003;101:4620–4629

30. Kottaridis PD, Milligan DW, Chopra R et al. In vivo CAMPATH-1H prevents graft-versus-host disease following nonmyeloablative stem cell transplantation. Blood 2000;96: 2419–2425

31. Hale G, Jacobs P, Wood L et al. CD52 antibodies for prevention of graft-versus-host disease and graft rejection following transplantation of allogeneic peripheral blood stem cells. Bone Marrow Transplant 2000;26:69–76

32. Plentz A, Hahn J, Holler E et al. Long-term parvovirus B19 viraemia associated with pure red cell aplasia after allogeneic bone marrow transplantation. J Clin Virol 2004; 31:16–19

33. Kawabata Y, Hirokawa M, Saitoh Y et al. Late-onset fatal Epstein-Barr virus-associated hemophagocytic syndrome following cord blood cell transplantation for adult acute lymphoblastic leukemia. Int J Hematol 2006;84:545–548

34. Steffens HP, Podlech J, Kurz S et al. Cytomegalovirus inhibits the engraftment of donor bone marrow cells by downregulation of hemopoietin gene expression in recipient stroma. J Virol 1998;72:5006–5015

35. Johnston RE, Geretti AM, Prentice HG et al. HHV-6-related secondary graft failure following allogeneic bone marrow transplantation. Br J Haematol 1999;105:4041–4043

36. Levy J, Wodell RA, August CS, Bayever E. Adenovirus-related hemophagocytic syndrome after bone marrow transplantation. Bone Marrow Transplant 1990;6:349–352

37. Potter MN, Foot AB, Oakhill A. Influenza A and the virus associated haemophagocytic syndrome: cluster of three cases in children with acute leukaemia. J Clin Pathol 1991;44:297–299

38. Storb R, Deeg HJ, Pepe M et al. Methotrexate and cyclosporine versus cyclosporine alone for prophylaxis of graft-versus-host disease in patients given HLA-identical marrow grafts for leukemia: long-term follow-up of a controlled trial. Blood 1989;73:1729–1734

39. Colby C, McAfee S, Sackstein R et al. A prospective randomized trial comparing the toxicity and safety of atovaquone with trimethoprim/sulfamethoxazole as Pneumocystis carinii pneumonia prophylaxis following autologous peripheral blood stem cell transplantation. Bone Marrow Transplant 1999;24:897–902

40. Moretti S, Zikos P, van Lint MT et al. Foscarnet vs ganciclovir for cytomegalovirus (CMV) antigenemia after allogeneic hemopoietic stem cell transplantation (HSCT): a randomised study. Bone Marrow Transplant 1998;22:175–180

41. Busca A, de Fabritiis P, Ghisetti V et al. Oral valganciclovir as preemptive therapy for cytomegalovirus infection post allogeneic stem cell transplantation. Transpl Infect Dis 2007;9:102–107

42. Mourad M, Malaise J, Chaib ED et al. Correlation of mycophenolic acid pharmacokinetic parameters with side effects in kidney transplant patients treated with mycophenolate mofetil. Clin Chem 2001;47:88–94

43. Agura ED, Vila E, Petersen FB et al. The use of ranitidine in bone marrow transplantation. A review of 223 cases. Transplantation 1988;46:53–56

44. Remberger M, Watz E, Ringden O et al. Major ABO blood group mismatch increases the risk for graft failure after unrelated donor hematopoietic stem cell transplantation. Biol Blood Marrow Transplant 2007;13:675–682

45. Martin PJ. Donor CD8 cells prevent allogeneic marrow graft rejection in mice: potential implications for marrow transplantation in humans. J Exp Med 1993;178:703–712

46. Bachar-Lustig E, Reich-Zeliger S, Reisner Y. Anti-third-party veto CTLs overcome rejection of hematopoietic allografts: synergism with rapamycin and BM cell dose. Blood 2003;102:1943–1950

47. Shaw BE, Russell NH, Devereux S et al. The impact of donor factors on primary non-engraftment in recipients of reduced intensity conditioned transplants from unrelated donors. Haematologica 2005;90:1562–1569

48. Bensinger WI, Martin PJ, Storer B et al. Transplantation of bone marrow as compared with peripheral-blood cells from HLA-identical relatives in patients with hematologic cancers. N Engl J Med 2001;344:175–181

49. Schrezenmeier H, Passweg JR, Marsh JC et al. Worse outcome and more chronic GVHD with peripheral blood progenitor cells than bone marrow in HLA-matched sibling donor transplants for young patients with severe acquired aplastic anemia. Blood 2007;110: 1397–1400

50. Aversa F, Terenzi A, Tabilio A et al. Full haplotype-mismatched hematopoietic stem-cell transplantation: a phase II study in patients with acute leukemia at high risk of relapse. J Clin Oncol 2005;23:3447–3454

51. Khoury HJ, Loberiza FR Jr, Ringden O et al. Impact of posttransplantation G-CSF on outcomes of allogeneic hematopoietic stem cell transplantation. Blood 2006;107:1712–1716

52. Ringden O, Labopin M, Gorin NC et al. Treatment with granulocyte colony-stimulating factor after allogeneic bone marrow transplantation for acute leukemia increases the risk of graft-versus-host disease and death: a study from the Acute Leukemia Working Party of the European Group for Blood and Marrow Transplantation. J Clin Oncol 2004;22:416–423

53. Nemunaitis J, Singer JW, Buckner CD et al. Use of recombinant human granulocyte-macrophage colony-stimulating factor in graft failure after bone marrow transplantation. Blood 1990;76:245–253

54. Helbig G, Stella-Holowiecka B, Wojnar J et al. Pure red-cell aplasia following major and bi-directional ABO-incompatible allogeneic stem-cell transplantation: recovery of donor-derived erythropoiesis after long-term treatment using different therapeutic strategies. Ann Hematol 2007;86:677–683

55. Diez-Martin JL, Gomez-Pineda A, Serrano D et al. Successful treatment of incipient graft rejection with donor leukocyte infusions, further proof of a graft versus host lymphohaemopoietic effect. Bone Marrow Transplant 2004;33:1037–1041

56. Larocca A, Piaggio G, Podesta M et al. Boost of CD34+-selected peripheral blood cells without further conditioning in patients with poor graft function following allogeneic stem cell transplantation. Haematologica 2006;91:935–940

57. Jabbour E, Rondon G, Anderlini P et al. Treatment of donor graft failure with nonmyeloablative conditioning of fludarabine, antithymocyte globulin and a second allogeneic hematopoietic transplantation. Bone Marrow Transplant 2007;40:431–435

58. Wolff SN. Second hematopoietic stem cell transplantation for the treatment of graft failure, graft rejection or relapse after allogeneic transplantation. Bone Marrow Transplant 2002;29:545–552

59. Le BK, Samuelsson H, Gustafsson B et al. Transplantation of mesenchymal stem cells to enhance engraftment of hematopoietic stem cells. Leukemia 2007;21:1733–1738

60. Ball LM, Bernardo ME, Roelofs H et al. Cotransplantation of ex vivo expanded mesenchymal stem cells accelerates lymphocyte recovery and may reduce the risk of graft failure in haploidentical hematopoietic stem-cell transplantation. Blood 2007;110:2764–2767

Acute graft-versus-host disease

H Joachim Deeg and Mary ED Flowers

CHAPTER 38

Introduction

Graft-versus-host disease (GvHD) is the most frequent complication after allogeneic hematopoietic cell transplantation (HCT). First described as 'secondary disease' in mice that had their marrow function ablated by total-body irradiation (TBI)[1] and were then given viable splenocytes from histoincompatible donors, the syndrome was soon shown to be caused by immunocompetent donor cells, specifically T-lymphocytes.[2–4] Arguably, the first case of human GvHD was observed after marrow cells were used to treat survivors of a nuclear accident in Yugoslavia.[5] As the scientific basis for human HCT was established around 1970, it became apparent that GvHD would be a formidable problem even with transplantation of marrow cells from sibling donors identical with the patient for the antigens of the major histocompatibility complex (MHC), termed human leukocyte antigens (HLA) in humans.

An early acute form of GvHD and a delayed chronic form have been described.[6] However, a clear distinction between acute and chronic GvHD is no longer tenable. Observations in patients transplanted with reduced-intensity conditioning regimens or in patients receiving donor lymphocyte infusions (DLI) at various time intervals after HCT indicate that patients may have acute GvHD several months after transplantation.[7] Conversely, GvHD with characteristics of the 'chronic' form can occur as early as 50 or 60 days after transplantation.[7,8] Some investigators have proposed to simply refer to life-threatening and non-life threatening GvHD, regardless of the time of presentation.[9] The recent NIH Consensus Conference suggested recognition of two categories of GvHD (Fig. 38.1): *acute* GvHD (absence of features consistent with chronic GvHD), comprising (1) classic acute GvHD (before day 100) and (2) persistent, recurrent or late acute GvHD (after day 100, often upon withdrawal of immunosuppression); *chronic* GvHD, comprising (1) classic chronic GvHD (diagnostic clinical features of chronic GvHD must be present) and (2) an overlap syndrome, in which features of both acute and chronic GvHD are present.[10]

GvHD can also occur following blood transfusions in immunodeficient recipients or in patients in whom histoincompatibility exists for the GvH but not for the host-versus-graft vector (generally with related transfusion donors).[11,12]

Pathophysiology

The basic requirements for GvHD were summarized by Billingham:[2]

- the graft must contain immunocompetent cells
- the recipient must express tissue antigens that are not present in (and therefore are novel to) the donor
- the recipient must be unable to reject or destroy the donor cells.

Research over the ensuing 40 years has generated a large amount of data and led to additional insights, e.g. that inappropriate recognition of self antigens (after reinfusion of autologous cells) can also lead to a GvHD-like disease (autologous GvHD);[13] however, the basic Billingham criteria are still valid.

A three-step process of GvHD development best reflects the current view (reviewed by Ferrara[14]). In this model, TBI or other cytotoxic therapy results in the release of inflammatory cytokines such as interleukin (IL)-1 and tumor necrosis factor (TNF)-α and apoptosis in endothelial cells; in the gut this may lead to translocation of lipopolysaccharide (LPS) and other breakdown products into the circulation, further enhancing cytokine release. In this milieu, donor cells, including T-lymphocytes, are activated and expand. Studies in mice have shown that host antigen-presenting cells, in particular dendritic cells, are essential,[15] and the cytokines released by tissue damage upregulate MHC gene products on those cells. CD4+ T-cells interact primarily with MHC class II molecules (and associated peptides), and CD8+ cells with MHC class I. Minor histocompatibility antigens (miHA) are also presented by MHC molecules. Numerous cytokines are released from activated T-cells, including interferon (IFN)-γ, IL-2, and TNF-α. IL-2 plays a central role in T-cell expansion; however, the overall response depends upon the polarization to a Th1 (IL-2, TNF-α, etc.) versus a Th2 (IL-10, IL-4, etc.) pattern. The interactions are complex and described in detail in recent reviews and monographs.[14]

These events are followed by the generation of cytotoxic effectors including (more) inflammatory cytokines, cytotoxic effector cells (using Fas- and perforin-mediated mechanisms), large granular lymphocytes (LGL), and nitric oxide. There is good evidence for interactions of innate (LGL/NK (natural killer) cells) and adaptive (alloreactive T-lymphocytes) immune responses that lead to end-organ damage. Additional complexity has been added by the recent description of NK T-cells, and regulatory T-cells (Treg). For a detailed review see reference 14.

Risk factors for and incidence of acute graft-versus-host disease

Risk factors for GvHD were identified for cohorts of patients, not for individuals. To overcome this problem, in vitro tests were developed, aimed at determining before HCT whether a given patient would develop GvHD if transplanted from a specific donor.[16] One test used skin biopsies from the patient in a co-culture system with lymphocytes from the prospective donor. The pattern of infiltration of skin tissue by lymphocytes and the resulting histologic changes were used to predict the development of GvHD. In the initial study there was a correlation of in vitro findings with the occurrence of GvHD of the

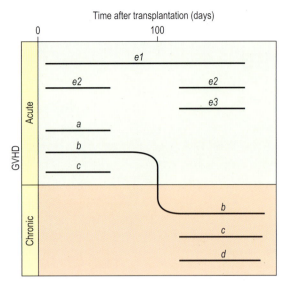

Figure 38.1
Categorization of GVHD combining the classification by Sullivan[213] and NIH Consensus Conference (Filipovich[10]).
Acute GvHD:
1. Classic acute GvHD: (a) responding spontaneously or with therapy; (b) progressing to chronic GvHD; (c) as for (a), but followed by chronic GvHD after a quiescent interval.
2. Persistent (e1), recurrent (e2) or late acute GvHD (e3).
Chronic GvHD:
3. Classic chronic GvHD, with progressive onset (b), with onset after a quiescent interval (c), with de novo onset (d).
4. Overlap syndrome: b, c, or d in combination with e(1, 2 or 3).

Table 38.1 Risk factors for the development of acute GvHD

Generally accepted
Histoincompatibility – HLA – non-HLA (miHA)
Alloreactive donor T cells
Patient age
Donor age
Donor–patient sex mismatch
Allosensitization of donor
Intensity of conditioning regimen
Source of stem cells PBPC > BM > cord blood
Donor lymphocyte infusion (DLI)
Controversial
HLA alleles
Splenectomy
Herpes virus immunity
ABO incompatibility
CD34 cell dose
Donor–patient cytokine gene polymorphism

ABO, ABO blood group; BM, bone marrow; HLA, human leukocyte antigen; PBPC, peripheral blood progenitor cells.

skin, but not other organs.[17,18] However, results with this and with other tests have been difficult to reproduce,[19,20] and they have not been widely adopted. Others have attempted to assign GvHD risk on the basis of donor and patient polymorphisms of CD31, IL-10 or TNF-α, but the predictive value of those tests has remained controversial.[21–25]

Important risk factors are summarized in Table 38.1.

Histocompatibility

The two major risk factors for GvHD are implied in the requirements for GvHD as formulated by Billingham:[2] histoincompatibility and the transfer of immunocompetent donor cells, specifically T-lymphocytes that recognize 'foreign' antigen in the recipient.

Histoincompatibility has the most profound effect when MHC, i.e. HLA, barriers are involved. Differences for class II antigens (HLA-DR, DP, DQ) are more relevant for GvHD, whereas differences for class I antigens (HLA-A, B and especially C) may interfere with engraftment.[26] Certain 'mismatches', for example isolated differences for HLA-DQ, are tolerated and do not negatively impact on transplant outcome.[27]

The development of GvHD in HLA-identical recipients, particularly with sibling donors where the same HLA haplotypes on the two parental chromosomes were inherited 'en bloc', is presumably due to differences in miHA outside MHC.[28] Despite progress over the past 15 years, we are still limited in our ability to assess miHAs. Male individuals express unique H-Y antigens encoded on the Y chromosome. These H-Y antigens are recognized by female donor cells in the context of HLA compatibility and trigger GvHD. The effect is most profound if the female donor is allosensitized, generally by pregnancy.[29–31] Other miHA include HA-1–5, and probably antigens that have not yet been characterized.[29,32]

Alloreactive donor cells

GvHD is triggered by alloreactive donor T-lymphocytes. In murine models, both CD4+ and CD8+ T-cells are involved, somewhat dependent upon the histocompatibility barrier involved.[33] The distinction in humans appears to be less clear. The potential benefit of both selective CD4 and CD8 depletion has been investigated, but no definitive conclusions could be drawn.[34–36] Depletion of CD3+ T-lymphocytes by two or three logs is effective in preventing or reducing the incidence of acute GvHD, although this approach has been associated with an increased risk of graft failure and, in patients with malignant diseases, an increased probability of disease recurrence.[37,38] T-cell reduction (rather than depletion) or graded add-back of T-lymphocytes may be able to circumvent these problems.[34,35] The value of limiting dilution analyses of anti-host specific donor T-helper and cytotoxic cells as predictors for the development of GvHD has remained controversial.[39–42]

Recent data show that a high degree of donor T-cell chimerism early (<day 28) after HCT is associated with an increased probability of acute GvHD, particularly in patients prepared with reduced-intensity conditioning regimens, although it is not clear whether the high degree of chimerism is a risk factor for or a reflection of GvHD.[43]

In addition, older age of the recipient is associated with an increased incidence of GvHD, and older age of the donor may also be a factor.[30,44] Donor–patient sex mismatch increased the risk of GvHD; with a female donor into a male recipient, the risk is increased about twofold compared to same-sex transplants. Allosensitization of the donor (see above), disease stage, and intensity of the conditioning regimen are further risk factors.[7,8,30,44–50] The latter in particular is of interest as recent reports suggest that acute GvHD, especially severe GvHD, is less frequent in patients conditioned with reduced-intensity conditioning (RIC) regimens.[7,51] More controversial is the impact of certain HLA alleles,[45,52] prior splenectomy,[47,53] exposure to herpes viruses,[54] ABO incompatibility,[55] and CD34 cell dose.[50] The CD34 cell dose is of considerable interest as recent trials, especially in children, suggest that massive doses of CD34+ cells may be associated with an acceptable incidence of acute GvHD.[56]

Incidence

Among patients transplanted from HLA-identical siblings with T-cell replete marrow, following conditioning with a conventional regimen (e.g. TBI plus cyclophosphamide, busulfan plus cyclophosphamide, or fludarabine plus busulfan) and given prophylaxis with ciclosporin (CSP) or tacrolimus (FK506; TAC) plus methotrexate (MTX) or mycophenolate mofetil (MMF), about 40–60% develop acute GvHD requiring therapy. The addition of steroids to such a combination in some studies has reduced the incidence to 10–20%. Among patients transplanted for non-malignant diseases, such as aplastic anemia, who are generally conditioned with less intensive regimens, the incidence has been lower, in the range of 20–40%.[57] In some T-cell depletion trials, incidence rates below 10% have been reported.[58] The use of a gnotobiotic environment has been effective in reducing GvHD incidence at some centers (see below).

In patients transplanted from unrelated donors, acute GvHD incidence rates as high as 60–80% have been reported. Among patients prepared with RIC regimens and transplanted from HLA-identical siblings, the incidence may be 40%.[7,51] In many studies the incidence of grade I GvHD was not reported.

Clinical presentation and diagnosis

Diagnosis of GvHD

Acute GvHD is a clinical syndrome involving primarily skin, liver, and gastrointestinal tract. Any target can be affected alone or in combination with other organs. The skin is most frequently involved and in most cases accompanies manifestations in other organs. However, the diagnosis of GvHD may be difficult. For instance, an elevated direct serum bilirubin, a relatively non-specific abnormality, is the principal parameter for hepatic GvHD. Short of a liver biopsy, hyperbilirubinemia may be ascribed to GvHD when it is actually related to infection or transplant-related toxicities. Diarrhea may be related to infections, conditioning, drug toxicity or GvHD. Similarly, GvHD skin rashes may be difficult to distinguish from drug eruptions, even on histology.

Martin and colleagues found substantial interobserver variability in assessing GvHD severity.[59] In a recent multicenter Phase III trial, the incidence (and severity) of GvHD as determined by an independent committee was substantially lower than reported by the investigators.[60] Nevertheless, an experienced clinician will generally be able to establish a working diagnosis of GvHD that is satisfactory for a meaningful prognostic assessment.[61]

Time of onset of GvHD

The onset of GvHD depends upon donor–recipient histoincompatibility, the number of donor T-cells infused, the intensity of the conditioning regimen, and the regimen used for GvHD prophylaxis. GvHD with fever, erythroderma and fluid retention may occur within a week of HCT in patients with severe HLA mismatches and in patients who receive T-cell replete transplants without or with inadequate in vivo GvHD prophylaxis.[62] This form of GvHD may be rapidly fatal. In patients receiving more conventional (in vivo) GvHD prophylaxis, e.g. a combination of CSP or TAC and MTX, the median onset of GvHD is 15–30 days after HCT; with in vitro T-cell depleted transplants the onset may be delayed.[63] Thus, a rash and diarrhea by 1 week after HCT would likely represent GvHD, particularly if minimal or

ineffective prophylaxis were administered. The same kinetics would be unlikely with CSP or TAC or in vitro T-cell depletion of the stem cell inoculum.

A less ominous syndrome of fever, rash, fluid retention and low-pressure pulmonary edema in the first 1–2 weeks after donor cell infusion has been termed 'engraftment syndrome' which may be seen with either allogeneic or autologous HCT.[64] The syndrome is thought to be due to a wave of cytokine production as the donor graft starts to recover, distinct from the 'cytokine storm'[65] which is thought to contribute to acute GvHD in that there is no concomitant T-cell mediated attack. Whether homeostatic proliferation of lymphocytes contributes to this clinical picture is a matter of speculation.[66] In most patients this syndrome responds promptly to steroids.[67] In autologous HCT, the differential diagnosis is of little relevance, but in allogeneic transplant recipients it must be distinguished from the hyperacute manifestations of GvHD. A prompt response to steroids would argue in favor of an engraftment syndrome, although some patients with GvHD will also improve.

Skin and mucosa

The most common manifestation of GvHD is a maculopapular, occasionally morbilliform, sometimes confluent, erythematous exanthema often involving palms and soles, a useful clinical hint since drug eruptions are less likely on the palms. However, a painful, blistering acral erythema, usually in the second week and resembling a second-degree burn, can also be related to conditioning therapy (e.g. busulfan).[68,69] Skin manifestations of GvHD may be asymptomatic, pruritic or painful. Erythema typically starts on shoulders, face and arms, most commonly in sun-exposed areas. A skin biopsy may be helpful in substantiating the diagnosis, but by itself will not prove the presence of GvHD. In its mildest manifestation, GvHD may involve less than 25% of the body surface, but it can progress to whole-body erythema, desquamation, bullae formation and sloughing of the skin. Mild skin GvHD often responds to modest doses of corticosteroids (1–2 mg/kg/day) or other immunosuppressants. In its severe forms GvHD can be difficult to distinguish from Stevens–Johnson syndrome or toxic epidermal necrolysis. It is noteworthy, however, that the conjunctivae are infrequently affected by acute GvHD.

The loss of integrity of the integument leads to an increased risk of infection with normal skin flora such as *S. aureus* and *S. epidermidis* and with gram-negative rods and fungi. In severe GvHD pain control, fluid and electrolyte replacement, metabolic support, and infection control are similar to the management of patients with severe burns. In fact, in patients with severe skin GvHD, consultation with a burn specialist is advisable.

Mucositis was not part of the classic description of acute GvHD. However, if infection is excluded, mucosal lesions that fail to heal with hematologic recovery may signify mucosal (oral, conjunctival, and vaginal) GvHD.

Liver

Hepatic GvHD is graded on the basis of total serum bilirubin levels, but alkaline phosphatase levels are often elevated; increases in transaminase are seen less consistently. Acute GvHD after DLI, i.e. with some delay after HCT, may take the form of 'hepatitic' GvHD, including transaminase elevations.[70] However, none of the routine serologic tests of liver injury is definitive. Bilirubin may be elevated only three- to fourfold or may reach levels of 10–20 mg/dl or higher; in extreme cases there may be a loss of liver synthetic function. Without a bona fide test the diagnosis of hepatic GvHD on clinical grounds may be tenuous. Drug toxicity, parenteral nutrition, hepatic sinusoidal obstruction syndrome, infection, cholangitis lenta, cholelithiasis, acalculous cholecystitis, and other unrelated conditions may co-exist or be confused with hepatic GvHD. In contrast to sinusoidal obstruction syndrome, hepatic GvHD only rarely leads to weight gain, capsular pain, or ascites.

Infections, especially with gram-negative organisms, can be associated with bilirubin elevations without direct hepatic involvement. The presence of cytomegalovirus (CMV) can be confusing, since CMV activation and infection often occur concomitantly with GvHD. Drugs such as CSP and estrogens are notorious hepatotoxins after HCT.

Thus, the diagnosis of acute GvHD of the liver is difficult. Transvenous biopsies are associated with a low morbidity and, if results are unequivocal, may lead to changes in the clinical diagnosis (and management) in as many as 50% of patients;[71,72] however, the small biopsy sample may still leave diagnostic uncertainty.

Intestinal tract

Involvement of the gut by GvHD may cause nausea, anorexia, pain, and watery, secretory diarrhea. In severe cases intestinal function may fail due to mucosal denudation, resulting in protein-losing enteropathy, with hypoalbuminemia, hemorrhage, or frank ileus. These manifestations, along with fluid losses through damaged skin and decreased hepatic synthetic function, render management difficult. Frequent evaluation of blood, urine, and stool electrolytes, and careful intake and output measurements are mandatory. Infection with C. difficile or other organisms, conditioning-related toxicity, lactose intolerance, and non-specific mucosal damage may mimic gut GvHD or may be present concurrently. In contrast to skin histopathology, the histology of rectal and gastric or duodenal mucosal biopsies is more distinct or even pathognomonic, and therapy can be targeted more narrowly.[73–75]

Isolated GvHD of the upper gastrointestinal tract is not uncommon, and Martin et al reported that the frequency has increased in recent years.[76] When upper gastrointestinal GvHD occurs alone, it is commonly the cause of otherwise unexplained nausea and vomiting. It must be distinguished from herpesvirus infection, candidiasis, and non-specific gastritis.[75,77,78] Esophagogastroduodenoscopy and mucosal biopsies will usually lead to the correct diagnosis. GvHD of the upper intestinal tract tends to be sensitive to corticosteroid therapy given systemically or topically in the form of beclomethasone.[79]

Radiographic findings of intestinal GvHD are non-specific but include increased bowel wall thickness (edema) and vascularity, and fluid-filled bowel loops. Transit time may be extremely rapid, and Doppler studies may show increased arterial flow to the inflamed organ. A magnetic resonance imaging (MRI) study may show generalized bowel wall enhancement after administration of gadolinium.[80,81]

Other organs

The involvement of other organs by acute GvHD has remained a matter of controversy. The most likely candidate is the lung.[82] Lung toxicity, including interstitial pneumonitis and alveolar hemorrhage, occurs in 20–60% of allogeneic but in few autologous transplant recipients. Causes of pulmonary damage other than GvHD include 'engraftment syndrome' (see above), infection, radiation pneumonitis, and chemotherapy-related toxicity (e.g. MTX, busulfan). At least one retrospective analysis failed to link severe pulmonary complications to clinical acute GvHD per se.[83] Mortality due to pneumonia increases with the severity of GvHD, although this association does not necessarily imply that GvHD, as opposed to immunosuppression given for therapy, is the cause. Lymphocytic bronchitis was attributed to GvHD in one study,[84] but has not been confirmed by others. Nevertheless, the lungs are likely targets of GvHD because of their extensive reticulo-endothelial system and direct exposure to the environment, and there is strong support from studies in murine transplant models.[85] Bronchi-

olitis obliterans organizing pneumonia or cryptogenic organizing pneumonia can be a manifestation of acute or chronic GvHD.

Renal and urinary tract symptoms are common, but are generally attributed to the conditioning regimen, immunosuppressive agents, or infection. There is no convincing evidence for a role of acute GvHD. Similarly, neurologic complications are common after transplantation, but most can be attributed to drug toxicity, infection, or vascular insults. Nevertheless, data on vasculitis of the CNS, possibly associated with GvHD, and peripheral neuropathy have been presented.[86–88]

Histopathology

The histopathology of GvHD has been described in detail elsewhere.[74] Programmed cell death (apoptosis) in the tissue layer responsible for proliferation and regeneration is a typical histologic feature of GvHD. In the skin, the dermoepidermal junction is most severely affected. There is epidermal and basal cell vacuolar degeneration, disorganization of epidermal cell maturation, eosinophilic body formation, and melanocyte incontinence.[74,89–91] Histopathologic changes consistent with acute GvHD are mimicked by the effects of chemoradiotherapy and drug reactions.[92] Hepatic small bile ducts may show segmental disruption, injury to the periductular epithelium, bile duct atypia, and cellular degeneration. Cholestasis may be present.[93,94] Mucosal ulcerations and crypt destruction are present in the intestinal tract. The crypt bases are most severely affected. The colon is more frequently involved than the ileum and shows crypt cell apoptosis and dropout with flattening of the villous architecture.[93,94] Often, mononuclear cell infiltrates are surprisingly mild in view of the degree of clinical illness. The involvement of the 'stem cell' layer of the organ, i.e. the base of the crypts in the gut and the dermoepidermal junction in the skin, results in a reduced ability to repopulate the damaged epithelium, with the consequence of blister formation, loss of villi, and associated dysfunction.

Staging and grading of acute GvHD

To provide prognostic guidance, assess treatment responses, and allow for comparison between different studies, investigators have attempted to quantify abnormalities of certain parameters for individual organs and generate overall grades to describe the severity of GvHD. The original grading system was proposed by Glucksberg;[6] it was modified subsequently into a 'consensus' system[95] (Table 38.2) and complemented by the International Bone Marrow Transplant Registry (IBMTR) GvHD Severity Index[61] (see Table 38.2). An important modification in the IBMTR index is the inclusion of upper gastrointestinal findings (nausea, vomiting, pain, positive biopsy). This IBMTR system has been validated in a retrospective analysis, and severity as determined by this system was reflected in the incidence of transplant-related mortality.[61] IBMTR levels A, B, C and D correspond approximately to Glucksberg grades I, II, III, and IV, respectively,[59] and a recent prospective trial indicates that both systems are comparable in their ability to assess GvHD severity and prognosis.[96] Another modification involves a division of grade II, originally proposed by Vogelsang,[97] into IIa (with a better prognosis) and IIb, dependent upon extent of skin involvement, bilirubin values, and amount of diarrhea. If further clinical studies provide compelling evidence for manifestations of acute GvHD in other organs such as the lungs[82] and an impact on prognosis, these features may have to be considered in future grading systems.

Mild-to-moderate GvHD (grades I or II (level A or B by IBMTR index)) is associated with limited morbidity but is a significant risk

Table 38.2 Grading of acute GvHD

Grade	Organ/extent of involvement					
	Skin (rash % BSA)		Liver (bilirubin; mg/dl)		Intestinal tract	
Consensus grading, modified[a]						
0	None		None		None	
I	<50%		None		None	
IIa	<50% not progressing rapidly		<3 mg/dl		Diarrhea <1000 ml/d (<20 ml/kg/d). No blood, no cramping	
IIb	≥50% or rapidly progressing		≥3 mg/dl[b]		Diarrhea ≥1000 ml/d ± blood, cramping	
III	–		≥6 and ≤15 mg/dl	or	Diarrhea ≥1500 ml/d. Abdominal pain ± ileus	
IV	Generalized erythema and bullae formation	or	>15 mg/dl		–	

IBMTR Severity Index[c]

Index	Organ/extent of involvement					
	Skin (rash % BSA)		Liver (bilirubin; mg/dl)		Gastrointestinal tract	
					Diarrhea (ml/day)	UGI
A	<25		<3.4		<500	–
B	25–50	or	3.5–7.9	or	500–1500	Nausea, vomiting or epigastric pain
C	>50	or	8.0–15.0	or	>1500	Positive biopsy
D	Bullae	or	>15.0	or	Severe pain, ileus	–

[a] Adapted from the Consensus Report by Przepiroka[95] with incorporation of a split of grade II into two subgroups.
[b] ≥6 mg/dl if other hepatic complications are present.
[c] Index is assigned on the basis of maximum involvement in any organ system (modified from Rowlings[61]).
Abbreviations: BSA, body surface area; UGI, upper gastrointestinal tract.

factor for the development of subsequent chronic GvHD.[98] As indicated above, subgrouping of grade II into a and b may be useful. Grades III and IV (levels C and D by IBMTR index) GvHD carry a grave prognosis. In patients with grade IV GvHD (Severity Index D), mortality is 90–100%.

One criticism of all these grading systems has been that they assess maximum severity but do not consider the disease course over time. Leisenring[99] recently presented an 'Acute GvHD Activity Index' (determined in a cohort of 386 patients, 193 each in the training and validation sets, with chronic myeloid leukemia (CML) transplanted from unrelated donors between 1987 and 1994) in which GvHD at 10-day intervals was assessed (Fig. 38.2). Factors considered were: skin rash, bilirubin, diarrhea, caloric intake, body temperature, medications administered, and performance level. Bilirubin values, uncontrolled anorexia (nausea, vomiting, caloric intake <40% of requirements), use of prednisone (or more intensive immunosuppressive therapy), and poor performance status were associated with an increased risk of non-relapse mortality by day 200. This activity index is awaiting validation in other disease cohorts.

Syngeneic and autologous graft-versus-host disease

Some 10–15% of autologous or syngeneic transplant recipients have been reported to develop a clinical picture that resembles GvHD, primarily of the skin, that usually responds promptly to corticosteroid therapy. There may be hepatic involvement.[100] Such a syndrome in the absence of allogeneic barriers may be interpreted as evidence of a loss of tolerance to 'self' (inappropriate recognition of self antigens) that occurs in the disrupted immune system. Hess and colleagues have proposed that infused T-cells recognize MHC class II antigens in

association with a peptide from the invariant chain (CLIP) (public determinants).[101,102] It is possible that some cases of syngeneic GvHD reflected a mistaken assumption that the donor was syngeneic without extensive molecular confirmation. Another hypothesis was proposed by Nelson and colleagues, who showed that in some individuals maternal cells transmitted during fetal development remain present throughout life.[103] This suggests the possibility that small numbers of HLA-incompatible cells (derived from the donor's mother) may be transmitted with 'HLA-identical transplants'. Transplacentally transferred maternal cells may also play a role in the development of neonatal GvHD.[104]

Transfusion-associated graft-versus-host disease

Most blood products administered to immunocompromised patients are irradiated or leukocyte depleted to avoid the transfusion of viable alloreactive T-cells.[11] Typically, MHC incompatibility between donor and recipient results in rapid clearance of transfused T-cells by the recipient's immune system. However, transfusions from donors who are homozygous for one of the recipient's MHC haplotypes may not be recognized as foreign by the recipient.[12] These cells can survive, 'engraft' and mount an immunologic attack against the unshared haplotype in the patient, resulting in transfusion-induced GvHD.[11,105]

Transfusion-associated GvHD differs from GvHD after HCT in regard to its kinetics and manifestations insofar as the recipient marrow is a major target, as also observed with DLI after HCT. Since the number of stem cells in the offending blood product is inadequate, there is no hematopoietic recovery from donor cells. This syndrome is generally fatal due to refractory pancytopenia.

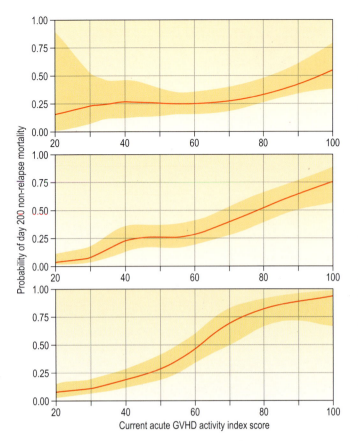

Figure 38.2
Predicted non-relapse mortality by day 200 as a function of current acute GvHD activity. Shown are index scores at three different time intervals after transplantation and their impact on mortality at day 200. Within each panel, the solid line represents the predicted median activity index scores, and the shaded areas represent 95% confidence intervals. (This research was originally published in Leisenring WM, Martin PJ, Petersdorf EW, Regan AE, Aboulhosn N, Stern JM, Aker SN, Salazar RC, McDonald GB. An acute graft-versus-host disease activity index to predict survival after hematopoietic cell transplantation with myeloablative conditioning regimens.[99] © American Society of Hematology.)

Prevention of graft-versus-host disease

Prevention of GvHD involves the elimination of recognized risk factors whenever possible and the minimization of the impact of those that are implicit in the transplant.

Donor selection

The preferred donor is a young HLA-identical sibling who has not had CMV exposure (CMVnegative), is not allosensitized, and is of the same sex as the patient, although it is noteworthy that stronger graft-versus-leukemia effects are observed with HLA non-identical or unrelated donors. In fact, some recent reports, particularly with RIC, suggest superior transplant outcome with unrelated donors in some disease categories.[106]

While HLA non-identical related donors may be acceptable, dependent upon the degree of mismatch, the disease to be treated and the willingness of the patient to enroll in investigational protocols, generally a search for an unrelated donor is initiated if an HLA-identical sibling is not available. With the growth of unrelated donor registries (more than 5 million individuals are registered) and the progress in molecular HLA typing, many unrelated donors identical for HLA at the DNA level are identified for patients.

Another potential source of stem cells is cord blood cells, which in virtually all cases will not be HLA identical with the patient but, due to their immaturity as well as cell composition and function, are associated with a lower incidence of GvHD than expected on the basis of HLA disparity.[107,108]

Selection of donors on the basis of certain cytokine (e.g. TNF-α, IL-10) polymorphisms is currently not a realistic option.

Host factors

Murine studies showed that transplantation in a gnotobiotic (i.e. sterile) environment prevented GvHD.[4] Studies in human patients who were placed in isolation (laminar air flow or other isolation rooms) and underwent intestinal and integumental decontamination have shown partial efficacy, particularly in patients with non-malignant diseases[109,110] and, at some centers, in all patients so treated.[111] While this approach has been abandoned by many investigators, it is noteworthy that two recent reports describe a reduced incidence of GvHD in patients treated prophylactically with metronidazole (combined with ciprofloxacin) and fluconazole, respectively.[112,113] There is also evidence in animal models that the use of LPS (or TNF-α) antagonists may decrease intestinal GvHD.[114] IL-11 and keratinocyte growth factor have been tested, but there is no evidence that either one provides potent anti-GvHD protection.[115,116]

Conditioning regimen

As described under Pathophysiology, intensive conditioning, especially with high-dose TBI, leads to endothelial injury and associated tissue damage. In agreement with preclinical observations, clinical results suggest that less toxic conditioning regimens (e.g. cyclophosphamide alone or various RIC regimens) are associated with a lower incidence of, and less severe acute GvHD.[7,51,110,117]

In vivo prophylaxis

Pharmacologic agents

Early studies used single-agent MTX (based on the seminal work by Uphoff, using α-aminopterin[118] or, less frequently, cyclophosphamide for GvHD prophylaxis. Pilot trials that omitted prophylaxis showed an incidence of acute GvHD close to 100%, often severe,[62] whereas patients given MTX (15 mg/m² on day 1, and 10 mg/m² on days 3, 6, 11 and weekly until day 102, based on studies in a canine model) experienced GvHD grades II–IV in 30–60% of cases;[119] abbreviated MTX regimens were less effective.[120]

The arrival of calcineurin inhibitors, first ciclosporin (CSP)[121] and then tacrolimus (TAC),[122] offered new possibilities. One advantage is the lack of myelosuppression. CSP is administered starting one to several days before transplantation, at doses of 1.5–2.5 mg/kg iv every 12 hours (or as a continuous infusion) with a switch to oral drug, 6 mg/kg, every 12 hours, when tolerated. Dependent upon the regimen and the method used to measure CSP, blood levels of 150–400 ng/ml have been targeted. Tapering typically starts on day 50 (earlier if necessitated by toxicity) and continues over 6–12 months.

TAC is often given as a continuous infusion, 0.03–0.04 mg/kg/day, and switched to an oral preparation when tolerated (0.15 mg/kg/day). Blood levels are targeted at or below 15 ng/ml. In a randomized Japanese trial, TAC was superior to CSP, with an incidence of acute GVHD of 13%/21% (HLA identical/non-identical) versus 41%/54% in patients given CSP.[123]

Based on preclinical studies which showed an advantage of a combination of MTX plus CSP over CSP (or MTX) as a single agent,[124] subsequent clinical trials tested single agents against drug combinations or combinations against each other. Some representative trials

Table 38.3 Randomized trials of combination immunosuppression for prevention of acute GvHD

Center (year, reference)	Disease groups	Patients (n)	Regimens compared	Median age (year)	Acute GvHD (%)
HLA-identical sibling donors					
Minneapolis (1982)[134]	Non-malignant and malignant diseases	32 35	MTX+ATG+PSE vs MTX	16 16	21 (p = 0.01) 48
Seattle (1989)[187]	AML in CR1 and CML in CP	43 50	MTX+CSP vs CSP	30 30	33 (p = 0.01) 54
City of Hope (1987)[188]	Acute leukemia and CML	53 54	MTX+PSE vs CSP+PSE	26 26	47 (p = 0.05) 28
Baltimore (1987)[189]	Non-malignant and malignant diseases	42 40	CSP+MP vs CY+MP	23 24	32 (p = 0.05) 68
Seattle (1990)[190]	Non-malignant and malignant diseases	59 63	MTX+CSP+PSE vs MTX+CP	32 28	46 (p = 0.02) 25
Stanford (1993)[191]	Malignant diseases	74 75	CSP+PSE vs MTX+CSP+PSE	32 28	23 (p = 0.02) 9
Multicenter (1998)[192]	Hematologic malignancies	164 165	MTX+CSP vs MTX+TAC	40 40	44 (p = 0.01) 32
Stanford (2000)[193]	Hematologic malignancies	96 90	MTX+CSP vs MTX+CSP+PSE	34 34	20 (n.s.) 18
Helsinki (2000)[194]	Hematologic malignancies Severe aplastic anemia	55 53	MTX+CSP vs MTX+CSP+PSE	41 42	56 (p = 0.001) 19
Cleveland (2005)[127]	Hematologic malignancies	21 19	MMF+CSP MTX[a]+CSP	NA NA	48 (p = 0.40) 37
HLA non-identical donors					
Multicenter (2000)[60]	Non-malignant and malignant diseases	90 90	MTX+CSP vs MTX+TAC	35 34	74 (p = 0.001) 56

[a] MTX at 5 mg/m^2 on days 1, 3, 6, and 11.
Abbreviations: AML, acute myeloid leukemia; ATG, antithymocyte globulin; BC, donor buffy coat cells; CML, chronic myeloid leukemia; CP, chronic phase; CR, complete remission; CSP, ciclosporin; CY, cyclophosphamide; GvHD, graft-versus-host disease; MP, methylprednisolone; MTX, methotrexate; n.s., not significant; NA, not applicable, PSE, prednisone; TAC, tacrolimus.

are summarized in Table 38.3. With MTX plus CSP combinations, the incidence rates of acute GvHD grades II–IV were 20–56% with HLA-identical sibling transplants. With the combination of CSP plus methylprednisolone (MP), at doses of 0.5–1.0 mg/kg, for various intervals after HCT, the incidence ranged from 23% to 32%, and with the triple combination MTX plus CSP plus MP, from 9% to 46%. The spread of these results reflects not only differences in the dose schedules, but also patient selection, patient age, the conditioning regimen used, and variations in the clinical grading of GvHD.[125] Importantly, even though drug combinations may have resulted in a lower incidence of GvHD, in many trials this was not reflected in improved survival. This was particularly true with the incorporation of MP as a third drug. Nevertheless, overall drug combinations are superior to single agents, and the use of TAC appears to have an advantage over CSP.[126]

The replacement of MTX by MMF has reduced the frequency and severity of mucositis; however, outcome, with regard to both GVHD and survival, was not superior to that observed with MTX.[127,128] Many investigators have reduced the amount of MTX administered,[129,130] and Przepiorka has reported a 'mini-MTX' regimen.[131] Such a strategy may reduce problems with mucositis and allow for better compliance with concurrently given CSP or TAC. Thus, many current regimens use MTX at doses of 7.5 (rather than 15 or 10) mg/m^2 or even lower,

and often give it only on days 1, 3 and 6. There is evidence, however, that omission of the day 11 dose is associated with an increase in the frequency of GvHD.[49]

Cutler et al replaced MTX by sirolimus (rapamycin) in a Phase II trial in combination with tacrolimus, and with HLA-identical sibling transplants showed an incidence of acute GvHD of 10%, and a day 100 relapse-free survival of 93%.[132] The same investigators then used a triple combination of TAC, sirolimus and low-dose MTX with unrelated donor transplants and observed an incidence of grades II–IV acute GvHD of 26%.[133] However, so far these results have not been reproduced by other investigators.

In vivo antibody prophylaxis

Several recent trials have used the antithymocyte globulin (ATG) preparation, thymoglobulin (rabbit), as part of the conditioning and GvHD regimen, resuming a strategy proposed by Ramsay et al in 1982.[134] These reports show that thymoglobulin given in the pre- and peritransplant period reduces the incidence of acute (and chronic) GvHD and may be associated with lower late morbidity.[135–140] Russell reported an incidence of acute GvHD of 8% with related and 19% with unrelated donors;[140] incidence figures reported by others have been higher.[135,137] Very high doses of thymoglobulin are associated with more infections.[135] A dose in the range of 6–8 mg/kg may be appropriate.

The use of large doses of intravenous immunoglobulins, despite initial promising results, is controversial. One undesired effect is interference with immune recovery.[141]

The most widely used monoclonal antibody given in vivo for GvHD prophylaxis is probably CAMPATH 1H (anti-CD52), which has been administered in various regimens and has been found to reduce the incidence of GvHD and non-relapse mortality in related and unrelated transplant recipients.[142] An added attraction is that this antibody has a 'graft-facilitating' activity. Antibodies to the IL-2 receptor (CD25) have shown some benefit.[143] The use of ricin-conjugated anti-CD5 antibody did not result in a significant advantage.[63,144,145]

In vitro T-cell depletion

Theoretically, removal of host-reactive donor T-cells should solve the problem of GvHD and, in fact, all T-cell depletion studies have shown a reduction in acute (albeit not in chronic) GvHD. However, failure of engraftment and disease relapse occurred in a larger proportion of patients than observed with T-cell replete transplants. Nevertheless, trials using various monoclonal antibodies with or without a non-human source of complement, E-rosetting/lectin methods, elutriation techniques or functional inactivation via phototherapy have continued.[142,144,146] In an attempt to prevent problems associated with global T-cell removal, various trials have carried out selective depletion of CD4+ or CD8+ cells or partial depletion of either subset.[35] Another strategy in a small study of HLA non-identical HCT has been the removal of activated T-cells by incubation with CTLA4-Ig (in the presence of donor antigen-presenting cells).[147]

Recently, Wagner et al presented the results of a randomized trial involving 15 centers comparing the use of MTX plus CSP (n = 204) to T-cell depletion plus CSP (n = 201) as GvHD prophylaxis. T-cell depletion used either elutriation or treatment of donor cells with the monoclonal antibody T10B9 (targeting the T-cell receptor αβ) plus rabbit complement.[58] The incidence of GvHD grades III–IV was 19% with T-cell depletion and 29% with MTX plus CSP (p = 0.017). However, there was no significant difference in long-term survival, and the incidence of relapse among patients with CML was 20%, versus 7% in patients given MTX plus CSP (p = 0.009); there was also a higher incidence of CMV infection with T-cell depletion (p = 0.023). Others have used T-cell depletion and, by design, administered additional DLI following HCT with the intent of obtaining the benefit of T-cell depletion without risking relapse.[146]

Recently, T-cell depletion has also been applied to peripheral blood progenitor cells (PBPC)[148] since they carry a higher risk of GvHD than marrow. One consideration here is the fact that following administration of granulocyte colony-stimulating factor (G-CSF) to the donor there is a shift in favor of type 2 dendritic cells (DC2).[149] DC2 cells activate Th2 cytokines IL-4 and IL-10 and are unable to initiate proliferation of naïve T-cells. Thus, the concept is that partial removal of CD3+ T cells, while maintaining the remainder of cells, will preserve the favorable DC2 action and reduce the risk of GvHD.[149,150]

Other methods

Ruutu et al reported on the use of ursodeoxycholic acid (UDCA), originally with the aim of reducing hepatotoxicity.[151] The study involved related and unrelated donor transplants. Patients were randomized to receive (n = 123) or not to receive (n = 119) UDCA, 12 mg/kg/day, from before conditioning until day 90. Non-relapse mortality (19% versus 34%, p = 0.01) was reduced, and survival (71% versus 55%) was improved. There was also a reduction in the inci-

dence of acute GVHD, which was significant for grades III–IV (p = 0.01).

Treatment of graft-versus-host disease

Some 10–90% of patients develop acute GvHD requiring therapy. Effective treatment is important since the probability of survival depends upon the response to therapy.[152–154] Table 38.4 summarizes the results of some RCTs in acute GvHD. A possible treatment algorithm is given in Figure 38.3.

Primary therapy

Corticosteroids (e.g. methylprednisolone (MP), 2 mg/kg/day for 14 days or longer) remain the mainstay of acute GvHD therapy. Lysis of lymphocytes during interphase and anti-inflammatory effects may lead to prompt improvement, including patients with hyperacute presentations. Complete responses occur in 20–25%, and useful responses in 40–50% of patients with grades II–IV acute GvHD. A prospective, randomized study comparing 2 mg/kg/day of MP to 10 mg/kg/day failed to show any advantage of the higher dose.[155] In a subsequent report[156] the same investigators presented results in 211 patients with grades I–IV GvHD treated with MP, 2 mg/kg/day. In 150 patients (71%) the dose could be tapered beginning after 5 days of therapy, whereas 61 patients (29%) required continuation of therapy. The non-responders were randomized to receive MP at 5 mg/kg/day for 10 days, alone or combined with thymoglobulin (6.25 mg over 10 days); 26% of patients had complete responses. Non-relapse mortality for the day-5 responders and non-responders was 27% and 49% (p = 0.009), and 5-year survival was 53% and 35%, respectively (p = 0.007). There was no significant difference between the two secondary therapies.

However, systemic therapy with high-dose steroids is associated with considerable toxicity, in particular infections. Therefore, there has been a keen interest in developing alternative strategies. A randomized trial in 60 patients with intestinal GvHD compared oral MP, at 1 mg/kg/day, plus placebo, to MP plus beclomethasone. Treatment responses by day 10 were 55% and 71%, respectively; the durable responses by day 30 were 41% and 71% for the two groups (p = 0.02).[157,158] A follow-up study by McDonald[79] describes 129 patients with gastrointestinal GvHD who received prednisone at 1–2 mg/kg/day and beclomethasone, 8 mg/kg/day, or placebo for 50 days; at study day 10 prednisone was tapered if GvHD had improved, and the study drug was continued. The day 200 survival was 92% for patients on beclomethasone and 76% for placebo-treated patients (p = 0.01). In a multivariate analysis, only the use of beclomethasone remained significant (p = 0.05) for day 200 survival. Patients with recurrent GvHD had greater steroid exposure and a higher risk of death. There was a 2% incremental increase in the risk of death for every 1.0 mg/kg increase in cumulative prednisone exposure relative to the lowest dose (p = 0.045).

CSP has been used with some success therapeutically in patients who had not received CSP prophylaxis. TAC, with a mechanism of action similar to CSP, provides effective therapy in some patients who have failed CSP prophylaxis,[159] although a retrospective analysis suggested a true benefit only in patients who were switched to TAC because of CNS toxicity.[160]

Equine (ATGAM) and rabbit ATG (thymoglobulin) are potent anti-T-cell agents that achieve responses in 20–30% of patients even after steroid failure.[152,154,161,162] However, infections and thrombocytopenia are common complications and in some trials patient survival was as low as 10%.[163] A combination of TAC and ATG has yielded promising results in one study.[164]

MMF and rapamycin (sirolimus) have recently been introduced for the treatment of acute GvHD.[165] MMF may be effective in some patients in combination with CSP and prednisolone.[166]

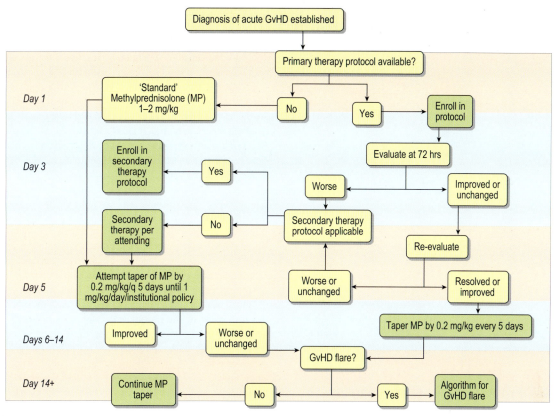

Figure 38.3
Treatment algorithm for acute GvHD. Protocol treatment is preferred. Days indicated at the left margin are intended to serve as a guide for the timing of therapeutic decisions.

Table 38.4 Treatment of acute GvHD – results of some RCTs

Investigator (year, reference)	Patients (n)	Regimens compared	Median age (year)	Response (flare) (%)	Overall Survival (%)
Seattle (1981)[195]	20 17	MP vs ATG	24 24	65 35	40 (n.s.) 24
Seattle (1985)[196]	39 38	MP vs CSP	27 26	41 (p = 0.039) 61	28 (n.s.) 24
Minneapolis (1993)[197]	16 14	MP long taper vs MP short taper	33 29	(13) (n.s.) (29)	81 (n.s.) 66
France (1995)[198]	34 35	MP+CSP+placebo vs MS+CSP+CD25 mAB	29 25	63 (n.s.) 70	59 (n.s.) 66
Seattle (1996)[168]	114 129	MP+placebo vs MP+CD5-IT	30 29	25 (p = 0.019) 40	(45) (n.s.) 49
Italy (1998)[156]	47 48	MP 2 mg/kg vs MP 10 mg/kg	26 28	68 (n.s.) 71	63 (n.s.) 62
Seattle (1998)[158] (enteric GVHD)	29 31	MP+placebo vs MP+Beclo	39 34	41 (p = 0.02) 71	NA NA
Minneapolis (2000)[169]	46 50	MP vs MP+ATG	28 23	55 (p = 0.02) 27	50 (n.s.) 40
Multicenter (2004)[199]	53 49	MP + Daclizumab vs MP+placebo	45 42	29 (p = 0.002) 60	25[a] (p = 0.005) 56

[a] Disease-free survival at 1 year.
Abbreviations: ATG, antithymocyte globulin; Beclo, beclomethasone; CSP, ciclosporin; GvHD = graft-versus-host disease; IT, immunotoxin; MAB, monoclonal antibody; MP, methylprednisolone; NA, not available; n.s., not significant.

Table 38.5 Treatment options for steroid-unresponsive acute GvHD

Agent/strategy	Selected references
PUVA	Furlong,[200] Wetzig[201]
ECP	Couriel,[202] Greinix[182]
Anti-TNF-α agents	Couriel,[203] Patriarca,[204] Wolff[205]
Human anti-CD3	Carpenter,[173] Carpenter[174]
Denileukin diftitox (ONTAK)	Ho[206]
Anti-IL-2 receptor antibody	Massenkeil,[207] Wolff[205]
Sirolimus	Benito,[165] Jacobsohn & Vogelsang[208]
Tacrolimus	Peters[209]
ATG	MacMillan,[152] Peters[209]
Pentostatin	Bolanos-Meade,[210] Margolis & Vogelsang[211]

Abbreviations: ATG, antithymocyte globulin; ECP, extracorporeal photopheresis; PUVA, psoralen sensitization and exposure to ultraviolet A light.

Toxin-conjugated monoclonal antibodies have also shown encouraging results.[167] However, a randomized trial comparing MP with MP plus a ricin A-conjugated anti-CD5 antibody, while showing a higher response rate (25% versus 40%; p = 0.019), revealed no significant difference in the incidence of chronic GvHD or survival.[168] The same was true for a comparison of MP and MP plus ATG.[169]

Secondary therapy (steroid-unresponsive GvHD) (Table 38.5)

CSP, TAC, ATG and MMF have all been used to treat steroid-unresponsive acute GVHD. A recent trial with rapamycin in 21 patients showed a response rate of more than 50%, and suggested improved survival compared to historic controls.[165]

A broad array of monoclonal antibodies in murine or humanized form with pan T- or T-subset reactivity has been used, often as secondary therapy of GvHD, in patients not responding to corticosteroids. Responses, sometimes sustained, are observed with anti-CD2, anti-CD3, anti-CD5 and other antibodies.[38,170,171] In a trial using the anti-CD147 antibody ABX-CBL, more than half of the patients with steroid-refractory acute GvHD responded, and survival was superior to that observed in a historical comparison group treated with horse ATG.[172] However, a subsequent Phase III trial comparing ABX-CBL with ATG (ATGAM) in 92 patients, with an endpoint of day 180 survival, failed to show a significant difference between the two arms (unpublished).

Intriguing results have been obtained with a humanized antibody, HuM291 (visilizumab, directed at the T-cell receptor zeta chain), by Carpenter.[173] Among 15 patients with steroid-refractory GvHD, seven and eight achieved complete and partial responses, respectively. Notably, sustained responses were achieved with a single dose of antibody. A follow-up study enrolled 44 patients, 86% of whom had grades III–IV acute GvHD. The overall response rate was 32%, complete responses 14% at 42 days. Survival at 6 months was 32%.[174] In both trials, 40–50% of patients experienced a rise in plasma titers of Epstein-Barr virus (EBV) DNA, which was controlled following the administration of the anti-CD 20 antibody, rituximab.

Another treatment strategy involves antibodies against cytokine receptors. A monoclonal antibody to the IL-2R (B-B10) was found to be effective experimentally and clinically.[175] Pilot trials using genetically engineered human monoclonal antibody specific for Tac, the α-subunit of the IL-2R (anti-Tac, dacliumzab), in patients who had failed to respond to corticosteroids showed responses in about 40%.[176,177] Experimental data suggest that blockade of other receptors, for example IL-1, may also be beneficial. However, a recent report shows

a lack of efficacy in patients.[116] One clinical report suggested efficacy of an anti-TNF-α monoclonal antibody (infliximab) in steroid-refractory acute GvHD.[178] This approach should be used cautiously, however, as a high incidence of tuberculosis reactivation was noted in patients with autoimmune diseases treated with this agent.[179]

PUVA treatment (photosensitization with 8-methoxypsoralen and UVA irradiation) is effective in the treatment of acute and chronic GvHD of the skin in some patients. Extracorporeal exposure of the recipient's peripheral blood mononuclear cells to the photosensitizing effect of 8-methoxypsoralen and UV light and their subsequent reinfusion is effective in treating acute (and chronic) GvHD refractory to conventional treatment.[180–182]

Summary

Acute GvHD is a complex clinical syndrome that occurs in a setting where the diagnosis may be difficult to establish. There are no simple laboratory tests. However, it is extremely important to recognize the disease, since the survival of patients may well depend on the accuracy of the clinical diagnosis and prompt institution of therapy. None of the prophylactic strategies currently available has been completely successful, and the most effective ones have been associated with other complications, in particular an increased incidence of relapse of the primary disease. There is some evidence that acute GvHD may be less frequent and less severe in patients conditioned with RIC regimens. However, chronic GvHD has not been affected.

Qualitatively new approaches such as risk-adapted first-line treatment or pre-emptive therapy might have an impact on outcome. A better definition of predictive parameters is needed. Endothelial cells have only recently been identified as important targets of GvHD,[183] and agents modulating endothelial activation have not been tested. Finally, the increasingly recognized role for regulatory T-cells such as CD4+CD25+ T-cells or T-regulatory type 1 cells[184–186] suggests that strategies aiming at modulation of subpopulations of cells or the therapeutic use of regulatory cells may be useful.

Acknowledgments

Supported by PHS grants HL36444, CA18029, and CA15704.

References

1. Lorenz E, Uphoff D, Reid TR et al. Modification of irradiation injury in mice and guinea pigs by bone marrow injections. J Natl Cancer Inst 1951;12:197–201
2. Billingham RE. The biology of graft-versus-host reactions. In: The Harvey Lectures. Academic Press 1966; New York, p 21–78
3. Elkins WL. Cellular immunology and the pathogenesis of graft versus host reactions (Review). Progress in Allergy 1971;15:78–187
4. van Bekkum DW, de Vries MJ. Radiation chimaeras. Logos Press, London, 1967
5. Mathé G, Jammet H, Pendic B et al. Transfusions et greffes de moelle osseuse homologue chez des humains irradiés a haute dose accidentellement. Revue Francaise d' Etudes Cliniques et Biologiques 1959;IV:226–238
6. Glucksberg H, Storb R, Fefer A et al. Clinical manifestations of graft-versus-host disease in human recipients of marrow from HL-A-matched sibling donors. Transplantation 1974;18:295–304
7. Mielcarek M, Martin PJ, Leisenring W et al. Graft-versus-host disease after nonmyeloablative versus conventional hematopoietic stem cell transplantation. Blood 2003;102:756–762
8. Mielcarek M, Burroughs L, Leisenring W et al. Prognostic relevance of 'early-onset' graft-versus-host disease following nonmyeloablative hematopoietic cell transplantation. Br J Haematol 2005;129:381–391
9. Flowers ME, Traina F, Storer B et al. Serious graft-versus-host disease after hematopoietic cell transplantation following nonmyeloablative conditioning [erratum appears in BMT 2005;35:535]. Bone Marrow Transplant 2005;35:277–282
10. Filipovich AH, Weisdorf D, Pavletic S et al. National Institutes of Health consensus development project on criteria for clinical trials in chronic graft-versus-host disease: I. Diagnosis and Staging Working Group report. Biol Blood Marrow Transplant 2005;11(12):945–956
11. Higgins MJ, Blackall DP. Transfusion-associated graft-versus-host disease: a serious residual risk of blood transfusion (review). Curr Hematol Rep 2005;4(6):470–476

12. Juji T, Takahashi K, Shibata Y et al. Post-transfusion graft-versus-host disease in immunocompetent patients after cardiac surgery in Japan (Letter to Editor). N Engl J Med 1989;321:56
13. Hess AD, Jones RJ. Autologous graft-versus-host disease. In: Thomas ED, Blume KG, Forman SJ (eds) Hematopoietic cell transplantation, 2nd edn. Blackwell Science, Boston, 1999: 342–348
14. Ferrara JL, Cooke KR, Deeg HJ (eds) Graft-vs.-host disease. Marcel Dekker, New York, 2005
15. Shlomchik WD, Couzens MS, Tang CB et al. Prevention of graft versus host disease by inactivation of host antigen-presenting cells. Science 1999;285(5426):412–415
16. Sviland L, Dickinson AM. A human skin explant model for predicting graft-versus-host disease following bone marrow transplantation. J Clin Pathol 1999;52(12):910–913
17. Theobald M, Nierle T, Bunjes D et al. Host-specific interleukin-2-secreting donor T-cell precursors as predictors of acute graft-versus-host disease in bone marrow transplantation between HLA-identical siblings. N Engl J Med 1992;327(23):1613–1617
18. Vogelsang GB, Hess AD, Berkman AW et al. An in vitro predictive test for graft versus host disease in patients with genotypic HLA-identical bone marrow transplants. N Engl J Med 1985;313:645–650
19. Dickinson AM, Sviland L, Wang XN et al. Predicting graft-versus-host disease in HLA-identical bone marrow transplant: a comparison of T-cell frequency analysis and a human skin explant model. Transplantation 1998;66(7):857–863
20. Wang XN, Taylor PR, Skinner R et al. T-cell frequency analysis does not predict the incidence of graft-versus-host disease in HLA-matched sibling bone marrow transplantation. Transplantation 2000;70(3):488–493
21. Cullup H, Dickinson AM, Jackson GH et al. Donor interleukin 1 receptor antagonist genotype associated with acute graft-versus-host disease in human leucocyte antigen-matched sibling allogeneic transplants. Br J Haematol 2001;113(3):807–813
22. Lin MT, Storer B, Martin PJ et al. Genetic variation in the IL-10 pathway modulates severity of acute graft-versus-host disease following hematopoietic cell transplantation: synergism between IL-10 genotype of patient and IL-10 receptor genotype of donor. Blood 2005;106(12):3995–4001
23. Nichols WC, Antin JH, Lunetta KL et al. Polymorphism of adhesion molecule CD31 is not a significant risk factor for graft-versus-host disease. Blood 88 1996;(12):4429–4434
24. Rocha V, Franco R F, Porcher R et al. Host defense and inflammatory gene polymorphisms are associated with outcomes after HLA-identical sibling bone marrow transplantation. Blood 2002;100(12):3908–3918
25. Takahashi H, Furukawa T, Hashimoto S et al. Contribution of TNF-alpha and IL-10 gene polymorphisms to graft-versus-host disease following allo-hematopoietic stem cell transplantation. Bone Marrow Transplant 2000;26(12):1317–1323
26. Petersdorf EW, Hansen JA, Martin PJ et al. Major-histocompatibility-complex class I alleles and antigens in hematopoietic-cell transplantation. N Engl J Med 2001;345(25):1794–1800
27. Petersdorf W, Kollman C, Hurley CK et al. Effect of HLA class II gene disparity on clinical outcome in unrelated donor hematopoietic cell transplantation for chronic myeloid leukemia: the US National Marrow Donor Program experience. Blood 2001;98(10):2922–2929
28. Dickinson AM, Wang XN, Sviland L et al. In situ dissection of the graft-versus-host activities of cytotoxic T cells specific for minor histocompatibility antigens. Nat Med 2002;8(4):410–414
29. Goulmy E, Schipper J, Pool J et al. Mismatches of minor histocompatibility antigens between HLA-identical donors and recipients and the development of graft-versus-host disease after bone marrow transplantation. N Engl J Med 1996;334:281–285
30. Kollman C, Howe CW, Anasetti C et al. Donor characteristics as risk factors in recipients after transplantation of bone marrow from unrelated donors: the effect of donor age. Blood 2001;98(7):2043–2051
31. Rufer N, Wolpert E, Helg C et al. HA-1 and the SMCY-derived peptide FIDSYICQV (H-Y) are immunodominant minor histocompatibility antigens after bone marrow transplantation. Transplantation 1998;66(7):910–916
32. Tseng L-H, Lin M-T, Hansen JA et al. Correlation between disparity for the minor histocompatibility antigen HA-1 and the development of acute graft-versus-host disease after allogeneic marrow transplantation. Blood 1999;94(8):2911–2914
33. Korngold R. Lethal graft-versus-host disease in mice directed to multiple minor histocompatibility antigens: features of CD8+ and CD4+ T cell responses. Bone Marrow Transplant 1992;9(5):355–364
34. Herrera C, Torres A, García-Castellano JM et al. Prevention of graft-versus-host disease in high risk patients by depletion of $CD4^+$ and reduction of $CD8^+$ lymphocytes in the marrow graft. Bone Marrow Transplant 1999;23:443–450
35. Martin PJ, Rowley SD, Anasetti C et al. A phase I-II clinical trial to evaluate removal of CD4 cells and partial depletion of CD8 cells from donor marrow for HLA-mismatched unrelated recipients. Blood 1999;94(7):2192–2199
36. Nimer SD, Giorgi J, Gajewski JL et al. Selective depletion of CD8+ cells for prevention of graft-versus-host disease after bone marrow transplantation. Transplantation 1994;57:82–87
37. Kernan NA. T-cell depletion for the prevention of graft-versus-host disease. In: Thomas ED, Blume KG, Forman SJ (eds) Hematopoietic cell transplantation, 2nd edn. Blackwell Science, Boston, 1999: 186–196
38. Soiffer RJ, Martin P. T-cell depletion of allogeneic hematopoietic stem cell grafts. In: Atkinson K, Champlin R, Brenner M et al (eds) Clinical bone marrow and blood stem cell transplantation: a reference book, 3rd edn. Cambridge University Press, Cambridge, UK, 2008
39. Healey G, Schwarer AP. The helper T lymphocyte precursor (HTLp) frequency does not predict outcome after HLA-identical sibling donor G-CSF-mobilised peripheral blood stem cell transplantation. Bone Marrow Transplant 2002;30(6):341–346
40. Keever-Taylor CA, Passweg J, Kawanishi Y et al. Association of donor-derived host-reactive cytolytic and helper T cells with outcome following alternative donor T cell-depleted bone marrow transplantation. Bone Marrow Transplant 1997;19(10):1001–1009
41. Kircher B, Niederwieser D, Gachter A et al. No predictive value of cytotoxic or helper T-cell precursor frequencies for outcome when analyzed from the graft after stem cell transplantation. Ann Hematol 2004;83(9):566–572
42. Pei J, Farrell C, Hansen J A et al. Evaluation of the limiting dilution cytotoxic T lymphocyte precursor frequency (fCTLp) assay in a multicenter study. In: Charron D (ed) HLA genetic diversity of HLA functional and medical implication, vol II. EDK, Paris, France, 1997: 577–579
43. Baron F, Baker JE, Storb R et al. Kinetics of engraftment in patients with hematologic malignancies given allogeneic hematopoietic cell transplantation after nonmyeloablative conditioning. Blood 2004;104(8):2254–2262
44. Weisdorf D, Hakke R, Blazar B et al. Risk factors for acute graft-versus-host disease in histocompatible donor bone marrow transplantation. Transplantation 1991;51:1197–1203
45. Bross DS, Tutschka PJ, Farmer ER et al. Predictive factors for acute graft-versus-host disease in patients transplanted with HLA-identical bone marrow. Blood 1984;63:1265–1270
46. Gale RP, Bortin MM, van Bekkum DW et al. Risk factors for acute graft-versus-host disease. Br J Haematol 1987;67:397–406
47. Hagglund H, Bostrom L, Remberger M et al. Risk factors for acute graft-versus-host disease in 291 consecutive HLA-identical bone marrow transplant recipients. Bone Marrow Transplant 1995;16(6):747–753
48. Nakai K, Mineishi S, Kami M et al. Antithymocyte globulin affects the occurrence of acute and chronic graft-versus-host disease after a reduced-intensity conditioning regimen by modulating mixed chimerism induction and immune reconstitution. Transplantation 2003;75(12):2135–2143
49. Nash RA, Pepe MS, Storb R et al. Acute graft-versus-host disease: analysis of risk factors after allogeneic marrow transplantation and prophylaxis with cyclosporine and methotrexate. Blood 1992;80:1838–1845
50. Przepiorka D, Smith TL, Folloder J et al. Risk factors for acute graft-versus-host disease after allogeneic blood stem cell transplantation. Blood 1999;94(4):1465–1470
51. Couriel DR, Saliba RM, Giralt S et al. Acute and chronic graft-versus-host disease after ablative and nonmyeloablative conditioning for allogeneic hematopoietic transplantation. Biol Blood Marrow Transplant 2004;10(3):178–185
52. Storb R, Prentice RL, Hansen JA et al. Association between HLA-B antigens and acute graft-versus-host disease. Lancet 1983;2:816–819
53. Baughan AS, Worsley AM, McCarthy DM et al. Haematological reconstitution and severity of graft-versus-host disease after bone marrow transplantation for chronic granulocytic leukaemia: the influence of previous splenectomy. Br J Haematol 1984;56(3):445–454
54. Gratama JW, Sinnige LGF, Zwaan FE et al. Marrow donor immunity to herpes simplex virus: association with acute graft-versus-host disease. Exp Hematol 1987;15:735–740
55. Seebach JD, Stussi G, Passweg JR et al. ABO blood group barrier in allogeneic bone marrow transplantation revisited. Biol Blood Marrow Transplant 2005;11(12):1006–1013
56. Handgretinger R, Klingebiel T, Lang P et al. Megadose transplantation of purified peripheral blood CD34(+) progenitor cells from HLA-mismatched parental donors in children. Bone Marrow Transplant 2001;27(8):777–783
57. Storb R, Blume KG, O'Donnell MR et al. Cyclophosphamide and antithymocyte globulin to condition patients with aplastic anemia for allogeneic marrow transplantations: the experience in four centers. Biol Blood Marrow Transplant 2001;7:39–44
58. Wagner JE, Thompson JS, Carter SL et al. Effect of graft-versus-host disease prophylaxis on 3-year disease-free survival in recipients of unrelated donor bone marrow (T-cell Depletion Trial): a multi-centre, randomised phase II-III trial. Lancet 2005;366(9487):733–741
59. Martin P, Nash R, Sanders J et al. Reproducibility in retrospective grading of acute graft-versus-host disease after allogeneic marrow transplantation. Bone Marrow Transplant 1998;21:273–279
60. Nash RA, Antin JH, Karanes C et al. Phase 3 study comparing methotrexate and tacrolimus with methotrexate and cyclosporine for prophylaxis of acute graft-versus-host disease after marrow transplantation from unrelated donors. Blood 2000;96(6):2062–2068
61. Rowlings PA, Przepiorka D, Klein JP et al. IBMTR Severity Index for grading acute graft-versus-host disease: retrospective comparison with Glucksberg grade. Br J Haematol 1997;97(4):855–864
62. Sullivan KM, Deeg HJ, Sanders J et al. Hyperacute graft-v-host disease in patients not given immunosuppression after allogeneic marrow transplantation (concise report). Blood 1986;67(4):1172–1175
63. Antin JH, Bierer BE, Smith BR et al. Selective depletion of bone marrow T lymphocytes with anti-CD5 monoclonal antibodies: Effective prophylaxis for graft-versus-host disease in patients with hematologic malignancies. Blood 1991;78:2139–2149
64. Lee CK, Gingrich RD, Hohl RJ et al. Engraftment syndrome in autologous bone marrow and peripheral stem cell transplantation. Bone Marrow Transplant 1995;16(1):175–182
65. Antin JH, Ferrara JL. Cytokine dysregulation and acute graft-versus-host disease. Blood 1992;80:2964–2968
66. Anderson BE, McNiff JM, Matte C et al. Recipient CD4+ T cells that survive irradiation regulate chronic graft-versus-host disease. Blood 2004;104(5):1565–1573
67. Spitzer TR. Engraftment syndrome following hematopoietic stem cell transplantation (review). Bone Marrow Transplant 2001;27(9):893–898
68. Crider MK, Jansen J, Norins AL et al. Chemotherapy-induced acral erythema in patients receiving bone marrow transplantation. Arch Dermatol 1986;122(9):1023–1027
69. Ruiz-Genao DP, Villalta MJ, Penas PF et al. Pustular acral erythema in a patient with acute graft-versus-host disease. J Eur Acad Dermatol Venereol 2003;17(5):550–553
70. Akpek G, Boitnott JK, Lee LA et al. Hepatitic variant of graft-versus-host disease after donor lymphocyte infusion. Blood 2002;100(12):3903–3907
71. Carreras E, Granena A, Navasa M et al. Transjugular liver biopsy in BMT. Bone Marrow Transplant 1993;11(1):21–26
72. Shulman HM, Gooley T, Dudley MD et al. Utility of transvenous liver biopsies and wedged hepatic venous pressure measurements in sixty marrow transplant recipients. Transplantation 1995;59(7):1015–1022
73. Kraus MD, Feran-Doza M, Garcia-Moliner ML et al. Cytomegalovirus infection in the colon of bone marrow transplantation patients. Mod Pathol 1998;11(1):29–36

74. Sale GE, Shulman HM, Hackman RC. Pathology of hematopoietic cell transplantation. In: Blume KG, Forman SJ, Appelbaum FR (eds) Thomas' hematopoietic cell transplantation. Blackwell Publishing, Oxford, 2004: 286–299
75. Weisdorf DJ, Snover DC, Haake R et al. Acute upper gastrointestinal graft-versus-host disease: clinical significance and response to immunosuppressive therapy. Blood 1990;76:624–629
76. Martin PJ, McDonald GB, Sanders JE et al. Increasingly frequent diagnosis of acute gastrointestinal graft-versus-host disease after allogeneic hematopoietic cell transplantation. Biol Blood Marrow Transplant 2004;10(5):320–327
77. Spencer GD, Hackman RC, McDonald GB et al. A prospective study of unexplained nausea and vomiting after marrow transplantation. Transplantation 1986;42:602–607
78. Wu D, Hockenbery DM, Brentnall TA et al. Persistent nausea and anorexia after marrow transplantation: a prospective study of 78 patients. Transplantation 1998;66(10): 1319–1324
79. Hockenbery DM, Cruickshank S, Rodell TC et al. A randomized, placebo-controlled trial of oral beclomethasone dipropionate as a prednisone-sparing therapy for gastrointestinal graft-versus-host disease. Blood 2007;109(10):4557–4563
80. Klein S A, Martin H, Schreiber-Dietrich D et al. A new approach to evaluating intestinal acute graft-versus-host disease by transabdominal sonography and colour Doppler imaging. Br J Haematol 2001;115(4):929–934
81. Mentzel HJ, Kentouche K, Kosmehl H et al. US and MRI of gastrointestinal graft-versus-host disease. Pediatr Radiol 2002;32(3):195–198
82. Watkins TR, Chien JW, Crawford SW. Graft versus host-associated pulmonary disease and other idiopathic pulmonary complications after hematopoietic stem cell transplant. Semin Respir Crit Care Med 2005;26(5):482–489
83. Ho VT, Weller E, Lee SJ et al. Prognostic factors for early severe pulmonary complications after hematopoietic stem cell transplantation (review). Biol Blood Marrow Transplant 2001;7(4):223–229
84. Beschorner WE, Saral R, Hutchins GM et al. Lymphocytic bronchitis associated with graft-versus-host disease in recipients of bone-marrow transplants. N Engl J Med 1978;299:1030–1036
85. Yanik G, Cooke KR. The lung as a target organ of graft-versus-host disease (review). Semin Hematol 2006;43(1):42–52
86. Greenspan A, Deeg HJ, Cottler-Fox M et al. Incapacitating peripheral neuropathy as a manifestation of chronic graft-versus-host disease. Bone Marrow Transplant 1990;5:349–352
87. Padovan CS, Bise K, Hahn J et al. Angiitis of the central nervous system after allogeneic bone marrow transplantation? Stroke 1999;30(8):1651–1656
88. Takatsuka H, Okamoto T, Yamada S et al. New imaging findings in a patient with central nervous system dysfunction after bone marrow transplantation. Acta Haematol 2000;103(4):203–205
89. Kohler S, Hendrickson MR, Chao NJ et al. Value of skin biopsies in assessing prognosis and progression of acute graft-versus-host disease. Am J Surg Pathol 1997;21(9):988–996
90. Massi D, Franchi A, Pimpinelli N et al. A reappraisal of the histopathologic criteria for the diagnosis of cutaneous allogeneic acute graft-vs-host disease. Am J Clin Pathol 1999;112(6):791–800
91. Zhou Y, Barnett MJ, Rivers JK. Clinical significance of skin biopsies in the diagnosis and management of graft-vs-host disease in early postallogeneic bone marrow transplantation. Arch Dermatol 2000;136(6):717–721
92. Sviland L, Pearson AD, Eastham EJ et al. Histological features of skin and rectal biopsy specimens after autologous and allogeneic bone marrow transplantation. J Clin Pathol 1988;41(2):148–154
93. Shulman HM, Sharma P, Amos D et al. A coded histologic study of hepatic graft-versus-host disease after human bone marrow transplantation. Hepatology 1988;8:463–470
94. Snover DC, Weisdorf SA, Ramsay NK et al. Hepatic graft versus host disease: A study of the predictive value of liver biopsy in diagnosis. Hepatology 1984;4:123–130
95. Przepiorka D, Weisdorf D, Martin P et al. 1994 Consensus conference on acute GVHD grading. Bone Marrow Transplant 1995;15(6):825–828
96. Cahn JY, Klein JP, Lee SJ et al. Prospective evaluation of 2 acute graft-versus-host (GVHD) grading systems: a joint Societe Francaise de Greffe de Moelle et Therapie Cellulaire (SFGM-TC), Dana Farber Cancer Institute (DFCI), and International Bone Marrow Transplant Registry (IBMTR) prospective study. Blood 2005;106(4):1495–1500
97. Vogelsang GB, Hess AD, Santos GW. Acute graft-versus-host disease: Clinical characteristics in the cyclosporine era. Medicine 1988;67(3):163–174
98. Remberger M, Kumlien G, Aschan J et al. Risk factors for moderate-to-severe chronic graft-versus-host disease after allogeneic hematopoietic stem cell transplantation. Biol Blood Marrow Transplant 2002;8(12):674–682
99. Leisenring WM, Martin PJ, Petersdorf E W et al. An acute graft-versus-host disease activity index to predict survival after hematopoietic cell transplantation with myeloablative conditioning regimens. Blood 2006;108(2):749–755
100. Saunders MD, Shulman HM, Murakami CS et al. Bile duct apoptosis and cholestasis resembling acute graft-versus-host disease after autologous hematopoietic cell transplantation. Am J Surg Pathol 2000;24(7):1004–1008
101. Hess AD, Horwitz L, Beschorner WE et al. Development of graft-vs.-host disease-like syndrome in cyclosporine-treated rats after syngeneic bone marrow transplantation. I. Development of cytotoxic T lymphocytes with apparent polyclonal anti-Ia specificity, including autoreactivity. J Exp Med 1985;161:718–730
102. Hess AD, Bright EC, Thoburn C et al. Specificity of effector T lymphocytes in autologous graft-versus-host disease: role of the major histocompatibility complex class II invariant chain peptide. Blood 1997;89(6):2203–2209
103. Nelson JL. Microchimerism: incidental byproduct of pregnancy or active participant in human health? Trends Mol Med 2002;8(3):109–113
104. Adams KM, Holmberg LA, Leisenring W et al. Risk factors for syngeneic graft-versus-host disease after adult hematopoietic cell transplantation. Blood 2004;104(6):1894–1897
105. Greenbaum BH. Transfusion-associated graft-versus-host disease: historical perspectives, incidence, and current use of irradiated blood products. J Clin Oncol 1991;9:1889–1902
106. Maris MB, Sandmaier BM, Storer BE et al. Allogeneic hematopoietic cell transplantation after fludarabine and 2 Gy total body irradiation for relapsed and refractory mantle cell lymphoma. Blood 2004;104(12):3535–3542
107. Gluckman E, Rocha V, Arcese W et al. Factors associated with outcomes of unrelated cord blood transplant: guidelines for donor choice. Exp Hematol 2004;32(4):397–407
108. Laughlin MJ, Eapen M, Rubinstein P et al. Outcomes after transplantation of cord blood or bone marrow from unrelated donors in adults with leukemia. N Engl J Med 2004;351(22):2265–2275
109. Heidt PJ, Vossen JM. Experimental and clinical gnotobiotics: influence of the microflora on graft-versus-host disease after allogeneic bone marrow transplantation (review). J Med 1992;23(3–4):161–173
110. Storb R, Prentice RL, Buckner CD et al. Graft-versus-host disease and survival in patients with aplastic anemia treated by marrow grafts from HLA-identical siblings. Beneficial effect of a protective environment. N Engl J Med 1983;308:302–307
111. Beelen DW, Elmaagacli A, Muller KD et al. Influence of intestinal bacterial decontamination using metronidazole and ciprofloxacin or ciprofloxacin alone on the development of acute graft-versus-host disease after marrow transplantation in patients with hematologic malignancies: final results and long-term follow-up of an open-label prospective randomized trial. Blood 1999;93(10):3267–3275
112. Guthery SL, Heubi JE Filipovich A. Enteral metronidazole for the prevention of graft versus host disease in pediatric marrow transplant recipients: results of a pilot study [erratum appears in Bone Marrow Transplant 2005;36(4):371]. Bone Marrow Transplant 2004;33(12):1235–1239
113. Marr KA, Seidel K, Slavin MA et al. Prolonged fluconazole prophylaxis is associated with persistent protection against candidiasis-related death and gut GVHD in allogeneic marrow transplant recipients: long-term follow-up of a placebo controlled trial. Blood 1999;94(suppl. 1)(10):394
114. Cooke KR, Gerbitz A, Crawford JM et al. LPS antagonism reduces graft-versus-host disease and preserves graft-versus-leukemia activity after experimental bone marrow transplantation. J Clin Invest 2001;107(12):1581–1589
115. Antin JH, Lee SJ, Neuberg D et al. A phase I/II double-blind, placebo-controlled study of recombinant human interleukin-11 for mucositis and acute GVHD prevention in allogeneic stem cell transplantation. Bone Marrow Transplant 2002;29:373–377
116. Antin JH, Weisdorf D, Neuberg D et al. Interleukin-1 blockade does not prevent acute graft-versus-host disease: results of a randomized, double-blind, placebo-controlled trial of interleukin-1 receptor antagonist in allogeneic bone marrow transplantation. Blood 2002;100(10):3479–3482
117. Vossen JM. Gnotobiotic measures for the prevention of acute graft-vs-host disease. In: Burakoff SJ, Deeg HJ, Ferrara J et al (eds) Graft-vs-host disease: immunology, pathophysiology, and treatment. Marcel Dekker, New York, 1990:403–414
118. Uphoff DE. Alteration of homograft reaction by A-methopterin in lethally irradiated mice treated with homologous marrow. Proc Soc Exp Biol Med 1958;99:651–653
119. Thomas ED, Storb R, Clift RA et al. Bone-marrow transplantation. N Engl J Med 1975;292(16, 17):832–843, 895–902
120. Sullivan KM, Storb R, Buckner CD et al. Graft-versus-host disease as adoptive immunotherapy in patients with advanced hematologic neoplasms. N Engl J Med 1989;320:828–834
121. Powles RL, Clink HM, Spence D et al. Cyclosporin A to prevent graft-versus-host disease in man after allogeneic bone-marrow transplantation. Lancet 1980;1:327–329
122. Fay JW, Wingard JR, Antin JH et al. FK506 (tacrolimus) monotherapy for prevention of graft-versus-host disease after histocompatible sibling allogeneic bone marrow transplantation. Blood 1996;87:3514–3519
123. Hiraoka A, Ohashi Y, Okamoto S et al. Phase III study comparing tacrolimus (FK506) with cyclosporine for graft-versus-host disease prophylaxis after allogeneic bone marrow transplantation. Japanese FK506 BMT Study Group. Bone Marrow Transplant 2001;28(2):181–185
124. Deeg HJ, Storb R, Weiden PL et al. Cyclosporin A and methotrexate in canine marrow transplantation: engraftment, graft-versus-host disease, and induction of tolerance. Transplantation 1982;34:30–35
125. Weisdorf DJ, Hurd D, Carter S et al. Prospective grading of graft-versus-host disease after unrelated donor marrow transplantation: a grading algorithm versus blinded expert panel review. Biol Blood Marrow Transplant 2003;9(8):512–518
126. Horowitz MM, Przepiorka D, Bartels P et al. Tacrolimus vs. cyclosporine immunosuppression: results in advanced-stage disease compared with historical controls treated exclusively with cyclosporine. Biol Blood Marrow Transplant 1999;5:180–186
127. Bolwell B, Sobecks R, Pohlman B et al. A prospective randomized trial comparing cyclosporine and short course methotrexate with cyclosporine and mycophenolate mofetil for GVHD prophylaxis in myeloablative allogeneic bone marrow transplantation. Bone Marrow Transplant 2004;34(7):621–625
128. Nash RA, Johnston L, Parker P et al. A phase I/II study of mycophenolate mofetil in combination with cyclosporine for prophylaxis of acute graft-versus-host disease after myeloablative conditioning and allogeneic hematopoietic cell transplantation. Biol Blood Marrow Transplant 2005;11:495–505
129. Deeg HJ, O'Donnell M, Tolar J et al. Optimization of conditioning for marrow transplantation from unrelated donors for patients with aplastic anemia after failure of immunosuppressive therapy. Blood 2006;108(5):1485–1491
130. Uberti JP, Ayash L, Braun T et al. Tacrolimus as monotherapy or combined with minidose methotrexate for graft-versus-host disease prophylaxis after allogeneic peripheral blood stem cell transplantation: long-term outcomes. Bone Marrow Transplant 2004;34(5):425–431
131. Przepiorka D, Khouri I, Ippoliti C et al. Tacrolimus and minidose methotrexate for prevention of acute graft-versus-host disease after HLA-mismatched marrow or blood stem cell transplantation. Bone Marrow Transplant 1999;24(7):763–768
132. Cutler C, Kim HT, Hochberg E et al. Sirolimus and tacrolimus without methotrexate as graft-versus-host disease prophylaxis after matched related donor peripheral blood stem cell transplantation. Biol Blood Marrow Transplant 2004;10(5):328–336

133. Antin JH, Kim HT, Cutler C et al. Sirolimus, tacrolimus, and low-dose methotrexate for graft-versus-host disease prophylaxis in mismatched related donor or unrelated donor transplantation. Blood 2003;102(5):1601–1605
134. Ramsay NK, Kersey JH, Robison LL et al. A randomized study of the prevention of acute graft-versus-host disease. N Engl J Med 1982;306:392–397
135. Bacigalupo A, Lamparelli T, Bruzzi P et al. Antithymocyte globulin for graft-versus-host disease prophylaxis in transplants from unrelated donors: 2 randomized studies from Gruppo Italiano Trapianti Midollo Osseo (GITMO). Blood 2001;98(10):2942–2947
136. Bacigalupo A, Lamparelli T, Barisione G et al. Thymoglobulin prevents chronic graft-versus-host disease, chronic lung dysfunction, and late transplant-related mortality: Long-term follow-up of a randomized trial in patients undergoing unrelated donor transplantation. Biol Blood Marrow Transplant 2006;12:560–565
137. Deeg HJ, Storer BE, Boeckh M et al. Reduced incidence of acute and chronic graft-versus-host disease with the addition of thymoglobulin to a targeted busulfan/cyclophosphamide regimen. Biol Blood Marrow Transplant 2006;12:573–584
138. Finke J, Schmoor C, Lang H et al. Matched and mismatched allogeneic stem-cell transplantation from unrelated donors using combined graft-versus-host disease prophylaxis including rabbit anti-T lymphocyte globulin. J Clin Oncol 2003;21(3):506–513
139. Remberger M, Svahn BM, Mattsson J et al. Dose study of thymoglobulin during conditioning for unrelated donor allogeneic stem-cell transplantation. Transplantation 2004;78(1):122–127
140. Russell JA, Tran HT, Quinlan D et al. Once-daily intravenous busulfan given with fludarabine as conditioning for allogeneic stem cell transplantation: study of pharmacokinetics and early clinical outcomes. Biol Blood Marrow Transplant 2002;8(9):468–476
141. Sokos DR, Berger M, Lazarus HM. Intravenous immunoglobulin: appropriate indications and uses in hematopoietic stem cell transplantation. Biol Blood Marrow Transplant 2002;8(3):117–130
142. Chakrabarti S, Hale G, Waldmann H. Alemtuzumab (Campath-1H) in allogeneic stem cell transplantation: where do we go from here? Transplant Proc 2004;36(5):1225–1227
143. Blaise D, Olive D, Hirn M et al. Prevention of acute GVHD by *in vivo* use of anti-interleukin-2 receptor monoclonal antibody (33B3.1): a feasibility trial in 15 patients. Bone Marrow Transplant 1991;8:105–111
144. Martin PJ, Pei J, Gooley T et al. Evaluation of a CD25-specific immunotoxin for prevention of graft-versus-host disease after unrelated marrow transplantation. Biol Blood Marrow Transplant 2004;10:552–560
145. Weisdorf D, Filipovich A, McGlave P et al. Combination graft-versus-host disease prophylaxis using immunotoxin (anti-CD5-RTA [Xomazyme-CD5]) plus methotrexate and cyclosporine or prednisone after unrelated donor marrow transplantation. Bone Marrow Transplant 1993;12:531–536
146. Papadopoulos EB, Carabasi MH, Castro-Malaspina H et al. T-cell-depleted allogeneic bone marrow transplantation as postremission therapy for acute myelogenous leukemia: freedom from relapse in the absence of graft-versus-host disease. Blood 1998;91:1083–1090
147. Guinan EC, Boussiotis VA, Neuberg D et al. Transplantation of anergic histoincompatible bone marrow allografts. N Engl J Med 1999;340(22):1704–1714
148. Cornelissen JJ, van der Holt B, Petersen EJ et al. A randomized multicenter comparison of CD34(+)-selected progenitor cells from blood vs from bone marrow in recipients of HLA-identical allogeneic transplants for hematological malignancies. Exp Hematol 2003;31(10):855–864
149. Arpinati M, Green CL, Heimfeld S et al. Granulocyte-colony stimulating factor mobilizes T helper 2-inducing dendritic cells. Blood 2000;95:2484–2490
150. Rissoan MC, Soumelis V, Kadowaki N et al. Reciprocal control of T helper cell and dendritic cell differentiation. Science 1999;283(5405):1183–1186
151. Ruutu T, Eriksson B, Remes K et al. Ursodeoxycholic acid for the prevention of hepatic complications in allogeneic stem cell transplantation. Blood 2002;100(6):1977–1983
152. MacMillan ML, Weisdorf DJ, Davies SM et al. Early antithymocyte globulin therapy improves survival in patients with steroid-resistant acute graft-versus-host disease. Biol Blood Marrow Transplant 2002;8(1):40–46
153. Martin PJ, Schoch G, Fisher L et al. A retrospective analysis of therapy for acute graft-versus-host disease: initial treatment. Blood 1990;76(8):1464–1472
154. Martin PJ, Schoch G, Fisher L et al. A retrospective analysis of therapy for acute graft-versus-host disease: secondary treatment. Blood 1991;77:1821–1828
155. van Lint MT, Uderzo C, Locasciulli A et al. Early treatment of acute graft-versus-host disease with high- or low-dose 6-methylprednisolone: a multicenter randomized trial from the Italian Group for Bone Marrow Transplantation. Blood 1998;92(7):2288–2293
156. van Lint MT, Milone G, Leotta S et al. Treatment of acute graft-versus-host disease with prednisolone: significant survival advantage for day +5 responders and no advantage for nonresponders receiving anti-thymocyte globulin. Blood 2006;107(10):4177–4181
157. Bertz H, Afting M, Kreisel W et al. Feasibility and response to budesonide as topical corticosteroid therapy for acute intestinal GVHD. Bone Marrow Transplant 1999;24(11):1185–1189
158. McDonald GB, Bouvier M, Hockenbery DM et al. Oral beclomethasone dipropionate for treatment of intestinal graft-versus-host disease: a randomized, controlled trial. Gastroenterology 1998;115(1):28–35
159. Ohashi Y, Minegishi M, Fujie H et al. Successful treatment of steroid-resistant severe acute GVHD with 24-h continuous infusion of FK506. Bone Marrow Transplant 1997;19(6):625–627
160. Furlong T, Storb R, Anasetti C et al. Clinical outcome after conversion to FK 506 (tacrolimus) therapy for acute graft-versus-host disease resistant to cyclosporine or for cyclosporine-associated toxicities. Bone Marrow Transplant 2000;26:985–991
161. Bacigalupo A, Oneto R, Lamparelli T et al. Pre-emptive therapy of acute graft-versus-host disease: a pilot study with antithymocyte globulin (ATG). Bone Marrow Transplant 2001;28(12):1093–1096
162. Graziani FV. Treatment of acute graft versus host disease with low dose-alternate day anti-thymocyte globulin. Haematologica 2002;87(9):973–978
163. Khoury H, Kashyap A, Brewster C et al. Anti-thymocyte globulin (ATG) for steroid-resistant acute graft-versus-host disease after allogeneic hematopoietic stem cell transplantation: a costly therapy with limited benefits. Blood 1999;94(suppl. 1)(10):668
164. Mollee P, Morton AJ, Irving I et al. Combination therapy with tacrolimus and anti-thymocyte globulin for the treatment of steroid-resistant acute graft-versus-host disease developing during cyclosporine prophylaxis. Br J Haematol 113(1):217–223
165. Benito AI, Furlong T, Martin PJ et al. Sirolimus (Rapamycin) for the treatment of steroid-refractory acute graft-versus-host disease. Transplantation 2001;72(12):1924–1929
166. Basara N, Blau WI, Romer E et al. Mycophenolate mofetil for the treatment of acute and chronic GVHD in bone marrow transplant patients. Bone Marrow Transplant 1998;22(1):61–65
167. van Oosterhout YV, van Emst L, Schattenberg AV et al. A combination of anti-CD3 and anti-CD7 ricin A-immunotoxins for the in vivo treatment of acute graft versus host disease. Blood 2000;95(12):3693–3701
168. Martin PJ, Nelson BJ, Appelbaum FR et al. Evaluation of a CD5-specific immunotoxin for treatment of acute graft-versus-host disease after allogeneic marrow transplantation. Blood 1996;88(3):824–830
169. Cragg L, Blazar BR, DeFor T et al. A randomized trial comparing prednisone with anti-thymocyte globulin/prednisone as an initial systemic therapy for moderately severe acute graft-versus-host disease. Biol Blood Marrow Transplant 2000;6(4A):441–447
170. Hebart H, Ehninger G, Schmidt H et al. Treatment of steroid-resistant graft-versus-host disease after allogeneic bone marrow transplantation with anti-CD3/TCR monoclonal antibodies. Bone Marrow Transplant 1995;15(6):891–894
171. Przepiorka D, Phillips GL, Ratanatharathorn V et al. A phase II study of BTI-322, a monoclonal anti-CD2 antibody, for treatment of steroid-resistant acute graft-versus-host disease. Blood 1998;92(11):4066–4071
172. Deeg HJ, Blazar BR, Bolwell BJ et al. Treatment of steroid-refractory acute graft-versus-host disease with anti-CD147 monoclonal antibody, ABX-CBL. Blood 2001;98(7):2052–2058
173. Carpenter PA, Appelbaum FR, Corey L et al. A humanized non-FcR-binding anti-CD3 antibody, visilizumab, for treatment of steroid-refractory acute graft-versus-host disease. Blood 2002;99(8):2712–2719
174. Carpenter PA, Lowder J, Johnston L et al. A phase II multicenter study of visilizumab, humanized anti-CD3 antibody, to treat steroid-refractory acute graft-versus-host disease. Biol Blood Marrow Transplant 2005;11:465–471
175. Hervé P, Wijdenes J, Bergerat JP et al. Treatment of corticosteroid resistant acute graft-versus-host disease by in vivo administration of anti-interleukin-2 receptor monoclonal antibody (B-B10). Blood 1990;75:1017–1023
176. Anasetti C, Hansen J A, Waldmann TA et al. Treatment of acute graft-versus-host disease with humanized anti-Tac: An antibody that binds to the interleukin-2 receptor. Blood 1994;84:1320–1327
177. Przepiorka D, Kernan NA, Ippoliti C et al. Daclizumab, a humanized anti-interleukin-2 receptor alpha chain antibody, for treatment of acute graft-versus-host disease. Blood 2000;95(1):83–89
178. Kobbe G, Schneider P, Rohr U et al. Treatment of severe steroid refractory acute graft-versus-host disease with infliximab, a chimeric human/mouse antiTNFalpha antibody. Bone Marrow Transplant 2001;28(1):47–49
179. Keane J, Gershon S, Wise RP et al. Tuberculosis associated with infliximab, a tumor necrosis factor alpha-neutralizing agent. N Engl J Med 2001;345(15):1098–1104
180. Besnier DP, Chabannes D, Mahé B et al. Treatment of graft-versus-host disease by extracorporeal photochemotherapy: a pilot study. Transplantation 1997;64(1):49–54
181. Dall'Amico R, Rossetti F, Zulian F et al. Photopheresis in paediatric patients with drug-resistant chronic graft-versus-host disease. Br J Haematol 1997;97(4):848–854
182. Greinix HT, Volc-Platzer B, Kalhs P et al. Extracorporeal photochemotherapy in the treatment of severe steroid-refractory acute graft-versus-host disease: a pilot study. Blood 2000;96(7):2426–2431
183. Biedermann BC, Sahner S, Gregor M et al. Endothelial injury mediated by cytotoxic T lymphocytes and loss of microvessels in chronic graft versus host disease. Lancet 2002;359(9323):2078–2083
184. Barao I, Hanash AM, Hallett W et al. Suppression of natural killer cell-mediated bone marrow cell rejection by CD4+CD25+ regulatory T cells. Proc Natl Acad Sci USA 2006;103(14):5460–5465
185. Hoffmann P, Ermann J, Edinger M et al. Donor-type CD4(+)CD25(+) regulatory T cells suppress lethal acute graft-versus-host disease after allogeneic bone marrow transplantation. J Exp Med 2002;196(3):389–399
186. Li L, Godfrey WR, Porter SB et al. CD4+CD25+ regulatory T-cell lines from human cord blood have functional and molecular properties of T-cell anergy. Blood 2005;106(9):3068–3073
187. Storb R, Deeg HJ, Pepe M et al. Methotrexate and cyclosporine versus cyclosporine alone for prophylaxis of graft-versus-host disease in patients given HLA-identical marrow grafts for leukemia: Long-term follow-up of a controlled trial. Blood 1989;73:1729–1734
188. Forman SJ, Blume KG, Krance RA et al. A prospective randomized study of acute graft-v-host disease in 107 patients with leukemia: Methotrexate/prednisone v cyclosporine A/prednisone. Transplant Proc 1987;19:2605–2607
189. Santos GW, Tutschka PJ, Brookmeyer R et al. Cyclosporine plus methylprednisolone versus cyclophosphamide plus methylprednisolone as prophylaxis for graft-versus-host disease: a randomized double-blind study in patients undergoing allogeneic marrow transplantation. Clin Transplant 1987;1:21–28
190. Storb R, Pepe M, Anasetti C et al. What role for prednisone in prevention of acute graft-versus-host disease in patients undergoing marrow transplants? Blood 1990;76:1037–1045
191. Chao NJ, Schmidt GM, Niland JC et al. Cyclosporine, methotrexate, and prednisone compared with cyclosporine and prednisone for prophylaxis of acute graft-versus-host disease. N Engl J Med 1993;329:1225–1230
192. Ratanatharathorn V, Nash RA, Przepiorka D et al. Phase III study comparing methotrexate and tacrolimus (Prograf, FK506) with methotrexate and cyclosporine for graft-versus-host-disease prophylaxis after HLA-identical sibling bone marrow transplantation. Blood 1998;92(7):2303–2314

193. Chao NJ, Snyder DS, Jain M et al. Equivalence of 2 effective graft-versus-host disease prophylaxis regimens: results of a prospective double-blind randomized trial. Biol Blood Marrow Transplant 2000;6(3):254–261

194. Ruutu T, Volin L, Parkkali T et al. Cyclosporine, methotrexate, and methylprednisolone compared with cyclosporine and methotrexate for the prevention of graft-versus-host disease in bone marrow transplantation from HLA-identical sibling donor: a prospective randomized study. Blood 2000;96(7):2391–2398

195. Doney KC, Weiden PL, Storb R et al. Treatment of graft-versus-host disease in human allogeneic marrow graft recipients: a randomized trial comparing antithymocyte globulin and corticosteroids. Am J Hematol 1981;11:1–8

196. Kennedy MS, Deeg HJ, Storb R et al. Treatment of acute graft-versus-host disease after allogeneic marrow transplantation: randomized study comparing corticosteroids and cyclosporine. Am J Med 1985;78:978–983

197. Hings IM, Filipovich AH, Miller WJ et al. Prednisone therapy for acute graft-versus-host disease: short- versus long-term treatment. A prospective randomized trial. Transplantation 1993;56(3):577–580

198. Cahn JY, Bordigoni P, Tiberghien P et al. Treatment of acute graft-versus-host disease with methylprednisolone and cyclosporine with or without an anti-interleukin-2 receptor monoclonal antibody. A multicenter phase III study. Transplantation 1995;60(9):939–942

199. Lee SJ, Zahrieh D, Agura E et al. Effect of up-front daclizumab when combined with steroids for the treatment of acute graft-versus-host disease: results of a randomized trial. Blood 2004;104(5):1559–1564

200. Furlong T, Leisenring W, Storb R et al. Psoralen and ultraviolet A irradiation (PUVA) as therapy for steroid-resistant cutaneous acute graft-versus-host disease. Biol Blood Marrow Transplant 2002;8:206–212

201. Wetzig T, Sticherling M, Simon JC et al. Medium dose long-wavelength ultraviolet A (UVA1) phototherapy for the treatment of acute and chronic graft-versus-host disease of the skin. Bone Marrow Transplant 2005;35(5):515–519

202. Couriel D, Hosing C, Saliba R et al. Extracorporeal photopheresis for acute and chronic graft-versus-host disease: does it work? Biol Blood Marrow Transplant 2006;12(1)(suppl 2):37–40

203. Couriel D, Saliba R, Hicks K et al. Tumor necrosis factor-alpha blockade for the treatment of acute GVHD. Blood 2004;104(3):649–654

204. Patriarca F, Sperotto A, Damiani D et al. Infliximab treatment for steroid-refractory acute graft-versus-host disease. Haematologica 2004;89(11):1352–1359

205. Wolff D, Roessler V, Steiner B et al. Treatment of steroid-resistant acute graft-versus-host disease with daclizumab and etanercept. Bone Marrow Transplant 2005;35(10):1003–1010

206. Ho VT, Zahrieh D, Hochberg E et al. Safety and efficacy of denileukin diftitox in patients with steroid-refractory acute graft-versus-host disease after allogeneic hematopoietic stem cell transplantation. Blood 2004;104(4):1224–1226

207. Massenkeil G, Rackwitz S, Genvresse I et al. Basiliximab is well tolerated and effective in the treatment of steroid-refractory acute graft-versus-host disease after allogeneic stem cell transplantation. Bone Marrow Transplant 2002;30(12):899–903

208. Jacobsohn DA, Vogelsang GB. Novel pharmacotherapeutic approaches to prevention and treatment of GVHD. Drugs 2002;62(6):879–889

209. Peters C, Minkov M, Gadner H et al. Statement of current majority practices in graft-versus-host disease prophylaxis and treatment in children. Bone Marrow Transplant 2000;26(4):405–411

210. Bolanos-Meade J, Jacobsohn D, Anders V et al. Pentostatin in steroid-refractory chronic graft-versus-host disease. Blood 2005;106(Part 1)(11):513

211. Margolis J, Vogelsang G. An old drug for a new disease: pentostatin (Nipent) in acute graft-versus-host disease. Semin Oncol 2000;27(2 suppl 5):72–77

Chronic graft-versus-host disease

Mary ED Flowers and H Joachim Deeg

Introduction

Chronic graft-versus-host disease (GvHD) is the major determinant of late non-relapse morbidity and mortality after allogeneic hematopoietic cell transplantation (HCT).[1,2] Chronic GvHD is associated with decreased quality of life (QOL), impaired functional status, and prolonged treatment with immunosuppressive agents,[3-6] but it also has a potent effect on eradicating malignant cells via the associated graft-versus-tumor (GvT) effect.[7-9] The incidence of chronic GvHD varies from 20% to 85%, depending on factors such as the stem cell source (blood stem cells versus marrow versus umbilical cord), donor type and other characteristics (previously pregnant female versus male donor), age (older versus younger), and others. Increasing rates of chronic GvHD in the past decades have been influenced by several factors including:

- decreased early transplant-related mortality (less toxic conditioning, more effective immunosuppressive prophylaxis of acute GvHD, improved infection control and less advanced diseases at transplant resulting in increased survival)
- transplantation for older recipients and with older donors
- increased use of peripheral blood as a source of stem cells
- expansion of donor pool (unrelated, mismatched)
- use of donor lymphocyte infusion (DLI) after HCT.

While prevention and treatment of *acute* GvHD have improved over the past three decades, similar progress in chronic GvHD has remained elusive.

Risk factors

Risk factors for the development of chronic GvHD

Previously reported risk factors for the development of chronic GvHD include preceding acute GvHD, older patient age, the use of female donors for male recipients, use of DLI, use of unrelated or HLA-mismatched donors, and, more recently, the use of granulocyte colony-stimulating factor (G-CSF) mobilized peripheral blood cells as opposed to marrow as a source of stem cells.[10-18]

Risk factors associated with increased non-relapse mortality

Factors associated with an increased risk of non-relapse mortality among patients with chronic GvHD include: involvement of multiple (organ) sites, clinical performance score, thrombocytopenia (platelet count <100,000/μl), progressive onset of chronic GvHD from prior acute GvHD, hyperbilirubinemia, and extent of skin involvement at the time of diagnosis, among others.[19-23] More recently, results of a multivariate retrospective analysis of 751 patients with chronic GvHD[24] confirmed that thrombocytopenia and hyperbilirubinemia of more than 2 mg/dl at the time of diagnosis of chronic GvHD were significantly associated with increased non-relapse mortality. Additional risk factors, including HLA mismatching, older patient age and use of older donors, were also identified. In addition, patients receiving higher doses of prednisone immediately before the diagnosis of chronic GvHD was established were found to have the highest risk of non-relapse mortality.[24] All the previously reported studies taken together indicate that characteristics consistently associated with an increased risk of non-relapse mortality among patients with chronic GvHD are thrombocytopenia and progressive onset of chronic GvHD from acute GvHD.

Risk factors and disease characteristics associated with duration of therapy for chronic GvHD

Risk factors and disease characteristics associated with the duration of immunosuppressive treatment for chronic GvHD have been examined in retrospective and randomized studies.[24-28] Results of at least one randomized study indicated the need for longer duration of prednisone treatment for chronic GvHD after transplantation of blood stem cells as compared to bone marrow cells.[25] Results of a multivariate analysis in a large retrospective cohort of patients with chronic GvHD also showed that immunosuppressive treatment was required for prolonged periods of time in patients who received peripheral blood cells, as well as in male patients with female donors, in patients with HLA mismatching in the graft-versus-host direction, and in patients with hyperbilirubinemia or multiple sites affected by chronic GvHD at the onset of disease.[24] Discontinuation of immunosuppressive therapy in the absence of recurrent malignancy has been used as a surrogate endpoint indicating resolution of chronic GvHD.[24-28]

Diagnosis and grading severity

Chronic GVHD can affect multiple organs or sites (Fig. 39.1). Advances in HCT and a better understanding of chronic GvHD have contributed to the refinement of the diagnosis of this syndrome first reported several decades ago.[21,29] Chronic GvHD presents with manifestations that may resemble scleroderma, Sjögren's syndrome, wasting syndrome, primary biliary cirrhosis, bronchiolitis obliterans, immune cytopenias, and chronic immunodeficiency disorders.[30,31] Chronic GvHD occurs virtually exclusively within 3 years after HCT, and approximately 50% of the patients are diagnosed within 6 months of transplantation. Manifestations of chronic GvHD can begin before day 100 after the transplant, and 'classic' manifestations of acute GvHD may develop, persist or recur long after day 100, for example after non-myeloablative HCT.[32] Moreover, chronic and acute GvHD features may present simultaneously, especially after DLI.[33] New criteria to categorize acute and chronic GvHD (Table 39.1) have been developed by the National Institutes of Health (NIH) Chronic GvHD Consensus Group that take into consideration the characteristic signs and symptoms of chronic GvHD (Table 39.2).[34]

How to diagnose chronic GvHD: proposed new criteria[34]

Signs and symptoms of chronic GvHD have been reviewed to standardize criteria for diagnosis and classification of chronic GvHD (see Table 39.2). The clinical diagnosis of chronic GvHD has no time restrictions and requires the presence of at least one *diagnostic* clinical sign of chronic GvHD (e.g. lichen planus-like features, sclerotic features, poikiloderma or esophageal web) or the presence of at least one *distinctive* manifestation (e.g. keratoconjunctivitis sicca, depigmentation) confirmed by pertinent biopsy or other relevant tests (e.g. Schirmer's test) in the same or other organs (see Table 39.2). Thus, the diagnosis of chronic GvHD requires the following:

- distinction from acute GvHD (see Table 39.1)
- presence of at least one diagnostic clinical manifestation *or* presence of at least one distinct manifestation confirmed by pertinent biopsy or other relevant tests (see Table 39.2)
- exclusion of other possible diagnoses that could account for the manifestation (e.g. infection, drug effect, others).

Histologic confirmation is necessary in the absence of diagnostic clinical or distinctive features confirmed by other pertinent tests (see Table 39.2).

How to score severity of chronic GvHD in each organ: proposed new scoring system[34]

A new scoring system (0–3) has been proposed to grade the severity of chronic GvHD in each organ or site, taking functional impact into account.[34] The pulmonary score uses both symptoms and pulmonary function testing (PFT) scale whenever possible (Table 39.3). When discrepancies exist between pulmonary symptoms and PFT scores, the higher value should be used for final scoring. Scoring by lung function score (LFS) is preferred, but if DLCO (carbon monoxide diffusion capacity corrected for hemoglobin) is not available, grading should be based on FEV1 (forced expiratory volume). The LFS is a global assessment of lung function after the diagnosis of bronchiolitis obliterans has already been established.[34] The percentage predicted FEV1 and DLCO (adjusted for hemoglobin but not alveolar volume) should be converted to a numeric score as follows:

$\geq$80% = 1; 70–79% = 2; 60–69% = 3; 50–59% = 4; 40–49% = 5; <40% = 6.

The LFS = FEV1 score + DLCO score, with a possible range of 2–12.

How to score global severity of chronic GvHD: proposed new classification[34]

Manifestations of chronic GvHD may be restricted to a single organ or site or may be widespread. Historically, chronic GvHD was classified as 'limited' or 'extensive' based on a small cohort of patients reported more than two decades ago.[21,29] Over time, this widely adopted chronic GvHD classification has shown its limitations.[30,34] A new global scoring system of chronic GvHD has been proposed by the NIH consensus group according to the numbers of organs involved and the degree of involvement in affected organs/sites (Table 39.4).[34]

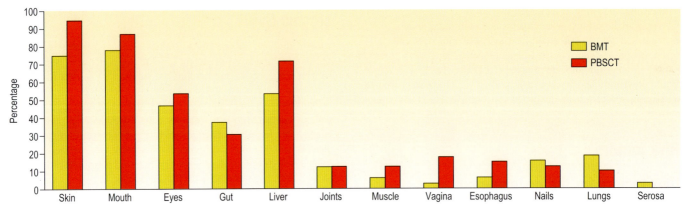

Figure 39.1
Sites affected by chronic GvHD after peripheral blood stem cell transplantation (PBSCT) compared to bone marrow transplantation (BMT). Skin and vaginal involvement was more prevalent after PBSCT. Columns show the proportions of patients with organs affected by chronic GvHD at any time. (This figure was originally published in *Blood*.[26] © The American Society of Hematology.)

Table 39.1 Categories of acute and chronic graft-versus-host disease

Category	Time of symptoms after HCT or DLI	Presence of acute GvHD features	Presence of chronic GvHD features[a]
Acute GvHD			
Classic acute GvHD	≤100 days	Yes	No
Persistent, recurrent or late-onset acute GvHD	>100 days	Yes	No
Chronic GvHD			
Classic chronic GvHD	No time limit	No	Yes
Overlap syndrome	No time limit	Yes	Yes

Abbreviations: HCT, hematopoietic stem cell transplant; DLI, donor lymphocyte infusion.
[a] See Table 39.2 for chronic GvHD features.

Table 39.2 Signs and symptoms of chronic graft-versus-host disease

Organ or site	Diagnostic (sufficient to establish the diagnosis of chronic GvHD)	Distinctive (seen in chronic GvHD but insufficient alone to establish a diagnosis of chronic GvHD)	Other features[a]	Common (seen with both acute and chronic GvHD)
Skin	• Poikiloderma • Lichen planus-like features • Sclerotic features • Morphea-like features • Lichen sclerosus-like features	• Depigmentation	• Sweat impairment • Ichthyosis • Keratosis pilaris • Hypopigmentation • Hyperpigmentation	• Erythema • Maculopapular rash • Pruritus
Nails		• Dystrophy • Longitudinal ridging, splitting or brittle features • Onycholysis • Pterygium unguis • Nail loss[b] (usually symmetric, affects most nails)		
Scalp and body hair		• New onset of scarring or non-scarring scalp alopecia, (after recovery from chemoradiotherapy) • Scaling, papulosquamous lesions	• Thinning scalp hair, typically patchy, coarse or dull (not explained by endocrine or other causes) • Premature gray hair	
Mouth	• Lichen-type features • Hyperkeratotic plaques • Restriction of mouth opening from sclerosis	• Xerostomia • Mucocele • Mucosal atrophy • Pseudomembranes[b] • Ulcers[b]		• Gingivitis • Mucositis • Erythema • Pain
Eyes		• New-onset dry, gritty or painful eyes[c] • Cicatricial conjunctivitis • Keratoconjunctivitis sicca[c] • Confluent areas of punctate keratopathy	• Photophobia • Periorbital hyperpigmentation • Blepharitis (erythema of the eyelids with edema)	
Genitalia	• Lichen planus-like features • Vaginal scarring or stenosis	• Erosions[b] • Fissures[b] • Ulcers[b]		
GI tract	• Esophageal web • Strictures or stenosis in the upper to mid third of the esophagus[b]		• Exocrine pancreatic insufficiency	• Anorexia • Nausea • Vomiting • Diarrhea • Weight loss/failure to thrive (children)
Liver				• Total bilirubin, alkaline phosphatase >2 × upper limit of normal[b] • ALT or AST >2 × upper limit of normal[b]
Lung	• Bronchiolitis obliterans diagnosed with lung biopsy	• Bronchiolitis obliterans diagnosed with PFTs and radiology[c]		• BOOP
Muscles, fascia, joints	• Fasciitis • Joint stiffness or contractures secondary to sclerosis	• Myositis or polymyositis[c]	• Edema • Muscle cramps • Arthralgia or arthritis	
Hematopoietic and immune systems			• Thrombocytopenia • Eosinophilia • Lymphopenia • Hypo- or hyper- gammaglobulinemia • Autoantibodies (AIHA, ITP)	
Other			• Pericardial or pleural effusions • Ascites • Peripheral neuropathy • Nephrotic syndrome • Myasthenia gravis • Cardiac conduction abnormality or cardiomyopathy	

[a] Can be acknowledged as part of the chronic GvHD features if diagnosis is confirmed.

[b] In all cases, infection, drug effect, malignancy or other causes must be excluded.

[c] Diagnosis of chronic GvHD requires biopsy or radiologic confirmation, or Schirmer's test for eyes (Schirmer's test with a mean value ≤5 mm (average of both eyes) at 5 minutes, or mean values of 6–10 mm in patients with keratoconjunctivitis sicca symptoms by slit-lamp examination), or pulmonary function tests for lungs.

Abbreviations: AIHA, autoimmune hemolytic anemia; ALT, alanine aminotransferase; AST, aspartate aminotransferase; BOOP, bronchiolitis obliterans organizing pneumonia; ITP, idiopathic thrombocytopenic purpura; GvHD, graft-versus-host disease; PFTs, pulmonary function tests. (Adapted with permission from Filipovich et al.[34])

Table 39.3 Chronic GvHD scoring scale to assess severity for each organ or site

	SCORE 0	SCORE 1	SCORE 2	SCORE 3
PERFORMANCE SCORE: KPS ECOG LPS	Asymptomatic and fully active (ECOG 0; KPS or LPS 100%)	Symptomatic, fully ambulatory, restricted only in physically strenuous activity (ECOG 1, KPS or LPS 80–90%)	Symptomatic, ambulatory, capable of self-care, >50% of waking hours out of bed (ECOG 2, KPS or LPS 60–70%)	Symptomatic, limited self-care, >50% of waking hours in bed (ECOG 3–4, KPS or LPS <60%)
SKIN *Diagnostic/ distinctive features:* ☐ Present ☐ Absent **% BSA____**	No symptoms	<18% BSA with disease signs but **NO** sclerotic features	19–50% BSA **OR** involvement with superficial sclerotic features 'not hidebound' (able to pinch)	>50% BSA **OR** deep sclerotic features 'hidebound' (unable to pinch) **OR** impaired mobility, ulceration or severe pruritus
MOUTH *Diagnostic/distinctive features* ☐ Present ☐ Absent	No symptoms	Mild symptoms with disease signs but not limiting oral intake significantly	Moderate symptoms with disease signs **with** partial limitation of oral intake	Severe symptoms with disease signs on examination **with** major limitation of oral intake
EYES Mean tear test (mm): ☐ >10 ☐ 6–10 ☐ ≤ 5 ☐ Not done	No symptoms	Mild dry eye symptoms not affecting ADL (requiring eyedrops <3 × per day) **OR** asymptomatic signs of keratoconjunctivitis sicca	Moderate dry eye symptoms partially affecting ADL (requiring drops >3 × per day or punctal plugs) **WITHOUT** vision impairment	Severe dry eye symptoms significantly affecting ADL (special eyewear to relieve pain) **OR** unable to work because of ocular symptoms **OR** loss of vision caused by keratoconjunctivitis sicca
GI TRACT	No symptoms	Symptoms such as nausea, vomiting, anorexia, dysphagia, abdominal pain or diarrhea without significant weight loss (<5%)	Symptoms associated with mild-to-moderate weight loss (5–15%)	Symptoms associated with significant weight loss >15%, requires nutritional supplement for most calorie needs **OR** esophageal dilation
LIVER	Normal LFT	Elevated bilirubin, AP, AST or ALT <2 × ULN	Bilirubin >3 mg/dl or bilirubin, enzymes 2–5 × ULN	Bilirubin or enzymes >5 × ULN
LUNGS *Pulmonary function test* **FEV1** **DLCO**	No symptoms FEV1 >80% **OR** LFS 2[a]	Mild symptoms (shortness of breath after climbing one flight of steps) FEV1 60–79% **OR** LFS 3–5[a]	Moderate symptoms (shortness of breath after walking on flat ground) FEV1 40–59% **OR** LFS 6–9[a]	Severe symptoms (shortness of breath at rest; requiring O_2) FEV1 <39% **OR** LFS 10–12[a]
JOINTS AND FASCIA	No symptoms	Mild tightness of arms or legs, normal or mild decreased range of motion (ROM) **AND** not affecting ADL	Tightness of arms or legs **OR** joint contractures, erythema thought due to fasciitis, moderate decrease ROM **AND** mild to moderate limitation of ADL	Contractures **WITH** significant decrease of ROM **AND** significant limitation of ADL (unable to tie shoes, button shirts, dress self, etc.)
GENITAL TRACT *Diagnostic/distinctive features:* ☐ Present ☐ Absent ☐ Not examined	No symptoms	Symptomatic with mild signs on exam **AND** no effect on coitus and minimal discomfort with gynecologic exam	Symptomatic with moderate signs on exam **AND** with mild dyspareunia or discomfort with gynecologic exam	Symptomatic **WITH** advanced signs (stricture, labial agglutination or severe ulceration) **AND** severe pain with coitus or inability to insert vaginal speculum

Abbreviations: ADL, activities of daily living; ALT, alanine aminotransferase; AP, alkaline phosphatase; AST, aspartate aminotransferase; BSA, body surface area; ECOG, Eastern Co-operative Oncology Group; KPS, Karnofsky Performance Status; LPS, Lansky Performance Status; LFS, lung function score; LFTs, liver function tests; ULN, upper limit of normal.
[a]See text for details regarding LFS. (Adapted with permission from Filipovich et al.[34])

Table 39.4 New proposed categorization of chronic GvHD: global severity[34]

Category	Numbers of organs	Maximum severity in all organs (scores according to Table 39.3)
Mild	≤2	1 (0 for lung)
Moderate (a)	≥3	1 (0 for lung)
Moderate (b)	Any	2 (1 for lung)
Severe	Any	3 (2 for lung)

The new global score of chronic GvHD (mild, moderate or severe) has been developed to replace the historical 'extensive/limited' classification.

Treatment

Optimal care of patients with chronic GvHD requires a multidisciplinary approach. Chronic GvHD can lead to debilitating conse-

quences, e.g. joint contractures, loss of sight, end-stage lung disease, psychologic impact, and increased mortality due to profound chronic immune dysregulation associated with GvHD or related to systemic treatment resulting in recurrent or life-threatening infections. Left untreated, fewer than 20% of patients with chronic GvHD survive without disability.[29] Karnofsky or Lansky clinical performance scores below 60%, weight loss of 15% or more, and recurrent infections are usually signs of poorly controlled chronic GvHD.

Indications for systemic treatment are summarized in Table 39.5. Topical therapy is often sufficient for patients with *mild* chronic GvHD unless they have platelet counts less than 100,000/μl or are receiving glucocorticoid treament already at the onset of chronic GvHD. Table 39.6 summarizes selected randomized trials reported for *primary* treatment of chronic GvHD, and Table 39.7 summarizes selected reports for *secondary* treatment of chronic GvHD.

Standard systemic treatment of chronic GvHD usually begins with daily administration of glucocorticoids (1 mg/kg) followed by a taper to an alternate-day regimen (Table 39.8), with or without daily ciclosporin or tacrolimus. The median duration of systemic treatment for

Table 39.5 Indications for systemic treatment of chronic GvHD

Chronic GVHD category	High risk[a]	Systemic therapy
Mild	No	No
Mild	Yes	Yes[b]
Moderate	Yes or No	Yes[b]
Severe	Yes or No	Yes

[a] High risk defined as thrombocytopenia (<100,000/μl) or receiving glucocorticoids at the onset of chronic GvHD.
[b] The benefit of graft-versus-leukemia/tumor effect versus the risk of delaying systemic treatment for chronic GvHD needs to be weighed based also on the risk of recurrent malignancy after transplantation.

chronic GvHD has been reported at 3.1 years after peripheral blood stem cell transplantation and 1.7 years after bone marrow transplantation.[24] Factors associated with duration of immunosuppressive treatment are presented under the Risk Factors section above. Approximately 40% of patients (who survive without relapse) require systemic immunosuppression for at least 4 years from the initial diagnosis of chronic GvHD. Enrollment in clinical trials should always be considered because current 'standard' therapies are associated with high morbidity and decreased survival in patients with high-risk chronic GvHD.

Table 39.6 Primary therapy for chronic GvHD: summary of results of selected randomized trials

Treatment	No. of patients per arm	Comments/conclusions	Reference
Prednisone (PDN) versus PDN + azathioprine	63/63	*Standard risk[a]* 40% in each arm had subclinical disease. No difference in response rate. Lower survival in the azathioprine arm (47% vs 61%) due to more infections	22
PDN versus PDN + ciclosporin (CSP)	145/142	*Standard risk[a]* No differences in transplant-related mortality, recurrence of malignancy, secondary therapy for chronic GvHD and discontinuation of all immunosuppressive therapy between the two arms. Disease-free survival was lower in the combination arm. Avascular necrosis was less frequent in the combination arm	27
PDN + CSP or tacrolimus (Tac) versus PDN + CSP or Tac + thalidomide	26/26	*Thrombocytopenia and progressive onset only (high risk)* Closed early after interim analysis showed slow accrual and only 42% probability of reaching statistical significance by enrolling remainder of patients. No difference in 3-year survival (47% vs 49%)	36
PDN + CSP + versus PDN + CSP + thalidomide	24/27	*50% high risk in each arm* Closed early after interim analysis showed slow accrual and higher response rates in both arms than projected. No significant difference in 2-year survival (54% vs 66%)	37

[a] Defined as platelet count equal to or above 100,000/μl.

Table 39.7 Summary of selected reports of secondary therapy for chronic GvHD

Treatment	No. of patients	Response rate		Survival (%) /follow-up[a]	Reference
		Complete	Overall[a]		
High-dose methylprednisolone	56	48%		81% 2-yr	38
Ciclosporin	21	52%	71%	67% 4-yr	39
Tacrolimus	39	35%		64% 3-yr	40
Mycophenolate mofetil Children only	26 15	8% 13%	46% 60%		41 42
Sirolimus	35	17%	63%	41%/3-yr	43
Extracorporeal photopheresis	71	14%	61%	51%/1-yr	44
	25	0%	64%		45
	15	80%	Skin response		46
Psoralen and UVA (PUVA)	11–40	40%	78%		47, 48, 49, 50, 51
Thalidomide	14–80	3–42%	20–71%		52, 53, 54, 55, 56
Hydroxychloroquine	32	9%	50%		57
Clofazimine	22		55%		58
Rituximab Case report	21	10%	70%		59 60
Ursodeoxycholic acid	12		33%		61
Etretinate (no longer available)	27		74%		62
2-deoxycoformycin	42		50%		63

Total lymphoid radiation (1 Gy)
    Reported in abstracts
    Case reports
	38		42%		64, 65
					66, 67

Etanercept	Case series				68
Intravenous lidocaine	Case report				69

[a] Where available.

Table 39.8 Standard '9 months' glucocorticoid treatment of chronic GvHD

Week	Dose of prednisone (mg/kg)
1–2	1.0 daily
3	1.0 alternating with 0.5 qod
4	1.0 alternating with 0.25 qod
5	1.0 alternating with 0.12 qod
6	1.0 alternating with 0.06 qod
7–20	1.0 qod
21–24	Taper within 4 weeks to 0.5 qod
25–40	0.5 qod
	After resolution of all reversible manifestations, taper prednisone by 10% every 2–4 weeks as tolerated

Abbreviations: qod, every other day.

Monitoring, ancillary treatment and supportive care

Close monitoring is necessary for early detection of chronic GvHD manifestations, to allow prompt institution or change of treatment and other supportive measures so as to prevent the serious outcome associated with advanced GvHD. Regular clinical assessment using the scoring system described in Table 39.3 can be helpful in identifying early manifestations of chronic GvHD. For instance, early fasciitis or sclerotic skin features of chronic GvHD can be recognized clinically by identifying declines in wrist extension ability (Buddha's hands praying position) or by identifying new rippling or grooving in the skin appearance (often more prominent with arms extended laterally and upwards). A subtle, lacy appearance of the oral mucosa can easily be detected and is often the first manifestation of chronic GvHD.

Antibiotic prophylaxis for encapsulated bacterial infections, *Pneumocystis jirovecii*, herpes zoster, and monitoring for late cytomegalovirus infections are necessary in patients treated for chronic GvHD.

A comprehensive review of ancillary therapy, supportive care, and monitoring of chronic GvHD was developed recently by the NIH consensus group.[35] These guidelines include recommendations for management of symptoms, prevention of severe manifestation, infections prophylaxis, and prevention and management of common treatment complications. Specific dispensary guidelines on ancillary care of chronic GvHD can be obtained at the American Society for Blood and Marrow Transplant website: www.asbmt.org/GvHDforms/.

Summary

Chronic GvHD is a frequent complication after allogeneic hematopoietic cell transplantation. The incidence has increased over the past decade and has not decreased with the use of reduced-intensity conditioning regimens. Management of patients with a multidisciplinary approach has enhanced treatment efficacy and reduced morbidity. New classification schemes should facilitate comparison of results obtained in different studies. The recent consensus development and collaborative efforts are expected to improve the management of chronic GvHD.

Acknowledgment

Supported by PHS grants HL36444, CA18029, and CA15704.

References

1. Goerner M, Gooley T, Flowers ME et al. Morbidity and mortality of chronic GVHD after hematopoietic stem cell transplantation from HLA-identical siblings for patients with aplastic or refractory anemias. Biol Blood Marrow Transplant 2002;8:47–56
2. Lee SJ, Klein JP, Barrett AJ et al. Severity of chronic graft-versus-host disease: association with treatment-related mortality and relapse. Blood 2002;100:406–414
3. Duell T, van Lint MT, Ljungman P et al. Health and functional status of long-term survivors of bone marrow transplantation. EBMT Working Party on Late Effects and EULEP Study Group on Late Effects. European Group for Blood and Marrow Transplantation. Ann Intern Med 1997;126:184–192
4. Socié G, Stone JV, Wingard JR et al. Long-term survival and late deaths after allogeneic bone marrow transplantation. Late Effects Working Committee of the International Bone Marrow Transplant Registry. N Engl J Med 1999;341:14–21
5. Sutherland HJ, Fyles GM, Adams G et al. Quality of life following bone marrow transplantation: a comparison of patient reports with population norms. Bone Marrow Transplant 1997;19:1129–1136
6. Syrjala KL, Chapko MK, Vitaliano PP et al. Recovery after allogeneic marrow transplantation: prospective study of predictors of long-term physical and psychosocial functioning. Bone Marrow Transplant 1993;11:319–327
7. Horowitz MM, Gale RP, Sondel PM et al. Graft-versus-leukemia reactions after bone marrow transplantation. Blood 1990;75:555–562
8. Sullivan KM, Weiden PL, Storb R et al. Influence of acute and chronic graft-versus-host disease on relapse and survival after bone marrow transplantation from HLA-identical siblings as treatment of acute and chronic leukemia. Blood 1989;73:1720–1728
9. Weiden PL, Sullivan KM, Flournoy N et al. Antileukemic effect of chronic graft-versus-host disease. Contribution to improved survival after allogeneic marrow transplantation. N Engl J Med 1981;304:1529–1533
10. Atkinson K, Horowitz MM, Gale RP et al. Risk factors for chronic graft-versus-host disease after HLA-identical sibling bone marrow transplantation. Blood 1990;75:2459–2464
11. Carlens S, Ringden O, Remberger M et al. Risk factors for chronic graft-versus-host disease after bone marrow transplantation: a retrospective single centre analysis. Bone Marrow Transplant 1998;22:755–761
12. Cutler C, Giri S, Jeyapalan S et al. Acute and chronic graft-versus-host disease after allogeneic peripheral-blood stem-cell and bone marrow transplantation: a meta-analysis. J Clin Oncol 2001;19:3685–3691
13. Kollman C, Howe CW, Anasetti C et al. Donor characteristics as risk factors in recipients after transplantation of bone marrow from unrelated donors: the effect of donor age. Blood 2001;98:2043–2051
14. Kondo M, Kojima S, Horibe K et al. Risk factors for chronic graft-versus-host disease after allogeneic stem cell transplantation in children. Bone Marrow Transplant 2001;27:727–730
15. Ochs LA, Miller WJ, Filipovich AH et al. Predictive factors for chronic graft-versus-host disease after histocompatible sibling donor bone marrow transplantation. Bone Marrow Transplant 1994;13:455–460
16. Przepiorka D, Anderlini P, Saliba R et al. Chronic graft-versus-host disease after allogeneic blood stem cell transplantation. Blood 2001;98:1695–1700
17. Ringden O, Paulin T, Lonnqvist B et al. An analysis of factors predisposing to chronic graft-versus-host disease. Exp Hematol 1985;13:1062–1067
18. Storb R, Prentice RL, Sullivan KM et al. Predictive factors in chronic graft-versus-host disease in patients with aplastic anemia treated by marrow transplantation from HLA-identical siblings. Ann Intern Med 1983;98:461–466
19. Akpek G, Lee SJ, Flowers ME et al. Performance of a new clinical grading system for chronic graft-versus-host disease: a multi-center study. Blood 2003;102:802–809
20. Arora M, Burns LJ, Davies SM et al. Chronic graft-versus-host disease: a prospective cohort study. Biol Blood Marrow Transplant 2003;9:38–45
21. Shulman HM, Sullivan KM, Weiden PL et al. Chronic graft-versus-host syndrome in man. A long-term clinicopathologic study of 20 Seattle patients. Am J Med 1980;69:204–217
22. Sullivan KM, Witherspoon RP, Storb R et al. Prednisone and azathioprine compared with prednisone and placebo for treatment of chronic graft-versus-host disease: prognostic influence of prolonged thrombocytopenia after allogeneic marrow transplantation. Blood 1988;72:546–554
23. Wingard JR, Piantadosi S, Vogelsang GB et al. Predictors of death from chronic graft versus host disease after bone marrow transplantation. Blood 1989;74:1428–1435
24. Stewart BL, Storer B, Storek J et al. Duration of immunosuppressive treatment for chronic graft-versus-host disease. Blood 2004;104:3501–3506
25. Flowers ME. Emerging strategies in the treatment of chronic graft-versus-host disease: traditional treatment of chronic graft-versus-host disease (symposium report). Blood Marrow Transplant Rev 2002;12:5–8
26. Flowers ME, Parker PM, Johnston LJ et al. Comparison of chronic graft-versus-host disease after transplantation of peripheral blood stem cells versus bone marrow in allogeneic recipients: long-term follow-up of a randomized trial. Blood 2002;100:415–419
27. Koc S, Leisenring W, Flowers ME et al. Therapy for chronic graft-versus-host disease: a randomized trial comparing ciclosporin plus prednisone versus prednisone alone. Blood 2002;100:48–51
28. Lee JH, Lee JH, Choi SJ et al. Graft-versus-host disease (GVHD)-specific survival and duration of systemic immunosuppressive treatment in patients who developed chronic GVHD following allogeneic haematopoietic cell transplantation. Br J Hematol 2003;122:637–644
29. Sullivan KM, Shulman HM, Storb R et al. Chronic graft-versus-host disease in 52 patients: adverse natural course and successful treatment with combination immunosuppression. Blood 1981;57:267–276
30. Lee SJ, Vogelsang G, Flowers ME. Chronic graft-versus-host disease. Biol Blood Marrow Transplant 2003;9:215–233
31. Sullivan KM. Graft-vs.-host disease. In: Blume KG, Forman SJ, Appelbaum FR (eds) Thomas' hematopoietic cell transplantation, 3rd edn.. Blackwell Publishing, Oxford, 2004:635–664

32. Mielcarek M, Martin PJ, Leisenring W et al. Graft-versus-host disease after nonmyeloablative versus conventional hematopoietic stem cell transplantation. Blood 2003;102: 756–762

33. Flowers ME, Leisenring W, Beach K et al. Granulocyte colony-stimulating factor given to donors before apheresis does not prevent aplasia in patients treated with donor leukocyte infusion for recurrent chronic myeloid leukemia after bone marrow transplantation. Biol Blood Marrow Transplant 2000;6:321–326

34. Filipovich AH, Weisdorf D, Pavletic S et al. National Institutes of Health consensus development project on criteria for clinical trials in chronic graft-versus-host disease: I. Diagnosis and Staging Working Group report. Biol Blood Marrow Transplant 2005;11: 945–956

35. Couriel D, Carpenter PA, Cutler C et al. Ancillary therapy and supportive care of chronic graft-versus-host disease: National Institutes of Health consensus development project on criteria for clinical trials in chronic graft-versus-host disease: V. Ancillary Therapy and Supportive Care Working Group report. Biol Blood Marrow Transplant 2006;12:375–396

36. Koc S, Leisenring W, Flowers ME et al. Thalidomide for treatment of patients with chronic graft-versus-host disease. Blood 2000;96:3995–3996

37. Arora M, Wagner JE, Davies SM et al. Randomized clinical trial of thalidomide, ciclosporin, and prednisone versus ciclosporin and prednisone as initial therapy for chronic graft-versus-host disease. Biol Blood Marrow Transplant 2001;7:265–273

38. Akpek G, Lee SM, Anders V et al. A high-dose pulse steroid regimen for controlling active chronic graft-versus-host disease. Biol Blood Marrow Transplant 2001;7: 495–502

39. Sullivan KM, Witherspoon RP, Storb R et al. Alternating-day ciclosporin and prednisone for treatment of high-risk chronic graft-versus-host disease. Blood 1988;72:555–561

40. Carnevale-Schianca F, Martin P, Sullivan K et al. Changing ciclosporin to tacrolimus as salvage therapy for chronic graft-versus-host disease. Biol Blood Marrow Transplant 2000;6:613–620

41. Mookerjee B, Altomonte V, Vogelsang G. Salvage therapy for refractory chronic graft-versus-host disease with mycophenolate mofetil and tacrolimus. Bone Marrow Transplant 1999;24:517–520

42. Busca A, Saroglia EM, Lanino E et al. Mycophenolate mofetil (MMF) as therapy for refractory chronic GVHD (cGVHD) in children receiving bone marrow transplantation. Bone Marrow Transplant 2000;25:1067–1071

43. Couriel DR, Saliba R, Escalon MP et al 2005 Sirolimus in combination with tacrolimus and corticosteroids for the treatment of resistant chronic graft-versus-host disease. Br J Hematol 2005;130:409–417

44. Couriel DR, Hosing C, Saliba R et al. Extracorporeal photochemotherapy for the treatment of steroid-resistant chronic GVHD. Blood 2006;107:3074–3080

45. Foss FM, DiVenuti GM, Chin K et al. Prospective study of extracorporeal photopheresis in steroid-refractory or steroid-resistant extensive chronic graft-versus-host disease: analysis of response and survival incorporating prognostic factors. Bone Marrow Transplant 2005;35:1187–1193

46. Greinix HT, Volc-Platzer B, Rabitsch W et al. Successful use of extracorporeal photochemotherapy in the treatment of severe acute and chronic graft-versus-host disease. Blood 1998;92:3098–3104

47. Eppinger T, Ehninger G, Steinert M et al. 8-methoxypsoralen and ultraviolet A therapy for cutaneous manifestations of graft-versus-host disease. Transplantation 1990;50: 807–811

48. Jampel RM, Farmer ER, Vogelsang GB et al. PUVA therapy for chronic cutaneous graft-vs-host disease. Arch Dermatol 1991;127:1673–1678

49. Kapoor N, Pelligrini AE, Copelan EA et al. Psoralen plus ultraviolet A (PUVA) in the treatment of chronic graft versus host disease: Preliminary experience in standard treatment resistant patients. Semin Hematol 1992;29:108–112

50. Redding SW, Callander NS, Haveman CW et al. Treatment of oral chronic graft-versus-host disease with PUVA therapy: case report and literature review (review). Oral Surg Oral Medi Oral Pathol Oral Radiol Endodont 1998;86:183–187

51. Vogelsang GB, Wolff D, Altomonte V et al. Treatment of chronic graft-versus-host disease with ultraviolet irradiation and psoralen (PUVA). Bone Marrow Transplant 1996;17:1061–1067

52. Browne PV, Weisdorf DJ, DeFor T et al. Response to thalidomide therapy in refractory chronic graft-versus-host disease. Bone Marrow Transplant 2000;26:865–869

53. Flowers ME, Martin PJ. Evaluation of thalidomide for treatment or prevention of chronic graft-versus-host disease. Leuk Lymphoma 2003;44:1141–1146

54. Parker PM, Chao N, Nademanee A et al. Thalidomide as salvage therapy for chronic graft-versus-host disease. Blood 1995;86:3604–3609

55. Rovelli A, Arrigo C, Nesi F et al. The role of thalidomide in the treatment of refractory chronic graft-versus-host disease following bone marrow transplantation in children. Bone Marrow Transplant 1998;21:577–581

56. Vogelsang GB, Farmer ER, Hess AD et al 1992 Thalidomide for the treatment of chronic graft versus host disease. N Engl J Med 1992;326:1055–1058

57. Gilman AL, Chan KW, Mogul A et al. Hydroxychloroquine for the treatment of chronic graft-versus-host disease. Biol Blood Marrow Transplant 2000;6(3A):327–334

58. Lee SJ, Wegner SA, McGarigle CJ et al. Treatment of chronic graft-versus-host disease with clofazimine. Blood 1997;89:2298–2302

59. Cutler C, Miklos D, Kim HT et al. Rituximab for steroid-refractory chronic graft-versus-host disease. Blood 2006;108:756–762

60. Ratanatharathorn V, Carson E, Reynolds C et al. Anti-CD20 chimeric monoclonal antibody treatment of refractory immune-mediated thrombocytopenia in a patient with chronic graft-versus-host disease. Ann Intern Med 2000;133:275–279

61. Fried RH, Murakami CS, Fisher LD et al. Ursodeoxycholic acid treatment of refractory chronic graft-versus-host of the liver. Ann Intern Med 1992;116:624–629

62. Marcellus DC, Altomonte VL, Farmer ER et al. Etretinate therapy for refractory sclerodermatous chronic graft-versus-host disease. Blood 1999;93:66–70

63. Bolanos-Meade J, Jacobsohn D, Anders V et al. Pentostatin in steroid-refractory chronic graft-versus-host disease. Blood 2005;106 (Part 1):513

64. Devergie A, Girinski T, Socié G et al. Immunosuppressive treatment with 1 Gy lymphoid irradiation for the treatment of severe chronic graft versus host disease. Blood 1996;88 (Part 1):644

65. Fung HC, Voss NJ, Barnett MJ et al. Low dose thoraco-abdominal irradiation for treatment of advanced chronic graft-versus-host disease. Blood 1995;86(suppl 1):390

66. Bullorsky EO, Shanley CM, Stemmelin GR et al. Total lymphoid irradiation for treatment of drug resistant chronic GVHD. Bone Marrow Transplant 1993;11:75–76

67. Socié G, Devergie A, Cosset JM et al. Low-dose (one gray) total-lymphoid irradiation for extensive, drug-resistant chronic graft-versus-host disease. Transplantation 1990;49: 657–658

68. Chiang KY, Abhyankar S, Bridges K et al. Recombinant human tumor necrosis factor receptor fusion protein as complementary treatment for chronic graft-versus-host disease. Transplantation 2002;73:665–667

69. Voltarelli JC, Ahmed H, Paton EJ et al. Beneficial effect of intravenous lidocaine in cutaneous chronic graft-versus-host disease secondary to donor lymphocyte infusion. Bone Marrow Transplant 2001;28:97–99

Management of relapse and minimal residual disease after stem cell allotransplantation

CHAPTER 40

Stephan Mielke and A John Barrett

Introduction

It is unfortunately the case that disease relapse is the most common cause of treatment failure following allogeneic stem cell transplantation (SCT). Data from the Center for International Blood and Marrow Transplant Research (CIBMTR) on transplants performed worldwide from 1998 to 2002 show that 38% of deaths after matched related transplants and 32% of deaths after matched unrelated transplants are from disease relapse (Fig. 40.1).[1]

Disease type and stage of disease at transplant are major factors influencing post-transplant relapse.[2] First chronic phase chronic myeloid leukemia (CML) and first remission acute leukemias carry the lowest chances for post-transplant relapse, while blastic-phase CML or refractory acute leukemias have the highest chances of relapsing. In addition to these factors, the transplant itself influences the outcome. The occurrence of graft-versus-host disease (GvHD) is associated with a lower risk for relapse,[3] while T-cell depletion carries a higher risk of relapse.[4] Although the introduction of reduced-intensity conditioning (RIC) regimens has helped to diminish transplant-related mortality (TRM),[5] relapse rates appear to be increased as compared to those seen after full-intensity conditioning regimens.[6]

In general, but with some notable exceptions, disease recurrence after SCT carries a poor prognosis,[2] reflecting the fact that subsequent treatment attempts are less effective than the transplant itself, designed as it is to be the best single attempt to cure the malignancy. The curative potential of allogeneic SCT relies on the conditioning regimen which debulks the malignant disease, followed by a continuing immunologically based graft-versus-leukemia (GvL) effect which, in successful cases, eliminates residual disease.[7] In reality, post-transplant immunosuppression, used to prevent severe GvHD, deprives the allograft of its full antileukemia potential, thereby favoring disease re-occurrence.

Minimal residual disease (MRD) can be tracked post transplant by molecular or flow cytometric screening, permitting early detection of relapse (Table 40.1).[8] Here, we describe the features of residual disease and relapsed hematologic malignancies, the methods used to monitor disease post SCT and the results of treatment, and provide guidelines for management of relapse.

Patterns of relapse

Figure 40.2 illustrates the possible outcomes of hematologic disease after allogeneic SCT. Acute leukemias usually have the most rapid recurrence, with relapse occurring as soon as a month from transplant, whereas patients with more chronic diseases (such as CML, chronic lymphatic leukemia (CLL), myeloma or lymphoma) show a slower evolution. Monitoring for MRD is more useful in these latter conditions, providing the opportunity for therapeutic intervention before overt clinical and hematologic manifestation of the disease. Timing is a major factor determining the prognosis of relapse: the longer after transplant the relapse occurs, the greater the prospect for a second attempt at disease control or cure.[9] This is partly related to disease pace but is also because the patient who has recovered from the initial transplant complications is more likely to tolerate intensive treatments such as chemotherapy, donor lymphocyte infusions (DLI) or a second transplant.[10]

Other factors which may determine outcome include whether the relapse is local or generalized and also individual susceptibility of the relapsed disease to chemotherapy or immunotherapy. Extramedullary relapse following allogeneic stem cell transplantation may occur in both lymphoid and myeloid malignancies.[11] Breast, testis and gut are common sites for acute myeloid leukemia (AML) extramedullary relapse. In CML patients, paravertebral chloromas have been described frequently. The acute lymphoblastic leukemia (ALL) sanctuary sites of CNS and testis are prone to extramedullary relapse post SCT. However, the disease can also spread in the lymph nodes and lymphatic organs, mimicking lymphoblastoid lymphoma. Critical to treatment decision making is whether the extramedullary relapse is isolated or whether the bone marrow is also involved.[12] It is much safer to assume that the extramedullary relapse is the tip of the iceberg of relapsed disease, and in most situations local treatment of the relapse should be accompanied by systemic treatment.

Relapse in donor cells

Up to 5% of all relapses may occur in transformed donor cells.[13] Donor relapse mimicking the original disease phenotype is described in both acute and chronic leukemias. The mechanism is unknown but the phenomenon implicates both an inherited susceptibility to leukemia in related donor–recipient pairs and a recipient milieu favoring the induction of leukemia. Relapse in donor cells is managed similarly to relapse of recipient leukemia.

Relapse and the immunologic milieu

Relapses occurring while the donor immune system is compromised by immunosuppression present an opportunity for initial immunotherapeutic intervention to boost the GvL effect by withdrawal of immunosuppression, whereas relapse in the context of full donor immune competence or tolerance accompanying mixed donor–recipient chimerism invites treatments to reset alloimmune effects with DLI[7] or a second transplant.[10] Relapses occurring in the presence of GvHD

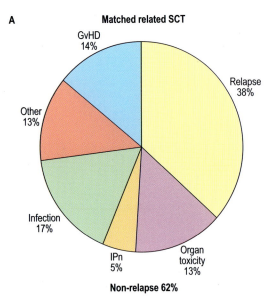

A Matched related SCT

- Relapse 38%
- GvHD 14%
- Other 13%
- Infection 17%
- IPn 5%
- Organ toxicity 13%

Non-relapse 62%

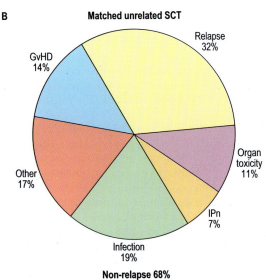

B Matched unrelated SCT

- Relapse 32%
- GvHD 14%
- Other 17%
- Infection 19%
- IPn 7%
- Organ toxicity 11%

Non-relapse 68%

Figure 40.1
CIBMTR data (1998–2002): causes of death after matched sibling and matched unrelated transplants. Data from Pasquini & Nugent.[1] (Reprinted with permission from CIBMTR.)

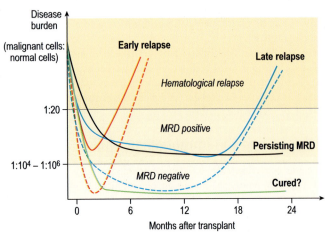

Disease burden (malignant cells: normal cells)

- Early relapse
- Late relapse
- Hematological relapse
- 1:20
- MRD positive
- $1:10^4 – 1:10^6$
- Persisting MRD
- MRD negative
- Cured?

Months after transplant (0, 6, 12, 18, 24)

Figure 40.2
Schematic pattern of relapse after allogeneic SCT.

Table 40.1 Common targets for MRD screening in different malignancies

Disease	MRD target
Myelodysplastic syndrome (MDS)	del(5q), monosomy 7, trisomy 8
Chronic myeloid leukemia (CML)	t(9;22) [p210]
Acute myeloid leukemia (AML)	t(8;21), inv(16)
Acute lymphoblastoid leukemia (B-ALL)	t(9;22) [p190, p210], FC
Acute lymphoblastoid leukemia (T-ALL)	t(4;11), t(8;14), TCR rearrangement, FC
Follicular lymphoma	t(14;18) IgH rearrangement
Mantle cell lymphoma	t(11;14), IgH rearrangement
Chronic lymphatic leukemia (CLL)	del(13q), del(11q), del (17p), trisomy 12
Multiple myeloma	del(13q), del(11q), IgH rearrangement

TCR, T-cell receptor; IgH, immunoglobulin heavy chain; FC, flow cytometry.

suggest that immune manipulation is unlikely to be successful in controlling the malignancy, largely precluding immune manipulations such as DLI.[10] Leukemia relapsing uniquely in extramedullary sites may represent a local escape from the GvL effect, but little is known currently about the relationship between immune sanctuaries and local relapse.

Relapse and marrow function

The quality of donor-derived marrow function is also critical in determining appropriate treatment options. Relapsing disease usually presents within at least a partially functioning donor marrow. Donor hematologic recovery is therefore possible without stem cell rescue. Nevertheless, reduced-intensity chemotherapy is advisable in relapses occurring within 3 months of SCT. In contrast, in CML the relapsing marrow progressively supplants donor hematopoiesis, leading to complete extinction of donor hematopoietic progenitors (but not of cellular immunity). In the absence of donor-derived marrow cells, treatment of the CML or advanced stages of acute leukemias with DLI may cause marrow failure because normal donor stem cells are lacking.[14,15] Growth factor support with granulocyte colony-stimulating factor (G-CSF) or stem cell rescue is advisable for patients with low levels of residual donor hematopoiesis measured by myeloid lineage-specific chimerism.

Diagnosis of persistent or recurrent disease

Low levels of malignant disease, undetected by conventional clinical or morphologic methods, are referred to as minimal residual disease (MRD). MRD can be identified by using molecular[16] or flow cytometric techniques.[17] The allogeneic setting further allows detection of residual or recurrent disease by linage-specific chimerism analysis performed using molecular techniques.[18] Techniques used to detect relapse are listed in Table 40.2. In cases of suspected extramedullary relapse a tissue biopsy is essential for proper diagnosis and differentiation from other causes such as Epstein–Barr virus (EBV) lymphomas (of donor origin).

Prospective post-transplant monitoring for MRD

The purpose of monitoring MRD after SCT is to track disease disappearance or, if disease burden increases, to start therapeutic interventions at the stage when they are most likely to be effective. Conventional cytogenetic studies have only a small place in disease monitoring because they are insensitive. Fluorescence in situ hybridization (FISH) using fluorescent probes binding to specific DNA sequences visualizes chromosomal aberrations with a detection level of 1 malignant cell in 100–1000 cells.[19,20] Flow cytometry reliably detects 1 malignant in 10,000 normal cells but may approach the sensitivity of polymerase chain reaction (PCR)-based assays if sufficient cells are acquired.[17] The PCR detects altered gene sequences specific for the malignant clone with a detection level as low as 1 malignant cell per 10^5 to 10^6 cells. Both genomic DNA and mRNA can be used as a source of genetic material.[16] When using genomic DNA for conventional PCR assays, results are reported as number of malignant cells in 100,000 total cells. Real-time PCR results are expressed as a percentage respective to a housekeeping gene such as *G6PD* or *abl*, expressed by normal and malignant cells. Clonal evolution with loss of phenotypes leading to false-negative results is a limitation to the measurement of MRD. Because of the diversity of techniques in use, MRD is best tracked by a single test in the same laboratory.[21]

Most clinical experience for monitoring MRD comes from the detection of CML cells using PCR for *bcr/abl* fusion transcripts. The prognostic impact of persisting *bcr/abl* transcripts in patients up to 6 months after allogeneic SCT is still subject to controversial discussion[22,23] while long-persisting transcript levels of *bcr/abl* appear to be associated with increased risk of relapse.[24] In about half of all patients with AML, specific translocations such as t(8;21) or inv(16) can be detected and used for MRD monitoring after allogeneic SCT.[16] In most patients with mantle cell lymphoma, PCR for the translocation t(11;14) can be used. In follicular lymphoma the use of molecular monitoring for t(14;18) translocations is compromised by the occurrence of t(14;18) cells in healthy controls.[16] As an alternative, follicular lymphoma can be molecularly screened for clone-specific heavy chain (IgH) rearrangement (which can be used in all B-cell malignancies).

Despite an abundance of these leukemia- and lymphoma-specific markers, many malignancies lack useful molecular markers to track MRD. Flow cytometric MRD diagnosis is useful in T-ALL using the marker combination CD3/CD5+ /CD34/TdT+ unique to leukemic T-cells.[17] Flow cytometry is only useful for B-ALL aberrantly co-expressing myeloid markers such as CD13 or CD33 with CD19+. Flow cytometric MRD diagnostics for AML can be challenging and usually targets early progenitor markers in context with the over- or underexpression of regularly present myeloid markers.[17]

Monitoring donor–recipient chimerism

In sex-mismatched transplants, FISH analysis of the sex chromosomes (XY-FISH) can be used for chimerism analysis. In all allogeneic SCT, PCR can be used to measure distinct donor and recipient patterns of highly polymorphic repetitive DNA sequences – either short tandem repeats (STR) or variable number of tandem repeats (VNTR) – to distinguish between donor and host.[18] When all analyzed cells are of donor origin, donor chimerism is full. Mixed chimerism refers to the co-existence of host and donor cells expressed as percentages. The detection limit for a minor population detected by STR- or VNTR-based chimerism is about 1%. More information can be obtained if chimerism is separately analyzed in lymphoid and myeloid cells rather than on whole blood or bone marrow (lineage-specific chimerism). Cells are selected by sorting or by magnetic separation using monoclonal antibodies against T-cell (e.g. CD3) or myeloid antigens (e.g. CD14/15). Lineage-specific chimerism analysis allows tracking of myeloid engraftment separately from lymphocyte engraftment. In a standard transplant, mature donor lymphocytes are transferred with the stem cells, promoting proper engraftment by controlling residual host-derived lymphocytes which could reject the allograft. Following successful engraftment, hematopoiesis is restored from the donor-derived lymphocytes. In RIC regimens, the transplanter is often confronted with the difficulties of interpreting mixed myeloid and lymphocyte chimerism resulting from the incomplete ablation of host marrow and lymphoid system characteristic of non-myeloablative conditioning.[8]

Beside important information about myeloid and lymphoid engraftment, lineage-specific chimerism screening may provide warning signs of impending relapse. Unfortunately, the sensitivity of chimerism analysis is not sufficient to be substituted for MRD diagnostics and thus its predictive value is low. Nevertheless, falling myeloid chimerism in a myeloid malignancy can reflect recurrence of disease, heralding hematologic relapse. The analysis of T-cell chimerism in the case of relapse or MRD makes it possible to determine whether the relapse is taking place in the presence or absence of donor immune cells.

Management of disease relapse

The outlook for many patients with relapsed leukemia following SCT is so poor that before any active treatment is pursued, a frank discussion with the patient and family is necessary to define likely outcomes and treatment objectives. Patients who have received intense attention during their transplant period can find it hard to adapt to the reality that further treatment may be ineffective, and thus it is important to emphasize to the patient that they are not being abandoned even if it is possible only to give supportive care. Aside from supportive care, active treatment revolves around the combination of three strategies: immunotherapy, chemotherapy, and molecular therapies (Fig. 40.3).

Table 40.2 Techniques used to detect relapse

Type of relapse	Material	Diagnostic tool
Minimal residual disease (MRD)	Peripheral blood, bone marrow biopsy	PCR, FISH, cytogenetics, flow cytometry
Dropping, lineage-specific chimerism	Peripheral blood, bone marrow biopsy	STR-PCR, VNTR-PCR, XY-FISH, after cell selection
Hematologic relapse	Peripheral blood, bone marrow biopsy	Cytology, (immuno)histology
Extramedullary relapse	Biopsy, punctuate	Clinical, radioimaging, cytology, histology

PCR, polymerase chain reaction; FISH, fluorescence in situ hybridization; STR, short tandem repeats; VNTR, variable number of tandem repeats.

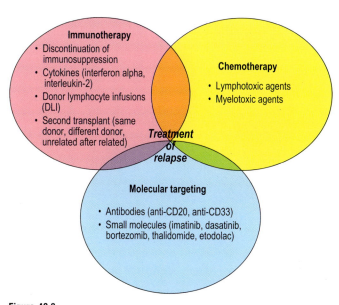

Figure 40.3
Components of relapse treatment after allografting.

Immunotherapy

Immunotherapy can be given in a series of graded steps of increasing complexity and risk: removal of immunosuppression and boosting alloreactivity, DLI, lymphoablation followed by DLI, and second stem cell transplant. However, since alloreactivity against relapsed disease overlaps with GvHD, the development of this complication is a likely consequence of all these maneuvers and may need treatment.

Withdrawal of immunosuppression

The graft alloimmune effect can be enhanced by reducing or stopping immunosuppression. GvL effects induced by removal of ciclosporin[25] or addition of cytokines[26] have been documented but these reports do not extend beyond anecdotal examples.

DLI

Since the first observation by Kolb and colleagues that DLI were effective in the treatment of relapsed CML,[7] there is now a broad experience in the use of this strategy in every form of relapsed malignancy. At best, DLI can induce permanent remissions of disease – notably in CML.[7] In other diseases, the beneficial effect is more often short-lived or incomplete, and in the majority of early relapses in acute leukemia, ineffective (Fig. 40.4). The dose of DLI given to HLA-identical recipients ranges between 1×10^6 and 1×10^8 CD3+ lymphocytes per kilogram body weight. The risk of GvHD is greatest from DLI given within 3 months of transplantation, and at least a low-dose calcineurin inhibitor is recommended to mitigate against the high risk of severe GvHD which can occur with the lowest DLI dose. In later relapses the strategy usually taken is to stop all immunosuppression and transfuse a series of DLI of increasing cell dose, given at least 6 weeks apart, until either GvHD prevents further escalation or the disease responds.

In the treatment of CML relapse, there are data supporting a dose of 10^7 CD3+ cells/kg as an optimum, capable of inducing remission while carrying a relatively low risk of GvHD.[27] Most investigators have adopted similar schedules for treatment of relapse in other conditions. In relapsed CML, the response to DLI has been found to be dose dependent.[28] In HLA-mismatched individuals, DLI should be used with extreme caution. Doses of CD3 cells as low as 10^4/kg are likely to induce severe GvHD, albeit with some GvL effect.

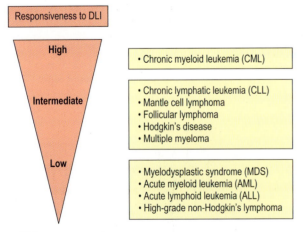

Figure 40.4
Schematic diagram illustrating the responsiveness of relapse to DLI treatment as estimated by probability to induce durable responses. Within a disease significant differences may apply with respect to stage and disease-specific risk factors (e.g. blastic-phase CML has usually low and accelerated-phase CML intermediate responsiveness to DLI).

DLI with adjuvant treatments

It has recently been appreciated that DLI given after a patient has been rendered lymphopenic create a more powerful alloimmune response, due to the incoming lymphocytes. Again, while the GvL effect may be enhanced by the prior administration of lymphosuppressive treatment (e.g. fludarabine 30 mg/m²/d for 3–5 days) there is a high risk of causing acute GvHD, even with DLI doses of around 10^6 CD3+ cells/kg. Alternatively, attempts have been made to boost GvL by enhancing antigen presentation of the malignancy with interferon-α (upregulates MHC) or GM-CSF (promotes antigen presentation by dendritic cells).

Second allografts

Second transplants can be used both as stem cell replacement to allow myeloablative treatment for the relapse and also to deliver a GvL effect.[10,29] Clearly, to have any chance of being more effective at controlling disease than the first transplant, it is best to use a strategy that is likely to enhance GvL via the second graft. Methods of escalating the GvL effect are to give peripheral blood instead of bone marrow,[30] to reduce or avoid all post-transplant immunosuppression, and to switch to a new donor,[31] perhaps less fully matched than the original donor. Second transplants are limited in their success because of the high risk of further relapse, treatment-related mortality and death from GvHD. However, an early study from the EBMT identified transplants inducing chronic GvHD as being more likely to result in prolonged remissions.[10] Before re-allografting, a chemotherapy and/or molecularly targeted therapy should be chosen to reduce the malignant burden, followed by the conditioning regimen (e.g. melphalan ± fludarabine or busulfan ± fludarabine) and the stem cells.

Chemotherapy

Chemotherapy may be simply used to palliate relapsing disease, or it may be used in an attempt to achieve a hematologic remission or at least a reduction in tumor burden which, in turn, will facilitate immunotherapeutic approaches.[32] Many malignancies retain susceptibility to chemotherapy after SCT. For example, ALL may respond well to relatively simple treatment with combinations of vincristine, prednisone and anthracyclines.[32] When choosing a chemotherapy schedule, a balance has to be struck between achieving the best tumor reduction and selecting a regimen that is tolerated by a patient who has already undergone a transplant procedure, possibly with GvHD, and who is no longer chemotherapy naïve. In this regard, the interval between transplant and further chemotherapy is the most important factor in selecting treatment of an appropriate dose intensity. Patients relapsing less than 6 months post transplant will usually require reduced doses of chemotherapy to induce remission. Chemotherapy treatment schedules for relapsed leukemia tend to be designed on an individual basis and there are no hard and fast rules. However, as a guideline, schedules used in our institute in preparation for immunotherapy are outlined in Table 40.3.

Molecular targeting

In recent years, the advent of non-classic chemotherapy agents which molecularly target hematologic malignancies has opened up a new era in combining immunotherapeutic strategies with agents which lack the limiting toxicities caused by chemotherapy and which may have high efficacy against the malignancy.[33] Molecularly targeted therapies include monoclonal antibodies such as anti-CD20 (rituximab) targeting B-cell malignancies,[34] and anti-CD33 (gemtuzumab) targeting myeloid malignancies,[35] small molecules such as imatinib, dasatinib and nilotinib (for bcr-abl-positive leukemias),[36] as well as bortezo-

Table 40.3 Examples of relapse regimens used for different malignancies with the intention of reducing the tumor burden and usually followed by either DLI or stem cell infusion

Disease group	Preferred regimen
Acute lymphoid leukemia (ALL)	d1,d7,d15, (d21): vincristine 2 mg absolute d1,d7,d15, (d21): daunorubicin 45–60 mg/m² d1–d28: prednisone 1 mg/kg/d
Myeloid malignancies (AML, MDS)	d1–d3: idarubicin 8–10 mg/m² d1–d3(5): fludarabine 25–30 mg/m² d1–d3(5): cytarabine 1 g/m²
Chronic lymphatic leukemia (CLL), follicular or mantle cell lymphoma	d1: rituximab* 375 mg/m² d2–d4: fludarabine 25–30 mg/m² d2–d4: cyclophosphamide 250 mg/m²

* May be repeated post DLI or stem cell infusion.

mib,[37] thalidomide[38] and lenalidomide[39] targeting myeloma and other lymphoid malignancies. These highly effective therapies can cause tumor lysis or cytokine release syndromes, so that appropriate precautions should be taken. Treatment approaches when combining these agents with immunotherapy have yet to be defined in most relapse situations.

Imatinib targets the fusion protein bcr-abl and promises cytogenetic response rates of up to 90% in early chronic phase CML patients.[36] When relapse occurs after allografting, bcr-abl inhibitors can be combined with DLI.[40] Pre-existing or newly acquired point mutations in the bcr-abl fusion gene can be associated with resistance against imatinib and may require the use of novel bcr-abl inhibitors such as dasatinib or nilotinib.[36]

The small molecules bortezomib, a proteasome inhibitor, and thalidomide have proven efficacy in the treatment of patients with progressive myeloma. Tipifarnib is an inhibitor of the farnesyltransferase-inducing antiproliferative and proapoptotic responses in myeloid leukemias and myelodysplastic syndromes. Up to 40% of acute myeloid leukemia patients carry fms-like tyrosine kinase 3 (FLT3) mutations associated with kinase activation of the downstream signaling pathway.[41] To date, four different inhibitors of FLT3 have been tested in early clinical trials.[42–46] Etodolac is a non-steroidal anti-inflammatory drug (NSAID) that has shown promising results in the treatment of refractory B-CLL patients.[47] It appears that etodolac selectively targets B-CLL cells but not normal B- and T-lymphocytes. The use of these small molecules as part of an improved conditioning regimen for relapsed patients undergoing a second transplant is yet to be addressed comprehensively.

Treatments for specific types of relapsed disease

Relapsed CML

The majority of patients with relapsed CML can be successfully treated with DLI, bcr-abl inhibitors or a combination of both. Kolb and colleagues reported the successful use of leukocyte transfusions from the original donor for the treatment of CML relapsing after bone marrow transplantation in 1995.[7] Since then, many studies have confirmed the efficacy of DLI treatment after allogeneic SCT, achieving up to 80% durable responses. Prognostic factors for successful relapse treatment are stage of disease, type of relapse and timing of relapse after transplant.[28]

- Chronic-phase (CP) CML is more susceptible to DLI treatment than accelerated- (AP) or blastic-phase (BP) CML, presumably reflecting leukemia evolution and increasing resistance of the malignant clone in advanced disease stages.[15]

- Hematologic relapse is associated with lower response rates following DLI treatment as compared to cytogenetic or molecular relapse, reflecting the leukemia burden.[48]
- Longer transplant-to-relapse time intervals represent another favorable factor.[49]

Mortality associated with DLI is low, ranging from 3% to 10%, and is mainly due to marrow failure and GvHD. Attempts to optimize DLI dosing schedules have led to the introduction of effective cell doses (ECD) based on dose escalation studies. It has been suggested by Mackinnon and colleagues that DLI doses of 1×10^7/kg are capable of delivering a potent GvL effect while reducing the risk of GvHD. Using progressively increasing lymphocyte doses from 1×10^7/kg to above 1×10^8/kg for matched related transplants, and doses from 1×10^6/kg to above 1×10^8/kg for matched unrelated transplants, 88% molecular remissions were achieved in 81 retrospectively studied patients with relapsed CML. In this study, doses of 1×10^7/kg or below were associated with lower molecular response rates, emphasizing the impact of dosing. At comparable dose levels and disease stages, patients receiving DLI from matched unrelated donors achieved significantly higher response rates than did those with matched related donors. This phenomenon reflects the higher degree of histoincompatibility between donor and recipient in unrelated transplants, increasing the probability of beneficial GvL effects. Immunotherapy with interleukin-2 in conjunction with DLI can ameliorate the immune milieu post transplant, favoring remissions, but it may also increase the risk of GvHD.[26]

The availability of bcr-abl inhibitors offers new opportunities for the treatment of CML relapsing after allogeneic SCT.[50] Imatinib may induce complete cytogenetic responses in patients failing DLI treatment. In a multicenter study of the Chronic Leukaemia Working Party of the European Group of Bone and Marrow Transplantation (EBMT), 128 patients with relapsed CML were treated with imatinib, leading to 58% complete cytogenetic responses in patients in CP as compared to 48% and 22% in patients with AP and BC.[51] Complete molecular responses were obtained in 26%.

Bcr-abl inhibitors offer the opportunity of relapse treatment without significantly increasing the risk of GvHD. Preliminary, retrospective data on the question of whether the combination of bcr-abl inhibitors and DLI is superior to single strategy treatment suggests a synergistic effect of imatinib and DLI.[40] In this study, patients receiving imatinib plus DLI achieved their molecular remission more rapidly (90% of the patients within 3 months) and had superior disease-free survivals. Interestingly, these patients maintained their molecular remission after discontinuation of imatinib, suggesting an ongoing GvL effect.

Combinations of DLI and imatinib are even successful in patients with advanced CML relapsing into blast crisis. Unfortunately, CML patients accepted for SCT with pre-existing or newly acquired point mutations in the *bcr-abl* fusion gene are increasingly found to have disease resistant to imatinib and may require the use of novel bcr-abl inhibitors such as dasatinib or nilotinib.[50]

Treatment of relapsed acute leukemia

In contrast to relapsed CML, the prognosis of relapsed acute leukemias is extremely poor.[2] DLI are often unsuccessful, with survival rates of 20% and lower,[7,15] and the successful use of cytokines is described in a few case reports only.[52] Results on the outcome of second transplants for relapsed acute leukemia are also very limited.[29,53,54] One of the very few studies evaluating outcome of relapsed AML after a second transplant alone quotes a further relapse rate of 76% and an overall survival of 10% 4 years post second transplant.[55]

Arellano and colleagues recently published their long-term, retrospective analysis on relapsed or refractory AML and ALL after allogeneic SCT in a total of 310 total patients treated at a single institution.[9]

In their study, 31% of patients with AML and 35% of patients with ALL relapsed after SCT. Regarding all patients, remission status (disease burden) at the time of transplant and unfavorable cytogenetics at diagnosis of leukemia were independent risk factors for relapse after transplant. Transplants from unrelated donors were associated with an increased risk for relapse on both univariate and multivariate analysis. Remission status at the time of transplant remained significant even when considering patients with AML and ALL separately. Cytogenetics were more important for the prediction of relapse in AML as compared to ALL patients. Attempted salvage therapy for these 100 relapsed patients consisted of chemotherapy, including radiation to extramedullary sites, and targeted therapies, supportive care, second transplants, DLI with or without chemotherapy, and the use of cytokines such as GM-CSF and interferon-α. In all relapsed patients immunosuppression was stopped at diagnosis of relapse. At the time of analysis only 7% of patients were still alive, reflecting the overall poor prognosis of relapse. Complete remissions were observed in 8% of patients receiving chemotherapy or supportive care, in 62% of patients receiving a second transplant, 45% of patients after DLI, and in 71% of patients receiving cytokines. Second transplants and the use of cytokines were associated with longer median survival times as compared to chemotherapy, supportive care or DLI. GvHD after relapse ranged from 71% in patients receiving cytokines to 8% in patients receiving chemotherapy or supportive care. A multivariate analysis showed that a longer period to post-transplant relapse, peripheral blood as a source of stem cells and the immunotherapeutic salvage approaches (second transplants, DLI or cytokines) were independently associated with improved post-relapse survival.

Post-transplant relapse of acute leukemias is universally associated with an extremely poor prognosis. As data on such outcomes are very limited, prospective trials focusing on the treatment of relapse after transplant are needed. Novel approaches with immunotherapy in these patients may improve this unfavorable situation.[56]

Treatment of relapsed lymphoid malignancies

While the use of allogeneic stem cell transplantation for the treatment of patients with CLL, follicular lymphoma, mantle cell lymphoma, high-grade lymphoma, myeloma and Hodgkin's disease has been studied to some extent, the literature on the treatment of post-transplant relapses in these disease is extremely limited. Different authors have reported beneficial effects of DLI for the treatment of post-transplant relapse in patients with low-grade lymphoma, CLL and Hodgkin's disease.[30,57] Russell and colleagues retrospectively studied the use of DLI for the treatment of 17 patients with relapsed or refractory chronic lymphatic leukemia, follicular lymphoma, mantle cell lymphoma and high-grade lymphoma.[30] In this study, 3/4 patients with CLL, 4/4 with mantle cell lymphoma, 3/4 with follicular lymphoma and none of the patients with high-grade lymphoma experienced a complete remission. Overall, quotes for post-DLI acute and chronic GvHD were 45% and 88% respectively, associated with long-lasting responses.

The use of DLI for post-transplant relapse in patients with multiple myeloma has been studied in larger cohorts. Lokhorst and colleagues reported 52% overall, and 17% complete responses in 54 myeloma patients after DLI treatment.[58] These responses were rather short-lived and their occurrence was associated with the development of acute and chronic GvHD (57% and 47% respectively).

Although a majority of patients with myeloma appears to be susceptible to DLI, the effects on overall survival are rather disappointing. Additional strategies are therefore needed. Novel molecular therapies such as bortezomib were able to induce 61% overall and 22% complete responses, as recently shown in a retrospective study on 23 patients with myeloma who relapsed after allografting.[37] Typical toxicities included thrombocytopenia and peripheral neuropathy. Thalidomide represents a further promising agent for the treatment of refractory or relapsed myeloma, where response rates of 30% have been reported.[38] Its unique immunomodulatory effects have shown promising results in other lymphoid malignancies. However, the effects of thalidomide for the treatment of post-transplant relapse in lymphoid malignancies still require assessment.

A common observation in the treatment of such lymphoid malignancies has been that low-grade and chronic diseases are more susceptible to DLI as compared to the more aggressive and fast-progressing diseases.[30] Furthermore, the beneficial effects of DLI appear to be largely linked to the appearance of acute or chronic GvHD. The manner in which this influences long-term survival of these patients requires addressing in larger cohorts of patients.

New approaches

Treatment of post-transplant relapse in malignancies other than CML remains challenging. As relapse after transplant mainly reflects failure of the donor immune system to control the malignant disease, attempts at boosting these apparently insufficient GvL effects should be undertaken. Reduction of immunosuppression, use of immune modulators, DLI and second transplant from an unrelated donor may increase GvL but may also result in severe GvHD, even further reducing the chances of relapse control. Future approaches therefore clearly need to focus on selective boosting of GvL while avoiding GvHD.

In HLA-matched transplantation, donor–recipient disparities of polymorphisms in minor histocompatibility antigens (miHA) may induce GvL, GvHD or both, as based on the miHA expression distribution in target tissues of the recipient.[59] The in vivo development of donor T-cell responses against disparities on host leukemia cells appears to be limited by the insufficient antigen presentation of leukemic antigens to donor T-cells. Donor or patient vaccination, ex vivo pulsing with leukemia-specific antigens, or the transfer of co-stimulatory molecules into leukemia cells may overcome limitations in antigen-presenting cell (APC) function of the leukemia and may result in potent antileukemia donor T-cell responses.

Isolation of miHA-specific antileukemic T-cell clones allows their expansion ex vivo as well as determination of their T-cell receptors (TCR) gene sequences. Since the transfer of ex vivo-expanded CMV- and EBV-specific T-cells for the treatment of viral infections has already been proven feasible[60,61] and successful, the ex vivo generation of miHA-specific, antileukemic donor T-cells could result in similar outcomes for the treatment of relapsed hematologic malignancies. Recently, miHA-specific TCRs have been successfully transferred into CMV-specific T-cells and have resulted in T-cells maintaining full antiviral and anti-miHA function.[62]

The overexpression of autoantigens such as Wilms tumor antigen (WT1) or proteinase 3 (PR1) on leukemia cells has been shown to be immunogenic and, unlike miHA, may offer broadly applicable targets for vaccination and adoptive T-cell transfer.[63] A pilot study of PR1 vaccination in patients with refractory or progressing myeloid leukemia including relapses after SCT reported encouraging preliminary results, demonstrating PR1-specific immune responses in the majority of patients, including a number of clinical responses.[64] A further study at our institution is currently investigating the efficacy of a combination of PR1 and WT1 vaccination in patients with refractory or progressing myelodysplastic syndrome or myeloid leukemia, including relapses after SCT.

Donor natural killer (NK) cell activity is well known to play a major role in disease control after mismatched (haploidentical) allogeneic stem cell transplantation.[65] Recent evidence suggests that NK cells also play an important role in controlling malignant diseases in the

HLA-matched setting.[66,67] The latter effects appear to be largely attributable to mismatches in the killer cell inhibitory receptors (KIR) between donor and recipient.[68,69] NK cells are thought to play a critical role in stem cell transplantation based on their ability to eliminate host APCs, thereby reducing the risk of GvHD as well as delivering a direct cytotoxic effect to leukemia cells. The effects of NK cells in HLA-matched transplants are most visible after T-cell depleted allotransplantation where T-cell effects are less evident.[70] In this setting, early NK cell recovery has been shown to impact upon the response of patients after transplantation. The use of ex vivo-expanded donor-derived NK cells for the treatment of relapsed leukemias therefore promises disease control without an increased risk of developing GvHD.[71–73]

As the use of post-transplant immunosuppression deprives the allograft of its full GvL effects and thereby contributes to the likelihood of disease recurrence, future transplant strategies should aim to avoid the appearance of relapse in the first place. This may be achieved by ex vivo removal of host-reactive T-cells from donor allografts, allowing transplantation in an uncompromised immune environment. This novel approach, usually referred to as selective allodepletion, has been shown to be feasible both experimentally and clinically.[74] To date, four studies have been reported using an anti-CD25 immunotoxin for the ex vivo depletion of donor T-cells reacting against recipient-derived APCs in matched[75,76] and mismatched transplants.[77,78] Further studies are exploring the use of a TH9402-based photodepletion strategy in mismatched and matched transplants, delivering selectively depleted lymphocytes at the time of transplant or as delayed lymphocyte add-back.[79,80] This strategy is aimed at avoiding GvHD and disease relapse, but it may be also used to optimize the effects of DLI when relapse occurs.

References

1. Pasquini MC, Nugent ML. Current use and outcome of hematopoietic stem cell transplantation: part I CIBMTR Summary Slides, 2005. CIBMTR Newsletter [serial online]. 2006;12:5–8. www.cibmtr.org/ABOUT/NEWS/2006MAY.pdf (accessed August 2007).
2. Dazzi F, Fozza C. Disease relapse after haematopoietic stem cell transplantation: risk factors and treatment. Best Pract Res Clin Haematol 2007;20:311–327.
3. Weiden PL, Sullivan KM, Flournoy N et al. Antileukemic effect of chronic graft-versus-host disease: contribution to improved survival after allogeneic marrow transplantation. N Engl J Med 1981;304:1529–1533.
4. Goldman JM, Gale RP, Horowitz MM et al. Bone marrow transplantation for chronic myelogenous leukemia in chronic phase. Increased risk for relapse associated with T-cell depletion. Ann Intern Med 1988;108:806–814.
5. Barrett AJ, Savani BN. Stem cell transplantation with reduced-intensity conditioning regimens: a review of ten years experience with new transplant concepts and new therapeutic agents. Leukemia 2006;20:1661–1672.
6. Alyea EP, Kim HT, Ho V et al. Comparative outcome of nonmyeloablative and myeloablative allogeneic hematopoietic cell transplantation for patients older than 50 years of age. Blood 2005;105:1810–1814.
7. Kolb HJ, Schattenberg A, Goldman JM et al. Graft-versus-leukemia effect of donor lymphocyte transfusions in marrow grafted patients. Blood 1995;86:2041–2050.
8. Perez-Simon JA, Caballero D, ez-Campelo M et al. Chimerism and minimal residual disease monitoring after reduced intensity conditioning (RIC) allogeneic transplantation. Leukemia 2002;16:1423–1431.
9. Arellano ML, Langston A, Winton E et al. Treatment of relapsed acute leukemia after allogeneic transplantation: a single center experience. Biol Blood Marrow Transplant 2007;13:116–123.
10. Barrett AJ, Locatelli F, Treleaven JG et al. Second transplants for leukaemic relapse after bone marrow transplantation: high early mortality but favourable effect of chronic GVHD on continued remission. A report by the EBMT Leukaemia Working Party. Br J Haematol 1991;79:567–574.
11. Au WY, Kwong YL, Lie AK et al. Extra-medullary relapse of leukemia following allogeneic bone marrow transplantation. Hematol Oncol 1999;17:45–52.
12. Koc Y, Miller KB, Schenkein DP et al. Extramedullary tumors of myeloid blasts in adults as a pattern of relapse following allogeneic bone marrow transplantation. Cancer 1999;85:608–615.
13. Stein J, Zimmerman PA, Kochera M et al. Origin of leukemic relapse after bone marrow transplantation: comparison of cytogenetic and molecular analyses. Blood 1989;73:2033–2040.
14. Dazzi F, Szydlo RM, Craddock C et al. Comparison of single-dose and escalating-dose regimens of donor lymphocyte infusion for relapse after allografting for chronic myeloid leukemia. Blood 2000;95:67–71.
15. Collins RH Jr, Shpilberg O, Drobyski WR et al. Donor leukocyte infusions in 140 patients with relapsed malignancy after allogeneic bone marrow transplantation. J Clin Oncol 1997;15:433–444.
16. Schuler F, Dolken G. Detection and monitoring of minimal residual disease by quantitative real-time PCR. Clin Chim Acta 2006;363:147–156.
17. Campana D, Coustan-Smith E. Minimal residual disease studies by flow cytometry in acute leukemia. Acta Haematol 2004;112:8–15.
18. Thiede C, Bornhauser M, Ehninger G. Strategies and clinical implications of chimerism diagnostics after allogeneic hematopoietic stem cell transplantation. Acta Haematol 2004;112:16–23.
19. Muhlmann J, Thaler J, Hilbe W et al. Fluorescence in situ hybridization (FISH) on peripheral blood smears for monitoring Philadelphia chromosome-positive chronic myeloid leukemia (CML) during interferon treatment: a new strategy for remission assessment. Genes Chromos Cancer 1998;21:90–100.
20. Buno I, Wyatt WA, Zinsmeister AR et al. A special fluorescent in situ hybridization technique to study peripheral blood and assess the effectiveness of interferon therapy in chronic myeloid leukemia. Blood 1998;92:2315–2321.
21. van der Velden V, Hochhaus A, Cazzaniga G et al. Detection of minimal residual disease in hematologic malignancies by real-time quantitative PCR: principles, approaches, and laboratory aspects. Leukemia 2003;17:1013–1034.
22. Radich JP, Gehly G, Gooley T et al. Polymerase chain reaction detection of the BCR-ABL fusion transcript after allogeneic marrow transplantation for chronic myeloid leukemia: results and implications in 346 patients. Blood 1995;85:2632–2638.
23. Olavarria E, Kanfer E, Szydlo R et al. Early detection of BCR-ABL transcripts by quantitative reverse transcriptase-polymerase chain reaction predicts outcome after allogeneic stem cell transplantation for chronic myeloid leukemia. Blood 2001;97:1560–1565.
24. Mughal TI, Yong A, Szydlo RM et al. Molecular studies in patients with chronic myeloid leukaemia in remission 5 years after allogeneic stem cell transplant define the risk of subsequent relapse. Br J Haematol 2001;115:569–574.
25. Collins RH Jr, Rogers ZR, Bennett M et al. Hematologic relapse of chronic myelogenous leukemia following allogeneic bone marrow transplantation: apparent graft-versus-leukemia effect following abrupt discontinuation of immunosuppression. Bone Marrow Transplant 1992;10:391–395.
26. Nadal E, Fowler A, Kanfer E et al. Adjuvant interleukin-2 therapy for patients refractory to donor lymphocyte infusions. Exp Hematol 2004;32:218–223.
27. Mackinnon S, Papadopoulos EB, Carabasi MH et al. Adoptive immunotherapy evaluating escalating doses of donor leukocytes for relapse of chronic myeloid leukemia after bone marrow transplantation: separation of graft-versus-leukemia responses from graft-versus-host disease. Blood 1995;86:1261–1268.
28. Simula MP, Marktel S, Fozza C et al. Response to donor lymphocyte infusions for chronic myeloid leukemia is dose-dependent: the importance of escalating the cell dose to maximize therapeutic efficacy. Leukemia 2007;21:943–948.
29. Bosi A, Laszlo D, Labopin M et al. Second allogeneic bone marrow transplantation in acute leukemia: results of a survey by the European Cooperative Group for Blood and Marrow Transplantation. J Clin Oncol 2001;19:3675–3684.
30. Russell NH, Byrne JL, Faulkner RD et al. Donor lymphocyte infusions can result in sustained remissions in patients with residual or relapsed lymphoid malignancy following allogeneic haemopoietic stem cell transplantation. Bone Marrow Transplant 2005;36:437–441.
31. Duus JE, Stiff PJ, Choi J et al. Second allografts for relapsed hematologic malignancies: feasibility of using a different donor. Bone Marrow Transplant 2005;35:261–264.
32. Litzow MR. The therapy of relapsed acute leukaemia in adults. Blood Rev 2004;18:39–63.
33. Adachi S, Leoni LM, Carson DA, Nakahata T. Apoptosis induced by molecular targeting therapy in hematological malignancies. Acta Haematol 2004;111:107–123.
34. Maloney DG, Grillo-Lopez AJ, White CA et al. IDEC-C2B8 (Rituximab) anti-CD20 monoclonal antibody therapy in patients with relapsed low-grade non-Hodgkin's lymphoma. Blood 1997;90:2188–2195.
35. Sievers EL, Appelbaum FR, Spielberger RT et al. Selective ablation of acute myeloid leukemia using antibody-targeted chemotherapy: a phase I study of an anti-CD33 calicheamicin immunoconjugate. Blood 1999;93:3678–3684.
36. Deininger M, Buchdunger E, Druker BJ. The development of imatinib as a therapeutic agent for chronic myeloid leukemia. Blood 2005;105:2640–2653.
37. Bruno B, Patriarca F, Sorasio R et al. Bortezomib with or without dexamethasone in relapsed multiple myeloma following allogeneic hematopoietic cell transplantation. Haematologica 2006;91:837–839.
38. Singhal S, Mehta J, Desikan R et al. Antitumor activity of thalidomide in refractory multiple myeloma. N Engl J Med 1999;341:1565–1571.
39. de Raeve H, Vanderkerken K. Immunomodulatory drugs as a therapy for multiple myeloma. Curr Pharm Biotechnol 2006;7:415–421.
40. Savani BN, Montero A, Kurlander R et al. Imatinib synergizes with donor lymphocyte infusions to achieve rapid molecular remission of CML relapsing after allogeneic stem cell transplantation. Bone Marrow Transplant 2005;36:1009–1015.
41. Stirewalt DL, Kopecky KJ, Meshinchi S et al. FLT3, RAS, and TP53 mutations in elderly patients with acute myeloid leukemia. Blood 2001;97:3589–3595.
42. Fabbro D, Buchdunger E, Wood J et al. Inhibitors of protein kinases: CGP 41251, a protein kinase inhibitor with potential as an anticancer agent. Pharmacol Ther 1999;82:293–301.
43. Weisberg E, Boulton C, Kelly LM et al. Inhibition of mutant FLT3 receptors in leukemia cells by the small molecule tyrosine kinase inhibitor PKC412. Cancer Cell 2002;1:433–443.
44. Fong TA, Shawver LK, Sun L et al. SU5416 is a potent and selective inhibitor of the vascular endothelial growth factor receptor (Flk-1/KDR) that inhibits tyrosine kinase catalysis, tumor vascularization, and growth of multiple tumor types. Cancer Res 1999;59:99–106.
45. Kelly LM, Yu JC, Boulton CL et al. CT53518, a novel selective FLT3 antagonist for the treatment of acute myelogenous leukemia (AML). Cancer Cell 2002;1:421–432.
46. Propper DJ, McDonald AC, Man A et al. Phase I and pharmacokinetic study of PKC412, an inhibitor of protein kinase C. J Clin Oncol 2001;19:1485–1492.

47. Nardella FA, LeFevre JA. Enhanced clearance of leukemic lymphocytes in B-cell chronic lymphocytic leukemia with etodolac. Blood 2002;99:2625–2626

48. van Rhee F, Lin F, Cullis JO et al. Relapse of chronic myeloid leukemia after allogeneic bone marrow transplant: the case for giving donor leukocyte transfusions before the onset of hematologic relapse. Blood 1994;83:3377–3383

49. Dazzi F, Szydlo RM, Cross NC et al. Durability of responses following donor lymphocyte infusions for patients who relapse after allogeneic stem cell transplantation for chronic myeloid leukemia. Blood 2000;96:2712–2716

50. Bocchia M, Forconi F, Lauria F. Emerging drugs in chronic myelogenous leukemia. Expert Opin Emerg Drugs 2006;11:651–664

51. Olavarria E, Ottmann OG, Deininger M et al. Response to imatinib in patients who relapse after allogeneic stem cell transplantation for chronic myeloid leukemia. Leukemia 2003;17:1707–1712

52. Singhal S, Powles R, Treleaven J, Mehta J. Sensitivity of secondary acute myeloid leukemia relapsing after allogeneic bone marrow transplantation to immunotherapy with interferon-alpha 2b. Bone Marrow Transplant 1997;19:1151–1153

53. Eapen M, Giralt SA, Horowitz MM et al. Second transplant for acute and chronic leukemia relapsing after first HLA-identical sibling transplant. Bone Marrow Transplant 2004;34:721–727

54. Mrsic M, Horowitz MM, Atkinson K et al. Second HLA-identical sibling transplants for leukemia recurrence. Bone Marrow Transplant 1992;9:269–275

55. Radich JP, Sanders JE, Buckner CD et al. Second allogeneic marrow transplantation for patients with recurrent leukemia after initial transplant with total-body irradiation-containing regimens. J Clin Oncol 1993;11:304–313

56. Blair A, Goulden NJ, Libri NA et al. Immunotherapeutic strategies in acute lymphoblastic leukaemia relapsing after stem cell transplantation. Blood Rev 2005;19:289–300

57. Anderlini P, Acholonu SA, Okoroji GJ et al. Donor leukocyte infusions in relapsed Hodgkin's lymphoma following allogeneic stem cell transplantation: CD3+ cell dose, GVHD and disease response. Bone Marrow Transplant 2004;34:511–514

58. Lokhorst HM, Wu K, Verdonck LF et al. The occurrence of graft-versus-host disease is the major predictive factor for response to donor lymphocyte infusions in multiple myeloma. Blood 2004;103:4362–4364

59. Falkenburg JH, Willemze R. Minor histocompatibility antigens as targets of cellular immunotherapy in leukaemia. Best Pract Res Clin Haematol 2004;17:415–425

60. Heslop HE, Ng CY, Li C et al. Long-term restoration of immunity against Epstein-Barr virus infection by adoptive transfer of gene-modified virus-specific T lymphocytes. Nat Med 1996;2:551–555

61. Riddell SR, Watanabe KS, Goodrich JM et al. Restoration of viral immunity in immuno-deficient humans by the adoptive transfer of T cell clones. Science 1992;257:238–241

62. Heemskerk MH, Hoogeboom M, Hagedoorn R et al. Reprogramming of virus-specific T cells into leukemia-reactive T cells using T cell receptor gene transfer. J Exp Med 2004;199:885–894

63. Barrett AJ, Rezvani K. Translational mini-review series on vaccines: peptide vaccines for myeloid leukaemias. Clin Exp Immunol 2007;148:189–198

64. Qazilbash MH, Wieder E, Rios R et al. Vaccination with the PR1 leukemia-associated antigen can induce complete remission in patients with myeloid leukemia. ASH Annual Meeting Abstracts 2004;104:259

65. Ruggeri L, Capanni M, Urbani E et al. Effectiveness of donor natural killer cell alloreactivity in mismatched hematopoietic transplants. Science 2002;295:2097–2100

66. Jiang YZ, Barrett AJ, Goldman JM, Mavroudis DA. Association of natural killer cell immune recovery with a graft-versus-leukemia effect independent of graft-versus-host disease following allogeneic bone marrow transplantation. Ann Hematol 1997;74:1–6

67. Sconocchia G, del Principe D, Barrett AJ. Non-classical antileukemia activity of early recovering NK cells after induction chemotherapy and HLA-identical stem cell transplantation in myeloid leukemias. Leukemia 2006;20:1632–1633.

68. Boyington JC, Motyka SA, Schuck P et al. Crystal structure of an NK cell immunoglobulin-like receptor in complex with its class I MHC ligand. Nature 2000;405:537–543

69. Brooks AG, Boyington JC, Sun PD. Natural killer cell recognition of HLA class I molecules. Rev Immunogenet 2000;2:433–448

70. Savani BN, Rezvani K, Mielke S et al. Factors associated with early molecular remission after T cell-depleted allogeneic stem cell transplantation for chronic myelogenous leukemia. Blood 2006;107:1688–1695

71. Passweg JR, Koehl U, Uharek L et al. Natural-killer-cell-based treatment in haematopoietic stem-cell transplantation. Best Pract Res Clin Haematol 2006;19:811–824

72. Koehl U, Esser R, Zimmermann S et al. Ex vivo expansion of highly purified NK cells for immunotherapy after haploidentical stem cell transplantation in children. Klin Paediatr 2005;217:345–350

73. Koehl U, Sorensen J, Esser R et al. IL-2 activated NK cell immunotherapy of three children after haploidentical stem cell transplantation. Blood Cells Mol Dis 2004;33:261–266

74. Mielke S, Solomon SR, Barrett AJ. Selective depletion strategies in allogeneic stem cell transplantation. Cytotherapy 2005;7:109–115

75. Solomon SR, Mielke S, Savani BN et al. Selective depletion of alloreactive donor lymphocytes: a novel method to reduce the severity of graft-versus-host disease in older patients undergoing matched sibling donor stem cell transplantation. Blood 2005;106:1123–1129

76. Mielke S, Rezvani K, Savani BN et al. Reconstitution of foxp3+ regulatory T cells (Tregs) after CD25-depleted allotransplantion in elderly patients and association with acute graft-versus-host disease (GvHD). Blood 2007;110(5):1689–1697

77. Andre-Schmutz I, Le Deist F, Hacein-Bey-Abina S et al. Immune reconstitution without graft-versus-host disease after haemopoietic stem-cell transplantation: a phase 1/2 study. Lancet 2002;360:130–137

78. Amrolia PJ, Muccioli-Casadei G, Huls H et al. Adoptive immunotherapy with allodepleted donor T-cells improves immune reconstitution after haploidentical stem cell transplantation. Blood 2006;108:1797–1808

79. Mielke S, Nunes R, Rezvani K et al. A clinical scale selective allodepletion approach for the treatment of HLA-mismatched and matched donor-recipient pairs using expanded T lymphocytes as antigen-presenting cells and a TH9402-based photodepletion technique. Blood 2008;111(8), in press

80. Roy DC, Cohen S, Busque L et al. Phase I clinical study of donor lymphocyte infusion depleted of alloreactive T cells after haplotype mismatched myeloablative stem cell transplantation to limit infections and malignant relapse without causing GVHD. ASH Annual Meeting Abstracts 2006;108:309

Bacterial infections

Unell Riley

Introduction

Infection is one of the most significant complications after stem cell transplantation. The stem cell transplant recipient is immunocompromised for a number of reasons and these occur at different time points during the transplantation process. Disruption of the anatomic barrier, neutropenia, dysfunction of cell-mediated immunity, dysfunction of humoral immunity and hyposplenism all render the transplant recipient susceptible to bacterial infections.

Disruption of the anatomic barrier

Intact skin and mucosa are vital for protection of the individual from bacterial infections. In the pre-engraftment and periengraftment phases which usually last for approximately 30 days, breakdown of the anatomic barrier and neutropenia are the most significant factors leading to susceptibility to infection. The skin and mucosal surfaces of the alimentary canal form the main barriers against microbial invasion. Both of these surfaces are colonized with a variety of micro-organisms.[1] When the surfaces are intact they are able to prevent colonization with potentially more pathogenic organisms which are in the immediate environment, particularly if the ecologic balance with indigenous flora is maintained. The skin, for instance, is usually a hydrophobic environment with a high salt content, where only certain organisms such as staphylococci, corynebacteria and lipophilic yeasts can flourish and constitute the normal skin flora. Antibiotics secreted in sweat can disturb the balance between commensal flora and therefore leave the surface more vulnerable to colonization with exogenous, gram-negative bacilli. Also, antibiotics can exert selected pressure, causing resistant organisms to emerge.[2–4] Irradiation and chemotherapy can bring about radical changes to healthy skin, causing hair loss, dryness and loss of sweat production. The normal skin barrier can be disrupted by needle punctures and intravascular catheters, allowing organisms to access the bloodstream.

Although intravascular devices are now considered essential for the management of transplant patients, they are associated with an increased instance of bacteremia with coagulase-negative staphylococci which often colonize the intraluminal or extraluminal surfaces of catheters or the exit site of these devices.[5,6] Other possible routes for entry of infection associated with intravascular catheters are the catheter/giving set/Y-junction during change of intravenous fluid, or a contaminated fluid container. Infection on the external surface of the catheter such as at the exit site or in the tunnel can cause serious soft tissue infection and lead to catheter-associated bacteremia or septicemia.[7,8] Intraluminal colonization is often caused by relatively non-virulent organisms such as coagulase-negative staphylococci, corynebacteria, *Bacillus* spp, *Pseudomonas* spp and so on, and once established these infections can be difficult to manage and cannot be treated without removal of the catheter.[9–12]

In the alimentary canal, anaerobic bacteria predominate in the lower gastrointestinal tract and also in the oral cavity. These bacteria play an important role in maintaining a healthy commensal flora by resisting colonization by exogenous bacteria, a process known as colonization resistance.[13,14] Colonization resistance can be disrupted by a variety of antibiotics, many of which would be used in the treatment of a febrile episode during the pre-engraftment phase.[15–17] Loss of normal commensal flora allows exogenous organisms such as *Candida* spp, *Klebsiella pneumoniae* and *Pseudomonas aeruginosa* to become established in the gut.[18] Also important in disrupting colonization resistance is loss of the gastric barrier caused by antacids used to counterbalance dyspepsia, combined with the excessive swallowing of mucus which occurs in the presence of mucositis. The potential sites for colonization by altered endogenous and exogenous flora therefore extend the full length of the alimentary canal.[19–21] Diarrhea caused by cytoxic agents, total-body irradiation and graft-versus host-disease (GvHD) also alters the ecology of bowel flora.[22–24]

Mucositis is the clinical manifestation of mucosal barrier injury and varies greatly in its severity.[25] It causes significant morbidity and markedly impairs quality of life for patients.[26,27] Mucosal barrier damage in the upper part of the digestive tract, such as the oral cavity, predisposes to infection with oral viridans streptococci, whereas infections caused by gram-negative organisms and neutropenic enterocolitis are manifestations of mucosal damage in the lower part of the digestive tract. The GI tract has been recognized as being the principal site of origin of infections due to enteric organisms such as *Escherichia coli* and *Klebsiella pneumoniae*.[28,29] In addition, neutropenic enterocolitis or typhilitis, a severe form of mucosal damage of the gut caused by cytotoxic therapy, can be a portal of entry for organisms such as *Staphylococcus aureus*, *Pseudomonas aeruginosa* and *Clostridia* species.[30,31] Finally, *Candida* colonization in this setting is associated with local mucosal damage which is a separate risk factor for invasive candidiasis.[32–34]

Neutropenia

Normally functioning neutrophils are important in dealing with infections and they usually congregate at the site of inflammation followed by macrophages. Stem cell transplantation affects the functioning of neutrophils in two ways. First, it causes the absolute numbers of neutrophils to fall; virtually all cytotoxic drugs used in the treatment of malignant disease cause a negative effect on normal hematopoiesis, leading to granulocytopenia and depletion of the bone marrow reserve. Total-body irradiation has the same effect. It is well recognized that neutropenia is associated with an increased risk of bacterial infection, particularly if the total neutrophil count has fallen below $0.5 \times 10^9/l$. The risk is greater still if neutropenia is prolonged (more than 7 days), profound ($< 0.1 \times 10^9/l$) and if the fall in the neutrophil count is rapid, all of which occur in the bone marrow transplant setting.[35,36]

Cell-mediated and humoral immunity

The cell-mediated immune system is important for ridding the host of intracellular bacterial pathogens and virus-infected cells. Macrophages are important for dealing with a number of organisms. However, they have a limited ability to curb these organisms by themselves and indeed, some micro-organisms can replicate and survive in inactivated macrophages. Macrophages must be activated, a complex process which is mediated by cytokines and healthy T-cells. The process can be easily disturbed by cytotoxic therapy, irradiation, and immunosuppressive agents including steroids, ciclosporin and mycophenolate, and purine analogs such as fludarabine. It is well recognized that allogeneic stem cell transplantation causes prolonged suppression of T- and B-cell function, especially in the presence of chronic graft-versus-host disease and its treatment.

Certain malignancies such as lymphomas can also have a direct effect on T- and B-cell function, and lymphoproliferative disorders such as chronic lymphocytic leukemia and myeloma may affect the ability of B-lymphocytes to produce antibody, therefore impairing humoral immunity.

Hyposplenism

The spleen is important in the removal of non-opsonized and encapsulated organisms such as *Streptococcus pneumoniae* and *Haemophilus influenzae*. Total-body irradiation and chronic GvHD lead to functional asplenia in the stem cell transplant patient and therefore allogeneic transplant patients are at risk from these organisms.[37,38]

Other factors that may be associated with infections in stem cell transplant patients include conditions such as diabetes, which lead in their own right to an increased risk of infection. Smoking damages the respiratory tract, predisposing to infection, and psychologic stress may affect host defense mechanisms. The nutritional status of the patient is important and will be affected during the period of pre-engraftment when the gut mucosa is damaged by mucositis. The protective role of platelets is overestimated, and thrombocytopenia is now thought to be an independent risk factor for bacteremia.[39] Thrombocytopenia also retards repair of damaged tissue.

Febrile neutropenia

In the pre-engraftment phase, neutropenia and breakdown of the anatomic barrier combine to greatly increase host susceptibility to infection. Most infections originate at the site where the concentration of commensal organisms colonizing the host is at its greatest. Predictably, most infections come from the oral cavity, skin, alimentary canal, particularly the lower GI tract, the perianal area, and the upper respiratory tract leading to lower respiratory tract infections. An infectious origin for febrile neutropenia can be confirmed microbiologically or clinically in only 30–50% of cases, and the normal features of infection such as pus formation do not always correspond to bacteremia.[40] It is therefore obligatory to take a very good clinical history and perform a thorough examination of the febrile patient to identify any possible source of infection.

The organisms

The majority of infections in neutropenic, mucosa-damaged patients are caused by *Pseudomonas aeruginosa*, *Escherichia coli*, *Klebsiella* spp, coagulase-negative staphylococci, *Staphylococcus aureus* and *Streptococcus* spp.

Sepsis caused by aerobic gram-negative bacilli such as the Enterobacteriaceae and *Pseudomonas aeruginosa* have traditionally been the most feared organisms, with their propensity to cause overwhelming sepsis in a neutropenic host, leading to toxemia. However, since the 1980s there has been a shift in the spectrum of bacterial infections such that infections due to gram-positive bacteria have become more common than those due to gram-negative bacilli.[41] This is probably due to a number of factors, including the widespread use of central venous catheters, possibly an increased use of cytotoxic agents causing more mucositis, and increased use of fluoroquinolones as prophylaxis. Quite recently some evidence has suggested that the ecologic pattern is shifting back again.[42]

Gram-negative infection usually manifests itself as a septicemia-like illness. However, enterobacteriaceases, in particular, can cause localized infection in the perianal area and repeated localized sepsis should prompt a search for perianal lesions such as a perianal fissure or hemorrhoids. The most serious localized infection in bone marrow transplantation is that due to *Pseudomonas aeruginosa*. This can take a number of forms, the most common being ecthyma gangrenosum lesions which are vasculitic skin lesions with a necrotic center, caused by subcutaneous invasion by the organism.[43] They can occur as a manifestation of metastatic *Pseudomonas aeruginosa* septicemia, or as a primary localized skin lesion. Similar lesions have been produced by *Aspergillus* spp,[44,45] mucormycosis[46] and *Candida* spp.[47] *Pseudomonas aeruginosa* has also been associated with buccal and orbital cellulitis.

Gram-positive bacterial isolates are now the most common during the neutropenia following bone marrow transplantation. They are usually due to *Staphylococcus epidermidis* and this is thought to be related to the wide use of long-term central venous catheters. *Staphylococcus epidermidis* can readily colonize these devices, producing a very thick glycocalyx[48] which is protective and makes eradication of the bacteria from the line by antibiotics very difficult. Although usually considered of low virulence, in this setting they can produce repeated bacteremias, tunnel catheter infections and even progress to large vessel thrombophlebitis, with occlusion and bacterial endocarditis.

Other bacteria associated with line infections are *Staphylococcus aureus*, *Corynebacterium jeikeium* and *Bacillus* spp, which can also cause serious sepsis in neutropenic patients. *Staphylococcus aureus* is an important cause of sepsis, as it can gain access through broken skin and mucosa, and can cause septicemia as well as localized lesions in the line, skin or lungs. It is important to note that although most infections caused by *Staphylococcus aureus* are acquired by patients endogenously, they can also acquire *Staphylococcus aureus* readily from exogenous sources in the form of a hospital-acquired infection. Such organisms as methicillin-resistant *Staphylococcus aureus* (MRSA) are commonly more resistant to antibiotics.

Line infection with *Corynebacterium jeikeium* can lead to metastatic abscesses in the subcutaneous soft tissue and muscle,[49–52] which can be difficult to treat since these bacteria are intrinsically highly resistant. The environmental pseudomonads can also cause line infections. These organisms are often multiply resistant to antibiotics. For example, *Stenotrophomonas maltophila*[53] is intrinsically resistant to carbapenems.

Alpha-hemolytic streptococci are now recognized as a significant cause of sepsis in the neutropenic patient.[19–21,54–57] *Streptococcus mitis* has been associated with adult respiratory distress syndrome (ARDS) and septic shock syndrome.[21,58] *Streptococcus sanguis* has been associated with severe oral mucositis. There is particular concern that these types of infections are often seen in patients receiving prophylaxis with ciprofloxacin.[59,60]

Diagnosis of infection

Fever still remains the main indicator for initiation of antibiotic therapy. The degree of fever which should trigger antibiotic treatment is ill defined but in general, a single oral temperature of 38.5°C, or a temperature of > 38°C for more than 1 hour when blood[61] products have not been given, should lead to initiation of therapy. Clinical evidence of an infection focus should also be sought, particularly in known risk areas such as the perianal area, lungs, skin, central venous catheter exit site and the oropharynx. Tachycardia, breathlessness and impaired organ function can also be indicators of infection. Adult respiratory distress syndrome can be a manifestation of sepsis. A chest X-ray taken at the onset of fever may not always show lung infiltrates and should therefore be repeated in the event of persistent fever,[62] and a CT scan should be considered. C-reactive protein may help in the differentiation of fever due to bacterial and fungal infection rather than other causes.[63,64] C-reactive protein is usually specific for bacterial and fungal infections, and thus a fall in C-reactive protein may indicate a response to treatment, and a rise, a persistent secondary infection or non-response to empirical therapy.

Microbiologic investigation should include taking blood cultures. Ideally, at least 20 ml of blood should be taken to detect low levels of bacteremia. The specificity of the blood culture may be reduced if the sample is taken through a catheter which may be colonized by coagulase-negative staphylococci. Sets of blood cultures should be taken peripherally and from each lumen of the central venous catheter, before commencement of empirical therapy.

Quantitative blood culture methods may be useful for differentiating bacteremia due to the central venous catheter or from a tissue source; however, this is labour intensive and expensive.[65] Microbiologic samples should also be taken from suspected sites of infection and may include exit site swabs, urine samples and sputum samples.

The role of surveillance cultures

Surveillance cultures have sometimes been used to monitor infection problems in bone marrow transplant patients and are most useful when selective bowel decontamination is being used. Since there is evidence that colonization precedes infection,[66] it is to be expected that surveillance cultures are able to predict causative organisms, influence empirical regimens which are used for treatment of febrile neutropenia, detect the presence of multiply resistant organisms (including MRSA and vancomycin-resistant enterococci) and monitor the efficacy of gut decontamination. However, information gained from surveillance has proved disappointing in that the causative agent of infection is rarely predicted.[67] Routine surveillance cultures are also time-consuming and expensive if performed properly and can involve a large number of samples being sent weekly from the same patient. The isolation of *Pseudomonas aeruginosa*, *Aspergillus* and non-albicans *Candida* spp,[68,69] however, may be helpful in the management of the neutropenic patient. Therefore, surveillance cultures should probably be limited to weekly samples from the nose to detect colonization due to *Staphylococcus aureus* and *Aspergillus* spp, catheter exit site swabs to detect heavy growth of staphylococci or environmental pseudomonads, and throat and stool samples to detect colonization with *Candida* spp, to check the efficacy of gut decontamination and to monitor resistance patterns of any isolated aerobic gram-negative bacilli.

Management of febrile neutropenia

Fever in neutropenia should always be considered as being due to infection until proven otherwise and always treated as a medical emergency. Febrile episodes in neutropenia can be classified according to the absence/presence of microbiologic or clinical documentation of infection.[70,71] The classification can be as:

- microbiologically documented infection with bacteremia, with a significant pathogen in normal blood cultures
- microbiologically documented infection without bacteremia, with isolation of an organism from another site not blood, such as urine, respiratory secretions, etc.
- clinically documented infection in the presence of a clinical picture clearly and objectively infectious in nature, with no microbiologic proof
- fever of known origin, where clinical and microbiologic proof is lacking but the clinical picture is compatible with infection.

There has been much reduction in the mortality rate associated with febrile neutropenia from that of the classic study performed in 1962[72] and from the International Antimicrobial Therapy Group (IATG) of the European Organization for Research and Treatment of Cancer (EORTC) study performed in 1978, when more than 20% of patients with gram-positive bacteremia and about 50% of patients with gram-negative bacteremia died. During the course of the 25 years during which studies and trials were performed by the IATG-EORTC on febrile neutropenic patients, the mortality rate has fallen to 10% for gram-negative and 6% in gram-positive bacteremias.[73–75]

Empiric antimicrobial chemotherapy

Since the 1960s, it has been realized that there can be significant mortality due to gram-negative sepsis in the neutropenic patient if antibiotic therapy is delayed. Such therapy should therefore be started promptly at the onset of fever.

Patients who are severely neutropenic with gram-negative sepsis have a mortality rate which can approach 40% if antimicrobial treatment is not initiated promptly.[76,77] This was the reason behind the rationale of using broad-spectrum antibiotics which are active against *Pseudomonas aeruginosa* in these patients, and has been the focus of therapy since this period. A vast number of empiric regimens have been evaluated in clinical trials. The earliest used, and probably still the most popular, is a β-lactam with antipseudomonas activity, in combination with an aminoglycoside.[74,75,78,79] The first β-lactams used consisted of ureidopenicillins, such as piperacillin. Various β-lactam antibiotics have been developed with broader activity against gram-negative agents and some gram-positive activity, and these have been examined by the IATG-EORTC trials in various combinations and as monotherapies. An interesting phenomenon has been seen, in that the success of empiric therapy has been decreasing trial by trial from 1995 through 2000 although the decrease in mortality has been maintained. The reason is not clear but it could be due to clinicians changing antimicrobials too early and not allowing time for them to work; however, increasing resistance cannot be excluded.[80]

The use of aminoglycosides as adjuvant therapy in febrile neutropenia is a contentious issue. The classic combination of a β-lactam and aminoglycosides has always been considered the treatment of choice in febrile neutropenia, mainly because of the wide spectrum of activity against facultative gram-negative organisms, the potential synergistic activity of aminoglycosides to combat gram-negative infection, and the potential for reducing the emergence of resistance in an individual patient while on treatment, although this has never been proven. The disadvantages of aminoglycoside therapy are the nephro- and ototoxicity, the relativity poor activity against staphylococci and streptococci and the historic need for multidosing. For these reasons, double β-lactam[85] combinations or a β-lactam-quinolone have been used with apparent success. Single-agent therapy became feasible and safer due to the development of broader spectrum cefalosporins such as ceftazidime and cefepime, and carbapenems such as imipenem and meropenem.

A recent study comparing piperacillin-tazobactam monotherapy with dual therapy with an aminoglycoside showed little difference between the success rates,[81] and a recent meta-analysis comparing the effectiveness of β-lactam monotherapy with β-lactam/aminoglycoside therapy showed that there was little difference between the two, and maybe even an advantage with monotherapy, with a low rate of adverse events, lower rates of failures and a trend for better survival.[82,83] The traditional method of multidose administration of aminoglycosides has been replaced by once-daily aminoglycoside dosing, thought to be as effective as multiple dosing while producing less nephrotoxicity. Although there is little documented evidence of any efficacy in bone marrow transplant recipients, this mode of administration may represent an advance.[84] Theoretically, the more modern way of using aminoglycosides would have less toxicity and better efficacy. The consensus is that monotherapy may be successful although many clinicians would still want to use dual therapy in their higher risk patients.[84–91]

There are conflicting ideas concerning the use of intravenous ciprofloxacin empirically, although a randomized study showed reasonable efficacy of monotherapy.[92] However, the IATG-EORTC was obliged to discontinue a study due to an unacceptably high mortality rate, and most failings were due to gram-positive infections.[93] These problems may be overcome by combining ciprofloxacin with either a glycopeptide or a ureidopenicillin.[88] The use of ciprofloxacin for empiric therapy will always be constrained by its use as a prophylactic agent.

The second contentious issue is the early inclusion of glycopeptide antibiotics such as vancomycin and teicoplanin in empiric antibiotic regimens, mainly because of the increase in incidence of gram-positive infections. Some studies have shown that use of these antimicrobials results in a reduction in gram-positive secondary infections, total febrile days, and more rapid defervescence of fever and the use of less amphotericin B.[94–96] However more reliable studies, including EORTC trials, have shown that there is little advantage in adding a glycopeptide to initial empiric therapy.[97–100] A further consideration is the increase in vancomycin-resistant enterococci in oncology and bone marrow transplant units.[101] These organisms are generally multiresistant and there are limited antibiotic treatment options if they cause clinical infection. There appears to be an association between heavy vancomycin usage and an increased incidence of vancomycin-resistant enterococci.[101,102] With the recent appearance of vancomycin-resistant staphylococci, the empiric use of glycopeptides should be reserved for persistently febrile neutropenic patients with lung infection, septic shock or clinically documented infection likely to be caused by gram-positive organisms such as catheter-associated or soft tissue infections.

Ultimately, the choice of an empiric regimen depends upon presentation of the infection and the resistance patterns of the organisms commonly seen in a particular institution. Modifications to the empiric therapy regimen may be needed depending upon the nature of the infection and fever presentation. When there is microbiologic evidence for the cause of infection, treatment should be tailored to treat this specifically when sensitivities are available. Again, modification in treatment depends upon the isolate and the suspected site of infection. For instance, in *Staphylococcus aureus* septicemia, treatment should include a specific antistaphylococcal agent for 14 days.[102,103]

The persistently febrile neutropenic patient who has not responded to a reasonable course of empiric antibiotic therapy with no microbio-

logically confirmed infection is a problem. These clinical situations are difficult to manage because clinicians are under pressure to change antibiotics and usually do this without any microbiological or clinical back-up. A patient may take days to defervesce even when receiving antimicrobials appropriate for the causative bacteria.

There should be specific reasons for changing antimicrobial therapy in febrile neutropenia. Other possible reasons for fever should be investigated and considered, such as fungal infection, viral infection with adenovirus, CMV or herpes simplex. If these are excluded, changes should only be made if there is:

- persistent fever greater than 39°C after 48–72 hours of therapy
- relapse of fever greater than 38°C after initial fever defervescence for 24 hours
- progression of sepsis syndrome
- development of DIC, acute respiratory distress syndrome or multiorgan failure
- persistence of positive blood cultures after 24 hours of therapy
- relapse of a primary infection
- appearance of a new infection.

Duration of treatment in patients with fever of unknown origin who have shown a good response to antimicrobials is also contentious. Some would suggest continuing antibiotic therapy for at least 14 days or until the patient's neutrophil count rises above $0.5 \times 10^9/l$. This, however, leaves the patient at risk of toxicity secondary to the antibiotic therapy and many would advocate a minimum of 7 days treatment with four consecutive afebrile days with no residual evidence of localized infection.

References

1. Roth RR, James WD. Microbial ecology of the skin. Ann Rev Microbiol 1988;42:441–464
2. Kotilainen P, Nikoskelainen J, Houovinen P. Emergence of ciprofloxacin-resistant coagulase-negative staphloccal skin flora in immunocompromised patients receiving ciprofloxacin. J Infect Dis 1990;161:41–44
3. Kern W, Jurrie E, Schmeiser T. Streptococcal bacteremia in adult patients with leukemia undergoing aggressive chemotherapy: a review of 55 cases. Infection 1990;18:138–145
4. Høiby N, Jarløv JO, Kemp M et al. Excretion of ciprofloxacin in sweat and multiresistant Staphylococcus epidermidis. Lancet 1997;349:167–169
5. Weightman NC, Simpson EM Speller DCE et al. Bacteremia related to indwelling central venous catheters: prevention, diagnosis and treatment. Eur J Clin Microbiol Infect Dis 1988;7:125–129
6. Raad II, Bodey GP. Infectious complications of indwelling vascular catheters. Clin Infect Dis 1992;15:197–208
7. Salzman MB, Isenbergy HD, Shapiro JF et al. A prospective study of the catheter hub as the portal of entry for microorganisms causing catheter-related sepsis in neonates. J Infect Dis 1993;167:487–490
8. Groeger JS, Lucas AB, Thaler HT et al. Infectious morbidity associated with long term use of venous access devices in patients with cancer. Ann Intern Med 1993;119:1168–1174
9. de Pauw BE, Novakova IR, Donnelly JP. Options and limitations of teicoplanin in febrile granulocytopenic patients. Br J Haematol 1990;2:1–5
10. Weems JJ. Candida parapsilosis: epidemiology, pathogenicity, clinical manifestations and antibiotic susceptibility. Clin Infect Dis 1992;14:756–766
11. Lecciones JA, Lee JW, Navarro EE et al. Vascular catheter-associated fungemia in patients with cancer: analysis of 155 episodes. Clin Infect Dis 1992;14:875–883
12. Morrison VA, Haake RJ, Weisdoft DJ. Non-candida fungal infections after bone marrow transplantation: risk factors and outcome. Am J Med 1994;96:497–503
13. van der Waaij D. The ecology of the human intestine and its consequences for over growth by pathogens such as Clostridium difficile. Annu Rev Microbiol 1989;43:69–87
14. Facklam R. What happened to the streptococci: overview of taxonomic and neomenclature changes. Clin Microbiol Rev 2002;15:613–630
15. Donnelly JP, Maschmeyer G, Daenen S. Selective oral antimicrobial prophylaxis for the prevention of infection in acute leukemia – ciprofloxacin versus co-trimoxazole plus colistin. The EORTC-Gnotobiotic Project Group. Eur J Cancer 1992;28A:873–878
16. Freifield AG, Walsh T, Marshall D et al. Monotherapy for fever and neutropenia in cancer patients: a randomized comparison of ceftazidime versus imipenem. J Clin Oncol 1995;13:165–176
17. Schimpff SC. Infection prevention during profound granulocytopenia: new approaches to alimentary canal microbial suppression. Ann Intern Med 1980;93:358–361
18. van der Waaij D. The colonization resistance of the digestive tract of man and animals. In: Fleidner TM (ed) Clinical and experimental gnotobiotics. Gustav Fischer, Stuttgart, 1979
19. van der Lelie H, van Ketel RJ, von dem Borne AEGK et al. Incidence and clinical epidemiology of streptococcal septicemia during treatment of acute myeloid leukemia. Scand J infect Dis 1991;23:163–168
20. Bochud PY, Calandra T, Francioli P. Bacteremia due to viridans streptococci in neutropenic patients: a review. Am J Med 1994;97:256–264

21. Elting LS, Bodey GP, Keefe BH. Septicemia and shock syndrome due to virdans streptococci: a case-control study of predisposing factors. Clin Infect Dis 1992;14:1201–1207
22. Peters WG, Villemze R, Colly LP, Guiot HFL. Side effects of intermediate and high dose cytosine arabinsodie in the treatment of refractory or relapsed acute leukemia and non-Hodgkin's lymphoma. Neth J Med 1987;30:64–74
23. Guiot HFL, Biemond J, Klasen E et al. Protein loss during acute graft-versus-host disease: diagnostics and clinical significance. Eur J Hematol 1987;38:187–196
24. Callum JL, Brandwein JM, Sutcliffe SB et al. Influence of total of total body irradiation on infections after autologous bone marrow transplantation. Bone Marrow Transplant 1991;8:245–251
25. Potten CS, Wilson JW, Booth C. Regulation and significance of apoptosis in the stem cells of the gastrointestinal epithelium. Stem Cells 1997;15:82–93
26. Sonis St, Oster G, Fuchas H et al. Oral mucositis and the clinical and economic outcomes of hematopoietic stem-cell transplantation. J Clin Oncol 2001;19:2001–2205
27. Rapoport AP, Miller Watelet LP, Linder T et al. Analysis of factors that correlate with mucositis in recipients of autologous and allogeneic stem-cell transplants. J Clin Oncol 1999;17:2446–2453
28. Schimpff SC. Gram-negative bacteremia. Support Care Cancer 1993;1:5–18
29. Schimpff SC. Infections in cancer patients: differences between developed and less developed countries? Eur J Cancer 1991;27:407–408
30. Pouwels MJ, Donnelly JP, Raemaekers JM et al. Clostridium septicum sepsis and neutropenic enterocolitis in a patient treated with intensive chemotherapy for acute myeloid leukemia. Ann Hematol 1997;74:143–147
31. Gomez L, Martino R, Rolaston KV. Neutropenic enterocolitis: spectrum of the disease and comparison of definite and possible cases. Clin Infect Dis 1998:27:695–699
32. Bow EJ, Loewen R, Cheang MS et al. Cytotoxic therapy-induced D-xylose malabsorption and invasive infection during remission-induction therapy for acute myeloid leukemia in adults. J Clin Oncol 1997;15:2254–2261
33. Bow EJ, Loewen R, Cheang MS, Schacter B. Invasive fungal disease in adults undergoing remission-induction therapy for acute myeloid leukemia: the pathogenetic role of the anti-leukemic regimen. Clin Infect Dis 1995:21:361–369
34. Nucci M, Anaissie E. Revisiting the source of candidemia: skin or gut? Clin Infect Dis 2001;33:1959–1967
35. Bodey GP, Buckley M, Sathe YS et al. Qualitative relationship between circulating leucocytes and infections in patients with acute leukemia. Ann Intern Med 1966;64:328–340
36. Schimpff SC. Therapy of infection in patients with granulocytopenia. Med Clin North Am 1978;61:1101–1118
37. van der Meer J. Defects in host defense mechanisms. In: Rubin R, Young LS (eds) Current approaches to infection in the compromised host. Plenum Medical, New York, 1994:3–46
38. Carlisle H, Saslaw S. Properdin levels in splenectomized persons. Pro Soc Exp Biol Med 1959;102:150–155
39. Viscoli C, Bruzzi P, Castagnola E et al. Factors associated with bacteremia in febrile, granulocytopenic cancer patients. The International Antimicrobial Therapy Cooperative Group (IATCG) of the European Organization for Research and Treatment of Cancer (EORTC). Eur J Cancer 1994:4:430–437
40. Sickles EA, Greene WH, Wiernik PH. Clinical presentation of infection in graulocytopenic patients. Arch Intern Med 1975;135:715–719
41. Pizzo PA, Ladisch S, Simon R et al. Increasing incidence of Gram-positive sepsis in cancer patients. Med Paed Oncol 1978;5:241–244
42. de Bock R, Cometta A, Kern W et al. Incidence of single agent gram-negative bacteremias (SAGNB) in neutropenic cancer patients (NCP) in EORTC-IATG trials of empirical therapy for febrile neutropenia. In: Proceedings of the 41st Interscience Conference on Antimicrobial Agents and Chemotherapy, Chicago, 2001
43. Bodey GP, Jadeja L, Elting L. Pseudomonas bacteremia: a retrospective analysis of 410 episodes. Ann Intern Med 1985;145:1621–1629
44. Walmsley S, Devi S, King S et al. Invasive aspergillus infections in a paediatric hospital: a ten year review. Pediatr Infect Dis 1993;12:673–682
45. Allo MA, Miller J, Townsend T et al. Primary cutaneous aspergillosis associated with Hickman intravenous catheters. N Engl J Med 1987;317:1105–1108
46. Anaissie E. Opportunistic mycoses in the immunocompromised host: experience at a cancer centre and review. Clin Infect Dis 1992;14 (suppl 1):S43-S53
47. Fine JD, Miller JA, Harrist TJ et al. Cutaneous lesions in disseminated candidiasis mimicking ecthyma gangrenosum Am J Med 1981;70:1133–1135
48. Tenney JH, Moody MR, Newman KA et al. Adherent micro-organisms on luminal surfaces of long-term intravenous catheters: importance of Staphylococcus epidermidis in patients with cancer. Ann Intern Med 1986;146:1949–1954
49. Pearson TA, Braine HG, Rathburn HK. Corynebacterium species in oncology patients. JAMA 1997;238:1737–1740
50. Gill VJ, Manning C, Lumsom M et al. Antibiotic-resistant group JK bacteria in hospitals. J Clin Microbiol 1981;13:472–477
51. Stamm WE, Thompkins LS, Wagner KF et al. Infection due to Corynebacterium species in marrow transplant patients. Ann Intern Med 1979;91:167–173
52. Dan M, Somer I, Knobel B et al. Cutaneous manifestations of infection with Corynebacterium JK. Rev Infect Dis 1988;10:1204–1207
53. Khadori N, Elting L, Wong E et al. Nosocomial infection due to Xanthomonas maltophila (Pseudomonas maltophila) in patients with cancer. Rev Infect Dis 1990; 12:997–1003
54. Awada A, van der Auwera P, Meunier F et al. Streptococcal and enterococcal bacteremia in patients with cancer. Clin Infect Dis 1992;15:33–48
55. Richard V, Meurnier F, van der Auwera P et al. Pneumococcal bacteremia in cancer patients. Eur J Epidemiol 1988;4:242–245
56. Valteau D, Hartmann O, Brugieres L et al. Streptococcal septicemia following autologous bone marrow transplantation in children treated with high-dose chemotherapy. Bone Marrow Transplant 1991;7:415–419
57. Villablanca JG, Steiner M, Kersey J et al. The clinical spectrum of infection with viridans streptococci in bone marrow transplant patients. Bone Marrow Transplant 1990;6:387–393
58. McWhinney DHM, Gillespie SH, Kibbler CC et al. Streptococcus mitis and ARDS in neutropenic patients. Lancet 1991;337:429 (letter)
59. Karp JE, Merz WG, Hendicksen C et al. Oral norfloxacin for prevention of gram-negative bacterial infection in patients with acute leukemia and granulocytopenia. Ann Intern Med 1987;106:1–7
60. Dekker AW, Rozenberg Arsaka M, Verhoef J. Infection prophylaxis in acute leukemia: a comparison of ciprofloxacin with trimethoprim-sulphamethoxazole and colistin. Ann Intern Med 1987;106:7–12
61. Hughes WT, Armstrong D, Bodey GP et al. IDSA guidelines: 2002 guidelines for the use of antimicrobial agents in neutropenic patients with cancer. Clin Infect Dis 2002;34:730–751
62. Dorowitz GR, Harman C, Pope T, Steward M. The role of the chest roentengram in the febrile neutropenic patient. Arch Intern Med 1991;151:701–704
63. Lightenborg PC, Hoepelman IM, Oude Sogtoen GAC et al. C-reactive protein in the diagnosis and management of infections in granulocytopenic and non-granulocytopenic patients. Eur J Clin Microbiol Infect Dis 1991;10:25–31
64. de Bel C, Gerritson E, de Maaker G et al. C-reactive protein in the management of children with fever after allogenic bone marrow transplantation. Infection 1991;19:92–96
65. Kiehn TE, Armstrong D. Changes in the spectrum of organisms causing bacteremia and fungemia in immunocompromised patients due to venous access devices. Eur J Clin Microbiol Infect Dis 1990;9:869–872
66. Schimpff SC. Surveillance cultures. J Infect Dis 1981;144:81–84
67. Kramer BS, Pizzo PA, Robichaud KJ et al. Role of serial microbiological surveillance and clinical evaluation in the management of cancer patients with fever and granulocytopenia. Am J Med 1982;72:561–568
68. Aisner J, Murillo J, Schimpff SC et al. Invasive aspergillosis in acute leukemia: correlation with nose cultures and antibiotic use. Ann Intern Med 1979;90:4–9
69. Wells CL, Ferrieri P, Weisdorf DJ et al. The importance of surveillance stool cultures during periods of severe neutropenia. Infect Control 1987;8:317–319
70. Consenus Panel of the Immunocompromised Host Society. The design, analysis and reporting of clinical trials on the empirical antibiotic management of the neutropenic patient. J Infect Dis 1990;161:397–401
71. Hughes W, Wade JC, Armstrong D et al. Evaluation of new anti-infective drugs for the treatment of febrile episodes in neutropenic patients. Clin Infect Dis 1992;15(suppl): S206-S215
72. McCabe WR, Jackson GG. Gram-negative bacteremia. II. Clinical, laboratory, and therapeutical observations. Arch Intern Med 1962;110:857–864
73. Viscoli C. Management of infection in cancer patients: studies of the EORTC International Antimicrobial Therapy Group (IATG). Eur J Cancer 2002;38(suppl):S83-S87
74. Schimpff SC, Saterlee W, Young VM et al. Empirical therapy with carbenicillin and gentamicin for febrile patients with cancer and granulocytopenia. N Engl J Med 1971;284:1061–1065
75. Love LJ, Schimpff SC, Schiffer CA et al. Improved prognosis of granulocytopenic patients with Gram-negative bacteremia. Am J Med 1980;68:643–648
76. Klastersky J. Concept of empiric therapy with antibiotic combinations: indications and limits. Am J Med 1986;80(suppl 5C):2–12
77. Schimpff S, Satterlee WM, Young VM. Empiric therapy with carbenicillin under gentamicin for febrile patients with cancer and granulocytopenia. N Engl J Med 1971;284: 1061–1075
78. EORTC International Antimicrobial Therapy Co-operative Group. Ceftazidime combined with short and long course amikacin for empirical therapy of Gram-negative bacteremia in cancer patients with granulocytopenia. N Engl J Med 1987;317:1692–1698
79. Hughes WT, Armstrong D, Bodey GP et al, Working Committee of the Infectious Disease Society of America. Guidelines for the use of antimicrobial agents in neutropenic patients with unexplained fever. J Infect Dis 1990;161:381–396
80. Baden LR, Rubin RH. Fever, neutropenia and the second law of thermodynamics. Ann Intern Med 2002;137:123–124
81. del Favero A, Menichetti F, Martino P et al. A multicenter, double-blind placebo controlled trial comparing piperacillin-tazobactam with and without amikacin as empiric therapy for febrile neutropenia. Clin Infect Dis 2001;33:1295–1301
82. Barza M, Ioannidis JPA, Cappelleri JC, Lau J. Single or multiple daily doses of aminoglycosides: a meta-analysis. BMJ 1996;312:338–344
83. Paul M, Soares-Weiser K, Leibovici L. Beta lactam monotherapy versus beta lactam aminoglycoside combination therapy for fever with neutropenia: systematic review and meta-analysis. BMJ 2003;326:1111
84. EORTC International Antimicrobial therapy Co-operative Group. Single daily dosing of amikacin and ceftriaxone is as efficacious and no more toxic than multiple daily dosing of amikacin and ceftazidime. Ann Intern Med 1993;115:584–593
85. Winston DJ, Ho WG, Bruckner DA et al. Beta-lactam antibiotic therapy in febrile granulocytopenic patients: a randomized trial comparing cefoperazone plus piperacillin, ceftazidime plus pipercillin, and imipenem alone. Ann Intern Med 1991;115:849–859
86. Bodey GP. Evolution of antibiotic therapy for infection in neutropenic patients: studies at MD Anderson hospital. Rev Infect Dis 1989;1 (suppl 7):S1582-S1590
87. Bodey GP, Fainstein V, Elting LS et al. Beta-lactam regimens for the febrile neutropenic patient. Cancer 1990;65:9–16
88. Philpott-Howard JN, Barker KF, Wade JJ et al. Randomised multi-centre study of ciprofloxacin plus azlocillin versus gentamicin and azlocillin in the treatment of febrile neutropenia patients. J Antimicrob Chemother 1990;26:549–559
89. Sanders JW, Pave NR, Moore RD. Ceftazidime monotherapy for empiric treatment of febrile neutropenic patients – a meta-analysis. J Infect Dis 1991;164:907–916
90. Cometta A, Calandra T, Gaya H et al. Monotherapy with meropenem versus combination therapy with ceftazidime plus amikacin in empirical therapy for fever in granulocytopenic patients with cancer. Antimicrob Agents Chemother 1996;40:1108–1115

91. Novakova IRO, Donnelly JP, de Pauw BE. Ceftazidime as monotherapy or combined with teicoplanin for initial empiric treatment of presumed bacteremia in febrile granulocytopenic patients. Antimicrob Agents Chemother 1991;35:672–678

92. Johnson PRE, Liu Yin JA, Tooth JA. High-dose intravenous ciprofloxacin in febrile neutropenic patients. J Antimicrob Chemother 1990;26:101–107

93. Meunier F, Zinner SH, Gaya H et al. Prospective randomized evaluation of ciprofloxacin versus piperacillin plus amikacin for empiric antibiotic therapy for febrile granulocytopenic cancer patients with lymphoma and solid tumours. Antimicrob Agents Chemother 1991;35:872–878

94. Shenep J, Hughes WT, Robertson PK et al. Vancomycin, ticarcillin and amikacin compared with ticarcillin-clavulanate and amikacin in the empirical treatment of febrile neutropenic children with cancer. N Engl J Med 1988:319:1053–1058

95. Karp JE, Dick C, Angelopulos C. Empiric use of vancomycin during prolonged treatment induced granulocytopenia: randomized double blind, placebo controlled trial in patients with acute leukemia. Am J Med 1986;81 :237–242

96. del Favero A, Menichetti F, Guerciolini R et al. Prospective randomised clinical trial of teicoplanin for empiric combined antibiotic therapy in febrile granulocytopenic acute leukemia patients. Antimicrob Agents Chemother 1987;31:1126–1129

97. EORTC-IATCG. Vancomycin added to empirical combination antibiotic therapy for fever in granulocytopenic cancer patients. J Infect 1991;163:951–958

98. Micozzi A, Nucci M, Venditti M et al. Piperacillin/tazobactam/amikacin versus piperacillin/amikacin/teicoplanin in the empirical treatment of neutropenic patients. Eur J Clin Microbiol Infect Dis 1003;12:1–8

99. Rubin M, Hathorn JW, Marshall D et al. Gram-positive infection and the use of vancomycin in 550 episodes of fever and neutropenia. Ann Intern Med 1988;108: 30–35

100. Viscoli C, Moroni C, Boni L et al. Ceftazidime plus amikacin versus ceftazidime plus vancomycin as empiric therapy in febrile neutropenic children with cancer. Rev Infect Dis 1991;13:397–404

101. Montecalvo MA, Horowitz H, Gedris C et al. Outbreak of vancomycin-, ampicillin-, and aminoglycoside-resistant Enterococcus faecium bacteremia in an adult oncology unit. Antimicrob Agents Chemother 1994;38:1363–1367

102. Nolan CM, Beaty HN. Staphylococcus aureus bacteremia: current clinical problems. Am J Med 1976;60:495

103. Iannini PB, Crossley K. Therapy of Staphylococcus aureus bacteremia associated with a removable focus of infection. Ann Intern Med 1976;84:558–560

Viral infections

Chrystal U Louis and Helen E Heslop

CHAPTER 42

Introduction

Following transplantation, reconstitution of the recipient immune system occurs with donor-derived cells and viral infections are a major cause of morbidity and mortality until this process is complete. All hemopoietic stem cell transplant (HSCT) recipients are at risk for the development of viral infections, but those patients who have received alternative donor grafts, especially haploidentical transplants, have a higher risk which can be attributed to the increased time to engraftment, increased T-cell dysfunction (due to either product manipulation, conditioning or immunosuppression regimens), and the increased presence of chronic graft-versus-host disease (GvHD).[1] Furthermore, the use of antithymocyte globulin (ATG) or alemtuzumab in conditioning regimens has also been associated with a significant increase in the incidence of viral infections.[2]

Reactivation of latent infection versus new infection

Patients contract viral infections either by primary contact with infected materials (i.e. secretions, blood products, donor graft) or through viral reactivation. Due to the inherent dangers of transmitting viral infections in transplant units, all facilities should have documented infection control procedures that cover topics such as strict hand washing, cleaning of stethoscopes, droplet precautions, and patient isolation techniques. Universal adherence to these rules should decrease the rates of nosocomial infectious spread.

Blood products and donor grafts should be tested for known viral agents prior to administration. All reasonable attempts should be made to deliver seroequivalent products (identical patient/donor serologic status) whenever transfusions or stem cell products are used. For example, patients who are cytomegalovirus (CMV) seronegative and receive a transplant from a CMV-seropositive donor (D+/R– transplant) are at a higher risk for developing severe, symptomatic CMV disease when compared to patients who receive D–/R– transplants.

An additional method by which patients develop infections after transplant is viral reactivation. Some viruses like CMV, herpes simplex viruses (HSV) 1 and 2, Epstein–Barr virus (EBV) and varicella zoster virus (VZV) remain latent in the host after an initial infection. Viral reactivation and increased virus replication can subsequently occur under times of extreme stress, systemic illness, immunocompromise and in the presence of GvHD.

Immune recovery and ability to control viral infections

The risk of developing and clearing infections post transplant is associated with time to immune system recovery. Generally, bacterial infections are common in the first few weeks after transplant due to severe neutropenia; however, patients remain at risk of contracting a viral infection for several months due to the length of time needed for adaptive immune response recovery. After transplant, natural killer (NK) cells typically return first, and CD8+ T-cells can recover within the first 3 months. However, it can take over 1 year for recovery of the CD4+ T-cell population.[3]

Murine and human studies have demonstrated that control of viral infections after transplantation is enhanced by the presence of virus-specific cytotoxic T-cells in the peripheral blood. These cells can be measured by a number of different assays, including tetramer staining or functional assays such as ELIspot or cytotoxicity assays (Fig. 42.1). Reusser et al noted that the lack of CMV-specific cytotoxic T-lymphocyte (CTL) activity after transplant was associated with fatal CMV pneumonia, while detection of CMV-specific CTL responses appeared to be protective against development of CMV disease.[4] Furthermore, they observed that the presence or absence of CMV-specific T-helper cell proliferation was directly related to CMV-specific CTL activity (see Fig. 42.1). Foster et al further looked at the pattern of CD8+ and CD4+ CMV-specific T-cell reconstitution after transplant and found that the reconstitution patterns were similar.[5] They suggested that both cell types were needed to combat infection since CD4+ cells are important for the regulation of cytotoxic T-cell activity via Th1 cytokine production and activation of antigen-presenting cells.[5]

In addition to the virus-specific T-cell subtypes, lymphopenia in and of itself is an important factor in the development and clearance of viral infections after transplant. In 2005, Heemskerk et al studied the immune reconstitution and clearance of adenoviral viremia in pediatric transplant patients.[6] They found that a low lymphocyte count at the onset of adenoviral infection was associated with progression to viremia. Furthermore, survival after documented viremia was directly related to the host's ability to mount a lymphocyte response.[6]

Due to the significant sequelae and risk of death often associated with viral infections, there has been a concerted effort to improve both the diagnostic tools and treatment strategies available for combating these infections in the post-transplant setting (Table 42.1).

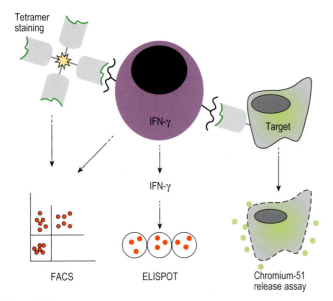

Figure 42.1
Methods for evaluating virus-specific CTL. There are a variety of methods used to evaluate the number and function of virus-specific CTL. FACS analysis can be used to phenotype CTL lines, quantify the number of virus-specific cells in CTL lines via the use of pentamer and/or tetramer staining, and sort cells based on cell surface markers. Elispot assays can be used to determine the functionality of CTL based upon the quantification of secreted factors such as IFN-γ and IL-2. The ability and specificity of CTL killing can be evaluated by the use of chromium release assays.

Table 42.1 Summary of viral infection diagnostic methods

Serology	Most effective prior to transplant
Culture	Gold standard; may take weeks before results available
Shell vial culture	Labor intensive; decreased use in clinical setting
Antigenemia assay	Historically used to guide treatment decisions; requires circulating neutrophils
PCR	Quick results; quantitative and qualitative data available; no historical guidelines to aid with data interpretation
Immunofluorescence	Quick results; results can be laboratory and specimen dependent
Histopathology and immunohistopathology	Used to detect invasive disease within tissue biopsy samples

Diagnostic methods

Serology

Prior to transplant, it is routine for both the donor and the recipient to undergo serologic testing to determine a history of viral infection exposure. This information is important to medical personnel who need to determine which infectious agents have the possibility of reactivating after transplant or if patients will need prophylactic therapy during the peritransplant period due to a history of exposure. However, after transplant, serologic testing is no longer the most accurate method to either diagnose disease or determine the possibility of new exposures as patients may not be able to mount an antibody response.

Viral culture

Viral cultures provide a standard method for determining the presence of disease in the peritransplant setting and culture samples can be generated from almost all biologic fluids and anatomic tissue samples. However, viral cultures routinely take days to weeks to return with positive results, making timely treatment difficult. Furthermore, cultures are limited in utility by the sample size provided, in vitro viral growth parameters, and the potential for cross-contamination.

Shell vial culture and antigenemia assay

Advancements in techniques to determine the presence or absence of viral disease are based on increasing the sensitivity and specificity while reducing the time needed to obtain results. For example, CMV-specific antigens produced in tissue cultures can be identified using the shell vial culture technique. However, shell vial cultures have been increasingly replaced by the CMV antigenemia assay in which the immunodominant pp65 CMV protein is detected in the nucleus of circulating neutrophils.[1,7–9] Since this method is reported as a proportion of antigen-positive cells per number of neutrophils counted, it has the benefits of diagnostic speed coupled with a quantitative measurement that can be followed over time. One drawback to this method is that it requires the presence of a significant number of circulating neutrophils (usually greater than 500/ul)[7] for diagnostic accuracy.

Polymerase chain reaction

An alternative approach is to use quantitative polymerase chain reaction (qPCR) methods to determine viral load measurements of pathogens like CMV, EBV and adenovirus. Several studies have found that PCR levels increase the overall sensitivity and specificity when used to follow viral load in post-transplant patients.[10–13] However, unlike opportunistic infection management in patients with HIV, there are no definitive data for most viruses to determine when pharmacologic interventions should be started. Therefore, most practitioners use a combination of the time post transplantation, the viral load, the rate of rise in the level and pertinent clinical symptoms to determine what interventions, if any, need to be undertaken.

Immunofluorescence

Lastly, techniques like immunofluorescence, in which viral antibodies are conjugated to fluorescent molecules (e.g. fluorescein isothiocynate), can be used to determine the presence of viruses like influenza and parainfluenza in nasal secretions and HSV in vesicular fluid.

Risk of viral infections during the transplant period

The risk of different types of viral infection can vary with time (Table 42.2).

Pretransplant

Pretransplant host-specific factors can increase a patient's risk for developing viral infections. For example, patients who are older, have had significant previous treatment, have been immunocompromised for a long period prior to transplant (either due to medications or the overall disease process), and/or have been infected with latent viruses like the herpes viruses are at increased risk for the develop-

Table 42.2 Most common viral infections encountered during the different stages of engraftment

	Pre-engraftment (days 0–30)	Postengraftment (days ~30–100)	Late postengraftment (days ≧100)
Immune status	Severe neutropenia	Decreased cell-mediated and humoral immunity; decreased phagocytic function	Recovery of cell-mediated and humoral immunity; complications associated with chronic GvHD
Frequency and types of infection seen	1. Bacterial 2. Fungal 3. Viral	1. Viral 2. Fungal 3. Bacterial	1. Viral 2. Bacterial 3. Fungal
Viral infections	HSV	CMV	CMV
		EBV	EBV
		Adenovirus	Adenovirus
		VZV	
		BK/JC viruses	
		Influenza, parainfluenza, RSV	
		HHV6	
		Picornaviruses	

ment of opportunistic infections in the peri- and post-transplant setting.[1,7]

Both donor and recipient should undergo serologic testing to determine a history of viral exposure and the resulting possibility of viral reactivation in the post-transplant setting. Donor testing should include screening for viral hepatitis B and C, HIV types 1 and 2, human T-cell lymphotrophic virus (HTLV) types 1 and 2, CMV and syphilis.[14,15] Transplant recipients should also be evaluated for prior exposure to viral hepatitis B and C, CMV, EBV, HSV types 1 and 2, and VZV.[15] Serologic data should then be used to determine which patients will need prophylactic antiviral therapy or are at risk of reactivation in the pre- and postengraftment periods.

Pre-engraftment (days 0–30)

The risk for various infections during this period is related most closely to neutropenia and lymphopenia and mucosal membrane damage from the conditioning regimens.[1] Due to the presence of prolonged neutropenia post transplant, the most common infections are bacterial, followed by fungal and then viral infections.[16] The virus most commonly seen in this period is HSV, usually as a reactivation rather than primary infection. Multiple studies have documented that HSV reactivation with concurrent disease can occur in up to 80% of patients not treated with prophylaxis.[17,18] Clinical manifestations of HSV reactivation include pneumonia, oral and/or genital ulcers, and stomatitis.[19]

Postengraftment (days ~30–100)

Infections during this period are typically related to the severe immunodeficiency that ensues while awaiting reconstitution of cellular and humoral immunity.[1] With improvements in neutropenia and mucosal damage from the pre-engraftment stage, the most common types of infections encountered during this phase are viral. CMV may present in this stage as either a reactivation of pretransplant disease or as a primary infection. Primary disease can occur in patients who were CMV negative prior to transplant and received either a stem cell product from a CMV-positive donor or CMV-positive blood products.[19] For this reason, CMV prophylaxis is recommended in recipients who are CMV positive or in recipients whose donors are CMV positive. Additionally, CMV-negative, or at a minimum CMV-safe, blood products should be used in all recipients whose serologies and donor serologies are CMV negative.

Other viruses encountered during this period that can lead to pulmonary disease include VZV, adenovirus, human herpes virus-6 (HHV-6),

and the community-acquired viruses, such as respiratory syncytial virus (RSV), influenza, parainfluenza, human metapneumovirus and the picornaviruses.[1,19–26] Respiratory viruses can lead to significant morbidity and mortality in the post-transplant setting, especially in pediatric patients. Other infections seen during this period include hemorrhagic cystitis due to either BK virus or adenovirus, and HHV-6 causing prolonged febrile illnesses and/or encephalitis.[1,19,27,28]

Late postengraftment (days >100)

This time frame is associated with eventual recovery of humoral and cellular immunity. While the typical time to normalization is approximately 1 year, immune reconstitution may take longer than 12 months in patients with chronic GvHD.[1] Chronic GvHD can lead to decreased opsonization, and corticosteroids, typically used to treat GvHD, can worsen the immune dysfunction by causing impaired phagocytosis and cellular immunity.[1]

Late-onset CMV disease can also manifest itself during this period. The immune dysfunction seen during this time frame has been associated with delayed recovery of both CMV-specific CD8+ CTLs and CMV-specific CD4+ T-helper cells needed for controlling CMV infections.[10,29–31]

EBV-associated post-transplant lymphoproliferative diseases (EBV-PTLD) occur more frequently in the first 6 months post transplant, although they can be detected prior to day +100 in patients who have received anti-T cell monoclonal antibodies or T-cell depleted grafts.[32–34] Those most at risk of developing EBV-PTLD also tend to have greater degrees of immune dysfunction.[33,34]

Viral infections commonly seen after stem cell transplantation

Human cytomegalovirus (CMV)

Human CMV is a DNA-virus member of the herpesvirus family. It can be transmitted from person to person via contact with virus-containing secretions, vertical transmission, blood transfusions and transplantation from CMV-seropositive donors. Since the virus is ubiquitous in the population, approximately 60–80% of healthy adults are CMV positive.[35] After a primary infection, CMV becomes latent in leukocytes and tissues. Therefore, during times of immunosuppression and decreased cell-mediated immunity, CMV can reactivate and lead to the development of disease.

Clinical presentation

Patients with a history of CMV, as well as those who are seronegative but receiving a seropositive product (D+/R−), are at an increased risk for the development of either reactivated or primary disease.

After transplantation, CMV disease can present as fever, malaise, pancytopenia, abnormal liver function, gastrointestinal disease, myelitis, chorioretinitis, and neurologic dysfunction.[35–38] One of the most severe and potentially fatal complications of CMV disease is the development of interstitial pneumonitis. Prior to the initiation of routine CMV antiviral prophylaxis/pre-emptive therapy for high-risk patients, one institution noted an 8.8% incidence of CMV pneumonia in their transplant patients.[39] Disease was more frequently seen in older patients or those who received allogeneic products, total-body irradiation, T-cell depleted grafts, and/or had evidence of CMV in either the urine or blood.[39] Ninety-three percent of those patients not treated died of disease. Furthermore, survival outcomes were poor if antiviral therapy was not initiated prior to the need for ventilatory support.[39]

Diagnosis

Due to the significant sequelae that can occur from CMV in the post-transplant setting, all patients and donors have serologic testing before transplant to assess disease risk. Historically, the shell vial technique and CMV antigenemia assays have been used to determine CMV status post transplant. An earlier study evaluating the utility of CMV antigenemia reported that by the first positive result, they were detecting a median of 4 granulocytes (range 1–48) per 2.5×10^5 cells in which pp65 protein could be identified in the nucleus.[40] Therefore, what became evident is that the risk of disease progression is multifactorial, based upon the actual antigenemia level, the time to conversion after transplant, the rate of rise and the response of the level to antiviral therapy.

PCR analysis for CMV-DNA levels has become an important evaluation tool due to rapid turn-around time and because it does not rely on granulocyte engraftment. Solano et al found that quantitative PCR in plasma samples, when compared to CMV antigenemia levels, had a 90% concordance rate.[41] For patients found to be viremic by both methods, PCR conversion occurred approximately 1 week prior to and resolved a median of 7 days later than antigenemia assays. However, these authors noted that basing pre-emptive treatment strategies on PCR detection alone would have caused 'unnecessary' treatment in 24% of viremic patients who never progressed to end-stage disease.[41]

A survey of the transplant centers that participate in the National Marrow Donor Program found that of all the methods of detection available, CMV antigenemia, PCR levels, and the shell vial culture technique are the tests most commonly used to initiate therapy.[42] However, no consensus currently exists as to the time for intervention or which pharmacologic agent should be used. As such, PCR levels should be used either in conjunction with or supplemental to CMV antigenemia levels when initiating interventions.

Therapy

The prevention of CMV disease in seronegative transplant patients should be attempted by the use of donor seronegative products, including CMV-negative and/or leukodepleted blood products, when possible.

Antiviral prophylaxis for high-risk patients and early pre-emptive antiviral therapy are the two methods currently used by different institutions to decrease the rates of CMV end-organ disease (Table 42.3). Initial studies evaluated aciclovir, but ganciclovir has been the most commonly used prophylactic drug since the early 1990s. Prospective studies found that prophylactic administration of ganciclovir during the peritransplant period decreased the rates of CMV infections and interstitial pneumonia in high-risk patients from 23% and 17%, respectively, to zero.[43] More recent studies have attempted to streamline therapy, but found that when comparing 3-day with 5-day prophylactic ganciclovir therapy, the 5-day regimen was associated with statistically less CMV infection and disease.[44]

One common dose-limiting side-effect seen with ganciclovir therapy is neutropenia. Since a percentage of patients will not be able to tolerate treatment with ganciclovir and with the development of ganciclovir-resistant CMV, the use of other agents such as foscarnet has been investigated. Foscarnet decreases the rates of CMV

Table 42.3 Prophylaxis, pre-emptive and treatment choices for CMV

Agent	Prophylaxis	Pre-emptive	Treatment	Reference
Aciclovir	500 mg iv q 8 hours 800 mg po bid × 1 year			Prentice et al 1994[145] Boeckh et al 2006[96]
Ganciclovir	5 mg/kg iv q 12 hours × 14 doses, then 6 mg/kg × 5 days each week	5 mg/kg iv q 12 hours × 28 doses, then once daily × 5 days a week	5 mg/kg iv q 12 hours for at least 28 doses, then once daily for 3–4 weeks	Winston et al 2003[46] Reusser et al 2002[146] Machado et al 2000[52] Boeckh et al 2003[147]
Foscarnet	90 mg/kg iv q 12 hours from day +11 to +16, then once daily 3 times a week	60 mg/kg iv q 12 hours × 14 days, if still positive then 90 mg/kg daily × 5 days a week for 14 days	60 mg/kg iv q 8 hours for at least 42 doses	Ordemann et al 2000[148] Reusser et al 2002[146] Aschan et al 1992[149]
Valaciclovir	2 g po q 6 hours			Winston et al 2003[46]
Valganciclovir		900 mg po bid		van der Heiden et al 2006[150]
IVIG			500 mg/kg iv q other day × 10 doses	Emanuel et al 1988[50] Machado et al 2000[52]
Cidofovir			3–5 mg/kg iv × 1, then q 2 weeks; all doses given with probenecid	Ljungman et al 2001[53] Chakrabarti et al 2001[151]
CTL	Per investigational protocol	Per investigational protocol	Per investigational protocol	Cobbold et al 2005[58] Leen et al 2006[57]
Leflunomide			Case report	Avery et al 2004[152]

infection and disease with increasing doses, but acute renal toxicity may lead to drug discontinuation in a significant number of patients.[45] Therefore, it is generally a second-line therapeutic option for patients who either cannot tolerate or do not respond to ganciclovir therapy.

Valaciclovir and valganciclovir are oral prodrugs of aciclovir and ganciclovir, respectively. Due to the success of prophylactic therapy with their iv counterparts, different groups have investigated the efficacy of these oral compounds with respect to CMV prophylaxis. One multicenter randomized trial found that prophylaxis with either oral valaciclovir or intravenous ganciclovir during the postengraftment phase provided similar protection from development of CMV infections and disease.[46] Another recent study evaluated the efficacy of oral versus iv ganciclovir prophylaxis and found that there were no cases of CMV disease during the study period in either group.[47] While more patients in the oral ganciclovir group (eight versus two in the IV cohort) were not able to complete the scheduled therapy, either method was a safe and effective form of CMV prophylaxis.[47] With the ease of oral administration and similar efficacy profiles, more institutions will be likely to move toward the use of oral agents as front-line prophylactic therapy.

Other centers have chosen to pre-emptively use antiviral therapy only upon early detection of CMV infection and until a defined time post resolution. In this strategy, only patients with documented CMV infection and/or disease are treated with antiviral agents rather than all at-risk patients. One group tested this theory by randomizing patients after engraftment to prophylactic or pre-emptive treatment with ganciclovir.[48] They found that treatment based on antigenemia levels resulted in more cases of CMV infection and disease by day +100. However, prophylaxis from the time of engraftment was associated with a higher rate of invasive fungal infections and increased late-onset CMV disease by day +180.[48] Another group compared foscarnet with ganciclovir for prophylactic treatment of CMV antigenemia in an open-labeled randomized study and found that there was no statistical difference between the two agents when comparing drug-specific side-effects, clearance of CMV antigenemia, treatment failures, CMV disease and CMV-related death.[49]

Since the institution of prophylaxis and aggressive pre-emptive therapy, the number of patients who develop CMV infections and disease after transplant has dramatically decreased. However, once patients contract CMV disease, the rates of significant secondary sequelae and death remain high. Treatment of CMV disease has traditionally been accomplished with a combination of intravenous immune globulin and ganciclovir.[50,51] Enright et al reported a survival rate of approximately 40% with this combination of agents if patients are treated prior to becoming ventilator dependent.[39] However, others have noted no survival advantage provided by the use of intravenous immunoglobulin (IVIG) in patients with CMV disease treated with ganciclovir.[52] In those patients who develop either CMV infections or end-stage disease that does not respond to ganciclovir, cidofovir has provided a curative treatment option for a subset of patients.[53]

T-cell mediated immunity is necessary for clearance and treatment of viral infections and several groups have shown that the risk of CMV reactivation and infection relates to recovery of the immune response to CMV. Therefore, an additional treatment option should be the administration of CMV-specific cytotoxic T-lymphocytes and several groups have shown that these T-cells can restore CMV immunity and confer protection from CMV disease.[54–57] One limitation of this approach is the time taken to generate CTL lines. To overcome this problem Cobbold et al purified CMV-specific CD8+ T-cells directly from the blood of HSCT donors using FACS sorting with HLA-restricted peptide tetramers. Adoptive transfer of this product was associated with a reduction of the viral load in all patients and clearance of CMV viremia in 8/9 patients.[58] However, the infused clones

only recognized one viral epitope. As such, this method may be associated with a higher risk of viral evasion in the long term.

Epstein–Barr virus (EBV)

EBV is a ubiquitous member of the herpesvirus family and more than 90% of adults have been infected with the virus by the age of 40. Transmission generally occurs through contact with the saliva of an infected person or with exposure to infected blood products. After contact, infection of mucosal epithelial cells causes the virus to replicate and eventually lyse the cell.[59,60] The virus can then infect B-cells where it may become latent; however, reactivation of EBV-infected memory B-cells can lead to lytic replication of the virus and reactivation to a proliferating lymphoblast expressing all latent cycle antigens. Normally, such cells would be rapidly eliminated by an EBV-specific T-cell response but if a recipient is highly immunosuppressed, the cells may grow unchecked and cause a post-transplant lymphoproliferative disorder (PTLD). After HSCT, risk factors for developing PTLD include the degree of mismatch between donor and recipient, manipulation of the graft to deplete T-cells and the degree of immunosuppression used to prevent GvHD.[61] In contrast to T-cell depletion, the incidence of PTLD is much lower when T- and B-cells are depleted, supporting the concept that the malignant outgrowth of EBV-positive B-cells is favored by an imbalance between EBV-infected B-cells and EBV-specific T-cells.[62]

Clinical presentation

Once EBV reactivation has occurred post transplant, patients may develop fever and malaise. However, the majority of patients do not have any clinical symptoms early after reactivation.[63] The most severe complication associated with reactivation is the development of EBV-PTLD. Clinically PTLD presents as fever, lymphadenopathy and/or disseminated lymphoproliferation of the liver, lungs, gastrointestinal tract, central nervous system and bone marrow.[59,64]

Diagnosis

Over the last decade progress has been made in better identifying high-risk patients and understanding the pathogenesis of PTLD.[65–67] PCR quantitative EBV-DNA levels are typically used to diagnose EBV reactivation; however, these levels do not always correlate with reactivation versus EBV-PTLD. Our group has suggested that EBV viral load should be used to guide prompt rather than pre-emptive treatment.[66] In support of this strat-egy, Annels et al described patients who were able to mount an EBV-specific T-cell response and clear elevated viral loads without medical intervention during EBV reactivation.[63]

Therapy

While most of the antiviral medications currently available have some activity against EBV, they do not modulate the growth of infected B-cells. Current therapeutic options include approaches targeting the malignant B-cells such as anti-CD20 monoclonal antibody or approaches aimed at reconstituting immunity to EBV such as EBV-specific CTL or unmanipulated donor lymphocyte infusions. Our group has shown that infusion of EBV-CTL generated from allogeneic donors is safe and can be used not only to treat patients with active PTLD but also to decrease the incidence of EBV-PTLD to approximately 0% when used as prophylactic therapy in high-risk patients.[68,69] Rituximab, a chimeric murine/human monoclonal anti-CD20 antibody, has also been used successfully as prophylaxis and treatment for PTLD post HSCT, with responses rates varying between 70% and 100%.[61,70,71]

Adenovirus

There are at least 51 different serotypes of this non-enveloped, lytic DNA virus. The human serotypes have been divided into six specific species (A–F). Due to the ubiquitous nature of this virus, the majority of adults have been exposed to adenovirus at least once during their lifetime. Adenovirus can be transmitted through respiratory secretions, fomites and via the fecal–oral route. In the transplant setting, patients with adenoviral infections may acquire them as a primary infection, through reactivation and possibly by transmission from the donor graft.[72,73]

Adenoviral infections can lead to significant morbidity and mortality in transplant patients. Infection can occur in up to 31% of patients post transplant;[24,74] however, up to 73% of infected patients may develop systemic disease.[72,75] Risk factors associated with the development of disease include the use of ATG or alemtuzumab (anti-CD52 monoclonal antibody) in the conditioning regimen, a T-cell depleted product, transplantation with matched unrelated donor or haploidentical donor products, the presence of adenovirus in the peripheral blood, and the severity of lymphopenia at the time of diagnosis.[75–77]

Clinical presentation

Clinical symptoms consistent with adenovirus range from asymptomatic infection to multisystem organ disease. Patients may present with respiratory tract infections, myocarditis, gastroenteritis, hepatitis, nephritis, hemorrhagic cystitis, and/or encephalitis.[78] The onset of infection differs based upon the age of the transplant recipient, with children having a shorter time to viral detection compared to adults (<30 days versus >90 days).[72]

Diagnosis

Samples from blood, urine, stool, nasopharyngeal secretions, CSF and tissues can be evaluated with the use of immunofluorescence assays and viral cultures. Additionally, real-time PCR can be used to quantify viral levels and distinguish between the different adenoviral species.[75]

Therapy

Three major risk factors for disseminated disease include severe lymphopenia at the time of infection, concurrent use of immunosuppressive agents and a positive PCR blood sample. Chakrabarti el al recommended observation for asymptomatic patients not receiving immunosuppressive medications with an absolute lymphocyte count (ALC) >300/mm^3; withdrawal of immunosuppression, if possible, in patients who were asymptomatic; and commencement of antiviral therapy in those patients who had an ALC <300/mm^3, positive blood PCR samples, or in those patients in whom immunosuppression could not be stopped.[77]

Antiviral medications have been used with variable success. Ribivarin was used in the past, but it consistently showed few clinical responses.[74,79,80] Recently, Yusuf et al reported that of 57 patients with documented adenovirus infection (eight of whom had disease), 98% had complete resolution of virus detection and symptoms after treatment with cidofovir[81] although infection in this study may have been overestimated as it was defined by PCR positivity.

As T-cell dysfunction is clearly associated with the risk of developing adenoviral infection and disease, several groups are evaluating whether ex vivo expanded, adenovirus-specific CTL can be used to treat adenoviral infection and disease. Clinical responses have been reported in patients with adenoviral disease using this approach.[57,82]

Herpes simplex virus (HSV)

HSV is a double-stranded, enveloped DNA virus with two major subtypes, which can be transmitted through contact with infected oral secretions or lesions, and through sexual intercourse. After a primary infection, HSV becomes latent in sensory ganglia, with the trigeminal and sacral ganglions being the most common locations, depending on the site of the primary infection.[36] Reactivation in the peri- and post-transplant setting led to significant and even fatal sequelae prior to the discovery that prophylaxis with aciclovir during the pre-engraftment phase significantly decreased the rates of HSV reactivation.[83,84] Prophylaxis has since become the standard of care when transplanting seropositive patients.

Clinical presentation

Prior to prophylaxis, the most common presentation of HSV was reactivation of the virus in mucous membranes leading to severe mucositis/gingivostomatitis, fever and pain. Vesicular or ulcerative skin lesions can occur in any location of the body, with the most typical sites located on the face, perioral region, and the genitals. Disseminated skin lesions can occur in patients who are severely immunocompromised. Patients can also be afflicted with conjunctivitis, keratitis and herpetic whitlow (lesions located on the distal portions of the fingertips). If the central nervous system becomes infected, patients may experience symptoms of fever, meningitis, encephalitis, seizures, altered mental status, Bell's palsy, trigeminal neuralgia and/or ascending myelitis.

Diagnosis

Serologic testing for the presence of antibody titers is now done on all patients prior to transplant. Primary or reactivated lesions can be scraped looking for multinucleated giant cells and eosinophilic intranuclear inclusions when Tzanck preparations are evaluated microscopically. Increased diagnostic sensitivity is produced when samples are sent for culture but it can take from 1 to 15 days for culture results to become positive.[36] Fluorescent antibody stains and enzyme immunoassays can permit rapid determinations of disease status. Additionally, PCR can be used to follow quantitative DNA levels and determine the presence of the virus in the CSF.

Therapy

In the first major study evaluating the efficacy of prophylaxis for transplant patients with HSV, no patients treated with aciclovir developed culture-positive lesions, as compared to 70% of seropositive patients in the placebo group.[83] Based upon this and other comparable prophylaxis data, the Centers for Disease Control (CDC) now recommends prophylaxis through at least the pre-engraftment phase and would consider longer therapy for those patients with either a history of multiple reactivations or GvHD.[36] Due to similar efficacy, cost and simpler dosing schedule, some institutions use valaciclovir rather than aciclovir for HSV prophylaxis.[85–87]

Once either primary or reactivated HSV has been identified, first-line treatment in transplant patients is aciclovir. However, the prevalence of aciclovir-resistant HSV strains is increasing.[88] Therefore, patients who cannot tolerate aciclovir therapy or have documented aciclovir-resistant HSV should be treated with either foscarnet or cidofovir.

Varicella zoster virus (VZV)

As a single serotype virus, VZV, a member of the herpesvirus family, causes chickenpox (i.e. varicella) with a primary infection and shingles (i.e. zoster) upon viral reactivation. Primary infection occurs mostly by contact with respiratory droplets, although contact with vesicular lesions and maternal-to-child transmission have also been documented.[36] After transmission, the virus infects the mucosa of the upper respiratory tract, spreads in the blood and tracks to the skin. Skin lesions are vesicular in appearance and biopsies are composed of multinucleated giant cells with intranuclear inclusions at the base of the lesions. Once the primary infection has resolved, the virus becomes latent in the dorsal root ganglia. With advancing age, infection, stress, trauma and/or episodes of immune dysfunction, the virus can reactivate as zoster.

Clinical presentation

As mentioned previously, primary infection with VZV typically manifests as a pruritic, generalized, vesicular rash and fever. Acute dissemination and death have been reported in patients taking corticosteroids, especially when administered during the incubation period or within 3 weeks of clinical symptoms.[36,89–92] Immunocompromised patients with T-cell dysfunction or B-cell abnormalities are also at greater risk for disseminated disease.[36]

Reactivation of VZV occurs in approximately 30% of patients after HSCT.[93–95] Painful, vesicular lesions clustered over 1–3 sensory dermatomes are the most common presentation of zoster. Many patients present with pain prior to the onset of skin lesions. Historically, those presenting with either severe abdominal or back pain prior to dermatitis have more severe disease.[89] Similar to primary infection, those taking corticosteroids near the time of presentation are at further risk for disseminated, severe disease. Immunocompromised patients may also present with atypical disease in the lung, gastrointestinal tract, liver, and CNS with or without skin lesions.[93]

Diagnosis

VZV can be diagnosed based on clinical symptoms if skin lesions are present. A vesicular biopsy or Tzanck smear of a vesicular lesion should have evidence of multinucleated giant cells with inclusion bodies. However, the presence of these cells is not specific for VZV. Tissue culture from the base of a lesion will allow for distinction between VZV and HSV, but direct fluorescent antigen (DFA) detection is much faster than standard tissue culture. Additionally, samples from the blood, bone marrow, CSF, and organ tissues can be evaluated via PCR.[36]

Therapy

Because of the potential severity of this infection in the transplant setting, once a patient has been exposed to or diagnosed with VZV they should be isolated in accordance with the hospital's airborne and contact precautions for VZV. According to the CDC, seronegative patients exposed to VZV should be treated with varicella zoster immune globulin within 96 hours of exposure.[14] Seropositive patients are at high risk for disease reactivation for 3–12 months post transplant.[96] Several groups have shown that prophylactic aciclovir in seropositive patients for 6–12 months post transplant has decreased the rates of VZV reactivation but has not decreased the overall rates of long-term reactivation.[96–98] One group noted the majority of patients with reactivation after 1 year of prophylactic aciclovir were those who required long-term immunosuppression and suggested this may be a population in which prolonged therapy should be considered.[96]

For patients with active VZV, treatment depends on the severity of the disease. In those with chickenpox or disseminated zoster, iv aciclovir is the treatment of choice. Patients who have either resistant disease or who cannot tolerate iv aciclovir should be treated with foscarnet.[99] Localized zoster has been treated successfully with aciclovir, by all routes, and valaciclovir.[99]

Human herpesvirus 6 (HHV6)

HHV6 is a member of the herpesviridae family of viruses, and humans are the only known carriers. HHV6 includes type A and type B variants and contains a large, double-stranded, DNA genome and disease. Transmission of the virus is typically from contact with secretions from asymptomatic carriers.[36] Most children are seropositive for HHV6 by the age of 2[36,100,101] and 95% of adults will have detectable DNA in peripheral blood mononuclear cells (PBMC) and in the saliva after a primary infection.[26]

Clinical presentation

Reactivation of HHV6, more commonly type B, typically occurs in the pre-engraftment phase and HHV6 can often be found in the blood of patients within the first 20–30 days post transplant.[100,102] Clinically, patients exhibit a wide variety of symptoms after reactivation. HHV6 can cause encephalitis, altered mental status and seizures if reactivation occurs primarily in the central nervous system.[7] Systemic reactivation has been associated with delayed platelet engraftment, bone marrow suppression, skin rashes, pneumonia, and hepatitis.[25,100–103]

Diagnosis

Due to the ubiquitous nature of this virus in the population, there is no clear-cut method for monitoring disease. Neither qualitative PCR nor serology is reliable due to the large number of patients who can become positive after transplantation.[104] Therefore, following viral load levels and clinical correlation (e.g. symptoms of encephalitis coupled with the presence of quantitative HHV6 levels in the CSF) are likely to provide the most useful diagnostic information.[7]

Therapy

There have been reports of in vitro activity of foscarnet, ganciclovir and cidofovir in the treatment of HHV6 infections.[7,100] While no prospective studies evaluating the utility of any of these antiviral agents have been undertaken, reports using each of the medications in the treatment of HHV6-induced encephalitis, pneumonia, thrombocytopenia and enteritis have provided encouraging results.[7,105–107]

BK and JC viruses

Both BK and JC viruses are classified as papovaviruses. Theses viruses are naked icosahedral pathogens composed of double-stranded, circular supercoiled DNA. In the post-transplant setting, both viruses can be excreted in the urine independent of associated disease.

Clinical presentation

BK virus can be serologically detected in up to 60–90% of adults[108] and can be found in the kidneys and the peripheral blood of normal hosts.[109] Reactivation of BK virus after transplant has been associated with hemorrhagic cystitis. Symptoms include bilateral lower quadrant abdominal pain, dysuria, frequency and hematuria. More severe cases can be associated with clot formation in the bladder, obstructive nephropathy and potential progression to renal insufficiency/failure.

JC virus is known to persist in the kidneys of immunocompetent individuals without causing disease. However, in patients with abnormal immune function, JC virus can migrate to the central nervous system, infect and destroy myelin-producing oligodendrocytes. This destruction leads to progressive multifocal leukoencephalopathy (PML), a rapidly developing neuromuscular disease. Symptoms of PML include visual field defects, extreme weakness, paralysis, mental impairment and possibly death.

Diagnosis

While JC and BK viruses can be identified by immunofluorescence microscopy, the use of PCR-based assays allows for efficient diagnosis and the quantification of viral load levels in urine, blood and brain tissue samples.[110,111]

Therapy

Both vidarabine and cidofovir have been used in the treatment of papopavirus infections.[7] One center recently reported the incidence, treatment and outcome of viral-induced hemorrhagic cystitis in transplant patients.[112] They noted resolution of cystitis in 78.9% of patients with at least grade 2 hemorrhagic cystitis (defined as at least macroscopic hematuria with small clots) treated with cidofovir.[112]

Parvovirus B19 (B19)

As a small, non-enveloped, single-stranded DNA virus, the B19 subtype is the only parvovirus that has been known to cause disease in humans. B19 has a worldwide distribution and can be transmitted via respiratory secretions, exposure to blood products and through vertical transmission between mother and child. Evaluation of immunocompetent host IgG levels has shown that approximately 60% of school-aged children have been previously exposed to parvovirus.[113,114] Lifelong persistence of parvovirus B19-specific IgG antibodies is thought to be one reason for decreased reactivation rates in immunocompetent hosts. However, dysfunctional humoral immunity post transplant is believed to be one of the reasons patients may exhibit either primary disease or recurrence/reactivation of B19.[113,115]

Clinical presentation

B19 typically infects either bone marrow, especially red blood cell precursors, or blood vessel endothelial cells. Immunocompromised patients, with either acute or chronic infection, may present after unexplained episodes of anemia, reticulocytopenia, fever, pancytopenia, hepatitis or myocarditis.[113,116]

Diagnosis

Parvovirus B19 infections can be determined by serologic titers in patients with intact immune systems. However, in the post-transplant immunocompromised setting, diagnosis is typically made by detection from immunoassays or PCR. It should be recognized that B19 DNA may be detected by PCR for up to 9 months after an acute infection.[36]

Therapy

Mild cases of B19 infection can be managed with supportive care and transfusion of blood products as needed. More severe cases of disease have been treated successfully with intravenous immunoglobulin, possibly from an IgG-specific B19 component[36,113,117] All immunocompromised patients diagnosed with B19 should be placed on droplet precautions to avoid the spread of disease to other patients.

Hepatitis B (HBV) and hepatitis C (HCV)

HBV is a DNA-containing hepadnavirus. HCV is a single-stranded RNA virus and member of the flavivirus family. Both viruses can be transmitted by contact with blood and HBV can also be transmitted via contact with body fluids. Due to the high prevalence of disease in some countries and the need for a graft in patients with no 'eligible' donors, some products used for transplantation will be obtained from HBV- and HCV-seropositive donors.

Patients positive for HBV surface antigen (HBsAg) prior to transplant are not at an increased risk for early transplant-related mortality when compared to their antigen-negative counterparts.[118,119] In fact, the use of stem cell grafts from donors that have HBV immunity was associated with sustained clearance of HBsAg and a decreased rate of liver cirrhosis.[120] Long term, however, more than 65% of patients positive prior to transplant will have reactivation of their HBV by 24 months post transplant.[121]

Unlike patients with HBV, those patients who were HCV RNA positive before HSCT are at increased risk for peritransplant complications. In a retrospective review of HCV-positive transplant recipients, one group found the presence of pretransplant HCV infection and elevated serum aspartate levels were strongly associated with the development of severe veno-occlusive disease (relative risk of 9.6). Some patients developed acute hepatitis flares prior to day +180; however, none progressed to fulminant liver failure or had an overall risk of increased mortality by 10 years post transplant.[122]

Clinical presentation

Hepatitis caused by either HBV or HCV can be asymptomatic or acutely present with abnormal liver enzyme tests, abdominal pain, jaundice, pruritus, arthritis or a macular rash.[36] In severe cases, patients can develop fulminant liver failure, veno-occlusive disease and/or die. Viral hepatitis can cause liver disease throughout the entire peri- and post-transplant period; however, the highest rates of hepatitis-induced liver disease occur in the late post-transplant period.[121,123] Long-term sequelae from HBV and HCV chronic infections are cirrhosis and hepatocellular carcinoma.

Diagnosis

Pretransplant evaluations of hepatitis status are typically done via serologic titers. Blood, serum, and liver biopsy samples can be used for diagnosis after transplant. HBsAg and other markers for evaluating HBV can be detected using enzyme immunoassays. PCR can also be used to quantify and follow HBV DNA levels. HCV status can be determined by the use of enzyme-linked immunosorbent assays (ELISA). Increased result sensitivity for HCV can be obtained by the use of reverse transcription PCR. PCR has also been used for quantification of HCV levels.

Therapy

If possible, the use of stem cell products from donors that are either HBsAg or HCV positive should be avoided. If these products must be used, then patients should be monitored for signs and symptoms consistent with viral hepatitis.

When an HBsAg-positive product is given to a seronegative patient, treatment with lamivudine and vaccination prior to transplant can decrease rates of HBV-associated hepatitis and death secondary to hepatitis-related hepatic failure.[124] Famciclovir therapy alone has also been used in this population and was associated with a decreased rate of post-transplant hepatitis.[125] Interferon-α therapy has been used in children who develop HBV post transplant. It provided therapeutic results comparable to those seen in patients without a history of cancer treatment or transplant.[126]

Treatment of an HCV-positive donor with interferon-α prior to collection and transplantation has been reported to prevent virus transmission.[127] If the patient has contracted the virus in the pretransplant setting and the donor is HCV negative, prophylaxis using oral ribivarin until engraftment was associated with seroconversion in three out of four patients in a small pilot study.[128] Lastly, patients who have seroconverted post transplant are currently being treated with interferon-α and ribivarin with similar results to immunocompetent patients treated with the same regimen.[126]

Respiratory syncytial virus (RSV)

Humans are the only known hosts of this single-stranded, enveloped RNA virus. A member of the paramyxovirus family, RSV can be transmitted through close contact with contaminated secretions, respiratory droplets or fomites. Most humans have been infected with RSV by 2 years of age and reinfection is common, independent of age. Community-acquired and nosocomial spread of RSV on transplant units has led to severe and even fatal outbreaks of the disease.[129,130] Mortality rates due to RSV in transplant patients range from 17% to 45%.[129,131,132]

Clinical presentation

Acute respiratory tract infections are the most common manifestations of RSV. However, in very young patients, apnea, poor feeding and irritability can precede respiratory symptoms.[36] Typical presentations include upper and/or lower tract disease, rhinorrhea, wheezing, bronchiolitis, pneumonia and respiratory distress or failure. Increased severity of disease and higher mortality rates are noted in patients who contract RSV during the pre-engraftment phase.[129,131,133]

Diagnosis

Identification of RSV can be conducted by a multitude of methods, including isolation from culture samples of nasopharyngeal secretions, bronchial alveolar lavages, sputum and lung tissue. Culture results are generally available within 5 days, but sensitivity of the results varies between different laboratories based on collection and viral isolation methods.[36] More rapid methods for viral determination include PCR, immunofluorescent and enzyme immunoassays.

Therapy

For those patients with active disease, contact precautions and respiratory droplet precautions should be used until the virus resolves. In very young infants, viral shedding may last as long as 3–4 weeks after the initial illness.[36] Although the initial data in transplant patients were mixed, most practitioners now treat RSV-infected patients with a combination of aerosolized ribivarin and IVIG.[7,129,134]

Palivizumab is a humanized respiratory syncytial virus monoclonal antibody that has been successful in the prevention of RSV in premature infants. In 2001, Boeckh et al reported the results of a Phase I study using the antibody in six patients without and 15 patients with active RSV post transplant.[135] They found that administration of the antibody was safe, and use in the patients with upper tract disease inhibited progression to the lower tract.[135]

Parainfluenza (HPIV)

Parainfluenza viruses are single-stranded RNA viruses spread by either respiratory droplets or contact with contaminated surfaces. HPIVs have been divided into four major serotypes (types 1–4), the majority of which have defined times of seasonal infectivity.[36]

Clinical presentation

In the post-transplant setting, HPIV can be associated with upper and lower respiratory tract disease and pneumonia. Of the individual subtypes, HPIV 3 tends to cause the most severe disease and is commonly associated with mortality.[7,136] Different studies have found that the incidence of parainfluenza infection ranges from 2% to 7%, and patients who have received unrelated donor transplants are at the highest risk for contracting HPIV.[136–138]

Diagnosis

The diagnostic gold standard for HPIV is positive identification of the virus in culture from nasopharyngeal washings. However, it may take several days before cultures become positive, leading many institutions to also obtain rapid diagnostic measurements such as reverse transcriptase PCR (RT-PCR) or immunofluorescence assays.

Therapy

Due to the highly infectious nature of parainfluenza viruses, once patients have a confirmed diagnosis they should be placed in respiratory isolation and strict hand washing should be observed. At this time, no antiviral agent has proven to be completely effective at eradicating HPIV infections. However, although published results evaluating efficacy have been mixed, the early use of ribivarin is the most common form of pharmacologic therapy.[136,138–140]

Influenza A and B

Although there are three antigenic subtypes of influenza (types A, B and C), only types A and B are known to cause epidemic and/or pandemic disease. These orthomyxoviruses are spread by direct contact with infected people, respiratory droplets or items containing nasopharyngeal secretions.[36] Epidemics generally occur in the fall and winter months, but influenza seasons can last longer if communities are afflicted with more than two or three subtypes.

Patients who have contracted the disease are contagious from approximately 24 hours prior to the onset of clinical symptoms until 5–7 days later once viral shedding is complete. Immunocompromised patients may continue to be symptomatic and shed viral particles for longer periods of time.

Clinical presentation

HSCT recipients with influenza can present with fever, chills, myalgia, upper respiratory tract symptoms, pneumonia, bronchiolitis, croup, wheezing or any combination thereof. Complications of this infection include, but are not limited to, the development of central nervous system abnormalities, myositis and Reye syndrome.[36]

Nichols et al reported their experience with influenza infections after stem cell transplant and noted that approximately 1% of their 4800 transplant patients were diagnosed with influenza within 120 days of receiving their graft.[141] Influenza A was responsible for 66% of the cases, and transplant during the influenza season, female gender, and advanced pretransplant disease were risk factors for contracting the virus. Progression from upper to lower respiratory tract disease/pneumonia was highest in patients lymphopenic at the time of diagnosis. Most importantly, 10% of the patients with influenza died secondary to their infection within 30 days of their initial diagnosis.[141]

Diagnosis

Nasopharyngeal secretions are the most common samples used when attempting to detect influenza. If samples are cultured, they should be obtained during the first 3 days of illness when viral shedding is the greatest. As culture results may not be available for 2–6 days, rapid identification measures using immunofluorescence and direct fluorescent antibody assays are also available.

Therapy

Primary prevention of influenza is carried out via immunization. All healthcare workers and carers of transplant patients should receive the flu vaccination. In the post-transplant patient, however, it takes at least 6 months to mount a protective immune response and patients are at increased risk for contracting influenza during this period.

Table 42.4 Vaccination recommendations after transplant

Vaccine	Time post transplant before first dose	Schedule/doses required	Other
Inactive			
Polio	1 year	12, 14 and 24 months post transplant	Given as inactivated polio vaccine
Influenza	≧6 months	Yearly	
Hepatitis A	6–12 months	3 doses	Recommended for patients in endemic areas or scheduled to travel in those areas
Hepatitis B	6–12 months	12, 14 and 24 months post transplant	Consider early vaccination in patients who are anti-HBs positive prior to transplant
Live virus			
MMR	24 months	1 dose	Not to be given to patients with chronic GvHD or continued use of immunosuppression
Varicella	24 months	Still under investigation	Not to be given to patients with chronic GvHD or continued use of immunosuppression; currently not recommended for use in transplant patients by the CDC
Yellow fever	24 months	1 dose	Not to be given to patients with chronic GvHD or continued use of immunosuppression; recommended use in travelers

MMR, Measles-mumps-rubella.
Adapted from Ljungman et al 2005[143] and CDC 2000.[14]

Currently, there are no randomized trials evaluating the necessity or efficacy of chemoprophylaxis during the 180 days post transplant; however, treatment is recommended for this population during an outbreak of influenza in the community.[14]

Immunocompromised patients should be treated within 48 hours with antiviral medications. Prior to the 2005–2006 influenza season, the four antiviral medications approved for treatment in the United States were amantadine, rimantadine, oseltamivir and zanamivir. Due to the relative ease of creating viral resistance to the adamantanes (amantadine and rimantadine) via a single point mutation and a 3-year increase in the global prevalence of adamantine-resistant influenza (1.9% to 12.3%), in January 2006 the CDC issued a Health Alert Notice that for an interim period neither drug should be used for chemoprophylaxis or treatment of influenza A. Instead, neuraminidase inhibitors, which are effective against both influenza A and B, should be utilized: oseltamivir for chemoprophylaxis and either oseltamivir or zanamivir for treatment.[142]

Immunizations post transplant

Following transplant, almost all patients lose the immunity to infections they acquired from prior immunizations. Additionally, due to the young age of some transplant recipients, there is a growing percentage of patients that never completed their primary and/or booster immunization series. Therefore, practitioners must stay aware of the current immunization schedules recommended for patients after transplant.

The most current recommendations from the CDC and European Group for Blood and Marrow Transplantation were published in 2000 and 2005, respectively[14,143] (Table 42.4). In both cases, recommendations were made based upon the clinical benefit, efficacy of the intervention and types of supporting evidence. Underlying the recommendations is the knowledge that responses to vaccination therapy begin to become consistent approximately 6 months after transplantation and that repeated doses may be needed to obtain a clinical response.[7,144] Furthermore, in patients with sustained immune dysfunction and/or chronic GvHD, serious consideration must be given to the risk/benefit ratio provided with each immunization.

Viral vaccinations that can be given safely in the post-transplant setting include those that are inactivated, subunit viruses and recombinant DNA vaccines. There is an increased risk accompanying the use of live-attenuated vaccines. For example, the measles, mumps and rubella (MMR) vaccine, with a booster 12 months later, is recommended for only immunocompetent patients at least 2 years post transplant.[14]

Serologic testing and clinical history can be used to identify the response to vaccine therapy. Vaccinations that historically elicit a good immune response (i.e. inactivated polio) or where no benefit is obtained with a second dose (i.e. influenza during each season) do not require serologic evaluations to determine response.[143] However, treatment with vaccines like hepatitis B and MMR, that may not provide adequate immunity with a single administration, do warrant consideration of serologic titer response to determine the necessity of additional doses.[143]

Chapter 35 gives a fuller account of issues related to reimmunization.

References

1. Wingard JR. Opportunistic infections after blood and marrow transplantation. Transpl Infect Dis 1999;1:3–20
2. Chakrabarti S, MacKinnon S, Chopra R et al. High incidence of cytomegalovirus infection after nonmyeloablative stem cell transplantation: potential role of Campath-1H in delaying immune reconstitution. Blood 2002;99(12):4357–4363
3. Reimer P, Kunzmann V, Wilhelm M et al. Cellular and humoral immune reconstitution after autologous peripheral blood stem cell transplantation (PBSCT). Ann Hematol 2003;82:263–270
4. Reusser P, Riddell SR, Meyers JD, Greenberg PD. Cytotoxic T-lymphocyte response to cytomegalovirus after human allogeneic bone marrow transplantation: pattern of recovery and correlation with cytomegalovirus infection and disease. Blood 1991;78:1373–1380
5. Foster AE, Gottlieb DJ, Sartor M et al. Cytomegalovirus-specific CD4+ and CD8+ T-cells follow a similar reconstitution pattern after allogeneic stem cell transplantation. Biol Blood Marrow Transplant 2002;8:501–511
6. Heemskerk B, Lankester AC, van Vreeswijk T et al. Immune reconstitution and clearance of human adenovirus viremia in pediatric stem-cell recipients. J Infect Dis 2005;191: 520–530
7. Ljungman P, Einsele H. Viral infections. In: Atkinson K, Champlin R, Ritz J et al (eds) Clinical bone marrow and blood stem cell transplantation, 3rd edn. Cambridge University Press, Cambridge, 2004:1180–1206
8. Boeckh M, Bowden RA, Goodrich JM et al. Cytomegalovirus antigen detection in peripheral blood leukocytes after allogeneic marrow transplantation. Blood 1992;80:1358– 1364
9. van der Bij W, Torensma R, van Son WJ et al. Rapid immunodiagnosis of active cytomegalovirus infection by monoclonal antibody staining of blood leucocytes. J Med Virol 1988;25:179–188
10. Yoshikawa T. Significance of human herpesviruses to transplant recipients. Curr Opin Infect Dis 2003;16:601–606
11. Yakushiji K, Gondo H, Kamezaki K et al. Monitoring of cytomegalovirus reactivation after allogeneic stem cell transplantation: comparison of an antigenemia assay and quantitative real-time polymerase chain reaction. Bone Marrow Transplant 2002;29:599–606

12. Mori T, Okamoto S, Watanabe R et al. Dose-adjusted preemptive therapy for cytomegalovirus disease based on real-time polymerase chain reaction after allogeneic hematopoietic stem cell transplantation. Bone Marrow Transplant 2002;29:777–782
13. Li H, Dummer JS, Estes WR et al. Measurement of human cytomegalovirus loads by quantitative real-time PCR for monitoring clinical intervention in transplant recipients. J Clin Microbiol 2003;41:1871–1891
14. Guidelines for preventing opportunistic infections among hematopoietic stem cell transplant recipients. MMWR Recomm Rep 2000;49(RR-10):1–7
15. Dummer JS, Ho M. Risk factors and approaches to infections in transplant recipients. In: Mandell G, Bennett J, Dolin R (eds) Principles and practice of infectious disease, 5th edn. Churchill Livingstone, Philadelphia, 2000:3126–3136
16. Sable CA, Donowitz GR. Infections in bone marrow transplant recipients. Clin Infect Dis 1994;18:273–281
17. Leather HL, Wingard JR. Infections following hematopoietic stem cell transplantation. Infect Dis Clin North Am 2001;15:483–520
18. van Burik JA, Weisdorf DJ. Infections in recipients of blood and marrow transplantation. Hematol Oncol Clin North Am 1999;13:1065–1089, viii
19. Chawala R, Davies H. Infections after bone marrow transplantation. E-medicine 2006. Available from: www.emedicine.com/ped/topic2850.htm
20. Whimbey E, Bodey GP. Viral pneumonia in the immunocompromised adult with neoplastic disease: the role of common community respiratory viruses. Semin Respir Infect 1992;7:122–131
21. Hertz MI, Englund JA, Snover D et al. Respiratory syncytial virus-induced acute lung injury in adult patients with bone marrow transplants: a clinical approach and review of the literature. Medicine (Baltimore) 1989;68:269–281
22. Whimbey E, Elting LS, Couch RB et al. Influenza A virus infections among hospitalized adult bone marrow transplant recipients. Bone Marrow Transplant 1994;13:437–440
23. Wendt CH, Weisdorf DJ, Jordan MC et al. Parainfluenza virus respiratory infection after bone marrow transplantation. N Engl J Med 1992;326:921–926
24. Flomenberg P, Babbitt J, Drobyski WR et al. Increasing incidence of adenovirus disease in bone marrow transplant recipients. J Infect Dis 1994;169:775–781
25. Carrigan DR, Drobyski WR, Russler SK et al. Interstitial pneumonitis associated with human herpesvirus-6 infection after marrow transplantation. Lancet 1991;338:147–149
26. Cone RW, Hackman RC, Huang ML et al. Human herpesvirus 6 in lung tissue from patients with pneumonitis after bone marrow transplantation. N Engl J Med 1993;329:156–161
27. Zerr DM, Gooley TA, Yeung L et al. Human herpesvirus 6 reactivation and encephalitis in allogeneic bone marrow transplant recipients. Clin Infect Dis 2001;33:763–771
28. Cone RW, Huang ML, Corey L et al. Human herpesvirus 6 infections after bone marrow transplantation: clinical and virologic manifestations. J Infect Dis 1999;179:311–318
29. Wolf DG, Lurain NS, Zuckerman T et al. Emergence of late cytomegalovirus central nervous system disease in hematopoietic stem cell transplant recipients. Blood 2003;101:463–465
30. Lacey SF, Diamond DJ, Zaia JA. Assessment of cellular immunity to human cytomegalovirus in recipients of allogeneic stem cell transplants. Biol Blood Marrow Transplant 2004;10:433–447
31. Reddehase MJ, Mutter W, Munch K et al. CD8-positive T lymphocytes specific for murine cytomegalovirus immediate-early antigens mediate protective immunity. J Virol 1987;61:3102–3108
32. Curtis RE, Travis LB, Rowlings PA et al. Risk of lymphoproliferative disorders after bone marrow transplantation: a multi-institutional study. Blood 1999;94:2208–2216
33. Hale G, Waldmann H. Risks of developing Epstein-Barr virus-related lymphoproliferative disorders after T-cell-depleted marrow transplants. CAMPATH users. Blood 1998;91: 3079–3083
34. Lucas KG, Burton RL, Zimmerman SE et al. Semiquantitative Epstein-Barr virus (EBV) polymerase chain reaction for the determination of patients at risk for EBV-induced lymphoproliferative disease after stem cell transplantation. Blood 1998;91:3654–3661
35. Zaucha-Prazmo A, Wojcik B, Drabko K et al. Cytomegalovirus (CMV) infections in children undergoing hematopoetic stem cell transplantation. Pediatr Hematol Oncol 2005;22:271–276
36. Committee on Infectious Diseases AAoP. Section 3: summary of infectious diseases. In: Pickering L, Peter G (eds) 2000 Red Book: Report of the Committee on Infectious Diseases, 25th edn. American Academy of Pediatrics, Elk Grove Village, 2000:161–643
37. Hernandez-Boluda JC, Lis MJ, Goterris R et al. Guillain-Barre syndrome associated with cytomegalovirus infection after allogeneic hematopoietic stem cell transplantation. Transpl Infect Dis 2005;7:93–96
38. Fiegl M, Gerbitz A, Gaeta A et al. Recovery from CMV esophagitis after allogeneic bone marrow transplantation using non-myeloablative conditioning: the role of immunosuppression. J Clin Virol 2005;34:219–223
39. Enright H, Haake R, Weisdorf D et al. Cytomegalovirus pneumonia after bone marrow transplantation. Risk factors and response to therapy. Transplantation 1993;55:1339–1346
40. Bacigalupo A, Tedone E, Isaza A et al. CMV-antigenemia after allogeneic bone marrow transplantation: correlation of CMV-antigen positive cell numbers with transplant-related mortality. Bone Marrow Transplant 1995;16:155–161
41. Solano C, Munoz I, Gutierrez A et al. Qualitative plasma PCR assay (AMPLICOR CMV test) versus pp65 antigenemia assay for monitoring cytomegalovirus viremia and guiding preemptive ganciclovir therapy in allogeneic stem cell transplantation. J Clin Microbiol 2001;39:3938–3941
42. Avery RK, Adal KA, Longworth DL, Bolwell BJ. A survey of allogeneic bone marrow transplant programs in the United States regarding cytomegalovirus prophylaxis and preemptive therapy. Bone Marrow Transplant 2000;26:763–767
43. Atkinson K, Downs K, Golenia M et al. Prophylactic use of ganciclovir in allogeneic bone marrow transplantation: absence of clinical cytomegalovirus infection. Br J Haematol 1991;79:57–62
44. Maltezou H, Whimbey E, Abi-Said D, Przepiorka D et al. Cytomegalovirus disease in adult marrow transplant recipients receiving ganciclovir prophylaxis: a retrospective study. Bone Marrow Transplant 1999;24:665–669
45. Bregante S, Bertilson S, Tedone E et al. Foscarnet prophylaxis of cytomegalovirus infections in patients undergoing allogeneic bone marrow transplantation (BMT): a dose-finding study. Bone Marrow Transplant 2000;26:23–29
46. Winston DJ, Yeager AM, Chandrasekar PH et al. Randomized comparison of oral valaciclovir and intravenous ganciclovir for prevention of cytomegalovirus disease after allogeneic bone marrow transplantation. Clin Infect Dis 2003;36:749–758
47. Szer J, Durrant S, Schwarer AP et al. Oral versus intravenous ganciclovir for the prophylaxis of cytomegalovirus disease after allogeneic bone marrow transplantation. Intern Med J 2004;34:98–101
48. Boeckh M, Gooley TA, Myerson D et al. Cytomegalovirus pp65 antigenemia-guided early treatment with ganciclovir versus ganciclovir at engraftment after allogeneic marrow transplantation: a randomized double-blind study. Blood 1996;88:4063–4071
49. Moretti S, Zikos P, van Lint MT et al. Foscarnet vs ganciclovir for cytomegalovirus (CMV) antigenemia after allogeneic hemopoietic stem cell transplantation (HSCT): a randomised study. Bone Marrow Transplant 1998;22:175–180
50. Emanuel D, Cunningham I, Jules-Elysee K et al. Cytomegalovirus pneumonia after bone marrow transplantation successfully treated with the combination of ganciclovir and high-dose intravenous immune globulin. Ann Intern Med 1988;109:777–782
51. Reed EC, Bowden RA, Dandliker PS et al. Treatment of cytomegalovirus pneumonia with ganciclovir and intravenous cytomegalovirus immunoglobulin in patients with bone marrow transplants. Ann Intern Med 1988;109:783–788
52. Machado CM, Dulley FL, Boas LS et al. CMV pneumonia in allogeneic BMT recipients undergoing early treatment of pre-emptive ganciclovir therapy. Bone Marrow Transplant 2000;26:413–417
53. Ljungman P, Deliliers GL, Platzbecker U et al. Cidofovir for cytomegalovirus infection and disease in allogeneic stem cell transplant recipients. The Infectious Diseases Working Party of the European Group for Blood and Marrow Transplantation. Blood 2001;97: 388–392
54. Walter EA, Greenberg PD, Gilbert MJ et al. Reconstitution of cellular immunity against cytomegalovirus in recipients of allogeneic bone marrow by transfer of T-cell clones from the donor. N Engl J Med 1995;333:1038–1044
55. Peggs KS, Verfuerth S, Pizzey A et al. Adoptive cellular therapy for early cytomegalovirus infection after allogeneic stem-cell transplantation with virus-specific T-cell lines. Lancet 2003;362:1375–1377
56. Einsele H, Roosnek E, Rufer N et al. Infusion of cytomegalovirus (CMV)-specific T cells for the treatment of CMV infection not responding to antiviral chemotherapy. Blood 2002;99:3916–3922
57. Leen A, Myers GD, Sili U et al. Monoculture-derived T lymphocytes specific for multiple viruses expand and produce clinically relevant effects in immunocompromised patients. Nat Med 2006;12:1160–1166
58. Cobbold M, Khan N, Pourgheysari B et al. Adoptive transfer of cytomegalovirus-specific CTL to stem cell transplant patients after selection by HLA-peptide tetramers. J Exp Med 2005;202:379–386
59. Cohen JI. Epstein-Barr virus infection. N Engl J Med 2000;343:481–492
60. Sixbey JW, Nedrud JG, Raab-Traub N et al. Epstein-Barr virus replication in oropharyngeal epithelial cells. N Engl J Med 1984;310:1225–1230
61. Gottschalk S, Rooney CM, Heslop HE. Post-transplant lymphoproliferative disorders. Annu Rev Med 2005;56:29–44
62. Cavazzana-Calvo M, Bensoussan D, Jabado N et al. Prevention of EBV-induced B-lymphoproliferative disorder by ex vivo marrow B-cell depletion in HLA-phenoidentical or non-identical T-depleted bone marrow transplantation. Br J Haematol 1998;103:543–551
63. Annels NE, Kalpoe JS, Bredius RG et al. Management of Epstein-Barr virus (EBV) reactivation after allogeneic stem cell transplantation by simultaneous analysis of EBV DNA load and EBV-specific T cell reconstitution. Clin Infect Dis 2006;42:1743–1748
64. Paya CV, Fung JJ, Nalesnik MA et al. Epstein-Barr virus-induced posttransplant lymphoproliferative disorders. ASTS/ASTP EBV-PTLD Task Force and The Mayo Clinic Organized International Consensus Development Meeting. Transplantation 1999;68:1517–1525
65. van Esser JW, van der Holt B, Meijer E et al. Epstein-Barr virus (EBV) reactivation is a frequent event after allogeneic stem cell transplantation (SCT) and quantitatively predicts EBV-lymphoproliferative disease following T-cell-depleted SCT. Blood 2001;98:972–978
66. Wagner HJ, Cheng YC, Huls MH et al. Prompt versus preemptive intervention for EBV lymphoproliferative disease. Blood 2004;103:3979–3981
67. Clave E, Agbalika F, Bajzik V et al. Epstein-Barr virus (EBV) reactivation in allogeneic stem-cell transplantation: relationship between viral load, EBV-specific T-cell reconstitution and rituximab therapy. Transplantation 2004;77:76–84
68. Rooney CM, Smith CA, Ng CY et al. Use of gene-modified virus-specific T lymphocytes to control Epstein-Barr-virus-related lymphoproliferation. Lancet 1995;345:9–13
69. Rooney CM, Smith CA, Ng CY et al. Infusion of cytotoxic T cells for the prevention and treatment of Epstein-Barr virus-induced lymphoma in allogeneic transplant recipients. Blood 1998;92:1549–1555
70. Milpied N, Vasseur B, Parquet N et al. Humanized anti-CD20 monoclonal antibody (Rituximab) in post transplant B-lymphoproliferative disorder: a retrospective analysis on 32 patients. Ann Oncol 2000;11(suppl 1):113–116
71. Kuehnle I, Huls MH, Liu Z et al. CD20 monoclonal antibody (rituximab) for therapy of Epstein-Barr virus lymphoma after hemopoietic stem-cell transplantation. Blood 2000;95:1502–1505
72. Leen AM, Bollard CM, Myers GD, Rooney CM. Adenoviral infections in hematopoietic stem cell transplantation. Biol Blood Marrow Transplant 2006;12:243–251
73. Runde V, Ross S, Trenschel R et al. Adenoviral infection after allogeneic stem cell transplantation (SCT): report on 130 patients from a single SCT unit involved in a prospective multi center surveillance study. Bone Marrow Transplant 2001;28:51–57
74. La Rosa AM, Champlin RE, Mirza N et al. Adenovirus infections in adult recipients of blood and marrow transplants. Clin Infect Dis 2001;32:871–876

75. Lion T, Baumgartinger R, Watzinger F et al. Molecular monitoring of adenovirus in peripheral blood after allogeneic bone marrow transplantation permits early diagnosis of disseminated disease. Blood 2003;102:1114–1120
76. Myers GD, Krance RA, Weiss H et al. Adenovirus infection rates in pediatric recipients of alternate donor allogeneic bone marrow transplants receiving either antithymocyte globulin (ATG) or alemtuzumab (Campath). Bone Marrow Transplant 2005;36:1001–1008
77. Chakrabarti S, Mautner V, Osman H et al. Adenovirus infections following allogeneic stem cell transplantation: incidence and outcome in relation to graft manipulation, immunosuppression, and immune recovery. Blood 2002;100:1619–1627
78. Kojaoghlanian T, Flomenberg P, Horwitz MS. The impact of adenovirus infection on the immunocompromised host. Rev Med Virol 2003;13:155–171
79. Bordigoni P, Carret AS, Venard V et al. Treatment of adenovirus infections in patients undergoing allogeneic hematopoietic stem cell transplantation. Clin Infect Dis 2001;32:1290–1297
80. Lankester AC, Heemskerk B, Claas EC et al. Effect of ribavirin on the plasma viral DNA load in patients with disseminating adenovirus infection. Clin Infect Dis 2004;38:1521–1525
81. Yusuf U, Hale GA, Carr J et al. Cidofovir for the treatment of adenoviral infection in pediatric hematopoietic stem cell transplant patients. Transplantation 2006;81:1398–1404
82. Feuchtinger T, Matthes-Martin S, Richard C et al. Safe adoptive transfer of virus-specific T-cell immunity for the treatment of systemic adenovirus infection after allogeneic stem cell transplantation. Br J Haematol 2006;134:64–76
83. Saral R, Burns WH, Laskin OL et al. Aciclovir prophylaxis of herpes-simplex-virus infections. N Engl J Med 198;305:63–67
84. Gluckman E, Lotsberg J, Devergie A et al. Prophylaxis of herpes infections after bone-marrow transplantation by oral aciclovir. Lancet 1983;2:706–708
85. Dignani MC, Mykietiuk A, Michelet M et al. Valaciclovir prophylaxis for the prevention of Herpes simplex virus reactivation in recipients of progenitor cells transplantation. Bone Marrow Transplant 2002;29:263–267
86. Eisen D, Essell J, Broun ER et al. Clinical utility of oral valaciclovir compared with oral aciclovir for the prevention of herpes simplex virus mucositis following autologous bone marrow transplantation or stem cell rescue therapy. Bone Marrow Transplant 2003;31:51–55
87. Liesveld JL, Abboud CN, Ifthikharuddin JJ et al. Oral valaciclovir versus intravenous aciclovir in preventing herpes simplex virus infections in autologous stem cell transplant recipients. Biol Blood Marrow Transplant 2002;8:662–665
88. Langston AA, Redei I, Caliendo AM et al. Development of drug-resistant herpes simplex virus infection after haploidentical hematopoietic progenitor cell transplantation. Blood 2002;99:1085–1088
89. Hill G, Chauvenet AR, Lovato J, McLean TW. Recent steroid therapy increases severity of varicella infections in children with acute lymphoblastic leukemia. Pediatrics 2005;116:e525-e529
90. Dowell SF, Bresee JS. Severe varicella associated with steroid use. Pediatrics 1993;92:223–228
91. Gershon A, Brunell PA, Doyle EF, Claps AA. Steroid therapy and varicella. J Pediatr 1972;81:1034
92. Kasper WJ, Howe PM. Fatal varicella after a single course of corticosteroids. Pediatr Infect Dis J 1990;9:729–732
93. Locksley RM, Flournoy N, Sullivan KM, Meyers JD. Infection with varicella-zoster virus after marrow transplantation. J Infect Dis 1985;152:1172–1181
94. Schuchter LM, Wingard JR, Piantadosi S et al. Herpes zoster infection after autologous bone marrow transplantation. Blood 1989;74:1424–1427
95. Steer CB, Szer J, Sasadeusz J et al. Varicella-zoster infection after allogeneic bone marrow transplantation: incidence, risk factors and prevention with low-dose aciclovir and ganciclovir. Bone Marrow Transplant 2000;25:657–664
96. Boeckh M, Kim HW, Flowers ME et al. Long-term aciclovir for prevention of varicella zoster virus disease after allogeneic hematopoietic cell transplantation – a randomized double-blind placebo-controlled study. Blood 2006;107:1800–1805
97. Ljungman P, Wilczek H, Gahrton G et al. Long-term aciclovir prophylaxis in bone marrow transplant recipients and lymphocyte proliferation responses to herpes virus antigens in vitro. Bone Marrow Transplant 1986;1:185–192
98. Selby PJ, Powles RL, Easton D et al. The prophylactic role of intravenous and long-term oral aciclovir after allogeneic bone marrow transplantation. Br J Cancer 1989;59:43443–43448
99. Enright AM, Prober C. Antiviral therapy in children with varicella zoster virus and herpes simplex virus infections. Herpes 2003;10:32–37
100. Boeckh M, Erard V, Zerr D, Englund J. Emerging viral infections after hematopoietic cell transplantation. Pediatr Transplant 2005;7(suppl):48–54
101. Zerr DM, Meier AS, Selke SS et al. A population-based study of primary human herpesvirus 6 infection. N Engl J Med 2005;352:768–776
102. Ljungman P, Wang FZ, Clark DA et al. High levels of human herpesvirus 6 DNA in peripheral blood leucocytes are correlated to platelet engraftment and disease in allogeneic stem cell transplant patients. Br J Haematol 2000;111:774–781
103. Drobyski WR, Dunne WM, Burd EM et al. Human herpesvirus-6 (HHV-6) infection in allogeneic bone marrow transplant recipients: evidence of a marrow-suppressive role for HHV-6 in vivo. J Infect Dis 1993;167:735–739
104. Wang FZ, Dahl H, Linde A et al. Lymphotropic herpesviruses in allogeneic bone marrow transplantation. Blood 1996;88:3615–3620
105. Wang FZ, Linde A, Hagglund H et al. Human herpesvirus 6 DNA in cerebrospinal fluid specimens from allogeneic bone marrow transplant patients: does it have clinical significance? Clin Infect Dis 1999;28:562–568
106. Zerr DM, Gupta D, Huang ML et al. Effect of antivirals on human herpesvirus 6 replication in hematopoietic stem cell transplant recipients. Clin Infect Dis 2002;34:309–317
107. Tokimasa S, Hara J, Osugi Y et al. Ganciclovir is effective for prophylaxis and treatment of human herpesvirus-6 in allogeneic stem cell transplantation. Bone Marrow Transplant 2002;29:595–598
108. Walker DL, Padgett BL. The epidemiology of human polyomaviruses. Prog Clin Biol Res 1983;105:99–106
109. Priftakis P, Bogdanovic G, Kokhaei P et al. BK virus (BKV) quantification in urine samples of bone marrow transplanted patients is helpful for diagnosis of hemorrhagic cystitis, although wide individual variations exist. J Clin Virol 2003;26:71–77
110. Hogan TF, Padgett BL, Walker DL et al. Rapid detection and identification of JC virus and BK virus in human urine by using immunofluorescence microscopy. J Clin Microbiol 1980;11:178–183
111. Arthur RR, Shah KV, Charache P, Saral R. BK and JC virus infections in recipients of bone marrow transplants. J Infect Dis 1988;158:563–569
112. Gorczynska E, Turkiewicz D, Rybka K et al. Incidence, clinical outcome, and management of virus-induced hemorrhagic cystitis in children and adolescents after allogeneic hematopoietic cell transplantation. Biol Blood Marrow Transplant 2005;11:797–804
113. Broliden K. Parvovirus B19 infection in pediatric solid-organ and bone marrow transplantation. Pediatr Transplant 2001;5:320–330
114. Cohen BJ, Buckley MM. The prevalence of antibody to human parvovirus B19 in England and Wales. J Med Microbiol 1988;25:151–153
115. Kurtzman GJ, Cohen BJ, Field AM et al. Immune response to B19 parvovirus and an antibody defect in persistent viral infection. J Clin Invest 1989;84:1114–1123
116. Schleuning M, Jager G, Holler E et al. Human parvovirus B19-associated disease in bone marrow transplantation. Infection 1999;27:114–117
117. Kurtzman G, Frickhofen N, Kimball J et al. Pure red-cell aplasia of 10 years' duration due to persistent parvovirus B19 infection and its cure with immunoglobulin therapy. N Engl J Med 1989;321:519–523
118. Reed EC, Myerson D, Corey L, Meyers JD. Allogeneic marrow transplantation in patients positive for hepatitis B surface antigen. Blood 1991;77:195–200
119. Lau GK, Liang R, Chiu EK et al. Hepatic events after bone marrow transplantation in patients with hepatitis B infection: a case controlled study. Bone Marrow Transplant 1997;19:795–799
120. Hui CK, Lie A, Au WY et al. A long-term follow-up study on hepatitis B surface antigen-positive patients undergoing allogeneic hematopoietic stem cell transplantation. Blood 2005;106:464–469
121. Locasciulli A, Bruno B, Alessandrino EP et al. Hepatitis reactivation and liver failure in haemopoietic stem cell transplants for hepatitis B virus (HBV)/hepatitis C virus (HCV) positive recipients: a retrospective study by the Italian Group for Blood and Marrow Transplantation. Bone Marrow Transplant 2003;31:295–300
122. Strasser SI, Myerson D, Spurgeon CL et al. Hepatitis C virus infection and bone marrow transplantation: a cohort study with 10-year follow-up. Hepatology 1999;29:1893–1899
123. Kim BK, Chung KW, Sun HS et al. Liver disease during the first post-transplant year in bone marrow transplantation recipients: retrospective study. Bone Marrow Transplant 2000;26:193–197
124. Hui CK, Lie A, Au WY et al. Effectiveness of prophylactic Anti-HBV therapy in allogeneic hematopoietic stem cell transplantation with HBsAg positive donors. Am J Transplant 2005;5:1437–1445
125. Lau GK, Liang R, Wu PC et al. Use of famciclovir to prevent HBV reactivation in HBsAg-positive recipients after allogeneic bone marrow transplantation. J Hepatol 1998;28:359–368
126. Gigliotti AR, Fioredda F, Giacchino R. Hepatitis B and C infection in children undergoing chemotherapy or bone marrow transplantation. J Pediatr Hematol Oncol 2003;25:184–192
127. Vance EA, Soiffer RJ, McDonald GB et al. Prevention of transmission of hepatitis C virus in bone marrow transplantation by treating the donor with alpha-interferon. Transplantation 1996;62:1358–1360
128. Ljungman P, Andersson J, Aschan J et al. Oral ribavirin for prevention of severe liver disease caused by hepatitis C virus during allogeneic bone marrow transplantation. Clin Infect Dis 1996;23:167–169
129. Whimbey E, Couch RB, Englund JA et al. Respiratory syncytial virus pneumonia in hospitalized adult patients with leukemia. Clin Infect Dis 1995;21:376–379
130. Jones BL, Clark S, Curran ET et al. Control of an outbreak of respiratory syncytial virus infection in immunocompromised adults. J Hosp Infect 2000;44:53–57
131. Harrington RD, Hooton TM, Hackman RC et al. An outbreak of respiratory syncytial virus in a bone marrow transplant center. J Infect Dis 1992;165:987–993
132. Abdallah A, Rowland KE, Schepetiuk SK et al. An outbreak of respiratory syncytial virus infection in a bone marrow transplant unit: effect on engraftment and outcome of pneumonia without specific antiviral treatment. Bone Marrow Transplant 2003;32:195–203
133. Small TN, Casson A, Malak SF et al. Respiratory syncytial virus infection following hematopoietic stem cell transplantation. Bone Marrow Transplant 2002;29:321–327
134. Ghosh S, Champlin RE, Ueno NT et al. Respiratory syncytial virus infections in autologous blood and marrow transplant recipients with breast cancer: combination therapy with aerosolized ribavirin and parenteral immunoglobulins. Bone Marrow Transplant 2001;28:271–275
135. Boeckh M, Berrey MM, Bowden RA et al. Phase 1 evaluation of the respiratory syncytial virus-specific monoclonal antibody palivizumab in recipients of hematopoietic stem cell transplants. J Infect Dis 2001;184:350–354
136. Nichols WG, Corey L, Gooley T et al. Parainfluenza virus infections after hematopoietic stem cell transplantation: risk factors, response to antiviral therapy, and effect on transplant outcome. Blood 2001;98:573–578
137. Dignan F, Alvares C, Riley U et al. Parainfluenza type 3 infection post stem cell transplant: high prevalence but low mortality. J Hosp Infect 2006;63:452–458
138. Elizaga J, Olavarria E, Apperley J et al. Parainfluenza virus 3 infection after stem cell transplant: relevance to outcome of rapid diagnosis and ribavirin treatment. Clin Infect Dis 2001;32:413–418
139. Lewis VA, Champlin R, Englund J et al. Respiratory disease due to parainfluenza virus in adult bone marrow transplant recipients. Clin Infect Dis 1996;23:1033–1037

140. Sparrelid E, Ljungman P, Ekelof-Andstrom E et al. Ribavirin therapy in bone marrow transplant recipients with viral respiratory tract infections. Bone Marrow Transplant 1997;19:905–908

141. Nichols WG, Guthrie KA, Corey L, Boeckh M. Influenza infections after hematopoietic stem cell transplantation: risk factors, mortality, and the effect of antiviral therapy. Clin Infect Dis 2004;39:1300–1306

142. Centers for Disease Control and Prevention. CDC recommends against the use of amantadine and rimantadine for the treatment or prophylaxis of influenza in the United States during the 2005–06 influenza season. Available from: www.cdc.gov/flu/han011406.htm

143. Ljungman P, Engelhard D, de la Camara R et al. Vaccination of stem cell transplant recipients: recommendations of the Infectious Diseases Working Party of the EBMT. Bone Marrow Transplant 2005;35:737–746

144. Parkkali T, Stenvik M, Ruutu T et al. Randomized comparison of early and late vaccination with inactivated poliovirus vaccine after allogeneic BMT. Bone Marrow Transplant 1997;20:663–668

145. Prentice HG, Gluckman E, Powles RL et al. Impact of long-term aciclovir on cytomegalovirus infection and survival after allogeneic bone marrow transplantation. European Aciclovir for CMV Prophylaxis Study Group. Lancet 1994;343:749–753

146. Reusser P, Einsele H, Lee J et al. Randomized multicenter trial of foscarnet versus ganciclovir for preemptive therapy of cytomegalovirus infection after allogeneic stem cell transplantation. Blood 2002;99:1159–1164

147. Boeckh M, Nichols WG, Papanicolaou G et al. Cytomegalovirus in hematopoietic stem cell transplant recipients: current status, known challenges, and future strategies. Biol Blood Marrow Transplant 2003;9:543–558

148. Ordemann R, Naumann R, Geissler G et al. Foscarnet – an alternative for cytomegalovirus prophylaxis after allogeneic stem cell transplantation? Ann Hematol 2000;79:432–436

149. Aschan J, Ringden O, Ljungman P et al. Foscarnet for treatment of cytomegalovirus infections in bone marrow transplant recipients. Scand J Infect Dis 1992;24:143–150

150. van der Heiden PL, Kalpoe JS, Barge RM et al. Oral valganciclovir as pre-emptive therapy has similar efficacy on cytomegalovirus DNA load reduction as intravenous ganciclovir in allogeneic stem cell transplantation recipients. Bone Marrow Transplant 2006;37:693–698

151. Chakrabarti S, Collingham KE, Osman H et al. Cidofovir as primary pre-emptive therapy for post-transplant cytomegalovirus infections. Bone Marrow Transplant 2001;28:879–881

152. Avery RK, Bolwell BJ, Yen-Lieberman B et al. Use of leflunomide in an allogeneic bone marrow transplant recipient with refractory cytomegalovirus infection. Bone Marrow Transplant 2004;34:1071–1075

Fungal infections

Carolyn Hemsley and Chris Kibbler

CHAPTER 43

Introduction

The fungal infections of concern in hemopoietic stem cell (HSCT) recipients can be divided into superficial or invasive infections. The vast majority are due to *Candida* and *Aspergillus* species which account for >85% of fungal infections. Invasive infections caused by the so-called 'newly emerging fungi' (e.g. *Fusarium*, the zygomycetes, *Scedosporium* spp and other dematiaceous fungi), *Pneumocystis jirovecii* (formerly *P. carinii*) and *Cryptococcal* spp are less common. Infection due to geographically restricted systemic mycoses (e.g. *Blastomyces dermatitidis, Histoplasma capsulatum* and *Coccidioides immitis*) is rare except with compatible travel/exposure history.

Epidemiology

Superficial infection

Superficial candidal infection was a major cause of morbidity prior to routine use of fluconazole prophylaxis in the early 1990s. Approximately one-third of all patients would have evidence of superficial candidal infection prior to azole use.[1] Introduction of azole prophylaxis resulted in a reduction of superficial fungal infections to 15–20% of the amount seen in those not receiving fluconazole, and this reduction was evident at each of the three most common sites of infection: the oropharynx, genital and rectal areas, and skin.[2–4] Oropharyngeal candidiasis was, and still is, the most common manifestation of superficial candidal infection. Esophageal disease is much less common and usually co-exists with oropharyngeal disease, but up to 30% cases have no visible oral lesions.

Skin and nail infections are not major problems in the HSCT population but occasionally paronychia and/or athlete's foot/onychomycosis may be a source of invasive fungal infection, e.g. *Fusarium*[5] (Fig. 43.1). *Aspergillus* infection has been described at sites of wound or line infection.[6]

Invasive infection

The incidence of invasive disease and its associated mortality varies with the hematology population studied, being highest in myeloablative unmatched allogeneic transplant recipients and least in autologous transplant recipients. There have been marked changes in the epidemiology of invasive fungal infections in the blood and marrow transplant population over the last two decades. These changes are probably due to a combination of factors, including changing antifungal prophylaxis practices, a wider patient population being offered transplantation, the use of different immunosuppressive regimens and aggressive medical intervention leading to increased early survival, resulting in more fungal infections being diagnosed later on post transplant.

In the 1980s, yeasts (particularly *Candida albicans*) were the most common causative agents. Superficial colonization was common (~50%) and invasive disease rates were as high as 10–20% in allogeneic transplant recipients.[7] The widespread routine use of fluconazole prophylaxis in the early 1990s has seen a dramatic reduction in invasive *Candida albicans* disease to <5% even in the highest risk individuals.[8] This reduction in invasive disease is despite similar rates of colonization[8] although the mortality associated with candidemia remains high, ~20–40%.[8–10] A number of centers have documented an increase in fluconazole-resistant *Candida* species, such as *C. glabatra* and *C. krusei*, in bone marrow transplant (BMT) recipients since the introduction of fluconazole,[11,12] although others have not.[8]

Invasive infection with molds, including *Aspergillus*, has become more frequent over a similar time period.[13–15] It is difficult to estimate the true incidence of invasive infection due to *Aspergillus* spp and other molds, as counting the number of cases where empiric antifungal treatment is used undoubtedly overestimates the number and counting only autopsy-identified cases will underestimate the case load. Based on European Organization for Research and Treatment of Cancer/Invasive Fungal Infections Cooperative Group and the National Institute of Allergy and Infectious Diseases Mycoses Study Group (EORTC/MSG) definitions for invasive disease, the reported incidence of invasive *Aspergillus* infection varies from 1–2% in autologous recipients to 5–20% in allogeneic transplant recipients, with higher rates in those with unrelated or HLA-mismatched than HLA-matched donors.[13,16–18]

The outcome of invasive aspergillosis remains poor and has changed little in the last decade. Disseminated or central nervous system disease carries a case fatality rate of >85%, whereas pulmonary disease and sinus disease have case fatality rates of 60% and 26%, respectively.[19,20] *Aspergillus fumigatus* remains the most common pathogen but a notable trend is the increasing frequency of isolation of *Aspergillus* spp other than *A. fumigatus*.[19] This is cause for concern as some species, e.g. *A. terreus*, are innately resistant to amphotericin B, the most commonly used empiric antifungal agent. *A. terreus* accounts for between 3% and 13% of all cases of invasive *Aspergillus* infection.[15]

The number of infections with molds other than *Aspergillus* remains low but there are increasing numbers of reports of infections caused by *Fusarium* sp, zygomycetes and *Scedosporium* spp.[17,21,22] The prognosis of infection with *Fusarium*, zygometes or other non-*Aspergillus* molds is extremely poor with high mortality rates (>80% in zygomycosis and *Fusarium* infection and up to 100% for *Scedosporium* infection), and a short mean survival from time of diagnosis[17,23]

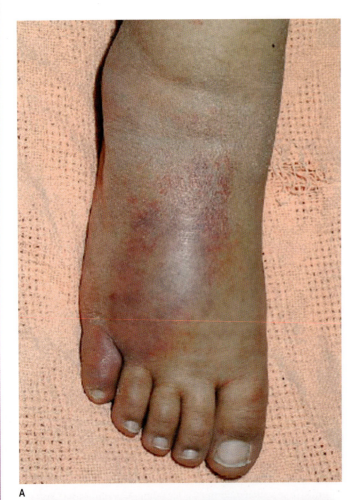

A

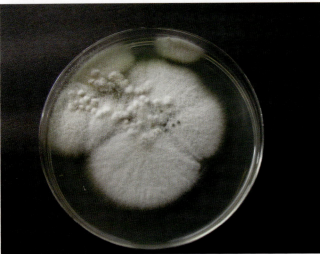

B

Figure 43.1
(a) Proven *F. dimerum* soft tissue infection of the foot. (b) Culture plate of *F. dimerum* at 7 days. (Ref. 5)

In recent years, the use of alternative sources of harvested stem cells, newer preparative regimens and the introduction of non-myeloablative conditioning for allogeneic transplantation have affected the epidemiology of invasive fungal infection.[14] Use of peripheral blood stem cells as opposed to bone marrow-derived cells has been shown to lead to faster regeneration, a reduction in the duration of neutropenia and reduction in frequency of early invasive fungal infection. The non-myeloablative approach uses a reduced-intensity condi-

tioning regimen, compared with conventional allogeneic stem cell transplantation. This results in more rapid engraftment with reduction in the period of neutropenia and less toxicity to host mucosal barriers. This type of transplant can, however, be associated with severe graft-versus-host disease (GvHD), often requiring high doses of corticosteroids and other immunosuppressive agents. There has been concern over an increasing incidence of invasive fungal infection, particularly with molds, in the non-myeloablative transplant population at later time periods (up to 23%).[24] This has not been borne out across all studies. Some have noted fewer invasive fungal infections, whereas others have found rates comparable (14–19%).[14,25] The reason for this discrepancy across units remains unclear. The case mix may be quite different from center to center, and conditioning regimens may differ. Non-myeloablative transplants do appear to be associated with a higher frequency of non-*Aspergillus* mold infection.[14,23,24]

Infection with *P. jiroveci* pneumonia (PCP) remains uncommon in those taking trimethoprim/sulfamethoxazole (TMP/SMX) prophylaxis (<1%) and typically only occurs in those in whom PCP prophylaxis has been discontinued[26,27] or those taking low-dose dapsone prophylaxis (5% in one study).[28] Infection with *Cryptococcus* spp is unusual in contrast to its frequent occurrence in the HIV population.

Chronology of fungal infection post transplantation and associated risk factors

Typically, there are three risk periods of immunologic deficiency that occur predictably in HSCT recipients: the pre-engraftment period, early postengraftment period (until day 100) and the late period (after day 100). These risk periods coincide with periods of peak incidence of many infections, including fungal infections (Fig. 43.2). Yeast infections typically occur early post transplantation (median 2 weeks post transplantation in the period of neutropenia). Invasive aspergillosis and other mold infections tend to have a bi or trimodal distribution of occurrence, with a peak of disease early and one or two later peaks. The first peak of invasive aspergillosis is immediately after transplantation while the patient is neutropenic, and the second around 100 days post transplant, primarily as a result of GvHD or its treatment, or as a result of graft failure. Late cases of aspergillosis, >1 year after receipt of HSCT, can occur.

Invasive disease with non-*Aspergillus* spp tends to present slightly later than invasive aspergillosis. The majority of cases of zygomycosis and fusariosis, for example, are diagnosed late after transplantation (>1 year) when none of these patients is neutropenic.[22] The exception is *Scedosporium* spp which are most common in the first 30 days after transplantation in the period of neutropenia.[23] It is possible that the control of other aggressive infections has allowed patients to live long enough to develop late fungal infection at a time when they are at risk because they are receiving therapy for GvHD and/or have severe T-cell mediated immunodeficiency.

Superimposed on this basic pattern are several other factors associated with an increased risk of invasive fungal infection (Table 43.1). As a whole, risk factors can be divided into three main areas.

1. Patient factors and factors affecting the net state of patient immunosuppression (including age, chemotherapeutic regimens, cytomegalovirus (CMV) disease, prolonged and profound neutropenia and lymphopenia).
2. Breaches in physical defenses and organ dysfunction (invasive lines or medical devices, mucositis, pulmonary dysfunction, severe GvHD).
3. History of previous fungal infection or colonization.

For practical purposes, distinguishing high-risk from low-risk individuals may be useful in guiding decisions regarding prophylaxis and empiric therapy protocols.[13]

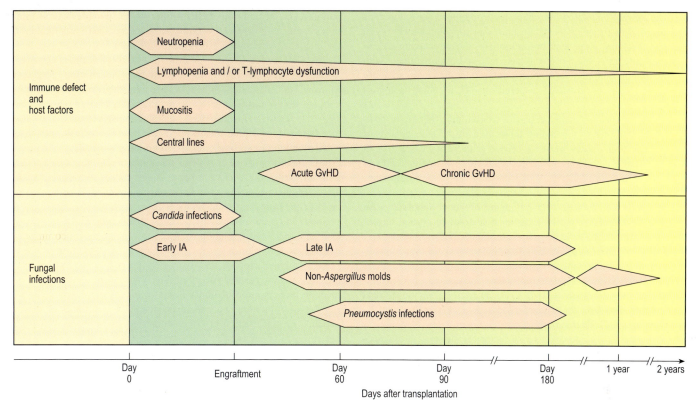

Figure 43.2
Chronology of and risk factors for predictable fungal infections in HSCT recipients. IA, invasive aspergillosis.

Table 43.1 Risk factors for invasive fungal infections in patients with hematologic malignancies

Fungi	Risk factor
Candida	
Patient factors	Older age
	Colonization
	Neutropenia
	Central venous catheterization
	Mucositis
	CMV disease
Chemotherapeutic regimen	Corticosteroid use
Aspergillus and other molds	
Patient factors	Older age
	Allograft
	BMT histoincompatibility
	Refractory hematologic disease
	Previous invasive aspergillosis
	Prolonged severe neutropenia (<0.5 × 10⁹ cells/l for>10 days)
	Lymphopenia
	GvHD and its treatment
Chemotherapeutic regimen	T-cell depleted or CD34-selected stem cells
	Melphalan/fludarabine
	Anti-CD52 antibody
	T-cell depleted or CD34-selected stem cells
	Corticosteroids >0.5 mg/kg/day

Neutropenia in the early post-transplant period is a major risk factor for invasive fungal infection (due to both yeast and molds) and the duration and degree of neutropenia are important. The risk is highest in those with prolonged severe neutropenia (<0.5 ×10⁹ cells/l for >10 days) and increases considerably with neutropenia >21 days.[29,30] Mechanical defects also play a major role in the risk of candidemia, as they do for the risk of bacteremia, the main two being the presence of invasive intravascular lines and disruption of mucosal barriers, with mucositis complicating the administration of chemotherapeutic agents. Lines and mucositis provide portals of entry for normal skin and gastrointestinal flora, including candidal species, to otherwise sterile body sites. Invasive candidal infection is almost always of endogenous origin, usually from the gastrointestinal tract. The relative contribution of venous catheters versus the gut as the primary source of candidemia is difficult to determine except in the case of candidemia due to *C. parapsilosis*, which appears to be associated with central intravenous catheter use.[31] Colonization with *Candida* spp at two or more sites is predictive of candidemia.[8,9] The positive predictive value of colonization is low but lack of colonization strongly militates against invasive candidiasis.

After recovery of peripheral blood cells there is a period of abnormal T-cell function. It is now recognized that T-cell dysfunction and dysregulated T-cell responses play key roles in the pathogenesis of invasive aspergillosis and other mycoses.[19] In the allogeneic transplant setting, T-cell dysfunction is most apparent in the first 100 days in those without significant GvHD. In patients who experience GvHD, T-lymphocyte dysfunction may be more severe and prolonged, and the presence of GvHD is a known continuing independent risk factor for invasive mold infections.[17,32] The late post-transplant risk period ends when the patient regains normal immunity. This is generally by 18 months after transplantation in patients who are not being treated with myelosuppressive medication and who remain free from GvHD.

Invasive mold infections are much less common in the autologous compared with the allogeneic transplantation population. However, patients receiving more than one transplant, those receiving CD34-enriched autografts and those who have received prior treatment with potent immunosuppressive regimens for refractory malignancy are at higher risk of invasive aspergillosis than other autograft recipients.[29,32]

The use of specific agents as part of conditioning therapy or post-transplantation therapy, including those used in the management of GvHD, has been shown to be associated with an increased risk of invasive fungal infections including molds and *P. jiroveci*. This is most likely as a consequence of their immunosuppressive properties. These agents include

- high-dose prednisolone (0.5–1.0 mg/kg of body weight/day) for GvHD prophylaxis and high cumulative doses of corticosteroids prior to transplant or in the post-transplant period
- the use of nucleoside analogs (e.g. cytarabine and fludarabine), particularly in combination with steroids
- the management of GvHD with potent immnosuppressive agents such as alemtuzumab (CAMPATH), an anti-CD52 monoclonal antibody that depletes peripheral blood T- and B-cells, or infliximab, an anti-TNF-α antibody.[33]

CMV disease is an independent risk factor for subsequent development of invasive candidal infection and other invasive mycoses.[8,32] A similar association between CMV disease and fungal infections has been noted in solid organ recipients.[34,35] It is not clear what the mechanism behind this association is. It is possible that CMV is purely a marker for a specific immunologic defect that predisposes to both CMV and fungal infection or that the virus itself has immunomodulatory effects that result in an increased risk for fungal infection.

The risk of *P. jiroveci* infection is greatest during the first 6 months post transplantation, with a median time of onset of 1–3 months post transplantation. Prior to routine use of prophylaxis the incidence of disease was ~7% with a mortality of 5%.[36] Prophylaxis with co-trimoxazole (Septrin) has resulted in a reduction in infection rates to negligible levels. Prophylaxis is in widespread use in high-risk individuals and infection is now typically seen as a much later complication in allogeneic transplant recipients in whom prophylaxis has been discontinued[27] or in those on alternative prophylaxis regimens such as dapsone (as high as 5% in one study) where the level of protection appears to be less.[28]

T-cell dysfunction and corticosteroid use are the major risk factors for cryptococcal infection. Isolated neutropenia is rarely associated with cryptococcal infection. The principal portal of entry is by inhalation, with spread to the blood and central nervous system and subsequent development of meningitis. As in the HIV population, meningitis is the most common manifestation of infection.

Prevention

The mortality associated with invasive fungal infection is high.[19,37] Fungal infections are difficult to diagnose and treatment that is initiated once infection is well established is not as successful as either prevention or pre-emptive therapy. For these reasons the standard practice is to attempt to prevent invasive fungal infections. Prevention can take the form of reduction or avoidance of exposure to the infectious agent and/or use of prophylaxis in the form of antifungals.

Sources and environmental controls

The main mode of transmission of most molds, such as *Aspergillus* spp, is by inhalation of spores. High efficiency particulate air (HEPA) filter systems are capable of filtering out 99.97% of 0.3 μm diameter particles and the addition of HEPA filters to positive pressure ventilation systems in bone marrow transplant units has led to a reduction in the incidence of invasive aspergillosis.[38–40]

The Centers for Disease Control (CDC), the Infectious Diseases Society of America (IDSA) and the American Society for Blood and Marrow Transplantation (ASBMT) have published guidelines for preventing opportunistic infections among HSCT recipients in the USA.[41–43] These evidence-based guidelines provide specific recommendations for hospital infection control issues in HSCT, including room ventilation and issues related to building work. They state that efforts should be made to protect transplant recipients from contact with air containing excessive spore counts and recommend that all allogeneic hematopoietic stem cell transplant recipients be housed in positive pressure ventilated rooms with more than 12 air exchanges per hour and point-of-use HEPA filters. HEPA-filtered rooms should also be considered for autologous transplant patients if there is an expectation of prolonged neutropenia. Hospital construction is recognized as a risk factor for invasive aspergillosis, as there may be disturbance and increased dispersal of fungal spores. Attempts should be made to prevent airborne transmission of fungal spores from sites of renovation or building work to areas occupied by immunosuppressed patients, by construction of effective barriers that prevent dust from entering patient areas.

Although invasive candidal infection is almost always of endogenous origin, the endogenous patient flora are modified in hospital and there is an increase in azole-resistant species. Transfer of *Candida* spp from person to person on the hands of medical personnel has been demonstrated and hand washing by medical personnel is strongly recommended to prevent this.[41]

It is well documented that fungal spores including *Aspergillus* can be found in domestic and hospital water supplies and commonly in many food stuffs such as vegetables and spices. Most BMT units have guidelines on appropriate diet, food storage and preparation, both in the highest risk neutropenic period (neutropenic diets) and in the later periods post transplantation, in an attempt to reduce patient exposure to potentially pathogenic microbial agents.

Antifungal therapy in the prevention of invasive fungal infection and prophylaxis

Primary prophylaxis refers to the giving of antifungal agents to those without evidence of infection to prevent its occurrence. Secondary prophylaxis refers to the giving of antifungal agents to those with a prior episode of mold infection who are at risk of relapse when receiving additional immunosuppression, with the aim of preventing significant disease.

Our armamentarium of antifungal drugs still does not match that of the antibacterial agents but there have been major advances in antifungal therapy in recent years. The availability of echinocandins and a second generation of triazoles such as voriconazole and posaconazole has had a significant impact on the management of fungal infection in the BMT population. Antifungal drugs can be divided into four main classes based on their mechanism of action: polyenes, azoles, fluoropyrimidines and echinocandins. Their licensed indications for use and antifungal profiles are illustrated in Table 43.2 and Figure 43.3. Even though it is not unusual for many of these agents (particularly the newer ones) to be used in clinical situations outside the primary indications for use, these licensed indications must be appreciated.

Polyenes

Amphotericin B is the most important polyene. It exerts its antifungal effect by binding to ergosterol in the fungal cell membrane, altering membrane permeability. It has activity against most fungi, although primary resistance is common for *Aspergillus terreus*, *Scedosporium*

Table 43.2 Licensed indications for antifungal agent use

Antifungal agent	Licensed indication
Amphotericin B deoxycholate (Fungizone)	Treatment of systemic fungal infections
Ambisome	Empirical treatment of presumed fungal infection in neutropenic patients Treatment of cryptococcal meningitis in HIV-infected patients Treatment of patients with invasive aspergillosis, candidal or cryptococcal infections that are refractory to amphotericin B deoxycholate or when renal impairment or unacceptable toxicity precludes the use of amphotericin B deoxycholate
Amphocil/Amphotec	Treatment of severe systemic or deep mycoses in patients refractory to amphotericin B deoxycholate or when renal impairment or unacceptable toxicity precludes the use of amphotericin B deoxycholate
Abelcet	Treatment of severe invasive candidiasis Treatment of severe systemic fungal infections in patients refractory to amphotericin B deoxycholate or when renal impairment or unacceptable toxicity precludes the use of amphotericin B deoxycholate, including invasive aspergillosis, cryptococcal meningitis and disseminated cryptococcosis in HIV patients
Ketoconazole	Treatment of systemic mycoses Treatment of serious chronic resistant mucocutaneous candidiasis, serious chronic resistant gastrointestinal mycoses and serious chronic resistant vaginal candidiasis Treatment of resistant dermatophyte infections of the skin or finger nails (but not toe nails) Prophylaxis of mycoses in immunosuppressed patients
Fluconazole	Treatment of vaginal candidiasis Treatment of mucosal candidiasis Treatment of tinea pedis, corporis, cruris, pityriasis versicolor and dermal candidiasis Treatment of invasive candidal infections Treatment of invasive cryptococcal infections Prevention of relapse of cryptococcal infections after completion of primary therapy in HIV patients Prevention of fungal infections in immunocompromised patients
Itraconazole	Treatment of oropharyngeal and/or mucosal candidiasis Treatment of tinea pedis, corporis, cruris, pityriasis versicolor and onychomycosis Treatment of histoplasmosis Treatment of systemic aspergillosis, candidiasis and cryptococcosis including meningitis where other antifungals are inappropriate or ineffective Maintenance of HIV patients to prevent relapse of underlying fungal infection Prophylaxis in neutropenia when standard therapy is inappropriate
Voriconazole	Treatment of invasive *Aspergillus* infections Candidemia in non-neutropenic adult patients Treatment of disseminated skin, intra-abdominal, kidney, bladder wall and wound infections Treatment of esophageal candidiasis Treatment of serious fungal infections caused by *Fusarium* spp, and *Scedoporium* spp
Posaconazole	Treatment of invasive aspergillosis refractory to amphotericin B or itraconazole, or in patients intolerant of those therapies Treatment of fusaricosis refractory to amphotericin B or in patients intolerant of amphotericin B Treatment of chromoblastomycosis and mycetoma refractory to itraconazole or in patients intolerant of itraconazole Treatment of coccidioidomycosis refractory to amphotericin B, itraconazole, fluconazole, or in patients intolerant to those products Treatment of oropharyngeal candidiasis Prevention of invasive *Aspergillus* and candidal infections in immunocompromised patients
Caspofungin	Treatment of invasive candidiasis in non-neutropenic adult patients Treatment of invasive *Aspergillus* infections that are refractory to alternative therapy Treatment of esophageal candidiasis Empirical treatment of presumed fungal infection in neutropenic patients Treatment of candidemia Treatment of candidal infections including: intra-abdominal, abscess, peritonitis and pleural space
Flucytosine	Systemic yeast and fungal infections Adjunct to amphotericin or fluconazole in treatment of cryptococcal meningitis Adjunct to amphotericin in treatment of severe systemic candidiasis
Anidulafungin	Treatment of esophageal candidiasis Treatment of candidal infections including intra-abdominal abscesses and peritonitis Treatment of candidemia
Micafungin	Treatment of candidemia Treatment of esophageal candidiasis Treatment of acute disseminated candidiasis and *Candida* peritonitis and abscesses Prophylaxis of *Candida* infections in HSCT recipients

spp and *Trichosporon* spp. There are four commercially available preparations: amphotericin B deoxycholate (Fungizone) and three lipid formulations, liposomal amphotericin (AmBisome), amphotericin B colloidal dispersion (Amphotec, Amphocil) and amphotericin B lipid complex (Abelcet). All preparations are for intravenous use. Amphotericin B deoxycholate (AmB) has been the mainstay of treatment of invasive fungal infections to date. Its major drawback is its side-effect profile, the most notable problem being nephrotoxicity. The common drug effects on the kidneys are a dose-dependent decrease in glomerular filtration rate, uremia, potassium and magnesium wasting, renal tubular acidosis and polyuria. Nephrotoxicity is usually reversible but permanent loss of renal function is related to high total dose. The nephrotoxicity is often exacerbated by co-administration of other nephrotoxic agents, which is a common problem in the HSCT population. Infusion-related toxicity is also a significant problem. Reactions such as fever, rigors and hypotension tend to occur within the first 45 minutes of infusion but can normally be managed with preadministration of paracetamol and/or co-administration of hydrocortisone.

PART 5 MANAGEMENT OF POST-TRANSPLANT COMPLICATIONS

	Fluconazole	Itraconazole	Voriconazole	Posaconazole	Amphotericin[a]	Caspofungin	Flucytosine
C. albicans	green	green	green	green	green	green	green
C. parapsilosis	green	green	green	green	green	yellow	green
C. lusitaniae	green	green	green	green	yellow	green	green
C. tropicalis	green	green	green	green	green	green	green
C. glabrata	yellow	yellow	green	green	green	green	green
C. krusei	red	yellow	green	green	green	green	yellow
Cryptococcus spp.	green	green	green	green	green	red	green
A. fumigatus	red	green	green	green	green	green	red
A. flavus	red	green	green	green	yellow	green	red
A. niger	red	yellow	green	green	green	green	red
A. terreus	red	green	green	green	yellow	green	red
Zygomycetes	red	red	red	green	green	red	red
Fusarium spp.	red	red	yellow	green	yellow	red	red
P. boydii	red	red	green	green	red	red	red
Trichosporon spp.	green	green	green	green	red	red	red
Scedosporium spp.	red	red	yellow	green	red	red	red

[a] Includes lipid formulations

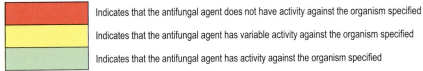

red — Indicates that the antifungal agent does not have activity against the organism specified

yellow — Indicates that the antifungal agent has variable activity against the organism specified

green — Indicates that the antifungal agent has activity against the organism specified

Figure 43.3
In vitro susceptibilities of fungi to antifungal agents.

The advantage of the lipid-associated formulations is that they are notably better tolerated than conventional amphotericin, with a reduction in severity and frequency of acute infusion reactions and reduction in chronic nephrotoxicty. These agents are, however, significantly more expensive and by no means free of adverse reactions. Association with nephrotoxicity is in the following order: amphotericin B deoxycholate > amphotericin B colloidal dispersion > amphotericin B lipid complex > liposomal amphotericin.

Azoles

The azoles include fluconazole, itraconazole, ketoconazole and the newer agents voriconazole, posaconazole and ravuconazole (not yet licensed). They affect synthesis of ergosterol, an essential component of the fungal cytoplasmic membrane. Fluconazole is well absorbed from the GI tract and has an excellent safety profile, but its main limitation is its narrow spectrum of activity. It is active against many *Candida* spp, but it is inactive against *C. krusei* and its activity against *C. glabrata* is variable and dose dependent. It has no activity against *Aspergillus* and other important molds. Itraconazole, voriconazole, posaconazole and ravuconazole have an extended spectrum of activity including *Aspergillus* spp and other molds. Use of these newer agents can be complicated by significant drug–drug interactions (resulting from inhibition of cytochrome P450 isoenzymes), and dose adjustment and/or close monitoring for toxicity is required when they are co-administered with certain agents. There are some agents with which co-administration should be avoided altogether, for example vinca alkaloids and cyclophosphamide (Table 43.3). Itraconazole use had been limited his-

Table 43.3 Important drug interactions of triazoles with chemotherapeutic agents

Chemotherapeutic agents	Azole	Effect on drug	Comments
Busulfan	Itraconazole Voriconazole	↑ ↑	Avoid azole
Vinca alkaloids	Itraconazole Voriconazole Posaconazole	↑ ↑ ↑	Avoid azole
Docetaxel	Itraconazole Voriconazole	↑ ↑	Avoid azole
Cyclophosphamide	Itraconazole	↑	Avoid co-administration but can introduce itraconazole 24 hours post cessation of cyclophosphamide
Methylprednisolone	Itraconazole	2–3×↑	Use dexamethasone as an alternative
Ciclosporin	Itraconazole Voriconazole Fluconazole Posaconazole	50%↑ 2×↑ 50%↑ ↑	Decrease ciclosporin dose by 50% and closely monitor levels and toxicity
Tacrolimus	Itraconazole Voriconazole Fluconazole Posaconazole	5×↑ 3×↑ ↑ 3×↑	Decrease tacrolimus dose by 50% and closely monitor levels and toxicity
Sirolimus	Itraconazole Voriconazole Fluconazole	↑↑ ↑↑ ↑↑	Azoles contraindicated

torically by poor oral bio-availability with capsule formulation, but this has been overcome by the availability of an oral solution and an intravenous formulation. Voriconazole is generally well tolerated but exhibits a similar toxicity pattern to itraconazole. It can cause transient visual disturbance, which is reversible on cessation of the drug.

Fluoropyrimidines

Flucytosine (5-fluorocytosine or 5-FC) is a synthetic fluorinated pyrimidine. It is metabolized within cells to fluorouracil, which can be incorporated into the RNA in place of uracil, leading to mistranslation. It also causes inhibition of DNA synthesis by blocking thymidalate synthetase. It is active against most *Candida* spp, *Cryptococcus neoformans* and some dematiaceous molds but should be used in combination with other antifungal agents and not as monotherapy because of the risk of emergence of resistance. It comes as an oral and iv preparation. It must be given with extreme caution in patients with renal impairment as it is excreted primarily by the kidneys and renal impairment can lead to drug accumulation. Blood concentrations should be monitored weekly in such patients to ensure that drug accumulation is detected. Gastrointestinal disturbance, hepatitis and hematologic disturbance are the most common recognized adverse effects. Bone marrow depression is recognized and may preclude its use in some HSCT patients.

Echinocandins

The echinocandins are the first new antifungal drug class introduced for 20 years. They inhibit synthesis of β-1,3 D-glucan, an essential component of the cell wall of certain fungi.[44,45] Activity is primarily against *Candida* and *Aspergillus* spp. They are cidal for *Candida* spp and bacteriostatic for *Aspergillus* spp. They are not active against *Cryptococcus* spp, *Fusarium* spp, dimorphic endemic molds, *Trichosporon* spp and the mucorales. Three echinocandins have been developed for use: caspofungin, micafungin and anidulafungin. All are available only as intravenous preparations. One advantage they have over other agents is that they have minimal side-effects and there are very few drug interaction issues, particularly when compared with the azoles. Elevation in serum liver enzyme levels has been reported in 10–24% of patients and it is therefore prudent to monitor serum liver enzyme levels in those receiving these drugs.[44]

Primary prophylaxis

The decision concerning which patient group should receive antifungal prophylaxis depends mostly on the risk of acquiring invasive fungal infection. There is a large body of evidence to show that primary antifungal prophylaxis should be given to patients at high risk of invasive fungal infection, particularly in the case of candidal infection, and there are published guidelines regarding prevention of opportunistic infection, including fungal infections, in transplant recipients.[31,42,43,46] The high-risk patients are those who have received allogeneic stem cell transplantation and those with acute leukemia who undergo protracted myelosuppressive chemotherapy with prolonged periods of neutropenia.[13,47,48] Those who receive autologous peripheral stem cells have a much lower incidence of invasive fungal disease and are usually considered to be low risk. Autologous HSCT recipients may therefore not need to be given routine antifungal prophylaxis.[43,47] Consensus opinion, however, recommends giving prophylaxis to a subgroup of autologous HSCT recipients who have underlying malignancies such as acute leukemia and those who have or will have prolonged neutropenia and severe mucosal damage from conditioning regimens or who have recently received T-cell suppressive purine analogs as these factors increase their risk of acquiring invasive fungal infection.[43]

Which agents and for how long?

Although it has become the standard of care to give systemic antifungal prophylaxis to high-risk patients, there continue to be varying practices in choice of drug and duration of prophylaxis.[46,49] Fluconazole, itraconazole, posaconazole and amphotericin B have all been shown to reduce the incidence of invasive fungal infections. The toxicity profile of amphotericin B and cost of lipid formulations of amphotericin, plus the added advantage of oral administration of the azoles, mean that fluconazole and/or itraconazole are the two most common agents in routine use.[47] Specifically which agent to use depends on several aspects such as patient risk for invasive aspergillosis and other molds, drug–drug interactions and patient tolerability.

Two placebo-controlled studies in the 1990s demonstrated the efficacy of fluconazole in reducing invasive fungal infection and mortality in allogeneic bone marrow transplant recipients.[1,3] Since then, fluconazole, 400 mg/day orally or intravenously, from the day of transplantation, has been the standard regimen for those at risk of invasive candidal infections.[31,43,46] A more recent meta-analysis demonstrated that fluconazole prophylaxis reduces the use of parenteral antifungal therapy, the incidence of superficial fungal infections, of invasive candidal infections and fungal infection-related mortality in HSCT recipients but there was no reduction in invasive aspergillosis.[4] Lower doses (50–200 mg/day) have also been studied, and although their efficacy in prophylaxis has not convincingly been shown, it is possible that they may be sufficient.[50] Fluconazole 400 mg/od therefore remains the preferred option for higher risk groups of autologous HSCT recipients and an option for allogeneic HSCT recipients.

Fluconazole is an attractive agent because of its ease of administration and excellent safety profile, but its main limitation is its narrow spectrum of activity. Although it provides cover against many *Candida* spp, it is inactive against *C. krusei* and its activity against *C. glabrata* is variable and may be dose dependent. It does not cover *Aspergillus* spp and other molds, which cause infection in 1–25% of allograft recipients.

Itraconazole has an extended spectrum, including activity against non-*albicans Candida* spp, *Aspergillus* and other molds. There is now increasing evidence for the use of itraconazole as prophylaxis in patients at high risk of invasive aspergillosis and other mold infections.[13,46,47,51,52] A meta-analysis in 2003 showed that itraconazole was only active in doses that were equivalent to at least 200 mg/day of bio-available drug. In the higher dose group there was a significant reduction in proven invasive fungal infection, fungal infection-related mortality and the rate of invasive aspergillosis.[51]

Appropriate levels are difficult to achieve consistently with itraconazole capsules. Intravenous loading followed by oral itraconazole to ensure adequate dosing has been evaluated against fluconazole in two open-label studies in allogeneic HSCT recipients.[52,53] Both studies showed a benefit with itraconazole use in preventing invasive mold infections. However Marr et al, using a higher dose of 600 mg/day, reported a 36% drop-out rate in the itraconazole arm due to toxicity and drug intolerance and unexpected liver toxicity when used concomitantly with cyclophosphamide in conditioning therapy.[53] The investigators amended their protocol to start itraconazole post conditioning to avoid this drug–drug interaction. Given the clear dose–response relationship with itraconazole use, it is also recommended that drug levels should be monitored to ensure adequate dosing, aiming for a trough level of at least 500 ng/ml.[46,47]

Itraconazole can be recommended for prophylaxis of those at high risk of invasive aspergillosis and it is in routine use in many centers. Although it reduces the incidence of invasive fungal infection, clearcut data to show a survival benefit when compared to fluconazole are still lacking. Levels should probably be measured and its use is contraindicated or it should be used with caution in some patients, dictated by their concomitant therapy (see Table 43.3).

The new triazole posaconazole[54] has also been shown to be an effective agent for prophylaxis, although additional trials are needed to evaluate its use further. In a double-blind multicenter trial for prophylaxis of invasive fungal infections, posaconazole was compared with fluconazole in patients with GvHD who had undergone HSCT. Posaconazole was superior to fluconazole in preventing aspergillosis and comparable to fluconazole in other invasive fungal infections. No survival benefit was seen in this study.

The use of various amphotericin formulations for prophylaxis has also been studied and the results reviewed.[4,47,55] These include aerosolized amphotericin B,[56] systemic low-dose amphotericin B[57,58] and lipid formulations.[59,60] Although there was an apparent reduction in the incidence of invasive fungal infection with the use of liposomal or low-dose amphotericin B, criticisms can be made of the studies in terms of the use of historical controls, insufficient power and the presence of various uncontrolled parameters. Amphotericin formulations are not therefore routinely recommended for prophylaxis.

The administration of topical non-absorbable antifungal agents such as clotrimazole, nystatin, and amphotericin B lozenges orally or to the skin has been shown to decrease the colonizing fungal burden, particularly yeasts, and probably to decrease superficial infection (oral thrush, pharyngeal and esophageal candidiasis). Topical therapy does not, however, reduce the incidence of invasive candidiasis or invasive mold infection in HSCT recipients.

Antifungal prophylaxis should start on the day of transplantation and continue until the neutrophil count is $> 0.5 \times 10^9/l$ or for approximately 100 days in the allogeneic transplantation setting[46,61] but well-designed trials looking at this specific issue are lacking. Patients with prolonged GvHD, and those receiving high-dose steroids or other immunosuppressive agents for treatment of GvHD are known to be at increased risk of invasive fungal infection for longer.[32,62] In this situation, antifungal prophylaxis should be extended to cover this high-risk period.

Pneumocystis prophylaxis

Co-trimoxazole (Septrin) (960 mg bd 2×/week) is the agent of choice for the prevention of PCP infection in those who can tolerate it.[43,63] However, because of the theoretical concern of myelosuppression, prophylaxis regimens typically avoid co-trimoxazole use prior to engraftment (Table 43.4). Alternative regimens are available for

Table 43.4 Suggested dosing schedule for antifungals (prophylaxis and treatment)

Drug	Dose	Comments
Prophylaxis		
Candida and molds		
Fluconazole	po: 400 mg/day	Recommended dose as per international guidelines but lower doses have been used successfully (see text)
Itraconazole	po: 200 mg bd	
	iv: 200 mg bd for 48 h od thereafter	Avoid iv formulation if CrCl[a] <30 ml/min
PCP		
Co-trimoxazole (TMP/SMX)	po: 960 mg bd 2×/week	Administer for week prior to HSCT until day −1, then alternative prophylaxis regime, e.g. nebulized pentamidine until engraftment and reinstitution of co-trimoxazole prophylaxis post engraftment
Dapsone with or without trimethoprim or pyrimethamine	po: 50–100 mg/day dapsone, 25–50 mg/week pyrimethamine or trimethoprim 100–200 mg/day	
Pentamidine	Nebulized: 300 mg every 3–4 weeks or 150 mg every 2 weeks	
Treatment		
Candida and molds		
Amphotericin B deoxycholate (Fungizone)	iv: 1–1.5 mg/kg	Toxicity commonly precludes the use of this preparation in the HSCT recipient population
Liposomal preparations Ambisome Amphocil/Amphotec Abelcet	iv: 3 mg/kg od iv: 3–5 mg/kg iv: 5 mg/kg	
Caspofungin	iv: 70 mg loading dose, 50 mg od thereafter	
Fluconazole	po: 6–12 mg/kg od	
	iv: 6–12 mg/kg od	
Voriconazole	po: 200 mg bd for 24 h, 100 mg thereafter	
	iv: 6 mg/kg bd for 24 h, 4 mg/kg bd thereafter	Avoid iv route if CrCl[a] <30 ml/min
PCP		
Co-trimoxazole (TMP/SMX)	iv: 15–20 mg/kg/day TMP + 75–100 mg/kg/day SMX in divided doses	Addition of steroids if significant hypoxia
Cryptococcus		
Amphotericin B deoxycholate plus flucytosine follow-on fluconazole	iv: 0.7 mg/kg od plus po flucytosine 25 mg/kg qds	Suggested 2 weeks dual therapy then po fluconazole 400 mg od for 10 weeks or until CSF sterile then consider long-term po 200 mg od fluconazole suppression
Liposomal amphotericin B plus flucytosine	iv: 4 mg/kg od plus po flucytosine 25 mg/kg qds	

[a] CrCl, creatinine clearance.

those who cannot tolerate co-trimoxazole but none provides the same level of protection.[28,63] These include aerosolized pentamidine (300 mg every 3–4 weeks) or dapsone with or without trimethoprim or pyrimethamine (50–100 mg/day dapsone, 25–50 mg/week pyrimethamine or trimethoprim 100–200 mg/day). Prophylaxis should be offered to allogeneic HSCT recipients throughout the period of significant T-cell suppression.[43,64] Prophylaxis should be routinely given until 6 months post transplant and continued for longer in those who are receiving prolonged immunosuppression or who have chronic GvHD.

Secondary prophylaxis

Patients with previously documented fungal infection (proven or probable) are at risk of reactivation and recurrent fungal infection during HSCT, and relapsing invasive fungal disease has a higher mortality than primary infection (ranging from 88% to 100%).[65,66] No prospective studies have examined the role of secondary antifungal prophylaxis or its role in preventing relapsing infection. The existing experience is based on small retrospective studies and case reports. Patients with a past history of proven or probable invasive aspergillosis should receive secondary prophylaxis during subsequent neutropenia, transplantation and GvHD.[67,68] Not giving secondary prophylaxis significantly increases the risk of relapse to unacceptable levels, 62% versus 15%,[67] although specifically which agent to use and for what duration is not clear. The availability of more antifungal agents with good activity against *Aspergillus* spp such as voriconazole, itraconazole, posaconazole and the echinocandins offers many options for secondary prophylaxis without the need for prolonged amphotericin administration and its associated toxicities. Amphotericin formulations, voriconazole and itraconazole have all been used successfully as secondary prophylaxis.[67]

Resection of residual lesions after primary infection might also help reduce the incidence of relapse during subsequent immunosuppression and should at least be considered for fit young patients in remission and who have solitary *Aspergillus* lesions. There are numerous reports of the successful use of a combination of surgery and antifungal agents before HSCT,[66,67,69,70] but whether a combination approach results in better outcome than medical therapy with secondary prophylaxis alone is not known.

Additional preventive measures

It is well recognized that CMV infection contributes to the overall state of immunosuppression, as the virus has immunomodulatory properties. As stated before, CMV disease is an independent risk factor for invasive fungal infection. Control of CMV replication and prevention of active CMV disease is important for not only its direct benefits but also its indirect effect on reducing incidence of invasive fungal infection.

Effective control of GvHD can also reduce the incidence of invasive fungal infection. A lesson from solid organ transplantation experience is that reduction in steroid use with steroid-sparing agents such as ciclosporin or mycophenolate mofetil (MMF) can impact on the incidence of invasive fungal disease.

Clinical features

Candidiasis

Mucosal candidiasis was extremely common prior to the use of routine azole prophylaxis, the most common sites being oropharyngeal, genital and perineal. Esophageal candidiasis usually co-exists with oropharyngeal disease, but up to 30% cases have no visible oral lesions.

Invasive candidal infection usually presents as fungemia, visceral or chronic disseminated candidiasis. Suspicion of invasive candidal infection relies strongly on the presence of fever as an indicator. Fever may be the only feature of invasive disease or fungemia because lack of the main effector cells of the inflammatory response reduces the likelihood of focal signs and symptoms.[10] *Candida* spp are the most common fungi isolated from blood cultures and candidemia is the most common manifestation of invasive candidal infection. Candidiemia can be associated with rigors, sepsis-type syndrome and septic shock.[10,71] Fundoscopy should be performed in patients with candidemia as endophthalmitis (which has a characteristic appearance on fundscopy) complicates a small proportion of cases. Skin lesions can be present in acute disseminated candidiasis, These are typically macronodular but can progress to form central necrosis. Visceral and disseminated candidiasis typically presents with upper abdominal pain, jaundice, hepatosplenomegaly and fever unresponsive to broad-spectrum antibiotics.[72] It is associated with candidal seeding of liver, spleen and other visceral organs. It is thought that visceral dissemination may be either a late manifestation of earlier candidemia or secondary passage of fungi from the gastrointestinal tract to the portal and systemic circulation.

Aspergillosis

Aspergillosis can affect almost any organ in an immunocompromised host but sinus and pulmonary disease are the most common manifestations. Early diagnosis of invasive aspergillosis is notoriously difficult and, as with candidemia, fever that does not respond to broad-spectrum antibacterial agents may be the only sign. Fever may, however, be absent in as many as 30% of patients with invasive fungal infection, at least in the initial stages of infection.

There are very few features that are classically associated with invasive aspergillosis (Table 43.5).[73] Angio-invasion by fungal hyphae can lead to vascular thrombosis and tissue infarction and necrosis. This underlies the ulceration and necrosis of lesions, which may occasion-

Table 43.5 Clinical features of invasive fungal infection

Organ/system	Features	Likely infection
Skin	Scattered lesions, often on the limbs: maculopapular progressing to central necrosis	Acute disseminated candidiasis
	Pustular lesions	Disseminated aspergillosis or *Fusarium* infection
Nose	Upper respiratory tract symptoms, necrotic or ulcerated areas	Invasive aspergillosis or zygomycosis
Chest	Signs are few and non-specific – all should be investigated	Invasive pulmonary aspergillosis, *P. jiroveci* pneumonitis, other fungal pneumonias
Eyes	Fundoscopy may reveal the 'cotton-wool ball' lesions of *Candida* endophthalmitis (rare in neutropenic patients)	Acute disseminated candidiasis
Central nervous system	Focal neurologic deficit Fits	Invasive aspergillosis or other mold infection
	Headache, confusion, reduced level of consciousness, fits, neck stiffness	Cryptococcal or candidal meningitis

Modified after Kibbler.[73]

ally be seen clinically on skin and mucosal surfaces and are suggestive of fungal infection. Respiratory or sinus symptoms with antibiotic refractory fever should prompt imaging and trigger attempts to obtain good samples for microbiological analysis. Symptoms of invasive pulmonary aspergillosis are non-specific and include progressive dry cough, dyspnea, pleuritic chest pain and hemoptysis. *Aspergillus* sinusitis may present simply as pressure, nasal congestion, or pain. Involvement of the ethmoid sinus carries a high risk of extension into the cavernous sinus and cavernous sinus thrombosis and signs of ophthalmoplegia should be carefully sought. The presence of eschars on the hard palate or on the nasal turbinates is highly suggestive of fungal disease. Brushings or biopsies of these lesions may show fungal elements or grow mold.

Other mycoses

Disseminated infection with non-*Aspergillus* molds is often clinically indistinguishable from invasive aspergillosis. Blood cultures may be positive in *Fusarium* infections and skin lesions are occasionally seen in *Fusarium* infection (less commonly in disseminated aspergillosis). Biopsy of such lesions can be very helpful in making the diagnosis. *P. jiroveci* typically manifests as pneumonia with dyspnea, cough, fever, bilateral infiltrates on chest X-ray and a 'mosaic' pattern on CT scan. *Cryptococcus neoformans* typically presents with meningitis in the postengraftment phase but is unusual, in contrast to its more frequent occurrence in those infected with HIV. The widespread use of anti-*Candida* fluconazole prophylaxis may contribute to this low frequency of infection.

Diagnostic methods

Diagnosis of invasive fungal infection is notoriously difficult. Cultures from blood, respiratory tract secretions and other sites lack sensitivity. Absolute confirmation of invasive infection requires histopathologic evidence from biopsy, or recovery of fungus from a normally sterile or a radiologically abnormal site. In reality, it may not be possible to obtain either of these and diagnosis is based on a combination of clinical, radiologic and microbiologic features (Fig. 43.4).

The members of the EORTC/MSG formed a consensus committee to develop standard definitions for invasive mycoses and published the first guidelines in 2002, which are now under revision.[74,75] Three levels of probability have been proposed: 'Proven', 'Probable' and 'Possible'. The definitions include host, clinical and microbiologic criteria (Table 43.6). Although the intention of the committee was to standardize the definitions of invasive fungal infections for clinical research and not specifically for clinical management, the definitions are of clinical value. They can guide the clinician's choice of appropriate diagnostic investigations and provide a framework on which to base empiric and targeted antifungal therapy.

Radiology

High-resolution computed tomography (HRCT) plays a crucial part in the diagnosis of invasive infection in the stem cell transplant population.[76] Studies in the 1990s demonstrated the increased sensitivity of CT scans over standard X-rays for investigation in this patient group.[77] HRCT can often help differentiate between invasive pulmonary mycoses and bacterial or viral infection.[78] The characteristic CT appearance of angio-invasive pulmonary aspergillosis is a nodule surrounded by a halo of ground-glass attenuation[79] (Fig. 43.5). Other typical features include wedge-shaped peripheral areas of consolidation usually extending to the pleural surface, or nodular areas of consolidation, often related to blood vessels. The appearance on CT scan is dependent on timing of the scan in relation to the start of the infec-

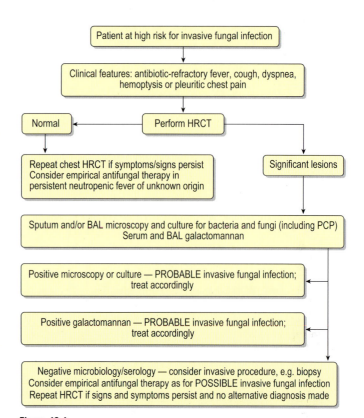

Figure 43.4
Diagnostic algorithm for investigation of individuals with suspected invasive fungal infection.

tion and the degree of neutropenia. Halo sign presence decreases in the first week of infection as the frequency of other appearances increases. By day 7 of the infection, approximately 50% of patients will have a non-contributory CT scan before the appearance of cavitation and air crescent sign with the recovery of neutrophils[79] (see Fig. 43.2).

Given the ever-changing practice in the use of antiprophylaxis and empiric antifungal therapy, the classic HRCT findings reported in the 1990s may be seen less frequently now, with non-specific CT appearances being a more typical finding. The HRCT appearances for cranial and sinus fungal infection have always been less specific but may aid diagnosis of invasive fungal infection. CT scanning and ultrasonography are also both helpful in diagnosing chronic disseminated candidiasis, with sensitivities of 96–100% but undefined specificity.[72]

HSCT patients who have a new cough, chest pain or hemoptysis, an abnormal chest X-ray, a new positive culture of *Aspergillus* spp or mold from any site, microscopic evidence of hyphae from any site, or an unresolved fever after 7 days of antimicrobials should have an HRCT of the chest (Table 43.7).[80] High-risk patients with negative CT scans but persistence of recurrent unexplained fever should be reimaged after a week or so.

Standard laboratory techniques including histology and microbiology

Visualization of fungal elements within the affected tissue is required to be absolutely confident that a patient has invasive local or disseminated fungal infection. However, there are problems with reliance on histologic diagnosis. Histology lacks sensitivity due to sampling error; the presence of fungal elements within tissue denotes infection, but it may not be possible to define the species or the species may be misinterpreted. Furthermore, tissue sampling is often precluded in this group of patients because of thrombocytopenia and the risk of bleed-

Table 43.6 Definitions of proven, probable and possible invasive infection (adaptation of revised EORTC/MSG definitions)

Proven invasive fungal diseases
Histopathologic, cytopathologic or direct microscopic examination of a needle aspiration or biopsy specimen showing yeast or hyphal forms with evidence of associated tissue damage OR Recovery of mold by culture from a sample obtained from a normally sterile site (including blood, CSF, excluding BAL, cranial sinus cavity washings and urine)

Probable invasive fungal disease
Defined by at least: One host AND one clinical AND one microbiologic criterion

Possible invasive fungal disease
Defined by at least: One host AND one clinical BUT no microbiologic criterion

Host criteria

1. Recent history of neutropenia ($<0.5 \times 10^9$ cells/l) for >10 days temporally related to the onset of fungal infection
2. Receipt of an allogeneic stem cell transplant
3. Prolonged corticosteroid use at an average minimum dose of 0.3 mg/kg/day prednisolone equivalent for >3 weeks
4. Treatment with other T-cell immune suppressant agents (e.g. ciclosporin, TNF-α blockers, specific monoclonal antibodies, nucleoside analogs) during the past 90 days
5. Inherited severe combined immunodeficiency

Clinical criteria

1. Presence of specific imaging signs on CT (well-defined nodule, air crescent sign, wedge-shaped infiltrate or cavity)
2. Presence of new non-specific focal infiltrate PLUS at least one of the following:
    i. Pleural rub
    ii. Pleural pain
    iii. Hemoptysis
3. Tracheobronchial ulceration, nodule, pseudomembrane, plaque or eschar seen on bronchoscopy
4. Imaging showing sinusitis PLUS at least one of the following:
    i. Acute localized pain
    ii. Nasal ulcer, black eschar
    iii. Extension from paranasal sinus across bony barriers, including into the orbit
5. Endophthalmitis as determined by ophthalmologic examination
6. CNS infection as defined by:
    i. Focal lesions on imaging
    ii. Meningeal enhancement on MRI or CT
7. Small, peripheral, target-like abscesses in liver and/or spleen typical of chronic disseminated candidiasis

Microbiologic criteria

1. Sputum, BAL and bronchial brush samples demonstrating the presence of fungal elements by culture or direct microscopy
2. Sinus aspirate demonstrating the presence of fungal elements by culture or direct microscopy
3. Skin ulcers, draining soft tissue lesions or fissure demonstrating the presence of fungal elements by direct microscopy AND culture
4. Positive galactomannan antigen EIA on a single plasma, serum, BAL, pleural fluid or CSF
5. Positive β-D-glucan on a single serum sample

Table 43.7 Recommendations for radiology imaging

1. All patients who have profound neutropenia ($<0.5 \times 10^9$ cells/l) with any of the following should have a high-resolution (or spiral) CT scan of the chest:
    a. A new cough, chest pain or hemoptysis
    b. An abnormal chest X-ray
    c. A new positive culture of *Aspergillus* or another mold from any site
    d. Microscopic evidence of hyphae in any invasive sample
    e. Unresolved temperature after 7 days of antibiotics and/or antifungals
2. All transplant patients with a new positive culture of *Aspergillus* or another mold should have a CT scan of the chest
3. All transplant patients with new neurologic features or possible or proven meningitis should have a CT or MRI imaging scan of the brain

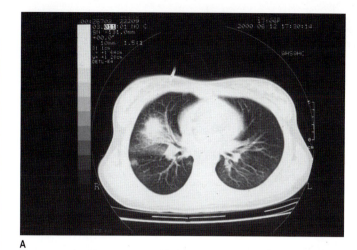

A

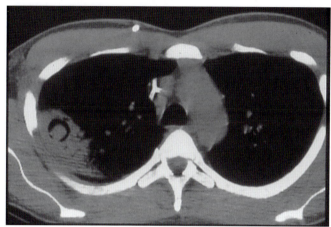

B

Figure 43.5
HRCT of the chest. (a) Halo sign with area of low attenuation surrounding a nodular lung lesion. (b) Air crescent sign with cavitation within a lung lesion. Courtesy of Dr J Cleverley.

ing. Immunohistochemistry may increase the specificity of tissue sample testing.[81] Molecular techniques including the use of PCR with pan-fungal primers on DNA extracted from tissue followed by southern blotting or sequencing, have also been shown to be useful.[82,83]

Even with improving molecular diagnostics, diagnosis still relies heavily on standard microscopy and culture of specimens (blood, respiratory tract secretions, fluid from sterile sites including CSF, urine and tissue) but there are known problems with sensitivity and/or specificity. Although bronchoalveolar lavage (BAL) cultures have a sensitivity of only 50%, in immunosuppressed individuals with focal pulmonary lesions[84] isolation of *Aspergillus* spp (Fig. 43.6) from respiratory tract specimens is highly predictive of invasive disease.[85,86] Microscopy on BAL specimens is more sensitive than culture, and microscopy for fungal elements should be performed on all BAL.[80] The diagnosis of PCP is made by BAL microscopy as the fungus cannot be cultured on standard media. Suspicious mucosal lesions should be biopsied, microscopy performed and the specimen cultured. All CSF samples with abnormal concentrations of glucose, protein or leukocytes from transplant patients should be tested for cryptococcal antigen and cultured on fungal media.

Serologic and molecular diagnostics – which test and when can they be helpful?

In recent years, efforts have been made to identify non-invasive markers for rapid and reliable diagnosis of invasive fungal infection,

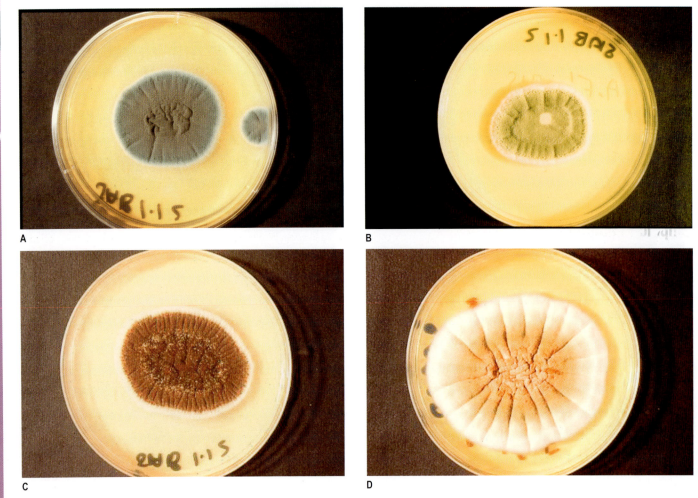

Figure 43.6
Colony morphology of the most common clinical *Aspergillus* isolates. (a) *A. fumigatus*. (b) *A. flavus*. (c) *A. niger*. (d) *A. terreus*.

particularly aspergillosis. These include detection of fungal antigens or nucleic acid from blood or other bodily fluids such as BAL or CSF. They have primarily been examined as a diagnostic adjunct or as a surveillance tool in high-risk patients to detect early invasive mycoses before overt clinical disease. Detection of two such antigens – galactomannan and 1,3 β-D-glucan – is now included in the microbiologic criteria in the EORTC/MSG consensus revised definitions for invasive fungal infections (see Table 43.6) but due to lack of external validation at present, detection of fungal nucleic acid by PCR will not be included.[75]

Galactomannan (GM) is a polysaccharide cell wall component of *Aspergillus* spp that is released into the blood during fungal growth in tissue. Circulating GM can be detected by commercially available sandwich ELISA. The assay has been approved by the United States Food and Drug Administration (FDA) as an adjunctive test for invasive pulmonary aspergillosis. Studies evaluating the role of the GM assay on serum samples in the diagnosis of invasive aspergillosis in hematology patients document a sensitivity of 33–100% and a specificity of 75–98.8%.[87,88] GM testing by ELISA on BAL fluid has been reported as having a higher sensitivity and specificity than serum in patients suspected of having invasive pulmonary aspergillosis.[89] When serially monitored, a positive serum GM result appears to precede the diagnosis of invasive aspergillosis by an average of 6–14 days.[90] The use of antifungal agents, however, may lower circulating GM levels by decreasing the fungal load, thus reducing the sensitivity of the test further in these patients.[19] False positives have been described in those consuming various foodstuffs or receiving certain antibiotics such as

piperacillin-tazobactam.[91,92] The timing of collection of the sample in relation to administration of piperacillin-tazobactam may influence the test results and for this reason the recommendation is for sample collection at trough levels or prior to drug administration.[93]

1,3 β-D-glucan is a component of cell walls in a number of yeasts and molds, including *Candida*, *Aspergillus*, *Fusarium*, *Acremonium* and *Saccharomyces* species. It has been less well studied than galactomannan and has only recently been licensed for clinical use. Sensitivities and specificities of tests in studies are in the range 67–100% and 84–100% respectively.[19] To date, PCR-based molecular diagnostic tests for invasive fungal infection remain largely unstandardized. It is hoped that the recent development of two commercial assays and a concerted UK and European effort to achieve a consensus on optimal DNA extraction, primer sets, amplification conditions and platforms will allow widespread use within the next 5 years.

These assays can certainly be of value in clinical practice in high-risk patients but care must be taken when interpreting a result. The prevalence of fungal disease is crucial when translating sensitivity and specificity into predictive value. In a setting where *Aspergillus* infection occurs at low prevalence (even in a high-risk group such as HSCT recipients with an incidence of approximately 15%) a test with 80% sensitivity and 80% specificity equates to a positive predictive value of only 31% and a negative predictive value of 97%. When prior probability of disease is increased because of the presence of clinical features, then these predictive values will also change. Tests detecting *Aspergillus* antigens should perhaps not necessarily be considered diagnostic but more as providing information regarding the probability of disease occurring given each patient's clinical scenario.[87] A second sample to confirm a positive result is recommended.

Treatment options

Timely initiation of treatment, reduction of immunosuppression and neutrophil recovery are the most important predictors of a successful outcome in invasive fungal infection. Antifungal treatment can take the form of empirical treatment in those with fever or directed therapy for those with probable or proven disease. It is important to involve the microbiology or infectious disease services in the choice and duration of therapy.

Empiric treatment – which agent?

Following studies from the 1980s comparing empiric amphotericin B deoxycholate (AmB) with no treatment, it is standard practice to start empiric antifungal therapy for neutropenic patients with a fever that is unresponsive to broad-spectrum antibiotics.[94–96] It is recommended that empiric therapy should be initiated in those patients with fever persisting despite >72 hours to 7 days of antibiotic therapy. The trials showed a reduction in death from invasive fungal infection and in time to defervescence of fever. The availability of echinocandins and second-generation triazoles, such as voriconazole and posaconazole, has impacted significantly on the management of fungal infection in the BMT population. Comparative trials over the last two decades, however, have not shown any clear superiority of one antifungal agent over another in terms of efficacy. In several studies nephrotoxicity occurred more frequently in those receiving AmB than in patients receiving liposomal amphotericin or other antifungal agents[97–99] and for this reason liposomal AmB, caspofungin or voriconazole may be preferred to AmB.[100] One study failed to show non-inferiority of voriconazole for empiric treatment when compared with liposomal AmB when assessing for overall response and defervescence. Secondary analysis of data from the same study, excluding resolution of fever as an endpoint, showed the two drugs to be equivalent.[98] Given the emergence of increasing numbers of fluconazole-resistant *Candida* spp and with the use of itraconazole prophylaxis, itraconazole cannot be as strongly recommended for empiric therapy as some of the alternative agents.[100]

Directed treatment

Candidiasis

Invasive candidiasis can be effectively treated by AmB preparations, caspofungin, oral or intravenous fluconazole, or a combination of fluconazole plus AmB.[31] The choice between these options depends upon knowledge of the *Candida* spp and known or predicted susceptibilities, the clinical state of the patient, the site involved and drug interactions. For high-risk and clinically unstable patients it is sensible to administer a broad-spectrum antifungal agent initially. Given that most HSCT patients develop candidemia as a breakthrough infection while receiving azole prophylaxis, the agents chosen for empiric therapy will usually be appropriate. This can be rationalized once species and sensitivity are known. Antifungal susceptibilities can be predicted to some degree by knowledge of the species (see Fig. 43.3). Intravascular catheters present at the time of candidemia should be removed or replaced if at all possible[101] as they can be a focus of continuing candidemia. Patients should undergo at least one ophthalmologic examination to exclude the possibility of candidal ophthalmitis. For candidemia, treatment should be continued for at least 2 weeks after the last positive blood culture and until recovery of the neutrophil

count.[94] Fluconazole (6 mg/kg/day) is the preferred option in patients with chronic disseminated candidiasis who are clinically stable, with amphotericin preparations being reserved for acutely ill patients or for azole-resistant organisms. Therapy should be continued until calcification or resolution of lesions as premature discontinuation of treatment in immunosuppressed patients may lead to recurrence/relapse of infection.[31]

Aspergillosis and other mycoses

AmB preparations were the drugs of choice for the treatment of invasive aspergillosis for many years. A randomized trial comparing voriconazole with AmB, has now shown voriconazole to be the treatment of choice for proven invasive aspergillosis.[102] Voriconazole was associated with significantly improved survival (71% vs 58% voriconazole vs AmB, respectively), although the poorest outcomes were in allogeneic HSCT recipients. It is not known whether voriconazole versus liposomal AmB from the outset of therapy would provide the same result. One non-*fumigatus Aspergillus* species, *A. terreus*, is notable for being resistant to AmB but sensitive to voriconazole. *Aspergillus terreus* accounts for 3–13% of all cases of invasive *Aspergillus* infection[15] in the transplant population and this is another reason to be cautious with the use of AmB preparations in proven invasive aspergillosis unless there is confirmation that it is a non-*terreus* species.

The exact length of antifungal therapy has not been well defined but the recommendation is that therapy should be continued for 10–12 weeks or for at least 4–6 weeks beyond resolution of radiographic abnormalities and resolution of immunosuppression.[103]

One caveat with voriconazole and caspofungin use is that they lack activity against the zygomycetes. As the clinical appearance of invasive infection by other molds, including the zygomycetes, can mimic those of invasive aspergillosis, an AmB preparation should be considered if microbiologic confirmation of *Aspergillus* infection cannot be made. There may also be practical issues regarding the use of voriconazole because of significant drug–drug interactions (see Table 43.3). Intravenous voriconazole is contraindicated in patients with a creatinine clearance of less than 50 ml/min, because of concerns about accumulation of voriconazole's renal excreted carrier. Caspofungin has in vitro activity against most *Candida* and *Aspergillus* spp, but not *Fusarium* spp, zygomycetes or *Cryptococcus neoformans*. Its use has been shown to be associated with a favorable response when given as salvage therapy for invasive aspergillosis, either alone[104] or in combination with voriconazole[105] or liposomal AmB.[106] Further studies are needed to establish its effectiveness as primary therapy for invasive aspergillosis.[107]

Combination therapy

There has been significant interest in combination therapy pairing an echinocandin with either an amphotericin B preparation or a triazole. Echinocandins target a site distinct from azoles and polyenes. The combination of an echinocandin with an azole or amphotericin B has neutral to synergistic activity in vitro and has improved efficacy over monotherapy in some animal models of invasive mycoses. Prospective randomized controlled trials comparing combination and monotherapy are lacking but there is promising experience with combination therapy for invasive mycoses, particularly in those failing standard monotherapy. The combination of caspofungin with liposomal amphotericin led to a favorable outcome in 40–60% of patients with invasive aspergillosis, and a survival advantage of caspofungin plus voriconazole over voriconazole alone was seen in retrospective analysis of salvage therapy for invasive aspergillosis.[19,76] Trials are required to definitively assess the benefit of combination therapy over monotherapy for treatment of invasive mycoses.

PCP and cryptococcus

Co-trimoxazole (15–20 mg/kg TMP + 75–100 mg/kg SMX daily divided into three or four doses) is the treatment of choice for *P. jiroveci*. In HIV-associated cryptococcal meningitis, amphotericin (0.7–1 mg/kg daily) plus 5-flucytosine (100 mg/kg daily) for the first 2 weeks, followed by long-term maintenance fluconazole therapy, has been recommended.[108] In the absence of modern randomized trials the same regimen is recommended for non-HIV associated cryptococcal meningitis (see Table 43.4).

Adjunctive/additional therapies

Even with timely initiation of therapy, invasive fungal infection is associated with significant mortality and a successful outcome is unlikely without recovery from neutropenia and lightening of immunosuppression. Despite this, there have been various attempts to find immune augmentation strategies that may be effective in treatment of invasive fungal infection.

Colony-stimulating factors (CSFs) (granulocyte-macrophage colony-stimulating factor and granulocyte colony-stimulating factor) can be used to accelerate myelopoiesis in neutropenic patients. They also augment phagocyte function, increasing fungicidal activity of phagocytes in vitro. GM-CSF may have the theoretical advantage against pathogens such as *Aspergillus* spp for which host defense is dependent on both neutrophil and macrophage function. Their role in treatment of invasive fungal disease in the immediate post-transplantation period is unclear as they have not been shown to produce a survival advantage in the majority of studies. Similarly, the rationale behind the use of granulocyte infusions is to provide supportive therapy for neutropenic patients by augmenting the number of circulating neutrophils until neutrophil recovery, but again survival benefit is not clear. For these reasons CSFs and granulocyte infusions are reserved for neutropenic patients with life-threatening infection refractory to conventional therapy.

Interferon-γ augments both innate and Th1-dependent immunity, both of which will contribute to host defense against mold infections. Data on its use in invasive aspergillosis are limited to case reports and small series, and no firm recommendation for its use in this setting can be made.[76] One concern is the potential for worsening GvHD in allogeneic HSCT. Other therapies are under study. A recent trial comparing lipid-associated amphotericin B alone versus in combination with an antibody-based inhibitor of heat shock protein 90 (Mycograb) in patients with invasive candidiasis showed promising results with an increased frequency of clinical and microbiologic resolution at day 10.[109]

The role of surgical resection post HSCT of lesions presumed to be secondary to invasive aspergillosis has not been established by randomized trial but there does not appear to be a clearcut survival advantage conveyed by operation. Surgery is not presently recommended except possibly in those with worsening lesions on medical therapy when technically feasible.[110]

References

1. Goodman JL, Winston DJ, Greenfield RA et al. A controlled trial of fluconazole to prevent fungal infections in patients undergoing bone marrow transplantation. N Engl J Med 1992;326:845–851
2. Pfeiffer CD, Fine JP, Safdar N. Diagnosis of invasive aspergillosis using a galactomannan assay: a meta-analysis. Clin Infect Dis 2006;42:1417–1427
3. Slavin MA, Osborne B, Adams R et al. Efficacy and safety of fluconazole prophylaxis for fungal infections after marrow transplantation – a prospective, randomized, double-blind study. J Infect Dis 1995;171:1545–1552
4. Bow EJ, Laverdiere M, Lussier N et al. Antifungal prophylaxis for severely neutropenic chemotherapy recipients: a meta analysis of randomized-controlled clinical trials. Cancer 2002;94:3230–3246
5. Bigley VH, Duarte RF, Gosling RD et al. Fusarium dimerum infection in a stem cell transplant recipient treated successfully with voriconazole. Bone Marrow Transplant 2004;34:815–817
6. Loudon KW, Coke AP, Burnie JP et al. Kitchens as a source of Aspergillus niger infection. J Hosp Infect 1996;32:191–198
7. Goodrich JM, Reed EC, Mori M et al. Clinical features and analysis of risk factors for invasive candidal infection after marrow transplantation. J Infect Dis 1991;164:731–740
8. Marr KA, Seidel K, White TC, Bowden RA. Candidemia in allogeneic blood and marrow transplant recipients: evolution of risk factors after the adoption of prophylactic fluconazole. J Infect Dis 2000;181:309–316
9. Verfaillie C, Weisdorf D, Haake R et al. Candida infections in bone marrow transplant recipients. Bone Marrow Transplant 1991;8:177–184
10. Viscoli C, Girmenia C, Marinus A et al. Candidemia in cancer patients: a prospective, multicenter surveillance study by the Invasive Fungal Infection Group (IFIG) of the European Organization for Research and Treatment of Cancer (EORTC). Clin Infect Dis 1999;28:1071–1079
11. Wingard JR, Merz WG, Rinaldi MG et al. Association of Torulopsis glabrata infections with fluconazole prophylaxis in neutropenic bone marrow transplant patients. Antimicrob Agents Chemother 1993;37:1847–1849
12. Wingard JR, Merz WG, Rinaldi MG et al. Increase in Candida krusei infection among patients with bone marrow transplantation and neutropenia treated prophylactically with fluconazole. N Engl J Med 1991;325:1274–1277
13. O'Brien SN, Blijlevens NM, Mahfouz TH, Anaissie EJ. Infections in patients with hematological cancer: recent developments. Hematology (Am Soc Hematol Educ Program) 2003:438–472
14. Junghanss C, Marr KA. Infectious risks and outcomes after stem cell transplantation: are nonmyeloablative transplants changing the picture? Curr Opin Infect Dis 2002;15:347–353
15. Wingard JR. The changing face of invasive fungal infections in hematopoietic cell transplant recipients. Curr Opin Oncol 2005;17:89–92
16. Richardson MD. Changing patterns and trends in systemic fungal infections. J Antimicrob Chemother 2005;56(suppl):i5-i11
17. Marr KA, Carter RA, Crippa F et al. Epidemiology and outcome of mold infections in hematopoietic stem cell transplant recipients. Clin Infect Dis 2002;34:909–917
18. Morgan J, Wannemuehler KA, Marr KA et al. Incidence of invasive aspergillosis following hematopoietic stem cell and solid organ transplantation: interim results of a prospective multicenter surveillance program. Med Mycol 2005;43(suppl 1):S49–58
19. Singh N, Paterson DL. Aspergillus infections in transplant recipients. Clin Microbiol Rev 2005;18:44–69
20. Lin SJ, Schranz J, Teutsch SM. Aspergillosis case-fatality rate: systematic review of the literature. Clin Infect Dis 2001;32:358–366
21. Nucci M, Anaissie E. Cutaneous infection by Fusarium sp in healthy and immunocompromised hosts: implications for diagnosis and management. Clin Infect Dis 2002;35:909–920
22. Nucci M, Marr KA, Queiroz-Telles F et al. Fusarium infection in hematopoietic stem cell transplant recipients. Clin Infect Dis 2004;38:1237–1242
23. Nucci M. Emerging molds: Fusarium, Scedosporium and zygomycetes in transplant recipients. Curr Opin Infect Dis 2003;16:607–612
24. Hagen EA, Stern H, Porter D. High rate of invasive fungal infections following nonmyeloablative allogenic transplantation. Clin Infect Dis 2003;36:9–15
25. Fukuda T, Boeckh M, Carter RA et al. Risks and outcomes of invasive fungal infections in recipients of allogeneic hematopoietic stem cell transplants after nonmyeloablative conditioning. Blood 2003;102:827–833
26. Chen C-S, Boeckh M, Seidel K et al. Infections post transplantation. Incidence, risk factors and mortality from pneumonia developing late after hematopoietic stem cell transplantation. Bone Marrow Transplant 2003;32:515–522
27. de Castro N, Neuville S, Sarfati C et al. Occurrence of Pneumocystis jiroveci pneumonia after allogeneic stem cell transplantation: a 6-year retrospective study. Bone Marrow Transplant 2005;36:879–883
28. Souza JP, Boeckh M, Gooley TA et al. High rates of Pneumocystis carinii pneumonia in allogeneic blood and marrow transplant recipients receiving dapsone prophylaxis. Clin Infect Dis 1999;29:1467–1471
29. Prentice HG, Kibbler CC, Prentice AG. Towards a targeted, risk-based, antifungal strategy in neutropenic patients. Br J Haematol 2000;110:273–284
30. Gerson SL, Talbot GH, Hurwitz S et al. Prolonged granulocytopenia: the major risk factor for invasive pulmonary aspergillosis in patients with acute leukemia. Ann Intern Med 1984;100:345–351
31. Pappas PG, Rex JH, Sobel JD et al. Guidelines for treatment of candidiasis. Clin Infect Dis 2004;38:161–189
32. Marr KA, Carter RA, Boeckh M et al. Invasive aspergillosis in allogeneic stem cell transplant recipients: changes in epidemiology and risk factors. Blood 2002;100:4358–4366
33. Marty FM, Lee SJ, Fahey MM et al. Infliximab use in patients with severe graft-versus-host disease and other emerging risk factors of non-Candida invasive fungal infections in allogeneic hematopoietic stem cell transplant recipients: a cohort study. Blood 2003;102:2768–2776
34. Husni R, Gordon S, Longworth DL. Cytomegalovirus is a risk factor for invasive aspergillosis in lung transplant recipients. Clin Infect Dis 1998;26:753–755
35. George MJ, Snydman DR, Werner BG et al. The independent role of cytomegalovirus as a risk factor for invasive fungal disease in orthotopic liver transplant recipients. Am J Med 1997;103:106–113
36. Saito T, Seo S, Kanda Y et al. Early onset Pneumocystis carinii pneumonia after allogeneic peripheral blood stem cell transplantation. Am J Hematol 2001;67:206–209
37. Gudlaugsson O, Gillespie S, Lee K et al. Attributable mortality of nosocomial candidemia, revisited. Clin Infect Dis 2003;37:1172–1177
38. Pizzo PA, Levine AS. The utility of protected-environment regimens for the compromised host: A critical assessment. In: Brown B (ed) Progress in hematology. Grune and Stratton, New York, 1997:311–332

39. Barnes RA, Rogers TR. Control of an outbreak of nosocomial aspergillosis by laminar air-flow isolation. J Hosp Infect 1989;14:89–94
40. Wald A, Leisenring W, van Burik JA, Bowden RA. Epidemiology of Aspergillus infections in a large cohort of patients undergoing bone marrow transplantation. J Infect Dis 1997;175:1459–1466
41. CDC, Infectious Disease Society of America, American Society of Blood and Marrow Transplantation. Guidelines for preventing opportunistic infections among hematopoietic stem cell transplant recipients: recommendations of CDC, the Infectious Disease Society of America, and the American Society of Blood and Marrow Transplantation. MMWR 2000;49(No. RR-10):1–125
42. Dykewicz CA, National Center for Infectious Diseases, Centers for Disease Control and Prevention, Infectious Diseases Society of America, American Society for Blood and Marrow Transplantation. Guidelines for preventing opportunistic infections among hematopoietic stem cell transplant recipients. Biol Blood Marrow Transplant 2001; 7(suppl):19–22
43. Dykewicz CA. Summary of the guidelines for preventing opportunistic infections among hematopoietic stem cell transplant recipients. Clin Infect Dis 2001;33:139–144
44. Denning DW. Echinocandins: a new class of antifungal. J Antimicrob Chemother 2002;49:889–891
45. Deresinski SC, Stevens DA. Caspofungin. Clin Infect Dis 2003;36:1445–1457
46. Maertens JA, Frère P, Lass-Flör C et al. European guidelines for primary antifungal prophylaxis in leukemia patients. Proceedings of the International Immunocompromised Host Society Conference, Crans-Montana, Switzerland, 2006
47. Glasmacher A, Prentice AG. Evidence-based review of antifungal prophylaxis in neutropenic patients with hematological malignancies. J Antimicrob Chemother 2005;56(suppl 1):i23–i32
48. McLintock LA, Jordanides NE, Allan EK et al. The use of a risk group stratification in the management of invasive fungal infection: a prospective validation. Br J Haematol 2004;124:403–404
49. Trifilio S, Verma A, Mehta J. Antimicrobial prophylaxis in hematopoietic stem cell transplant recipients: heterogeneity of current clinical practice. Bone Marrow Transplant 2004;33:735–739
50. Cornely OA, Ullmann AJ, Karthaus M. Evidence-based assessment of primary antifungal prophylaxis in patients with hematologic malignancies. Blood 2003;101:3365–3372
51. Glasmacher A, Prentice A, Gorschluter M et al. Itraconazole prevents invasive fungal infections in neutropenic patients treated for hematologic malignancies: evidence from a meta-analysis of 3,597 patients. J Clin Oncol 2003;21:4615–4626
52. Winston DJ, Maziarz RT, Chandrasekar PH et al. Intravenous and oral itraconazole versus intravenous and oral fluconazole for long-term antifungal prophylaxis in allogeneic hematopoietic stem-cell transplant recipients. A multicenter, randomized trial. Ann Intern Med 2003;138:705–713
53. Marr KA, Crippa F, Leisenring W et al. Itraconazole versus fluconazole for prevention of fungal infections in patients receiving allogeneic stem cell transplants. Blood 2004;103:1527–1533
54. Torres HA, Hachem RY, Chemaly RF et al. Posaconazole: a broad-spectrum triazole antifungal. Lancet Infect Dis 2005;5:775–785
55. Johansen HK, Gotzsche PC. Amphotericin B versus fluconazole for controlling fungal infections in neutropenic cancer patients. Cochrane Database Systematic Reviews 2002;CD000239
56. Schwartz S, Behre G, Heinemann V et al. Aerosolized amphotericin B inhalations as prophylaxis of invasive aspergillus infections during prolonged neutropenia: results of a prospective randomized multicenter trial. Blood 1999;93:3654–3661
57. Rousey SR, Russler S, Gottlieb M, Ash RC. Low-dose amphotericin B prophylaxis against invasive Aspergillus infections in allogeneic marrow transplantation. Am J Hematol 1991;91:484–492
58. Perfect JR, Klotman ME, Gilbert CC et al. Prophylactic intravenous amphotericin B in neutropenic autologous bone marrow transplant recipients. J Infect Dis 1992;165: 891–897
59. Kelsey SM, Goldman JM, McCann S et al. Liposomal amphotericin (AmBisome) in the prophylaxis of fungal infections in neutropenic patients: a randomised, double-blind, placebo-controlled study. Bone Marrow Transplant 1999;23:163–168
60. Tollemar J, Ringden O, Andersson S et al. Randomized double-blind study of liposomal amphotericin B (Ambisome) prophylaxis of invasive fungal infections in bone marrow transplant recipients. Bone Marrow Transplant 1993;12:577–582
61. Marr KA, Seidel K, Slavin MA et al. Prolonged fluconazole prophylaxis is associated with persistent protection against candidiasis-related death in allogeneic marrow transplant recipients: long-term follow-up of a randomized, placebo-controlled trial. Blood 2000; 96:2055–2061
62. Grow WB, Moreb JS, Roque D et al. Late onset of invasive aspergillus infection in bone marrow transplant patients at a university hospital. Bone Marrow Transplant 2002;29:15–19
63. Fisherman JA. Prevention of infection caused by Pneumocystis carinii in transplant recipients. Clin Infect Dis 2001;33:1397–1405
64. Tuan IZ, Dennison D, Weisdorf DJ. Pneumocystis carinii pneumonitis following bone marrow transplantation. Bone Marrow Transplant 1992;10:267–277
65. Fukuda T, Boeckh M, Guthrie KA et al. Invasive aspergillosis before allogeneic hematopoietic stem cell transplantation: 10-year experience at a single transplant center. Biol Blood Marrow Transplant 2004;10:494–503
66. Offner F, Cordonnier C, Ljungman P et al. Impact of previous aspergillosis on the outcome of bone marrow transplantation. Clin Infect Dis 1998;26:1098–1103
67. Sipsas NV, Kontoyiannis DP. Clinical issues regarding relapsing aspergillosis and the efficacy of secondary antifungal prophylaxis in patients with hematological malignancies. Clin Infect Dis 2006;42:1584–1591
68. Martino R, Parody R, Fukuda T et al. Impact of the intensity of the pre-transplant conditioning regimen in patients with prior invasive aspergillosis undergoing allogeneic hematopoietic stem cell transplantation: a retrospective survey of the infectious diseases working party of the european group for blood and marrow transplantation. Blood 2006;108(9):2928–2936
69. McWhinney PH, Kibbler CC, Hamon M et al. Progress in the diagnosis and management of aspergillosis in bone marrow transplantation: 13 years' experience. Clin Infect Dis 1993;17:397–404
70. Sevilla J, Hernandez-Maraver D, Aguado MJ et al. Autologous peripheral blood stem cell transplant in patients previously diagnosed with invasive aspergillosis. Ann Hematol 2001;80:456–459
71. Kibbler CC, Seaton S, Barnes RA et al. Management and outcome of bloodstream infections due to Candida species in England and Wales. J Hosp Infect 2003;54:18–24
72. Pagano L, Mele L, Fianchi L et al. Chronic disseminated candidiasis in patients with hematological malignancies. Clinical features and outcomes of 29 episodes. Haematologica 2002;87:535–541
73. Kibbler CC. Defining invasive fungal infections in neutropenic or stem cell transplant patients. J Antimicrob Chemother 2005;56(suppl. S1):i12-i16
74. Ascioglu S, Rex JH, de Pauw B et al. Defining opportunistic invasive fungal infections in immunocompromised patients with cancer and hematopoietic stem cell transplants: an international consensus. Clin Infect Dis 2002;34:7–14
75. EORTC/BAMSG. EORTC/BAMSG consensus revised definitions. www.doctorfungus.org/lecture/EOTRC_MSG_rev06.htm
76. Segal BH, Walsh TJ. Current approaches to diagnosis and treatment of invasive aspergillosis. Am J Respir Crit Care Med 2006;173:707–717
77. Graham NJ, Muller NL, Miller RR, Shepherd JD. Intrathoracic complications following allogeneic bone marrow transplantation: CT findings. Radiology 1991;181:253–259
78. Worthy SA, Flint JD, Muller NL. Pulmonary complications after bone marrow transplantation: high-resolution CT and pathologic findings. Radiographics 1997;17:1359–1371
79. Caillot D, Couaillier JF, Bernard A et al. Increasing volume and changing characteristics of invasive pulmonary aspergillosis on sequential thoracic computed tomography scans in patients with neutropenia. J Clin Oncol 2001;19:253–259
80. Denning DW, Kibbler C, Barnes RA. British Society for Medical Mycology proposed standards of care for patients with invasive fungal infections. Lancet Infect Dis 2003;3:230–240
81. Fenelon LE, Hamilton AJ, Figueroa JI et al. Production of specific monoclonal antibodies to Aspergillus species and their use in immunohistochemical identification of aspergillosis. J Clin Microbiol 1999;37:1221–1223
82. Paterson PJ, Seaton S, McLaughlin J, Kibbler CC. Development of molecular methods for the identification of aspergillus and emerging molds in paraffin wax embedded tissue sections. Mol Pathol 2003;56:368–370
83. Paterson PJ, Seaton S, McHugh TD et al. Validation and clinical application of molecular methods for the identification of molds in tissue. Clin Infect Dis 2006;42:51–56
84. Levine SJ. An approach to the diagnosis of pulmonary infections in immunosuppressed patients. Semin Respir Infect 1992;7:81–95
85. Yu VL, Muder RR, Poorsattar A. Significance of isolation of Aspergillus from the respiratory tract in diagnosis of invasive pulmonary aspergillosis. Results from a three-year prospective study. Am J Med 1986;81:249–254
86. Horvath JA, Dummer S. The use of respiratory-tract cultures in the diagnosis of invasive pulmonary aspergillosis. Am J Med 1996;100:171–178
87. Marr KA, Leisenring W. Design issues in studies evaluating diagnostic tests for aspergillosis. Clin Infect Dis 2005;41(suppl 6):S381-S386
88. Pfeiffer CD, Fine JP, Safdar N. Diagnosis of invasive aspergillosis using a galactomannan assay; A meta-analysis. Clin Infect Dis 2006;42:1417–1427
89. Musher B, Fredricks D, Leisenring W et al. Aspergillus galactomannan enzyme immunoassay and quantitative PCR for diagnosis of invasive aspergillosis with bronchoalveolar lavage fluid. J Clin Microbiol 2004;42:5517–5522
90. Maertens J, van Eldere J, Verhaegen J et al. Use of circulating galactomannan screening for early diagnosis of invasive aspergillosis in allogeneic stem cell transplant recipients. J Infect 2002;189:1297–1306
91. Viscoli C, Machetti M, Cappellano P et al. False-positive galactomannan platelia Aspergillus test results for patients receiving piperacillin-tazobactam. Clin Infect Dis 2004;38: 913–916
92. Ansorg R, van den Boom R, Rath PM. Detection of Aspergillus galactomannan antigen in foods and antibiotics. Mycoses 1997;40:353–357
93. Singh N, Obman A, Husain S et al. Reactivity of platelia Aspergillus galactomannan antigen with piperacillin-tazobactam: clinical implications based on achievable concentrations in serum. Antimicrob Agents Chemother 2004;48:1989–1992
94. Hughes WT, Armstrong D, Bodey GP et al. 2002 guidelines for the use of antimicrobial agents in neutropenic patients with cancer. Clin Infect Dis 2002;34:730–751
95. Pizzo PA, Robichaud KJ, Gill FA, Witebsky FG. Empiric antibiotic and antifungal therapy for cancer patients with prolonged fever and granulocytopenia. Am J Hematol 1982;72:101–111
96. Anonymous. Empiric antifungal therapy in febrile granulocytopenic patients. EORTC International Antimicrobial Therapy Cooperative Group. Am J Med 1989;86:668–672
97. Walsh TJ, Finberg RW, Arndt C et al. Liposomal amphotericin B for empirical therapy in patients with persistent fever and neutropenia. National Institute of Allergy and Infectious Diseases Mycoses Study Group. N Engl J Med 1999;340:764–771
98. Walsh TJ, Pappas P, Winston DJ et al. Voriconazole compared with liposomal amphotericin B for empirical antifungal therapy in patients with neutropenia and persistent fever. N Engl J Med 2002;346:225–234
99. Walsh TJ, Teppler H, Donowitz GR et al. Caspofungin versus liposomal amphotericin B for empirical antifungal therapy in patients with persistent fever and neutropenia. N Engl J Med 2004;351:1391–1402
100. Cordonnier C, Calandra T, Meunier F. Guidelines from the First European Conference on Infections in Leukaemia: ECIL-1. EJC Supplements 2007;5(2):1–60
101. Walsh TJ, Rex JH. All catheter-related candidemia is not the same: assessment of the balance between the risks and benefits of removal of vascular catheters. Clin Infect Dis 2002;34:600–602

102. Herbrecht R, Denning DW, Patterson TF et al. Voriconazole versus amphotericin B for primary therapy of invasive aspergillosis. N Engl J Med 2002;347:408–415

103. Walsh TJ, Anaissie EJ, Denning DW et al. Treatment of aspergillosis: clinical practice guidelines of the Infectious Diseases Society of America. Clin Infect Dis 2008;46:327–360

104. Maertens J, Raad I, Petrikkos G et al. Efficacy and safety of caspofungin for treatment of invasive aspergillosis in patients refractory to or intolerant of conventional antifungal therapy. Clin Infect Dis 2004;39:1563–1571

105. Marr KA, Boeckh M, Carter RA et al. Combination antifungal therapy for invasive aspergillosis. Clin Infect Dis 2004;39:797–802

106. Kontoyiannis DP, Hachem R, Lewis RE et al. Efficacy and toxicity of caspofungin in combination with liposomal amphotericin B as primary or salvage treatment of invasive aspergillosis in patients with hematologic malignancies. Cancer 2003;98:292–299

107. Maertens J. Caspofungin: an advanced treatment approach for suspected or confirmed invasive aspergillosis. Int J Antimicrob Agents 2006;27:457–467

108. Saag MS, Graybill RJ, Larsen RA et al. Practice guidelines for the management of crypto-coccal disease. Infectious Diseases Society of America. Clin Infect Dis 2000;30:710–718

109. Pachl J, Svoboda P, Jacobs F et al. A randomized, blinded, multicenter trial of lipid-associated amphotericin B alone versus in combination with an antibody-based inhibitor of heat shock protein 90 in patients with invasive candidiasis. Clin Infect Dis 2006;42:1404–1413

110. Yeghen T, Kibbler CC, Prentice HG et al. Management of invasive pulmonary aspergillosis in hematology patients: a review of 87 consecutive cases at a single institution. Clin Infect Dis 2000;31:859–868

Parasitic infections

Jennifer Treleaven

CHAPTER 44

Introduction

In addition to being present in the host or transmitted from the stem cell donor, a number of parasitic diseases are known or suspected to be transmitted by blood transfusion. Of greatest concern are malaria and Chagas' disease but babeosis, a parasite infection similar to malaria, and leishmania and toxoplasmosis are also a particular risk in the immunocompromised host. Thus, the infections outlined below should always be suspected in patients who develop unexplained symptoms and signs, particularly if their background endorses the possibility of a parasitic infection.

Toxoplasmosis

Toxoplasma gondii is a ubiquitous obligate intracellular protozoal parasite whose definitive host is cats, but it can be carried by most warm-blooded animals, including humans. It is very widespread in distribution. The disease caused by this organism, toxoplasmosis, is usually minor and self-limiting but can have serious or even fatal effects in a fetus whose mother first contracts the disease during pregnancy or in an immunocompromised human. Hence, toxoplasmosis, although rare, can often be fatal in allogeneic stem cell transplant recipients, in whom it commonly manifests as reactivation of a latent infection. The incidence after bone marrow transplant (BMT) is 0.3–5%, and it usually occurs 60–150 days after BMT, commonly causing cerebral abscesses (Fig. 44.1). Candidates for allogeneic hematopoietic stem cell transplant (HSCT) can be tested for IgG antibody to determine whether they are at risk for disease reactivation after HSCT, although it should be borne in mind that this test is not entirely accurate. Autologous transplant recipients are at negligible risk for toxoplasmosis reactivation, and no prophylaxis or screening for toxoplasmosis infection is recommended for such patients.

The advent of reduced-intensity conditioned transplants and transplants, in which a panlymphocyte monoclonal antibody such as CAMPATH IH has been used in the preparative regimen, may well result in an increased incidence of toxoplasma infection in these patients. Polymerase chain reaction (PCR) offers the possibility of making the diagnosis earlier than by conventional techniques, and is expected to improve the prognosis.[1,2] Historically, the length of time taken to obtain evidence for toxoplamsa infection has meant that in many cases the disease has progressed too far by the time therapy is initiated, and a very high death rate of up to 66% has been the result.[3] The worst prognosis is seen in disseminated toxoplasmosis, where many patients die without therapy, and the diagnosis is often made post mortem. In the transplant setting, most patients will present with the classic symptoms of aphasia and hemiparesis,[4] in addition to fever.

Other serious manifestations include chorioretinitis and pneumonitis with acute respiratory or multiorgan failure.[5] Table 44.1 shows the EBMT-IDWP definitions for toxoplasmosis infection after stem cell transplantation, adapted from Martino et al.[1]

Treatment

If ring-enhancing lesions are present on MRI examination of the brain, empiric treatment is recommended with pyrimethamine, plus sulfadiazine/clindamycin and folinic acid (atovaquone if intolerant in combination). There is usually a 50% reversal in clinical neurology within 7–10 days of starting treatment, which should be continued for 4–6 weeks after resolution of all signs and symptoms. Patients should then receive maintenance therapy at half dose for life, or until immunosuppression ceases.

It should be borne in mind that:

- serology in both donor and recipient should be checked pretransplant to ascertain patients at risk of developing the disease
- IgG antibodies rise after 12 weeks of infection, and remain positive for life
- IgM antibodies are often falsely positive for a variable duration and are more useful if negative.

In patients who are at risk of developing toxoplasmosis, weekly prophylaxis with Fansidar should be given; in 90 cases receiving this prophylaxis, no cases of toxoplasmosis were seen.[6] Following engraftment, pyrimethamine and sulfadiazine 1.5 g every 6 hours can be used although these can be myelotoxic. Azithromycin (1.5 g daily) and clindamycin may also have a role in treatment.

Amebiasis

Disseminated *Acanthamoeba* infections are rare, but occur in both the solid organ[7] and marrow stem cell transplant settings.[8] They are almost invariably fatal, with no universally accepted treatment approach. *Acanthamoeba* infection may be identified in transplant recipients who have had exposure to contaminated water and who develop non-healing cutaneous ulcers with granulomatous inflammation. The cutaneous lesions are the initial manifestation of infection and represent a reservoir for subsequent dissemination. Early institution of combination antimicrobial therapy is therefore necessary for effective treatment and prevention of lethal spread to the central nervous system, although finding an effective therapy can be problematic.[9] A combination of pentamidine, 5-fluorocytosine, itraconazole, and topical chlorhexidine gluconate/ketoconazole cream has proven effective in the transplant setting,[7] as have 5-fluorocytosine, sulfadiazine and isethionate.

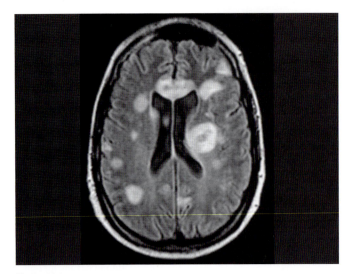

Figure 44.1
Toxoplasmosis affecting the brain.

Table 44.1 EBMT-IDWP definitions for toxoplasmosis after stem cell transplantation[1]

Toxoplasmosis disease	Criteria	
Definite	Tachyzoites histology or cytology	Biopsy Bronchoalveolar lavage Post mortem (culture parasite)
Probable	Clinical/radiologic + PCR	History and examination Blood/CSF/BAL
Possible	CT/MRI highly suggestive and response to anti-toxo therapy	
Evidence of infection	PCR positive in blood Seroconversion in a previously seronegative patient	No organ involvement

Nocardia

In the United States, *Nocardia* is estimated to be responsible for 500–1000 infections per year, 13% of which occur in transplant organ recipients.[10,11] *Nocardia* rarely causes clinical disease except in immunocompromised individuals, especially organ transplant recipients. Ninety percent of such patients manifest pulmonary symptoms, including cough, pleuritic chest pain, dyspnea, and radiologic abnormalities such as nodules and nodular infiltrates. About 20% of patients with nocardiosis present with cutaneous lesions, either localized or disseminated, and/or central nervous system involvement.

Three species of *Nocardia* are responsible for most human infections. *Nocardia* cells have been isolated from organic material and domestic animals. Human infection usually results from the inhalation of airborne bacilli or the traumatic inoculation of organisms into the skin. The infection is not transmissible between individuals.

In immunocompromised hosts, pulmonary infection may result in the formation of abscesses and, rarely, granulomas. Owing to the debilitated nature of the infected patients, mortality is up to 45%.

Diagnosis

Nocardia can be identified by gram and acid-fast stains and culture from appropriate clinical specimens. Sputum culture is useful for patients with a productive cough. The presence of branching, weakly acid-fast organisms in histologic sections, pus or sputum suggests the clinical diagnosis, although more invasive procedures such as thoracocentesis, transtracheal aspiration, or bronchial biopsy may be necessary to obtain material for staining and culture of *Nocardia*.

Treatment

Antimicrobial therapy with sulfa drugs such as trimethoprim-sulfamethoxazole is the treatment of choice. The duration of therapy ranges from 2–3 months for minor infections to 1 year for major infections.

Malaria

Malaria has quite commonly been reported after stem cell or solid organ transplantation.[12–15] It may either arise in a host who has suffered a previous infection, or it may be transmitted by an infected donor[12,13] or, less commonly, by transfusion of infected blood products.[14,16] Donors and recipients at risk pre-BMT should routinely be given specific treatment before marrow harvesting and conditioning, independent of the appearance of blood smears. It should be borne in mind that malaria infection in the immunocompromised transplant recipient may be even more life-threatening than would be the case in a normal patient.

Treatment

In uncomplicated cases, chloroquine or a chloroquine-based regimen is acceptable but it should be borne in mind that the organism could be resistant. The WHO guidelines[17] on treatment suggest appropriate alternatives in this situation.

Strongyloidiasis

This disease is caused by the parasitic helminth *Strongyloides stercoralis*. It is a nematode which is able to complete its life cycle in humans. It may cause infection over a period as long as several decades. Individuals with an intact immune system may have minimal or no symptoms. In contrast, those with a compromised immune system may develop a rapidly fatal infection (e.g. hyperinfection syndrome, disseminated strongyloidiasis). It has been described a number of times in recipients of either an autologous or allogeneic stem cell transplant procedure.[18–21] Allogeneic recipients should avoid cutaneous exposure to soil or other surfaces that might be contaminated with human feces.

Pathophysiology

Strongyloidiasis is typically acquired when the infective filariform larvae penetrate the skin during contact with contaminated soil, although ingestion of filariform larvae via the fecal–oral route can also result in infection. The larvae are transferred through the circulation to the lungs. In immunocompromised hosts, larvae may migrate beyond the normally controlled internal pathways, with widespread dissemination to the extraintestinal regions, including the CNS, heart, urinary tract, endocrine organs, and skin.

Frequency

Strongyloidiasis is uncommon in the USA but it is endemic in tropical and subtropical countries. The worldwide prevalence is approximately 35 million cases, and rates are as high as 40% in certain regions, including Southeast Asia, Latin America, and the Caribbean basin.

Definitive diagnosis depends on the microscopic demonstration of *S. stercoralis* larvae in the feces. Although serologic analysis with an enzyme-linked immunosorbent assay is the most sensitive test for strongyloidiasis (sensitivity, 84–92%), it is not specific and cross-reactions with other nematode infections are possible. Microscopic analysis of at least three stool samples is necessary to confirm the diagnosis.

Treatment

This is with anthelmintic agents such as ivermectin (Stromectol, Mectizan) or albendazole (Albenza).

Chagas' disease

This is also called American trypanosomiasis and is a human tropical parasitic disease which occurs in the Americas, particularly in South America. Its pathogenic agent is a flagellate protozoan named *Trypanosoma cruzi*, which is transmitted to humans and other mammals mostly by blood-sucking bugs of the subfamily Triatominae. Other forms of transmission are possible, including ingestion of food contaminated with parasites, blood transfusion and fetal transmission. The acute phase always requires treatment with benznidazole.[22] However, a significant proportion of cases may be resistant to this group of drugs. Evidence of Chagas' disease should be sought in all BMT patients coming from endemic areas because parasitemia and reactivation are potential complications during the period of neutropenia and immunosuppression.[23–25] Such HSCT candidates should be screened for serum IgG anti-*Tr. cruzi* antibody. *Trypanosoma cruzi* seropositivity is not a contraindication to HSCT, but if an acute illness occurs in a *Tr. cruzi*-seropositive HSCT recipient, *Tr. cruzi* reactivation can then be excluded. A case has recently been described in the recipient of a cord blood transplant.[26]

References

1. Martino R, Bretagne S, Einsele H et al. Early detection of *Toxoplasma* infection by molecular monitoring of *Toxoplasma gondii* in peripheral blood samples after allogeneic stem cell transplantation. Clin Infect Dis 2005;40:67–78
2. Bretagne S, Costa JM, Foulet F et al. Prospective study of toxoplasma reactivation by polymerase chain reaction in allogeneic stem-cell transplant recipients. Transpl Infect Dis 2000;2:127–132
3. de Medeiros BC, de Medeiros CR, Werner B et al. Disseminated toxoplasmosis after bone marrow transplantation: report of 9 cases. Transpl Infect Dis 2001;3:24–28
4. Mele A, Paterson PJ, Prentice HG et al. Toxoplasmosis in bone marrow transplantation: a report of two cases and systematic review of the literature. Bone Marrow Transplant 2002;29:691–698
5. Power M, McCann S, O'Connor M et al. Retinal and cerebral toxoplasmosis following nonmyeloablative stem cell transplant for chronic lymphocytic leukaemia. Bone Marrow Transplant 2005;36(11):1019–1020
6. Foot AB, Garin YJF, Ribaud P et al. Prophylaxis of toxoplasmosis with pyrimethamine/sulfadoxine (Fansidar) in bone marrow transplant recipients. Bone Marrow Transplant 1994;14:241–245
7. Duarte A, Sattar F, Granwehr B et al. Disseminated acanthamoebiasis after lung transplantation. J Heart Lung Transplant 2006;25:237–240
8. Castellano-Sanchez A, Popp AC, Nolte FS et al. *Acanthamoeba castellani* encephalitis following partially mismatched related donor peripheral stem cell transplantation. Transplant Infect Dis 2003;5:191–194
9. Schuster FL, Visvesvara GS. Opportunistic amoebae: challenges in prophylaxis and treatment. Drug Resist Updates 2004;7:41–51
10. Kennedy GA, Durrant S. Nocardia infection following bone marrow transplantation. Intern Med J 2005;35:688
11. Carradice D, Szer J. Nocardia infection following bone marrow transplantation. Intern Med J 2006;36:402
12. Raina V, Sharma A, Gujral S, Kumar R. Plasmodium vivax causing pancytopenia after allogeneic blood stem cell transplantation in CML. Bone Marrow Transplant 1998;22:205–206
13. Lefrère F, Besson C, Datry A et al. Transmission of Plasmodium falciparum by allogeneic bone marrow transplantation. Bone Marrow Transplant 1996;18:473–474
14. Dharmasena F, Gordon-Smith EC. Transmission of malaria by bone marrow transplantation (letter). Transplantation 1986;42:228
15. Villeneuve L, Cassaing S, Magnaval JF et al. *Plasmodium falciparum* infection following allogeneic bone-marrow transplantation. Ann Trop Med Parasitol 1999;93:533–535
16. Dodd RY. Transmission of parasites by blood transfusion (review). Vox Sang 1998;74(suppl 2):161–163
17. WHO Guidelines for the treatment of malaria. www.who.int/malaria/docs/ TreatmentGuidelines2006.pdf
18. Qazilbash MH, Ueno NT, Hosing C et al. Strongyloidiasis after unrelated nonmyeloablative allogeneic stem cell transplantation. Bone Marrow Transplant 2006;38:393–394
19. Gupta S, Jain A, Fanning TV et al. An unusual cause of alveolar hemorrhage post hematopoietic stem cell transplantation: a case report. BMC Cancer 2006;6:87
20. Schaffel R, Portugal R, Maiolino A, Nucci M. Strongyloidiasis pre and post autologous peripheral blood stem cell transplantation. Bone Marrow Transplant 2004;33:117
21. Orlent H, Crawley C, Cwynarski K et al. Strongyloidiasis pre and post autologous peripheral blood stem cell transplantation. Bone Marrow Transplant 2003;32:115–117
22. Dictar M, Sinagra A, Verón MT et al. Recipients and donors of bone marrow transplants suffering from Chagas' disease: management and preemptive therapy of parasitemia. Bone Marrow Transplant 1998;21:391–393
23. Moraes-Souza H, Bordin JO. Strategies for prevention of transfusion-associated Chagas' disease. Transfus Med Rev 1996;10:161–170
24. Altclas J, Sinagra A, Jaimovich G et al. Reactivation of chronic Chagas' disease following allogeneic bone marrow transplantation and successful pre-emptive therapy with benznidazole. Transplant Infect Dis 1999;1:135–137
25. Altclas J, Jaimovich G, Milovic V et al. Chagas' disease after bone marrow transplantation. Bone Marrow Transplant 1996;18:447–448
26. Forés R, Sanjuán I, Portero F et al. Chagas' disease in a recipient of cord blood transplantation. Bone Marrow Transplant 2007;39:127–128

Multiple organ failure and intensive care

Charles Craddock and Gavin D Perkins

CHAPTER

45

Introduction

Advances in supportive care have played a central role in decreasing the morbidity and mortality of stem cell transplantation (SCT) over the past decade.[1,2] It is important to remember that whilst modifications of the conditioning regimen, principally the introduction of reduced-intensity conditioning (RIC) protocols, have underpinned our ability to extend the potentially curative benefit of transplantation to older patients,[3,4] our increased ability to provide effective treatment for patients with multiorgan failure has also played a vital role.[5,6] Central to these advances has been an increased awareness of the importance of identifying patients at risk of developing severe organ toxicity and the benefits of early intervention, whether in the setting of a high-dependency or intensive treatment unit (ITU).

At the same time as developing more effective strategies to identify and treat patients at risk of multiorgan failure, there has been significant progress in the accurate identification of patients for whom further intensification of support is medically futile. Retrospective analysis of large databases has helped to define situations where the continued provision of intensive care is of no benefit. This information is of real importance both in determining which patients will not benefit from transfer to an ITU but also in identifying at what point it may be appropriate to discontinue therapy in those receiving intensive care.[7–9] The careful integration of these data into discussion with relatives and, when possible, patients can spare many the indignity of prolonged and futile intervention.[10] It also provides the basis for an evidence-based and constructive dialog between the transplant team and the ITU. This can help circumvent many of the frustrations of the past in which intensivists felt themselves forced to provide expensive, emotionally draining care to patients whose likelihood of benefiting was negligible.

The requirement for intensive care in patients undergoing autologous and allogeneic SCT

The likelihood of developing organ failure requiring admission to the ITU after stem cell transplantation varies widely according to patient demographics, transplant type and institutional criteria for ITU admission. Recent studies suggest a reduction in the proportion of patients requiring ITU admission but even so, between 11% and 40% of patients require intensive care at some stage during their treatment.[5,11] By far the most important factor predicting the likelihood of developing life-threatening complications post transplant relates to whether the patient has undergone an autologous or allogeneic transplant procedure. The risk of life-threatening complications and death is sub-

stantially higher in patients who have undergone allogeneic SCT.[12–14] Other important factors predisposing to the development of multiple organ failure include: age, pretransplant co-morbidities, degree of human leukocyte antigen (HLA) disparity, intensity of the conditioning regimen and the presence of acute graft-versus-host disease (GvHD) (Table 45.1).[15,16]

Historically, the outcome for patients admitted to an intensive care unit in the first 100 days after stem cell transplantation has been very poor.[7,12,17] However, the last 10 years has seen a significant improvement in the prospects for transplant patients admitted to intensive care.[1,11,18,19] While part of this progress undoubtedly reflects better patient selection, there has also been progress in the early identification of patients who require intensification of supportive care and advances in our ability to deliver effective organ support. The increasing use of peripheral blood stem cells as opposed to bone marrow, cytokine support and improved antifungal and antiviral prevention and treatment strategies have undoubtedly also played a part in improving outcome. These advances have been underpinned by the growing recognition of the importance of hematologists working with intensivists to provide a more integrated service. As a result, many large transplant units now benefit from the advice of an outreach ITU team who assess and advise on patients who develop early signs of organ failure.

Early identification of patients who may require intensive care

The decision to admit a patient to intensive care following SCT is difficult and can at times be controversial. Recent data showing improved outcomes in these patients are starting to reverse some of the pessimism previously associated with this population of patients.[1] To achieve maximum benefit from admission to intensive care, referral should be made early in the course of critical illness, necessitating early decisions about the appropriateness of referral for intensive care.

One of the most important developments assisting early identification of patients at risk of developing organ failure has been the introduction of physiologic track and trigger systems which facilitate the early recognition of the acutely ill patient.[20] These systems track routinely measured physiologic variables (such as respiratory rate, heart rate, blood pressure and urine output) to identify early signs of critical illness. Figure 45.1 depicts a typical adult observation chart. Based on predetermined abnormalities in well-defined physiologic signs, a response from the critical care team is triggered (e.g. review by the critical care outreach team). A number of different scoring systems have been developed which include the modified early warning system

Forename		Surname	
Consultant		Hospital No.	
Ward	D.O.B		Age

Sandwell and West Birmingham Hospitals NHS Trust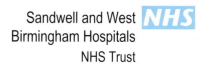

Adult Observation Chart

If you are concerned about the patient's condition you can call for medical assistance or Outreach at any time.

Green Observations

Continue established observations and treatment plan.

Any One Amber Observation

1

- Check observations manually and inform Nurse in Charge.
- Take any appropriate actions as required / prescribed.
- Increase frequency of patient observations.
- Inform medical staff/Nurse Practitioner if concerned about patient.

Any Two Amber Observations

2

- Check observations manually and inform Nurse in Charge.
- Take any appropriate actions as required / prescribed.
- Bleep House Officer (HO)/Nurse Practitioner.
  Ask doctor or Nurse Practitioner to review patient within 30 minutes.
- Continue to monitor patient. Hourly observations and fluid balance until stable.

Any Three or More Amber Observations

3

- Check observations manually and inform Nurse in Charge.
- Take any appropriate actions as required / prescribed.
- Bleep Senior House Officer (SHO). Ask doctor to review immediately.
- If no medical review within 30 minutes inform registrar.
- Continually monitor patient with 30 minute observations until stable.

Any Red Observations
CALL E.M.R.T. now!
Call 2222

A

Figure 45.1
Adult observation chart.

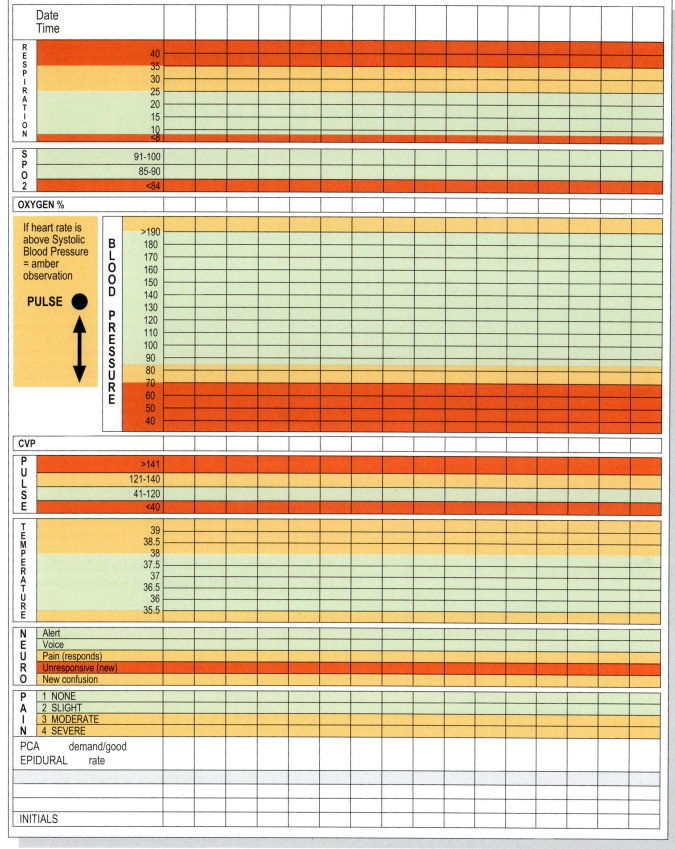

B

Figure 45.1, cont'd

Table 45.1 Predictors of admission to ITU[13]

Allogeneic transplant
Degree of HLA disparity
Age
Conditioning regimen
Pretransplant co-morbidities

Table 45.2 Clinical assessment

Daily assessment of vital signs coupled with scrutiny of biochemistry test results are crucial in optimizing outcome of transplant patients and play an important role in both preventing referral to ITU and also identifying patients at high risk of developing multiorgan failure promptly. The formal review of vital signs and laboratory results on a daily basis is of overwhelming importance in optimizing outcome, particularly in the peritransplant period.

Clinical and laboratory features requiring daily assessment	Features which should trigger review by ITU team
Systolic blood pressure	Hypotension unresponsive to fluid replacement and commencement of broad-spectrum antibiotics
Oxygen saturations	Sustained hypoxia (<90%) confirmed by arterial blood gases despite FiO$_2$ > 40%. An increasing respiratory rate is also an important predictor of impending respiratory failure
Daily weight	Sustained increase in weight (>10%) Refractory to fluid restriction or diuretics
Urine output	Oliguria (<40 ml/h) or rising serum creatinine

Table 45.3 Predictors of increased mortality after admission to ITU

Intubation and mechanical ventilation
Allogeneic transplant
Steroid-refractory graft-versus-host disease
Multiorgan failure especially concomitant renal and hepatic impairment
Hemodynamic shock
High serum lactate at admission
Age
High APACHE score

(MEWS),[21] the patient at risk team criteria (PART) and medical emergency team (MET) calling criteria.[22,23] These systems facilitate accurate identification of patients at risk of requiring intensive care support, allowing their prompt referral.

Even without the use of such a formal score, all transplant physicians should ensure that the bedrock of their clinical care is meticulous assessment of the clinical state of the patient on a daily basis. In many patients who are transferred to the ITU, it is possible to identify clinical features which were present days before the patient deteriorated which would have been apparent from scrutinizing the clinical parameters. The core features of the clinical assessment which can identify patients at high risk of transfer to the ITU are identified in Table 45.2. It is important to remember that none of these is sophisticated and much of the information required to predict incipient organ failure is present on the nursing chart.

Predictors of outcome in transplant patients admitted to intensive care

Outcome analyses have provided invaluable information which allows identification of patients with multiorgan failure who may benefit from intensive care. Further sophistication in defining who will benefit from admission to the intensive care unit has been provided by the application of scoring systems. These include the acute physiology and chronic health evaluation (APACHE II and III) mortality prediction models and simplified acute physiology (SAPS) prognostic systems.[24] Although these tools are useful for comparing outcomes in populations of patients receiving intensive care, none of them has sufficient precision to be used reliably for determining whether to admit an individual patient to intensive care.[1,25] Scoring systems or prediction models cannot replace dialog between the patient (when possible),

relatives, hematologist and intensive care physician when contemplating admission to intensive care. Consideration of patient wishes, the likely success of the SCT in treating the underlying condition, patient co-morbidities, severity of the disease and degree of organ dysfunction at presentation will all influence the decision to admit the patient to intensive care. Defining any limits to treatment at admission (for example, ventilation, vasopressors, renal replacement therapy) and early re-evaluation of the success of treatment/evolution of organ failure will assist in making the transition from intensive therapy to palliation in the face of continued deterioration when further treatment may be futile.

While it is possible to identify a cohort of patients who are unlikely to benefit from admission to the ITU, such as patients with relapse and rapid progression of their underlying malignant disease or patients with steroid-refractory GvHD, other preadmission characteristics are not sufficiently reliable to be used as the sole criteria for determining suitability for admission to the ITU. It is therefore generally considered wise to offer admission to the ITU to all patients requiring it unless there are compelling reasons why it would not be in the patient's best interest. However, there are now a number of studies which identify parameters predicting for a low chance of survival after admission to the ITU (Table 45.3), which can further guide the admission decision.[7,14]

Technological improvements in supportive care for stem cell transplant patients

A major contribution to the recent improvement in outcome for patients admitted to the ITU after SCT has been due to advances in contemporary management strategies. This is underlined by the fact that the improvement in outcome of transplant patients has followed similar improvements in outcome of non-transplant patients with similar degrees of organ dysfunction, and the increased recognition that the outcome of transplant patients is more dependent on the degree of organ dysfunction than on any inherent complications consequent upon their status as transplant patients. Specific interventions that may contribute to the trends in improved outcome include increasing use of non-invasive ventilation, lung-protective ventilation strategies and improvements in the management of patients with sepsis.

The risk of death is substantially increased in patients requiring mechanical ventilation following SCT. Non-invasive positive pressure ventilation (NIPPV) has been shown to reduce the need for endotracheal intubation and ventilation, and to improve outcomes in patients with hematologic malignancies and respiratory failure.[26] Improvements in ventilator technology and patient–ventilator interfaces (e.g. full face masks, nasal masks and helmets) and increased availability of equipment make this a viable treatment option in patients with early evidence of respiratory failure. The benefits of NIPPV are likely to be attributable to reducing the need for endotracheal intubation and invasive ventilation which are associated with ventilator-induced lung injury and ventilator-associated pneumonia.

The implementation of lung-protective ventilation strategies for patients with acute lung injury (ALI) or the acute respiratory distress syndrome (ARDS) has been shown to improve survival. In a large multicenter study from the ARDSnet investigators in the USA, patients were randomized to receive mechanical ventilation with traditional tidal volumes of 12 ml/kg or a protective ventilation strategy comprising low tidal volume ventilation (6 ml/kg) and limiting plateau airway pressures to less than 30 cm H_2O. Patients treated with the protective ventilation strategy had significantly lower mortality (31% vs 40%) and reduced duration of ventilation.[27] Although SCT patients were excluded from the study, it is likely that the application of protective ventilation strategies would be similarly beneficial in this group. The use of conservative fluid management strategies in patients with ALI/ARDS has also been shown to improve lung function and shorten the duration of mechanical ventilation and intensive care without increasing non-pulmonary organ failures.

Recent advances in the management of critically ill patients with sepsis have been summarized in international guidelines from the Surviving Sepsis Campaign (www.survivingsepsis.com).[28] Specific recommendations include the need for early goal-directed therapy (designed to optimize systemic oxygen delivery in the first 6 hours after the onset of sepsis), broad-spectrum antibiotic cover until the causative pathogen is identified, maintenance of glycemic control, low-dose corticosteroids in the presence of septic shock and deep vein thrombosis, and peptic ulceration prophylaxis.

Organ failure after stem cell transplant

Respiratory failure

Respiratory failure represents the most common reason for admission to the ITU post transplant and accounted for 48% of admissions in a recent analysis.[11] The most common causes of respiratory failure after stem cell transplantation are pulmonary infection, ARDS, idiopathic interstitial pneumonitis and pulmonary hemorrhage.[29] The causes of life-threatening pulmonary complications after SCT are summarized in Table 45.4.

Table 45.4 Life-threatening pulmonary complications in stem cell transplant patients

Infections
Bacterial
S. pneumoniae
S. aureus
Ps. aeruginosa
K. pneumoniae
E. coli
Viral
Cytomegalovirus
Respiratory syncytial virus
Parainfluenza
Fungal
Aspergillus spp
Pneumocystis pneumonia
Other
Pulmonary edema
Idiopathic pneumonia syndrome
Diffuse alveolar hemorrhage
Engraftment syndrome

Infectious pulmonary complications

The etiology of life-threatening pulmonary infection can often be difficult to define, and treatment frequently has to be empiric. A number of clinical features, however, can be helpful in identifying the most likely causative pathogen underlying a post-transplant pneumonic process. The most important of these are: type of transplant (autologous vs allogeneic), time from transplant and clinical presentation.

The clinical features of the most common post-transplant pneumonias are outlined below.

Bacterial pneumonia

Bacterial pneumonias typically occur, in both autologous and allogeneic transplant recipients, during the neutropenic period in the first 20 days post transplant. The bacteria commonly causing a life-threatening pneumonia post transplant include *S. pneumoniae*, *E. coli* and *Ps. aeruginosa*.[30] Bacterial pneumomias in the neutropenic patient classically present abruptly, in association with fever, pleuritic pain and cough and lobar changes on the chest X-ray. They may, however, present with less well-defined pneumonic symptoms or even isolated, abrupt-onset hypoxemia in neutropenic patients post transplant, particularly in patients receiving high-dose corticosteroids. Bronchoalveolar lavage (BAL) can be effective in identifying the etiology of bacterial pneumonias post transplant.[31] Patients may require mechanical ventilation, but with appropriate antibiotics and ventilatory support there is a good chance of recovery.

Fungal pneumonia

Fungal pneumonias are a relatively common cause of respiratory failure, particularly after allogeneic transplantation, and typically occur in the first 100 days post transplant in the context of either prolonged neutropenia or high-dose corticosteroid therapy for the treatment of acute graft-versus-host disease.[32] The widespread use of fluconazole prophylaxis has substantially decreased the incidence of severe yeast infections post transplant, and life-threatening *Candida* infections are now rare. However, mold infections, principally caused by *Aspergillus* species but increasingly by other molds such as *Fusarium* spp, represent a major cause of life-threatening pulmonary infections post transplant. Invasive pulmonary aspergillosis (IPA) can present indolently, and in the early stages of infection may only be associated with fever and an elevated C-reactive protein. Progressive disease is associated with the development of hypoxemia, and in advanced cases hemoptysis, pleurisy or wheeze. Chest X-ray (CXR) usually demonstrates non-specific pulmonary infiltrates, although nodularity can sometimes be identified later in the course of the infection. Suspected IPA merits an urgent high-resolution computed tomography (HRCT) scan which may demonstrate typical features including peripherally located nodules or areas of consolidation, cavitation and the formation of a 'halo' sign.[33]

Pneumocystis pneumonia (PCP)

PCP is a rare but potentially devastating complication of SCT, most commonly observed in allograft recipients. Although it can be very effectively prevented by the use of prophylactic co-trimoxazole, it should be remembered in the differential diagnosis of all patients with an interstitial pneumonitis post transplant.[34,35] It typically occurs after engraftment in patients still receiving immunosuppression (steroids or ciclosporin) who did not tolerate co-trimoxazole and in patients who have received alternative forms of PCP prophylaxis, usually nebulized pentamidine or dapsone.[36,37] It is also rarely seen in patients supposedly receiving prophylactic co-trimoxazole who have been non-compliant. Patients present with high fever, a prominent cough and profound hypoxemia. Although CXR changes are often initially subtle, bilateral basal streaking is common, which rapidly develops into perihilar infiltrates. Diagnosis can be confirmed by examination of induced sputum although this has less sensitivity than silver staining of BAL washings. Treatment with high-dose co-trimoxazole should be commenced as soon as this diagnosis is suspected.[34] The addition of corticosteroids in patients with profound hypoxemia may also be of value.

Cytomegalovirus (CMV) pneumonia

CMV pneumonitis is now a rare complication of allogeneic transplantation. It was one of the most common causes of post-transplant death until the development of effective screening strategies allowing early detection of CMV infection. However, the advent of polymerase chain reaction (PCR) technology which allows early and rapid detection of low-level CMV reactivation has allowed the early institution of antiviral therapy and substantially reduced the risk of CMV pneumonitis.[38] It should, however, always be considered in any patient with CMV infection who develops hypoxemia in association with an interstitial infiltrate on CXR. It typically develops in the second and third months post transplant but can occasionally occur before neutrophil engraftment.[39] CMV pneumonitis should also be suspected in any patient at risk of CMV infection (i.e. any CMV-positive patient, or patient with a CMV-positive donor) who develops a diffuse pulmonary infiltrate, typically in association with 'tree and bud' abnormalities on CT scan.[40] BAL is a useful part of the diagnostic work-up of patients with suspected CMV pneumonitis, firstly by excluding other infectious causes of interstitial pneumonitis and secondly by the demonstration of CMV infection in lavage fluid, although this alone is not diagnostic of CMV disease.

While ganciclovir and foscarnet are effective agents for the treatment of CMV infection, they are often ineffective in preventing progression of CMV pneumonitis. Recent data suggest an important role for cidofovir in the management of CMV pneumonitis, with salvage rates in the region of 50% in patients with established CMV disease.[41]

Toxoplasmosis

Toxoplasma infection is a rare but often fatal complication of allogeneic transplantation. However, approximately 5% of patients who have not received co-trimoxazole prophylaxis and who demonstrate pretransplant positive IgG serology develop toxoplasmosis which can present as either an interstitial pneumonitis or CNS disease.[42] It is therefore important that this diagnosis is always borne in mind in at-risk patients who present with hypoxemia, fever and pulmonary infiltrates or symptoms suggestive of a cerebral space-occupying lesion.

Non-infectious pulmonary complications

Pulmonary edema

Fluid overload is common in patients undergoing SCT, usually as a consequence of the large volumes of fluid and blood products infused either during the conditioning regimen or post transplant. It is quite common for such patients to develop features of pulmonary edema which can present rapidly and evolve into a florid clinical presentation, with severe hypoxemia, cough or hemoptysis and bilateral pulmonary infiltrates. It is absolutely vital, therefore, for meticulous attention to be paid to simple nursing principles of ensuring accurate records of fluid balance and daily weight measurements. It is also important to remember to administer furosemide to all patients with pulmonary infiltrates in whom fluid overload might be a possible contributing factor to their clinical presentation, even young patients with no apparent cardiac compromise.

Idiopathic pneumonia syndrome

Idiopathic pneumonia syndrome (IPS) is characterized by the development of clinical features of lung injury after stem cell transplantation in which an infectious etiology cannot be demonstrated. IPS typically presents with dyspnea, hypoxemia, fever and clinical features of a pneumonitis in the first 100 days post transplant and has been reported in up to 10% of post-transplant patients.[43,44] An essential component of the diagnostic work-up for IPS is a BAL which fails to demonstrate any evidence of an infectious organism. Risk factors for IPS include older age, malignancy other than leukemia, lower performance status before transplantation, positive donor CMV serology, high-dose chemotherapy, total-body irradiation, severe acute GvHD and multiorgan failure. Treatment is primarily supportive. The role of corticosteroids in the management of IPS is controversial, with no unequivocal evidence existing of their benefit in this syndrome.[45] The outcome of IPS is extremely poor in patients with progressive hypoxemia who require ventilatory support, with reported mortality rates in the region of 60–85%.[5,45]

Diffuse alveolar hemorrhage

Diffuse alveolar hemorrhage (DAH) is a rare but potentially fatal complication of stem cell transplantation occurring in approximately 5% of patients post transplant. It appears to be equally common after autologous and allogeneic transplantation and is more common in older patients receiving total-body irradiation (TBI).[46,47] DAH usually occurs in the first 30 days post transplant and typically presents with dyspnea, cough, hypoxemia and, in some patients, hemoptysis. CXR demonstrates alveolar infiltrates which can often be florid and appear out of proportion to the severity of the clinical presentation. HRCT often demonstrates diffuse ground-glass opacification. Diagnosis can be confirmed by BAL which will reveal hemorrhagic pulmonary secretions and hemosiderin-laden macrophages. Serial BALs often demonstrate progressively greater degrees of hemorrhage in lavage fluid. The recommended treatment is corticosteroids but this is often ineffective.[47,48]

Engraftment syndrome

Engraftment syndrome refers to a poorly defined constellation of symptoms characteristic of acute lung injury whose development coincides with the period of stem cell engraftment. It is characterized clinically by a swinging fever, pulmonary infiltrates and hypoxemia and can be associated with diarrhea and rash. Symptoms usually resolve after a short course of high-dose corticosteroids. It has variously been described in patients undergoing any form of stem cell transplantation, but appears to be more commonly associated with autologous peripheral blood stem cell transplantation and cord blood transplantation.

Cardiac complications post transplant

Cardiac complications are rare after SCT, occurring in fewer than 10% of transplants.[49–51] Historically, one of the most common causes of cardiac failure after stem cell transplantation is cardiotoxicity secondary to drugs in the preparative regimen, principally cyclophosphamide.[49,52] Typically presenting as global and profound left ventricular dysfunction within a few days of the administration of high-dose cyclophosphamide, this complication is very rarely seen now that the maximum dose of cyclophosphamide is limited to 120 mg/kg.[53] However, more subtle long-term depression of left ventricular function has been described up to 5 years after high-dose cyclophosphamide administration.[51,54]

In older patients undergoing autologous and, increasingly, allogeneic transplantation, cardiac arrhythmias, principally atrial fibrillation, represent the most common cause of cardiac toxicity and can occur in patients with no history of prior cardiac dysfunction.[51,55] These may also be precipitated by volume overload and sepsis. Bradyarrhythmias as well as supraventricular arrhythmias are also reported in association with infusion of stem cells cryopreserved with dimethyl sulfoxide.[56] Pericarditis is quite common in the first days post transplant and is associated with characteristic ST segment changes.[57] However, clinically significant pericardial effusions are rare in this setting.

Renal failure

Renal failure is a well-recognized complication of stem cell transplantation, particularly in patients undergoing allogeneic stem cell transplantation, although its incidence has fallen significantly in the past decade. This is likely to reflect increased understanding of how to administer and monitor nephrotoxic drugs, principally ciclosporin, and emphasizes the fact that the most common cause of renal impairment is drug related. Other important causes of acute renal failure in patients on the intensive care unit include sepsis, hypotension, veno-occlusive disease and microangiopathic hemolytic anemia consequent upon ciclosporin administration.[58]

Ciclosporin toxicity represents by far the most common cause of significant renal impairment in patients undergoing allogeneic transplantation.[59] Although regular monitoring of ciclosporin levels to some degree limits the incidence of severe renal toxicity, it should be remembered that severe renal impairment can be seen in patients receiving ciclosporin at therapeutic levels, particularly if concurrent nephrotoxic drugs are administered. In patients with deteriorating renal function in the setting of acute illness, it is often wise to defer ciclosporin administration for 24 hours or more and the 'space' this provides can limit the incidence of severe renal toxicity.

Other drugs which commonly cause renal impairment in transplant recipients include amphotericin (including liposomal preparations), aminoglycoside antibiotics and vancomycin, foscarnet, cidofovir and aciclovir. It is therefore vitally important that the drug chart is scrutinized in any patient presenting to the ITU and nephrotoxic agents omitted in patients with incipient or established multiorgan failure.[60]

Hepatic failure

Liver failure is a well-recognized problem requiring admission to the intensive care unit in patients who have undergone stem cell (particularly allogeneic) transplantation. The most common cause of life-threatening hepatic failure, as opposed to a transient disturbance of liver function, is either sepsis or as part of a syndrome of multiorgan failure. Other well-recognized causes of hepatic failure post transplant are veno-occlusive disease (VOD), drug-induced hepatotoxicity, hepatic GvHD and fungal or viral hepatitis.[61] Hepatic GvHD is typically a relatively late manifestation occurring in patients with severe acute GvHD in the second or third month post transplant, classically after the initial manifestation of skin or gut GvHD.

VOD is characterized by a triad of hyperbilirubinemia, weight gain and renal impairment which typically occurs in the first 3 weeks post transplant.[62] The reported incidence of VOD varies widely but appears to have decreased substantially in the past decade, probably because of the advent of intravenous formulations of busulfan with more predictable pharmacokinetics, and the realization that many of the early cases of VOD were manifestations of ciclosporin toxicity.[63,64] Many of the clinical features of ciclosporin toxicity mirror VOD and it is therefore important to discontinue ciclosporin for at least 48–72 hours to assess whether this results in symptom resolution, in patients with progressive hyperbilirubinemia, with or without weight gain. VOD is fatal in up to 25% of patients and its severity can be accurately predicted using an algorithm incorporating weight gain, degree of hyperbilirubinemia and time of onset of symptoms.[65] The other major cause of life-threatening hepatic dysfunction is viral hepatitis, which typically occurs 3–6 months post transplant.

Rarely, CMV can cause hepatitis, and fungal and bacterial causes of hepatitis, particularly in the first 100 days post allograft, are also recognized. Medications commonly causing hepatic failure after stem cell transplantation include ciclosporin (principally hyperbilirubinemia), fluconazole, amphotericin B and total parenteral nutrition.

Post-transplant thrombotic microangiopathy

The syndrome of microangiopathic hemolysis associated with renal failure, neurologic impairment or both represents an important cause of morbidity and mortality after stem cell transplantation.[66] The syndrome usually occurs within the first 100 days after stem cell transplantation and is associated with advanced recipient age, female sex, unrelated or HLA-mismatched donor grafts, GvHD, viral or fungal infections and the use of calcineurin inhibitors such as ciclosporin.[67] The syndrome has been called hemolytic uremic syndrome (HUS)/thrombotic thrombocytopenic purpura (TTP) in the past as it shares many of the clinical features of these conditions. However, to differentiate between the various pathophysiologic processes and outcomes associated with stem cell-associated HUS/TTP, the term post-transplant thrombotic microangiopathy (TMA) is now recommended. The Bone Marrow Transplant Clinical Trials Network Toxicity Committee have developed a consensus definition for TMA[66] comprising:

- RBC fragmentation and >2 schistocytes per high-power field on peripheral smear
- concurrent increase in serum lactate dehydrogenase
- concurrent renal and/or neurologic dysfunction without other explanations
- negative direct and indirect Coombs test results.

TMA complicates 5–15% of stem cell transplants. The incidence is higher after allogeneic than autologous stem cell transplant. The clinical spectrum of TMA can range from life-threatening neurologic or renal complications to asymptomatic anemia and mild renal dysfunction. Mortality associated with TMA and organ dysfunction is high, with a recent review of over 5000 stem cell transplant recipients reporting a median 3-month mortality of 75%.[68]

Therapies for the treatment of TMA are extremely limited. The first-line treatment after diagnosing TMA should be discontinuation of calcineurin inhibitors. Many clinicians start corticosteroids or other immunosuppressive treatments to cover the withdrawal of the calcineurin inhibitor. Whether this is beneficial for treating TMA is unknown. Although plasmapheresis can be an effective treatment in classic HUS/TTP, it is less effective in stem cell transplant-associated microangiopathy and is not recommended for routine use in current guidelines.[66]

Conclusion

The increasing complexity of stem cell transplantation coupled with the rising age of eligible patients has resulted in a greater proportion of patients experiencing life-threatening complications. However, technologic improvements in intensive care medicine coupled with a more integrated pattern of care provision between hematologists and intensive care physicians have improved the prospects for patients who develop multiple organ failure post transplant. These advances have clarified management strategies in patients referred to intensive care and facilitated the development of a rational process allowing the rapid identification of patients who will benefit from prolonged support. As a consequence, it is now reasonable to hope that further work allowing the targeted delivery of advances in intensive care to transplant patients will continue to improve outcome after stem cell transplantation.

References

1. Pene F, Aubron C, Azoulay E et al. Outcome of critically ill allogeneic hematopoietic stem-cell transplantation recipients: a reappraisal of indications for organ failure supports. J Clin Oncol 2006;24:643–649

2. Kew AK, Couban S, Patrick W et al. Outcome of hematopoietic stem cell transplant recipients admitted to the intensive care unit. Biol Blood Marrow Transplant 2006;12:301–305

3. Giralt S, Estey E, Albitar M et al. Engraftment of allogeneic hematopoietic progenitor cells with purine analog-containing chemotherapy: harnessing graft-versus-leukemia without myeloablative therapy. Blood 1997;89:4531–4536

4. McSweeney PA, Niederwieser D, Shizuru JA et al. Hematopoietic cell transplantation in older patients with hematologic malignancies: replacing high-dose cytotoxic therapy with graft-versus-tumor effects. Blood 2001;97:3390–3400

5. Afessa B, Tefferi A, Hoagland HC et al. Outcome of recipients of bone marrow transplants who require intensive-care unit support. Mayo Clin Proc 1992;67:117–122

6. Paz HL, Crilley P, Weinar M, Brodsky I. Outcome of patients requiring medical ICU admission following bone marrow transplantation. Chest 1993;104:527–531

7. Crawford SW, Schwartz DA, Petersen FB, Clark JG. Mechanical ventilation after marrow transplantation. Risk factors and clinical outcome. Am Rev Respir Dis 1988;137:682–687

8. Rubenfeld GD, Crawford SW. Withdrawing life support from mechanically ventilated recipients of bone marrow transplants: a case for evidence-based guidelines. Ann Intern Med 1996;125:625–633

9. Shorr AF, Moores LK, Edenfield WJ et al. Mechanical ventilation in hematopoietic stem cell transplantation: can we effectively predict outcomes? Chest 1999;116:1012–1018

10. Bach PB, Schrag D, Nierman DM et al. Identification of poor prognostic features among patients requiring mechanical ventilation after hematopoietic stem cell transplantation. Blood 2001;98:3234–3240

11. Soubani AO, Kseibi E, Bander JJ et al. Outcome and prognostic factors of hematopoietic stem cell transplantation recipients admitted to a medical ICU. Chest 2004;126:1604–1611

12. Ewig S, Torres A, Riquelme R et al. Pulmonary complications in patients with haematological malignancies treated at a respiratory ICU. Eur Respir J 1998;12:116–122

13. Diaz MA, Vicent MG, Prudencio M et al. Predicting factors for admission to an intensive care unit and clinical outcome in pediatric patients receiving hematopoietic stem cell transplantation. Haematologica 2002;87:292–298

14. Faber-Langendoen K, Caplan AL, McGlave PB. Survival of adult bone marrow transplant patients receiving mechanical ventilation: a case for restricted use. Bone Marrow Transplant 1993;12:501–507

15. Jackson SR, Tweeddale MG, Barnett MJ et al. Admission of bone marrow transplant recipients to the intensive care unit: outcome, survival and prognostic factors. Bone Marrow Transplant 1998;21:697–704

16. Price KJ, Thall PF, Kish SK et al. Prognostic indicators for blood and marrow transplant patients admitted to an intensive care unit. Am J Respir Crit Care Med 1998;158(3):876–884

17. Crawford SW, Peterson FB. Long-term survival from respiratory failure after marrow transplantation for malignancy. Am Rev Respir Dis 1992;145(3):510–514

18. Naeem N, Reed MD, Creger RJ et al. Transfer of the hematopoietic stem cell transplant patient to the intensive care unit: does it really matter? Bone Marrow Transplant 2006;37:119–133

19. Soubani AO. Critical care considerations of hematopoietic stem cell transplantation. Crit Care Med 2006;34:S251–267

20. Gao H, McDonnell A, Harrison DA et al. Systematic review and evaluation of physiological track and trigger warning systems for identifying at-risk patients on the ward. Intens Care Med 2007;33:667–679

21. Subbe CP, Kruger M, Rutherford P, Gemmel L. Validation of a modified Early Warning Score in medical admissions. Q J Med 2001;94:521–526

22. Goldhill DR, Worthington L, Mulcahy A et al. The patient-at-risk team: identifying and managing seriously ill ward patients. Anaesthesia 1999;54:853–860

23. Lee A, Bishop G, Hillman KM, Daffurn K. The medical emergency team. Anaesth Intens Care 1995;23:183–186

24. Gunning K, Rowan K. ABC of intensive care: outcome data and scoring systems. BMJ 1999;319:241–244

25. Afessa B, Tefferi A, Dunn WF et al. Intensive care unit support and Acute Physiology and Chronic Health Evaluation III performance in hematopoietic stem cell transplant recipients. Crit Care Med 2003;31:1715–1721

26. Hilbert G, Gruson D, Vargas F et al. Noninvasive ventilation in immunosuppressed patients with pulmonary infiltrates, fever, and acute respiratory failure. N Engl J Med 2001;344:481–487

27. ARDSnet. Ventilation with lower tidal volumes as compared with traditional tidal volumes for acute lung injury and the acute respiratory distress syndrome. The Acute Respiratory Distress Syndrome Network. N Engl J Med 2000;342:1301–1308

28. Dellinger RP, Carlet JM, Masur H et al. Surviving Sepsis Campaign guidelines for management of severe sepsis and septic shock. Crit Care Med 2004;32:858–873

29. Scaglione S, Hofmeister CC, Stiff P. Evaluation of pulmonary infiltrates in patients after stem cell transplantation. Hematology 2005;10:469–481

30. Lossos IS, Breuer R, Or R et al. Bacterial pneumonia in recipients of bone marrow transplantation. A five-year prospective study. Transplantation 1995;60:672–678

31. Hofmeister CC, Czerlanis C, Forsythe S, Stiff PJ. Retrospective utility of bronchoscopy after hematopoietic stem cell transplant. Bone Marrow Transplant 2006;38:693–698

32. Marr KA, Carter RA, Boeckh M et al. Invasive aspergillosis in allogeneic stem cell transplant recipients: changes in epidemiology and risk factors. Blood 2002;100:4358–4366

33. Escuissato DL, Gasparetto EL, Marchiori E et al. Pulmonary infections after bone marrow transplantation: high-resolution CT findings in 111 patients. Am J Roentgenol 2005;185:608–615

34. Tuan IZ, Dennison D, Weisdorf DJ. Pneumocystis carinii pneumonitis following bone marrow transplantation. Bone Marrow Transplant 1992;10:267–272

35. Lyytikainen O, Ruutu T, Volin L et al. Late onset Pneumocystis carinii pneumonia following allogeneic bone marrow transplantation. Bone Marrow Transplant 1996;17:1057–1059

36. Vasconcelles MJ, Bernardo MV, King C et al. Aerosolized pentamidine as pneumocystis prophylaxis after bone marrow transplantation is inferior to other regimens and is associated with decreased survival and an increased risk of other infections. Biol Blood Marrow Transplant 2000;6:35–43

37. Souza JP, Boeckh M, Gooley TA et al. High rates of Pneumocystis carinii pneumonia in allogeneic blood and marrow transplant recipients receiving dapsone prophylaxis. Clin Infect Dis 1999;29:1467–1471

38. Goodrich JM, Mori M, Gleaves CA et al. Early treatment with ganciclovir to prevent cytomegalovirus disease after allogeneic bone marrow transplantation. N Engl J Med 1991;325:1601–1607

39. Limaye AP, Bowden RA, Myerson D, Boeckh M. Cytomegalovirus disease occurring before engraftment in marrow transplant recipients. Clin Infect Dis 1997;24:830–835

40. Gasparetto EL, Ono SE, Escuissato D et al. Cytomegalovirus pneumonia after bone marrow transplantation: high resolution CT findings. Br J Radiol 2004;77:724–727

41. Ljungman P, Deliliers GL, Platzbecker U et al. Cidofovir for cytomegalovirus infection and disease in allogeneic stem cell transplant recipients. The Infectious Diseases Working Party of the European Group for Blood and Marrow Transplantation. Blood 2001;97:388–392

42. Martino R, Cordonnier C. Toxoplasmosis following allogeneic hematopoietic stem cell transplantation. Bone Marrow Transplant 2003;31:617–618; author reply 619

43. Meyers JD, Flournoy N, Thomas ED. Nonbacterial pneumonia after allogeneic marrow transplantation: a review of ten years' experience. Rev Infect Dis 1982;4:1119–1132

44. Fukuda T, Hackman RC, Guthrie KA et al. Risks and outcomes of idiopathic pneumonia syndrome after nonmyeloablative and conventional conditioning regimens for allogeneic hematopoietic stem cell transplantation. Blood 2003;102:2777–2785

45. Crawford SW, Hackman RC. Clinical course of idiopathic pneumonia after bone marrow transplantation. Am Rev Respir Dis 1993;147:1393–1400

46. Nevo S, Swan V, Enger C et al. Acute bleeding after bone marrow transplantation (BMT) – incidence and effect on survival. A quantitative analysis in 1,402 patients. Blood 1998;91:1469–1477

47. Afessa B, Tefferi A, Litzow MR et al. Diffuse alveolar hemorrhage in hematopoietic stem cell transplant recipients. Am J Respir Crit Care Med 2002;166:641–645

48. Chao NJ, Duncan SR, Long GD et al. Corticosteroid therapy for diffuse alveolar hemorrhage in autologous bone marrow transplant recipients. Ann Intern Med 1991;114:145–146

49. Baello EB, Ensberg ME, Ferguson DW et al. Effect of high-dose cyclophosphamide and total-body irradiation on left ventricular function in adult patients with leukemia undergoing allogeneic bone marrow transplantation. Cancer Treat Rep 1986;70:1187–1193

50. Bearman SI, Petersen FB, Schor RA et al. Radionuclide ejection fractions in the evaluation of patients being considered for bone marrow transplantation: risk for cardiac toxicity. Bone Marrow Transplant 1990;5:173–177

51. Kupari M, Volin L, Suokas A et al. Cardiac involvement in bone marrow transplantation: electrocardiographic changes, arrhythmias, heart failure and autopsy findings. Bone Marrow Transplant 1990;5:91–98

52. Hertenstein B, Stefanic M, Schmeiser T et al. Cardiac toxicity of bone marrow transplantation: predictive value of cardiologic evaluation before transplant. J Clin Oncol 1994;12:998–1004

53. Goldberg MA, Antin JH, Guinan EC, Rappeport JM. Cyclophosphamide cardiotoxicity: an analysis of dosing as a risk factor. Blood 1986;68:1114–1118

54. Braverman AC, Antin JH, Plappert MT et al. Cyclophosphamide cardiotoxicity in bone marrow transplantation: a prospective evaluation of new dosing regimens. J Clin Oncol 1991;9:1215–1223

55. Hidalgo JD, Krone R, Rich MW et al. Supraventricular tachyarrhythmias after hematopoietic stem cell transplantation: incidence, risk factors and outcomes. Bone Marrow Transplant 2004;34:615–619

56. Alessandrino P, Bernasconi P, Caldera D et al. Adverse events occurring during bone marrow or peripheral blood progenitor cell infusion: analysis of 126 cases. Bone Marrow Transplant 1999;23:533–537

57. Bock J, Doenitz A, Andreesen R et al. Pericarditis after high-dose chemotherapy: more frequent than expected? Onkologie 2006;29:321–324

58. Gruss E, Bernis C, Tomas JF et al. Acute renal failure in patients following bone marrow transplantation: prevalence, risk factors and outcome. Am J Nephrol 1995;15:473–479

59. Parikh CR, McSweeney PA, Korular D et al. Renal dysfunction in allogeneic hematopoietic cell transplantation. Kidney Int 2002;62:566–573

60. Zager RA. Acute renal failure in the setting of bone marrow transplantation. Kidney Int 1994;46:1443–1458

61. McDonald GB, Shulman HM, Sullivan KM, Spencer GD. Intestinal and hepatic complications of human bone marrow transplantation. Part I. Gastroenterology 1986;90:460–477

62. Bearman SI, Anderson GL, Mori M et al. Venoocclusive disease of the liver: development of a model for predicting fatal outcome after marrow transplantation. J Clin Oncol 1993;11:1729–1736

63. Scott B, Deeg HJ, Storer B et al. Targeted busulfan and cyclophosphamide as compared to busulfan and TBI as preparative regimens for transplantation in patients with advanced MDS or transformation to AML. Leuk Lymphoma 2004;45:2409–2417

64. de Lima M, Couriel D, Thall PF et al. Once-daily intravenous busulfan and fludarabine: clinical and pharmacokinetic results of a myeloablative, reduced-toxicity conditioning regimen for allogeneic stem cell transplantation in AML and MDS. Blood 2004;104:857–864

65. Bearman SI. The syndrome of hepatic veno-occlusive disease after marrow transplantation. Blood 1995;85:3005–3020

66. Ho VT, Cutler C, Carter S et al. Blood and marrow transplant clinical trials network toxicity committee consensus summary: thrombotic microangiopathy after hematopoietic stem cell transplantation. Biol Blood Marrow Transplant 2005;11:571–575

67. Cutler C, Henry NL, Magee C et al. Sirolimus and thrombotic microangiopathy after allogeneic hematopoietic stem cell transplantation. Biol Blood Marrow Transplant 2005;11:551–557

68. George JN, Li X, McMinn JR et al. Thrombotic thrombocytopenic purpura-hemolytic uremic syndrome following allogeneic HPC transplantation: a diagnostic dilemma. Transfusion 2004;44:294–304

Late effects

Gérard Socié, Smita Bahtia and André Tichelli

Introduction

Large numbers of patients now survive long term following stem cell transplantation (SCT), and the late clinical effects of SCT are thus of major concern in the 21st century. *Secondary malignant diseases* are of particular clinical concern as more patients survive the early phase after transplantation and remain free of their original disease.[1,2] *Non-malignant late effects* are heterogeneous and although often non-life threatening, they significantly impair the quality of life of long-term survivors.[3]

The main aims of this chapter are to present an overview of these malignant and non-malignant late complications and to provide some recommendations regarding their prevention and early treatment. Extensive reviews with references have already been published.[1,2] Thus, only main references are included in this chapter. Recommendations for screening are those derived from a joint publication by international experts,[4] summarized in Tables 46.1 and 46.2.

The major risk factors for late complications post SCT are chronic graft-versus-host disease (c-GvHD) and/or its treatment and the use of irradiation in pretransplant conditioning. The inter-relationships between c-GvHD, total-body irradiation (TBI), and non-malignant late effects are summarized in Figure 46.1.

Non-malignant late effects

Late effects of chronic graft-versus-host disease

Chronic GvHD and its associated immune deficiency state are the prime causes of transplant-related mortality late after marrow grafting, and contribute directly or indirectly to most late complications. Since c-GvHD is reviewed elsewhere in this book, only the main points relating to late complications will be highlighted here.

Despite the advent of new treatment modalities, the incidence of c-GvHD is being sustained by changes in clinical SCT practice[5,6] as follows:

- the expanded use of matched unrelated as well as mismatched related donors
- the increasing use of SCT in older patients
- the increasing use of donor lymphocyte infusions to treat relapsed disease or to achieve full donor chimerism after non-myeloablative transplantation
- the increasing use of peripheral blood stem cells instead of bone marrow.

Immune reconstitution has a pivotal role in the long-term outcome of allogeneic SCT. Chronic GvHD is the major factor influencing immune reconstitution of B-cells and CD4- and CD8- T-cells.[5,6] Donor source (marrow versus peripheral blood), unrelated versus sibling transplant, and the degree of human leukocyte antigen (HLA) compatibility between donor and recipient also affect the pace of immune reconstitution. Low B-cell count, reversed CD4/CD8 ratio and a decreased IgA level are all risk factors associated with late infections. Factors contributing to post-SCT immune deficiency are summarized in Figure 46.2.

Late bacterial and viral infections have been extensively reviewed, and guidelines for preventing and treating these opportunistic infections after SCT have been proposed in a document published under the auspices of the Centers for Disease Control (CDC), the Infectious Disease Society of America and the American Society of Blood and Marrow Transplantation.[7] Susceptibility to encapsulated bacteria (*S. pneumoniae*, *H. influenzae*, and *N. meningitidis*) has been well documented, especially in patients with current or previous c-GvHD. Late (>2 years) fungal or cytomegalovirus (CMV) infections are rare, and almost invariably occur in patients with ongoing immune suppression from GvHD. Varicella zoster, in contrast, is extremely frequent even in patients without GvHD, but usually occurs within a few months of SCT, after aciclovir prophylaxis has been discontinued.

Finally, of the parasitic infections, late *Pneumocystis carinii* (PCP) and *Toxoplasma gondii* infections are more common in patients receiving active treatment for c-GvHD. Since PCP prophylaxis with trimethoprim-sulfamethoxazole is highly active, this regimen should be given to all patients receiving treatment for c-GvHD and/or those with CD4+ cells below 0.2×10^9/l. PCP prophylaxis should probably be continued for several weeks after the cessation of immunosuppressive therapy, in view of the long-lasting T-cell defects characteristic of patients who have developed c-GvHD. Also, as described later, c-GvHD is the main risk factor for squamous cell cancer occurring after SCT.

Late ocular effects

Ocular complications of the posterior segment

These can be divided into microvascular retinopathy, optic disk edema, hemorrhagic complications and infectious retinitis. Ischemic retinopathy, with cotton-wool spots and optic disk edema, has been described in 10% of patients following SCT. Microvascular retinopathy occurs mainly after TBI-conditioned allogeneic SCT, in patients receiving ciclosporin as GvHD prophylaxis. Visual acuity is decreased in most patients, but recovers when ciclosporin is withdrawn. In most cases, retinal lesions resolve with withdrawal or reduction of immunosuppressive therapy.[8]

Table 46.1 EBMT/CIBMTR/ASBMT summary recommendations for screening and prevention in long-term HCT survivors

Tissues/organs	Late complications	Risk factors	Monitoring tests and preventive measures
Immune system	Infections	Donor source HLA disparity T-cell depletion Graft-versus-host disease (GvHD) Venous access devices	Antibiotic prophylaxis targeting encapsulated organisms for duration of immunosuppressive therapy for c-GvHD. Some experts recommend antifungal prophylaxis for those receiving chronic corticosteroids Administration of prophylactic antibiotics for oral procedures should follow American Heart Association guidelines for endocarditis prophylaxis PCP prophylaxis for initial 6 months for all HCT recipients, or duration of immunosuppressive therapy to treat or prevent c-GvHD Some experts recommend continued CMV antigen or PCR testing for allogeneic recipients with chronic immunosuppression or chronic GvHD. Some experts recommend prophylaxis for HSV in patients receiving chronic immunosuppression for c-GvHD Immunizations per CDC or EBMT guidelines initiated at 1 year after HCT. Delayed initiation beyond 1 year may be considered in situations where recipients are unlikely to respond
Oral	Sicca syndrome Caries	GvHD Radiotherapy	Dental assessment at 6–12 months, individualized follow-up schedule thereafter according to dental professional. Subsequent dental/oral follow-up care should occur at least annually. Particular attention to intraoral malignancy evaluation in c-GvHD patients and recipients of radiotherapy
Liver	GvHD Viral hepatitis Iron overload	Cumulative transfusion exposure	Liver function testing (LFT) every 3–6 months in 1st year, then individualized but at least yearly Monitor HbsAg and viral load by PCR for patients with known hepatitis B or C, with liver and infectious disease specialist consultation Liver biopsy to assess cirrhosis should be considered for those with chronic HCV infection after 8–10 years Serum ferritin at 1 year after transplant, with consideration of confirmatory liver biopsy for abnormal results based upon magnitude of elevation and clinical context. Subsequent monitoring is suggested for patients with elevated LFTs, continued RBC transfusions or presence of hepatitis C infection
Muscle and fascia	Myopathy Myositis fasciitis	Corticosteroids GvHD	Frequent (monthly) clinical screening for corticosteroid myopathy. Physical therapy consultation for patients with prolonged corticosteroid exposure, fasciitis or sclerodermatous GvHD may minimize loss of function
Respiratory	Interstitial pneumonitis Bronchiolitis obliterans Chronic obstructive disease	Intensive conditioning regimen Radiation exposure Infectious agents GvHD	Clinical assessment for all patients at 6 months, 1 year and annually thereafter Avoidance of smoking tobacco should be recommended for all patients PFT and focused radiologic assessment for allogenic recipients at 1 year for signs or symptoms of compromise, or earlier as clinically indicated. Annual testing for those with deficits or appropriate clinical circumstances. Some experts suggest screening PFT evaluation every 3–6 months in the first 2 years, particularly in patients with c-GvHD PFTs should be performed for autologous recipients with known pretransplant deficits, or exposure to radiation or other lung toxic agents Radiographic evaluation as determined by diagnostic PFT testing or based on symptoms
Endocrine	Hypothyroidism Hypoadrenalism Gonadal failure Growth	Radiotherapy to head, neck, mantle TBI Prolonged corticosteroid usage TBI Intensive chemotherapy Young age Intensive prior chemoradiotherapy CNS radiotherapy Hypothyroidism Gonadal insufficiency	Thyroid function testing yearly post transplant in all patients, or if relevant symptoms develop Slow terminal tapering of corticosteroids for those with prolonged exposure Consider stress doses of corticosteroids during acute illness for patients who had received chronic corticosteroids Annual clinical and endocrinologic gonadal assessment for postpubertal women Clinical and endocrinologic gonadal assessment for prepubertal women within 1 year of transplant, with further follow-up as determined by pediatric endocrinologist in the peripubertal period Gonadal function in men including FSH, LH, testosterone should be assessed as warranted by symptoms (lack of libido, erectile dysfunction) Monitor growth velocity in children annually, assessment of thyroid, and growth hormone function if growth velocity is abnormal

Ocular	Cataracts Keratoconjunctivitis sicca Microvascular retinopathy	TBI, corticosteroids GvHD, TBI Ciclosporin Radiotherapy	Routine clinical evaluation at 6 months, 1 year and yearly thereafter, with instruction regarding sicca and cataract risk Schirmer's testing for those with c-GvHD Some experts recommend routine ocular exam (visual acuity, fundus exam) at 1 year for all patients, subsequent frequency of screening individualized according to symptoms or predisposing factors Prompt ophthalmologic examination in all patients with visual symptoms
Skeletal	Osteopenia Avascular necrosis	Corticosteroids TBI Inactivity Gonadal insufficiency Male gender	Dual-photon densitometry at 1 year for adult women, or any patient with prolonged corticosteroid or calcineurin inhibitor exposure. Subsequent densitometry testing determined by defects or to assess response to therapy Exercise, calcium and vitamin D supplementation and bisphosphonates are treatment options for osteopenia, and may help prevent loss of bone density. Clinicians should assess role of gonadal and thyroid function in patients with decreased bone density Some experts recommend use of bisphosphonates as prophylaxis for patients at high risk due to chronic corticosteroid usage. Screening for avascular necrosis is not recommended
Second cancers	Solid tumors Hematologic malignancies Post transplant lymphoproliferative disorders	Chemotherapy Radiotherapy Immunodeficiency Chronic GvHD EBV infection	Risk awareness counseling annually Screening clinical assessment annually Routine self-examination of breasts and skin, as per healthcare maintenance section Pap smear and mammogram annually as per healthcare maintenance section. Some experts recommend screening mammography earlier than age 40 for women with radiation exposure Avoidance of tobacco or excessive, unprotected UV exposure
Nervous system	Leukoencephalopathy Late infections Calcineurin neurotoxicity Peripheral neuropathy	Cranial radiotherapy Intrathecal chemotherapy Fludarabine GvHD Chemotherapeutic exposure	Clinical evaluation for symptoms and signs of neurologic dysfunction at 1 year Diagnostic testing (radiographs, nerve conduction, etc.) for those with symptoms or signs
Kidney and bladder	Nephropathy Bladder dysfunction	TBI, platinum exposure Adenovirus, CMV Cyclophosphamide	Blood pressure assessment at every clinic visit, with aggressive hypertension management Screening assessment of blood pressure, urine protein, BUN, creatinine at 6 months, 1 year, and annually if abnormalities on earlier studies Ultrasonography and/or renal biopsy as warranted to diagnose etiology of renal insufficiency
Vascular	Coronary disease Cerebrovascular disease	Gonadal failure	Routine clinical assessment of cardiovascular risk factors as per health maintenance Clinical assessment for vascular complications at regularly scheduled follow-up visits Testing for hypercoagulability for patients with significant thrombosis history
Quality of life	Depression Anxiety Fatigue Sexuality	Prior psychiatric Gonadal failure	Clinical assessment and psychosocial throughout recovery period, adjustment at 6 months, 1 year and annually thereafter, with mental health professional counseling recommended for those with recognized deficits. Encouragement of robust support networks Query adults about sexual function at 6 months and yearly
General health			Recommended screening as per general population (see text)

Table 46.2 EBMT/CIBMTR/ASBMT abbreviated summary recommendations for screening and prevention in long-term HCT survivors organized by time after transplantation

Recommended screening/prevention	6 months	1 year	Annually
Immunity			
Encapsulated organism prophylaxis	3	3	3
PCP prophylaxis	1	3	3
CMV testing	3	3	
Immunizations		1	1
Oral complications			
Dental assessment	1	1	1
Liver			
Liver function testing	1	1	+
Serum ferritin testing		1	+
Respiratory			
Clinical pulmonary assessment	1	1	1
Smoking tobacco avoidance	1	1	1
Pulmonary function testing		2	+
Chest radiography	+	+	+
Endocrine			
Thyroid function testing		1	+
Growth velocity children		1	1
Gonadal function assessment (prepubertal men and women)	1	1	1
Gonadal function assessment (postpubertal women)		1	1
Ocular			
Ocular clinical symptom evaluation	1	1	1
Schirmer's test		3	3
Ocular fundus exam		1	+
Skeletal			
Bone density testing (women and patients with prolonged corticosteroid, calcineurin use)		1	+
Second cancers			
Second cancer vigilance counseling		1	1
Breast/skin/testes self-exam		1	1
Clinical screening second cancers		1	1
Pap smear/mammogram (over age 40 years)		1	1
Nervous system			
Neurologic clinical evaluation		1	+
Kidney			
Blood pressure screening	1	1	1
Urine protein screening	1	1	+
BUN/creatinine testing	1	1	1
Vascular			
Cardiovascular risk factor assessment		1	1
Psychosocial			
Psychosocial/QOL clinical assessment	1	1	1
Sexual function assessment	1	1	1

1 = Recommended for all transplant patients.
2 = Recommended for allogeneic patients only.
3 = Recommended for any patient with ongoing c-GvHD or immunosuppression.
+ = Reassessment recommended for abnormal testing in a previous time period or new signs/symptoms.

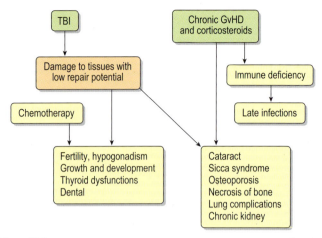

Figure 46.1
Inter-relationship between total body irradiation and chronic graft-versus-host disease in the genesis of late complications after allogeneic stem cell transplantation.

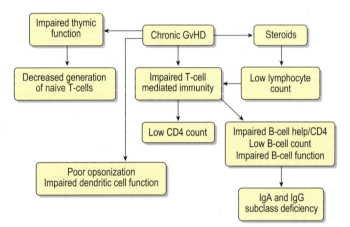

Figure 46.2
Factors contributing to late immune deficiency and late infection following allogeneic stem cell transplantation.

Ocular complications of the anterior segment

The two most common late complications affecting the anterior segment are cataract formation and keratoconjunctivitis sicca syndrome.

Cataract formation, particularly posterior subcapsular cataracts, has long been recognized in recipients of SCT as one of the most frequent late complications of TBI.[9–11] After single-dose TBI, almost all patients develop cataracts within 3–4 years, and most, if not all, need surgical intervention. Although the probability of developing cataracts after fractionated TBI lies at around 30% at 3 years, the incidence may reach over 80% 6–10 years post SCT (Table 46.3). On multivariate analysis, use of TBI in a single dose, rather than fractionated, and the use of steroid treatment for longer than 3 months were associated with a significant risk of cataract development. The effect of dose rate of irradiation on subsequent cataract development is also established. In the largest series evaluating a cohort of 1064 patients, factors independently associated with an increased risk of cataracts were older age (>23 years), higher dose rate (>0.04 Gy/min), allogeneic SCT and steroid administration. Finally, in prospective studies comparing cataract incidence and risk factors, it has been shown that patients who receive cyclophosphamide and TBI (Cy/TBI) have a higher incidence of cataract formation than do those treated with busulfan and cyclophosphamide (Bu/Cy).[12] The only treatment for cataracts is to surgically remove the lens from the eye to restore transparency of the visual

Table 46.3 Cataract after stem cell transplantation

Type of study	Number of patients	Probability of cataract formation			Remarks
		sTBI	fTBI	No TBI	
Single center (Seattle)	277	80% at 6 years	18% at 6 years	19% at 6 years	Sparing effect of fTBI
Single center (Basel)	197	100% at 3.5 years Surgery 96%	29% at 3.3 years 83% at 6 years		TBI Single dose Corticosteroids >3 months
Single center (Seattle)	492	85% at 11 years	Risk at 11 years 50% (>12 Gy) 34% (12 Gy)	19% at 11 years	Need of surgical repair – 59% sTBI – 33% fTBI – 23% no TBI Highest yearly hazard of cataract formation earlier with sTBI than fTBI
Single center (Paris)	494	34% at 5 years	11% at 5 years		High dose rate, main risk factor
EBMT registry	1063	Risk at 10 years 60% Surgery 32%	Risk at 10 years 43% Surgery 3%	–	Risk factors: – older age – higher dose rate – allogeneic SCT – no heparin
4 randomized studies	488	–	Risk at 7 years AML 12.4% CML 47%	Risk at 7 years AML 12.3% CML 16%	Comparison TBI versus Bu/Cy – increased risk for CML patients with TBI

TBI, total-body irradiation; sTBI, single-dose TBI; fTBI, fractionated TBI; BuCy, conditioning with busulfan/cyclophosphamide; Gy, gray.

axis. Today, cataract surgery is a low-risk procedure and improves visual acuity in 95% of eyes which have no other pathology. Results of surgical repair in transplanted patients are not yet available.

Keratoconjunctivitis sicca syndrome is usually part of a more general syndrome with xerostomia, vaginitis and dryness of the skin. All these manifestations are closely related to c-GvHD which may lead in its most extensive forms to a Sjögren-like syndrome. Ocular manifestations include reduced tear flow, keratoconjunctivitis sicca, sterile conjunctivitis, corneal epithelial defects, and corneal ulceration. The incidence of late-onset keratoconjunctivitis sicca syndrome may reach 20% 15 years after SCT , but reaches nearly 40% in patient with c-GvHD, compared to less than 10% in those without GvHD.[13] Risk factors for late-onset keratoconjunctivitis include c-GvHD, female sex, age >20 years, single-dose TBI, and the use of methotrexate for GvHD prophylaxis. Treatment is based on the management of c-GvHD with repeated use of topical lubricants. Topical corticosteroids may improve symptoms but can cause sight-threatening complications if used inappropriately when herpes simplex virus or bacterial keratitis are present. Topical ciclosporin A or retinoic acid may also be used.

Pulmonary late effects

Significant late toxicity involving both the airways and lung parenchyma affects 15–40% of patients after SCT. Most studies have been performed on adult patients and results are still conflicting due to varying selection and evaluation criteria, limited sample size, and short follow-up. Moreover, clinical syndromes are not well defined or definable because of overlapping mechanisms and/or because they represent a continuum rather than a distinct disorder. Sensitivity to cytotoxic agents and irradiation, infections, and immune-mediated lung injury associated with GvHD are the most prominent factors which contribute to late respiratory complications. Impaired growth of both lungs and chest can be additional factors in children.

Restrictive lung disease

Restrictive lung disease is frequently observed 3–6 months after SCT in patients conditioned with TBI and/or receiving allogeneic SCT, but in most cases it is not symptomatic. Restrictive disease is often stable and may recover, partially or completely, within 2 years. However, some patients do develop severe late restrictive defects and may eventually die from respiratory failure (reviewed in reference 3).

Chronic obstructive lung disease

Chronic obstructive pulmonary disease with reduced FEV_1/FVC and FEV_1 can be detected in up to 20% of long-term survivors after SCT.[14] Its pathogenesis is not yet well understood. It has been mainly associated with c-GvHD, but other potential risk factors including TBI, hypogammaglobulinemia, GvHD prophylaxis with methotrexate, and infections have been described.[15] While direct immune-mediated damage by donor T-lymphocytes and cytokines is classically the main mechanism, airflow obstruction can also be due to indirect consequences of c-GvHD, for example aspiration secondary to esophageal GvHD, sicca syndrome, abnormal mucociliary transport, and recurrent infections. Mortality is high among these patients, particularly in those with an earlier onset and rapid decline of FEV_1. Symptoms consist of non-productive cough, wheezing and dyspnea; chest radiography is normal in most cases. High-resolution computed tomography (CT) scanning may reveal non-specific abnormalities. Symptomatic relief can be obtained in some patients with bronchodilators; however, in most cases obstructive abnormalities are not improved by this treatment. Patients with low IgG and IgA levels should receive immunoglobulin to prevent infections, which may further damage the airways. Immunosuppressive therapy may be of benefit but typically, improvements occur in less than 50% of cases, probably because damage has already become irreversible or because other pathogenetic factors persist. Asymptomatic patients with abnormal pulmonary function tests (PFT) should be closely monitored for the development of respiratory symptoms; early recognition of airflow obstruction allows the initiation of treatment at a potentially reversible stage (reviewed in reference 3).

Obliterative bronchiolitis (OB), the best characterized obstructive syndrome, has been reported in 2–14% of allogeneic SCT recipients and carries a mortality rate of 50%.[3,15,16] OB is strongly associated with c-GvHD and low levels of immunoglobulin. GvHD is probably responsible for the initial epithelial injury to small airways, with further damage caused by repeated infections. Initial symptoms often resemble those of recurrent upper respiratory tract infections, and then persistent cough, wheezing, inspiratory rales and dyspnea appear. PFT gradually deteriorate, with severe and non-reversible obstructive abnormalities. Chest radiographs and CT scanning may reveal hyperinflation with or without infiltrates and vascular attenuation. However, radiologic findings do not correlate with lung function changes, probably because of the patchy nature of the disease. Bronchoscopy with transbronchial biopsy can help to rule out infection and may reveal obliteration of bronchioles with granulation tissue, mononuclear cell infiltration or fibrosis.

It is not clear to what extent combined immunosuppressive treatment can be effective in the treatment of this disease, which typically does not respond to treatment with steroids. Azathioprine and mycophenolate may lead to improvement in symptoms in some cases. Prophylaxis and prompt treatment of infections are the most important elements of clinical management and may help to alter the clinical course of a disease whose pace can vary from slow progression to rapidly fatal respiratory failure. Single or double lung transplantation has been suggested for patients with advanced disease, although the transplanted lung may also be a target for immune-mediated damage.

Late liver complications

Late liver complications may be difficult to assess in cancer survivors, because patients are often asymptomatic. Several causes of liver dysfunction may co-exist, and the pattern of viral serology may be atypical. Hepatitis B (HBV) or C (HCV) infections play a central role in late survivors.[17] The hepatitis may be asymptomatic, progress to fulminant hepatitis or evolve to chronic active hepatitis and cirrhosis. Before the systematic screening of blood products commenced in 1990, the rate of post-transfusion hepatitis exceeded 20%, although even for cancer patients treated since 1990 the prevalence of HBV+ and HCV+ transplanted recipients is 3.1% and 6%, respectively. Long-term studies of cancer survivors usually show a chronic pattern of liver disease with a mild course. In some patients, discontinuation of chemotherapy favors spontaneous arrest of virus replication. However, in patients with a follow-up of more than 10 years, a significant number are at risk of such adverse outcomes as impaired quality of life, liver cirrhosis, and liver carcinoma.[18,19]

Transplanted patients infected with HBV usually exhibit mild liver disease on long-term follow-up, and progression to cirrhosis has not been reported to date. Chronic hepatitis C is often asymptomatic, with fluctuating transaminase levels for many years after SCT. However, in HCV+ long-term survivors, cirrhosis is a common late complication. Even asymptomatic patients with persistently normal alanine aminotransferase levels may eventually progress to cirrhosis; the cumulative incidence of cirrhosis after allogeneic HSCT is 11% and 24% at 15 and 20 years post transplant, respectively. The risk of cirrhosis in transplant recipients is significantly higher, and median time to diagnosis is significantly shorter compared to a control population.[20] An increased risk of cirrhosis appears in long-term survivors after more than 10 years of follow-up. The role of possible risk factors for fibrosis, such as iron overload, viral genotype or histologic pattern, has not yet been elucidated.

Iron overload in cancer patients is essentially related to multiple transfusions and is therefore most commonly found in long-term survivors of acute leukemia or after SCT.[21] In addition to transfusion, prolonged dyserythropoiesis and increased iron absorption contribute to accumulation of iron.[22] These patients may present with hepatic dysfunction due to iron overload. Therapeutic phlebotomy can reduce iron overload, and normalize ferritin and liver function tests. After SCT, up to 88% of long-term survivors have iron overload with high ferritin levels and a high liver iron content. A clear correlation exists between iron overload and persistent hepatic dysfunction. However, the clinical consequences of iron overload and therapeutic

iron depletion in transplant recipients have not been extensively evaluated. In heavily transfused patients, such as those with thalassemia, iron accumulation may contribute to the development of liver fibrosis, cirrhosis and liver carcinoma.[23] A similar evolution can be expected decades after SCT in healthy long-term survivors with iron overload.

Thus, in long-term survivors liver function should be monitored yearly. Patients with known HBV or HCV infection should be monitored for HBs and viral load by polymerase chain reaction (PCR). Liver biopsy and determination of alpha-fetoprotein level should be considered in patients with chronic hepatitis C infection, to determine the extent of cirrhosis and detect hepatocellular carcinoma. Long-term results of treatment with ribavirin and/or interferon to prevent cirrhosis are not available.[24] In long-term survivors at risk of iron overload, serum ferritin and transferrin saturation should be monitored. Patients should be counseled to avoid excessive iron intake, and alcohol. Those with a documented liver iron content of greater than 7 mg/g dry weight should be treated with phlebotomy and/or chelation therapy. The use of erythropoietin may facilitate phlebotomy in patients with a low hemoglobin level.

Late complications of bones and joints

Avascular necrosis of bone (AVN)

The published incidence of AVN varies from 4% to over 10% in the largest series.[25–28] The mean time from transplant to AVN is 18 months (range 4–132 months), and pain is usually the first sign. Early diagnosis can rarely be made using standard radiography alone and magnetic resonance imaging is the investigation of choice. The hip is the affected site in over 80% of cases, with bilateral involvement occurring in more than 60% of patients. Other locations described include the knee (10% of patients with AVN), wrist and ankle. Symptomatic relief of pain and orthopedic measures to decrease pressure on the affected joints are of value, but most adult patients with advanced damage require surgery. The probability of total hip replacement following a diagnosis of AVN is approximately 80% at 5 years.[28] While short-term results of joint surgery are excellent in the majority (>85%) of cases, it is clear that long-term follow-up of the prostheses is needed in young patients who have a long life expectancy. Studies evaluating risk factors for AVN have clearly identified steroids (both total dose and duration) as the strongest risk factor.[25,29,30,] Thus, unnecessary long-term low-dose steroids for non-active chronic GvHD should be avoided. The second major risk factor for AVN is TBI, the highest risks being associated with single doses of 10 Gy or higher, or >12 Gy in fractionated doses.

Osteoporosis

Hematopoietic SCT (HSCT) can induce bone loss and osteoporosis via the toxic effects of TBI, chemotherapy, and hypogonadism (see reviews in references 31, 32). Osteopenia and osteoporosis are both characterized by a reduced bone mass and increased susceptibility to bone fracture.[33] These conditions are further distinguished by the degree of reduction in bone mass and can be quantified on dual-photon densitometry. The cumulative dose and number of days of glucocorticoid therapy and the number of days of ciclosporin or tacrolimus therapy showed significant associations with loss of bone density.[12,33,34] Non-traumatic fractures occurred in 10% of patients. Using WHO criteria, nearly 50% of patients have a low bone density, a third have osteopenia and roughly 10% have osteoporosis 12–18 months post transplant. Preventive measures for osteoporosis must include sex hormone replacement in patients with gonadal failure. The efficacy of new treatments for osteoporosis in long-term survivors of SCT requires evaluation.

Dental late effects

Both TBI-based regimens and those without irradiation can result in severe damage to the enamel organ and developing teeth. These defects may be prolonged or permanent. After TBI in children, underdevelopment of the mandible and anomalies in the mandibular joint may also occur. In children, long-term clinical and radiologic follow-up reveals hypoplasia and microdontia of the crowns of erupted permanent teeth and thinning and tapering of the roots of erupted permanent molars or incisors. Caries are found more frequently in transplanted patients compared to age-matched healthy children. The defects in dental elements post SCT may occur at any age of tooth development, and only the severity seems to depend on age at SCT.

Recommendations to minimize this adverse effect aim to preserve the enamel layer and prevent, by active oral hygiene, dental plaque, periodontal and oral mucosal infections and xerostomia, all of which contribute to the development of caries. Specialist dental consultation before SCT and yearly post transplant should be requested to register any specific dental problems, to provide treatment, and to give instruction on oral and dental care. In the long term, three key elements to reduce dental complications are brushing teeth, application of fluoride and the use of antiseptic mouth washes. Brushing teeth should be done twice daily, with a soft brush and fluorinated toothpaste.

Endocrine function after SCT

Thyroid dysfunction

After allogeneic SCT, 7–15% of patients develop subclinical hypothyroidism.[35,36] The incidence of hypothyroidism requiring L-thyroxine replacement therapy is highly variable and depends on the type of pretransplant conditioning therapy given. Single-dose TBI has a higher incidence than do fractionated TBI and conditioning without irradiation. Onset of thyroid organ dysfunction varies. It usually starts approximately 5 years after irradiation, although its appearance has been observed as late as 20 years after cancer treatment. Thus, patients treated with TBI should be evaluated for thyroid function throughout their remaining life. Treatment with L-thyroxine is indicated in all cases of frank hypothyroidism (elevated thyroid-stimulating hormone (TSH) with low free T4 blood levels). Thyroid hormone levels should be measured after commencement of replacement therapy, and dosage should be tailored thereafter to the individual patient and adjusted accordingly. Older patients should have an electrocardiogram prior to commencing treatment to exclude associated ischemic heart disease and/or arrhythmias.

Growth

Linear growth is an intricate process that may be influenced by several factors including genetic (i.e. mid-parental height), nutritional, hormonal and psychologic. Children who undergo SCT form a heterogeneous group due to the different treatment protocols employed. In addition, post-transplant factors such as GvHD and its treatment, especially the use of long-term steroids, may induce growth failure in childhood.

Final height achievement has been reported in some studies.[37–40] Impaired growth has been described in patients who underwent SCT during childhood. Growth deficiency is more pronounced in children transplanted at a younger age (less than 10 years) and in those who have received irradiation. In contrast, children who are conditioned with non-TBI regimens, such as cyclophosphamide or busulfan-cyclophosphamide, usually grow normally.[40] Patients who have been exposed to cranial radiotherapy (CRT) prior to conditioning with TBI show a greater retardation in growth. The role of growth hormone (GH) deficiency as a cause of growth failure and its substitution in children after SCT is still controversial; the reduced growth observed in irradiated patients may be explained by the direct effect of irradiation on the gonads, the thyroid gland, and/or the bone epiphyses.

Puberty and gonadal failure

Gonadal failure (both testicular and ovarian) is a common long-term consequence of the chemotherapy given prior to SCT, and of the pretransplant conditioning. The major cause of gonadal damage leading to hypergonadotropic hypogonadism is irradiation. Similar damage can also be caused by busulfan.

Male gonadal function

Radiation to the testes is known to result in germinal loss, with decreases in testicular volume and sperm production and increases in follicle-stimulating hormone (FSH). Radiation therapy may also be toxic to Leydig cells, although at doses higher than those which are toxic to germ (Sertoli) cells. Alkylating agents decrease spermatogenesis in a dose-dependent manner.[41,42] Gonadal damage following cumulative doses of cyclophosphamide lower than 200 mg/kg, as used in SCT, has been shown to be reversible in up to 70% of patients after therapy-free intervals of several years. In contrast to their prominent effects on germ cell epithelium, chemotherapy effects are less striking on slowly dividing Leydig cells and may be age related. Following exposure to alkylating agents in prepubertal boys, normal pubertal progression and normal adult levels of testosterone are the rule.

Screening for problems related to male gonadal function in survivors includes an annual age-appropriate history with specific attention to problems with libido, impotence or fertility and examination for gynecomastia, Tanner staging of body hair, and assessment of penile and testicular size. Hormonal evaluation, including at least a single measurement of serum luteinizing hormone (LH), FSH and testosterone levels, is recommended as a baseline. At age 14 years patients should be counseled for pretransplant sperm cryopreservation whenever possible, and may benefit from semen analysis post transplant; honest and sensitive discussions of fertility should be part of their follow-up visit. When abnormalities in testicular function are detected, close co-operation with an endocrinologist is essential in planning hormone replacement therapy or in monitoring patients for spontaneous recovery. When no abnormalities are noted on history and physical examination but sexual maturity has not been completely attained, these studies should be repeated every 1–2 years. Conversely, in light of the potential for recovery of spermatogenesis and interpatient variations in gonadal toxicity, reminders about contraception should be given.

Female gonadal function

In contrast to the process in male survivors, germ cell failure and loss of ovarian endocrine function occur concomitantly in females. Radiation effects are both age and dose dependent. In women older than 40 years at the time of treatment, irreversible ovarian failure is an almost universal result of 4–7 Gy of conventionally fractionated radiation delivered to both ovaries. In contrast, prepubertal ovaries are relatively radioresistant. Increasing age at the time of TBI has been found to predict ovarian failure. Premature menopause is very frequent in the setting of HSCT.

Ovarian failure has been associated with chemotherapy, especially the alkylating agents, and the gonadotoxicity is dose and age dependent.[37,43] Following myeloablative doses of alkylating agents such as busulfan and cyclophosphamide, permanent ovarian failure can be expected at all ages. Diagnostic evaluation of ovarian dysfunction relies on history (primary or secondary amenorrhea, menstrual irregularity, and pregnancies or difficulties becoming pregnant), and Tanner staging of breast and genital development. Serum gonadotropin (FSH, LH) and estradiol levels should be obtained in children as a baseline at age 13 years and systematically in adults. In the absence of clinical evidence of puberty (menarche, development of secondary sexual characteristics), in order to assess the need for hormone therapy to induce puberty, these tests are obviously mandatory. In addition, because young women who have received gonadotoxic therapy and have progressed through puberty may experience early onset of menopause, they should also undergo assessment of gonadotropin and estradiol levels if there are clinical symptoms of estrogen deficiency (irregular menses, amenorrhea, hot flashes and vaginal dryness). Survivors with concerns regarding fertility are urged to seek a consultation with a reproductive endocrinologist.

Fertility following stem cell transplantation

Despite the potential gonadotoxicity of pretransplant conditioning, gonadal recovery and pregnancies following SCT are well described. The precise incidence of fertility following SCT is hard to establish. The Bone Marrow Transplant Survivor Study used a mailed survey to describe the magnitude of compromise in reproductive function and investigate pregnancy outcomes in 619 women and partners of men treated with autologous (n = 241) or allogeneic (n = 378) hematopoietic cell transplantation (HCT) between 21 and 45 years of age, and surviving 2 or more years. Median age at HCT was 33.3 years and median time since HCT 7.7 years. Thirty-four patients reported 54 pregnancies after HCT (26 males, 40 pregnancies; eight females, 14 pregnancies), of which 46 resulted in live births. Factors associated with reporting no conception included older age at HCT (≥30 years: odds ratio (OR) = 4.8), female sex (OR = 3.0), and TBI (OR = 3.3). Prevalence of conception and pregnancy outcomes in HCT survivors were compared to those of 301 nearest-age siblings. Although the risk for not reporting a conception was significantly increased among HCT survivors (OR = 36), survivors were not significantly more likely than siblings to report miscarriage or stillbirth (OR = 0.7).[44]

Data from the EBMT Late Effects Working Party (LEWP) relating to incidence of pregnancy in patients transplanted prior to 1994 who survived for a minimum of 2 years indicated that the overall incidence of pregnancy is low (<2%) except for patients transplanted for severe aplastic anemia (SAA), and this is in accordance with the available literature.[45] Such data are limited in their ability to accurately predict the likely return of fertility post SCT, however, because many patients do not wish to become parents following the diagnosis of a potentially life-threatening illness, may have already completed their family before transplantation or may have partners beyond the normal biologic age of conception.

Fertility following SCT for non-malignant disease

Return of gonadal function following cyclophosphamide conditioning for SAA was noted in 56 of 103 adult female survivors in Seattle (as indicated by return of menstruation and normal gonadotropin and estradiol levels); 28 (27%) women subsequently conceived.[46] Of 109 adult male survivors in the same study, 61% had return of sperm production and 28 (26%) subsequently fathered children. Previous data from this and from other centers indicate that gonadal recovery is usual in women less than age 25 at the time of transplant but sharply decreases thereafter.

Fertility following SCT for malignant disease

The majority of patients who have received TBI experience gonadal failure. Recovery of gonadal function occurs in 10–14% of the women and the incidence of pregnancy is less than 3%.[45,46] In men, recovery of gonadal function has been reported in less than 20% of patients and use of increasing doses of TBI may be associated with considerably lower recovery. Parenting a child following TBI is a rare event in men.

Busulfan and cyclophosphamide (Bu/Cy) are also associated with a high incidence of gonadal failure in women, and there have been no pregnancies reported using Bu/Cy for patients with leukemia.[45,46] In men, this conditioning appears to be associated with return of gonadal function in approximately 17% of cases, which is similar to the recovery after TBI conditioning.

Pretransplant counseling and treatment options

Ideally, the pretransplant counseling process should include data on the incidence of gonadal failure and should assess the relevance of this to the patient. If the patient is of reproductive age and wishes to parent a child following SCT, it may be possible to alter the choice of conditioning protocol without compromising other factors such as survival. Clearly this is not always an option and discussion of management approaches for gonadal failure is thus essential. This should include explanation of assisted conception techniques and, in women, management of premature menopause.

In women with no residual ovarian function following SCT, implantation of embryos cryopreserved prior to SCT is currently the only option for parenting their own genetic child. This, however, requires that prior to SCT the underlying disease can tolerate a minimum 4–6 weeks delay in treatment for controlled stimulation of the ovary and egg collection. It also requires that the patient has a committed partner to provide sperm. In situations where treatment cannot be delayed or there is no committed partner, consideration can be given to freezing ovarian tissue prior to SCT. Centers in some countries provide this service for young women, but patients must be aware that currently this is a research rather than clinical tool and that to date there have been no successful pregnancies in human subjects using this methodology. Although the incidence of assisted conception increases annually there are few published reports of pregnancy outcome following assisted conception in SCT recipients

Sperm cryopreserved prior to SCT may be used post SCT for artificial insemination, in vitro fertilization (IVF) and embryo transfer, or for in vitro injection into the cytoplasm of the oocyte (ICSI). Semen collection should ideally occur at diagnosis before chemotherapy has been given. Concurrent administration of chemotherapy is not an absolute contraindication to storage, but the patient must be informed of potential risks.

Post-transplant management should routinely include symptomatic and biochemical monitoring of gonadal function. While the patient should be prepared for infertility, the possible need for contraception soon after SCT must also be emphasized, particularly in women who resume menstruation or in patients who do not wish to become parents. Patients have conceived within 6 months of SCT and an unexpected pregnancy may result in requests for termination.

Distressing vasomotor symptoms may commence acutely post SCT but this may be prevented by initiating hormone replacement therapy (HRT). Alternatively, HRT can be initiated at the onset of symptoms or when gonadotropin levels indicate ovarian failure. HRT does not suppress ovulation and will not, therefore, prevent recovery of gonadal function or pregnancy. It is therefore important to withdraw HRT intermittently and to assess gonadotropin levels. If there are signs of gonadal recovery, patients may benefit from contraceptive advice. Alternatively, since recovery in women is likely to be followed by a premature menopause, this period may be perceived by the patients as a window of opportunity to conceive naturally. Only regular follow-up will identify this point in time.

Quality of life and neuropsychologic function

The psychosocial effect of cancer has been well studied during the past few years. Psychosocial and quality-of-life late effects include aspects relating to adaptation of the patient to the personal consequences of cancer diagnosis and adjustment to the social consequences of the disease. People who have cancer experience the effect of the disease in many different ways and at different times. In turn, these issues exert an effect on perceived quality of life of the patient. At any age, disruption of function, even when temporary, becomes disturbing if it involves valued life activities. Few studies on quality of life with a specific questionnaire on long- term cancer survivors have been published. These questionnaires differ from the cancer-specific quality of life assessments designed for use during therapy, which include treatment-specific concerns such as nausea and vomiting that are not relevant in a healthy long-term survivor population. On the other hand, questionnaires developed for a healthy population may omit symptoms and concerns that continue to be important to long-term cancer survivors.

Many survivors continue to experience negative effects of cancer and treatment on their daily lives, resulting in a decreased quality of life well beyond completion of therapy. However, it is important to assess positive as well as negative psychosocial effects of cancer and its treatment. Positive psychologic effects of cancer and its treatment include feelings of being grateful and fortunate to be alive, an enhanced appreciation of life, and increased self-esteem. Documented negative psychosocial effects include concerns about the future, heightened sense of vulnerability, a sense of loss for what might have been (e.g. loss of fertility) and increased health worries or hypervigilance.

Large HSCT survivor studies conclude that less than half of survivors report normal functional status in most domains. Fatigue and sleep disturbances are common for both autologous and allogeneic patients. Many specific physical symptoms and limitations persist, particularly for allogeneic recipients. Continued improvement over time, with readaptation and return to some form of normalcy, has been observed. Within the first 3 years after HSCT, quality of life is significantly worse compared to the general population, while long-term survivors of more than 3 years declare improvement particularly in social functioning, mental health and vitality.

At a minimum, screening for depression is recommended. Clinical assessment for psychologic symptoms should be maintained annually, with mental health professional counseling for those with recognized deficits. Attention should also be given to the partner of the patient, who often reports loneliness, and the patient's children, who may suffer from separation from one of the parents.

Secondary malignancies

Secondary malignancies are a known complication of conventional chemotherapy and radiation treatment for patients with a variety of primary cancers and are now being increasingly recognized as a complication among HCT recipients. The magnitude of risk of secondary malignancies after HCT has ranged from fourfold to 11-fold that of the general population. The estimated actuarial incidence is reported to be 3.5% at 10 years, increasing to 12.8% at 15 years among recipients of allogeneic HCT.[1,2,47–50]

Risk factors for the development of secondary malignancies include exposure to chemotherapy and radiation prior to transplant, use of TBI and high-dose chemotherapy for myeloablation, infection with viruses such as Epstein–Barr virus (EBV) and HBV and HCV, immunodeficiency after transplant, aggravated by the use of immunosuppressive drugs for prophylaxis and treatment of graft-versus-host disease, including monoclonal and polyclonal antibodies, HLA non-identity,

and T-cell depletion, type of transplant (autologous versus allogeneic), type of hematopoietic stem cell (HSC), and the primary malignancy. However, global assessment of risk factors for all secondary malignancies in aggregate is somewhat artificial because of the heterogeneous nature of secondary malignancies, their differing clinicopathologic features, distinct pathogeneses, and hence very distinct risk factors associated with their development (reviewed in references[1,2]).

It has become conventional practice to classify secondary malignancies after HCT into three distinct groups:
• myelodysplasia and acute myeloid leukemia
• lymphoma, including lymphoproliferative disorders
• solid tumors.
Leukemia and lymphomas develop relatively early in the post-transplant period. On the other hand, solid cancers have a longer latency period, and are being increasingly described because of improved survival after HCT and longer follow-up.

Myelodysplasia and acute myeloid leukemia after autologous SCT

Autologous HCT has become the treatment of choice for patients with Hodgkin's disease (HD) and non-Hodgkin's lymphoma (NHL) who have a suboptimal response to initial therapy, those with refractory or relapsed disease or for those at high risk of relapse after conventional therapy. Autologous HCT is also being increasingly used in specific clinical situations among patients with multiple myeloma, breast cancer and advanced-stage germ cell tumors.

With improvement in survival following autologous SCT, therapy-related myelodysplasias (t-MDS) and therapy-related acute myeloid leukemias (t-AML) are emerging as serious long-term complications. The cumulative probability of t-MDS/t-AML reported in the literature has ranged from 1.1% at 20 months to 24.3% at 43 months after autologous transplant.[51–56] The median time to development of t-MDS/t-AML is 12–24 months after transplant (range, 4 months to 6 years). t-MDS/t-AML have also been observed after conventional chemotherapy, and to a lesser extent radiotherapy, for HD and NHL. The incidence of t-MDS/t-AML following conventional chemotherapy or radiation therapy ranges from 0.8% at 20 years to 6.3% at 30 years. The median time to development of t-MDS/t-AML has been reported to be 3–5 years, with the risk decreasing markedly after the first decade. It therefore appears that the magnitude of risk of t-MDS/t-AML is higher after HCT when compared to conventional chemotherapy and radiation therapy. In addition, the time to development of t-MDS/t-AML is shorter after HCT, as compared to that after conventional chemoradiotherapy.

Factors associated with an increased risk of t-MDS/t-AML include host factors such as older age at transplant, pretransplantation therapy with alkylating agents, topoisomerase II inhibitors and radiation therapy, method of stem cell mobilization (use of peripheral blood stem cells, priming with etoposide for stem cell mobilization) and transplant conditioning with TBI. Some other factors reported recently include a lower number of CD34+ cells infused at transplant, and a history of multiple transplants. Therefore, t-MDS/t-AML appears to be related to pretransplant chemotherapy and radiotherapy, transplant-related factors such as the stem cell priming and transplant conditioning regimens, or the cumulative effect of all these exposures.

The significant impact of primary chemotherapy and radiotherapy on the risk of t-MDS and t-AML after transplantation points toward an origin of events prior to transplant. Moreover, the nature of the pretransplant cytotoxic exposure (alkylating agent versus topoisomerase II inhibitor) has a significant impact on the type of t-MDS/t-AML which evolves post transplant, reinforcing this observation. A role for pretransplant exposures is supported by the observation that specific cytogenetic abnormalities are observed in the pretransplant marrow or peripheral blood stem cell product among patients who develop t-MDS/t-AML after transplant. Several studies support a role for genetic abnormalities induced by prior cytotoxic chemotherapy in the etiology of t-MDS/AML. However, prospective studies of larger groups of patients are warranted to determine the significance of these observations.

The use of TBI in the conditioning regimen has been reported to be associated with an increased risk of t-MDS/t-AML after autologous HCT, although other studies fail to confirm this association. An association of TBI with increased risk for t-MDS/t-AML raises the possibility that the disease may arise from residual stem cells that persist in the patient despite myeloablative treatment, rather than from reinfused stem cells, although it is also possible that TBI-induced alteration in the hematopoietic microenvironment may contribute to the development of t-MDS/t-AML. Therefore, it is unclear whether t-MDS/t-AML arises from the infused marrow (or peripheral blood) stem cells, from residual cells in the patient or as a result of a damaged microenvironment.[51-56]

A higher risk of t-MDS/t-AML has been demonstrated among recipients of CD34-enriched cells isolated from peripheral blood after chemotherapy priming and growth factors, as compared to autologous transplant using CD34+ cells from the bone marrow without pretreatment. Potential explanations offered for this observation include harvesting of hematopoietic precursor cells damaged by chemotherapy at a time before they have completed DNA repair, or an over-representation of damaged cells in the mobilized product. Supporting this hypothesis is the study by Krishnan et al, demonstrating an increased risk of t-AML with 11q23 abnormalities among patients with HD and NHL mobilized with high doses of etoposide for collection of stem cells prior to autologous HCT.[54]

Friedberg et al reported an increased risk of t-MDS among patients who received a significantly smaller number of cells reinfused per kilogram of body weight.[57] In the setting of low stem cell numbers, reconstitution of bone marrow clearly represents a great proliferative stress, which may increase susceptibility to irreversible DNA damage associated with t-MDS. These findings are corroborated by in vitro data suggesting that an increased proliferative stress is placed upon committed progenitors at the expense of the primitive progenitors.

It therefore seems that, in addition to the important role of pretransplant exposure to cytotoxic agents, the transplant process itself may potentiate the risk of t-MDS/t-AML through several mechanisms, including stem cell mobilization, collection and storage, chemotherapy and radiation used for myeloablation, and the stress on hematopoietic precursors of engraftment and hematopoietic regeneration.[58-60]

The prognosis of t-MDS after autologous SCT is uniformly poor, with a median survival of 6 months. Because of the poor response to conventional chemotherapy, allogeneic transplantation has been attempted, with an actuarial survival ranging from 0% to 24% reported at 3 years. Witherspoon et al reviewed data from patients transplanted for t-MDS/t-AML with the aim of identifying patient characteristics that are associated with a better long-term disease-free survival after an allogeneic transplant.[61] The probability of survival after transplantation for all patients was 13%. By stage of disease this was 33% for refractory anemia, 20% for refractory anemia with excess blasts, and 8% for refractory anemia with excess blasts in transformation or acute leukemia. The overall probability of non-relapse mortality was 78%, divided equally among infection or organ failure-related cause of death. Patients with t-AML tended to have lower disease-free survival (8.3%) and a higher relapse rate (43%) than did patients whose leukemia was not therapy related. There was no statistically significant difference in outcome in the results of these previously untreated patients compared to 20 patients (12 therapy related, eight myelodys-plasia-related) transplanted with chemotherapy-sensitive disease after induction chemotherapy.

In a subsequent report, results of related or unrelated hematopoietic stem-cell transplants in 111 patients with treatment-related leukemia or myelodysplasia performed consecutively at the Fred Hutchinson Cancer Research Center between December 1971 and June 1998 were reviewed.[62] The 5-year disease-free survival was 8% for TBI, 19% for Bu/Cy, and 30% for Bu/Cy-t (targeted dose Bu/Cy) conditioning regimens. The 5-year cumulative incidence of relapse was 40% for secondary AML, 40% for refractory anemia with excess of blasts in transformation (RAEB-T), 26% for refractory anemia with excess of blasts (RAEB), and 0% for refractory anemia (RA) or refractory anemia with ringed sideroblasts (RARS). The 5-year cumulative incidence of non-relapse mortality after TBI was 58%; after Bu/Cy, 52%; and after Bu/Cy-t, 42%.

Yakoub-Agha et al analyzed the predictors of survival, relapse and treatment-related mortality among 70 patients with t-MDS/AML undergoing allogeneic HCT. Older age (greater than 37 years), male sex, positive recipient CMV serology, absence of complete remission (CR) at HCT and intensive conditioning schedules were independently associated with poor outcome.[63] These studies indicate that in spite of the significant treatment-related mortality, disease-free survival was better when transplantation was undertaken earlier in the evolution of the disease because it resulted in a lower relapse rate.

Treatment of t-MDS/t-AML should include consideration of the likelihood of success of inducing remission with chemotherapy and, depending on availability of an appropriate donor, the likelihood of a successful outcome with an allogeneic transplant. The few patients with favorable cytogenetics may have a better chance of attaining remission with chemotherapy. However, patients with unfavorable cytogenetics without a high peripheral blast count may be considered for immediate transplant. It is important to follow patients at risk of developing t-MDS closely to identify any myelodysplasia early. Prompt transplantation should be considered after diagnosing secondary AML or high-risk myelodysplasia, particularly in patients with low peripheral blood blast cell counts. Innovative transplant strategies are needed to reduce the high risks of relapse and non-relapse mortality seen in this patient population. Since the poor outcomes of allogeneic transplant for t-MDS/t-AML are related in part to the high risk of treatment-related mortality, it is appropriate to consider reduced-intensity conditioning approaches, since preliminary reports suggest that these are feasible and may result in improved outcomes in patients who have had a previous autologous HCT, compared to a conventional allogeneic transplant.

Lymphomas

Lymphoproliferative disorders are the most common secondary malignancy in the *first year* after allogeneic HCT. Most of these cases are related to compromised immune function and EBV infection. The large majority of the post-transplant lymphoproliferative disorders (PTLD) have a B-cell origin, although some T-cell PTLD have been described.[64,65] These malignancies are thus excluded from this chapter on late effects and have been extensively reviewed elsewhere.

Several cases of late-occurring lymphoma have been reported. It is believed that these represent an entity that is distinct from the early-occurring B-cell PTLD.[66-70] In a large study of 18,000 HCT recipients, the only risk factor associated with the development of the late-occurring lymphoma was extensive chronic graft-versus-host disease.[66]

Hodgkin's disease developing among SCT recipients has also been described. SCT recipients followed as part of a large cohort were at a sixfold increased risk of developing HD when compared with the general population.[71] Most of the reported cases were of the mixed cellularity subtype, and most of the cases contained the EBV genome.

These cases differed from the EBV-associated PTLD by the absence of risk factors commonly associated with EBV-associated PTLD, by a later onset (>2.5 years), and relatively good prognosis. The increased incidence of HD among SCT recipients can possibly be explained by exposure to EBV and overstimulation of cell-mediated immunity.

Solid tumors

Solid tumors have been described after syngeneic, allogeneic and autologous HSCT. The magnitude of the increased risk of solid tumors has ranged from 2.1-fold to 2.7-fold when compared to an age-and sex-matched general population.[72,73] The risk increases with lengthening follow-up and among those who have survived 10 or more years after transplantation, this was reported to be 8.3 times as high as expected in the general population. Types of solid tumors reported in excess among HCT recipients when compared to the general population are those typically associated with exposure to radiation therapy. They include melanoma, cancers of the oral cavity and salivary glands, brain, liver, uterine cervix, thyroid, breast, bone and connective tissue.

Although most studies have focused on allogeneic transplant recipients, there is emerging evidence for an increased incidence of new solid malignancies among patients conditioned with TBI and receiving autologous transplants. There is therefore a need to follow this cohort of patients long term in order to ascertain the risk of new solid malignancies with precision. Sites significantly at increased risk of second cancers include: oral cavity, salivary glands, liver, skin, brain, thyroid, breast, bone and connective tissues.[48,49,73–77]

Thus, the risk of solid tumors increases sharply over time, and has been reported to be higher among children who have undergone SCT at less than 10 years of age.[78] TBI is associated with an increased risk of solid tumors. The risk of solid tumors rises with the dose of radiation, with three to four times the risk at the highest dose levels, as compared to those who have not received radiation therapy.

Pathogenesis of solid tumors after HCT

Little is known about the pathogenesis of solid tumors. An interaction between cytotoxic therapy, genetic predisposition, viral infection, and graft-versus-host disease with the consequent antigenic stimulation and use of immunosuppressive therapy, all seem to play a role in the development of new solid tumors.[12,79]

Radiogenic cancers generally have a long latent period, and the risk of such cancers is frequently high among patients undergoing irradiation at a young age. Both thyroid cancer and brain tumors have been reported after exposure to radiation to the craniospinal axis and the neck used as part of the conventional therapy for childhood acute lymphoblastic leukemia, HD and other primary brain tumors. Similarly, osteogenic sarcoma and other connective tissue tumors have been reported as secondary malignancies developing among patients receiving radiation therapy as part of conventional therapy for other primary malignancies such as retinoblastoma, and other bone tumors. Studies indicate the presence of a strong dose–response relationship for radiation exposure, in addition to an increased risk with increasing exposure to alkylating agents. The increased risk of thyroid, breast, brain and bone and soft tissue cancers seen after HCT appears to be related to cumulative doses of radiation exposure, both as a result of the pretransplant treatment regimen and the conditioning regimen used for transplant.[74,75,78]

Immunologic alterations may predispose patients to squamous cell carcinoma of the buccal cavity, particularly in view of the association with c-GvHD. Patients transplanted for aplastic anemia have been reported to be at increased risk of solid tumors, predominantly tumors of the buccal cavity and skin. The risk of these tumors was significantly increased after the administration of azathioprine for c-GvHD.[80]

In immune-suppressed patients, oncogenic viruses such as human papillomaviruses may contribute to the development of squamous cell cancers of the skin and buccal mucosa after transplantation. The observation of the excess risk of squamous cell cancers of the buccal cavity and skin in males is unexplained, but may be indicative of an interaction between ionizing radiation, immunodeficiency, and other risk factors more prevalent among men than women.

The increased risk of new solid tumors after HCT is thus likely to be related to the TBI used for pretransplant myeloablation, altered immune function in association with viral infections (HBV, HCV or human papillomavirus), and prior treatment for the primary disease.

Patients with a family history of early-onset cancers have been shown to be at an increased risk of developing a secondary cancer. Genetic predisposition also has a substantial impact on risk of secondary cancers. Studies exploring genetic predisposition and gene-environment interactions have focused thus far on patients exposed to non-transplant conventional therapy for cancer. Future studies are needed in the transplant population to clarify the roles of an interaction between genetic predisposition and myeloablative chemotherapy, TBI and the attendant post-transplant immune suppression in the development of secondary solid tumors.

Treatment strategies for patients developing solid tumors after transplantation are not well defined.[81,82] Concerns regarding limited bone marrow reserve and excessive organ toxicity because of prior therapy preclude the use of intensive approaches. However, some small case series indicate favorable outcomes after an intensive approach, and others note aggressive tumor growth and early relapse after standard therapy. A comprehensive study of a large number of patients with second solid tumors will help determine the nature of these tumors and their outcomes as compared to de novo tumors.

Extending the follow-up of SCT recipients to 20 years after transplantation will help clarify the risks for radiation-associated cancers such as breast, lung, and colon cancers. These epithelial cancers typically develop a median of 15–20 years after exposure to radiation therapy and are now beginning to emerge among cancer survivor populations treated with conventional therapy. These data indicate that SCT survivors face an increasing risk of solid cancers with time from transplantation, thus supporting the need for life-long surveillance. Preventive measures which need to be considered include programs to educate clinicians and survivors about the risk of secondary malignancies, and measures should be taken to decrease the morbidity associated with secondary malignancies, such as adopting healthy lifestyle choices. Other measures include intervention programs for smoking cessation, periodic and aggressive screening for breast, lung, skin, colorectal, prostate, thyroid and cervical cancers, chemoprevention for specific cancers, and avoidance of unnecessary exposure to sunlight, especially among patients who have received radiation. By understanding the risk factors for secondary malignancies and taking measures to avoid them, it may be possible to decrease the incidence of the most devastating consequences of surviving cancer while maintaining the high cure rates in this population.

References

1. Deeg HJ, Socie G. Malignancies after hematopoietic stem cell transplantation: many questions, some answers. Blood 1998;91:1833–1844
2. Ades L, Guardiola P, Socie G. Second malignancies after allogeneic hematopoietic stem cell transplantation: new insight and current problems. Blood Rev 2002;16:135–146
3. Socie G, Salooja N, Cohen A et al. Nonmalignant late effects after allogeneic stem cell transplantation. Blood 2003;101:3373–3385
4. Rizzo JD, Wingard JR, Tichelli A et al. Recommended screening and preventive practices for long-term survivors after hematopoietic cell transplantation: joint recommendations of the European Group for Blood and Marrow Transplantation, the Center for International Blood and Marrow Transplant Research, and the American Society of Blood and Marrow Transplantation. Bone Marrow Transplant 2006;37:249–261
5. Vogelsang GB. How I treat chronic graft-versus-host disease. Blood 2001;97:1196–1201
6. Lee SJ, Vogelsang G, Flowers ME. Chronic graft-versus-host disease. Biol Blood Marrow Transplant 2003;9:215–233

7. CDC, IDSA, ASBMT. Guidelines for preventing opportunistic infections among hematopoietc stem cell transplant recipients, 2000. www.cdc.gov/mmwr/preview/mmwrhtlm, pp. 659–741

8. Bernauer W, Gratwohl A, Keller A, Daicker B. Microvasculopathy in the ocular fundus after bone marrow transplantation. Ann Intern Med. 1991;115:925–930

9. Tichelli A, Gratwohl A, Egger T et al. Cataract formation after bone marrow transplantation. Ann Intern Med 1993;119:1175–1180

10. Deeg HJ, Flournoy N, Sullivan KM et al. Cataracts after total body irradiation and marrow transplantation: a sparing effect of dose fractionation. Int J Radiat Oncol Biol Phys 1984;10:957–964

11. Belkacemi Y, Labopin M, Vernant JP et al. Cataracts after total body irradiation and bone marrow transplantation in patients with acute leukemia in complete remission: a study of the European Group for Blood and Marrow Transplantation. Int J Radiat Oncol Biol Phys 1998;41:659–668

12. Socie G, Clift RA, Blaise D et al. Busulfan plus cyclophosphamide compared with total-body irradiation plus cyclophosphamide before marrow transplantation for myeloid leukemia: long-term follow-up of 4 randomized studies. Blood 2001;98:3569–3574

13. Tichelli A, Duell T, Weiss M et al. Late-onset keratoconjunctivitis sicca syndrome after bone marrow transplantation: incidence and risk factors. European Group for Blood and Marrow Transplantation (EBMT) Working Party on Late Effects. Bone Marrow Transplant 1996;17:1105–1111

14. Clark JG, Crawford SW, Madtes DK, Sullivan KM. Obstructive lung disease after allogeneic marrow transplantation. Clinical presentation and course. Ann Intern Med 1989;111:368–376

15. Freudenberger TD, Madtes DK, Curtis JR et al. Association between acute and chronic graft-versus-host disease and bronchiolitis obliterans organizing pneumonia in recipients of hematopoietic stem cell transplants. Blood 2003;102:3822–3828

16. Santo Tomas LH, Loberiza FR Jr, Klein JP et al. Risk factors for bronchiolitis obliterans in allogeneic hematopoietic stem-cell transplantation for leukemia. Chest 2005;128:153–161

17. Locasciulli A, Testa M, Valsecchi MG et al. The role of hepatitis C and B virus infections as risk factors for severe liver complications following allogeneic BMT: a prospective study by the Infectious Disease Working Party of the European Blood and Marrow Transplantation Group. Transplantation 1999;68:1486–1491

18. Strasser SI, Myerson D, Spurgeon CL et al. Hepatitis C virus infection and bone marrow transplantation: a cohort study with 10-year follow-up. Hepatology 1999;29:1893–1899

19. Strasser SI, Sullivan KM, Myerson D et al. Cirrhosis of the liver in long-term marrow transplant survivors. Blood 1999;93:3259–3266

20. Peffault de Latour R, Levy V, Asselah T et al. Long-term outcome of hepatitis C infection after bone marrow transplantation. Blood 2004;103:1618–1624

21. Strasser SI, Kowdley KV, Sale GE, McDonald GB. Iron overload in bone marrow transplant recipients. Bone Marrow Transplant 1998;22:167–173

22. Mariotti E, Angelucci E, Agostini A et al. Evaluation of cardiac status in iron-loaded thalassaemia patients following bone marrow transplantation: improvement in cardiac function during reduction in body iron burden. Br J Haematol 1998;103:916–921

23. Muretto P, del Fiasco S, Angelucci E et al. Bone marrow transplantation in thalassemia: modifications of hepatic iron overload and associated lesions after long-term engrafting. Liver 1994;14:14–24

24. de Latour RP, Asselah T, Levy V et al. Treatment of chronic hepatitis C virus in allogeneic bone marrow transplant recipients. Bone Marrow Transplant 2005;36:709–713

25. Socie G, Selimi F, Sedel L et al. Avascular necrosis of bone after allogeneic bone marrow transplantation: clinical findings, incidence and risk factors. Br J Haematol 1994;86:624–628

26. Atkinson K, Cohen M, Biggs J. Avascular necrosis of the femoral head secondary to corticosteroid therapy for graft-versus-host disease after marrow transplantation: effective therapy with hip arthroplasty. Bone Marrow Transplant 1987;2:421–426

27. Enright H, Haake R, Weisdorf D. Avascular necrosis of bone: a common serious complication of allogeneic bone marrow transplantation. Am J Med 1990;89:733–738

28. Bizot P, Nizard R, Socie G et al. Femoral head osteonecrosis after bone marrow transplantation. Clin Orthop 1998;357:127–134

29. Fink JC, Leisenring WM, Sullivan KM et al. Avascular necrosis following bone marrow transplantation: a case-control study. Bone 1998;22:67–71

30. Schulte CM, Beelen DW. Avascular osteonecrosis after allogeneic hematopoietic stem-cell transplantation: diagnosis and gender matter. Transplantation 2004;78:1055–1063

31. Weilbaecher KN. Mechanisms of osteoporosis after hematopoietic cell transplantation. Biol Blood Marrow Transplant 2000;6(2A):165–174

32. Schimmer AD, Minden MD, Keating A. Osteoporosis after blood and marrow transplantation: clinical aspects. Biol Blood Marrow Transplant 2000;6(2A):175–181

33. Schulte CM, Beelen DW. Bone loss following hematopoietic stem cell transplantation: a long-term follow-up. Blood 2004;103:3635–3643

34. Stern JM, Sullivan KM, Ott SM et al. Bone density loss after allogeneic hematopoietic stem cell transplantation: a prospective study. Biol Blood Marrow Transplant 2001;7:257–264

35. Sklar CA, Kim TH, Ramsay NK. Thyroid dysfunction among long-term survivors of bone marrow transplantation. Am J Med 1982;73:688–694

36. Boulad F, Bromley M, Black P et al. Thyroid dysfunction following bone marrow transplantation using hyperfractionated radiation. Bone Marrow Transplant 1995;15:71–76

37. Sanders JE. The impact of marrow transplant preparative regimens on subsequent growth and development. The Seattle Marrow Transplant Team. Semin Hematol 1991;28:244–249

38. Sanders JE, Pritchard S, Mahoney P et al. Growth and development following marrow transplantation for leukemia. Blood 1986;68:1129–1135

39. Sanders JE, Guthrie KA, Hoffmeister PA et al. Final adult height of patients who received hematopoietic cell transplantation in childhood. Blood 2005;105:1348–1354

40. Michel G, Socie G, Gebhard F et al. Late effects of allogeneic bone marrow transplantation for children with acute myeloblastic leukemia in first complete remission: the impact of conditioning regimen without total-body irradiation – a report from the Societe Francaise de Greffe de Moelle. J Clin Oncol 1997;15:2238–2246

41. Sarafoglou K, Boulad F, Gillio A, Sklar C. Gonadal function after bone marrow transplantation for acute leukemia during childhood. J Pediatr 1997;130:210–216

42. Rovo A, Tichelli A, Passweg JR et al. Spermatogenesis in long-term survivors after allogeneic hematopoietic stem cell transplantation is associated with age, time interval since transplantation, and apparently absence of chronic GvHD. Blood 2006;108:1100–1105

43. Sanders JE, Buckner CD, Amos D et al. Ovarian function following marrow transplantation for aplastic anemia or leukemia 57. J Clin Oncol 1988;6:813–818

44. Carter A, Robison LL, Francisco L et al. Prevalence of conception and pregnancy outcomes after hematopoietic cell transplantation: report from the bone marrow transplant survivor study. Bone Marrow Transplant 2006;37:1023–1029

45. Salooja N, Szydlo RM, Socie G et al. Pregnancy outcomes after peripheral blood or bone marrow transplantation: a retrospective survey. Lancet 2001;358:271–276

46. Sanders JE, Hawley J, Levy W et al. Pregnancies following high-dose cyclophosphamide with or without high- dose busulfan or total-body irradiation and bone marrow transplantation. Blood 1996;87:3045–3052

47. Socie G. Secondary malignancies. Curr Opin Hematol 1996;3:466–470

48. Witherspoon RP, Deeg HJ, Storb R. Secondary malignancies after marrow transplantation for leukemia or aplastic anemia. Transplantation 1994;57:1413–1418

49. Witherspoon RP, Fisher LD, Schoch G et al. Secondary cancers after bone marrow transplantation for leukemia or aplastic anemia. N Engl J Med 1989;321:784–789

50. Deeg HJ, Witherspoon RP. Risk factors for the development of secondary malignancies after marrow transplantation. Hematol Oncol Clin North Am 1993;7:417–429

51. Stone RM, Neuberg D, Soiffer R et al. Myelodysplastic syndrome as a late complication following autologous bone marrow transplantation for non-Hodgkin's lymphoma. J Clin Oncol 1994:2535–2542

52. Traweek ST, Slovak ML, Nademanee AP et al. Clonal karyotypic hematopoietic cell abnormalities occurring after autologous bone marrow transplantation for Hodgkin's disease and non-Hodgkin's lymphoma. Blood 1994;84:957–963

53. Miller JS, Arthur DC, Litz CE et al. Myelodysplastic syndrome after autologous bone marrow transplantation: an additional late complication of curative cancer therapy. Blood 1994;83:3780–3786

54. Krishnan A, Bhatia S, Slovak ML et al. Predictors of therapy-related leukemia and myelodysplasia following autologous transplantation for lymphoma: an assessment of risk factors. Blood 2000;95:1588–1593

55. Darrington DL, Vose JM, Anderson JR et al. Incidence and characterization of secondary myelodysplastic syndrome and acute myelogenous leukemia following high-dose chemo-radiotherapy and autologous stem-cell transplantation for lymphoid malignancies. J Clin Oncol 1994:2527–2534

56. Andre M, Henry-Amar M, Blaise D et al. Treatment-related deaths and second cancer risk after autologous stem-cell transplantation for Hodgkin's disease. Blood 1998;92:1933–1940

57. Friedberg JW, Neuberg D, Stone RM et al. Outcome in patients with myelodysplastic syndrome after autologous bone marrow transplantation for non-Hodgkin's lymphoma. J Clin Oncol 1999;10:3128–3135

58. Pedersen-Bjergaard J, Andersen MK, Christiansen DH, Nerlov C. Genetic pathways in therapy-related myelodysplasia and acute myeloid leukemia. Blood 2002;99:1909–1912

59. Pedersen-Bjergaard J, Andersen MK, Christiansen DH. Therapy-related acute myeloid leukemia and myelodysplasia after high-dose chemotherapy and autologous stem cell transplantation. Blood 2000;95:3273–3279

60. Stone RM. Myelodysplastic syndrome after autologous transplantation for lymphoma: the price of progress. Blood 1994;83:3437–3440

61. Witherspoon RP, Deeg HJ. Allogeneic bone marrow transplantation for secondary leukemia or myelodysplasia. Haematologica 1999;84:1085–1087

62. Witherspoon RP, Deeg HJ, Storer B et al. Hematopoietic stem-cell transplantation for treatment-related leukemia or myelodysplasia. J Clin Oncol 2001;19:2134–2141

63. Yakoub-Agha I, de la Salmoniere P, Ribaud P et al. Allogeneic bone marrow transplantation for therapy-related myelodysplastic syndrome and acute myeloid leukemia: a long-term study of 70 patients – report of the French Society of Bone Marrow Transplantation. J Clin Oncol 2000;18:963–971

64. Curtis RE, Travis LB, Rowlings PA et al. Risk of lymphoproliferative disorders after bone marrow transplantation: a multi-institutional study. Blood 1999;94:2208–2216

65. Cohen JI. Epstein-Barr virus lymphoproliferative disease associated with acquired immunodeficiency. Medicine (Baltimore) 1991;70:137–160

66. Zutter MM, Durnam DM, Hackman RC et al. Secondary T-cell lymphoproliferation after marrow transplantation. Am J Clin Pathol 1990;94:714–721

67. Verschuur A, Brousse N, Raynal B et al. Donor B cell lymphoma of the brain after allogeneic bone marrow transplantation for acute myeloid leukemia. Bone Marrow Transplant 1994;14:467–470

68. Meignin V, Devergie A, Brice P et al. Hodgkin's disease of donor origin after allogeneic bone marrow transplantation for myelogeneous chronic leukemia. Transplantation 1998;65:595–597

69. Rivet J, Moreau D, Daneshpouy M et al. T-cell lymphoma with eosinophilia of donor origin occurring 12 years after allogeneic bone marrow transplantation for myeloma. Transplantation 2001;72:965

70. Schouten HC, Hopman AH, Haesevoets AM, Arends JW. Large-cell anaplastic non-Hodgkin's lymphoma originating in donor cells after allogenic bone marrow transplantation. Br J Haematol 1995;91:162–166

71. Rowlings PA, Curtis RE, Passweg JR et al. Increased incidence of Hodgkin's disease after allogeneic bone marrow transplantation. J Clin Oncol 1999;17:3122–3127

72. Bhatia S, Louie AD, Bhatia R et al. Solid cancers after bone marrow transplantation. J Clin Oncol 2001;19:464–471

73. Bhatia S, Ramsay NK, Steinbuch M et al. Malignant neoplasms following bone marrow transplantation. Blood 1996;87:3633–3639

74. Deeg HJ, Socie G, Schoch G et al. Malignancies after marrow transplantation for aplastic anemia and Fanconi anemia: a joint Seattle and Paris analysis of results in 700 patients. Blood 1996;87:386–392

75. Lowsky R, Lipton J, Fyles G et al. Secondary malignancies after bone marrow transplantation in adults. J Clin Oncol 1994;12:2187–2192

76. Socie G, Henry-Amar M, Cosset JM et al. Increased incidence of solid malignant tumors after bone marrow transplantation for severe aplastic anemia. Blood 1991;78:277–279

77. Socie G, Kolb HJ, Ljungman P. Malignant diseases after allogeneic bone marrow transplantation: the case for assessment of risk factors. Br J Haematol 1992;80:427–430

78. Socie G, Curtis RE, Deeg HJ et al. New malignant diseases after allogeneic marrow transplantation for childhood acute leukemia. J Clin Oncol 2000;18:348–357

79. Socie G, Scieux C, Gluckman E et al. Squamous cell carcinomas after allogeneic bone marrow transplantation for aplastic anemia: further evidence of a multistep process. Transplantation 1998;66:667–670

80. Curtis RE, Metayer C, Rizzo JD et al. Impact of chronic GVHD therapy on the development of squamous-cell cancers after hematopoietic stem-cell transplantation: an international case-control study. Blood 2005;105:3802–3811

81. Favre-Schmuziger G, Hofer S, Passweg J et al. Treatment of solid tumors following allogeneic bone marrow transplantation. Bone Marrow Transplant 2000;25:895–898

82. Socie G, Henry-Amar M, Devergie A et al. Poor clinical outcome of patients developing malignant solid tumors after bone marrow transplantation for severe aplastic anemia. Leuk Lymphoma 1992;7:419–423

PART **6**

THE WIDER PERSPECTIVE

Starting a hemopoietic stem cell transplant unit

Anthony P Schwarer

CHAPTER 47

Introduction

Hematopoietic stem cell transplantation (HSCT) is a complex and multifaceted medical procedure with substantial risks to the patient. It behoves all physicians wishing to commence a new and successful HSCT program at their institution to consider all the aspects of the many components that form part of this potentially life-ending as well as life-saving treatment modality. This should be true for institutions wishing to establish an HSCT program in an existing hematology/oncology ward as well as institutions wishing to construct a new purpose-built HSCT unit. Best practice principles should be considered and established prospectively before the first patient is admitted to the program.

There are published guidelines (discussed below) that should be read in conjunction with this chapter. Relevant local legislation should be identified and complied with. The goal of this chapter is to provide a basis, in a more practical way, of what should be considered for the nascent HSCT program.

Published guidelines

A number of professional organizations have generated guidelines stating minimum standards for facilities and individuals performing HSCT, with the goal of promoting high-quality care in the performance of HSCT. These guidelines are essential reading for anyone contemplating establishing an HSCT program. This chapter will not recapitulate the guidelines outlined in these publications but will attempt to expand on those practical points that may not necessarily be addressed in those guidelines.

In 1992 the American Society of Clinical Oncology (ASCO) published recommendations for the performance of transplantation.[1] This one-page document briefly outlines criteria for patient volume, facilities, personnel and quality control.

In 1995, the American Society of Blood and Marrow Transplantation (ASBMT) published their recommended guidelines for clinical transplant centers.[2] This two-page document is similar to the ASCO document although it provides a little more detail. These guidelines are also available online at www.asbmt.org/policystat/policy_op.html.[3]

North America

In December 1994, the Laboratory Standards of the International Society of Hematotherapy and Graft Engineering (ISHAGE), now known as the International Society of Cellular Therapy (ISCT), were merged with the Clinical Standards of the ASBMT into a single document covering the collection, processing and transplantation of hematopoietic stem cells. In 1996, the ASBMT and ISCT established the Foundation for Accreditation of Hematopoietic Cell Therapy (FAHCT) (now known as the Foundation for the Accreditation of Cellular Therapy or FACT) for the purposes of voluntary inspection and accreditation of institutions involved in HSCT. In 1997 FACT began providing accreditation to centers involved in HSCT, whether it be patient management, hematopoietic stem cell (HSC) collection or processing, that successfully passed all aspects of an inspection. In addition, FACT standards require ongoing assessments of the program.

Europe

In 1998, the European Group for Blood and Marrow Transplantation (EBMT) and ISCT formed the Joint Accreditation Committee-ISCT and EBMT (JACIE), based on the FACT program, with the goal of creating a standardized accreditation process officially recognized across Europe that would promote quality in all areas of HSCT. These standards extend and detail the pre-existing standards of EBMT. JACIE will provide a certificate of accreditation to those programs and facilities that meet the minimum standards. Ongoing inspections will also be undertaken.

International guidelines

In February 2006, FACT and JACIE published online, for public review, a draft version of the *International standards for cellular therapy, product collection, processing and administration*, 3rd edition.[4] The ratified guidelines should be available by the time this chapter reaches print. The goal of the FACT-JACIE standards is to create a standardized system of guidelines and accreditation that is officially recognized worldwide and to encourage all centers involved in all aspects of HSCT to voluntarily seek compliance with these standards.

Other useful publications

Visit the website of the Centers for Disease Control and Prevention (CDC), www.cdc.gov, particularly for two recommendations and reports: the *Guidelines for preventing opportunistic infections among hematopoietic stem cell transplant recipients – recommendations of CDC, the Infectious Disease Society of America, and the American Society of Blood and Marrow Transplantation*, published October 2000 (MMWR 49 No RR-10 2000),[5] and the *Guidelines for environmental infection control health-care facilities – recommendations of CDC and the Healthcare Infection Control Practices Advisor Com-*

mittee (HICPAC), published June 2003 (MMWR 52 No RR-10 2003).[6] The former guidelines are also available in print (Centers for Disease Control 2000).[7] These two documents provide the detailed information that forms the basis of the infection control guidelines that would be relevant to anyone involved in the establishment of a new HSCT program.

General requirements

General facilities

The establishment of a new HSCT facility requires considerable forethought and planning. This is true whether the program is to be housed in a new, purpose-built facility or existing premises are to be modified to house the nascent program. It will of course be considerably easier to deal with the various hurdles if they have been considered before they occur, and not after buildings are built or refurbished, budgets established or less than ideal practices become accepted as the norm.

An HSCT program is best established as part of a modern, tertiary referral hospital that has an established service managing patients with acute leukemia and other high-grade hematologic malignancies. This will ensure that the units and departments necessary for the management of the HSCT patient, such as the infectious diseases service, the intensive care unit, the blood bank and many others, will have had experience managing neutropenic patients with leukemia – clearly experience that is highly relevant to the HSCT patient. A program contemplating allogeneic HSCT would be best served building on an established autologous HSCT program.

Support services

Routine laboratory support

Basic hematologic and biochemical investigations must be available on an urgent basis 24 hours per day every day of the year. A same-day service for the measurement of ciclosporin and tacrolimus levels should be a goal. A microbiology service experienced in the diagnosis of opportunistic infection and a histopathology service experienced in the diagnosis of graft-versus-host disease (GvHD) are essential. Flow cytometry is essential for the measurement of CD34+ cells in peripheral blood and bone marrow stem cell collections.

Molecular laboratory support

Monitoring for cytomegalovirus (CMV) reactivation and infection remains important in the allogeneic HSCT setting; quantitative polymerase chain reaction (Q-PCR) is very sensitive and, of the available tests, is probably the most useful clinically.[8] Results will need to be available in a timely manner – one or two runs per week. Molecular techniques for diagnostic and monitoring purposes of mold infections, such as *Aspergillus*,[9] remain under development but, almost certainly, will have a similarly important role in HSCT as they currently do for CMV. A diagnostic molecular service can be very useful for the diagnosis of many other infectious organisms such as BK virus, Epstein–Barr virus (EBV), various respiratory viruses, tuberculosis and others.[10,11] Molecular techniques for the diagnosis and monitoring of minimal residual disease for many hematologic malignancies, such as chronic myelogenous leukemia and acute promyelocytic leukemia, are now standard practice.

Blood bank support

A 24-hour per day onsite blood bank is needed for the urgent supply of platelets, red blood cells, fresh frozen plasma, cryoprecipitate and human serum albumin when such products are required.

Filtration by the collection center (prestorage filtration) of all platelets and red blood cells is important to remove contaminating white blood cells and so decrease the chance of the patient developing antibodies directed against human leukocyte antigen (HLA) and the incidence of alloimmunization that leads to poor platelet increments.[12] In addition, prestorage filtration, particularly of platelets, will decrease the incidence of the very unpleasant transfusion reactions secondary to various cytokines released by white blood cells during storage.[13] Filtration performed with inline filters at the bedside is considerably less effective.[13,14]

Most importantly, all cellular blood products – red blood cells, platelets and granulocytes – will require adequate irradiation to prevent transfusion-associated GvHD. The most commonly recommended dose is 2500 cGy.[15] The irradiation may take place offsite at the central blood bank or at the onsite blood bank. CMV-negative red blood cells and platelets should be available if needed. Appropriate storage of platelets at 22°C on an agitator onsite in the blood bank is essential.

Diagnostic and interventional radiology, and nuclear medicine

As well as all routine diagnostic radiology and ultrasound services, access to a computed tomography (CT) scanner is essential and access to magnetic resonance imaging (MRI) is often very useful. The latter is considerably more sensitive for detecting intracerebral infections, ciclosporin toxicity, leukemic infiltration of the meninges and other central nervous system (CNS) complications.

Most patients undergoing HSCT will require a permanent central venous access device. Many hospitals nowadays have a radiology department with interventional radiologists trained in the insertion of a variety of central venous access devices under ultrasound guidance. This is often quicker and more reliable than hoping for busy surgeons to find space on full surgical lists to insert devices. A transjugular liver biopsy in a thrombocytopenic or otherwise coagulopathic patient can be the only way to differentiate between veno-occlusive disease (VOD), GvHD, hepatitis or drug-induced liver abnormalities. This procedure is usually performed by an interventional radiologist under radiologic visualization.

Nuclear medicine can provide the frequently useful services of gated cardiac blood pool scans, positron emission tomography (PET) scans and radiolabeled white blood cell scans.

Other laboratory support

Access to HLA typing, including DNA-based typing HLA class I and class II, is essential for allogeneic HSCT programs.

Ancillary medical services

Infectious diseases

Infectious diseases physicians are crucial to the success of any HSCT program. One or a small group of infectious diseases physicians, with experience in the diagnosis and management of opportunistic infections, should be an integral part of the team that manages the HSCT patient on a day-to-day basis. Importantly, the infectious diseases physicians will need to develop, implement and monitor the effectiveness of policies established for infection control, infection prophylaxis and the treatment of infection. Infectious diseases input will be particularly important for programs performing allogeneic HSCT although it remains relevant to programs performing only autologous HSCT.

Intensive care unit (ICU)

The nature of HSCT dictates that a certain proportion of patients will require a level of medical support that cannot be provided by the

HSCT unit. This proportion has ranged from 10.6% to 44% in the series that have been reported although 15–20% has been the more recent experience.[16] Clearly, allogeneic HSCT patients are more likely to experience the complications that require ICU admission. Respiratory support or inotrope support, or perhaps hemofiltration/hemodialysis, often in the setting of sepsis, are the usual reasons for transfer to the ICU. Survival to discharge from hospital and long-term survival have improved substantially over the past decade.[16]

Admission to the ICU is extremely stressful for the patient and family. As a significant proportion of patients will require ICU support at some stage, the possibility of admission to the ICU and the ramifications of such an admission need to be discussed with the patient and family. Realistic goals of an ICU transfer and the very real limitations of the ICU should be discussed.

Nephrology

Renal complications will be commonly encountered in the patients of any HSCT program.[17] Opinions on the etiology and proposed management of renal abnormalities will often be needed. A significant proportion of allogeneic HSCTs will require renal replacement therapy, either hemodialysis or hemofiltration. It should be kept in mind that, due to a weakening mains water pressure, hemodialysis and ultrafiltration using standard machines may not be possible above the fourth floor of a building.

Pulmonary medicine

Complications involving the lung are frequent after HSCT and a pulmonary medicine opinion will often be useful. The facility to perform pulmonary function tests and bronchoscopies will be essential.[18]

Psychiatry and psychology

Undergoing a life-threatening treatment for a life-threatening disease will be a stressful time for the patient and the family. Psychiatric input from a professional with knowledge of hematology and HSCT, prior to the HSCT, will be useful to deal with any issues present as well as to identify patients at risk so that preventive measures can be put into place or warning signs highlighted so that pre-emptive therapy can begin. Ongoing psychiatric input post HSCT will be important to help recognize and deal with the long-term problems that can occur in patients with chronic complications such as GvHD.

Gastroenterology

Complications involving the gastrointestinal tract are frequent after HSCT. Endoscopy is an important diagnostic tool; gastroscopy and colonoscopy are essential procedures to help differentiate GvHD from infection and other gastrointestinal complications. Small bowel endoscopy or capsule endoscopy can, on occasions, be useful for investigating complications of the small bowel that are outside the reach of the gastroscope or colonoscope.

Radiation oncology

A radiation oncology service is essential. Their expertise and facilities will be needed for involved field radiation before or after autologous HSCT for Hodgkin and non-Hodgkin lymphoma as well as the bony complications of myeloma. Total-body irradiation (TBI) is an important component of many allogeneic and some autologous HSCT conditioning regimens. Particularly for TBI, it is important that it be performed on site. Sending the HSCT patient any significant distance to another facility, particularly if an inpatient stay is required at that other facility, should be avoided. Such patients are often unwell and unstable.

Surgery

On occasion, general surgery will be needed for the management of acute abdomens, and cardiothoracic surgeons will be needed to perform open lung biopsies in patients with lung pathology that needs a diagnosis. Neurosurgery is occasionally necessary for a diagnostic biopsy of an intracerebral lesion or the insertion of an Ommaya reservoir.

Cardiology

Cardiac arrhythmias are common in sick HSCT patients. Cardiologic opinion can be valuable. Infectious endocarditis is a common differential considered in the HSCT population – urgent access to echocardiography is important.

Endocrinology

Steroid-induced hyperglycemia is a frequent occurrence in the HSCT patient population. The expertise of the endocrinology service will be useful particularly when the blood sugars prove difficult to control with simple measures.

Urology

Hemorrhagic cystitis is a reasonably common complication, related to chemotherapy and/or viral infection. Clot retention, requiring urologic intervention, occasionally occurs.

Otolaryngology

Sinus infections, particularly with *Aspergillus* and other molds, are quite common, particularly in the allogeneic HSCT setting. Access to an ENT service will be needed for invasive diagnostic procedures and surgical debridement in some patients with invasive fungal infections.

Other services

Other services that may be needed on occasion include gynecology, dermatology, ophthalmology, anesthetics, orthopedics and neurology.

Inpatient requirements

Inpatient facilities

The service

It is much easier to start an HSCT program in an institution that has an established hematology service which is very familiar with the management of patients with acute leukemia. Experience in the scenarios and complications encountered in patients with acute leukemia receiving aggressive chemotherapy will provide a sound basis for the management of the very similar scenarios and complications that will be encountered in the HSCT patient population.

Ideally, the institution should have a purpose-built unit. If, for pragmatic reasons, this is not possible, HSCT patients may be managed in an established, dedicated hematology/oncology unit. A small program might have only two dedicated beds to manage the expected minimum of 10 HSCTs to be performed each year, although the average-sized unit will have 10 beds to perform 60 or so HSCTs per year. Importantly, this will allow readmissions to the HSCT unit, a common occurrence with patients undergoing allogeneic HSCT.

The ASCO guidelines[1] recommend that a minimum of 15–20 HSCTs should be performed each year to maintain the skill levels of the unit. These guidelines also suggest that the number of HSCTs performed each year should ensure that the unit is never empty and that it is allowable for new programs to take up to 2 years to reach these numbers. The ASBMT recommends that if a program performs only one type of HSCT (autologous or allogeneic), at least 10 HSCTs of that type must be performed each year, and that programs performing both types of HSCT should perform at least 10 of each kind each year.[2] The draft FACT-JACIE guidelines will consider accreditation for allogeneic HSCT for the program that has performed 10 allogeneic HSCTs in the preceding 12 months and annually thereafter, and for the autologous HSCT program that has performed five autologous HSCTs in the preceding 12 months and annually thereafter.[4]

Isolation rooms

The unit should have, wherever possible, all single isolation rooms. If this is not possible, adequate numbers of single rooms to house the allogeneic HSCT patients is a reasonable goal. Patients undergoing autologous HSCT are considerably less immunocompromised and hence single isolation rooms for this patient population are less important. Indeed, many programs routinely have their autologous HSCT patients spending part or all of their pre- and post-HSCT time as an outpatient. The single rooms must have ensuite facilities. Each room must have oxygen and suction facilities. Resuscitation equipment should be immediately available in the unit. The beds should tilt at both ends. Horizontal dust-accumulating blinds should be avoided, and vertical blinds or blinds within two sealed glass panels should be used. The floor should not be carpeted and porous ceiling tiles should be avoided. All walls and horizontal surfaces should be smooth and non-porous to prevent trapping of dust and to facilitate easy cleaning on a daily basis. Facilities for relatives to stay with the patient overnight in the patient's room should be available. A fold-out bed is all that is necessary.

The single most important infection control measure will be to prevent the direct transfer of infectious organisms from one patient to another via the hands or a fomite of a healthcare worker. Good hand hygiene and hand-washing practices are essential for all caregivers and visitors. To facilitate this, antimicrobial hand-washing solutions should be placed in highly visible and easily accessible positions that make it very easy for the healthcare worker to make use of the solutions, and hard for them to forget to use them. For example, a bottle should be placed at the entry to the unit, outside each room, at the foot of each bed and on every dressing trolley. Each room should have a dedicated sphygmomanometer, oximeter, thermometer and stethoscope.

Patients should be encouraged to bring in personal items such as TV, music player, computer and books, although old or dusty books should be left at home. The unit should have a designated kitchen area available to the patient and their relatives.

Minimization of exposure to infectious organisms

It is of considerable importance that HSCT patients be protected from the many potential infectious organisms to which they are susceptible. Infection control measures must be considered when constructing and managing a brand new facility or adapting a pre-existing facility for the management of HSCT patients. Examples include simple strategies such as the prevention of birds gaining access to hospital air-intake ducts, and ensuring that those ducts are directed away from any cooling towers to minimize the risk of *Legionella* infection. The most important consideration is the prevention of infections with molds, particularly *Aspergillus* spp. Also important are measures to limit the spread of resistant bacteria as well as preventing the introduction of respiratory viruses into the unit. Two publications from the CDC[5,6] deal with the many issues of infection control that should be considered when constructing a facility that will house immunocompromised patients.

The design and construction of the HSCT facility should aim to decrease the HSCT patient's exposure to fungal spores. One useful measure is to ban flowers and potted plants from the unit. Fungal spores are ubiquitous in the environment and their spread is facilitated by building construction, a common occurrence in most hospitals. Hence, the unit should be isolated from the outside environment to minimize the patient's exposure to fungal spores. There is considerable circumstantial evidence suggesting the benefits of isolation and all official guidelines recommend isolation, although the benefits of isolation nowadays have been questioned.[19] The degree of isolation can be less stringent for units undertaking only autologous HSCTs because such patients are considerably less susceptible to fungal infections compared to patients undergoing allogeneic HSCT. Indeed, some such patients are now managed partly or entirely in the home.

All doors and windows to the outside should be permanently shut with airtight seals. Entrances to the unit should be through an anteroom that has automatic doors that remain closed unless someone is entering or leaving. All other potential leaks, such as electrical outlets, must be sealed. The unit should use high efficiency particulate air (HEPA) filters.[20] By definition, a HEPA filter is one that removes 99.97% of all particles of ≥ 3 μm in diameter. Such a filter will remove most fungal spores from air passed through it. Ideally, the entire ward should have HEPA-filtered air, although practically, it is often only possible to have the individual rooms filtered. The airflow should be directed across the patient – the air-intake and exhaust ports should be placed such that room air comes from one side of the room, flows across the patient's bed and exits on the opposite side of the room. The air pressure in patients' rooms should be positive relative to the air pressure in the corridor and the air pressure in the corridors and the remainder of the unit should be positive relative to the rest of the hospital. This can be achieved so that the amount of HEPA-filtered supply air exceeds the amount of air exhausted by at least 10%. There should be at least 12 room-air changes per hour. An anteroom can help maintain the positive pressure of the isolation room. If the entire unit receives filtered air, this allows patients to leave their rooms on occasions, to walk around the unit for exercise. Time out of the room may be important psychologically for the longer stay patients as 4–6 weeks confined to a single room is a long time. Equipment for the continuous monitoring of the positive pressure areas, with appropriate alarms, should be installed.

The HSCT patient with varicella zoster infection (shingles) requires special consideration. Such a patient requires the usual isolation afforded to all HSCT patients but needs to be isolated from the remainder of the unit; the patient cannot be in a single room under positive pressure that vents into the corridor because this will expose those in the corridor to the virus. Hence, it would be useful to have at least one single room that is under positive pressure that vents not to the corridor but to the outside or some other appropriate area such as an anteroom with an independent exhaust. This will allow the patient to be protected from the environment and for the remainder of the unit to be protected from the patient.

During times of construction and renovation, additional guidelines and monitoring requirements need to be established.[21] Such guidelines should define the appropriate barriers and techniques required to prevent the spread of dust. It is particularly important to protect inpatients from this dust on those occasions when the patient leaves the protected environment of the unit. For example, the route to the diagnostic radiology department or to the surgical operating suites should avoid corridors or areas that may be exposed to the dust. Outpatients and day patients should have routes of access, from arrival at the hospital to their respective areas, that avoid proximity to the construction areas and avoid areas that may have been exposed to dust from the construction site. On these occasions, the use of particulate filter respirator masks for the patient should be considered.

The maintenance of water quality is necessary to minimize infections from contaminated water. Special considerations will be needed to prevent the spread of not only *Legionella* but also other waterborne pathogens.[6]

Marinella et al performed aerobic and anaerobic cultures on 40 randomly selected stethoscopes.[22] Eleven different organisms were isolated including coagulase-negative *Staphylococcus* from 100% of stethoscopes and *Staphylococcus aureus* from 38%, and even *Aspergillus niger* from one stethoscope. A 70% isopropyl alcohol prep was found to be an effective cleaning agent for the stethoscopes. Not only should hands be washed between patients but stethoscopes should be cleaned with an isopropyl alcohol prep, although ideally, as mentioned earlier, each patient/room should have a dedicated stethoscope.

The most important mode of transmission of methicillin-resistant *Staphylococcus aureus* (MRSA), and probably many other bacteria, is poor hand hygiene. Boyce[23] and Johnson et al[24] both showed that the introduction of an alcohol/chlorhexidine solution and an associated ongoing education program decreased nosocomial infections. They also targeted the cleaning of shared equipment between uses. Bottles of alcohol/chlorhexidine were put at the foot of every patient's bed and outside each room, on iv trolleys and wound dressing trolleys, and at nurses' stations. Bottles were replaced promptly when empty. The authors also indicated that the product used must be very accessible and non-irritant with frequent use, that education of new staff was essential, and periodic quality assessments were needed.

Inpatient staff

Medical staff

The HSCT clinical program should have a program director who has qualifications and experience appropriate to the clinical requirements of the program. The clinical director should be familiar with all the aspects of the HSCT program. In addition to the director, there must be at least one senior physician appropriately trained in autologous and/or allogeneic HSCT. Physicians should maintain knowledge and skill levels by an appropriate continuing education program.

A senior physician should be available for advice to the junior medical staff and, if necessary, to attend to sick patients 24 hours per day 365 days a year. Loberiza et al[25] surveyed 163 transplant centers in the United States and noted a decreased 100-day mortality at centers where there was a higher patient-per-physician ratio and at centers where the senior physicians answered calls after office hours. The effects were most noticeable with allogeneic HSCT and weaker with autologous HSCT. Therefore, particularly for allogeneic HSCT, greater physician involvement in patient care is important in producing favorable outcomes.

The unit should be covered 24 hours per day by appropriately trained and experienced junior medical staff who are able to attend to the patient immediately when required. The junior medical staff should have experience in the management of sick patients and particularly sick hematologic patients with neutropenia. There must be adequate supervision of the junior medical staff. The attending senior physician should round on a daily basis, particularly for allogeneic HSCT patients.

There should be a detailed handbook for junior medical staff new to the unit which outlines their duties as well as the routines and basics on the functioning of the HSCT program, related disciplines and the hospital. There should be an educational program for junior medical staff.

Nursing staff

HSCT programs should have formally trained and experienced nursing staff. The ASCO has stated that the single most important aspect of a successful HSCT program is the quality of the nursing staff.[1] The nurse-to-patient ratio should be appropriate to the complexity of the patient population undergoing HSCT: three or four to one for autologous HSCTs, and no more than two to one for allogeneic HSCTs are commonly accepted ratios. There should be an adequate number of experienced nursing staff on each shift, including the overnight shift. Junior nursing staff must have adequate supervision by the senior nursing staff. Nursing staff should be trained in the management of patients receiving HSCTs – specifically, training in the care of the hematology/oncology patient, the administration of cytotoxic chemotherapy, the management of neutropenic and other immunocompromised patients. There should be a formal education program for nursing staff which should include input from the senior nursing staff and the medical staff. 'Burnout' is common amongst nurses managing patients undergoing HSCT, especially allogeneic HSCT. Measures should be in place to recognize and manage this problem.

Transplant co-ordinator/s

One or more transplant co-ordinators are necessary for the smooth running of the HSCT program. The co-ordinator serves as a facilitator, educator and point of contact for the patient and their family from the time the transplant is being considered until the time the patient is admitted to hospital. The co-ordinator should make the path to HSCT as smooth as possible for the patient and family. The co-ordinator may continue to be involved during the inpatient stay and will often be involved in the co-ordination of the post-HSCT follow-up. The transplant co-ordinator will usually be responsible for the establishment and maintenance of the HSCT waiting list.

Donor search co-ordinator

Most allogeneic HSCT programs benefit from having a donor search co-ordinator who will be responsible for HLA typing of the patient, immediate family, extended family and the initiation and following through of searches of the unrelated donor registries. Duties often include organizing the logistics of getting hematopoietic cells from the donor, related or unrelated, to the patient, and on those occasions when the hospital is acting as a donor center, organizing hematopoietic stem cells to go to a patient in another hospital which may be local, in another state or province, or in another country.

Dietetics

Weight loss commonly occurs in the period prior to HSCT, as well as during and after HSCT. Underweight patients have an increased transplant-related mortality.[26] Significant weight loss presumably decreases the reserve of the patient and their ability to recover from the many insults that can occur during the transplant period. The benefits of professional dietary advice and assistance to help patients maintain or gain weight prior to HSCT and maintain weight during the post-HSCT period should not be underestimated.

Social services

Undergoing an HSCT is a major life event for the patient and family with significant social, psychologic and financial implications. Every patient and their family should be seen by the program's social worker during the pre-HSCT period and intermittently, as required, during and after the HSCT.

Psychology

Very few patients and families go through a treatment program for a hematologic malignancy with subsequent HSCT without acquiring a number of psychologic scars. An experienced psychologist is an important resource for the program.

Physiotherapy

Patients undergoing HSCT are often confined to a single room for weeks at a time with little possibility of exercising. Hence, most HSCT patients will rapidly become deconditioned. The program's physiotherapist will provide advice and assistance to minimize the deconditioning during this confined period and assist the patient's recovery after the HSCT. Advice on minimizing the risk of lung infections is also important.

Oncology pharmacist

A trained oncology/hematology pharmacist is essential to ensure the safe and appropriate management of chemotherapy agents as well as other medications. The pharmacist should also check all chemotherapy orders and should review all the chemotherapy protocols of the program. There must be a proper cytotoxic dispensing facility.

Pastoral care

Appropriate pastoral care should be available for all patients who request it.

Inpatient procedures and guidelines

All aspects of the clinical program will require written and detailed documents and protocols, preferably electronic (for ease of access), that cover the entire routine and emergency care of the HSCT patient, as well as the day-to-day running of the program. This should include appropriate documents and protocols for medical and nursing staff. The junior medical staff will appreciate the availability of a comprehensive handbook covering the relevant aspects of the program.

Regular meetings can ensure the safe and smooth running of the program. A meeting involving all the relevant staff should be held weekly to discuss the soon-to-be-admitted patients, the current inpatients and the recently discharged patients.

Day center and outpatient requirements

Day center and outpatient facilities

A dedicated day center is an essential requirement for a successful HSCT program. It provides the important link between the inpatient and the true outpatient. On discharge from the ward, patients will often need to be reviewed on a daily or alternate-daily basis, particularly patients undergoing allogeneic HSCT. The day center should provide a one-stop service: the patient arrives to be assessed by appropriately trained nursing staff who will facilitate blood collection and venous access device care, arrange medical review as well as provide blood product support and electrolyte replacement. The appropriate number of recliner chairs, beds and single rooms will depend on the expected volume of patients that will be treated in the day center.

Proximity of the inpatient, day patient and outpatient facilities can help foster regular interaction between these somewhat separate but overlapping areas.

Acute medical care should be available to the patient on a 24-hour basis via an emergency department that is familiar with the management of HSCT patients and particularly the management of febrile neutropenic patients. Patients should be provided with an appropriate alert card that identifies them as HSCT patients.

An appropriate outpatient department will be necessary for the follow-up of the patients beyond the acute phase of the HSCT.

Day center staff

Medical staff

The day center is often best served by having junior medical staff based in the area full time. This will ensure that the patients are reviewed promptly. Relying on the ward staff will frequently mean delays for the day patients while the sick inpatients are receiving attention.

Nursing staff

The day center commonly has the responsibility of looking after not only HSCT patients but also general hematology and oncology patients. Hence, the nursing staff for this area will require skills appropriate for these patient groups.

Day center procedures and guidelines

Written policies and guidelines, preferably electronic, for the medical and nursing staff covering all aspects of the day center are essential.

Apheresis

Apheresis facilities

The apheresis facility may be part of the day center and HSCT program or it may be an administratively and physically separate collection facility. What is important is that the successful clinical HSCT program has a convenient and reliable apheresis service. A minimum of two cell separators should be the goal, even in a small program, the second to act as back-up for the inevitable machine repairs or routine servicing. Alternatively, back-up could be provided at a neighboring institution. Emergency resuscitation equipment and staff must be immediately available at all times that the facility is active.

FACT-JACIE standards require that a minimum of 30 apheresis procedures are performed each 12 months for reaccreditation.

Patient/donor education prior to apheresis is important. A mechanism needs to be in place that provides adequate education and assessment of the patient/donor prior to apheresis. An education session may be conducted on the first day of G-CSF administration and, at that time, the patient/donor can also have their venous access assessed to decide whether central venous access is required. It is important to have a system in place that ensures that central venous devices will be inserted in a timely manner – usually the day of apheresis or the day before.

Apheresis staff

Medical staff

The apheresis facility will require a medical director who may either be the medical director of the HSCT clinical program or the medical director of the collection facility. The medical director should have qualifications and experience appropriate to the clinical requirements of the facility. Appropriately trained and experienced medical staff should be available immediately for care or advice of the patients undergoing apheresis.

Nursing staff

Apheresis requires nursing staff with an appropriate level of training and experience. Junior nursing staff will require adequate supervision. An ongoing education program should be in place.

Apheresis co-ordinator

It will be advantageous to have an individual responsible for generating and maintaining the apheresis waiting list. This is particularly relevant for the larger apheresis programs.

Apheresis procedures and guidelines

There should be written, preferably electronic, guidelines and policies covering all routine and emergency aspects of apheresis. There should also be written criteria for donor selection and management, both autologous and allogeneic.

Cellular therapy product processing requirements

The cellular therapy product processing facility may be part of the collection facility or it may be a separate facility. There must be co-operative liaison between the collection facility and the processing facility.

Cellular therapy product processing facilities

The processing facility will require a designated and dedicated area for the processing of cellular products such as peripheral blood stem cells or bone marrow. It will need to be secure to prevent access by unauthorized personnel and should have adequate areas of adequate size to prevent improper labeling or product contamination. This specifically designed laboratory will require appropriate lighting, ventilation and air conditioning.

The minimum equipment required will include a class II laminar flow biohazard hood, a controlled-rate freezer, liquid nitrogen storage tank/s, a refrigerated bench-top centrifuge and a blood product processing centrifuge such as a Cobe 2991. All freezers and refrigerators should have a system to monitor and record the temperature. The storage tanks must be alarmed to detect any problem with the storage conditions. The alarm must be sited in an area that is staffed 24 hours per day to ensure prompt attention to any equipment malfunction or other technical failures. Clearly, it would be an irretrievable disaster should the cryopreserved HSCs thaw due to unrecognized equipment failure. The area that houses the liquid nitrogen storage tanks and controlled-rate freezer must have adequate ventilation and be set up with oxygen meters with alarms to prevent staff from potentially fatally walking into a nitrogen-filled atmosphere.

A user-friendly inventory system for the liquid nitrogen storage tanks is important. Searching for hours to find the product required would be frustrating at best and potentially disastrous at worst. If space is not at a premium, it is a reasonable practice to cryopreserve each individual's HSCs in a minimum of two bags in case one is damaged. Aliquots of cells stored separately will allow ready access to a sample for testing in the future if required. It is useful to have a portable cryogenic container for the transport of cryopreserved cellular products. It is also appropriate to have containers for the transport of non-frozen cellular products, particularly if these products are to travel long distances.

On occasion, it may be necessary to remove the red blood cells or plasma from an ABO blood group-incompatible, usually bone marrow, donor product. This may be performed by hydroxyethyl starch (HES) sedimentation or, more easily, with a blood product processing centrifuge.

Ready and timely access to flow cytometry for the enumeration of CD34+ cells and other cells, such as T-cells, is required.

A plan for the disposal of cellular products that are no longer needed is essential, unless the facility has unlimited storage capacity. How long should cellular products be stored? Each program should develop a policy to deal with this question. The policy should be discussed with the patient/donor prior to the collection and a written agreement between the donor/patient and the storage facility should be routinely obtained. This process should involve the internal review board.

Cellular therapy product processing staff

The cellular therapy product processing facility must have a medical director with appropriate experience in the preparation and clinical use of cellular therapy products who will be responsible for all medical aspects of the facility.

The processing laboratory should be staffed by an adequate number of scientists and technicians appropriate to the workload of the facility. Ideally, there should be a minimum of two individuals with the experience to be able to independently undertake cellular product manipulation and cryopreservation.

Cellular therapy product processing procedures and guidelines

It is essential that the cellular therapy product processing facility has detailed written guidelines covering the processes and procedures to be undertaken by that facility. There must be a well-considered process to prevent mix-ups and contamination. There should be a written quality management system ensuring that high-quality materials are used and that standard procedures are followed, in order to produce a cellular therapy product that best conforms to specifications where possible, given the variable nature of the original cellular product.

Bone marrow harvest requirements

Bone marrow remains the preferred cellular product for certain patients undergoing allogeneic HSCT and the preferred option for some donors. Occasionally, an autologous bone marrow collection will be needed. The FACT-JACIE document requires a minimum of three bone marrow harvests to be performed each 12 months for reaccreditation.

Bone marrow harvest facilities

Bone marrow harvesting requires access to an operating theater and its facilities. Appropriate equipment for the harvesting procedure will be needed; a closed system is preferable.

Bone marrow harvest staff

A bone marrow harvest usually requires two harvesters, the anesthesiologist and other standard operating theater staff, and usually a laboratory scientist to attend to the marrow once it has been removed from the donor and placed into the collection bag.

Bone marrow harvest procedures and guidelines

Written documents, preferably electronic, are needed for the various procedures and guidelines are required for the bone marrow harvest procedure.

Patient and family accommodation

Patients and families of most HSCT programs will benefit from the availability of accommodation proximate to the hospital. The magnitude of this need will depend on the nature of the HSCT program – whether the program services just the local community or acts as a referral center for regions some distance away and whether it undertakes HSCT in the outpatient setting. In addition, it may also depend on the level of expertise of the referral center – an allogeneic HSCT patient may need to stay close to the program center for a longer period of time if the referral center has minimal experience handling this type of patient.

Each patient and their carers should be housed in accommodation that has a separate bathroom facility to minimize transmission of infection.

Some HSCTs are amenable to the outpatient setting, particularly autologous HSCTs and particularly melphalan-only autologous HSCTs, for patients with myeloma. Such transplants require sophisticated outpatient support facilities: a day center familiar with the management of such patients, accommodation nearby, 24-hour access to the hospital should the patient require attention or advice, and trained staff (particularly nursing staff) to attend the patient in the accommodation facility on a daily or more frequent basis. The patient, in this setting, will require a carer or carers who are available 24 hours a day and who are familiar with some of the basic nursing requirements that the patient will need. Written (and understood) guidelines or criteria for when to call the nurse or doctor or hospital should be supplied.

Patient population

Which patients should undergo HSCT? A deceptive question – apparently simple on the surface but, in reality, considerably more complex. What type of HSCTs, what diseases, what stages of those diseases, what ages, what co-morbidities are allowable and the timing of HSCT are all questions that should be answered before the first patient is admitted to the unit. The development of criteria for accepting patients for HSCT should allow input from all interested parties. Once established, the written criteria should be available to all who wish to view them.

Initially, the new autologous HSCT program may be best served by confining its patient population to well-accepted criteria such as younger patients with Hodgkin and non-Hodgkin lymphoma in first or second partial remission or second complete remission, or patients with multiple myeloma but without significant co-morbidities. The new allogeneic HSCT program, however, may be best served by confining its patient population to younger patients, with HLA-identical sibling donors, who have acute leukemia with poor-risk features in first complete remission, acute leukemia in second complete remission, severe aplastic anemia or chronic myelogenous leukemia in chronic phase resistant to tyrosine kinase inhibitors. Most new allogeneic HSCT programs should be established in the setting of an existing autologous HSCT program. This approach allows all the members of the program – medical, nursing, allied health and others – to gain experience and confidence before the program moves on to the more difficult types of HSCT or experimental forms of HSCT. The steps taken to expand the complexity of the program should probably be small.

It is useful to have a working meeting each week or so to discuss the HSCT waiting list – which patients should be added to the list, which patients are coming up for HSCT and their special requirements. All interested parties should be invited to this meeting. A written version of the waiting list should be made available to those who are not able to attend the meeting.

Referral base

A successful HSCT program will require a regular throughput of patients to maintain the skills of the HSCT staff, and hence a reliable referral base is essential. Links with referring hospitals and physicians should be actively fostered and maintained. Regular feedback, updates and education will be useful. Establishing satellite clinics at the referring centers for ease of patient access and follow-up should be considered.

Getting the patient and family to transplant, and after the transplant

Prior to undergoing HSCT, the patient and family must be fully informed and appropriately educated regarding HSCT. They must understand the rationale for HSCT and the alternatives to it. The success rate expected for the patient's particular scenario, the various morbidities that may be encountered and, most importantly, the mortality risk of the procedure must be understood. This information should come from a number of sources over a period of time – sources should include the physician in charge of the patient, written material either from the HSCT program or other sources, perhaps visual material such as an in-house DVD or third-party DVD, as well as input from nursing, social work and psychology. This will entail preferably more than one meeting with the physician and the other members of the team, as well as time to read, view and discuss the information.

Clearly, the transplant involves many individuals other than the patient. Hence, it is crucial that not only the patient but also family and involved friends are very well informed. The period prior to admission for HSCT, the inpatient stay and the immediate and long-term post-HSCT course need to be discussed. It is crucial that both patient and family have a realistic expectation of the HSCT itself, of the risks and outcomes, as well as information on any potential long-term complications. This is particularly true for allogeneic HSCT. Certain aspects of HSCT should be highlighted such as admission to the ICU so that patients and families are aware of the goals and limitations of the ICU. Also, the prolonged recovery time needs to be stressed. Autologous HSCT patients require 3–6 months and not infrequently longer to return to normal levels of activity, whereas allogeneic HSCT patients often take a good 12 months, and frequently 2–3 years, to return to normal levels of activity. A sizeable proportion of patients will never entirely return to normal because of ongoing problems, particularly chronic GvHD.

There must be a written and comprehensive plan of post-HSCT follow-up. The CIBMTR, EBMT and ASBMT have developed recommendations to offer care providers suggested screening and prevention practices for autologous and allogeneic HSCT survivors.[27] This includes a post-HSCT vaccination program according to either the CDC guidelines[5] or the EBMT guidelines.[28,29]

Data management and quality control

The FACT-JACIE standards require that all clinical, collection and processing programs evaluate and report clinical outcomes, and that each program should have a written plan for quality assessment. Most importantly, a mechanism is needed to detect errors and adverse events so that these can be assessed and investigated to identify measures that will minimize the risk of them occurring again in the future.

Databases

Clearly, each HSCT program should keep complete and accurate patient records. A database containing all relevant patient data should be established and maintained. The database should only contain information relevant for quality assurance and research to evaluate and improve the outcomes of the program. The patient should give informed, written consent prior to their details being included in the database. The CIBMTR or EBMT MED-A forms constitute the minimum data that need to be collected on HSCT recipients. The database should undergo quality assurance checks on a regular basis.

For ease of use, a relational database design, such as MS ACCESS or Stem Soft, that has the capacity to link relevant databases, should be considered. In addition, a database could be considered for the storage of the HSC collection data.

Data management should be conducted in accordance with local internal review board requirements and should be compliant with local privacy legislation. An up-to-date knowledge of any changes to these requirements is essential.

Registries

Data should be submitted to relevant local as well international registries such as the CIBMTR and EBMT. Prior to submission to any registry, internal review board approval and written informed consent from the patient should be obtained. Data transfer must comply with local privacy laws as well as the privacy laws of the country of the registry to which the data are being submitted. All data must be submitted in a de-identified manner.

Clinical research

Every HSCT program should be actively involved in clinical research. This may be small in-house trials or pilot studies, larger trials involving a few centers or large multicenter national and international trials. This approach remains crucial for the advancement of medical knowledge. Clearly, all trials, investigational treatment protocols, and the associated patient consent forms must be reviewed and approved by the internal review board.

It is worthwhile considering establishing a tissue bank for blood, bone marrow and/or serum. This may be particularly important for centers that will have a research laboratory.

References

1. ASCO. Recommended criteria for the performance of bone marrow transplantation. Oncology 1992;6:114
2. Phillips G, Armitage J, Bearman S et al. American Society for Blood and Marrow Transplantation guidelines for clinical centers. Biol Blood Marrow Transplant 1995;1:54–55
3. ASBMT. Policy statement, guidelines and reviews, 2006. www/asbmt.org/policy_op.html
4. FACT-JACIE. International standards for cellular therapy product collection, processing and administration (draft), 2006. www.jacie.org 0 3rd ed FACT-JACIE Standards.pdf
5. Centers for Disease Control and Prevention. Guidelines for preventing opportunistic infections among hematopoietic stem cell transplant recipients: recommendations of CDC, the Infectious Disease Society of America, and the American Society of Blood and Marrow Transplantation. MMWR 2000;49 (No. RR-10)
6. Centers for Disease Control and Prevention. Guidelines for environmental infection control health-care facilities: recommendations of CDC and the Healthcare Infection Control Practices Advisor Committee (HICPAC). MMWR 2003;52 (No. RR-10)
7. Centers for Disease Control and Prevention. Guidelines for preventing opportunistic infections among hematopoietic stem cell transplant recipients: recommendations of CDC, the Infectious Disease Society of America, and the American Society of Blood and Marrow Transplantation. Biol Blood Marrow Transplant 2000;6:659–734
8. Cortez KJ, Fischer SH, Fahle GA et al. Clinical trial of quantitative real-time polymerase chain reaction for detection of cytomegalovirus in peripheral blood of allogeneic hematopoietic stem-cell transplant recipients. J Infect Dis 2003;188:967–972
9. Halliday C, Hoile R, Sorrell T et al. Role of prospective screening of blood for invasive aspergillosis by polymerase chain reaction in febrile neutropenic recipients of haematopoietic stem cell transplants and patients with acute leukaemia. Br J Haematol 2005;132:478–486
10. Angeles Marcos M, Camps M, Pumarola T et al. The role of viruses in the aetiology of community-acquired pneumonia in adults. Antiviral Ther 2006;11:351–359
11. Rebollo MJ, San Juan Garrido R, Folqueira D et al. Blood and urine samples as useful sources for the direct detection of tuberculosis by polymerase chain reaction. Diagnost Microbiol Infect Dis 2006;56(2):141–146
12. Trial to Reduce Alloimmunization to Platelets Study Group. Leukocyte reduction and ultraviolet B irradiation of platelets to prevent alloimmunization and refractoriness to platelet transfusions. N Engl J Med 1997;337:1861–1869
13. Pruss A, Kalus U, Radtke H et al. Universal leukodepletion of blood components results in a significant reduction of febrile non-hemolytic but not allergic transfusion reactions. Transfus Apheresis Sci 2004;30:41–46
14. Williamson LM, Wimperis JZ, Williamson P et al. Bedside filtration of blood products in the prevention of HLA alloimmunization – a prospective randomized study. Blood 1994;83:3028–3035
15. Schroeder ML. Transfusion-associated graft-versus-host disease. Br J Haematol 2002;117:275–287
16. Naeem N, Reed MD, Creger RJ et al. Transfer of the hematopoietic stem cell transplant patient to the intensive care unit: does it really matter? Bone Marrow Transplant 2006;37:119–133
17. Pulla B, Barri YM, Anaissie E. Acute renal failure following bone marrow transplantation. Renal Failure 1998;20:421–435
18. Glazer M, Breuer R, Berkman N et al. Use of fiberoptic bronchoscopy in bone marrow transplant recipients. Acta Hematologica 1998;99:22–26
19. Hayes-Lattin B, Leis JF, Maziarz RT. Isolation in the allogeneic transplant environment: how protective is it? Bone Marrow Transplant 2005;36:373–381
20. Passweg JR, Rowlings PA, Atkinson KA et al. Influence of protective isolation on outcome of allogeneic bone marrow transplantation for leukemia. Bone Marrow Transplant 1998;21:1231–1238
21. Walsh TJ, Dixon DM. Nosocomial aspergillosis: environmental microbiology, hospital epidemiology, diagnosis and treatment. Eur J Epidemiol 1989;5:131–142
22. Marinella MA, Pierson C, Chenoweth C. The stethoscope. A potential source of nosocomial infection? Arch Intern Med 1997;157:786–790
23. Boyce JM. MRSA patients: proven methods to treat colonization and infection. J Hosp Infect 2001;48:S9–S14
24. Johnson DR, Martin R, Burrell LJ et al. Efficacy of an alcohol/chlorhexidine hand hygiene program in a hospital with high rates of nosocomial methicillin-resistant *Staphylococcus aureus* (MRSA) infection. Med J Aust 2005;183:509–514
25. Loberiza FR, Zang M-J, Lee S et al. Association of transplant center and physician factors on mortality after hematopoietic stem cell transplantation in the United States. Transplantation 2005;105:2979–2987
26. Deeg HJ, Seidel K, Bruemmer B et al. Impact of patient weight on non-relapse mortality after marrow transplantation. Bone Marrow Transplant 1995;15:461–468
27. Rizzo JD, Wingard JR, Tichelli A et al. Recommended screening and preventative practices for long-term survivors after hematopoietic cell transplantation: joint recommendations of the European Group for Blood and Marrow Transplantation, Center for International Blood and Marrow Transplantation Research, and the American Society for Blood and Marrow Transplantation (EBMT/CIBMTR/ASBMT). Bone Marrow Transplant 2006;37:249–261
28. Ljungman P. Immunization of transplant recipients. Bone Marrow Transplant 1999;23:635–636
29. EBMT transplant guidelines. www.ebmt.org/8TransplantGuidelines/tguide6.html

Ethical and legal considerations in stem cell transplantation

Simon Meller

Introduction

In the context of allogeneic hematopoietic stem cell transplantation (SCT), there are two patients rather than one. The recipient is a hospital patient who, typically, will have achieved a chemotherapy-induced remission after treatment for a malignant blood disorder and is predicted to be at high risk of a relapse, whereas the potential donor is usually a healthy person, either a sibling or a non-family member, who may or may not wish to volunteer to donate stem cells. Sometimes a family donor will be unable to give valid consent to the donation procedure, on account of age or learning difficulty. On the other hand, an unrelated donor will have been identified by a computer search of national or international tissue banks and will always be over 18 years of age and capable of giving consent. Such a person will have volunteered, sometime in the past, to provide a sample of blood for human leukocyte antigen (HLA) typing, and an attempt will be made to trace the person to confirm their suitability and willingness to act as a stem cell (SC) donor.

The indications for performing SCT vary from an established treatment of known risk and benefit, through to a more experimental scenario where the balance of doing good (beneficence) versus doing harm (maleficence) may be relatively uncertain. A SCT may offer a patient the only chance of cure, but often no better than a 50/50 chance; for some patients there may be alternative less toxic treatments available, albeit with a lesser chance of a successful outcome. It is important to realize that today's established indications were at some time in the past regarded as experimental. The amount of information that is currently regarded as sufficient for a potential recipient to be able to give valid consent will be discussed both where there is a well-established indication for SCT and in the more experimental contexts.

Consenting to be a donor is altogether a different matter because the 'patient' is neither sick nor do they stand to benefit in any physical sense from the procedure proposed. The law relating to organ donation distinguishes between the donation of regenerative and non-regenerative tissues. As a result, the donation of blood or bone marrow stem cells by competent related adults is much less regulated than non-regenerative solid organ transplantation and will seldom give rise to any legal objection, provided that the consent obtained before donation is valid. However, there may be ethical issues that need careful consideration even when the donor is an adult relative and has given valid consent in the eyes of the law. There are a number of dangers and drawbacks in acting as a SC donor. The physical dangers are small but measurable and are well documented.[1] The psychologic drawbacks are individual to a particular case and can occasionally be of overriding importance. The setting up of donor registries worldwide has resulted in an exponential growth of donations from unrelated volunteers that give rise to additional issues around confidentiality and anonymity. Separate medical advice for the donor in all matters, including consent, effectively excludes conflicts of interest and international guidelines that provide rigorous protection to unrelated donors have been drawn up by the Ethics Working Group of the World Marrow Donor Association.[2]

An adult within the sick person's family, usually a sibling, is just as capable as a non-family member of deciding whether to volunteer to donate marrow or peripheral blood stem cells (PBSC) and, as in any other important life decision, such a person should be well informed of the risks and not coerced into having the procedure. Family donors, unlike unrelated donors from a SC bank, are relatively unprotected because their source of information is either from family members, who will have a strong vested interest, or from the patient's treating medical team, who will have already recommended SCT as the treatment of choice. It is argued here that voluntariness may be compromised if agreement to the procedure is pledged at an early stage before the donor has received all the relevant medical information. Altruism is seldom unconditional, even within families, and will often depend on a number of medical and non-medical factors, including the risk–benefit ratio both to the donor and to the recipient. In the context of live tissue and organ donation, it has been said that forced altruism is not altruism at all.[3]

A potential adult donor within the recipient's family may lack the capacity to consent and will therefore draw the family and their medical and legal advisors into the difficult area of surrogate consent and best interest decision making. In England and Wales, the codes of practice associated with the Human Tissue Act 2004[4] and the Mental Capacity Act (MCA) 2005[5] now provide statutory guidance in an area that previously had been subject to common law principles derived from decided cases. Particular attention must be given to those who lack the necessary capacity, either by reason of a learning disability or on account of their age. At first sight, it may appear a relatively straightforward matter for parents, guided by a physician, to make a best interests decision on behalf of their child. It will often be argued that, in the eyes of the beholder, the potential psychologic benefits clearly outweigh (or 'trump') any physical dangers or potential disadvantages to the donor. The potential for bias is compounded when the recipient and potential donor are both children of the same family and under the care of the same medical team, who are also subject to a similar conflict of interests. A decision may be made using what has been called 'altruism by proxy'.[6] The age and degree of understanding of the child enter into the equation. An infant sibling will sometimes be placed under the care of a separate medical team, often including a pediatric anesthetist, who are well placed to act as impartial guardians of a young donor's interests and a case can be made for this approach to be taken whenever a potential donor lacks full adult competence.

Ethical issues also arise if parents decide that they wish to attempt to create a 'savior sibling'. The lottery-type situation of conceiving another baby in the hope that it will turn out to be HLA matched is usually viewed as being a matter solely within the parents' domain. But if the parents express a wish for an HLA-matched fetus to be created by in vitro fertilization (IVF) and preimplantation genetic diagnosis (PGD), no longer can the medical profession simply leave it all up to the parents, because they will require a great deal of technical assistance to achieve their aim, This slippery slope towards designer babies will soon become more commonplace in the UK since the Human Embryology and Fertilization Authority (HEFA) in 2004 declared that this particular type of genetic manipulation was legal.[7] Commentators in this field of medical ethics have been pronouncing their views and clinicians must be prepared to address a range of issues that are engaged by using these children created to be donors by positive embryo selection and volunteered for this purpose by their parents.[8–12]

The nature and purpose of consent

The basic definition of patient consent is: 'an agreement (usually by the patient him/herself or, in certain circumstances, by a proxy) for a health professional to provide care'.[13]

There are several separate purposes for obtaining consent. First, there is the clinical purpose of enlisting the patient's faith and confidence in the efficacy of treatment. Second, there is the ethical purpose of recognizing and respecting a patient's right to self-determination. Third, there is the legal purpose of providing those concerned in the treatment with a defence against a criminal charge of battery or a civil claim for damages for trespass to the person. Consent does not provide a defence against a claim in negligence for advising a particular treatment or negligently carrying it out. The ethical purpose of consent underpins the judicial approach on both sides of the Atlantic. The 1914 American dictum of Judge Cardoso in *Schloendorff v New York Hospital* is much quoted in legal texts: 'Every human being of adult years and sound mind has a right to determine what should be done with his own body; and the surgeon who performed an operation without his patient's consent performs an assault for which he is liable in damages'.[14]

The three cornerstones of valid consent are the requirements of capacity, voluntariness and information. The ascent of patient autonomy and the decline of medical paternalism have been a 50-year process of change and now leave little or no residual place for withholding information, when the patient is a competent adult. For a doctor to treat a competent patient in a particular way just because he thinks it would be in the patient's best interests is no longer acceptable. The leading English case on the required standard of disclosure of medical information was *Sidaway*, which came before the House of Lords in 1985.[15] Lord Scarman, albeit in a minority judgment, reflected the changing tide of public opinion by promoting the concept that it was the patient, not the doctor, who should determine what the patient needed to know before he or she gave consent to a medical procedure. Lord Scarman's statement effectively sounded the death knell for medical paternalism in the UK.

It has to be acknowledged that there have been major changes in the conduct of the medical profession for the better in the past 50 years but some remnants of paternalism, sometimes camouflaged or driven partially underground by prohibition, remain extant throughout the practice of western medicine. Have the critics of medical paternalism achieved what they wanted? O'Neill in a series of Reith Lectures in 2002 pointed out that, sadly, the public has not come to trust doctors more, and rather the reverse seems to be the case.[16]

Although medical paternalism has not really been eliminated from all medical settings, it is indisputable that one important aspect of a doctor's duty of care is to provide a patient with all the necessary information about a proposed treatment or procedure. The law has struggled with devising a satisfactory test for the adequacy of a doctor's disclosure. A physician may find the law's liking for a 'reasonable man' or a 'prudent patient' test too constraining when confronted by the rich variety of patients encountered in medical practice. One difficult issue is to know how much information is actually required by an individual patient and, of course, not all patients have identical requirements. In some jurisdictions, much attention has been given to so-called 'fully informed' consent, but attempting to fully inform a patient may not always achieve the desired effect because the patient may lose the plot on account of information overload and/or the doctor may adopt an inappropriately defensive stance. This expression has not found so much favor in the UK as it has in North America, and Jones has questioned whether the term is useful or whether it is a recognizable legal entity, and suggests that the information given simply has to be 'sufficient' (for the individual patient) in order for his consent to be valid.[17]

MCA 2005[5] gives statutory effect to the principle previously spelt out by Lord Donaldson in the case of *Re T*: 'Prima facie, every adult has the right and capacity to decide whether or not he will accept medical treatment, even if refusal may risk permanent injury to his health or even lead to premature death'.[18] MCA 2005 also defines how an individual should be assessed to determine whether he has the capacity to be granted the rights and benefits of fully autonomous decision making.

Legalistic thinking may distract the medical practitioner from the fundamental ethical purpose of consent, which is to protect the patient; it is the patient's choice that needs to be informed, so the information must be sufficient to permit the patient to be self-determining in that choice. Clearly, a doctor will want to protect himself from the risk of litigation but, unfortunately, the deterrent effect of the law may act on a doctor's disclosure behavior in a way that may not benefit the doctor–patient relationship.

The law is sometimes thought to protect the patient but, in practice, non-disclosure of a risk that is important enough for the patient to know about in order to make an informed choice can only be subject to an action in negligence in limited circumstances. The law of tort can compensate the patient only if it can be shown that:

- the kind of harm that should have been disclosed actually occurred and
- if the disclosure had been made, the patient would have withheld his consent to treatment.

At the end of the day, successful actions in negligence can only compensate individual patients financially and any spill-over deterrent effect gives scant protection to other patients who come to no harm as a result of medical treatment. It is the ethical perspective on consent that offers protection to the patient. All medical practitioners in the UK are obliged to follow the generic good practice guidelines published by the General Medical Council,[19] which go well beyond the rather narrow legal requirements for valid consent. Practice guidelines for consent to hemato-oncology procedures exist at both institutional and national levels.[20]

Unrelated donors

The marrow donor programs that are now up and running in most developed countries have explicit policies and procedures in place, designed to respect the privacy and autonomy of volunteer donors. The World Marrow Donor Association (WMDA) was established in the 1990s for this purpose.[21,22] There is worldwide collaboration for the collection and dispersal of SC donated by volunteers, and the detailed guidelines produced by the Ethics Working Group of the WMDA are particularly welcome and place proper constraints to protect confidentiality and to minimize the risk of coercion of donors.[2]

The protocol for a potential unrelated donor starts at the time of recruitment. Oral and written information must be provided in language that can be fully understood by the volunteer. Paragraph 2 of the WMDA protocol states: 'the volunteer must be provided with information on the principles, general procedures, restrictions and risks of providing blood samples and hematopoietic stem cells (either by marrow or peripheral blood donation). At no time should the information be coercive'.[2] The volunteer has the right to withdraw at any time from the registry. Before the volunteer agrees to join the registry, he should understand the principles and risks of hematopoietic stem cell donation and be asked to sign a simple comprehensible consent form of agreement. It must be explained to the volunteer that blood samples will be used for histocompatibility testing, blood grouping and infectious disease marker (IDM) analyses. Furthermore, a plan must be made for information to the donor about serious positive IDM results or other abnormal medical findings, which should include:

- how each particular donor wishes to receive such information.
- who has the responsibility to do this.
- recommendations for follow-up care in such an eventuality.

At the time of confirmatory histocompatibility testing, the volunteer must have an information session with a qualified representative of the donor center, which will include information about all procedures, restrictions and risks involved. Sufficient time should be allowed for the volunteer to ask all questions as necessary. The information given must not be coercive.

Paragraph 3 states that 'at no time must the volunteer be told that he/she is the only match for a patient'.[2] With regard to the alternatives of bone marrow aspiration under anesthesia or peripheral blood stem cell collection following G-CSF mobilization, the volunteer should be informed about all aspects of the procedures and be asked to consider both forms of donation. A volunteer retains the right to withdraw at any stage. The probability of the treatment being successful for the recipient should be presented using general terms only. The possibility of further donation requests following the initial stem cell donation should be discussed briefly. All the foregoing oral information must also be contained in an information sheet and, in signing consent, the volunteer should confirm that he/she has read, understood and agrees to all the procedures detailed.

Paragraph 4 recommends that the medical consultation prior to stem cell harvesting should provide 'sufficient time and a relaxed environment for detailed discussions with the volunteer'.[2] Before informed consent is obtained, the volunteer should be offered the opportunity to talk to one or more volunteers who have already donated, and the donor center has a responsibility to ensure that volunteers selected to talk to potential donors have a balanced view of the experience. Furthermore, a donor advocate should be available to discuss the approaching donation with the volunteer – such an advocate must be an independent third party and conversant with hematopoietic stem cell donation; the role of the advocate is to enable the volunteer to reach his/her decision. This session should be conducted with the aid of a comprehensive checklist which should be signed by the person conducting the information session and countersigned by the volunteer, with a copy provided to the donor.

With regard to the anonymity issue, the donor signs an understanding that the SC donation will go to an anonymous patient, who can opt to remain anonymous permanently if he so wishes. The patient's identity may only be provided to the donor if the patient requests this and if it is the registry and transplant center's policy to allow patient–donor contact.[2]

Although patient autonomy is a well-established and legally protected ethical concept, Bakken et al discuss the less well-understood concept of autonomy in the context of voluntary donation.[23] Their view is that autonomy should ensure that the donor's well-being and integrity are maintained and that the donor is fully informed about the consequences pertaining to both donor and patient. Those employed by a donor registry should understand and respect the donor's rights, integrity and autonomy at every stage of donor evaluation. Not only has the donor the right to withdraw at any stage, but he/she is also not obligated to reveal the reasons for withdrawal. The donor's autonomy, however, does not include a right to donate, and, if the registry chooses to proceed with a different donor, the volunteer must accept the decision. Rosenmayr et al also discuss the benefits and pitfalls of donor expectations and obligations.[2]

It is established practice that the recipient patient must be eligible for SCT as defined under WMDA standards. It is also recommended that the donor should be informed whether the planned stem cell procedure is going to be within a well-established clinical protocol or, alternatively, is of a more experimental nature. These guidelines are comprehensive and admirable for the protection that they provide for the unrelated donor's autonomy, integrity and rights and stand in stark contrast to the virtually unregulated area of intrafamily stem cell donation.

Adult related donors

'Sentenced to die by my sister. Leukemia victim refused her only chance of a transplant.' This was a headline in the *Daily Mail* and the subject of an annotation in the *BMJ* in 1997.[24] Ten years later, the *Daily Mail* ran an almost identical story exposing and criticizing an HLA-matched sister of another patient with relapsed acute myeloid leukemia (AML) for whom there was no available matched unrelated donor (MUD). While it seems inevitable that stories about body parts and transplants will make headlines, because the public are fascinated by these topics, the distortion of facts by the media serves little useful purpose.

The most striking difference between competent related and unrelated donors is that family donors are seldom afforded the right of choosing for themselves or, if they are granted this privilege, the right to confidentiality is not properly respected and the resulting freedom of choice is very restricted. As Davies points out, the potential donor becomes a patient as soon as she consents to a blood test, but does not appear to be granted the associated right of confidentiality that is the norm in medical practice. Davies suggests that the donation of blood or blood products within a family is a much more emotive situation that appeals to the tabloids compared to the anonymous altruism of unrelated donation.[24] A lack of altruism in family matters often makes the headlines when it concerns a refusal to agree to SC donation. The beleaguered sibling gets publicly lambasted by her family and the press, who treat the decision as a crime, without respecting her privacy or considering all the facts. Individuals, regardless of whether they are blood relatives or not, are not obliged to give any reasons for their autonomous choice to refuse an invasive non-therapeutic procedure. Any attempt to force altruism on an individual cannot be condoned in a democratic society.

Dame Elizabeth Butler-Sloss said in the leading obstetric case of *Re MB*: 'a competent woman, who has the capacity to decide, may, for religious reasons, other reasons, for rational or irrational reasons or for no reason at all, choose not to have medical intervention, even though the consequence may be the death or serious handicap of the child she bears, or her own death'.[25] Such a person refusing cesarean section should be accorded the privacy and confidentiality which is afforded to all patients. A pregnant woman, akin to a potential sibling SCT donor, is not a sick person but becomes a patient on account of her particular circumstance, namely pregnancy. It would be unusual for the press to invade the privacy of a pregnant woman, who was upholding her right of self-determination and remaining within the law.

Why should the reluctant family donor be exposed and vilified by the media, when the reluctant non-family donor has her privacy protected? Those who believe that altruism can still be altruism when the person is coerced talk about 'forced' and 'unforced altruism', just as others may attempt to defend 'weak' paternalism and distinguish it from 'strong' paternalism.[26] So where are we going wrong when adults of full capacity exercise their right to choose and in so doing refuse to be tissue-typed or later refuse to donate stem cells? We would not dream of forcing an unrelated volunteer to give a blood sample for tissue typing and serologic testing for IDM and yet little counseling takes place before the majority of potential family donors hold out their arm to have a blood sample taken that is the first step on the slippery slope to SC donation. On one side of the slippery track, family members are egging on the noble but reluctant volunteer and, on the other, healthcare professionals are reassuring him that he doing the right thing.

If the donor succumbs to the pressure, it meets the description of forced altruism so why does it happen? We may be making an assumption that all right-minded siblings would wish to donate and therefore they are often not afforded the time or the privacy to make their own decision without coercion. The first approach should not be made by a member of the family and certainly not by the sibling in need of SCT donation. It is accepted that this may be very difficult to achieve if the potential donor already knows that her sibling is in hospital and suffering from a serious blood disorder for which SCT may be the treatment of choice. The potential donor deserves to be presented with an impartial analysis of the alternatives available for the treatment of her sibling as well as an honest appraisal of the potential risks and benefits of the procedure to both parties. It has been the author's experience only too often that a sibling donor has been wittingly or unwittingly coerced into making a donation either because she believes that it is the only form of treatment which can offer a cure or, more worrying still, that SCT guarantees a cure for the blood disorder from which the sibling is suffering.

It is suggested that the correct way to approach a potential sibling donor is by an independent healthcare professional and, preferably, one who is not looking after the potential recipient; the first discussion should be held in confidence and prior to any blood tests for HLA typing. The codification of consent by adults with capacity in MCA 2005[5] will oblige counselors to draw the sibling's attention to the law of consent as it now stands in England and Wales. There is little evidence from countries with a more rigorous approach to fully informed consent, such as North America, that a potential sibling donor is afforded any more opportunity to express her autonomy and right of self-determination. It may be because society values other rights – such as privacy within families, altruism and lack of selfishness – so highly that, as a result, the evils of paternalism and coercion pale into relative insignificance.

A 'best interests' decision by a surrogate third party has no place where a capable adult is called upon to reach a decision of this kind. However, if the adult lacks capacity and is being called upon to act as a sibling donor, a judicial decision is necessary before proceeding and will be made by means of a broad interpretation of best interests of not only the incompetent donor, but also the potential recipient, and this may include wider third party family interests.

The English courts have only had to consider sibling bone marrow donation from an incompetent adult on one occasion. In the case of *Re Y*,[27] the judge made a declaration that a bone marrow donation from Y, a 25-year-old severely learning-disabled woman, to her 36-year-old sister, who was dying of leukemia, was lawful. The relationship between the sisters themselves was not especially close; however, the relationship between Y and her mother was very close, as was the relationship between the mother and her older sick daughter, who had

provided her with a grandchild. The judge accepted that if the older sister died, her death would have an adverse impact on the mother and, indirectly, on Y herself: she would be overburdened by caring for her grandchild and consequently less able to visit Y. On the other hand, if the transplant went ahead, hypothetically the positive relationship between Y and her mother might be enhanced, as might the relationship between the sisters. It was held that the risk and discomfort to Y would be minimal and, accordingly, it was in Y's best interests to allow the bone marrow transplant to go ahead. Brazier questions whether the judge should have sanctioned a transplant which amounted to enforced donation and commented that the benefit to Y would seem to be rather remote, based on the facts of the case.[28] Nonetheless, at present, this remains the English common law precedent for SC donation by incompetent adults and applies to donation of fresh marrow or PBSC.

Tissue and organ donation have come under the statutory authority of the Human Tissue Act 2004[4] and are regulated by the Human Tissue Authority (HTA). Issues around consent are contained in Chapter 6 of the Code of Practice associated with the Act.[29] Although this guidance primarily concerns itself with consent for post-mortem removal of tissues, it also applies to the removal of tissues from a living person, if the tissue is to be stored; the scope of the guidance specifically includes bone marrow, PBSC and lymphocytes, whether removed for transplantation or for some other purpose. However, the removal of tissues from a living person, providing there is no storage involved, is governed by the common law and is outside the scope of the Act. For this purpose, the Code of Practice refers transplant physicians to the Department of Health's *Reference guide to consent for examination and treatment* 2001 as the appropriate code of practice.[13]

Since September 2006, when the Act came into force in England and Wales, whenever any tissue is removed from a donor and stored prior to transplantation, it is mandatory to check that the appropriate consent has been obtained. To this end the Code of Practice contains seven excellent pages of detailed guidance on matters of consent by donors, whether the potential donor is adult, child, competent or lacking capacity. This guidance does not appear to distinguish between family and non-family donors and is even-handed in respecting the rights of all donors. Although this Code of Practice strictly only applies when SC are stored between donation and infusion, this guidance is highly commendable and, it is suggested, is the appropriate standard required to give proper respect and protection to all SC donors.

It seems inappropriate to have a different set of rules if the SC obtained from the donor are employed 'fresh' and transplanted without prior storage. The interesting point in the consent guidance is that it does not single out any particular relationship between the donor and recipient – whether family or only HLA type – for a greater or lesser standard of consent. The guidance states, for example, at para 36: 'their (i.e. the donor's) right to be free of any kind of coercion or threat against them or anyone else (for example, family or friends) . . . Consent deemed to be given under any such pressure will not be validated by the accredited assessor'.

There is of course a need for caution whenever the State seeks to regulate sensitive areas of personal and family life (issues such as reproduction and ownership of body parts clearly come into this category) but, it is proposed, common international guidelines for all donors would be the best way forward. If the approach of the HTA were to be extended to all donors this would solve the discrepancies in the standards of consent which currently exist for related and unrelated donors.

Gillick-competent sibling donors

In most jurisdictions, it is acknowledged that, as young people acquire knowledge, they should also have a proportionate degree of autonomy granted to them in the arena of medical decision making. The turning point in this evolution in the UK followed the case of *Gillick*[30] and, subsequently, the phrase 'Gillick competent' has become used in the context of consent to treatment by adolescents. The determination of the capacity of (and hence the degree of autonomy that should rightly be granted to) young persons under 16 years of age has been set incrementally in common law since Lord Scarman stated that a child who 'has sufficient understanding and intelligence to enable him or her to understand fully' what is involved in a proposed treatment has the capacity to consent. As the understanding required for different interventions and procedures varies considerably, a child under 16 may therefore have the capacity to consent to some interventions but not to others. If the child is Gillick competent and able to give her voluntary consent after receiving the appropriate information, that consent will be valid and additional consent from a person with parental responsibility is not strictly required. In practice, however, the hematologist would be unlikely to feel comfortable about proceeding with a SC harvest or transplant involving a person under the age of 16 without the tacit agreement of a person with parental responsibility.[13]

Subsequent development of the common law has imposed restrictive interpretations on Gillick competence and there is a somewhat controversial anomaly in English law that, when a young person under the age of 18 or a Gillick-competent person under the age of 16 refuses treatment of a potentially life-saving nature, they may not be granted the right of self-determination. In *Re W*, a 17-year-old girl with anorexia nervosa was ordered by the court to comply with an order to transfer her care to a specialist unit, in response to an application made by those who held parental responsibility and against her expressed wish.[31] The courts have not yet been asked to adjudicate either in case of a young person refusing to accept SCT or in case of a refusal to donate stem cells to a sibling and it is thought to be unlikely that such a case will arise because adolescents in this situation tend to agree both to give and to receive. Is this a reflection of their altruism or is it the result of compliance in response to pressure exerted by others? The latter is not a typical characteristic of the teenage years, so perhaps it is truly an expression of their unforced altruism.

To illustrate some of the tricky issues that may arise in sibling tissue and organ donation, a possibly unique case from the 1990s will be recounted and discussed, which occurred prior to routine use of PBSC as a source of stem cells. A 17-year-old boy (who we will call A) developed AML. The hematologist advised A and his parents that an HLA-matched allograft would be the treatment of choice once he was in remission. His only sibling was a 15-year-old Gillick-competent girl (who we will call C) who suffered from cystic fibrosis, bronchiectasis and persistent *Pseudomonas* colonization of the lungs. The family were advised to consult C's pediatrician before subjecting C to a blood test for HLA typing; the pediatrician advised that a general anesthetic would be contraindicated because of her chest condition but he noted that, although C and A, as is the case with most siblings, did not always get along very well together, on this occasion, C seemed to have a genuine desire to help her brother.

On the leukemia ward, there were discussions about how to harvest bone marrow from an anxious yet determined young woman, without general anesthesia, and it was decided to present her and her parents with the proposal of performing bilateral posterior iliac crest aspirations under spinal anesthesia with a preoperative anxiolytic, but to avoid strong analgesia, which could depress respiration. The challenge was to describe this to her in a balanced way so that she could make her own autonomous decision, without parental or professional interference or coercion, one way or the other. The health professionals on the cystic fibrosis team consisted of a pediatrician, a pediatric outreach nurse and a social worker, all of whom C had known for several years. The interview took place not on the leukemia unit where A was an inpatient, but at the children's hospital where C had always attended for CF treatment. These three health professionals were joined by a consultant anesthetist associated with the leukemia unit at the hospital where A was being treated; he expressed a willingness to do this but said that it would be a novel experience for, although he was experienced in obstetric epidural practice, he had never before been asked to administer a spinal anesthetic to a teenager for the purpose of bone marrow harvesting.

The whole focus of this meeting was on the risks that C would be undertaking if she agreed to this invasive and non-therapeutic procedure; the meeting did not attempt to measure the possible benefit to her brother or any feel-good factors within the family. Her parents, acutely aware of their vested interests, had agreed to support her in whatever decision she reached and, at C's request, her mother sat in and listened during the consultation. C decided that she would consent to the procedure if she turned out to be HLA matched and not only gave consent, but also asked for the blood sample to be taken there and then. She was a full HLA match and a month later, the bone marrow harvest and transplant took place, without any complications to the donor. The marrow engrafted with a mild degree of graft-versus-host disease (GvHD) and A achieved stable marrow chimerism. Twelve years later, he remains well in continuing first remission. As far as can be determined, at no time was C exposed to any coercion, either by the health professionals or her family, but she knew what was at stake and may have felt that there was no alternative to altruism, although this differs from forced altruism.

There are several aspects of this narrative that may provoke comment or criticism by the reader. For instance, with the benefit of hindsight, it is reasonable to question why no search was undertaken for a matched unrelated donor, in order to spare C any risk. The story has had a happy outcome for A, but some years later C's lung condition deteriorated and she received a cadaver heart-lung transplant, with her heart being donated in a domino procedure. Although C has remained reasonably well, some years later, she has progressed to end-stage renal failure consequent upon ciclosporin administration for immunosuppression. A expressed a desire to give his sister a kidney and the assessment of A's renal function revealed a normal plasma creatinine, but a glomerular filtration rate (GFR) just below reference range. A was disappointed to be rejected as an organ donor, because he had thought that this could be his 'payback time'. C has gone onto hemodialysis and is awaiting a cadaver kidney.

Anecdotes such as this may represent rare clinical examples, but moral philosophers must appreciate that they are not just thought experiments. It might be questioned why, a decade ago, medical wisdom regarded severe lung disease as no contraindication to bone marrow donation, when this was genuinely what the donor wanted to do. But later medical opinion, in its wisdom, regarded a reduced GFR as a contraindication to live kidney donation.

The initial consent by a sibling to act as a body part donor may have totally unforeseen consequences that can continue for years down the line for both adults and children. Nowhere does the issue create more controversy than when the initial consent for the minor to donate is made by a surrogate – a parent, another person with parental responsibility or a judge in court. Reference is made to this same issue in the section on savior siblings elsewhere in this chapter and to Jodie Picoult's contemporary and not altogether fictional novel *My sister's keeper*.[32]

Young sibling donors (lacking capacity)

The Department of Health's *Reference guide to consent for examination or treatment* contains advice under the heading: Using Children Lacking Capacity as Bone Marrow Donors.[33] The choice of the verb 'to use' sets the tone for the three paragraphs of clearly expressed guidance, which are reproduced verbatim below.

> *Paragraph 16: 'Donation of bone marrow can be painful and carries some significant risks. It is not a minimal intervention. Children lacking capacity have on some occasions provided bone marrow to assist in the treatments of a sibling. To have such a transplant may clearly be in the best interests of the sibling. However, in relation to medical interventions it is not acceptable for the needs of one sibling to be balanced against the needs of another. The legal test is whether donating bone marrow is in the best interests of the healthy child.'*

> *Paragraph 16.1: 'It may be extremely difficult for a person with parental responsibility who has one dying child to take a dispassionate view of the best interests of that child's healthy sibling . . . Health professionals may also find it difficult to assess the needs of the children independently. However, without such dispassionate assessment the treatment may not be lawful.'*

> *Paragraph 16.2 (written prior to the Human Tissue Act 2004) states: 'Best practice requires some form of independent scrutiny of the healthy child's best interests. Examples might include use of an assessor who is independent of the team responsible for the sick child, or consideration of the case by a hospital clinical ethics committee or other multidisciplinary board convened for the purpose. If there is any doubt about the healthy child's best interests, a ruling from the court should be sought before undertaking the intervention.'*

There is a broad consensus that it is necessary to involve even the youngest sibling donors in the consent process in the some way which is age appropriate. For instance, seeking the assent of children over the age of 7 or 8 years has been repeatedly recommended in the pediatric literature.[34,35] Delany et al used the term 'altruism by proxy' and started a debate about whether parents can justifiably make the moral claim that they know their child so well as to be certain that, if he were older and competent, he would want to be altruistic and help his sick sibling.[6] The legality and ethical justification for parents to give consent to SC harvesting from a minor are not universally accepted, and Delany holds that it should strictly be illegal to perform a medical procedure of this nature, which can, by its very nature, never be in the medical best interests of the child donor.

Experience tells us that altruism varies between individuals in an unpredictable way, even within families, and also that parents find they are progressively less successful in projecting their own values onto their children as they get older. It is doubtful whether proxy altruism can be said to exist as an entity; we may wish our children to be just like us, but in practice they seldom are. Commentators, while decrying medical paternalism (by expert doctors), may act as advocates for medical parentalism (by expert parents) on the grounds that medical decisions for children are usually made by parents in their best interests and that a decision to allow a young children to act as an SC donor for sick child in the family is just another example of appropriate parental decision making. Delany rebuffs this view and contends that parents are not well suited to give such consent, due to the conflict of interests created by the sick child.

In the same multi-author article, Month disagrees with Delany and ascribes relatively greater weight to the overall benefit to the whole family and argues that the risks of donation are minimal when compared to the risks of not donating marrow, i.e. the almost certain death of a sibling. This view might be valid if it could be said that the death of the sibling would be inevitable without the donation, and that saving the life of the sibling is guaranteed by the donation. Month argues from the premise that SCT is an accepted treatment that can be life-saving and often offers the best chance of cure. Savelescu, another co-author, goes to the heart of the matter and argues that although a SC donation, by definition, cannot be in the donor's medical best interest; it may be in his/her overall best interests when other (non-medical) considerations are taken into account. Savelescu's conclusion, which concurs with a majority view amongst medical ethicists, is that because parents so often have conflicting interests when making decisions about their children, and because they have a commitment to the overall good of the family, they are as likely to make as good a decision as any third party.[6] This view would perhaps be true in an ideal world with ideal parents who could fully understand the issues, weigh them in the balance and reach a reasoned conclusion without bias or conflict of interests. If there are two parents with parental responsibility, the law requires both of them to reach agreement on such an important decision, and for both of them to give their consent, in order for the consent to be valid; should there be disagreement, the correct procedure would be to seek a declaration from the court.[13]

There is a paucity of information about the policies and practices of transplant centers in both Europe and the USA. A survey of 70 transplant centers in North America was reported in 1996 and revealed that the majority of centers allow parents to be surrogate decision makers and only a minority involve independent child advocates alongside the parents.[35] In the case of disagreement between parents, eight centers said they would cancel the transplant and the remainder said that they would seek a variety of proxy decision makers to assist in finding a satisfactory resolution. This survey was conducted by pediatricians at the MD Anderson in Houston, who had felt uncomfortable when requested to harvest bone marrow from a 2-year-old child, which was to be used as a partially mismatched transplant for the child's mother who had relapsed AML (the child being one-fifth the weight of her mother). It is implied that if the recipient had been a sibling they would have gone ahead; was it therefore the doubt about the likely effectiveness and medical benefit to the recipient that made them think twice? Could it have been something else about this child-to-parent transplant that provoked them to question the use of a young child as the donor and why should the particular recipient of the proposed transplant make any difference as to whether surrogate consent could be valid? Holm has drawn attention to the possible reason behind the societal primordial response to child-to-parent organ and tissue transplantation; he explains this as a form of non-oral cannibalism and suggests that it is because children can be said to be the 'flesh of their parents' that what he calls a 'societal archi-prohibition' stirs subconsciously in our minds.[36]

The symposium 'Children as Organ Donors' in 2004 started with a review of the previous 30 years by Sheldon,[37] since Levine first coined the expression 'informed consent' in the context of bone marrow transplantation in childhood.[38] The contributors addressed the ethical problems around both solid organ and tissue transplants, and the report of the symposium is recommended to the reader. The symposium concluded with some cautionary remarks by Fleck about parents as surrogate decision makers: 'there is in fact a strong moral and psychologic pressure to endorse . . . donations, so much so that it might not be unfair to say that there is a presumptive duty of parents to permit such donations unless they could offer some compelling moral reason or excuse for not doing so'.[39]

Also included in the report from the same symposium is an institutional protocol from the MD Anderson Center, Houston, that is designed to be applicable to all cases of organ and tissue donation by young children.[40] An independent pediatrician, social worker and anesthetist individually interview the parties and weigh up the validity of consent by the proxy decision maker(s) while, at the same time, taking into account the best interests of the young child donor. If these three persons, together acting as judge and jury, do not raise any concerns then the transplant goes ahead but if any concerns are raised, the case is then referred to the hospital's clinical ethics committee. It would be laudable if other transplant centers around the world followed a model procedure of this kind.

There is little published information about what other transplant centers are doing in this sensitive area of donation within a family. Again, this contrasts with the degree of respect and protection afforded to non-family donors, where donations by persons under the age of 18 years are simply prohibited. It may be the reluctance of the state to intervene in private family matters that is inhibiting the careful evaluation of whether young family members can and should act as SC donors for their first-degree relatives.

Little has been written about SCT in patients with learning disability, but a survey in 1989 only identified 16 leukemic children with Down's syndrome in the USA who had been transplanted; this was estimated to be only 20–25% of the expected eligible number of cases based on incidence. As the outcome was not significantly different from that expected in a similar cohort of patients without Down's syndrome, the author and the accompanying editorial concluded that there was no reason not to offer transplantation to these children.[41] With regard to learning-disabled donors, the adult in *Re Y* is discussed above[27] but medical journals do not contain any references to children with severe learning disability acting either as organ or tissue donors for their siblings. A meeting in Melbourne in the 1990s discussed the ethics of using anencephalic newborns as a source of tissue or organs for allografting and raised a storm of controversy.[42]

The need for independent medical, psychologic and social advice on behalf of a potential child donor is more often recognized for infants. When a potential child donor is older and has acquired greater understanding, it may seem paradoxical that she and her family are less likely to be afforded advice that is independent of the team treating the recipient, before it is agreed that she will act as a sibling donor. Consenting a minor as a donor assumes greater importance when the indication for SCT is marginal, or if it is uncertain whether the recipient will obtain a greater benefit from SCT than could accrue from an alternative option. It is acceptable for well-informed parents to give valid consent for a sick child to take part in a well-constructed protocol that addresses a research question that cannot be answered by extrapolation from research in adults. But, by the nature of the procedure, it would also be necessary for them to give permission for the well sibling to be exposed to risks for uncertain gain.

Opinion is divided on how to approach the difficult issues that arise in this situation and whether parental altruism by proxy has any validity. What is often missing from the equation is the age-appropriate agreement of the donor sibling. The hematologist and the team acting for both recipient and donor may be able to find a consensus with both parents that does not conflict with the wishes of the donor sibling; in this situation a joint 'best interests' decision can be made with relative comfort and without seeking further opinions. A degree of bias and well-meaning paternalism cannot be entirely eliminated from anyone's 'best interest' decision making for children. In those rare cases where two parents fail to agree between themselves, or if one parent disagrees with the hematology team, or if the appropriately informed donor sibling has reservations, it is advisable to seek a second medical opinion about the indication for the SCT procedure and to arrange an independent pediatric, child psychology and social work opinion on behalf of the potential donor before seeking the advice of the court. The court will in any case require these independent opinions, when taking all the circumstances into account, before reaching a legal best interests decision.

The conception of a 'savior sibling'

When a child in a family needs HLA-matched stem cells and no donor can be found after testing the family and searching all available donor

banks, it is perhaps not surprising that desperate parents might want to conceive and bring into the world a 'savior sibling'. In the early days, prenatal genetic testing was offered to couples in order to positively select a healthy fetus that would lack a defective gene, known to be present in the family because of an already affected child, by analysis of amniotic fluid obtained by amniocentesis at around 16 weeks of gestation. Subsequently, it became possible to obtain fetal DNA by chorionic villous sampling (CVS) at 10–12 weeks of pregnancy. A fetus of the wrong HLA type would be aborted and only the right kind of fetus would be allowed to continue its existence in the hope that it would become the much-wanted savior sibling.

In 1989, Clark et al reported a case concerning a couple who already had a child with Wiskott–Aldrich syndrome and presented to a prenatal genetic diagnosis clinic in California wanting positive fetal selection by HLA typing.[43] The parents' position was that they would be prepared to abort as many fetuses as necessary until they conceived one that was both female and of the same HLA type as their existing child, who needed an HLA-matched donor for bone marrow transplantation. At the time, the genetic diagnosis clinic in question was able to offer prenatal gender diagnosis to couples who had a child suffering from a serious X-linked genetic abnormality such as Wiskott–Aldrich syndrome, but they would not offer sex selection on any other grounds. After a careful and ethically informed debate the clinic decided that prenatal HLA typing would be incompatible with their indications at the time for amniocentesis and termination of an unwanted fetus.

Positive embryo selection can now be performed by means of a technique known as preimplantation genetic diagnosis (PGD). It is a technically complicated and expensive technique with a limited success rate, which involves the creation of a number of embryos by IVF, extracting a nucleus and performing DNA analysis by PCR for each. Suitable embryos are chosen to be placed into the woman and others are discarded, thus obviating the need for termination of an unsuitable fetus. The first successful SCT of this kind for Fanconi anemia was reported by Wolf et al in 2001.[44] In 2004, the HFEA granted a license to an IVF clinic in the UK, permitting this technique to be used to assist a family to conceive a baby who would be a tissue match for their son, who suffered from Diamond–Blackfan anemia. This baby was born in July 2005 and cord blood stem cells were collected.[45,46]

It is of interest to examine the reasons why opinion seems to have changed since 1989, when it was considered unethical in the USA to create a savior sibling for a child with Wiskott–Aldrich syndrome and yet, by 2001, it was deemed ethical for a child with Fanconi anemia. One also has to ask why, by 2004, HFEA held that it would be both legal and ethical for an IVF clinic to attempt to create an HLA-matched baby by PGD to 'save' an older sibling with a condition such as Diamond–Blackfan anemia.[7] Could it be that the newer techniques have changed the ethics of the situation? The debate now is whether positive embryo selection following PGD and HLA typing, which cannot be of any medical benefit to those embryos selected, is a step too far down the slippery slope towards trivial or frivolous criteria for the selection of a so-called designer baby.

This is an area of reproductive technology which is heavily regulated by the HFEA in the UK. Section 3 of the Human Fertilization and Embryology Act 1990 states that 'no person shall bring about the creation of an embryo, or keep or use an embryo, except in pursuance of a licence'.[49] The HFEA was challenged in 2001, soon after PGD for HLA typing became available to couples, by two important test cases. The first was the Hashmi family, who had a son with thalassemia major, and the second was the Whitaker family who had a son with Diamond–Blackfan anemia. The courts at the time determined that the Hashmis were permitted to attempt to create a savior sibling, free of thalassemia and of the correct tissue type for their son, but subsequently they have been unable to achieve this desired result. On the other hand, the Whitakers were denied treatment in the UK but, paradoxically, succeeded in obtaining treatment in Chicago, and their son has been treated with stem cells from his brother's cord blood. Not surprisingly, both decisions have proved to be controversial. The HFEA's decision to license PGD and HLA typing in the case of the Hashmi family was challenged in the courts by Josephine Quintavalle on behalf of CORE (a pro-life organization) and the final appeal decision in the House of Lords[48] held that the HFEA had lawfully licensed the PGD procedure under the terms of Schedule 2 of the Human Fertilization and Embryology Act 1990, which says that 'practices designed to secure that embryos are in a suitable condition to be placed in a woman ought to determine whether embryos are suitable to that purpose'.[47] This particular interpretation of the Act, drafted as it was when the issues concerning embryo selection by HLA typing could not been anticipated, has been criticized.

The regulation of PGD for HLA typing by the HFEA has come in for criticism and, in particular, some jurists have considered their distinction between the cases of Hashmi and Whitaker to be unjustifiable and misguided.[49] The UK is compared to Canada by Nelson,[50] and Gitter compares the UK with the USA,[51] the three jurisdictions having different approaches to PGD regulation. It is not the intention here to discuss the issue of discarding four or more healthy embryos of the wrong HLA type for every one of the right HLA type but, at a symposium in Stanford in 2004, Hudson expressed the view that the national debate about technologies like PGD in the USA is 'stunted because it is currently cast in the same terms as the debate over abortion rights'.[52]

A criticism of the use of PGD with tissue typing is that 'it is treating the offspring to be born as a commodity', a description attributed to Winston, a pioneer in the field and co-author of the first description of PGD in the *Lancet* in 1989.[53] Winston has also drawn attention to the possibility that a donor sibling might face 'the spectre of being born for someone else's benefit throughout his whole life'.[54] These concerns are well expressed in this quotation from the team in Minnesota who reported the first successful savior sibling SCT in Fanconi anemia following PGD tissue typing:

Children conceived to be HLA matched face the possibility of donation throughout their lives. The initial cord blood donation could fail for any of several reasons: inadequate cord blood cell dose, graft failure after cord blood transplant, or the recipient child experiencing a recurrence of leukemia after transplantation. If the cord blood transplant fails, the next step is bone marrow harvest and transplant. This, too, might not engraft or leukemia may recur, requiring yet another bone marrow transplant. Further, once an HLA-matched donor is created, the need for tissues beyond bone marrow may arise. Indeed, after bone marrow transplant, toxicities related to chemotherapy and irradiation or immunosuppressive drugs could produce organ failure involving the kidneys, liver, or other organs. Then the question would arise of whether to harvest a solid organ from the donor child. The HLA-matched child created in the Nash case has thus far escaped further need for tissue or organs by his sister. However, he is quite young. He and all children created as donors face the potential of requests for donation throughout their lives.

Wolf et al go on to propose a system of nine safeguards to protect children conceived by means of PGD from serving as perpetual donors.[44]

This theme is also taken up by Jody Picoult in her novel *My sister's keeper*[32] and the events she describes are within the bounds of possibility. The savior sibling in her book is repeatedly called upon, after the initial donation of cord blood, to provide blood transfusions and bone marrow stem cells and to undergo peripheral blood cell separation procedures until, at the age of 12, she exerts her teenage autonomy when volunteered again by her mother, this time to be a kidney donor for her sister. The girl maintains that she never would have consented to any of the earlier procedures, if anyone had taken the trouble to explain the possible implications to her; she was angry that her mother had taken her altruism for granted and had simply used her body as a spare-part factory in the repeated attempts to save her older sister's life.

The HFEA were sensitive to this issue when granting a license to the clinic treating the Hashmi family in 2001, because they hoped to be able to limit the donation of stem cells, after the birth of any savior baby, to cord blood collection only. It was later held that this proscription was outside the jurisdiction of the HFEA, which is only charged with the regulation of fertility and the creation of embryos.[7] The best interests of any savior sibling created would have to be a matter of judgment by the appropriate person or the court, when and if that time should come. As events transpired, Mr and Mrs Hashmi eventually had to abandon hope of creating an HLA-matched child after six IVF cycles; this is a tragedy after all their efforts to create a savior sibling and highlights the limited ultimate success rate of PGD for HLA typing. Their son continues to be treated conventionally with red cell transfusion and iron chelation therapy. Winston is well aware of the frustrations that accompany IVF and warns that the combination of 'patient desperation, medical hubris and commercial pressures' can lead to unethical decision making about the use of reproductive technologies.[55]

Most commentators do not accept that a savior sibling would be a means to an end and it has been pointed out that Immanuel Kant's famous dictum was 'never use a person *solely* as a means'.[56] The prevailing view of contemporary consequentialist moral philosophers is that, as very little harm is likely to arise from PGD and as the sick sibling stands to gain a great deal, this, when taken in conjunction with the power of procreative rights, 'trumps' any possible adverse consequences to the donor baby. Boyle & Savulescu summarize: 'we must avoid the trap of interfering with individual liberty by preventing such procedures for no good reason, simply out of the "genophobia" that grips much of society today'.[9] Bellamy, in taking a deontologic stance, nevertheless concludes that the technique 'would not involve unacceptable commodification, instrumentality or psychologic damage to the resulting child'. He regards the reactive nature of a couple's request for embryo selection, born of medical necessity and a compassionate desire to heal a seriously ill child, and distinguishes it from the alternative proactive parental request for a 'designer baby' resulting from whim.[57]

Stem cell recipients

In some respects, hematopoietic SCT is just like any other high-risk medical procedure for which a competent adult patient is required to give valid consent. Before the physician seeks the consent of the patient to undergo the procedure, a medical decision-making process needs to be undertaken. Seldom is an allogeneic SCT the only form of treatment that can be offered and sometimes there is doubt as to whether this form of treatment will prove to be any more successful than an alternative that would not involve a third party having to make a donation of living issue. The transplant-related morbidity and mortality (TRM) is often greater than that resulting from non-myeloablative chemotherapy, or SCT that utilizes autologous stem cells to achieve marrow reconstitution. There are multiple 'trade-offs' in the risk–benefit equation.

It is an unfortunate fact that, in some quarters, SCT has acquired a reputation for being extremely potent and therefore a most desirable treatment, or a panacea perhaps, for life-threatening disease. This, of course, may or may not be the case in a given clinical situation, but has resulted in SCT acquiring celebrity status as the ultimate treatment that everyone should aspire to if they are able to afford it; it is not unknown for patients to think they are being given second-rate treatment if SCT is not served up on the therapeutic menu. It may well have been necessary for the early pioneering SC transplanters to elevate their product into this position in order to persuade patients to take risks, but even if this was once the case, it is argued that such considerations should no longer apply and the medical profession should play its part in educating the public and the media, in order to reduce the hype and spin associated with the whole SCT scene. The prudent patient in the 21st century wants and deserves the truth from healthcare professionals, if he is to make an informed, autonomous choice for himself without coercion.

The indications for allogeneic SCT in different disease settings have been addressed elsewhere in this book. Where there is a graft-versus-disease effect, the magnitude of this benefit will often outweigh the risks of TRM and result in better disease-free and overall survival rates than conventional chemotherapy alone or high-dose chemotherapy with autologous stem cell rescue. Chronic myeloid leukemia (CML) is an example of a disease where the best available medical treatment has been constantly evolving and changing. At one point in the evolution of treatment for CML, SCT was regarded as the most effective treatment for a younger patient with a matched sibling donor. However, the development of novel molecular therapies has now relegated SCT into second place (see Chapter 4).

CML may be taken as a model for the kind of complex and difficult medical decision making which is required before seeking the consent of the patient to undergo an SCT procedure. For example, consider the therapeutic dilemma that existed in the pre-Glivec era, when a 50-year-old presented in chronic phase with no sibling donor and for whom only a one haplotype-mismatched, CMV-positive unrelated donor could be identified after an international search of donor panels. Some physicians in the 1990s would have offered an allograft, and others would not. Some physicians might have held a conference with their colleagues before reaching a decision and some might have referred for a second opinion. Yet others might have felt it appropriate to take into account non-clinical criteria such as bed pressures, private insurance funding or state funding priorities in making their decision.

One ethical decision-making process that many bone marrow transplant units adopt is for the attending physician to lead a discussion and make the case for SCT for an individual patient at an in-house conference of expert peers. An objective evidence-based recommendation will then hopefully emerge and the reasoned decision can be minuted in the hospital record. The patient himself would have been told in advance that a conference of experts would convene to decide whether SCT should be seriously considered as an option, after a consensus had been reached about the relative risks and benefits and, hence, the advisability of the procedure. An appeal mechanism, possibly in a different forum or at another hospital, should exist for patients who are unwilling to accept the recommendation of the transplant committee.

It is argued that this approach goes some way to eliminate individual physician bias; critics might say that this kind of democratic medical decision making may be fair, just and ethical but would stifle the individual transplanter from making further progress – the argument that is heard is 'we didn't get where we are today by denying patients access to experimental and risky procedures'. This can be countered by commenting that as long as there is a clear demarcation between the experimental and established use of SCT, then there is no objection to a competent adult patient agreeing altruistically to please his physician and possibly to benefit others by consenting to undergo

an experimental medical procedure that might benefit others in the future. If, for example, the procedure is expected to carry a 40% risk of TRM, a 50% risk of failing to eradicate the underlying disease, and no more than a 10% chance of producing a cure, the patient should be told these facts. If such a procedure is not one that all specialists would recommend or if it is novel or experimental, the attending physician must say so, and if the experimental procedure is not part of an approved clinical trial there must be a rationale approved by the institutional research ethics committee for this kind of 'compassionate' use of an unpleasant medical procedure, which would be of dubious benefit to the patient himself.

Resource issues

Resource issues per se are not ethical or legal considerations, but when a patient or a group of patients is denied medical treatment on the grounds of poor cost-effectiveness, the aggrieved party is likely to have recourse to law in an attempt to reverse a decision made by a doctor, an insurance company or a public body vested with the task of rationing healthcare. Snyder defines the challenges faced by those who deliver treatment and ration healthcare: 'The ethical principle of justice requires caregivers and insurers to provide potentially life-saving, yet high-risk, procedures to HCT candidates in an open and equitable manner'.[58]

A study reported in 1997 that there are inequalities of access to bone marrow transplantation for leukemia and lymphoma in the USA. Americans of Afro-Caribbean origin, those covered by Medicaid and self-paying patients were less likely to receive a SCT than insured patients.[59]

In a world where medical resources are increasingly rationed, how should private insurance companies and public healthcare funding bodies operate in an open and equitable manner? Should they have standard, universal operating procedures that can be applied to all SCT candidates? SCT is a very expensive treatment if the patient is unlucky enough to suffer complications such as infection, rejection or GvHD. The indications for SCT can be controversial in the sense that the interpretation of risk–benefit ratio and cost–benefit ratio may not neatly tally up and they are likely to depend on the perspective of the adjudicator. There are several stakeholders: the patient and their family, the donor, the healthcare professionals, the hospital managers and either the private insurer or the state. Various state-regulated rationing systems are in operation. The current arrangement in the UK is that the Department of Health is centrally informed by National Institute for Clinical Excellence (NICE) guidelines[60] and decision making is then devolved down to be locally administered by primary care trusts (PCTs), who have to consider all competing health needs within a local community; this may result in funding variations between PCTs, which is sometimes popularly referred to as a 'post-code lottery'. An individual or a group action, appealing against a PCT decision, will generally take the format of judicial review, a legal process that declares on the legality of a local decision to refuse to fund treatment by means of a detailed examination of the process adopted by the public body in terms of fairness, proportionality and procedural propriety.

Where SCT is only one of a number of available treatment options, the alternatives may carry risk–benefit coefficients that vary over time and may be difficult for the hematologist to weigh in the balance when advising the recipient patient. For example, in the treatment of childhood AML in first remission, the improved results of chemotherapy in the 1990s meant that SCT was no longer the treatment of choice for the majority of patients. In a number of life-threatening diseases where SCT is a contender as a treatment option, the superiority of SCT over the alternatives will not have been established by the available evidence. Doctors and the institutions with which they are associated will tend to polarize into two camps – those who do and those who do not advocate SCT for the particular condition of the patient. If the indication is uncertain, in an ideal world, there should be a research protocol in the treating institution, which would have been scrutinized by an ethics committee, and the consent procedure would make the experimental nature of the proposed treatment clear to the patient.

Conclusion

The world of SCT is constantly evolving; the technology is changing, the indications and contraindications become modified and yesterday's experimental treatment might be adopted as mainstream treatment tomorrow or could just as well become virtually redundant and replaced by a new targeted molecular therapy, as happened with Glivec for CML a few years ago. It is hard enough for medical practitioners working in the field to keep up to date and very difficult for the public, the media and the internet to portray a balanced view of a multifaceted and complex array of competing treatments. It is a major concern that media spin and hype might cloud the issues for the two people at the center of any SCT: the donor and the recipient. Both these persons require clear information presented orally and in writing which is appropriate to their level of understanding; too much information can obscure the truth as much, if not more, than judicious explanation of the salient facts. There is a paradox that the unrelated donor is afforded greater respect and privacy, as a result of tight regulation of donor stem cell banking procedures, than is a sibling who may be a potential donor. Minors and persons lacking the capacity to consent are excluded as unrelated donors, but very often provide the best HLA match within a family.

The birth of modern bio-ethics in the 1960s produced an explosion of rhetoric proclaiming an unalienable right of autonomy for patients, and decried paternalism and coercion by healthcare professionals. For a while, there was a backlash from a reactionary medical profession against this new breed of medical ethicists. However, at the time, public opinion was ready to embrace the concept of self-determination in many different areas of life, and the tide of support for medical paternalism gradually dwindled. Most medical practitioners would now agree that the patient should determine what he wants to know. The physician should be a partner in this process and the information imparted should be sufficient for the resulting consent to be valid. It does not matter whether a particular jurisdiction has tightly regulated procedures for obtaining consent for organ or tissue donation, because the essence of consent to medical procedures is to be an expression of ethical respect for persons and constructed on the three pillars of capacity, sufficient information and voluntariness.

References

1. Horowitz MM, Confer DL. Evaluation of hematopoietic stem cell donors. Hematology Am Soc Hematol Educ Program 2005;469–475
2. Rosenmayr A, Hartwell L, Egeland T, on behalf of the Ethics Working Group of the World Marrow Donor Association. Informed consent – suggested procedures for informed consent for unrelated hematopoietic stem cell donors at various stages of recruitment, donor evaluation, and donor workup. Bone Marrow Transplant 2003;31:539–545
3. Zink S, Wertlieb SL. Forced altruism is not altruism. Am J Bioethics 2004;4:29–31
4. Human Tissue Act 2004. www.opsi.gov.uk/acts/acts2004/pdf/ukpga_20040030_en.pdf
5. Mental Capacity Act 2005. www.opsi.gov.uk/acts/acts2005/pdf/ukpga_20050009_en.pdf
6. Delany L, Month S, Savulescu J et al. Altruism by proxy: volunteering children for bone marrow donation. BMJ 1996;312:240–243
7. HFEA. Preimplantation tissue typing, 2004. www.hfea.gov.uk/cps/rde/xbcr/SID-3F57D79B-9129F1E3/hfea/PreimplantationReport.pdf
8. Holm S. Ethical issues in pre-implantation genetic diagnosis. In: Holm S, Harris J (eds) The future of human reproduction: ethics, choice and regulation. Clarendon Press, Oxford, 1998
9. Boyle RJ, Savulescu J. Ethics of using preimplantation genetic diagnosis to select a stem cell donor for an existing person. BMJ 2001;323:1240–1243
10. Sheldon S, Wilkinson S. Should selecting saviour siblings be banned? J Med Ethics 2004;30:533–537
11. Brownsword R. Reproductive opportunities and regulatory challenges. Modern Law Rev 2004;67:304–321
12. Scott R. Choosing between possible lives: legal and ethical issues in preimplantation genetic diagnosis. Oxf J Legal Stud 2006;26:153–178
13. Department of Health. Reference guide to consent for examination and treatment. Department of Health, 2001.www.dh.gov.uk/policyandguidance/healthandsocialcaretopics/consent/consentgeneralinformation/
14. Schloendorff v New York Hospital (1914) 105 NE 92
15. Sidaway v Board of Governors of the Bethlem Royal Hospital and the Maudsley Hospital [1985] 1 All ER 1018
16. O'Neill O. BBC Radio 4 Reith Lectures 2002. A Question of Trust. www.bbc.co.uk
17. Jones MA. Informed consent and other fairy stories. Med Law Rev 1999;7:103–134
18. Re T (Adult: Refusal of Treatment) [1992] 4 All ER 649
19. General Medical Council. Seeking patient's consent: the ethical considerations. General Medical Council, 1998. www.gmc-uk.org/guidance/current/library/consent.asp
20. Treleaven J, Cullis JO, Maynard R et al. British Committee for Standards in Haematology. Obtaining consent for chemotherapy Br J Haematol 2006;132:552–559
21. Goldman JM, for the Executive Committee of the World Marrow Donor Association. Special report: bone marrow transplants using volunteer donors – recommendations and requirements for a standardized practice throughout the world – 1994 update. Blood 1994;84:2833–2839
22. Cleaver SA, Warren P, Kern M et al. Donor work-up and transport of bone marrow. Recommendations and requirements for a standardized practice throughout the world from the Donor Registries and Quality Assurance Working Groups of the World Marrow Donor Association (WMDA). Bone Marrow Transplant 1997;20:621–629
23. Bakken R, van Walraven A, Egeland T, for the Ethics Working Group of the World Marrow Donor Association. Donor commitment and patient needs. Bone Marrow Transplant 2004;33:225–230
24. Davies S. Bone marrow transplant raises issues of privacy. BMJ 1997;314:1356
25. Re MB (Caesarean Section) [1997] 38 BMLR 175
26. Beauchamp T, Childress J. Principles of biomedical ethics, 5th edn. Oxford University Press, Oxford, 2001:178
27. Re Y (Mental Patient: Bone Marrow Donation) [1996] 2 FLR 787
28. Brazier M, Cave E (eds). Medicine, patients and the law, 4th edn. Penguin, London,2007:455
29. Bone Marrow Donation. Chapter 6 in Code of Practice – Consent. The Human Tissue Act 2004. www.hta.gov.uk/_db/_documents/2006-07-04_Approved_by_Parliament_-_Code_of_Practice_1_._Consent.pdf
30. Gillick v West Norfolk & Wisbech AHA [1986] AC 112
31. Re W (A Minor)(Medical Treatment) [1992] 4 All ER 627
32. Picoult J. My sister's keeper. Hodder and Stoughton, London, 2004
33. Department of Health. Using children lacking capacity as bone marrow donors. In: Reference guide to consent for examination and treatment. Department of Health, 2001. www.dh.gov.uk/policyandguidance/healthandsocialcaretopics/consent/consentgeneralinformation/
34. Serota F, August CS, O'Shea AT et al. Role of a child advocate in the selection of donors for pediatric bone marrow transplantation. J Pediatr 1981;98:847–850
35. Chan K-W, Gajewski JL, Supkis D et al. Use of minors as bone marrow donors: current attitude and management. J Pediatr 1996;128:644–648
36. Holm S. The child as organ and tissue donor: discussions in the Danish Council of Ethics. Cam Q Healthcare Ethics 2004;13:156–160
37. Sheldon S. Children as organ donors: a persistent ethical issue. Cam Q Healthcare Ethics 2004;13:119–122
38. Levine MD, Camitta M, Nathan D, Curran WJ. The medical ethics of bone marrow transplantation in childhood. J Pediatrics 1975;86:145
39. Fleck LM. Children and organ donation: some cautionary remarks. Cam Q Healthcare Ethics 2004;13:161–166
40. Pentz RD, Chan K-W, Neumann JL et al. Designing an ethical policy for bone marrow donation by minors and others lacking capacity. Cam Q Healthcare Ethics 2004;13:149–155
41. Arenson EB Jr, Fotbe MD. Bone marrow transplantation for acute leukemia and Down syndrome: report of a successful case and results of a national survey. J Pediatr 1989;114(l):69–72
42. Singer P. Rethinking life and death. The collapse of our traditional ethics.. Oxford University Press, Oxford, 1995
43. Clark RD, Fletcher J, Peterson G. Conceiving a fetus for bone marrow transplantation: an ethical problem in prenatal diagnosis. Prenatal Diagn 1989;9:329–334
44. Wolf SM, Kahn JP, Wagner JE. Using preimplantation genetic diagnosis to create a stem cell donor: issues, guidelines and limits. J Med Ethics 2003;31:327
45. Designer baby gets go-ahead. Daily Mail, September 7, 2004
46. Designed for life. Daily Mail, July 16, 2005
47. Human Fertilization and Embryology Act 1990. www.opsi.gov.uk/acts/acts1990/Ukpga_19900037_en_1.htm
48. Quintavalle v Human Fertilization and Embryology Authority [2005] UKHL 28
49. Sheldon S, Wilkinson S. Hashmi and Whitaker: an unjustifiable and misguided distinction. Med Law Rev 2004;12:137–163
50. Nelson EL. Comparative perspectives: regulating preimplantation genetic diagnosis in Canada and the United Kingdom. Fertil Steril 2006;6:1646–1652
51. Gitter DM. Am I my brother's keeper? The use of preimplantation genetic diagnosis to create a donor of transplantable stem cells for an older sibling suffering from a genetic disorder. Geo Mason Law Rev 2006;13:975–1035
52. Hudson KL. Pre-implantation genetic diagnosis: public policy and public attitudes. Fertil Steril 2006;6:1638–1645
53. Handyside AH, Pattinson JK, Penketh RJ et al. Biopsy of human preimplantation embryos and sexing by DNA amplification. Lancet 1989;1:347–349

54. Boseley S. As the age of the saviour sibling dawns, pressure mounts inexorably to change embryo rules. Guardian, June 20, 2003

55. Winston RML, Hardy K. Are we ignoring potential dangers of in vitro fertilization and related treatments? Nat Cell Biol 2002;4(suppl):S14–S18

56. Alghrani A, Harris J. Reproductive liberty: should the foundation of families be regulated? Child Fam Law Q 2006;18:191

57. Bellamy S. Lives to save lives – the ethics of tissue typing. Hum Fertil 2005;8: 5–11

58. Snyder DS. Ethical issues in hematopoietic cell transplantation. In: Blume KG, Forman SJ, Applebaum FR (eds) Thomas's hematopoietic cell transplantation, 3rd edn. Blackwell, Massachusetts, 2004:488–496

59. Mitchell JM, Meehan KR, Kong J, Schulman K. Access to bone marrow transplantation for leukemia and lymphoma: the role of sociodemographic factors. J Clin Oncol 1997;15:2644–2651

60. National Institute for Clinical Excellence. Improving outcomes in haematological cancers. National Institute for Clinical Excellence, 2003. www.nice.org.uk

How to build and use a stem cell transplant database

Bipin N Savani and A John Barrett

Data collection essentials

A stem cell transplant database is an essential component of the transplant unit. As well as the requirement for reporting data to international transplant registries such as the European Group for Blood and Marrow Transplantation (EBMT) and the Center for International Blood and Marrow Transplant Research (CIBMTR) (see Chapter 50), data may be needed locally for purposes of budgeting and local review board oversight. Furthermore, transplant teams have a responsibility to collect data on their patients for quality control and identification of complications that require remedial action. Whether or not patients are entered into formal transplant trials, outcomes following modification to transplant protocols must be documented to ensure that outcome and survival data are within the anticipated ranges. As with any database, however, the accuracy of the data has to be close to perfect for valid conclusions to be drawn from the results. The key features of a functional database are itemized below.

Consecutive reporting

A transplant series has to be complete to avoid selection bias. Any patient who receives a transplant must be assigned a unique patient number (UPN) whether they succumb within a few days or become a long-term survivor. It may also be useful to record separately data on all patients screened for transplant with an explanation of why they were not transplanted.

Comprehensive documentation of essential data

The database should contain a minimum of three data categories:
- patient and donor characteristics
- transplant details
- outcomes.

Electronic spreadsheets are invaluable because more variables can be added successively to the basic set. It is better to create a complete database of a small number of essential variables than to attempt to be comprehensive and create an incomplete and patchy database. A suggested list of essential transplant data is given in Table 49.1.

Regular data entry by dedicated personnel

A transplant database is never static; not only are new patients continually being added to the list, but new events occur all the time requiring documentation by a specific date. The easiest time to enter data is when an event has just occurred. This avoids the need to track back in the medical records to identify when a complication such as graft-versus-host disease (GvHD) was first identified. Data entry should be performed by a small group of competent individuals whose dedicated task is to regularly add data to the database, ideally at least weekly. This implies that several data access points are available. Team members should be discouraged from establishing their own mini databases – there should be only one data source for the unit. Also, data entry personnel should be discouraged from collecting values on paper and transcribing them in a second step to the database, because this increases the risk of error in translation.

Acquisition of electronic data

Where possible, numerical data such as laboratory results should be downloaded electronically directly onto the transplant database without any intermediary.

Consistency of nomenclature

A single format must be agreed upon to avoid confusion. Data entry staff should have access to guidelines such as those set out by the CIBMTR which assure consistency of reporting of diagnostic subtypes, GvHD grading, etc.

Database manager

One individual should have overall responsibility for managing the database and troubleshooting problems with data entry.

Security

For protection of patient confidentiality the database should be password protected and accessible only by a few identified individuals. Only data entry personnel and the data manager should be able to change or add new data to avoid corruption of the database.

Using spreadsheets

Excel is an ideal spreadsheet – easy to use, easy to expand, downloadable into statistical software and universally available. Descriptive entries should be avoided in favor of categoric descriptions. Descriptive data should be broken down into a series of specific features and assigned a yes (1) or no (0) score. Dates should follow a single format (e.g. MM/DD/YYYY). Spreadsheets can be readily used to calculate days between dates and derive the often-required 'days post transplant' information.

Table 49.1 Important transplantation variables list for datasheet

Baseline data	Chronic GvHD organs involved/severity for each organ system, date of onset
UPN	Disease relapse
Name	Death, cause of death (eg relapse/non-relapse mortality)
Date of birth	CMV reactivation date of each positive result
Sex	Immunosuppression start/stop, agents used
Pretransplant weight	Donor lymphocyte infusions (dates, dose, indication)
Protocol #	*Day 100 disease assessment* (blood, BM, cytogenetics, molecular studies, chimerism)
Diagnosis, disease subcategory, risk category molecular studies, cytogenetics	**Long-term follow-up**
Disease status immediately prior to transplant (remission, active, primary refractory, relapsing refractory, others)	Weight
Patient co-morbidities	Chronic GvHD by organ system and grade
Blood count, chemistry profile	Tests for residual disease (e.g. cytogenetics, molecular studies)
Pulmonary function tests	Chimerism
Donor name/number, relationship, sex, date of birth	Routine labs (blood count, chemistry profile)
HLA typing – patient and donor, degree of match	Quantitative immunoglobulin levels
Blood group (patient, donor)	Viral serology (hepatitis A, B, C)
CMV status (patient, donor)	Endocrine: thyroid function tests; antithyroid and thyroglobulin panels
Hepatitis serology (patient, donor)	Adrenal function tests (screening with cortisol levels and further work-up as indicated)
Transplant variables	Gonadal functions (estradiol, testosterone, LH, FSH, semen analysis, etc.)
Conditioning regimen details	Gynecologic exam
Stem cell source (marrow/blood/cord blood) and manipulations (T-cell depletion, etc.)	Dental examination
CD34 dose	Ophthalmologic examinations
CD3 dose	Pulmonary function
Post transplant	Cardiac function (EKG, echocardiogram, etc.)
Toxicities (mucositis, febrile neutropenia, renal, liver, cardiac, pulmonary, etc.)	Lipid profile
Engraftment day for neutrophils and platelets (date)	Radiology (CXR, CT chests and disease evaluation as indicated)
Duration of hospitalization (date discharge, hospital days in first 100 days)	Bone density scan
Graft failure – date of onset	Screening for second malignancies (skin, prostate, genitourinary, breast, oral cavity, etc.)
Acute GvHD organ/tissue, grade, date of onset, date of peak severity	Quality of life evaluations

Using the database to describe transplant data

Competence in these areas should make it possible for the reader to prepare and analyze standard transplant data for publication. For more sophisticated transplantation statistics the reader is referred to Klein et al.[1,2]

The process of data analysis involves four steps:

1. assembling and verifying data
2. presentation of descriptive data – patient, donor and transplant characteristics, selection of variables
3. descriptive outcome analysis – the actuarial survival, relapse, GvHD, non-relapse mortality (NRM), etc.
4. statistical comparisons of outcome between groups and identification of risk factors by univariate and multivariate analysis (Fig. 49.1).

Assembling and verifying data

The importance of defining the dataset and validating data entries before beginning an analysis cannot be overemphasized. The first issue is to decide what patient cohort will be studied (e.g. all human leukocyte antigen (HLA)-identical sibling transplants or all HLA-identical matched and mismatched transplants? Single disease entities? The last 5 years' transplants?). Will there be any exclusions (e.g. identical twin transplants, mismatched transplants, patients receiving a unique conditioning regimen)? Use the spreadsheet ranking function to identify extreme values and check that they are correct and not numerical errors. Similarly with days from transplant, errors can show up as negative values. Some values such as laboratory results transferred electronically will be more reliable than those requiring clinical judgment such as the date of onset and severity grading of GvHD. Missing values should be sought and entered. If an accurate date is not available it may be possible to substitute the 15th day of the month in question. Once the database is assembled and analyses begun, it is tedious to have to go back and enter more data and rerun the analysis. Therefore, time taken in optimizing the dataset is well rewarded.

Presentation of descriptive data

A review of publications of stem cell transplant data in specialist journals gives the best idea of how to present the key data describing the patient group under study. Examples are given in Tables 49.2 and

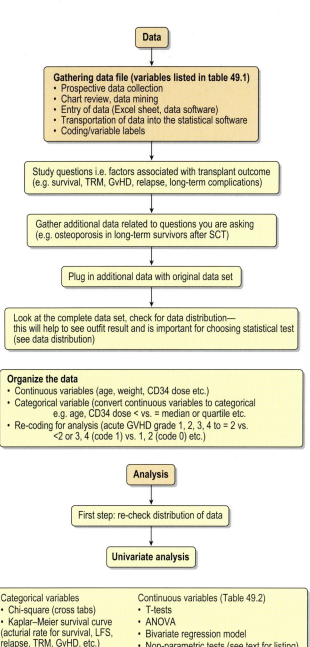

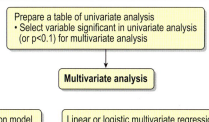

Figure 49.1
Basic steps in outcome analysis of transplant database.

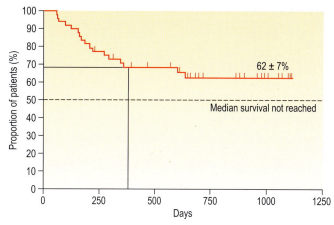

Figure 49.2
An example of an actuarial survival curve.

49.3. Continuous variables can be presented as median and range (e.g. median age and range), discontinuous variables as numbers and percent (e.g. number of male and number of female patients).

Calculating actuarial outcomes and drawing survival curves

A complete description of transplant outcome requires some form of actuarial analysis. Simply put, actuarial analysis takes care of the problem that a transplant series includes some patients who have reached one of the major endpoints (such as relapse, GvHD, transplant-related mortality) and others who have not experienced the endpoint but are still at future risk of an endpoint occurrence.

For example (Fig. 49.2), a series of 50 patients transplanted between 02/2004 and 10/2006 are analyzed for survival. Seventeen patients have died 56, 60, 64, 97, 121, 153, 159, 167, 183, 206, 208, 272, 293, 345, 357, 602 and 637 days after their transplant. The percentage survival for the series is 66% but this is not the figure that best describes the situation, because we know that if some patients died 1 year or more post transplant and there are patients in the series transplanted less than 1 year ago, the latter are still at risk from dying, and the percentage of patients dying is likely to continue to rise as time goes on. Actuarial survival, as used by insurance companies, examines survivorship at fixed data points, while the Kaplan–Meier analysis (the usual method applied to transplant data)[3] recalculates the probability of an event (e.g. survival) at each occurrence of the event according to the number of evaluable individuals who have reached that timepoint. For small patient series actuarial survival can be calculated, but a variety of software can rapidly perform these iterative calculations. In our examples using SPSS software, actuarial survival of the group is 62 ± 7%.

A complete description of an actuarial survival curve also includes confidence limits. Since the actuarial outcome at any moment is only a probability and not a definite figure, it is subject to variability due to chance. The right-hand end of the curve has greater variability because the number of individuals who have reached that timepoint is less. A complete description of a survival curve includes standard errors of the estimated survival function calculated using Greenwood's formula (available on most statistical software). At each relapse timepoint the percentage of relapsed patients is calculated for the number of survivors at that timepoint.[4] The median survival time, the timepoint which half the patients have reached, also adds a useful description of the maturity of the dataset. In our example the median survival is not yet reached (see Fig. 49.2).

Table 49.2 Selecting a test for non-actuarial data analysis

Query	Test	Type	Independent variable	Dependent variable
If 2 means are different	t-test	Independent Paired	1 categoric 2 levels	1 continuous
If means are different	ANOVA	Between subjects Within subjects	1 or more categoric 2 or more levels	1 continuous
If means are different	Mann–Whitney U	Between subjects	1 categoric 2 levels	1 ordinal (ranked)
If the observed frequencies (or proportions) same as expected	Chi-square	Goodness of fit	1 categoric	1 or more categoric
If the observed frequencies (or proportions) same for each group		Test of independence	2 or more levels	2 levels
If the frequencies (or proportions) same for each group	Fisher's exact	Between subjects	1 categoric 2 levels	1 categoric 2 levels
Whether variables related	Correlation	Pearson r Spearman rho	1 continuous 1 ordinal (ranked)	1 continuous 1 ordinal (ranked)
Variable independently predicting outcome	Regression	Linear Logistic	1 or more continuous or dichotomous 1 or more continuous or dichotomous	1 continuous 1 categoric 2 or more levels

Calculating actuarial probability of non-relapse mortality

The investigator must be clear at the outset whether this outcome will include all deaths not due to relapse (non-relapse mortality, NRM) or deaths due to transplant-related causes (transplant-related mortality, TRM). The former is clearly an unambiguous measure including deaths from all causes. The TRM, while commonly used, is subject to interpretative bias and may misrepresent outcome in, for example, older patient series where there is a significant contribution to mortality from co-morbidities. Here, the issue becomes whether the death was due entirely to co-morbidity (e.g. heart failure) or whether the transplant process precipitated the mortality. If a patient dies in an accident and had developed cataracts due to the conditioning regimen, can we simply dismiss the death as accidental (NRM) or was it due to the transplant (TRM)? Unless deaths in a transplant series can be unambiguously attributed only to relapse or transplant, the NRM is the safest measure to apply.

Calculating TRM and NRM requires Kaplan–Meier (KM) statistics. At each timepoint when a patient dies from TRM the calculation is made of the proportion of dead patients in the existing population at that timepoint. Patients who die from relapse before that timepoint do not contribute to the survival calculation – they are 'censored' at the time of last follow-up or death from relapse but no survival calculation is performed at the timepoint of their death. Similarly, if TRM is being calculated, patients who die from any cause that is not transplant related will be censored. Thus, the KM plot describes a probability for occurrence of only one event out of a series of competing events.

Calculating actuarial probability of GvHD

A similar approach is made for calculating the incidence of GvHD. Since acute GvHD occurs early after transplant when survival typically falls off rapidly, there is often a wide discrepancy between calculating the percentage of patients developing acute GvHD and the actuarial probability of developing GvHD. For example, in a series of 100 patients, the 100-day mortality was 30%. Acute GvHD grade II or more occurred in 50. The percentage of the cohort developing acute GvHD is 20%, but because patients may have died before developing GvHD, the actuarial incidence is going to be higher than 20% and could be as high as 27% ($100/70 \times 20\%$) if every patient destined to develop GvHD died before developing it. Another competing factor is graft failure – rejection and GvHD are (usually) mutually exclusive. Thus, a transplant series where a large proportion of patients reject the graft is likely to have a low incidence of GvHD. Data are best calculated only for engrafted patients.

Accurate description of GvHD incidence and severity is dogged by many inherent problems: diagnosis of GvHD onset is notoriously inaccurate, a patient may develop a rash which goes unnoticed for several days, and despite well-described grading criteria there is much subjective variation. Time to maximum GvHD severity is needed to calculate probabilities of specific grades of GvHD, but these dates can be complicated by the challenge of trying to compare, for example, two successive episodes of GvHD and correctly ascribing the data to the more severe occurrence. In calculating chronic GvHD which typically occurs beyond 100 days from transplant, the patients dying from TRM or relapse do not contribute to the actuarial chronic GvHD probability. A landmark analysis (using day 100 or the first occurrence of chronic GvHD) can be performed in this situation, calculating actuarial GvHD risk only for the cohort surviving beyond the landmark.

Calculating actuarial probability of relapse

The KM estimate of relapse is performed by censoring deaths and time of last follow-up of non-relapsed patients and performing the actuarial calculation at each timepoint an individual develops relapse. Problems with relapse calculation stem from the difficulty of defining precisely the moment of relapse; for example, the platelet count begins to fall 3 weeks before a bone marrow aspirate identifies relapse, but had the marrow been examined sooner, the relapse would have been diagnosed days to weeks earlier. Another related problem stems from the fact that relapses, for example in CML, cover five types of event (molecular, karyotypic, hematologic chronic phase, transformation to accelerated or blastic phase), each with different implications for treatment and survival. Furthermore, how should we handle patients who have had a relapse and have been successfully treated with imatinib or donor lymphocyte infusions (DLI), and are surviving disease free many years later? The only approach to the former dilemma is to calculate risk for defined relapse events, e.g. hematologic relapse (including chronic phase and blast phase, but excluding molecular or molecular and karyotypic relapse). For a better description of successfully treated relapse the 'current disease-free survival' has been introduced. The KM for relapse is calculated at each relapse event as above, but in addition, patients who had formerly relapsed and are now in remission are newly censored from the time they re-entered remission.

Table 49.3 Choosing a data format and commonly used statistical methods

Categoric data

Examples
A. Ordinal (grade of acute GvHD – I, II, III, IV; feeling – better, same, worse; agreement – agree, disagree, neutral, etc.)
B. Nominal (gender – male, female; obesity – yes, no; acute GvHD – yes, no, etc.)

Statistical tests
Choose contingency tables
Chi-squared tests, e.g. abnormal PFT yes or no and acute GvHD
Exact tests, e.g. comparing TRM in high- and low-risk disease
Logistic regression, e.g. probability of relapse after allo-SCT as a function of age, disease risk, type of conditioning regimen, cGvHD, etc.

Non-categoric (quantitative) data

Examples
A. Measured (age, weight, height, albumin levels, blood pressure, etc.)
B. Counted (number of DLI, number of molecular relapses in CML, number of hospitalizations in 100 days post transplantation, etc.)

Statistical tests
A. Are you comparing groups? (compare groups)
Choose compare measurement, enter each group into a column, e.g. t-tests on difference between mean response between two groups (time to neutrophil engraftment after allo-SCT on two types of conditioning regimens: unpaired comparisons)
Simple linear regression, e.g. day 30 absolute NK cell counts and relapse, acute GvHD rate, etc.
B. Are you comparing how two variables relate to each other? (choose 'X and Y') OR how multiple variables (e.g. age and weight) affect CD34+ cell collection (choose 'Y and 2 or more X' variables for multiple regression)
Correlation analysis (Kendall's, Spearman's, Pearson's) to determine the strength of associations between two variables
Non-parametric tests for comparing two or more groups (sign test, Kruskal–Wallis test, Wilcoxon–Mann–Whitney test)
Examples: Day 30 absolute lymphocyte, absolute NK cell numbers and CD34+ cell dose correlations
Correlations between FEV1, DLCO and VC (% predicted)

Time to event data (survival, actuarial, cumulative data)

Data entry: enter days/months/years (survival, time to relapse, time to aGvHD, etc.) and then events (score either '0 or 1' but be consistent), censor if patient is alive for survival or no events, e.g. no relapse, no aGvHD, etc. (by scoring '0 or 1', again be consistent) and should be different from event score (e.g. if event is scored '0', score censored subject as '1' and vice versa). Software will perform analysis for you, when you enter data with X axis column with days (time to event date) and for censor subjects till last follow-up; Y axis column (single for KM analysis and multiple for Cox regression analysis)

Examples:
Actuarial survival or disease/leukemia free survival (with SEM or 95% CI interval)
Cumulative incidence, e.g. relapse, a-GvHD, TRM, etc.
Occurrence of events (estimation/comparison), e.g. hazard ratio between favorable and unfavorable factors
Multiple Cox regression, logistic regression, relative risk analysis: independent factors associated with survival, relapse, aGvHD, etc.

Finally, there is the problem of calculating relapse in patients with progressive disease from transplant. In a sense, every patient who relapses with the original disease has the disease at transplant. With hematologic malignancies there is usually a period when the disease is undetectable. In other situations (e.g. transplant for solid tumors where responses are more modest) the more relevant calculation is the time to partial or complete remission.

Calculating actuarial disease-free survival (DFS)

The DFS is the 'bottom line' for transplant outcome, describing not simply the probability of survival (which could include survival with the original disease) but the co-existence of the two desired outcomes: survival without disease. The patients censored here are those who fulfill both states – survival and freedom from relapse. Otherwise the calculation remains the same as for survival.

Statistical analysis of transplant data

Figure 49.1 presents the stepwise statistical methods to approaching actuarial and non-actuarial transplant data.

Statistical analysis of actuarial outcomes

Univariate analysis

The Kaplan–Meier method is used to calculate actuarial rates. The statistical significance of the difference in actuarial outcomes between groups of patients can be calculated using the log-rank test. The log-rank test can be applied to multiple sets of survival data. For example, it can be used to see if there is a significant trend in survival in transplants performed in the eras 1990–1995, 1996–2000 and 2001–2006.

Example 1

We recently explored the relationship between transplant outcome and the day 30 post transplant natural killer (NK) cell count (NK30).[5] We hypothesized that NK30 correlates directly with engraftment, and inversely with acute GvHD and relapse rates. Apart from the NK30, we considered multiple factors that may have contributed to transplant outcome: disease type, age, gender, donor–patient sex match (female to male vs others); disease risk, type of transplant (bone marrow transplant (BMT) vs peripheral blood stem cell transplant (PBSCT)), CD34 dose, CD3 dose, ciclosporin (CSA) dose and conditioning regimen. We also wanted to determine whether NK killer immuno-globulin-like receptor (KIR) genetics and the degree of NK alloreactivity affected outcome. To analyze each of these factors, we chose categorical variables (e.g. standard versus high-risk disease type, sex match vs sex mismatch). Numerical series, such as NK30 and CD34 dose, were separated into two subcategories – above and below the median value (Table 49.4).

We then performed a univariate analysis, comparing outcome for each subcategory (above vs below median, high vs standard risk, etc.). We found that a number of variables, including higher NK30, were associated with less acute GvHD, NRM, relapse and better survival. We used the KM survival estimates and log-rank tests statistic to determine whether there was a statistical difference between subcategories for each outcome (acute GvHD, relapse, etc.). Statistical software automatically calculates a two-tailed p-value. From an inspection of Table 49.4 it can be seen that seven factors emerged as significantly affecting relapse, resulting in better outcome in patients with: (1) SR disease, (2) higher NK30 ($>150/\mu l$), higher numbers of (3) activating and (4) inhibitory (5) and total KIR (6) donor + KIR-2DL5A or 2DS1 or 3DS1 and (7) + 2DS5.

Multivariate analysis

The univariate analysis identified multiple factors affecting outcome. What it did not tell us is whether the factors are linked, i.e. whether one factor is a surrogate for another or truly independent. Multivariate analysis is the way to identify the independent variables. For actuarial data we use a Cox regression model.[6] All the factors significant on univariate analysis are entered in the multivariate analysis model. The significance cut-off for selecting a variable depends on the size of the series. Selections of variables with a significance of $p < 0.05$ are appropriate for small series. As a rule of thumb, a ratio of one variable per 10 patients is suitable for a multivariate Cox regression model, because smaller subsets are likely to yield a non-significant result.

The Cox proportional hazard regression analysis works by simultaneously exploring the effect of several independent variables on the outcome. It identifies which independent factor is significantly associated with better or poor outcome and the hazard ratio (HR). Hazard

Table 49.4 Univariate analysis of actuarial data using Kaplan–Meier log-rank

Factor (n)	n	%	p
Acute GvHD (grade II–IV) (n = 27); cumulative incidence 50.4 ± 6.8 %			
Disease risk			0.0039
High (n = 33)	22	67.8 ± 8.3	
Standard (n = 21)	5	23.8 ± 9.3	
NK30			0.0023
<150/µl (n = 26)	19	73 ± 8.6	
>150/µl (n = 28)	8	28 ± 8.6	
Number of KIR (total) in donor			0.03
<10 (n = 27)	15	65.2 ± 9.9	
≥10 (n = 23)	10	37.8 ± 9.5	
Number of activating KIR in donor			0.04
<4 (n = 27)	17	63 ± 9.3	
≥4 (n = 23)	8	35.6 ± 10.1	
Number of inhibitory KIR in donor			0.08
<7 (n = 18)	12	66.7 ± 11.1	
≥7 (n = 32)	13	41.2 ± 8.8	
Favorable KIR* in donor			0.053
Absent (n = 27)	17	62.9 ± 9.2	
Present (n = 27)	8	35.5 ± 10.1	
Relapse (n = 19); cumulative incidence 40.8 ± 7.5 % (myeloid leukemias)			
Disease risk			0.0003
High (n = 20)	11	63.1 ± 12	
Standard (n = 19)	1	6.6 ± 6.4	
NK30			0.0001
<150/µl (n = 20)	11	70.5 ± 12.8	
>150/µl (n = 19)	1	5.3 ± 5.1	
Number of KIR (total) in donor			0.0038
<10 (n = 15)	9	65 ± 13.4	
≥10 (n = 20)	3	17.5 ± 9.2	
Number of activating KIR in donor			0.0018
<4 (n = 16)	10	68.3 ± 12.6	
≥4 (n = 19)	2	11.2 ± 7.5	
Number of inhibitory KIR in donor			0.005
<7 (n = 11)	7	75 ± 14.9	
≥7 (n = 24)	5	22.4 ± 8.9	
Favorable KIR* in donor			0.0003
Absent (n = 17)	11	70.1 ± 12.3	
Present (n = 18)	1	6.3 ± 6	
Donor KIR 2DS5			0.001
Absent (n = 16)	10	70.2 ± 13	
Present (n = 19)	2	11.8 ± 7.8	
Survival (n = 28); actuarial survival 49.3 ± 7.3%			
Disease risk			<0.0001
High (n = 33)	9	23.4 ± 8.1	
Standard (n = 21)	19	90.5 ± 6.4	
NK30			0.0002
<150/µl (n = 26)	7	21.9 ± 9	
>150/µl (n = 28)	21	75 ± 8.2	
Number of KIR (total) in donor			0.013
<10 (n = 23)	7	25.2 ± 10.5	
≥10 (n = 27)	19	70.4 ± 8.8	
Number of activating KIR in donor			0.037
<4 (n = 27)	10	31.6 ± 10.5	
≥4 (n = 23)	16	69.6 ± 9.6	
Number of inhibitory KIR in donor			0.0002
<7 (n = 18)	3	13.9 ± 8.7	
≥7 (n = 32)	23	71.9 ± 7.9	
Favorable KIR in donor			0.02
Absent (n = 27)	10	29.6 ± 11.2	
Present (n = 23)	16	69.6 ± 9.6	
Chronic GvHD			0.002
No (n = 15)	5	25.9 ± 13.6	
Yes (n = 26)	21	57.1 ± 18.7	

is defined as the slope of the survival curve, a measure of how rapidly subjects are dying or an event occurring. Most statistical software reports HR and 95% confidence intervals (CI). For example if the HR is 2.0, then the rate of death (events such as TRM, GvHD, relapse, etc.) in one treatment group is twice the rate in the other group. The comparison of HR assumes that the ratio is consistent over time and that any differences are due to random sampling. If the two survival curves cross, the 95% CI interval will cross zero and the p-value will be non-significant. Another term used for HR is the odds ratio (OR) or relative risk (RR). RR is mainly used for larger studies.

Cox multivariate analysis: step-by step procedure

The analysis is performed with the SPSS statistical software. To obtain an unbiased effect of independent variables, it is necessary to adjust for competing variables before performing the analysis.

1. First select the variables significant in univariate analysis according to a chosen p-value (e.g. <0.05). All variables to be tested in multivariate analysis should be converted to categoric variables and coded as '0' or '1'.
2. Open the Cox regression model window and enter the time to the event (death, NRM, relapse, GvHD, etc.).
3. Enter status code '0' for censored data, '1' for the event (e.g. GvHD, relapse, death, etc.).
4. Enter all test variables in the covariates window stepwise. For example, enter disease risk data, then press 'enter'. In this way, enter stepwise all the variables, pressing 'enter' with each set. In the examples in Table 49.4 we entered seven variables significant in univariate analysis for relapse. Total number entered can be seen as '7 of 7' in the Cox regression window.
5. Next check for adjustment of competing variables, e.g. while testing factors associated with acute GvHD, death before day 100 is a competing risk. To adjust for these competing variables, competing covariates are entered together with the covariate in the window before pressing 'enter'. You can check whether a competing variable affects the result by comparing the p-value and HR with and without competing risk factors. Change in p-value implies that there is an effect of the competing factor on the tested variable and the data should be presented as a competing risk factor. The competing variable need not necessarily be a categoric variable; for example, age can be entered as a continuous variable.
6. Once all test variables are entered, press the 'option' key and check 95% CI (required for transplant data result presentation). Interpreting a Cox model also involves examining the coefficient for each independent variable. A positive regression coefficient for an independent variable means that the hazard is higher for a high value. A negative coefficient means that the two variables are inversely correlated.
7. Press 'OK'. The final results will be displayed as a stepwise regression model and at the end, a summary of Cox multivariate analysis results. In our study example, a typical result is shown in Table 49.5. Of all seven variables significant on univariate analysis (see Table 49.4), only NK30 emerged as an independent factor affecting relapse, with a HR of 18 and CI of 1.151–292.88 (see Table 49.5).

Statistical analysis of non-actuarial transplant data

Univariate analysis

Table 49.2 lists the tests used for analysis of non-actuarial data, and Table 49.3 presents typical examples using tests for non-actuarial data.

Table 49.5 Multivariate Cox regression models for relapse in AML/CM**L**

Variable list*	p-value	HR Exp(B)	95.0% CI for Exp(B)	
			Lower	Upper
Risk group (HR vs SR)	0.104	7.698	0.657	90.172
NK30 (<vs ≥ 150/μl)	0.039	18.357	1.151	292.881
Activating KIR (unfavorable <4 KIR vs favorable ≥ 4)	0.250	4.117	0.370	45.840
Inhibitory (unfavorable <7 KIR vs favorable ≥ 7)	0.250	4.518	0.347	58.896
Donor + favorable KIR (2DL5A or 2DS1 or 3DS1)	0.145	0.044	0.001	2.951
Total KIR (unfavorable <10 KIR vs favorable ≥ 10)	0.652	0.524	0.032	8.698
Donor + 2DS5	0.763	0.651	0.040	10.551

* Significant factor on univariate analysis included in multivariate Cox regression model.

Parametric tests are used only where a normal distribution is assumed. The most widely used tests are the t-test (paired or unpaired), ANOVA (one-way non-repeated, repeated; two-way, three-way), linear regression and Pearson rank correlation.

Non-parametric tests are used when continuous data are not normally distributed or when dealing with discrete variables. Most widely used are chi-squared, Fisher's exact tests, Wilcoxon's matched pairs, Mann–Whitney U-tests, Kruskal–Wallis tests and Spearman rank correlation.

Multivariate analysis

Logistic and linear regression methods are used when the dependent variable is categoric or continuous (see Table 49.2). Enter the tested categoric dependent variable in the logistic regression window and then enter all tested variables in the 'covariates' window. For any variable requiring adjustment, enter in the same covariates window before pressing the enter key. For linear regression, enter the tested dependent variable (continuous) and then enter the independent variable which, like logistic regression, can be continuous or dichotomous. Press the 'option' and 'statistic' keys and check the desired additional statistics you want (in addition to standard default setting).

Linear regression

To better understand the methodology of linear regression, we present examples of linear regression analysis from a recently published study 'Prediction and prevention of pulmonary mortality after transplantation'.[7] In the SPSS software linear regression model window, the outcome variable is called the *dependent variable* and the predictor variables are called *independent variables*. The goal in the multiple regression model is to find significant independent variables affecting the tested outcome (dependent variable).

Bivariate linear regression is used when it is desired to predict outcome from values of a single predictor (independent variable). In this example NK30 recovery is the outcome (dependent variable) and CD34+ cell dose the predictor/independent variable.[5]

In *multiple* linear regressions, the relationship between a single, dependent variable (continuous) and a series of two or more predictor/independent variables (continuous or categoric) is calculated. With multiple linear regression models, outcome effect (e.g. in this example, decrease in carbon monoxide diffusing capacity (DLCO) (continuous)) is tested with several independent variables, e.g. CD34 cell dose as a continuous variable or in a cut-off model with < vs ≥ median; CD3 cell dose; CSA dose, no vs low dose vs standard dose, to identify significant factors associated with decline in DLCO value.[7]

Steps in analysis are the same as described in the Cox regression model above. Start entering important variables first and adjust for competing factors/variables by entering together in the same window before pressing the 'next' button. For example, poor pre-SCT pulmonary function test (PFT) was found to be a significant predictor of post-SCT deterioration but here, when history of smoking (yes or no) was entered, pretransplant PFT was found to be correlated with a history of smoking. Sample size is a critical factor in linear regression modeling. If the sample size is too small and the ratio of predictor variable to patient number is greater than 1 : 10, there is a risk of overfitting the model, with a non-significant result. Conversely, if the sample size is large, the differences may be significant but the percentage difference between outcomes according to the value of the variable described may be trivial.

Logistic regression

An example of logistic regression is illustrated in a recent study, 'Increased risk of bone loss without fracture risk in long-term survivors after allogeneic stem cell transplantation'.[8] Logistic regression modeling is a very flexible tool to study the relationship between a set of variables that can be continuous or categoric with the categoric outcome. In the study, the outcome variable is bone loss 'yes' or 'no' and factors associated with bone loss are age, as a continuous or discontinuous variable; gender; diagnosis; BMT vs PBSCT; total-body irradiation (TBI) vs no TBI; disease risk (standard or high); follow-up, continuous, < vs ≥ median; 10 vs < 10 years follow-up; acute GvHD, yes vs no; chronic GvHD, yes vs no; prolonged immunosuppressive therapy (IST), yes vs no. Logistic regression analysis showed age (oldest quartile vs first quartile OR 3.5, p = 0.03; age < vs ≥ median, OR 2.7, p = 0.45) and prolonged IST (OR 5.3, p = 0.01) were independently associated with increased risk of osteoporosis. Logistic regression is useful for a range of experimental designs, including cross-sectional or retrospective studies.

Multiple linear regression analysis poses technical difficulties, when dependent variables can have only two values (event occurred or not occurred, survival yes or no). Here, logistic regression analysis is used to directly estimate the probability that one of two events occurs, based on values of sets of independent variables that can be either categoric or continuous (e.g. bone loss, yes vs no, and age, continuous variable).

References

1. Klein JP, Rizzo JD, Zhang MJ, Keiding N. Statistical methods for the analysis and presentation of the results of bone marrow transplants. Part I: unadjusted analysis. Bone Marrow Transplant 2001;28:909–915
2. Klein JP, Rizzo JD, Zhang MJ, Keiding N. Statistical methods for the analysis and presentation of the results of bone marrow transplants. Part 2: Regression modeling. Bone Marrow Transplant 2001;28:1001–1011
3. Kaplan EL, Meier P. Non-parametric estimation from incomplete observations. J Am Stat Assoc 1965;53:457–481
4. Klein JP, Moeschberger ML. Survival analysis – techniques for censored and truncated data. Springer-Verlag, New York, 1997
5. Savani BN, Mielke S, Adams S et al. Rapid natural killer cell recovery determines outcome after T-cell-depleted HLA-identical stem cell transplantation in patients with myeloid leukemias but not with acute lymphoblastic leukemia. Leukemia 2007;21(10:2145–2152
6. Cox DR. Regression models and life tables [with discussion]. J R Stat Soc B 1972;34:187–220
7. Savani BN, Montero M, Wu C et al. Prediction and prevention of transplant related mortality from pulmonary causes following total body irradiation and allogeneic stem cell transplantation. Biol Blood Marrow Transplant 2005;11:223–230
8. Savani BN, Donohue T, Kozanas E et al. Increased risk of bone loss without fracture risk in long-term survivors after allogeneic stem cell transplantation. Biol Blood Marrow Transplant 2007;13(5):517–520

Additional reading

Books

Agresti A. Categorical data analysis. John Wiley, New York, 1990 (review of numerous issues in examining categorical data)

Chatterjee S, Hadi AS, Price B. Regression analysis by example, 3rd edn. John Wiley, New York, 2000 (excellent discussion of model fitting and handling assumption violations in linear regression)

Conover WJ. Practical nonparametric statistics, 3rd edn. John Wiley, New York, 1999 (excellent general non-parametric statistics with excellent brief descriptions of many tests)

Friedman L, Furberg C, DeMets D. Fundamentals of clinical trials, 3rd edn. Springer-Verlag, New York, 1998 (good introduction to the many issues involved in clinical research)

Grimm L. Yarnold P (eds). Reading and understanding multivariate statistics. American Psychological Association, Washington, DC, 1995 (an applied introduction to multivariate statistics, including multiple regression, logistic regression, factor analysis, and meta-analysis)

Hosmer D, Lemeshow S. Applied logistic regression, 2nd edn. John Wiley, New York, 2000

Norusis MJ. SPSS 12.0 Statistical procedures companion. SPSS Inc, Chicago, 2003

Norusis MJ. SPSS 11.0 Guide to data analysis. SPSS Inc, Chicago, 2002

Rosner B. Fundamentals of biostatistics, 4th edn. Duxbury Press, New York, 2000 (information on special cases and corrections)

Schulman R. Statistics in plain English with computer applications. Van Nostrand Rheinhold, New York, 1992 (good introduction to statistics in 'plain English' with chapters on factorial designs and multiple regression, as well as discussion of SPSS, SAS, and Minitab syntax and output which is dated)

Sprent P, Smeeton N. Applied nonparametric statistical methods, 3rd edn. Chapman & Hall/CRC, New York, 2001 (introduction to nonparametric statistics with lots of information on confidence intervals)

Stevens J. Applied multivariate statistics for the social sciences, 3rd edn. Lawrence Erlbaum Associates, New Jersey, 1996

van Belle G. Statistical rules of thumb. John Wiley, New York, 2002 (interesting practical advice on dealing with applied statistical issues)

Web resources

Software

http://home.clara.net/sisa/index.htm
Overviews and calculators on a variety of statistical procedures, including a great note on Bonferroni adjustments.

http://tigger.uic.edu/~hedeker/
Donald Hedeker's site on longitudinal analysis and mixed modeling.

www.ats.ucla.edu/stat/
Extensive collection of resources for learning and using SPSS, SAS, and Stata.

www.cebm.utoronto.ca/
Center for Evidence Based Medicine site from Canada.

www.intmed.mcw.edu/clincalc.html
Interesting clinically related calculators, especially for sensitivity and specificity.

www.medsch.wisc.edu/landemets/
Programs for computing group sequential boundaries using Lan-DeMets method.

http://pages.infinit.net/rlevesqu/
Numerous collection of tips and techniques for using SPSS.

www.sas.com/
SAS homepage.

www.smallwaters.com/amos/
Site from AMOS developer on path analysis.

www.spc.univ-lyon1.fr/~mcu/easyma/
Popular program for running meta-analysis.

www.spss.com/
SPSS homepage.

www.stat.sc.edu/webstat/
WebStat is a web-based statistical package for basic statistics and control charts.

www.stat.ucla.edu/calculators/
Statistical calculators from UCLA, including some for power and sample size.

Learning clinical application of statistics

http://it.stlawu.edu/~rlock/tise98/onepage.html
Resources for teaching statistics.

http://members.aol.com/johnp71/javastat.html
Organized display of statistical calculators, free software, texts, and tutorials.

http://psych.colorado.edu/~mcclella/java/zcalc.html

Applets for demonstrating statistical concepts from a novel text.

www.amstat.org/publications/jse/
The *Journal of Statistics Education* provides many suggestions on teaching statistics.

www.ats.ucla.edu/stat/spss/library/spssmixed/mixed.htm
Tutorial of linear mixed models in SPSS.

www.graphpad.com/instatman/instat3.htm
Guide for choosing statistics with help interpreting results and answering common questions.

www.graphpad.com/www/Book/Choose.htm
Basic guide for choosing statistics.

www.dartmouth.edu/~chance/teaching_aids/books_articles/probability_book/bookapplets/index.html
Applets for calculation and education, includes demonstrations of regression and confidence intervals.

www.kuleuven.ac.be/ucs/java/index.htm
Applets for calculation and education, including especially good ones for regression and hypothesis testing.

www.ruf.rice.edu/~lane/rvls.html
Applets for calculation and education, including especially good ones for regression and effect size.

www.shef.ac.uk/~scharr/ir/nnt.html
Resource of links to information on number needed to treat.

www.stat.berkeley.edu/~stark/SticiGui/index.htm
Tools for teaching statistics.

www.stat.sc.edu/rsrch/gasp/
Applets for calculation and education, includes nice demonstrations of confidence intervals, outliers (in correlation/regression), and power.

www.stat.sc.edu/~west/javahtml/
Applets for teaching statistical concepts.

www.utexas.edu/cc/stat/
University of Texas at Austin statistical site with tutorials for LISREL and hierarchical linear modeling.

Texts

http://faculty.vassar.edu/lowry/webtext.html
On-line basic statistics text from Vassar.

http://ubmail.ubalt.edu/~harsham/stat-data/opre330.htm
On-line basic statistics text.

www.bmj.com/collections/statsbk/index.shtml
Introductory statistics text with a chapter on survival analysis.

www.sportsci.org/resource/stats/index.html
Nice on-line statistics text with regular, helpful updates and additions.

www.statsoft.com/textbook/stathome.html
Text with huge variety of statistical topics including techniques such as factor analysis, survival analysis, time series analysis. Includes statistical advisor to help choose statistics.

Web guides

http://ourworld.compuserve.com/homepages/Rainer_Wuerlaender/stathome.htm
Rainer's Website for Statisticians starts with a table of contents and offers resources on news groups, associations, schools, software, quotes, people, etc.

www.execpc.com/~helberg/statistics.html
Statistics on the Web begins with a table of contents and lists statistical resources of organizations, consulting, education, books, software, people, etc.

www.graphpad.com/www/welcome.html
Go to the recommendations section to get many suggestions on good resources and demonstrations, texts, software, articles.

www.helsinki.fi/~jpuranen/links.html
Resources for teaching statistics.

www.stat.ufl.edu/vlib/statistics.html
The Virtual Library of statistics gives lots of resources on jobs, schools, government, research, software, news groups, etc.

Other
www.amstat.org/
American Statistical Association site.

www.fedstats.gov/
Link to huge number of federal sites with statistical information on health and other topics.

Blood and marrow transplant organizations

Armand Keating, Jane Apperley, Mary Horowitz, Edwin Horwitz, Phyllis Warkentin and Daniel Weisdorf

Introduction

The field of blood and marrow transplantation has generated a number of thriving organizations that have been of enormous influence in improving patient care, advancing research and enhancing education. This chapter describes several, but by no means all of the most influential.

American Society for Blood and Marrow Transplantation

The ASBMT is a North American professional association that promotes education, research and clinical affairs to advance the field of cellular therapy and blood and marrow transplantation (www.asbmt. org). Members are individuals in clinical practice and/or conducting research with expertise in blood and marrow transplantation or cell therapy-related research.

History

In 1993, Dr Richard Champlin proposed the idea of forming an organization for clinicians and investigators in blood and marrow transplantation. The goals of the society would be to foster the development of the field, support clinical research, provide professional and patient education, establish guidelines for clinical practice and training, and act as an advocate for appropriate regulation of the field. On February 27 1993, an organizational meeting was held in Oak Brook, Illinois, and in attendance were Joseph Antin MD, James Armitage MD, Bart Barlogie MD, Richard Champlin MD, Nancy Collins PhD, Joseph Fay MD, John Hansen MD, Mary Horowitz MD, Armand Keating MD, John Kersey MD, Richard O'Reilly MD, Robertson Parkman MD, Keith Sullivan MD, Jeffrey Wolf MD, and legal counsel Bruce Mackler PhD.

The ASBMT was incorporated on September 7 1993, in the District of Columbia, as a not-for-profit 501(c)3 professional association with Dr Champlin as the first president.

Organizational structure

The leadership of the society is elected from the membership and consists of six officers (president, president-elect, vice president, immediate past president, secretary, treasurer), nine directors and the editor in chief of *Biology of Blood and Marrow Transplantation*, the society journal.

Objectives

ASBMT activities have been in seven broad areas, representing the interests of the membership in interactions with their medical and scientific peers, private and governmental agencies, industry and the general public.

Research

Fostering research and the development of bone marrow transplant (BMT), both as a science and as a therapy.

Representation

Responding to and representing the interests of BMT clinicians, investigators and ancillary personnel to the public, the media, lawmakers and related medical fields. The society has taken a leadership role in co-ordinating public policy with allied organizations in the field such as the International Society for Cellular Therapy (ISCT), National Marrow Donor Program (NMDP), American Association of Blood Banks, Foundation for the Accreditation of Cellular Therapy (FACT), and the Center for International Blood and Marrow Transplant Research (CIBMTR). In addition, it has formed a task force to develop policy on storage of stem cells for personal use, and a committee is developing logistics and protocols for handling patients after an accidental or terrorist detonation of a nuclear device.

Clinical standards

Identifying commonly accepted medical practice and developing standards of patient care in autologous and allogeneic transplants.

The ASBMT has developed evidence-based reviews of the indications for blood and marrow transplantation for specific diseases. The purpose is to provide authoritative information for reimbursement decisions in managed care, for public policy decisions by legislators and regulators, and as a guide for practicing clinicians.

The first evidence-based review was on non-Hodgkin's lymphoma, published in 2001. The second review concerning multiple myeloma was published in January 2003. The third review on adult and pediatric acute lymphocytic leukemia (ALL) was published in 2005.[1] A review on adult acute myeloid leukemia is nearing completion.

Regulation

Conducting and co-ordinating analyses for effective regulation of autologous and allogeneic transplantation and interacting with the Food and Drugs Administration (FDA) and other regulatory authorities.

Communications

Sponsoring publications and meetings for the exchange of scientific and clinical information.

Accreditation

Developing guidelines for transplant facilities and for professional training in blood and marrow transplantation. The ASBMT, working with the International Society for Cellular Therapy (ISCT), created the Foundation for Cellular Therapy (FACT), an independent accreditation agency (see below).

Reimbursement

Providing guidelines and improving transplantation reimbursement by third-party payers.

The society's official journal, *Biology of Blood and Marrow Transplantation*, was established in 1995, indexed by the National Library of Medicine in 1997 and publishes basic, preclinical and clinical research in blood and marrow transplantation and cell-related therapy. The society also publishes two widely circulated periodicals, *Blood and Marrow Transplantation Reviews*, which tracks developments in blood and marrow transplantation, and *ASBMT eNEWS* (www.news-source.org/ASBMT/asbmtonline.htm), a monthly email newsletter that provides updates on the latest developments in cellular therapy, BMT, and related fields.

The ASBMT holds an annual meeting in conjunction with the Center for International Blood and Marrow Transplant Research, commonly known as the BMT Tandem Meetings, the largest gathering of worldwide experts in blood and marrow transplant patient care, clinical investigation and laboratory research in North America. A feature of the meetings, in addition to the scientific and clinical presentations, is related conferences and courses that run in parallel including: BMT Pharmacists; Clinical Research Data Management Workshops; BMT Center Medical Directors; BMT Center Administrators; Transplant Nursing; Pediatric BMT Special Interest Group; and a Medical Trainees Workshop. The annual meeting is also the venue for the annual E Donnall Thomas Lecture, the ASBMT Public Service Award and the ASBMT Lifetime Achievement Award.

In 2007, the ASBMT inaugurated an in-residence BMT Clinical Research Training Course in Keystone, Colorado, to provide an opportunity for fellows and junior faculty to receive formal training in the field, including in the scientific principles of BMT, stem cell biology, biostatistics, translational research and research protocol development.

Center for International Blood and Marrow Transplant Research

The CIBMTR is a clinical research program whose major mission is to provide a resource of data and statistical expertise to the hematopoietic stem cell transplant (HCT) community.

History

The CIBMTR was formed in July 2004 through an affiliation of the International Bone Marrow Transplant Registry (IBMTR) of the Medical College of Wisconsin and the research arm of the United States (US) National Marrow Donor Program (NMDP-Research). The IBMTR was a voluntary organization involving > 400 transplant centers in 47 countries collaborating to share patient data and conduct scientific studies since 1972. The NMDP was established in 1987 to provide unrelated donors for patients in need of HCT; NMDP-Research had responsibility for analyzing data from these transplants to assess and improve results. The NMDP also maintained a large repository of donor–recipient biologic samples. The CIBMTR affiliation brought together the research efforts of both organizations, each with complementary strengths, to provide a single point of focus for support of HCT-related clinical research.

Organizational structure

CIBMTR activities are funded primarily by grants and contracts from the US government, including the National Cancer Institute (NCI), the National Heart Lung and Blood Institute (NHLBI), the National Institute for Allergy and Infectious Disease, and the Health Resources and Services Administration (HRSA). The organizational structure of the CIBMTR is shown in Figure 50.1. The Affiliation Board and Executive Director have managerial oversight. The Chief Scientific Director has primary responsibility for administrative and scientific operations. CIBMTR Scientific Working, Executive and Advisory Committees provide policy and scientific oversight for this work. The CIBMTR committee structure is designed to ensure that the activities of the CIBMTR are consistent with the priorities of the scientific community it serves.

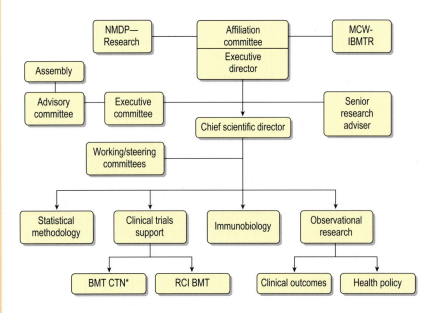

Figure 50.1
CIBMTR organizational chart. *The CIBMTR collaborates with the NMDP and the EMMES Corporation to serve as the Data and Co-ordinating Center of the BMT CTN. NMDP, National Marrow Donor Program; IBMTR, International Bone Marrow Transplant Registry; MCW, Medical College of Wisconsin; BMT CTN, Blood and Marrow Transplant Clinical Trials Network; RCI BMT, Resource for Clinical Investigations in Blood and Marrow Transplantation.

Scientific working committees set priorities for observational studies that use the large clinical databases of the IBMTR and NMDP. There are 18 working committees: Acute Leukemia; Chronic Leukemia; Lymphoma; Plasma Cell Disorders; Solid Tumors; Pediatric Cancer; Non-malignant Marrow Disorders; Immune Deficiencies/Inborn Errors of Metabolism; Autoimmune Diseases; Graft Sources and Manipulation; Graft-versus-Host Disease; Late Effects and Quality of Life; Immunobiology; Infection and Immune Reconstitution; Regimen-related Toxicty and Supportive Care; Health Services and Psychosocial Issues; Donor Health and Safety; Cellular Therapy. Each working committee is headed by 2–4 chairs appointed by the Advisory Committee to non-renewable 5-year terms. Membership of working committees is open to anyone willing to take an active role in studies using CIBMTR resources. Proposals for CIBMTR observational studies are submitted to the appropriate working committee and evaluated by the committee chairs and membership.

Two CIBMTR *steering committees* provide additional oversight for use of certain resources. The Immunobiology Steering Committee reviews and approves use of donor–recipient specimens from the NMDP repository for conducting CIBMTR studies approved by the working committees that link outcome data with biologic and genetic factors derived from analyses of these biologic materials. A Clinical Trials Advisory Committee (CTAC) formally reviews requests for CIBMTR resources to assist in planning and implementing clinical trials through a program established in 2005, the Resource for Clinical Investigations in Blood and Marrow Transplantation (RCI BMT). Of note, the CIBMTR, together with the NMDP and the EMMES Corporation, also functions as the Data and Co-ordinating Center of the US Blood and Marrow Transplant Clinical Trials Network (BMT CTN), a clinical trials network with its own oversight and governing mechanism (see below).

The CIBMTR *Assembly* is the voting membership, composed of a single representative from each CIBMTR research center. The CIBMTR *Advisory Committee* meets biannually to review scientific and other activities of the CIBMTR. Most Advisory Committee members and officers are elected by the CIBMTR Assembly. It also includes appointed members representing donor centers (n = 1), collection centers (n = 1), patients (n = 2) and individuals with expertise in business (n = 1), ethics (n = 1) and information systems (n = 1), as well as representatives from the NCI, NHLBI, NIAID and HRSA. The CIBMTR *Executive Committee* is a subcommittee of the Advisory Committee that provides ongoing advice and counsel to the CIBMTR Statistical Center between meetings of the Advisory Committee.

There are two additional standing committees: the *Consumer Advocacy Committee* (CAC) and the *International Studies Committee*. The CAC helps provide the patient and donor perspective in developing the CIBMTR's research agenda and helps communicate important information from CIBMTR studies to the non-medical community. The International Studies Committee's major charge is to facilitate communication between non-US centers and the CIBMTR leadership (as well as other national and international organizations), and to design and conduct studies dealing with questions specific to geographic regions.

Accomplishments

The CIBMTR has information on more than 260,000 HCT recipients and adds more than 12,000 new transplants to its database yearly. In 2006, the US government selected the CIBMTR to serve as the Stem Cell Therapeutic Outcomes Database charged with collecting outcome data on all allogeneic HCTs performed in the US and with assessing optimal registry size, US cord blood inventory and center-specific outcomes. In the context of this charge, the CIBMTR is working with other national and international organizations to achieve consensus on

a common data set for outcomes reporting. The CIBMTR has published more than 350 papers in the biomedical literature and there are more than 190 studies currently being conducted by the working committees using these data. Through either the BMT CTN or the RCI BMT, the CIBMTR has helped to initiate more than 15 prospective clinical trials that have enrolled more than 2000 patients over the past 3 years. Additional information can be found at www.cibmtr.org.

Blood and Marrow Transplant Clinical Trials Network

The field of hematopoietic cell transplantation merges cell biology, molecular genetics, clinical hematology/oncology, and critical care. The initial successes of hematopoietic cell transplantation in the 1960s have broadened to the widespread application of many thousands of transplants yearly throughout the US and the world. Numerous patients with otherwise lethal hematologic malignancies, marrow failure or non-malignant marrow and immune disorders have been saved by successful re-establishment of hematopoiesis and immune competence through the procedure of hematopoietic cell transplantation. The complexities of care, the individualized procedures developed in each center, and the relatively few procedures performed yearly at each center have all fostered creativity, but limited the availability of definitive clinical evidence to identify which procedures and practices are optimal.

While it is accepted that prospective clinical trials provide the best clinical evidence to validate and verify the utility of new treatment procedures, only limited numbers of prospective randomized trials in the field of hematopoietic cell transplantation have been performed. Recognizing interest in the transplant community and following validation of its importance through a series of State of the Science symposia, the National Heart, Lung and Blood Institute (NHLBI) and the National Cancer Institute (NCI) established the Blood and Marrow Transplant Clinical Trials Network (BMT CTN) in order to design, develop, and execute prospective clinical trials to improve the safety, applicability, and effectiveness of hematopoietic cell transplant therapy. With the establishment of the BMT CTN, 16 core centers were awarded co-operative agreements with the NHLBI/NCI and a broader network of over 60 transplant centers has facilitated 12 prospective trials, enrolling over 2000 patients in the first 5 years of patient accrual into BMT CTN trials. At present, 15 studies continue to evaluate regimen-related toxicity, protection against relapse, graft-versus-host disease, infections and immune reconstitution, non-malignant marrow disorders as well as quality of life and recovery from transplant treatment.[2] Regular BMT CTN Steering Committee meetings outline the scientific agenda for the Network, and monitor pro-gress in trial development and accrual. The first publication of their scientific findings is expected in the near future.

In its sixth year and following its first competitive renewal of funding, the BMT CTN initiated plans for another State of the Science symposium in hematopoietic cell transplantation, bringing leading investigators from across the US and internationally to outline the most critical issues needing clinical translation and amenable to prospective clinical trial testing over the next several years. This symposium established the framework for the ongoing portfolio of Network studies.

The principles of the BMT CTN establishment allow active participation by all who can contribute. The Network accepts proposals for trials and participation in protocol teams from all investigators able to contribute expertise, commitment, and willingness to further the clinical science of transplantation. Bringing the best evidence from single-center trials to multicenter feasibility and replication and finally to prospective formal clinical testing in Phase III trials is the translational pipeline bringing new treatments with greater safety to patients in need. The network of basic, translational, and clinical scientists who support the BMT CTN are committed to this goal and to its success.

European Group for Bone Marrow Transplantation

History

Over the past three decades the EBMT has grown from a small group of enthusiasts to a society representing more than 500 teams from 57 countries.

In 1975, teams from Paris, Leiden, London and Basel met for the first time to discuss general problems and individual patients, and to draw up protocols with a view to improving results. They continued to meet regularly in the Swiss or French Alps and the group, then called the European Co-operative Group for Bone Marrow Transplantation, attracted an ever-increasing number of participants. In 1979, the European Foundation for Bone Marrow Transplantation (EBMT) was formally established with legal status in Leiden, in The Netherlands. Four working parties were created, each with its own registry: Aplastic Anemia, Acute Leukemia, Inborn Errors and Transplantation Immunology. In 1989, a new constitution created the European Group for Bone Marrow Transplantation, the abbreviation EBMT being retained. Subsequently, the working parties were restructured and new ones added, i.e. Acute Leukemia, Aplastic Anemia, Autoimmune Disease, Chronic Leukemia, Immunobiology, Inborn Errors, Infectious Diseases, Late Effects, Lymphoma, Nursing, Pediatrics and Solid Tumors. In 1995 the name of the group was changed once more to the European Group for Blood and Marrow Transplantation, though the acronym EBMT again remained.

Each year an annual meeting is organized, the main purpose of which is to provide a forum for interaction, presentation of data, discussion of future projects and exchange of personal experiences. Most recently, the EBMT has developed a critical role as a stakeholder and advisor to national and international regulatory authorities as the field of transplantation has become subject to increasing scrutiny and legislation.

The overall objective of the EBMT is to improve the outcome of hemopoietic stem cell transplantation (HSCT) by a number of connected activities. The most long-standing of these activities is the collection, validation and analysis of outcome data of all transplants performed by member teams. However, the work of the group has expanded to include accreditation, education and outreach, prospective clinical trials and regulatory affairs.

EBMT members may be full members, associate members, individual members or corporate patrons. Full and associate memberships are granted to teams rather than individuals. EBMT members have the right to propose and elect office holders, stand for election, attend annual meetings and participate in the working parties and EBMT studies. Full membership implies a duty to report individual transplant data to the EBMT registries.

Organizational structure

The EBMT Board is composed of elected individuals including the president, secretary, treasurer and the working party chairpersons. The Board co-ordinates EBMT activities and is responsible for the budget. The major part of the work of the EBMT is performed by the working parties which are the heart of the EBMT, performing retrospective and prospective studies relating to their particular disease or other interest. However, the Board of the EBMT has long recognized the need for activities that cross working party activities. This led to the develop-

Table 50.1 EBMT committees

Committee	Responsibilities
Accreditation	JACIE, audit and activity survey (see text)
Registry	Co-ordination of individual registry activities, data collection, processing and management
Education	Training courses, handbook (jointly with ESH), outreach initiatives
Nuclear accident	Establishment of network of units with hematologic expertise to respond to the need for care of neutropenic patients in the event of nuclear accidents
Clinical trials	Prospective clinical trials
Stem cell quality	Standardization of assessment of hematopoietic cell product quality
Developmental	Broadening the definition of transplant to include all cellular therapy for hematologic and non-hematologic disorders.

ment of EBMT committees. Unlike the working party chairs, who are elected by the member centers and who have permanent positions on the EBMT Board, the chairs of the committees are appointed by the Board. They do not have positions or voting rights on the Board but are asked to report their activities and suggestions for Board approval. Committees are designed to be responsive to the needs of the organization and can be dissolved when there is no longer any requirement for the particular activity.

The current committees are shown in Table 50.1. The work of some of these committees will be discussed in more detail below.

Education and outreach

The Education Committee was established in 1995 with the intention of providing a more structural approach to training in HSCT. Together with the European School for Haematology (ESH), it has successfully organized the annual residential training course in which senior transplant physicians and scientists interact in formal and informal settings with less experienced colleagues. This course is regularly oversubscribed and has been successful in obtaining central funding from the European Commission to support scholarships in conjunction with the course. The committee has issued an ESH-EBMT transplant manual, now in its third edition.

Most recently, this committee has taken the initiative in the development of an outreach project to assist transplant units in economically disadvantaged countries. The EBMT is not alone in this concept and is actively integrating its ideas with the ESH, and is aware of similar programs within the American Society of Hematology (ASH), CIBMTR, the European Haematology Association (EHA) and the World Health Organization (WHO). This project supports educational initiatives including training courses in clinical and laboratory techniques, exchange programs, fellowships, clinical trial participation and twinning programs.

Prospective clinical trials

This committee was established in 2003 to assist the EBMT in its progress from a retrospective study organization to a prospective clinical trials group. The EBMT exploits its role as a data collection agency but feels that many unanswered questions in transplantation are best served by prospective studies. The introduction into European legislation of the EU Directive on Clinical Trials (2001/20/EC) has highlighted the necessity of creating an appropriate infrastructure for the conduct of these trials. Initial areas of discussion include the development of ProMISe-2 to develop an internet-based reporting system for clinical trials, compliance with data protection, formalizing insurance coverage, and addressing issues of 'sponsorship' and 'data monitoring'.

Accreditation

The Accreditation Committee has a number of diverse functions which have developed over many years. The committee was originally responsible for a simple form of accreditation for allogeneic sibling transplantation in which centers requested accreditation on the basis of performance of a minimum number of transplants annually. This process then necessitated annual audits of individual centers for the purposes of data and center validation. At the start of each year, one-third of centers are chosen at random and are alerted to the possibility of an audit. Later, a proportion of these centers are visited by senior transplant physicians and data are checked at source.

One of the most valuable activities of this committee and indeed of the EBMT is also one of the simplest. In 1990, Professor Alois Gratwohl began to collect information relating to the annual transplant activity of all transplant centers in Europe (including those centers that are not EBMT members). As a result, the EBMT now holds important data relating to activity, geographic variation, changing trends and the development of new technologies. Activity is published annually and has proven invaluable to the funding agencies (public and private) in identifying transplant needs.

More recently, the bulk of the work of the Accreditation Committee has been the development and introduction of the JACIE Accreditation Program for all transplant units. The Joint Accreditation Committee of ISCT-EBMT (JACIE) is a non-profit body established for the purposes of assessment and accreditation in the field of hematopoietic cell transplantation. The committee was founded in 1998 by the EBMT and the International Society for Cellular Therapy (ISCT), the two leading scientific organizations involved with HSCT in Europe. The JACIE modeled itself on the US-based Foundation for the Accreditation of Cellular Therapy (FACT), established in 1996 by the ISCT and the ASBMT. The JACIE actively collaborates with the FACT in establishing standards for the provision of quality medical and laboratory practice in HSC transplantation. The JACIE conducts inspections, accredits programs and encourages health institutions and facilities performing HCT to voluntarily meet these standards in order to demonstrate their high levels of quality of care. The organizational structure ensures wide consultation, with 20 European countries now represented on the Board in addition to nursing, pediatrics and cord blood representatives.

The primary aim of the JACIE is to improve the quality of HCT in Europe by providing a means whereby transplant centers, HSC collection facilities and processing facilities can demonstrate high-quality practice. This is supported by co-ordinating training courses in quality management for applicant centers and courses for inspectors. An additional and wider aim is to ensure harmonization between JACIE standards and other national and international standards, including the EU Tissues and Cells Directive (Directive 2004/23/EC) and the related implementing directives.

Since its inception, the essence of the EBMT has been to evaluate and optimize the outcome of patients treated by stem cell transplantation. In order to do this, it was always deemed necessary to collect patient data and so the EBMT registry was formed. Currently, the registry holds information on over 265,000 transplants performed by the member teams, and this has proven an invaluable resource in the analysis of factors affecting transplant outcome, in identifying complications and their optimal treatment, in determining trends in management and in evaluating new technologies.

Member teams are required to report all their transplant activity. 'Minimal essential data' (MED) are collected on a number of different forms. MED-A data form the basis of the registry. Relatively simple and limited data collected in this way allow the analyses of overall survival, disease-free survival, transplant-related mortality, and relapse risk. These data are identical to those collected by the CIBMTR on its Transplant Essential Data (TED) form, and the facility exists to allow cross-reporting to both registries.

More detailed information is collected on MED-B forms which relate to the specific disease and to the procedure (allograft and autograft). The submission of these data by members is voluntary, as opposed to MED-A data which are obligatory. Information relating to specific studies is collected via MED-C forms.

Until recently the term 'form' literally referred to hard copy in virtually all cases. Paper forms were sent to the EBMT and transcribed onto a central electronic database, but the complexity of the program and the relative lack of familiarity with computers at the time precluded widespread use of this approach. Over the past 10 years, Ronald Brand, based in the Department of Medical Biostatistics at the University of Leiden, has developed an on-line internet-based reporting system, Project Manager Internet Server or ProMISe. Data reported in this way are received simultaneously by the EBMT registries but can also be downloaded for local use. The second version of the system, ProMISe-2, was introduced in 2004. Added benefits include the ability to adapt the database for local, national and international prospective and retrospective studies. This system has revolutionized data reporting, with increasing numbers of centers adopting ProMISe. In 2006, 458 users from 364 centers accessed the database to enter data for more than 25,000 transplants.

Full member teams report their data via ProMISe but still have the facility to send paper forms. All Med-A and Med-B data are collated, transcribed if necessary and checked by the EBMT data office in Paris. The ProMISe helpdesk and database design activities are in London. Once the data are entered into ProMISe, they are immediately available to all EBMT registries currently based in Genoa, London, Leiden and Paris. In addition, the EBMT has welcomed the development of national transplant societies and has understood the desire of some of these groups to have their own national databases. In the past, for member centers in countries with national registries, data flowed from the center to the national registry and then to the EBMT. Centers in countries without a national registry reported directly to the EBMT. Now, if the center is utilizing ProMISe, the data are deposited simultaneously in the national and EBMT registries. The work of the registries is overseen and co-ordinated by one of the EBMT committees, the Registry Executive.

International Society for Cellular Therapy

The ISCT is a professional non-profit organization of members of the cell therapy community, including clinical physicians, clinical and laboratory investigators, cell processing laboratory technologists, legal and regulatory specialists. While largely focused on hematopoietic cells, the society seeks to encompass the vast array of emerging cell-based therapies. Accordingly, the mission of the ISCT is to serve as the global voice and resource for developing and promoting innovative cellular therapies through communication, education, training, and advocacy for the benefit of patients. In 2007, the Society had over 1200 members from six continents. The society journal, *Cytotherapy*, is focused on all aspects of cell therapy – preclinical, clinical and regulatory issues that govern research and practice in the field. The ISCT organizes an annual meeting of diverse groups of investigators, practitioners, and technologists, with a focus on research and education. Additional highly focused meetings are organized periodically to provide opportunities for brief but intensive discussions and education in new or rapidly changing areas.

The ISCT originally emerged from the rapidly growing practice of bone marrow and mobilized peripheral blood cell transplantation in which laboratory manipulations of the clinical graft were becoming increasingly popular. Throughout the 1980s, T-cell depletion, marrow purging, and other graft manipulations became increasingly popular and required the specialized expertise of investigators and laboratory technologists. At the Third International Symposium on Bone Marrow Purging and Processing in 1991, Drs Adrian Gee, Nancy Collins, and Diana Worthington-White formed the International Society of Hematotherapy and Graft Engineering (ISHAGE), which was incorporated in 1992. The purpose was, in part, to provide an educational forum for the therapeutic benefits of the rapidly emerging discipline of transplantation and to establish minimum laboratory standards for marrow processing. The ISCT also sought to stimulate the exchange of ideas in the then-emerging field of cell therapy and in related cell processing issues. With increasing recognition of related cell therapies such as mesenchymal cells and the use of hematopoietic cells for non-hematopoietic disorders, the society expanded its focus to the broad discipline of cell therapy, and in 2002, changed its name to the International Society for Cellular Therapy.

An aspect of the ISCT that makes it unique among professional societies is that it is designed to include *all* members of the cell therapy field, from the preclinical investigators who develop the scientific principles, to the processing lab scientific directors and the technologists who prepare the products, to the quality control and regulatory specialists who ensure the safety and legal compliance of the processing procedure and the trials, to the clinical investigators who conduct the cell therapy trials and care for the patients. The annual meeting, smaller focused meetings, and the journal reflect this broad interest of the society.

The ISCT is composed of several standing committees, representing all facets of ongoing activities of the society, and short-term working groups, designed to address immediate concerns within cell therapy, drafting position statements and guidance for broad dissemination or submission to the FDA. The committees on (i) hematopoietic stem cells, (ii) mesenchymal and tissue stem cells, (iii) immunotherapy and dendritic cells, (iv) gene therapy, and (v) cell and tissue evaluation are the core scientific groups. These committees facilitate discussion in their respective fields of study by organizing plenary sessions, workshops and technical sessions at the annual meetings, and educate and lead their fields by publishing editorials and position statements about controversial issues.[3]

The *Lab Practices Committee* serves to develop, standardize and disseminate laboratory practices for clinical applications of cellular therapy. The committee also participates in the translation of novel cell therapies from the laboratory to the clinic and encourages and fosters the participation of laboratory practitioners in all aspects of the society.

The ISCT recognized that commercial entities play a vital role in translating cell therapy from the bench to the bedside. The *Cell Therapy and Commercialization Committee* is responsible for facilitating the translation of successful cell therapies that require large-scale production to industry when appropriate. Additionally, industry often plays a substantial role in the earliest development of cell therapy, and this committee fosters academic–corporate relationships to accelerate the pace of new product development.

The *Legal and Regulatory Affairs Committee* provides information regarding compliance with federal, local, and professional regulations and represents the views of practitioners in the field to regulatory agencies. Because regulatory requirements vary among different countries, the Legal and Regulatory Affairs Committee is currently divided into one subcommittee for North America and another for Europe. As the regulatory environment in other areas of the world becomes more complex, the ISCT plans to create new subcommittees for these geographic areas.

The ISCT maintains temporary committees, termed working groups, designed to focus on issues of immediate concern. These groups serve as a platform for discussion and consensus building among the thought leaders in the specific domain and on occasion publish guidelines for the cell therapy community or submit recommendations to national regulatory agencies. As issues are resolved, the working groups may dissolve; however, new concerns can lead to the creation of new working groups. Hence, the organization generates a dynamic working group structure to maintain immediate relevance to the society's efforts.

In addition to the annual society meeting, the ISCT organizes focused meetings on the 'hot' topics in cell therapy. For example, it has co-sponsored four meetings on mesenchymal and tissue stem cells since 2001. These meetings were organized when increasing numbers of investigators new to the field became interested in mesenchymal cells and provided a forum for the burgeoning field. The ISCT also organizes an annual Somatic Cell Therapy Meeting which is focused on the regulatory issues facing investigators seeking to translate their work to the clinic.

Foundation for the Accreditation of Cellular Therapy

History

The FACT was founded in 1995 as a partnership between the ASBMT, representing physicians and investigators involved in the clinical conduct of hematopoietic cell transplantation, and the ISCT, representing scientists and physicians working in the area of cellular therapy product processing and manipulation. These founders determined that both quality standards and voluntary professional accreditation for the procurement, manipulation and transplantation of hematopoietic cellular products were necessary to promote quality patient care and laboratory practices and to preserve the flexibility required to nurture continued rapid scientific evolution of the field. The merger of the clinical standards proposed by the ASBMT with the cell collection and processing standards developed by the ISCT formed the foundation for the first edition of the FACT S*tandards for hematopoietic progenitor cell collection, processing and transplantation*, published in 1996.

FACT standards apply to all sources of hematopoietic progenitor cells, defined as stem and multipotent progenitor cells capable of self-renewal and/or maturation into any of the hematopoietic lineages, including committed and lineage-restricted progenitor cells isolated from any tissue source. These standards also include therapeutic cells, defined as nucleated cells from any tissue source (marrow, peripheral blood, umbilical cord blood) collected for therapeutic use other than as hematopoietic progenitor cells. FACT standards apply to all phases of collection, processing, storage, and administration of these cells that have been derived from marrow or peripheral blood, including various manipulations such as removal or enrichment of various cell populations, expansion of hematopoietic cell populations, and cryopreservation.

FACT standards also apply to the administration of hematopoietic progenitor cells derived from cord blood. However, additional standards are required for the complexities of cord blood collection and banking. In collaboration with members of NetCord,[4] an international organization of independent cord blood banks, these additional standards were promulgated, and a parallel accreditation program was developed. The first edition of NetCord-FACT *International standards for cord blood collection, processing, testing, banking, selection and release* was developed by consensus, circulated for member and public comment, adopted by the boards of NetCord and FACT, and published in June 2000. Now in their third edition, these international standards require all cord blood banks to maintain a comprehensive quality management program, to document training of all collection and processing staff, to utilize validated methods, supplies, reagents and equipment, to maintain product tracking, and to maintain details of clinical outcome.[3] These standards form the basis for the voluntary accreditation of cord blood banks worldwide. Twelve cord blood banks from the US, Europe, and the United Kingdom have achieved NetCord-FACT accreditation.

FACT representatives have also worked with colleagues from the EBMT and ISCT-Europe to establish the Joint Accreditation Committee of ISCT-Europe and EBMT (JACIE). The JACIE adopted the FACT standards in 1999. There followed joint inspector training courses and joint FACT and JACIE review of the second edition of the standards. Most recently, the third edition of the standards, published in 2006, was jointly developed and entitled *FACT-JACIE international standards for cellular therapy product collection, processing, and transplantation.*[5] The JACIE has developed an accreditation program in Europe similar, but not identical, to the FACT process. The JACIE is responsible for ensuring that standards remain constant and are updated as appropriate, and works with national co-operative blood and marrow transplant groups and national regulatory agencies in countries where these resources are available for the training of inspectors and on-site inspections.

FACT-JACIE international standards

FACT-JACIE standards are designed to provide minimum guidelines for facilities and individuals performing hematopoietic cell transplantation and related cellular therapies. Standards are developed by consensus by the FACT Standards Committee, composed of experts active in clinical, collection, and/or laboratory aspects of cellular therapy. The Standards Committee receives and considers comments from ASBMT, EBMT and ISCT members, other practitioners in cellular therapy, and the public, prior to final approval by the Boards of Directors. FACT-JACIE standards require that all clinical, collection, and processing facilities develop and maintain a comprehensive quality management plan that includes at least the following components: defined organizational structure, personnel requirements, process development, agreements, outcome analysis, audits, management of errors, accidents and adverse events, document control, product tracking, and, where appropriate, validation and qualification. The current edition also includes many of the regulatory requirements from the FDA and the Directives of the European Union, including donor eligibility and product labeling. The product proper names have been revised to be consistent with the names and definitions proposed for inclusion in the official language of *ISBT 128*.

Clinical standards define a blood and marrow transplant program; describe facility, standard operating procedures, and personnel requirements, including minimum skills, education, training and experience; enumerate support staff; cover donor evaluation, selection, eligibility, and consents; provide minimal guidelines for administration of cellular product therapy, including the preparative regimen of high-dose therapy; describe the appropriate management of clinical research and IRB-approved protocols; and require the maintenance of complete and accurate records. Comprehensive laboratory standards detail requirements for personnel, process controls, inventory management, validation and qualification of facilities, supplies, reagents and equipment, labels and labeling, storage, transport, and records. Communication between laboratory and clinical service is emphasized. Laboratory personnel are expected to follow clinical outcome as one measure of product safety and efficacy.

FACT accreditation

The goal of the FACT accreditation program is to raise the quality of performance for all cellular therapy programs and services in the expectation that such improvements will lead to better patient out-

comes. The process is intended to be educational rather than punitive, to allow capable and committed personnel to achieve accreditation.

FACT accreditation is voluntary and based on documented compliance with the current edition of the standards through submission of written documents and an on-site inspection. Facilities eligible to apply for accreditation are clinical transplant programs, hematopoietic progenitor cell (HPC) collection facilities and/or HPC processing laboratories. To achieve accreditation, a clinical program must utilize a collection service and a cell processing laboratory that both meet FACT standards. The on-site inspection is the responsibility of a team of volunteer inspectors, each of whom is active and expert in the field of hematopoietic cell therapy and meets the minimum qualifications of education and training – at least 2 years' experience in the area to be inspected, completion of FACT inspector training, a written exam, and at least one on-site inspection as a trainee. A checklist format is used to ensure completeness, consistency, and to emphasize reliance on the standards.

Inspector reports are reviewed by trained and experienced accreditation specialists in the FACT national office and by an Accreditation Committee, composed of persons in leadership roles in the field of hematopoietic cell therapy. Citations and recommendations are reviewed to maintain consistency throughout the process. Facilities with deficiencies at the end of this review are given the opportunity to correct these deficiencies, and subsequently to achieve accreditation. The Board of Directors retains accountability for the accreditation, and acts to resolve discrepancies or disagreements, or to make precedent-setting decisions. Accredited programs are published in the newsletters of the ISCT, ASBMT, and FACT, and are posted on the FACT website at www.factwebsite.org. The first blood and marrow transplant programs in North America were FACT-accredited in March 1998. Currently, there are 152 accredited programs accounting for an estimated 90% of eligible programs in North America.

Results of recent on-site inspections demonstrate that most programs have addressed the majority of the standards. Deficiencies observed generally represent failure to completely address a standard. The most commonly observed deficiencies have been tabulated for the past year and include the following:
- collection facility lacking some standard operating procedures (SOPs)
- collection facility lacking validation or qualification of significant products or processes
- omissions in the quality management plan
- missing SOPs in the processing facility
- data management errors in the clinical facility
- labels that lack required elements
- no evidence of record review by collection facility director or medical director.

Accreditation of cord blood banks follows a similar process. Experienced inspectors spend 2 days at each cord blood bank, and visit both laboratory and collection sites. A separate Cord Blood Bank Accreditation Committee reviews the reports of each inspection. Twelve cord blood banks in seven countries have achieved accreditation. Accredited banks are also published and listed at www.factwebsite.org.

FACT standards for cellular therapy products and for cord blood banking have gained international acceptance. FACT cellular therapy standards have been adopted in Australia for cell collection and processing. In the US, co-operative clinical trials groups, several states, and many insurance companies require or recommend FACT accreditation for participation. Cord blood standards have been adopted by the Therapeutic Goods Administration in Australia, by the World Marrow Donor Association, and AsiaCord. In this era of rapid advances in cellular therapies, both regulations and voluntary standards co-exist and hopefully contribute to the safety and efficacy of such therapies. Clinical outcomes remain the highest standard of quality care.

National Marrow Donor Program (NMDP)

The NMDP provides an invaluable service to patients in the United States and throughout the world. It facilitates the search, identification, and procurement of volunteer unrelated donor hematopoietic stem cells either as bone marrow, stimulated peripheral blood progenitor cells, or umbilical cord blood to support hematopoietic stem cell transplantation for patients in need.

The initiation of unrelated donor (URD) marrow transplantation followed early successes using related donors. After development of improved tools to understand the HLA system (1960s–1970s) for defining and matching the relevant factors of tissue typing, occasional patients had searches, usually through local blood bank registries, to identify a closely matched donor and proceed with transplantation. By the mid-1980s, registries of HLA-typed potential volunteers were established in large blood centers in Milwaukee, St Paul, Seattle, and Iowa City, mostly from regional lists of HLA-typed platelet donors. In 1984 with passage of the National Organ Transplant Act, the US Congress identified the need to evaluate URD marrow transplantation and recognized the feasibility of establishing a national donor registry. This led, in 1986, to establishment of the National Bone Marrow Donor Registry. In 1988 Congress formally authorized the establishment of the National Marrow Donor Program which has administered the growing pool of donors and the network of donor centers able to provide support and stem cell grafts for patients.

The NMDP registry has grown remarkably, and the NMDP has taken on various additional roles. Understanding and recognizing limitations of a conventionally recruited donor pool to provide suitably matched donors for patients with rarer tissue types, particularly those from racial and ethnic minorities, the NMDP launched efforts to identify many more donors, particularly those from less well-represented populations. These include American Indian and Alaskan Native populations, Black, African-American, Hispanic, Latino, Asian, Native Hawaiian, and Pacific Islander donors, who are directly recruited to expand opportunities for successful identification and delivery of needed marrow stem cells for patients appropriate for transplantation. At present, patients can search more than 6 million volunteer donors and over 50,000 cord blood units available through the NMDP registry as well as linking to an additional 4 million potential donors and many thousands of additional cord blood units through international connections between co-operative donor registries throughout the world. Each month, well over 200 patients receive transplants through the NMDP, and more than 25,000 transplants have been performed since initiation of NMDP operations in 1987. Improvements in HLA typing, expansion of histocompatibility matching techniques, and understanding factors beyond HLA which are important to donor selection have all been enhanced by procedures developed through the NMDP.

Beyond facilitating transplants through the network of many transplant centers and donor centers, the NMDP also operates a patient education and support facility through the Office of Patient Advocacy. This office answers questions, guides patients through the search process, supports confirmation of insurance approval, and helps in numerous ways to allow patients and families to seek and secure the appropriate support for their needed transplant therapy.

Through physician education efforts, the NMDP provides ongoing medical educational materials, conferences, and webcasts to improve the knowledge and available resources for hematologists, oncologists, and primary care physicians. This broadens understanding about the transplant procedure and judgment about when URD hematopoietic cell transplantation may be appropriate. In conjunction with the ASBMT, the NMDP publishes guidelines indicating appropriate timing for referral and consultation regarding hematopoietic cell transplantation, and has assisted the ASBMT in sponsoring the develop-

ment of evidence-based guidelines to understand better the role, timing, and appropriateness of transplant procedures.

In 2006, the NMDP responsibility broadened further as the congressionally authorized CW Bill Young Transplant Program was developed. This program provides the National Marrow Donor Registry, the National Cord Blood Program, the extension of the ongoing NMDP network of donor and collection centers, a new network of cord blood banks, and a single point of access for patients and physicians to initiate searches and identify appropriate hematopoietic cell donors. The NMDP was awarded contracts by the Health Resources and Service Administration (HRSA) to administer the bone marrow donor registry, and the cord blood program. It was also the single point of access, while the Center for International Blood and Marrow Transplant Research (CIBMTR) was awarded the contract to establish and administer the Stem Cell Therapeutic Outcomes Database (SCTOD) which prospectively collects relevant information on all allotransplants performed in the US in order to study further, understand, and foster improvements in the application and successes of hematopoietic cell transplantation.

Throughout its history, the NMDP has also been committed to supporting ongoing outcomes research to understand the optimum timing, techniques, and procedures needed to improve the safety and efficacy of hematopoietic cell transplantation. Additional research to understand how to offer donors a positive and supportive experience, maximize donor recruitment and retention into the network, and importantly, to maximize donor safety through the altruistic donation procedure have all been areas of NMDP research. With integration of the NMDP Research Department and the CIBMTR in 2005, research in hematopoietic cell transplantation was fostered even further to improve data collection techniques, establish an electronic network for data submission, validation and sharing, and accelerate the evaluation and dissemination of new scientific information regarding the growing field of transplantation.

The NMDP remains committed to advancing the field, and to supporting patients and their families as well as transplant centers and their physicians through the broad and essential network of donors, donor centers, and cord blood banks which provide this vital and needed resource.

World Marrow Donor Association

The WMDA is a voluntary organization of representatives of HCT donor registries, cord blood banks, and other organizations and individuals striving to improve and simplify stem cell donation for donors and patients. The WMDA was created in 1994 to address obstacles faced when transplantation involved donors and recipients in different countries. The organization fosters international discussion of all issues regarding the clinical use of hematopoietic stem cells from unrelated donors across national boundaries and has developed guidelines for interactions related to such use. An organizational chart is found in Figure 50.2. WMDA meetings take place at least twice yearly and are usually held in conjunction with other international HCT meetings.

Most of the work of the WMDA is done through its working groups (see Fig. 50.2), including establishment of WMDA guidelines. The working groups are concerned with recommending the best practice in terms of medical, ethical, technical, quality and financial aspects of international HCT. The working groups have developed template forms for all aspects of donor registry operation, including donor search processes.

Additionally, the WMDA established an accreditation program for donor registries in 2003, to certify adherence to WMDA standards for

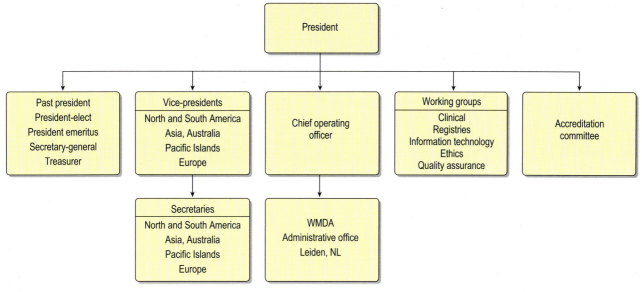

Figure 50.2
WMDA organizational chart.

registry operation. These standards cover the general organization of the registry, donor recruitment and consent procedures, donor characterization and evaluation, information technology, facilitation of search requests, second and subsequent donations, graft procurement and transport, assessment of donor and transplant outcomes and financial and legal liabilities. In addition, through an international effort named Alliance for Harmonization of Cellular Therapy Accreditation (www.ahcta.org), the standards of the WMDA and other international organizations are being harmonized with the objective of creating a single set of quality, safety and professional requirements for cellular therapy including HCT.

The WMDA publishes an annual report that summarizes global activity in unrelated donor HCT and provides a variety of forums to discuss issues related to international facilitation of HCT. The organization also provides data and expertise to national and international bodies addressing regulatory issues in HCT. Additional information can be found at www.worldmarrow.org.

References

1. Hahn T, Wall D, Camitta B et al. The role of cytotoxic therapy with hematopoietic stem cell transplantation in the therapy of acute lymphoblastic leukemia in adults: an evidence-based review. Biol Blood Marrow Transplant 2006;12:1–30

2. Weisdorf D, Carter S, Confer D et al. Blood and Marrow Transplant Clinical Trials Network (BMT CTN): addressing unanswered questions. Biol Blood Marrow Transplant 2007;13:257–262

3. Horwitz E, LeBlanc K, Dominici M et al. Clarification of the nomenclature for MSC: the International Society for Cellular Therapy position statement. Cytotherapy 2005;7:393–395

4. NETCORD, Foundation for the Accreditation of Cellular Therapy. International standards for cord blood collection, processing, testing, banking, selection and release, 3rd edn. NETCORD and the Foundation for the Accreditation of Cellular Therapy, Omaha, Nebraska, 2006

5. FACT-JACIE. International standards for cellular therapy product collection, processing and transplantation, 3rd edn. Foundation for the Accreditation of Cellular Therapy and Joint Accreditation Committee of EBMT and Euro-ISCT, Omaha, Nebraska, 2006

Stem cell transplantation – future prospects

A John Barrett

The current status of stem cell transplantation

It is more than a quarter of a century since E Donnall Thomas described the first series of 100 allogeneic stem cell transplantations (SCT) for leukemia[1] and established a myeloablative treatment schema which has served as the predominant approach for allografts for malignant disease. Since that time, the outcome for recipients of allogeneic stem cell transplants has improved at a rate of about 5–10% increased survival each decade. Currently, the transplant-related mortality (TRM) for transplants for human leukocyte antigen (HLA)-identical sibling donors is around 5%. However, the TRM is considerably higher for less than fully matched donor–recipient pairs and for patients with co-morbidities from disease or old age.

This progress is due to better supportive care – new and improved antibiotics and antifungals, and potent antiviral agents, better transfusion support, and a general accumulation of expertise in transplant teams facilitating early recognition and better control of potentially lethal transplant complications. There has been modest improvement in the prevention and management of graft-versus-host disease (GvHD) with the introduction in the mid-1980s of the combination of 'short' methotrexate (MTX) and ciclosporin (CYA), an immunosuppressive compromise which largely prevents serious GvHD while retaining some graft-versus-leukemia (GvL) activity. Reduced-intensity preparative regimens introduced in the 1990s have emboldened transplanters to extend allogeneic SCT to patients well over the age of 60 years with some remarkable successes. More transplants are being performed using non-family donors, either from an unrelated donor pool, which exceeds 5 million volunteers worldwide, or from a growing contribution from umbilical cord blood banks.

The repertoire of diseases potentially curable by SCT has also continued to expand. Currently, SCT has some place in treatment of nearly all hematologic malignancies and is being explored for the treatment of non-hematologic malignancies such as metastatic renal cell cancer. For non-malignant diseases, SCT has been used to correct a huge variety of congenital immunologic and hematologic deficiencies as well as a diverse group of lysosomal storage diseases. More recently, SCT has begun to find a place in the treatment of autoimmune diseases.

Against this optimistic record, it is also clear that SCT still has limited success and restricted applicability; SCT does not cure all the malignant or non-malignant diseases that it is used for, and it is still largely restricted to patients with HLA-identical or closely identical donors because of high TRM if the donor is mismatched. It is sobering to note that the relapse rate for standard-risk and high-risk leukemias

following SCT from a matched sibling donor has not changed appreciably from the 20% and 60% relapse rates first achieved in the 1970s, and also that the TRM for unrelated donor transplants is still double that of HLA-identical sibling transplants despite more refined compatibility testing.[2] SCT remains expensive because of the high-intensity medical care needed for patient support as well as the requirement for an integrated team of support staff.

Thus, even if fully successful, SCT is liable to take second place when simple and effective treatments become available, such as has occurred following the introduction of imatinib to treat chronic myelogenous leukemia (CML). In the field of non-malignant disorders, SCT is also challenged by new non-transplantation treatments. One example is the switch from performing allogeneic SCT for Gaucher disease with the advent of enzyme treatment; despite highly successful results from SCT, transplantation is hardly ever used now to treat Gaucher disease.

Challenges for the 21st century

SCT therefore faces some major limitations to its success, and indeed its survival, as a useful treatment approach. The success or failure of research to overcome these limitations, together with the success or failure of competing non-transplant treatments, will largely determine the place of SCT in the next decade or two. These treatment challenges and possible remedies are listed in Table 51.1 and discussed in detail below.

Prevention of GvHD without immune suppression

Current methods to prevent GvHD require the use of either immunosuppression or T-cell depletion with the consequence that immune recovery is compromised, GvL effects are mitigated and TRM from infection is increased. New techniques to selectively prevent GvHD are now at the early stages of clinical development, as listed in Table 51.2. They are all based on selection methods that remove T-cell subsets causing GvHD.[3] Ideally, these approaches should dispense with the need for immunosuppression. One of their shortcomings is that it is not yet clear whether any of these methods can specifically remove GvHD reactivity and preserve GvL and immune recovery. Most promising are techniques which deplete the alloresponse that causes GvHD, either in vivo, using a 'suicide' gene approach[4] to eliminate GvHD-reacting T-cells by treatment with ganciclovir, or in vitro by eliminating alloreacting donor cells stimulated by host targets bearing GvHD-related antigens.[5] A successful selective depletion

Table 51.1 Limitations of SCT as currently used to treat malignant and non-malignant disorders

Problem	Remedy
Transplant-related mortality	*Selection of the appropriate regimen*
Older or debilitated patients Recipients of mismatched transplants Genetic susceptibility for complications	Continued improvement in supportive care, co-morbidity scores to tailor treatment intensity Gene analysis to guide tailored SCT approach
Failure to control malignant disease	*Optimize GvL/GvT*
Relapse in refractory leukemias and lymphomas Modest GVT effects of transplants for solid tumors	Prevention of GvHD without immune suppression, boost GvL/GvT – vaccines Adoptive immune cell transfer Combine with non-transplant targeted therapy NK cell transfusions
Limited availability and shortcomings of mismatched donors	*Optimize SCT from alternative stem cell sources*
Limited numbers of related and unrelated matched donors High mortality from mismatched donors and UCB Poor engraftment of UCB	Autologous SCT corrected by gene insertion for non-malignant disease Larger panels, new matching strategies Prevention of GvHD without immune suppression In vitro cell expansion

Table 51.2 Strategies to selectively prevent GvHD

Selective depletion of alloactivated T-cells[3]
Suicide gene insertion[4]
Adoptive transfer of GvL and antiviral T-cells[5]
Transfer of specific T-cell subsets Tregs, Th2, naïve cell depletion[7]
Depletion of host APC[7]
Rerouting donor T-cells to prevent localization at sites of GvHD[8]
Manipulating engraftment with NK NKT cells[9]

approach would eliminate post-SCT GvHD prophylaxis and it would also provide a platform for vaccination of the transplant recipient to boost immunity against infectious agents and malignant diseases.

Optimizing conditioning regimens

The last decade has seen an explosion in the diversity of conditioning regimens and new conditioning agents.[6] It is now possible to select regimens of specific intensity with chosen bias towards immunoablation (to promote engraftment) and myelosuppression (to eliminate marrow disease). While progress will continue to be made in selecting regimens of appropriate intensity to minimize morbidity and mortality in older or debilitated individuals, the field still awaits the development of regimens which target malignant disease intensively while sparing healthy tissues. Some progress has been made with antibody-targeted radioactive compounds, but practical strategies to safely deliver intensive therapy to refractory malignancies are much needed. Transplanters face the growing problem of an increasingly aging population, and the need to adapt transplant treatments for malignant disease in the elderly. Chemotherapy for patients with acute myeloid leukemia (AML) over 70 years old has less than a 5% 1-year survival. The challenge will be to apply appropriately tailored conditioning regimes coupled with non-toxic strategies to boost GvL effects.

Table 51.3 Boosting the antimalignant effect of SCT

Vaccines for WT1 PR1[11]
Adoptive transfer of tumor-specific T-cells[5]
Allo-NK cell infusions[8]
Genetically modified effectors[12]
Combination of SCT with new biologics

Conditioning:
  Allogeneic transplantation: tumor or marrow targeted radiotherapy conditioning
  Autologous transplantation: lymphopenic conditioning to boost expansion of transferred lymphocytes[11]

Tailoring transplant design to compensate for specific genetically determined risks

Current research into the discovery of genetic polymorphisms of cytokine genes, receptors, and infection susceptibility genes predictive of particular transplant outcomes is likely to continue with an ever-widening array of genetically defined prognostic factors. Ultimately, it may be possible to tailor the transplant approach to these genetic variations so as to minimize the risks posed by adverse polymorphisms, and maximize the chances of beneficial effects from favorable polymorphisms.[7]

Optimizing the antitumor component of SCT

The main cause of treatment failure after SCT for malignant disease is disease recurrence. If SCT is to remain a competitive treatment for malignant disease, major improvements in the ability of SCT to cure aggressive and advanced malignancies are needed. Improved methods of targeting the conditioning regimen to the disease, as discussed above, may come from radioimmunotherapy, but perhaps a more promising area will be the association of novel, disease-specific drugs with the transplant. The classic example of a favorable association of SCT with targeted therapy is the combination of imatinib and SCT to treat CML, the imatinib providing leukemia burden reduction and the transplant providing immunologic control of residual disease.[10] In the future we can anticipate many more examples of a favorable synergy between SCT and 'small molecules'.

Another area of development that has the possibility of significantly enhancing graft-versus-tumor (GvT) effects is the use of tumor-specific vaccines to boost immunity after transplantation. These approaches are likely to advance more rapidly when the objective of specifically eliminating GvHD has been achieved (see Table 51.2). Several strategies will be explored increasingly: vaccination of the donor so as to transfer immune memory with the graft, and vaccination of the patient early after SCT to provide benefit from the massive lymphocyte expansion that occurs.[11] This strategy might also be increasingly applied to generate GvT-like effects in autologous SCT. Current techniques to adoptively transfer immune cells with strong antitumor activity are limited by the practicalities of bulk cell culture and inherent variability of cell products between individuals. In future, adoptive cell therapy may come of age when it is possible to deliver 'off-the-shelf' cell products with universal applicability, gene modified to target malignant cells (Table 51.3).[12] It is difficult to predict in the field of immunotherapy whether the less complicated approach using vaccines or the more sophisticated cell therapies will triumph. Alternatively, either cell therapy or vaccine strategies could be developed on an individual disease basis.

Enthusiasts for 'small molecule' treatments targeting specific malignancies believe that similar advances in understanding the biology of other malignant diseases will pave the way for intelligently designed molecules with few or no side-effects, which have powerful antitumor efficacy. Such treatments could progressively narrow the spectrum of diseases in which SCT is the first option. It might be that SCT will become increasingly reserved for more advanced disease and treatment failures, as has already been observed with CML. Alternatively, it may emerge that single, targeted treatments are never fully effective in any disease state. SCT would continue to be needed, and might have greater therapeutic effect when combined with a novel treatment agent. With continuing improvement in the safety of the transplant procedure, there would be a greater tendency to promote the transplant to treat less advanced disease states.

Extending 'safe' transplantation to suboptimal donor–recipient combinations

Currently, the lack of donor availability means that SCT with a fully matched related or unrelated donor is restricted to less than half of the patients in whom an SCT is indicated. While transplants can be successfully performed using less than fully matched donors, the chance of treatment success is greatly diminished. Thus, a major challenge for the future is to improve the availability of suitably matched donors while at the same time developing transplant approaches that are safe and effective, even with less than perfectly matched donors. Techniques to selectively prevent GvHD described in Table 51.2 may transform the field by making it possible to safely perform transplants with haploidentical family donors. Umbilical cord blood is already a promising source of stem cells, comparing favorably with better matched unrelated donors. This readily available stem cell source will fulfill an ever increasing role in future as the size and diversity of cord blood banks increase. However, the biggest improvement in the applicability of CBT will be realized when techniques to expand both hematopoietic stem cells and cord blood lymphocytes allow us to deliver the larger cell doses required for optimal adult SCT.

Another area of development is the identification of 'permissible' mismatches which allow safe engraftment without GvHD.[13] Looking further ahead, we may eventually see the modification of stem cell products with universal compatibility to reconstitute individual lineages (T-cells, NK cells and hematopoietic cells).

Application of stem cell transplant technology to new areas

Autoimmune diseases

While the clinical field of allogeneic and autologous SCT for autoimmune diseases (AID) is growing and producing promising results, most investigators would agree that the mechanistic basis for using SCT to correct AID is sketchy. A common finding in AID is the lack of functional regulatory T-cells. Thus, in addition to or instead of SCT to correct these disorders, there may be a role for cell therapy with in vitro selected and expanded regulatory T-cells. The ability to replace the defective immune system with that of a healthy donor by a stem cell allograft may nevertheless become more acceptable if reductions in TRM make such transplants safer.

Gene therapy

In the 1990s, gene therapy was heralded as the next major therapeutic advance for a number of disorders currently treated by allogeneic SCT such as the hemoglobinopathies and severe combined immune deficiency (SCID). However, the occurrence of genetically triggered leukemias in infants with otherwise successfully corrected SCID was a major setback to the field.[14] Current research is beginning to address

Table 51.4 Potential applications of non-hematopoietic cells for tissue repair[17,18]

Cell	Application
Bone cells	Osteoporosis
Cartilage cells	Osteoarthritis
Heart muscle cells	Myocardial infarcts, congestive heart failure
Insulin-producing cells	Diabetes
Liver cells	Hepatitis, cirrhosis
Nerve cells	Stroke, Parkinson's disease, Alzheimer's disease, spinal cord injury, multiple sclerosis
Retinal cells	Macular degeneration
Skeletal muscle cells	Muscular dystrophy
Skin cells	Burns, wound healing
Mesenchymal stem cells	Endothelial injury, GvHD

these shortcomings with new vectors that do not randomly integrate into the genome. It is therefore likely that gene therapy will eventually come of age as an attractive treatment option for large numbers of stem cell-based diseases, as well as allowing the construction of immune cells with enhanced ability to target cancer cells, control autoimmunity or repair non-hematopoietic tissue.[15,16] SCT techniques will still be required for some forms of gene therapy, but these future protocols may bear very little resemblance to current allo- or auto-transplant strategies.

Alternative stem cells for tissue repair

One of the greatest revolutions in stem cell biology has been the realization that aside from the hematopoietic stem cell, many tissues have specific progenitor cells which can repopulate in a recipient and be used for tissue repair. Furthermore, the ability of some of these progenitors (including hematopoietic stem cells) to generate a diversity of mature cell lineages opens up numerous prospects for this form of cell therapy. In addition to these developments in adult stem cell biology, there is a strong possibility that embryonic stem cells could also serve as a source for diverse cell types.

Currently, imagination surpasses actual practical possibilities – many cells are not comprehensively classified and a significant limitation is our lack of understanding of how to ensure the transplanted cells reach the appropriate site and establish themselves in the correct organ or tissue without changing their characteristics. Hematopoietic stem cells appear to play a role in cardiac muscle repair, but earlier indications that they transform into cardiac muscle have been refuted in favor of the theory that they improve revascularization. Future treatments with stem cells will share few similarities with current SCT methodologies.[17,18] Nevertheless, the problem of immunologic rejection of these novel cell transplant methods will remain and will have to be overcome by conventional immunosuppression, gene modification of autologous cells or by design of cells which evade immune recognition. Table 51.4 illustrates the wide potential of these new forms of cell therapy in the treatment of diverse disorders.

Conclusion

Stem cell transplantation as it is practiced today has little chance of surviving long into the 21st century. However, far from signaling the death of SCT, new developments in basic immunology and stem cell science and treatment, together with the beginnings of translational research to make sophisticated cell therapy a reality, should continue to move the field forward. These developments should ultimately render obsolete current preoccupations with GvHD, rejection, infection, disease relapse, and donor selection. There is every reason to expect SCT of the future to be performed more cheaply than at present, mainly on an outpatient basis, with few complications and with a low level of treatment failure. So daunting are the challenges medicine still faces with malignant disease and degenerative diseases in an increasingly older aged population that it is unlikely SCT will be replaced by small molecule 'magic bullets' (of which imatinib still remains the best example). Rather, it is more likely that diseases will continue to be treated as they are today, with a combination of integrated treatment approaches in which SCT will remain playing a key role.

References

1. Thomas ED, Buckner CD, Banaji M et al. One hundred patients with acute leukemia treated by chemotherapy, total body irradiation and allogeneic bone marrow transplant. Blood 1977;49:511–520

2. Barrett J. Allogeneic marrow transplantation: dinosaur or bird? Cytotherapy 2002;4:201–202

3. Mielke S, Solomon SR, Barrett AJ. Selective depletion strategies in allogeneic stem cell transplantation. Cytotherapy 2005;7:109–115

4. Ciceri F, Bonini C, Gallo-Stampino C, Bordignon C. Modulation of GvHD by suicide-gene transduced donor T lymphocytes: clinical applications in mismatched transplantation. Cytotherapy 2005;7:144–149

5. Barber LD, Madrigal JA. Exploiting beneficial alloreactive T cells. Vox Sang 2006;91:20–27

6. Barrett AJ, Savani BN. Stem cell transplantation with reduced-intensity conditioning regimens: a review of ten years experience with new transplant concepts and new therapeutic agents. Leukemia 2006;20:1661–1672

7. Barrett AJ, Rezvani K, Solomon S et al. New developments in allotransplant immunology. Hematology Am Soc Hematol Educ Program 2003:350–371

8. Sackstein R. A revision of Billingham's tenets: the central role of lymphocyte migration in acute graft-versus-host disease. Biol Blood Marrow Transplant 2006;12(suppl1):2–8

9. Passweg JR, Koehl U, Uharek L et al. Natural-killer-cell-based treatment in haematopoietic stem-cell transplantation. Best Pract Res Clin Haematol 2006;19:811–824

10. Goldman J, Gordon M. Why do chronic myelogenous leukemia stem cells survive allogeneic stem cell transplantation or imatinib: does it really matter? Leuk Lymphoma 2006;47:1–7

11. Molldrem JJ. Vaccination for leukemia. Biol Blood Marrow Transplant 2006;12(1 suppl 1):13–18

12. Morris E, Hart D, Gao L et al. Generation of tumor-specific T-cell therapies. Blood Rev 2006;20:61–69

13. Mullighan CG, Petersdorf EW. Genomic polymorphism and allogeneic hematopoietic transplantation outcome. Biol Blood Marrow Transplant 2006;12(1 suppl 1):19–27

14. Gaspar HB, Thrasher AJ. Gene therapy for severe combined immunodeficiencies. Expert Opin Biol Ther 2005;5:1175–1182

15. Sinn PL, Sauter SL, McCray PB Jr. Gene therapy progress and prospects: development of improved lentiviral and retroviral vectors – design, biosafety, and production. Gene Ther 2005;12:1089–1098

16. Dotti G, Heslop HE. Current status of genetic modification of T cells for cancer treatment. Cytotherapy 2005;7:262–272

17. Polak JM, Bishop AE. Stem cells and tissue engineering: past, present, and future. Ann NY Acad Sci 2006;1068:352–366

18. Keating A. Mesenchymal stromal cells. Curr Opin Hematol 2006;13:419–422

Index